Fundamentals of

COMPLEMENTARY AND ALTERNATIVE MEDICINE

Fifth Edition

MARC S. MICOZZI, MD, PhD
Adjunct Professor
Department of Physiology & Biophysics
and Department of Pharmacology
Georgetown University School of Medicine
Washington, DC;
Former Director
Center for Integrative Medicine
Thomas Jefferson University Hospital
Philadelphia, Pennsylvania

With forewords by

C. EVERETT KOOP, MD, ScD
(1916–2013)
Former Surgeon General of
the United States

AVIAD HARAMATI, PhD
Professor, Department of Biochemistry,
Cellular and Molecular Biology and
Department of Medicine
Georgetown University School of Medicine
Washington, DC;

GEORGE D. LUNDBERG, MD
Former Editor-in-Chief, *Journal of the
American Medical Association*, 1982-1999;
and *The Medscape, Journal of Medicine and
eMedicine* from WebMD, 1999-2009;
Consulting Professor, Stanford University
President and Chair, The Lundberg
Institute

ELSEVIER
SAUNDERS

3251 Riverport Lane
St. Louis, Missouri 63043

Notices

Knowledge and best practice in this field are constantly changing. As new research and experience broaden our understanding, changes in research methods, professional practices, or medical treatment may become necessary.

Practitioners and researchers must always rely on their own experience and knowledge in evaluating and using any information, methods, compounds, or experiments described herein. In using such information or methods they should be mindful of their own safety and the safety of others, including parties for whom they have a professional responsibility.

With respect to any drug or pharmaceutical products identified, readers are advised to check the most current information provided (i) on procedures featured or (ii) by the manufacturer of each product to be administered, to verify the recommended dose or formula, the method and duration of administration, and contraindications. It is the responsibility of practitioners, relying on their own experience and knowledge of their patients, to make diagnoses, to determine dosages and the best treatment for each individual patient, and to take all appropriate safety precautions.

To the fullest extent of the law, neither the Publisher nor the authors, contributors, or editors, assume any liability for any injury and/or damage to persons or property as a matter of products liability, negligence or otherwise, or from any use or operation of any methods, products, instructions, or ideas contained in the material herein.

Library of Congress Cataloging-in-Publication Data

Fundamentals of complementary and alternative medicine / [edited by] Marc S. Micozzi ; with forewords by C. Everett Koop, Aviad Haramati, and George D. Lundberg. – Fifth edition.
    p. ; cm.
    Includes bibliographical references and index.
    ISBN 978-1-4557-7407-4 (hardcover : alk. paper)
    I. Micozzi, Marc S., 1953- , editor.
    [DNLM: 1. Complementary Therapies.   WB 890]
    R733
    615.5–dc23
                        2014039588

Content Strategist: Kellie White
Publishing Services Manager: Jeff Patterson
Senior Project Manager: Anne Konopka
Design Direction: Christian Bilbow

Printed in the U.S.A.

Last digit is the print number: 9   8   7   6   5   4   3   2   1

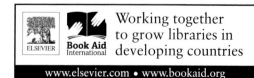

Dedicated to

Baruch S. Blumberg, MD, PhD (1925–2011)
C. Everett Koop, MD, ScD (1916–2013)

Acknowledgment to Jennifer Gehl for editorial assistance

An Anatomy of the World
And new philosophy calls all in doubt
The element of fire is quite put out
The sun is lost, and the earth, and no man's wit
Can well direct him where to look for it
And freely men confess that this world's spent
When in the Planets, and the Firmament
They seek so many new; they see that this
Is crumbled out againe to his Atomies
'Tis all in pieces, all cohaerence gone;
All just supply, and all relation

John Donne (1572–1631),
Physician and Metaphysician

Contributors

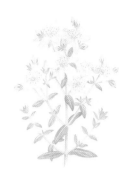

MONES S. ABU-ASAB, PHD
Senior Scientist
Laboratory of Immunopathology
National Eye Institute
National Institutes of Health
Bethesda, Maryland

HUNTER "PATCH" ADAMS, MD
Executive Director of Gesundheit
    Institute
Urbana, Illinois

HAKIMA AMRI, PHD
Associate Professor
Co-Director, Physiology and CAM
    Graduate Program
Department of Biochemistry, Cellular,
    and Molecular Biology
Division of Integrative Physiology
Georgetown University School of
    Medicine
Washington, DC

DONALD A. BISSON, Q.REFLEX,
OCR-CR, Q.MED, RRPR
Dean and Professor of Reflexology
Ontario College of Reflexology
New Liskeard, Ontario, Canada

GERARD C. BODEKER, EDD
Department of Primary Care Health
    Sciences
Division of Medical Sciences
University of Oxford
Oxford, UK
Department of Epidemiology
Mailman School of Public Health
Columbia University
New York, New York

CLAIRE M. CASSIDY, PHD, DIPL
AC, LAC
Licensed Acupuncturist
Medical and Nutritional Anthropologist
Executive Editor, *Journal of Alternative and
    Complementary Medicine*
Bethesda, Maryland

PATRICK COUGHLIN, PHD
Retired Professor, Department of
    Anatomy
Philadelphia College of Osteopathic
    Medicine
Philadelphia, Pennsylvania

JUDITH DELANY, LMT, CNMT
Director, Curriculum Developer
Neuromuscular Therapy Center
St. Petersburg, Florida

KEVIN V. ERGIL, MA, MS, LAC
Professor
Finger Lakes School of Acupuncture and
    Oriental Medicine
New York Chiropractic College
Seneca Falls, New York

MARNAE C. ERGIL, MA, MS, LAC
Professor
Finger Lakes School of Acupuncture and
    Oriental Medicine
New York Chiropractic College
Seneca Falls, New York

LAUREL S. GABLER, PHD, MSC
Harvard Medical School
Boston, Massachusetts

JENNIFER GEHL, BA, MHS(C)
Certified Acutonics® Practitioner
CEU Instructor
Altoona, Pennsylvania

SHERRY W. GOODILL, PHD,
BC-DMT, NCC, LPC
Clinical Professor and Chairperson
Department of Creative Arts Therapies
Drexel University
Philadelphia, Pennsylvania
Past President
American Dance Therapy Association
Columbia, Maryland

HOWARD HALL, PHD, PSYD, BCB
Professor of Pediatrics, Psychiatry, and
    Psychological Sciences
University Hospitals, Case Medical Center
Rainbow Babies & Children's Hospital
Cleveland, Ohio

MARIANA G. HEWSON, PHD
Author
Madison, Wisconsin

JOHN A. IVES, PHD
Senior Director, Brain, Mind, and Healing
Samueli Institute
Alexandria, Virginia

MICHAEL A. JAWER, CAE
Director of Government and Public
    Affairs
American Association of Naturopathic
    Physicians
Washington, DC

WAYNE B. JONAS, MD
President and CEO
Samueli Institute
Alexandria, Virginia

JOHN M. JONES, DO, MED
Professor of Clinical Medicine
Chair, Department of Osteopathic
  Principles and Practice
William Carey University College of
  Osteopathic Medicine
Hattiesburg, Mississippi

DAVID LARSON

RHIANNON LEWIS, FIFPA
Editor-in-Chief, *International Journal of
  Clinical Aromatherapy*
Director of Essential Oil Resource
  Consultants
Provence, France

DAVID MAYOR, MA, BAC, MBACC,
HON MEMBER AACP
Acupuncture Practitioner
Welwyn Garden City
Visiting Research Associate
(formerly Hon Research Fellow)
Department of Physiotherapy
School of Health and Social Work
University of Hertfordshire
Hertfordshire, UK

DONALD MCCOWN, PHD,
MAMS, MSS, LSW
Assistant Professor, Health
Co-Director, Center for Contemplative
  Studies
Program Director, Minor in
  Contemplative Studies
West Chester University
West Chester, Pennsylvania

LISA MESEROLE, MS, ND
Sage Healing
Seattle, Washington
Coupeville, Washington

ALICIA M. MICOZZI, BA, WEMT
Survey Researcher
University of Maryland Medical Center
Baltimore, Maryland

DANIEL E. MOERMAN, PHD
William E. Stirton Professor Emeritus of
  Anthropology
University of Michigan-Dearborn
Dearborn, Michigan

PAUL NOLAN, MCAT, MT-BC, LPC
Director of Music Therapy Programs
Hahnemann Creative Arts in Therapy
  Program
Drexel University
Philadelphia, Pennsylvania

CAROLE A. O'LEARY, PHD
Senior Adviser
Michael Moran & Associates (MMA)
Chevy Chase, Maryland
Denver, Colorado

JOSEPH E. PIZZORNO, JR., ND
Editor-in-Chief, *Integrative Medicine, A
  Clinician's Journal*
Seattle, Washington
President Emeritus
Bastyr University
Kenmore, Washington

SALOME RAHEIM, PHD, ACSW
Dean and Professor
The University of Connecticut
School of Social Work
West Hartford, Connecticut

DANIEL REDWOOD, DC
Associate Professor
Cleveland Chiropractic College
Overland Park, Kansas

PAMELA SNIDER, ND
Executive and Senior Editor
Foundations of Naturopathic Medicine
  Project
Associate Professor
National College of Natural Medicine
Portland, Oregon

KEVIN SPELMAN, PHD, MCPP
Research Scientist and Natural Products
  Industry Consultant
Health, Education and Research in
  Botanical Medicine (HERB Med)
Ashland, Oregon

JULIE K. STAPLES, PHD
Adjunct Assistant Professor
Department of Biochemistry and
  Molecular & Cellular Biology
Georgetown University School of
  Medicine
Washington, DC
Principal
Awareness Technologies, Inc.
Placitas, New Mexico

ROBERT T. TROTTER II, PHD
Regent's Professor and Chair
Department of Anthropology
Northern Arizona University
Flagstaff, Arizona

RICHARD W. VOSS, DPC, MSW,
MTS
Professor of Social Work
Undergraduate Social Work Department
West Chester University
West Chester, Pennsylvania
Visiting Professor and Researcher
Friedensau Adventist University
School of Social Work & Social Sciences
Möckern, Germany

MICHAEL I. WEINTRAUB, MD,
FACP, FAAN, FAHA
Clinical Professor of Neurology and
  Internal Medicine
New York Medical College
Valhalla, New York
Adjunct Clinical Professor of Neurology
Mt. Sinai School of Medicine
New York, New York

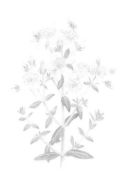

In Memory of C. Everett Koop, MD, ScD

For more than 50 years I have tried to identify the mix of personal attributes and technical skills that make one an outstanding doctor. I am sure that most physicians in the United States have pondered the same question. Now, through the work of the C. Everett Koop Institute at Dartmouth I have an opportunity to influence the way medical students are trained. The Institute, working in partnership with the Dartmouth Medical School and the Dartmouth-Hitchcock Medical Center, is actively engaged in training physicians for the new century.

Because doctors must remain abreast of a growing volume of new information, our medical schools help both their graduates and society by producing physicians who are computer literate and comfortable with telemedicine. As a scientific pursuit, medicine should take advantage of the technologic innovations that allow us to better serve the lifetime learning needs of physicians as well as the health education needs of patients. Nonetheless, because medicine is also an art, doctors still need to listen to their patients. This aspect of medical practice has not changed.

As I travel across the country, many of the people I meet are eager to share their ideas for improving the nation's health care system. The most common complaint I hear focuses on poor communication in the doctor–patient relationship. Too many patients feel that their physician does not really listen to them. When the patient attempts to explain his or her problem, the doctor interrupts. Subsequently, when the doctor tries to explain what conditions the patient has and attempts to outline a treatment regimen, the patient is confused because the physician does not communicate to the level of the patient's understanding.

From my perspective, medical students need to master the art of listening to and communicating with their patients just as much as they need to learn the fundamentals of human biology. We have found at the Koop Institute that a student's communication skills are greatly improved by having to explain the first principles of health promotion and disease prevention to second graders. Medical students who choose to participate in programs sponsored by the Koop Institute work in and with local communities from their very first year. Some choose to advise junior high and high school students on the risks associated with alcohol, tobacco, and sexually transmitted diseases; others help rural physicians take better advantage of the computer revolution.

Just as a physician should be sensitive to the feelings of a patient and the needs of the community, he or she must be conversant with major trends and developments in society. I would like to tell you about one current trend that is of interest to me. Studies conducted at Harvard Medical School and reported in the *New England Journal of Medicine* focused on attitudes toward complementary and alternative medicine in the United States. They indicate that one-third of adult Americans regularly use some kind of complementary or alternative treatment even though it was not covered by insurance and they had to pay for it themselves. This is an opportune time for us to take a second look at such alternative treatment approaches as acupuncture, botanical medicine, homeopathy, and others—not to offer these treatment modalities blindly but to expose them to the scientific method. Physicians have to depend on facts—on empirical data—when they determine treatment strategy for a particular patient. Today we do not have enough data on the potential of alternative approaches to help or harm human health. It is time to discover the value of these treatment regimens. We can conduct the necessary studies and assemble the data that doctors and health policy makers need, a type of biomedical research that would be a prudent long-term investment.

In my lifetime we have achieved great successes in the fight against infectious diseases. We have more work to do in our effort to improve quality of life and make people more comfortable as they endure chronic health problems such as cancer, heart disease, and arthritis. Drugs and surgery can be useful tools in the effort to treat these diseases, but when possible I would like to see us increase the range of approaches that can be used. My experience as a doctor has taught me that often a mix of different approaches is necessary to achieve success. We need to be flexible and adaptable because the diseases that challenge us certainly are not static.

A recent trend that concerns me is the growth of drug-resistant bacteria. Today it is easy to forget that prior to the development of antibiotics in the 1940s, a child's ear infection could be a frightening and fatal experience. I well remember patients with serious complications and death caused by the lack of antibiotics. If drugs we have depended on for decades are compromised, we may return to a time when even routine infections could be dangerous. As both a grandfather and a physician, I would hate to see that happen.

There is an element of good news in this picture. If some of the synthetic drugs we have developed are no longer as dependable as they once were, studies have shown that the botanical substances these drugs are based on are still effective in treating disease. I have never claimed to be an expert on botany or ecology, but current trends suggest that we need to do more. We need to conserve the plants that may contain the medicines of the future and, more importantly, we need to learn what local experts seem to understand about the pharmacological properties and uses of these medicines.

Reduced health care costs are an important by-product of the work we are doing at the Koop Institute. Our students know that the physician of the future must be a health educator first and foremost. Today, the challenge is to treat the patient once he or she has gone to the hospital. Tomorrow, the challenge will be to keep the patient out of the hospital in the beginning.

Preventive medicine means education, empowerment, and personal responsibility. Many patients want alternatives to invasive medical procedures and long stays in the hospital. Physicians can conserve time and resources by teaching patients how to reduce their risk of cancer, heart disease, and other life-threatening diseases. As our students know, the most inexpensive treatment is to keep the patient from becoming sick in the first place. Demand reduction in the health care system is the most immediate cost-saving effort.

I think that alternative/complementary therapies may potentially be an important part of this overall educational process. One must have an open mind about complementary therapies and understand belief systems that emphasize the mind–body connection. At a time when many Americans complain of stress, make poor nutritional choices, and are increasingly concerned about environmentally induced illnesses, these messages could not be more timely.

Many people are confused about alternative medicine, and I do not blame them. For many Americans alternative therapies represent a *new* discovery, but in truth, many of these traditions are hundreds or thousands of years old and have been used by millions of people worldwide. To ease the uncomfortableness of the word *alternative*, one must realize that while treatments may look like alternatives to us, they have long been part of the medical mainstream in their cultures of origin.

When I worked in Washington as Surgeon General for eight years, President Reagan had an important credo in his approach to foreign policy: "Trust but verify!" So it is with complementary and alternative medicine. So many people have relied on these approaches for so long that they may have something of value to offer. Let us begin the necessary research so that we could have substantive answers in the near future.

One reason such research is worth doing is that 80% of the world's people depend on these alternative approaches as their primary medical care. For years, we have attempted to export Western medicine to the developing world. The sad truth is that the people we are attempting to help simply cannot afford it. I have doubts about how much longer we can afford some of it ourselves. It is possible that in this new millennium, we may be more ready to ask the peoples of the developing world to share their wisdom with us.

During the nineteenth century, American medicine was an eclectic pursuit, where a number of competing ideas and approaches thrived. Doctors were able to draw on elements from different traditions in attempting to make people well. Perhaps there is more to this older model of American medicine than we in the twentieth century had been willing to examine. My experience with physicians has convinced me that they are healers first. As such, they are willing to use any ethical approach or treatment that has been proven to work. However, in the opinion of many doctors, there is not yet a definitive answer on the value of complementary and alternative medicine. I would like us to undertake the study and research that will provide definitive answers to prudent questions about the usefulness of complementary and alternative medicine for society at large.

C. Everett Koop, MD, ScD (1916–2013)
Surgeon General of the United States (1982–1989)

Foreword from the Fourth Edition

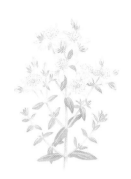

As I write these words in early February 2010, I am returning from my first trip to India. The purpose of my visit was to lead a delegation of six prominent leaders in complementary and integrative medicine from prestigious academic medical centers in the United States, at the invitation of the Ministry of Health in India, Department of AYUSH (Ayurveda, Yoga, Unani, Siddha, and homeopathy). The expressed goal of the Indian government was to inform our delegation about the evidence base for Ayurvedic medicine and to give us first-hand exposure to the use of traditional Indian medicine in clinical practice and in education and to explore potential research projects in this area. My own specific objective was to determine whether anything we saw or heard about traditional Indian medicine should eventually be included in the curriculum for physicians and other health professionals in the United States.

What struck me during this intense, seven-day visit was the chasm, even in India, between those trained in traditional medical practices and those trained in Western allopathic medicine. Many of the traditionalists feel that centuries of continued practice provides sufficient rationale for the use of various medical approaches (what in Europe constitutes "historic use" in terms of regulatory approval), irrespective of whether these therapies have been "proven" by modern scientific means, whereas most of those who are conventionally trained express a healthy skepticism and demand clear and unambiguous data to support the use of any therapy or medicinal plant.

This tension is very familiar to me. A decade ago, I helped launch a public lecture series on complementary and alternative medicine (CAM) at Georgetown University School of Medicine. At that time, a fellow colleague and I established a "mini-medical school" series at Georgetown University aimed at informing the public about the advances in medical science and health. For several years, over 200 men, women, and young adults, ranging in age from 16 to 83, would come to the medical center on eight Tuesday nights in the fall and spring semesters to hear some of our finest faculty teachers lecture on a myriad of medical issues. In response to our surveys inviting suggestions for future topics, many participants kept requesting lectures on CAM. Initially, we did not know what to make of these requests, but eventually we invited our fellow faculty member, Dr. Hakima Amri, to develop an eight-lecture series on CAM.

Thus began my education into this field, and I quickly realized that the public was eager to learn more about these treatment approaches and ancient medical systems. In contrast, the academic medical community was, in general, wary of venturing into areas many deemed unproven and unscientific. Our purpose in offering the public lecture series on CAM was to provide the best evidence available for what was harmful, what was safe and beneficial, and what aspects of CAM were simply unknown or untested.

This initial foray into a rather controversial field bore fruit. In December 1999, in an effort that demonstrated considerable courage, the leadership at the National Center for Complementary and Alternative Medicine at the National Institutes of Health issued a call for grant proposals from allopathic schools (conventional medicine and nursing) to develop curricular modules that would integrate CAM into the conventional training of physicians and other health professionals. The initiative led to important interactions between like-minded academic leaders of integrative medicine who were interested in determining, in an objective fashion, what aspects of CAM ought to be part of a medical curriculum. Those initial efforts led to a landmark series of articles that were published in the October 2007 issue of *Academic Medicine*, which addressed such topics as rationale for CAM education in health professions training programs, what should students learn about CAM, and instructional strategies for integrating CAM into the medical curriculum.

At Georgetown University School of Medicine, in addition to introducing CAM-relevant material into the medical and nursing curricula, our faculty in the Department of Physiology and Biophysics created an innovative graduate degree program of study in CAM. The mission of the program is to provide advanced study in the science and philosophy of predominant CAM therapies and disciplines and to train students to objectively assess the safety and efficacy of various CAM modalities. The program seeks to understand the mechanistic basis for CAM therapies such as acupuncture, massage, herbs and supplements, and mind–body interactions. By embedding CAM principles and paradigms firmly into a conventional, basic clinical sciences context, our intent is to prepare a new generation of health care providers, educators, and researchers for the challenging task of delivering the health care of the future—namely, a multidisciplinary approach to improved wellness, emphasizing health maintenance and disease prevention.

However, literacy in CAM, for students and faculty in our program, as well as for others around the nation, depends on an authoritative, comprehensive textbook that can provide the basic information regarding the philosophy and science for many of the CAM therapies. Fortunately, Dr. Marc Micozzi has done the field a great service by producing an outstanding text, entitled *Fundamentals of Complementary and Alternative Medicine*. Joined by a list of distinguished experts in the field, Dr. Micozzi introduces the reader to the foundations of CAM, the contexts for the use of CAM, and thorough, evidence-based descriptions of the predominant CAM therapies and traditional medical systems. The writing is easy to understand and the focus is sharp. Each chapter is referenced appropriately, and the reader is directed to several suggested additional readings. For the past few years, my colleagues at Georgetown have relied on this excellent work and have made it required reading for our program. In the new, fourth edition, Dr. Micozzi has made significant additions to the scope of the textbook, including a new and important section on mind–body–spirit.

It is essential that the health care practitioner of the future, either in the United States or elsewhere in the world, be able to bridge the current chasm between conventional and traditional medicine. Recently, the Consortium of Academic Health Centers for Integrative Medicine (www.imconsortium.org) defined *integrative medicine* as "the practice of medicine that reaffirms the importance of the relationship between practitioner and patient, focuses on the whole person, is informed by evidence, and makes use of all appropriate therapeutic approaches, healthcare professionals and disciplines to achieve optimal health and healing." If we are to produce practitioners who can truly address the needs of their patients, they must be knowledgeable about all therapeutic approaches, both conventional and those from other traditions, and be willing and interested to develop working relationships with practitioners from various disciplines. This textbook by Dr. Micozzi goes a long way in providing the reader with a fundamental understanding of complementary and integrative medicine. It is a journey worth taking and on which we at Georgetown University have seriously embarked.

Aviad Haramati, PhD
February 2010

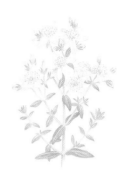

Foreword

Your "Good Medicine" Guide to CAM

There is no complementary or alternative medicine (CAM); there is only medicine. Medicine that has been tested and found to be safe and effective: use it; pay for it. Medicine that has been tested and found not to be safe and effective: don't use it; don't pay for it. And medicine that is plausible but has not been tested: test it and then place it into one of the two prime categories. If it's safe and effective, integrate it into mainstream medicine. Strange as it may seem to some readers, this prescription for action applies equally to medical practices taught in standard Western medical schools and practiced by licensed U.S. MDs and also to all those practices taught in those "other" health education institutions and practiced by so-called alternative practitioners. Sadly, there are many diagnostic and therapeutic practices in both camps yet to be properly tested and acted on.

The landmark theme issue of *JAMA* published in late 1998 demonstrated that it was possible, and responsible, to apply well-established scientific methods to the study of many CAM practices and begin that great parsing into "safe and effective" or "not safe or effective." That *JAMA* issue also convincingly illustrated that it was respectable for U.S. MDs to talk seriously with their patients about CAM. The science of CAM (yes or no) is much clearer now—some CAM works; much does not.

Americans, and people of all countries, use the methods and products called CAM for better or worse. They deserve such medical treatments to be informed by "best evidence." Doctors of many types and the public observe patients improving, even recovering, after an encounter with a "healer," regardless of the modality that healer applied. Such anecdotal experiences lead patients and practitioners to believe, even fervently, that the modality applied caused the therapeutic success, when actually only time and biology produced the success.

There is a vast historical, cultural, experiential, and increasingly clinical and evidentiary literature about that body of practice termed *CAM*. I know of no other one place where the interested reader can find a better collection of accurate and objective information about such CAM as the Micozzi text, *Fundamentals of Complementary and Alternative Medicine*, now into its fifth edition (first edition, 1996). Those who are biased (and there are still many), both for and against CAM in general and with specific CAM modalities, may or may not be swayed by the voluminous content in this 720-page tome. But the editor, Marc Micozzi, MD, PhD, and his 37 assembled authors deserve our thanks and praise for bringing us this detailed and compelling updated product to clarify this field of increasing importance as it becomes more and more integrated into the mainstream.

George D. Lundberg, MD
April 2014

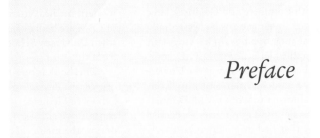
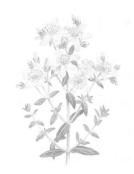

Preface

Background

During the U.S. Bicentennial year of 1976/77, I had the opportunity to live, study, and work in East and Southeast Asia, during which I was exposed to a much broader perspective on health and healing compared to what I had theretofore been able to observe in Western pre-medical and medical education. I was among just the second annual group awarded a one-year scholarship by the Henry Luce Foundation in New York, which has now sent 40 consecutive groups of 15 students each year to live and work in Asia. The Luce Scholars are comprised of students in law, journalism, architecture, fine arts, finance, philosophy, and other topics, including medicine. My exposure to students and young professionals outside medicine was equally enlightening in developing a broader perspective on medicine as a social institution as well as a science.

Pointedly, while I was in my hotel room in New York (at the old St. Regis-Sheraton), where the final interviews were being held to select the Luce Scholars for 1976, Ivan Illich, MD (1926-2002), appeared on *Good Morning America* to discuss his new book, *Medical Nemesis: The Expropriation of Health*. Here is a then-startling quote from his book:

> The medical establishment has become a major threat to health. The disabling impact of professional control over medicine has reached the proportions of an epidemic. *Iatrogenesis*, the name for this new epidemic, comes from *iatros*, the Greek word for "physician" and *genesis*, meaning "origin." Discussion of the disease of medical progress has moved up on the agendas of medical conferences, researchers concentrate on the sick-making powers of diagnosis and therapy, and reports on paradoxical damage caused by cures for sickness take up increasing space in medical dope-sheets.

His timely arguments helped bring home to me, at a very early point in my career, the need to find alternatives to the invasive, high cost, high-tech medicine of the twentieth century, even while Asian and indigenous medical systems provided me the opportunity to observe real choices in healing, providing a balance to the excesses of Western biomedicine.

In the Field

When I first arrived in Manila, Philippines, in September 1976, en route to my final destination on the island of Mindanao to the south, I was literally blown off course when a deadly typhoon grounded us. It had just claimed the lives of the USAID representatives in the Philippines in an aircraft accident, and my host, the Asia Foundation, kept us grounded in Manila until the weather cleared. To occupy this time, they arranged to send me to a conference organized by the Caliraya Foundation in nearby Laguna de Bay, on the famous Filipino faith healers Junie Kalaw and Peggy Green. (Incidentally, I also had the opportunity to work nearby as an "extra" in the USO show scene for the filming of Francis Ford Coppola's classic film *Apocalypse Now*, which had also been delayed due to the typhoon.)

Although I had gone to Southeast Asia with the original idea of studying tropical diseases, I was suddenly in contact with researchers and practitioners of an entirely different approach to disease and healing. This conference was about serious science, involving sensational "cures." Participants ranged from Elmer Green, PhD, of the Menninger Foundation; to pain expert C. Norman Shealy, MD; to Alan Landsburg, producer of the first season of a new TV show, *In Search Of . . .* hosted by Leonard Nimoy, which then ran in syndication from 1976 to 1984.

Studying these faith healers up close gave me another way to think about some startling, unexplained observations I had witnessed as a child. My great-grandparents and grandfather in Europe prepared and used various herbal remedies, as well as watching the "spontaneous" movements of a pendulum for the purposes of diagnosis, and "transferring" the heat of a high fever from an ill patient into a distant pot of water that had suddenly begun boiling.

Shortly thereafter, while I was living and working in Mindanao, the Nobel Prize in Medicine or Physiology was awarded jointly to Baruch S. Blumberg, MD, PhD (1925-2011), for the discovery of the hepatitis B virus, and to Carleton Gajdusek, MD (1923-2008), for the discovery of "slow viruses" that cause infectious dementia. (Blumberg died since the last edition of this text, and this new edition is dedicated to him.)

Blumberg and Gajdusek both made their critical discoveries by leaving the comfortable confines of the domestic research laboratory and going out into the great laboratory of nature. Incidentally, they both traveled to the South Pacific: Gajdusek to Papua New Guinea, where he conducted autopsy investigations by hurricane lamp during typhoons; and Blumberg around the world and the Pacific to Australia (what had been considered as a genetic marker, "the Australia antigen," turned out to be the hepatitis B virus surface antigen), eventually conducting clinical trials in Korea and Japan. Dr. Blumberg later personally told me that the evidence was so strong that the "Australia antigen" was not a genetic marker (but was actually the marker for the infectious hepatitis B virus) that they stopped the clinical trials before they were completed—so that he was awarded the Nobel Prize for research that he never actually completed. There was considerable consternation among laboratory virologists that two of the greatest discoveries about viruses during the twentieth century were made by nonvirologists. Both Blumberg and Gajdusek later personally confided to me that their investigations had essentially consisted of field work in medical anthropology. In keeping with this view, in 1977, Blumberg established a new MD/PhD combined degree program in Biomedical Anthropology at the University of Pennsylvania, where I was a student. After returning from Asia in 1977, I stopped off in California to work for McDonnell Douglas (now part of Boeing) as a clinical applications chemist adapting "space age" technology that had originally been developed for the NASA space shuttle, Exobiology, and Skylab programs. By the time I returned to finish my medical and graduate studies at Penn in 1978, I was able to become one of the first students in the new MD/PhD combined degree program in Biomedical Anthropology under Blumberg in the School of Medicine, and Solomon Katz and Francis E. Johnston in the Department of Anthropology.

Blumberg went on to become the first director of NASA's Astrobiology program, knowing that important discoveries could not be expected to come from the confines from the "same old" research approaches and settings that now dominate biomedical research when the world (and potentially the universe) is full of experiments of biology and nature.

When I finished my medical, graduate, and residency training in 1984, I received a research appointment at the National Institutes of Health and soon had the opportunity to work with Blumberg again on a research project on nutrition and cancer based on an experiment of nature in the People's Republic of China. The great Yangtze River washes down soil from the interior of China to form new lands in the river delta 1000 miles away. The nutrient content of the soil from the interior is very different for growing crops and foraging livestock. During Mao Zedong's Cultural Revolution of the 1960s, intellectuals and scientists had been relocated to the new lands in the river delta, including an island called Chongming (the "isle of wisdom"). With very different nutritional content in the soil, the inhabitants had very different cancer rates compared to adjacent Jiangsu to the north, or Shanghai to the south. After a successful start, our work was interrupted by the events at Tiananmen Square in Beijing during June 1989, when funding for our research was withdrawn, providing a stark example of the influence of politics over medical research. While not all examples of political interference with medical science are so obvious, they are ubiquitous.

Creating a Text on Complementary and Alternative Medicine

All these experiences have profoundly influenced my work, especially the creation of these texts, over the past 30 years. When interest (and frequently consternation) over complementary and alternative medicine (CAM) was heightened 20 years ago, I saw the need and opportunity to present the sciences that support CAM in terms of what anthropologists call *ethnomedicine*, as well as reconnect with the holistic health movement of the 1960s and 70s. While many figures in mainstream medicine were acting as if CAM had suddenly landed in their backyards (or front yards) from another planet, I understood that many of these traditions are based upon hundreds or thousands of years of experience among other cultures or societies, as part of our global patrimony, while many others are in fact part of our own history in the United States, which is usually conveniently forgotten.

Today, students are able to learn about these healing traditions without traveling to Asia, studying traditional societies, or

studying medical history or anthropology (a real oversight in our modern medical curricula). New curricula in the authentic study of CAM are being offered, such as the degree program at Georgetown University School of Medicine, as discussed in the foreword from the prior (fourth) edition of this text, reprinted here.

This book is now being used in programs such as the master's degree in Physiology, CAM track, at Georgetown University School of Medicine, which has now graduated more than a dozen consecutive classes. This program, and others, provide examples of how the medical curriculum is being supplemented ("complemented"?) to give health professions students the tools to understand a broader perspective in medicine and to be prepared to work in a post-biomedical paradigm. Students take science-based courses, acquire CAM-related knowledge, and learn the skills to critically analyze the available kinds of evidence on CAM studies. I acknowledge the inspiration that comes from teaching these students each year and the creativity of the faculty members working together under the directorship of Dr. Adi Haramati (who contributes a foreword to this text) and Dr. Hakima Amri (co-author of two chapters) as well as all those who have supported and nourished this program.

Benefit to All Health Professions

The need for more *science* is often identified as an issue in understanding alternative and complementary therapies. In this textbook we address that issue and also answer the need for more *sciences* in the study of CAM. For example, the social sciences are also critical for an understanding of the foundations of human knowledge and experience that underlay and support the practice of ancient and historic healing traditions, which we call here *complementary and alternative medicine* (and which social scientists, such as medical anthropologists, call *ethnomedicine*). For the many readers of this textbook, now in its fifth edition, it may be useful to see this work also as a complete textbook of medical approaches to healing. New chapters on the world's ethnomedical healing traditions now cover the globe and enhance and round out our knowledge and understanding of the world's great healing traditions. This text brings forward the best scholarship on ancient and historic healing traditions in application to our understanding of contemporary CAM. Some of the earliest translations of classical medical texts were not very sophisticated in terms of the medical terminology used for translation into English. With contemporary scholarship and translations, we now see that it was not the ancient healing traditions that appeared unsophisticated but the old English translations.

For those with an orientation to understanding from where this knowledge originates and how it has been promulgated as part of our global cultural patrimony, we move beyond the standard basic science curriculum of modern medical education and the clinical trials, protocols, and "cookbook recipes" of "integrative medicine."

Contents and Organization

This book is presented in six sections. The first section serves as an introduction to the field of complementary and alternative medicine, discussing the history, characteristics, translation, as well as issues and challenges in what is called "integrative" medicine. A new chapter presents the dimensions of CAM that exist outside what is defined as the health care system itself, as so much of what CAM offers is in the larger community outside medical facilities per se.

The sections next move into the subjects of ecology, vitalism, psychoneuroimmnology, mind–body approaches, spirituality, creative art therapies and humor contributed by the popular physician "Patch" Adams. The topics of energy medicine as well as electricity, light, sound, magnetism, and biophysical devices are presented next. Given this foundation, the book then moves the reader into thorough descriptions of the development and key concepts of the most prevalent complementary and alternative therapies being used in the United States Topics covered include massage, manual therapies and bodywork, yoga, chiropractic, osteopathy, herbal medicine, aromatherapy and essential oils therapy, "nature cure," naturopathy and naturopathic medicine, and nutrition and hydration. There is also unique content on herbal medicine: common herbs in clinical practice, East and Southeast Asian herbs, and Native North and South American herbs.

The sections on mind-body-spirit and on energetics, manual healing, and bodywork include overviews of all mind-body medical modalities, including relevant background on neurohumoral physiology and psychoneuroimmunology (PNI), energy healing, biophysical modalities and devices, creative arts and movement therapies, and humor.

The final two sections introduce and provide comprehensive overviews of traditional medical systems. The fifth section presents the medical systems of Chinese medicine (acupuncture, Qigong, and Tibetan medicine) and Ayurveda (a traditional medicine of India), as well as Siddha, Sufi healing, and Unani medicine. The sixth and final section continues the global perspective with new chapters and discussions of healing systems from Southeast Asia, the Pacific, Africa, and the Americas, as well as worldwide shamanism and neo-shamanism and contemporary global health care.

Where appropriate, new clinical guides have been added for the application of selected alternative healing traditions for common medical problems where they can substitute.

Covering All the Relevant Sciences

In addition to providing background from the biological sciences, this book takes a much broader approach compared to other texts on complementary, alternative, and integrative medicine. The social sciences, including social history and cultural anthropology (often called *cultural history* by social historians), provide the origins of the underlying science that informs one unique approach of this text to the study of CAM. In this edition, the preface and the introduction to Section Six (Chapter 34) can serve as a primer for those students and faculty who wish to use this work as a foundational text in the "basic sciences" of health and healing.

The behavioral and social sciences generally, and medical anthropology in particular, provide a disciplined approach (literally, as academic disciplines and as fields of practice) to understanding human biology and culture, and human nature in the context of nature, as particularly relevant to the naturalistic approaches of alternative and complementary medicine (and what is, in fact, often called *natural medicine*). These approaches have tremendous value in helping to understand which aspects of medical practice and health care are compelled, or chosen, which are based upon authentic science, and which aspects represent true alternatives on a global basis. Although biomedical science and clinical trials provide many answers to human medicine, we here offer an approach whereby other kinds of knowledge about health and healing may additionally be brought to bear in a serious and disciplined manner. Thus, this expanded fifth edition of *Fundamentals of Complementary and Alternative Medicine* presents the world's healing traditions, including those from the Western world, that continue to offer real alternatives and choices for health and healing to both practitioners and patients in the twenty-first century.

Notes to the Reader

While recovering and reinterpreting the ancient and traditional knowledge and wisdom about health and healing as now proven by contemporary scientific investigations, it is also important to take what we have learned about medicine in the twentieth century and form a new synthesis that represents a whole, or truly "holistic," approach for the twenty-first century. We must be prepared to live in a postbiomedical paradigm. Consumers described by social scientists as "cultural creatives" (numbering over 50 million people) are already there, voting with their feet and pocketbooks. This text provides the health professions with the fundamentals to be prepared to meet them, and help lead them, to a better, more optimistic, more complete kind of health care that recognizes the limits of biomedical technology as well as the limitless possibilities of human capabilities and the boundless human spirit.

The years since publication of the prior (fourth) edition of this text witnessed the deaths of two key mentors, Baruch S. Blumberg, MD, PhD (1925-2011), and C. Everett Koop, MD, DSc (1916-2013). Dr. Koop's foreword to the third edition of this text is reprinted here. Dr. Blumberg, in his roles as outlined above, taught me to look beyond statistical associations (today's fashion in "evidence-based medicine") to always consider biological plausibility. This new fifth edition is dedicated to them both.

FINIS

Marc S. Micozzi, MD, PhD
Longboat Key, Florida
March 2014

About the Author

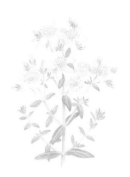

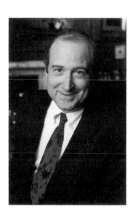

Marc Micozzi is a physician-anthropologist who has worked to create broadly science-based tools for the health professions to be better informed and productively engaged in the fields called complementary and alternative (CAM) and integrative medicine. He was the founding editor-in-chief of the first U.S. journal in CAM, *Journal of Alternative and Complementary Medicine: Research on Paradigm, Practice, and Policy* (1994), and the first review journal in CAM, *Seminars in Integrative Medicine* (2002). As well as editing this textbook for 20 years through four prior editions, he served as series editor for Churchill-Livingstone/Elsevier's *Medical Guides to Complementary and Alternative Medicine*, with 18 titles on a broad range of CAM therapies and therapeutic systems. He is co-editor of *Energy Medicine East and West* with Elsevier, and co-author of *Teaching Mindfulness* with Springer Publishers, among other current textbooks. He organized and chaired six international continuing education conferences on the theory, science, and practice of CAM from 1991 to 2001.

Dr. Micozzi published original research on diet, nutrition, and chronic disease as a senior investigator in the Intramural Cancer Prevention Studies program of the National Cancer Institute from 1984 to 1986. He continued this line of research when he was appointed associate director of the Armed Forces Institute of Pathology and founding director of the National Museum of Health and Medicine in 1986. His early work on carotenoids (including lutein and lycopene), iron and cancer (collaborating with Nobel laureate Baruch Blumberg), anthropometric methods for time-related assessment of nutritional status, and other research made important contributions to this field. He was recognized for his work as the recipient of the John Hill Brinton Young Investigator Award at Walter Reed Army Medical Center in 1992, at which time he was jointly appointed as a Distinguished Scientist in the American Registry of Pathology. He edited and co-edited two comprehensive technical volumes on application of clinical trials methods to new investigations of the role of nutrients in cancer. He has published 275 articles in the medical, scientific, and technical literature.

From 1995 to 2002, he served as executive director of the College of Physicians of Philadelphia. He revitalized all aspects of the college's programs, operations, and physical infrastructure. There, he opened the C. Everett Koop Community Health Information Center (Koop CHIC), which provided information to consumers on health and wellness, including CAM. The White House Commission on CAM recognized his work on behalf of consumer health in 2001.

Dr. Micozzi also actively collaborated with former U.S. Surgeon General C. Everett Koop for over 25 years. As a medical and scientific advisor to Dr. Koop LifeCare Corporation, he worked on new developments with the FDA regarding review of dietary supplements. Over the past several years Dr. Micozzi has developed his own formulations for dietary, herbal, and nutritional supplements for a variety of applications and has reviewed thousands of publications on hundreds of nutritional supplements and herbal remedies, including bringing to light little-known herbal remedies from the Southern African continent.

In 2002, he became founding director of the Policy Institute for Integrative Medicine in Washington, DC, educating the U.S. Congress, policy makers, the health professions, and the general public about needs and opportunities for CAM and integrative medicine. From 2003 to 2005, he accepted an additional interim appointment as executive director of the Center for Integrative Medicine at Thomas Jefferson University Hospital in Philadelphia. He is an Adjunct Professor in the Department of Medicine at the University of Pennsylvania and in the Departments of Pharmacology and Physiology & Biophysics at Georgetown University. In 2012 he became editor-in-chief at www.drmicozzi.com, where he writes a daily column on health and medicine, a monthly newsletter, and periodic monographs and special reports on current health care issues. Contact e-mail: marcsmicozzi@gmail.com.

Contents

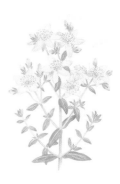

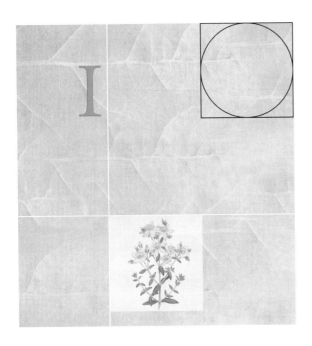

FOUNDATIONS

This section provides an introduction to the overall topic of complementary and alternative medicine (CAM), its themes and terminology, and the various contexts relative to its proper interpretation. In addition, this section addresses issues in what is now being called "integrative medicine," which represents an attempt to bring authentic CAM therapies into the continuum of mainstream health care. The chapters provide a social and cultural contextualization of CAM.

As an introduction to CAM, these chapters discuss social and cultural factors, an integrative medical model, and the dimensions of CAM practice. The cultural and social history of the use of CAM traditions is discussed in terms of intellectual, medical, and scientific discourse, which is important to the understanding of the common themes of bioenergy and self-healing. The ubiquitous use of plants and natural products among alternatives is introduced through underlying themes from both the social and the biological sciences.

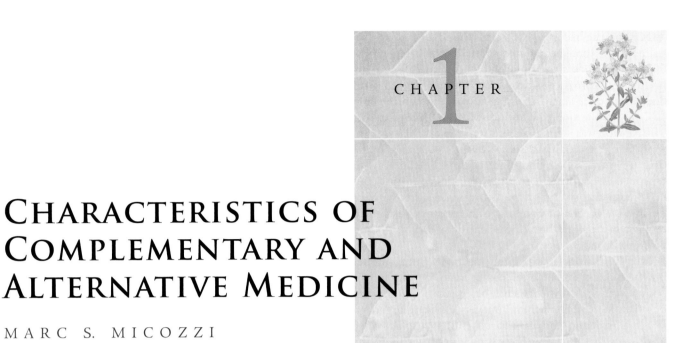

CHAPTER 1

CHARACTERISTICS OF COMPLEMENTARY AND ALTERNATIVE MEDICINE

MARC S. MICOZZI

The different medical systems subsumed under the category *complementary and alternative* are many and diverse, but these systems have some common ground in their views of health and healing. Their common philosophy can be considered as *a new ecology of health,* or sustainable medicine.

ROLE OF SCIENCE AND THE SCIENCES

Allopathic medicine is considered the "scientific" healing art, whereas the alternative forms of medicine have been considered "nonscientific." However, what is needed for proper interpretation is not *less science* but *more sciences* in the study of complementary and alternative medicine (CAM). Some of the central ideas of biomedicine are very powerful but may have become static philosophically. The study of dead tissue cells, components, and chemicals to understand life processes, and the quest for "magic bullets" to combat disease are based on a reductionist, materialist view of health and healing. Tremendous advances have been made over the past 100 years by applying these concepts to medicine. However, the resulting biomedical system is not always able to account for and use many important observations in the realms of clinical and personal experience, natural law, and human spirituality.

Contemporary biomedicine utilizes models from Newtonian physics and pre-evolutionary biology. Newtonian physics explains and can reproduce many observations on mechanics at the level of everyday experience. The biomedical model often employs a conceptual projection of Newtonian mechanics into the microscopic and molecular realms.

Contemporary fundamental physics (quantum mechanics, relativity, etc.) recognizes aspects of reality beyond Newtonian mechanics, such as matter–energy duality, "unified fields" of energy and matter, and wave functions (see Chapters 14 and 15). Quantum physics and contemporary biology-ecology (Chapter 27) may be needed to better understand alternative systems.

Nuclear medicine uses the technology of contemporary physics, for example, but biomedicine does not yet incorporate the concepts of quantum physics in its fundamental approach to human health and healing. Contemporary biomedicine measures the body's energy using electrocardiography, electroencephalography, and electromyography for diagnostic purposes, but it does not explicitly enlist the body's energy for the purposes of health and healing.

A MODEL FOR EVERYTHING

As a model for everything, Newtonian mechanics has limitations. It works within the narrow limits of everyday experience. It does not always work at a *macro* (cosmic) level, as shown by Einstein's theory of relativity, or at a *micro* (fundamental) level, as illustrated by quantum physics. However useful Newton's physics has been in solving mechanical problems, it does not explain a vast preponderance of nature: the motion of currents; the growth of plants and animals (Chapter 27); or the rise, functioning, and fall of civilizations (Chapter 5).

Per Bak (1947–2002) at the Niels Bohr Institute, Copenhagen, Denmark, was an expert on the physics of complex systems, chaos theory, and fractals who developed the now widely recognized theory of self-organizing criticality

(SOC) for the recurring patterns found in nature (for example, the dimensional and spatial ratios based on the Fibonacci numbers as employed by Leonardo Da Vinci in his widely reproduced, classic depiction of the human body). Bak once stated that Newtonian mechanics could explain why the apple fell but not why the apple existed or why Newton was thinking about it in the first place.

In fact, it is said that Isaac Newton was sitting under that apple tree in the first place because he had gone to Lincolnshire countryside to escape the plague of the 1660s in London and at Cambridge University. He left without finishing his degree at Cambridge and perhaps was able to retain his paradigm-breaking scientific creativity for not having finished.

Mechanics works in explaining machines. But no matter how popular this metaphor has become for the human body (with acknowledgment of *National Geographic*'s popular "incredible machine" imagery), a living organism is *not* a machine and cannot be entirely explained by mechanics. It is becoming increasingly clear that an understanding of energetics is required. This duality between the mechanical and the energetic, which has been accepted in physics for the past century now, is illustrated by the fact that J.J. Thomson won the Nobel Prize for demonstrating that the electron is a particle. His son, George P. Thomson, won the Nobel Prize a generation later for demonstrating that the electron is a wave (see Chapter 14 for more on this paradox).

Those styled as "hard scientists," such as physicists and molecular scientists, accept the duality of the electron but biomedical and clinical scientists often have difficulty accepting this duality as applied to the human body. Those so-called soft sciences, or psychological and social sciences, attempt to be inclusive in their study of the phenomena of life and nature, but are often looked on with disdain according to the folklore of the self-styled "real" scientists. However, real science must account for all of what is observed in nature, not just the conveniently reductionistic, materialist part.

The biological science of contemporary medicine can be seen, to an extent, as pre-evolutionary in that it typically emphasizes typology rather than individuality and variation. Each patient is defined as a clinical entity by a "type" diagnosis, given a prescribed code for tracking and billing purposes, and with treatment prescribed accordingly, as per the "standard dosage form" of a drug, for example. The modern understanding of the mechanics of the human genome does not make this approach to biomedical science less pre-evolutionary but it is potentially making it even more reductionistic.

The late Victor McKusick, Chairman of Medicine at Johns Hopkins University, often described as the founder of modern medical genetics, once expressed to me that the Human Genome Project was actually the ultimate projection of human dissection to type the genome right down to the level of the individual genes and chromosomes. (He was serving as chair of a panel I had convened at Walter Reed Army Medical Center—formerly the U.S. Army Medical Museum—to study the technical and ethical issues involved in testing the 1865 autopsy samples from Abraham Lincoln for the presence of the primary genetic disorder of Marfan's syndrome.)

Both the fundamental principles of inheritance (Gregor Mendel) and those of natural selection (Charles Darwin and Alfred Russel Wallace—see Chapters 27 and 35) were explained a century before the discovery of the physical structure of the gene itself. While contemporary biology-ecology continues to explore the phenomena of how living organisms and systems interact at the level of the whole—which cannot be seen under a microscope or in a test tube—molecular genetics continues to dissect the human genome in an effort to discover new cures. In the process, these investigations into genes and their regulation is actually demonstrating the long-sought "mechanisms of action" as to how natural approaches and nutrients, such as vitamin D (Chapter 26), actually manifest their multitudinous effects on human health, well beyond old ideas about chemical "antioxidants." Gene regulation is now even explaining what happens with regulation at the molecular genetic level with mind–body techniques such as relaxation therapy to bring about specific healthful physiologic responses (Chapters 9 and 10).

It may seem forbiddingly complex to construct a medical system based on the concepts of modern physics and biology-ecology while maintaining a unique diagnostic and therapeutic approach to each individual. This would indeed be complex if not for the fact that the body inherently manages its own complexity, as part of this whole nature, including an innate ability to heal itself.

ONE WAY

One way of studying and understanding complementary and alternative medicine is to view it in light of contemporary physics and biology-ecology and to focus not just on the sometimes subtle manipulations of alternative practitioners, but also on the physiological and homeostatic responses of the human body. When acupuncture or energetic healing is observed to result in a physiological or clinical response that cannot be explained by the current biomedical model, it is not the role of the scientist to deny this reality. Science does not advance from statements such as, "It doesn't work because it can't work," as was once essentially claimed by a former editor of the prestigious British journal *Nature*. When a stripped-down, "formulary" or "integrative" approach to herbal medicine, acupuncture, or any other therapy—as adapted from another cultural tradition (see Chapter 3)—actually yields a demonstrable healing response (despite being devoid of any traditional cultural meaning or "belief"), we must look to the physiology of the body and not just a putative effect of autosuggestion or placebo (as potent as they may be; see Chapter 9).

Rather, authentic science works to modify explanatory models to account for all empirical observations. In this way, science itself progresses. In the end, there is one "unified" reality. Complementary (or alternative) medical systems, many of which are relatively "old" in terms of human intellectual history, are themselves largely empirical (rather than experimental) systems of knowledge. Since their origins, they have always been trying to describe, understand, and work (within their own cultural terms) with the same reality of health and healing as biomedicine. Whereas contemporary biomedicine uses new technologies in the service of relatively fixed ideas about health and healing, alternative methods use relatively old technologies whose fundamental character may reflect new scientific ideas on physical and biological nature (Box 1-1).

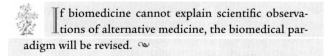

If biomedicine cannot explain scientific observations of alternative medicine, the biomedical paradigm will be revised. ✧

Science must account for *all* of what is observed, not just the convenient part of it. Physics has gone beyond Newtonian mechanics—and biology-ecology beyond typology. Is it possible for a valid biomedical model to be constructed that includes observations from CAM? Although it may be necessary to wait for further insights from physics and biology to understand aspects of CAM in terms of biomedicine, clinical pragmatism dictates that successful therapeutic methods should not be withheld while mechanisms are being explained—or debated. We live in a world filled with opportunities to observe the practice of complementary and alternative medicine; all that remains is to continue to apply appropriate scientific standards (from all the sciences) to its study and practice. In the meantime, patients are not waiting for physicians and scientists to more fully understand the mechanisms of CAM. As former U.S. Surgeon General C. Everett Koop, George Lundberg (former editor-in chief of the *Journal of the American Medical Association*), and I have all pointed out over the past two decades, "What works is not complementary or alternative. What works is good medicine."

Further, as students and scholars of health and healing, we can come to understand the underlying intellectual content and history of alternative forms of medicine as complete systems of thought and practice. These sources of information about CAM are properly part of human knowledge. Not every idea, thought, or construct that is useful in health and medicine need arise only from the controlled, clinical trial (the so-called gold standard) or from the narrow, biased perspective of so-called evidence-based medicine (see Chapter 3).

WELLNESS

The CAM systems generally emphasize what might be called "wellness" by the mainstream medical model or the popular wisdom. The goal of preventing disease is shared by alternative/complementary, integrative, and mainstream medicine alike. In the mainstream, biomedical model, this goal can involve using drugs, medical procedures, and/or surgery to prevent disease in those who are only at risk, rather than reserving these powerful methods for the treatment of disease.

I have called this trend the *medicalization* of prevention. In this approach, there is a dangerous perception that one may continue to engage in risky lifestyle behaviors while medicine provides "magic bullets" to prevent diseases that it cannot cure. Wellness in the context of complementary medicine is more than the prevention of disease. It is a focus on engaging the inner resources of each individual as an active and conscious participant in the maintenance of

BOX 1-1 *A Note About Nomenclature*

Although the term *complementary and integrative medicine (CIM)* was used in the third edition, *complementary and alternative medicine* was used in the title of the first two editions, and again resumed for the fourth edition, no longer a victim of fashion. The word *alternative,* or the term *complementary and alternative medicine,* now seems to be culturally encoded in the English language. In our view, the concept, organization, and practice of what is called "integrative medicine" has become too problematic and obscure to be countenanced in a text-book attempting to present medical knowledge (see Chapter 3).

"Alternative medicine" had been used to refer to those practices explicitly used for the purpose of medical intervention, health promotion, or disease prevention, which are not routinely taught at U.S. medical schools nor routinely underwritten by third-party payers within the existing U.S. health care system.

Such a definition seems to be a diagnosis of exclusion, meaning that alternative medicine is everything not presently being promoted in mainstream medicine. This definition may remind us of a popular song from the 1960s called "The Element Song," which offers a complete listing of the different elements of the periodic table (set to the tune of "I Am the Very Model of a Modern Major General" from Gilbert and Sullivan's *The Pirates of Penzance*). It ends with words to this effect: "These are the many elements we've heard about at Harvard. And if we haven't heard of them, they haven't been discovered."

I have likened the relatively recent "discovery" of alternative medicine to Columbus's discovery of the Americas. Although his voyage was a great feat that expanded the intellectual frontiers of Europe, Columbus could not really discover a world already known to millions of indigenous peoples who had complex systems of social organization and subsistence activities, including medical practices (see p. 9). Likewise, the definitional statement that alternative forms of medicine are not within the existing U.S. health care system is a curious observation for the tens of millions of Americans who routinely use them today and every day.

BOX 1-2 *Prevention versus Acute versus Chronic Disease*

In Western allopathic medicine, careful distinctions are often made among modalities for preventing disease, for treating acute disease, and for treating chronic disease.

Because complementary and alternative medicine (CAM) modalities are generally directed at the underlying causes rather than the symptoms of disease, CAM strategies for prevention, for treatment of acute disorders, and for treatment of chronic disorders may often be the same or similar.

Ambulatory CAM Care versus Residential CAM Care

CAM modalities are now widely available in the United States in both health care and non–health care settings. However, they are generally offered only as ambulatory care. Although there is much that can be accomplished by a CAM practitioner in a clinical setting, ambulatory care clients often experience a "reduced" form of the full potential benefits (Chapter 3). Traditional Chinese, Ayurvedic, naturopathic, and other CAM "cures" involve the client's being "admitted" for residential care in a healthful environment over prolonged periods in which all aspects of the client's experience are directed toward a healing response. Here, for example, diet is part of therapy and not something assigned to institutional food services, or "dieticians," as in modern hospitals. Although CAM modalities are generally gentler and less potent than modern biomedical technology, the potency of a full residential CAM cure can be remarkable (see Chapters 2 and 3).

his or her own health. By the same token, the property of being healthy is not conferred on an individual by an outside agency or entity, but rather results from the balance of internal resources with the external natural and social environments. This latter point relates to the "alternative" yet basic approach that relies on the abilities of the individual to get well and stay healthy, or "self-healing" (Box 1-2).

SELF-HEALING

The body heals itself. This might seem to be an obvious statement, because we are well aware that wounds heal and blood and tissue cells routinely replace themselves over time. Nonetheless, this concept is central and profound among CAM systems, because self-healing is the basis of *all* healing. External "medical" manipulations simply mobilize the body's inner healing resources. Instead of wondering why the body's cells are sick, alternative systems ask why the body is not replacing its sick cells with healthy cells. The body's ability to be well or ill is largely tied to inner resources, and the external environment—social and physical—has an impact on this ability.

What is the evidence for self-healing? The long and common history of clinical observations of the "placebo

effect" (see Chapter 9), the "laying on of hands," or "spontaneous remissions" may be included in this category. To paraphrase Carl Jung: Summoned or not summoned, self-healing will be there (but generally more so when summoned—see Chapter 9). Self-healing is so powerful that biomedical research methodology must design randomized, double-blind, controlled clinical trials to see what (usually small) percentage of benefit a potent drug can add to the healing encounter. While long considered the "gold standard" for medical research, this method actually has serious limitations in studying both drug and especially non-drug therapies (see Chapter 3).

Troubling is a contemporary analysis from Harvard University showing that of new drugs approved by the FDA over the past quarter-century, only 10% show greater effectiveness than the drugs they were designed to replace, whereas fully 50% are less safe than those older drugs (Light et al, 2013). This finding does not herald progress in terms of the therapeutic profile of most new drugs.

HEALING ENERGY

A related concept to self-healing is that the body has energy (see Chapters 14 and 15; see also Mayor & Micozzi, 2011). Accordingly, as a living entity, the body is an energetic system. Disruptions in the balance and flow of energy contribute to illness, and the body's response to energetic imbalance leads to perceptible disease. As the mind–body can heal itself, the mind–body may ultimately also make itself sick when out of balance. Restoring or facilitating the mind–body to recover its own balance restores health. The symptoms of a cold, flu, or allergy are caused by physiologic responses to rid the body of the offending agent. For example, by raising the body's temperature, a fever reduces bacterial reproduction (like an antibiotic, fever is literally bacteriostatic), and, of course, sneezing physically expels offending agents (see Figure 2-3, p. 19, and Chapter 2).

Pathologists know that there are only so many ways that cells can "look sick," because cellular reactions have a defined and limited repertoire for manifesting malfunction. There are only so many way cells can respond (essentially efforts to adapt) to injury, infection, or illness (Chapter 2). Biomedicine has learned a great deal over the past 100 years by systematically correlating the appearance of artefactually stained, dead tissue cells under the microscope with clinical diagnosis and prognosis. However, studying such devitalized tissues and cells for clinical significance does not allow direct observation of the dynamic energy of living cells, systems, organisms, and communities. Correlation of the appearance of stained tissue cells under a microscope to clinical conditions was long the most powerful concept and tool in diagnostic medicine.

By the time illness causes cells to become so damaged as to appear "pathologically abnormal" under the microscope, the patient has a disease—literally by definition. Alternative forms of medicine appear to provide a possible path to study the energy of living systems for health and healing and to detect and correct imbalances and illnesses before the onset of fixed diseases and "pathologies." The real goal of health care is to detect imbalances and disorders prior to the development of overt pathology and frank disease. In contemporary medical practice, patients without a "disease" by any pathologic definition are very frequently encountered (about 50% of patient visits). These many "functional complaints," which show no abnormalities in laboratory studies or pathological tests, include common conditions, such as migraine and other headaches, irritable bowel, chronic pain syndromes, menstrual dysfunction, etc. (see Chapter 2).

Alternative approaches to detect and treat such functional complaints are quite clinically useful because they are based on the premise that all things exist *in relationship* to everything else. This fact is one reason why the reductionist, singular focus becomes less relevant within the context of CAM. All things in the universe exist in relationship to everything else. Hippocrates said: "There is one common flow, one common breathing, all things are in sympathy."

Modern society, embedded and invested in technology, has led us away from the natural environment and the relations we as human organisms have with our own planet and the universe beyond (see Chapter 27). We need to better understand the relations among the cells, organs, and tissues in the human body, but also how we as organisms living on this planet are affecting our external environment and our health. Plants constitute a predominant part of the terrestrial environment in which humans evolved and live.

NUTRITION AND NATURAL PRODUCTS

The reliance on nutrition and natural products is fundamental to CAM and does not play merely a supportive or adjunctive role. Plant life formed a predominant part of the terrestrial environment in which animal life and humans evolved. Nutrients and plant products are taken into the body and incorporated in the most literal sense. They provide the body with energy in the form of calories and with the material and structural resources to grow and maintain cells, tissues and organs.

The basic plan of the body, as a physical entity and as an energetic system, evolves and exists in an ecological context. What the body needs it obtains from the environment in which it grew. Lao Tzu said that "what is deeply rooted in nature cannot be uprooted." The human organism evolved and is designed to obtain nutrients from natural food sources present in the natural environment, and the body is often best suited to obtain nutrients in their natural forms (see Chapter 26).

PLANTS

Plants are an important part of nature relative to health and a dominant part of the nature in which humans evolved. In addition to producing the oxygen that we breathe, plants are seen as sources of nutrients, medicines (e.g., phytochemicals), and essential oils (e.g., volatiles for inhalation and transdermal absorption); some systems also view plants as sources of vibrational energy. Many systems see the use of plants as sources of nutrients in continuity with their use as sources of medicine, paralleling some contemporary biomedical guidelines for nutrition as disease prevention. As in Chinese medicine, for example, foods exist in continuity with medicines among plant sources (see Chapters 26 and 28).

INDIVIDUALITY

The emphasis of CAM is on the whole person as a unique individual with his or her own inner resources. Therefore, the concepts of normalization, standardization, and generalization may be more difficult to apply to research and clinical practice compared with the allopathic method. Some believe that alternative/complementary forms of medicine restore the role of the individual patient and practitioner to the practice of medicine; the biomedical emphasis on standardization of training and practice to ensure quality may leave something lost in translation back to restoring the health of the individual.

> The focus on the whole person as a unique individual provides new challenges to the scientific measurement of the healing encounter. Mobilizing the resources of each individual to stay healthy and become well also provides new opportunities to move health care toward a model of wellness. Such awareness would also move "health care reform" toward authentic models for helping solve the current health care crisis—a crisis driven by politics and costs and a shortage of imagination and will for implementing alternative solutions that make scientific and economic sense.

HUMILITY

As the body heals itself, has its own energy, and is uniquely individual, then the focus is not on the healer but on the healed. Although this concept is humbling to a heroic role of practitioner as healer, it is liberating to realize that, in the end, each person heals himself or herself. If the healer is not the sole source of health and healing, there is room for humility and room for both patient and practitioner to participate in the interaction.

With all due emphasis on humility in healing, it is interesting to note that the practice of CAM in the United States has largely been sustained by the "healthy" egos of alternative practitioners who have not necessarily undergone the humbling (and frequently humiliating) experiences of four years of premed, four years of medical school, and four or more years of specialization and servitude as resident hospital physicians, followed by having their practices increasingly dictated by government bureaucrats and insurance company clerks. Often having benefited by "dropping out" of a system that is largely a matter of custom and economics, the struggle of the alternative practitioner, rather, has been against professional indifference and ridicule, and frequent harassment and sanctions from state licensing boards and federal agencies.

FUNCTIONAL DEFINITION

For the purposes of this book, a functional definition of CAM is offered, limited here to what may be called *alternative/complementary medical systems.* Complementary medical systems are characterized by a developed body of intellectual work that (1) underlies the conceptualization of health, healing and its precepts; (2) has been sustained over generations by many practitioners among many communities; (3) represents an orderly, rational, conscious system of empirical knowledge and thought about health and medicine; (4) relates more broadly to a way of life (or lifestyle) that is not all delimited by the modern concept of what is referenced as "medicine" (Chapter 4); and (5) has been widely observed to have definable results as practiced.

HOLISTIC

Although the term *holistic* has been applied to the approach to the "body as person" among CAM systems, I apply holism to the medical system itself as a complete system of thought and practice (what I have called "health beliefs and behaviors"; see Chapter 2). This system of knowledge is therefore shared by patients and practitioners—the active, conscious engagement of "patients" is relative to the focus on *self-healing* and *individuality* that are among the common characteristics of these systems.

In this regard it might be considered that this text is documenting the "classic" practices of CAM systems. In trying to build a bridge between a well-developed system of allopathic medicine and complementary medical systems, it is necessary to have strong foundations on both sides of this bridge. It is not possible to apply these criteria to the work of individual alternative practitioners who have unilaterally developed their own unique techniques over one or two generations (what might be called "unconventional"), just as it is not possible to build a bridge to nowhere.

This definition is meant to apply to systems of *thought* and not just techniques of practice. Often an underlying philosophy of individual practitioners surrounds new techniques they have developed, or new techniques may be subsumed under existing systems of practice. Holistic philosophy also posits that within each one thing is contained all; the microcosm is the macrocosm. Because the connection is already there, there is no need to impose a specific technique onto any modality, but simply educate each to the already existing connection they all hold in common.

ECLECTICISM

Eclecticism is used to refer to historical forms of medicines that would now be considered "alternative," and it drew from different traditions that were popular in the United States for a century or more. In such systems, treatment is guided by the affinities, preferences, and needs of each individual patient, not limited to what one given system or technique has to offer. Today in the United States, a chiropractor may practice in an Ayurveda clinic; osteopaths may practice in allopathic clinics; and chiropractors, osteopaths, or allopaths may all use acupuncture.

NATUROPATHY

Naturopathy, in some ways the most recent of homegrown alternatives from the European–North American tradition, consciously employs a variety of traditions ranging from acupuncture to herbal medicine. I have informally termed naturopathy as *neo-eclecticism,* with the unifying, underlying philosophy that the body heals itself using resources found in nature (see Chapter 22). When the fundamental principles and organization of Naturopathic Medicine is properly considered, it may in fact offer an authentic approach to genuine integrative medicine (Chapters 3 and 23).

Ultimately, any given medical system develops in answer to human health needs, just as agriculture develops to serve nutritional needs. Alternatives vary widely, but their characteristics cluster around the self-healing capabilities of the human organism and the human organism's ability to use (and rely on) resources present in nature. What is constant and at the center of such CAM systems is the individual human. Therefore, if the focus is not on the medical system itself but on the person at the center, there is really only one system.

SOME FUNDAMENTALS OF MEDICAL SCIENCE

Contemporary biomedicine is a scientific paradigm with a particular history and philosophy, as much influenced by cultural and social history and economics as by scientific laws (see Chapter 5). In the laudable effort to make medicine scientific, we have emphasized that knowledge about the world, including nature and human nature, must be pursued using the following criteria: (1) *objectivism*—the observer is separate from the observed; (2) *reductionism*—all complex phenomena are fully explainable in terms of simpler, component phenomena; (3) *positivism*—all relevant information can be derived from physically measurable data; and (4) *determinism*—all phenomena can be predicted from a knowledge of scientific law and initial starting conditions.

We all work and live our lives every day with an inherent understanding that this approach is not the only way of "knowing" things, but it became the twentieth-century test to determine whether knowledge is "scientific." In fact, science simply requires *empiricism*—making and testing models of reality by what can be observed, guided by certain values, and based on certain metaphysical assumptions. Any science itself is a system of human knowledge built over time by collecting observations, testing hypotheses, and constructing theories. Scientists can often detect distinctions between metaphysical reality and the scientific models constructed through human intellectual activity. The new thoughts engendered by CAM regarding the nature of medicine do not represent a "new science" so much as they represent a new philosophy.

The four criteria for the scientific paradigm just listed above are not always applicable. In the science of physics, *objectivism* is ultimately not possible at the fundamental level because the *Heisenberg uncertainty principle* states that the act of observing phenomena necessarily influences the behavior of the phenomena being observed (Chapter 14). Contemporary biological and ecological science has produced a wealth of observations about interactions among living organisms and their environments in transactional, multidirectional, and synergic ways that are not ultimately subject to *reductionist* explanations (Chapter 27). For *positivism* and *determinism* to be able to provide complete explanations, we must assume that science has all the physical methods and intellectual tools to ask all the right questions. However, the questions we ask, and the methods available, are based on the history of science itself as part of the history of human intellectual inquiry.

Spheres of Influence

One of the other important characteristics of what we now call complementary/alternative medicine is that it is not just "foreign." Some mainstream observers seem to react as if CAM had suddenly landed in our midst from another planet in the late twentieth century. In fact, many of the concepts of "alternative" healing traditions are inextricably linked with the history of Western societies, including that of the ancient Greeks, including Pythagoras, who is now known more for being a mathematician, although he was also a learned musician and healer in his own right. In fact, Pythagoras understood and taught the relations of math to music and the cosmos, what he originally called the *music of the spheres*, and taught methods of sound healing to his students. Pythagoras' methods became lost, destroyed, or abandoned.

Related traditions regarding the harmonies among the organization of nature and human affairs were ultimately intrinsic to the development of European Enlightenment thinkers. When the European Enlightenment reached Scotland, one result was the establishment of a school of "rational medicine" at the University of Edinburgh (also the location of the original publisher of this textbook). Rational medicine held that the interventions of the physician must be empirically observed to result in alleviation of suffering and/or the prolongation of life. Those outcomes were the rational tests of the effectiveness of medical care.

This approach to rational medicine was brought to Colonial America when Drs. Hutchinson and Morgan from the University of Edinburgh petitioned British colonial governor Thomas Penn of Pennsylvania to issue a charter for the College of Philadelphia (now the University of Pennsylvania) for a medical curriculum in 1765, the first medical school in what was to become the United States.

European Legacy

During the Middle Ages in Europe, knowledge and teaching were based on the "seven liberal arts" from the manner in which all knowledge had been assembled, codified, and preserved. This heritage was found in a religious work by Augustine, Bishop of Hippo (later canonized as Saint Augustine), and in a civil digest assembled by Roman Proconsul Martianus Capella, both residing in Roman Carthage, North Africa, at the end of the Roman Empire in the fifth century. Grammar was actually considered the foundation of science insofar as it permitted accurate and precise description, classification, and comparison—what today is called "systematics" (something we attempt to provide for CAM systems in this text).

Logic differentiated true from false. Rhetoric was the source of "laws." Arithmetic was the foundation of "order." Geometry was the science of measurement. Astronomy connected science with theology and divinity. Music was the seventh liberal art. Medicine, although not originally included as one of the liberal arts, was considered analogous to music because its object was the "harmony" of the human body. (Today, a sculpture of the seven liberal arts—together with another showing the "learned professions"—is prominent on the main staircase of the central hall of the University of Pennsylvania School of Medicine.)

Physicians, however, struggling with theory and empirical evidence, could not break away from the terminology of astronomy to which they believed all human physiology was subject. Medicine during the Middle Ages, perhaps because of its links with Arabic knowledge, was the one aspect of life that did not become shaped by Christian doctrine. In 1348, while struggling with the devastating effects of the Great Plague (or Black Death, which permanently altered the demographics and social organization of Europe), the medical faculty of the University of Paris reported to Philip VI of France that the cause was a triple conjunction of Jupiter, Mars, and Saturn in the 40th degree of Aquarius.

In the following century to come, the stars became of more practical use by enabling European explorers to "discover" Africa and the Americas.

"Complementary and Alternative" Medicine in America, 1492–1942

In what was to become a new nation in the New World called America, the Founding Fathers (including Washington, Adams, Jefferson, and others—see Chapter 7) were strongly influenced by concepts relating to the harmony of the cosmos and what was known as the "music of the spheres." The unique "American Experience" became characterized by the Enlightenment principles of developing a rational, ordered system for governing human affairs as conceptualized by the Founders in harmony with a divine cosmos.

In addition, the position of the new America, perched on the edge of successive frontiers to the West, and continuously in contact with indigenous peoples of the "New World," dramatically influenced culture in general as well as medical philosophy, arguably as late as World War II. The fact that there were not many "regular" physicians around as the frontiers expanded and were settled made room, literally and figuratively, for new philosophies and practices to arise, develop, and take root—made all the more necessary by the relative vacuum in standard medical practice and infrastructure.

Among the early exchanges to occur between European explorers (then settlers) and Native Americans were diseases and medical treatments. In the New World, Europeans were not surprised to find Native American remedies effective in light of the sixteenth-century "law of correspondences," which held that remedies could be found in the same locales where diseases occur. In the New World, most Europeans, and thence Americans, found themselves for most of the period from 1492 until as late as 1942 on the frontier, where there was often no doctor. And often that was not such a bad thing.

Native Americans also readily adopted "big medicine" from European "physick" and early surgical practices as well, starting from the early Spanish conquistador Cabeza de Vaca (1530), eventually taking the French word for physician (*médecin*), and incorporating it into their own languages to express something previously unknown to them.

Europeans could in turn be impressed by Native American reliance on the healing power of nature and spiritual healing. Nature in the New World provided a bounty of new medicinal plants and foods (whereas in Europe there had been only 16 cultivars—before chocolate, corn, squash, pumpkins, tomatoes, peppers, potatoes, and other foods of the Americas).

Colonial physician Benjamin Rush (a signer of the Declaration of Independence and often considered one of the Founders of the new American republic) recommended that colonists grow their own medicinal plant gardens, adapted from the traditional European folk remedies, that would grow in the new land, together with local Native American remedies that had been incorporated into medical practice (see the section "'Herb' and Other Words" in Chapter 24). In the English colonies beginning at Jamestown (1607), herbs such as sassafras were readily adopted. In Pennsylvania, William Penn (1680) himself became well acquainted with native herbs and other healing-spiritual practices such as the sweat lodge of the Delaware Indians (see Chapter 37).

EARLY HERBALS

Many of the earliest books to originate from the English colonies were natural histories, serving as "herbals," that documented the occurrence of medicinal plants in various parts of the colonies: John Josselyn (1671) on New England; and John Lederer (1670), Robert Beverley (1705), John Lawson (1709), and John Brickell (1737) on Virginia and the Carolinas. John Wesley, later founder of the Methodist Church in England, wrote a similar book on Georgia (1737) during his two-year service as chaplain in Savannah. These regions are very biodiverse with many plant species because they represent the southern edge at altitude of the most recent geologic glaciations, including both preglaciation and postglaciation species (see Chapter 27).

Later, the best known of such herbal chronicles was *Travels through North and South Carolina, Georgia, East and West Florida, the Cherokee Country, the Extensive Territories of the Muscogulges or Creek Confederacy, and the Country of the Chactaws. Containing an Account of the Soil and Natural Productions of Those Regions; Together with Observations on the Manners of the Indians* by William Bartram, professor of botany at the College of Philadelphia (later, the University of Pennsylvania) who was consulted by Lewis and Clark prior to their own travels in 1803. (*Bartram's Travels* is the one book carried by the fictional Confederate Civil War character Inman—not only for its practical value but because "it made him happy"—throughout his journey to Cold Mountain in the 1997 National Book Award winner of the same name by Charles MacDonald Frazier.)

Regular physicians were rare on the expanding frontier, which prevented "regular medicine" (such as bleeding by lancet, leeches, and cupping; and blistering, puking, and purging—of which Francis Bacon had said, "The remedy is worse than the disease") from taking root where there were effective natural and home remedies. The American "self-help" book first took hold on the frontier with the publication in 1734 of *Every Man His Own Doctor: Or, The Poor Planter's Physician* by John Tennent of rural Spotsylvania County, Virginia, describing many Native American herbal remedies. The potent American ginseng of Appalachia quickly became an international commodity with exportation to China. Frontiersman Daniel Boone for a time earned a living as a "sanger," gathering the herb in the wild ("wild crafting"). Perhaps the most popular self-help book of all was *Gunn's Domestic Medicine: Or Poor Man's Friend,* by Dr. John C. Gunn of Knoxville, Tennessee, continuously in print for nearly a century, from 1830 to 1920. It is mentioned, for example, in Mark Twain's *Huckleberry Finn* (1885) and in John Steinbeck's *East of Eden* (1952).

NATURE, WILDERNESS AND CIVILIZATION

In 1774, the leading American physician, Benjamin Rush (see Chapter 37), published a treatise on the importance of Native American remedies, and he later advised Lewis and Clark in 1803. Amazingly, only one man died on their expedition, which implied that living in raw nature was healthier than remaining behind in civilization. Charles Dickens described the unhealthy conditions of urban, "civilized" areas of America in grim detail in his *American Notes* (1842). The "West cure, rest cure, and nature cures" developed by Philadelphia neurologist and novelist Silas Weir Mitchell became the recommended means of recuperating from the illnesses of nineteenth-century civilization. This "West cure" was used to good effect in the Dakotas by future president Theodore Roosevelt, for example.

Other journeys of exploration that expanded the frontier and the reach of natural medicine included those of Zebulon Pike (1806; before Lewis and Clark had even returned). Hugh Campbell set out in 1833 with Dr. John Scott Harrison, who was son of President William Henry Harrison and father of President Benjamin Harrison—and who died of alcoholism just prior to his father's election in 1840. Other expeditions were mounted by John C. Frémont (1836–1848) and John Wesley Powell (named for the aforementioned Methodist minister), sometimes accompanied by colorful "mountain men" like Jedediah Smith, Jim Bridger, and Kit Carson.

Andrew Jackson's election in 1828 had provided a second American revolution with the ascendency of the common man along with his medicines. A backlash against the regular medicine of the elites was accompanied by the formal organization of natural healing by Samuel Hahnemann (see Chapter 22), Samuel Thomson (see Chapter 22), Franz Joseph Gall, and later John Harvey Kellogg (see Chapter 22). By the middle of the nineteenth century, the natural remedies of frontier medicine represented a well-established and widely available form of health care throughout America.

During the Civil War (1861-1865), after the Union naval blockade of the South began taking effect in 1862, the Confederacy found it difficult to obtain manufactured medicines and returned to natural remedies, publishing a pamphlet listing native herbs that could be used for treatment: snakeroot, sassafras, partridgeberry, lavender, dogwood, tulip tree, and red and white oak. Confederate Medical Corps kits contained many of these remedies toward the end of the war. After the Civil War came the heyday of patent (herbal) remedies, including Dr. Pepper, Dr. John Pemberton's Coca-Cola, and Dr. Hire's Root Beer, still enormously popular today as "soda," "pop," "tonic," and "root beer."

The term *quack* (from the German *quacksalver*, "quicksilver" or "mercury," which was actually a toxic regular medical treatment of the time) began to be applied to the practitioners of natural remedies. Although natural remedies had been considered useful and even essential on the American frontier from the 1500s to the 1850s, they suddenly became "quackery" at about the same time the American Medical Association was organized in 1847 (which was actually accomplished at least partially in reaction to the prior formation of the American Homeopathic Association in 1842).

Physicians and scientists who made real health advances with the use of natural healing in the mid- to late nineteenth century (Samuel Thomson; Vincent Priessnitz, the water cure; Russell Trall, the nature cure; Nikola Tesla, pioneer of electromagnetism) were rounded up in the judgment of twentieth-century history together with true charlatans like Thomas Alva Edison, Jr. (son of the inventor, who had done his best to put Tesla, the true genius of electricity and energy, out of business), John Romulus Brinkley, Dr. C. Everett Field, and Norman Baker. This pejorative label came to include hypnotists and "magnetic" healers (e.g., Franz Anton Mesmer) and the emerging manual therapists of osteopathy and chiropractic, originally "magnetic healers" in the tradition of Mesmer (e.g., Andrew Taylor Still, Daniel David Palmer) of the nineteenth century who originated in and were also initially a phenomenon of the rural frontier. In retrospect, the exploits of nineteenth-century and early twentieth-century charlatans can seem quaint in comparison with the organized havoc wreaked on the public health during the last quarter-century by the drug and insurance industries and the government.

The great unexamined assumption for today's reader is that natural healing in the late nineteenth century suddenly became "quackery." This attitude betrays something of a triumphalist approach to the wonders of twentieth-century medicine, whereas twenty-first-century American health care in many ways has become nothing to celebrate. The majority of post-WWII Americans were once able to leave "frontier medicine" for two or three generations, and enjoy medical practice and health care marked by well-trained physicians they knew and trusted, and the widespread availability of compassionate health services in hospitals that were accountable only to their own communities.

THE NEW FRONTIER

In the twenty-first century, Americans now subsidize and sustain with trillions of dollars each year—accounting for 18% of gross domestic product—the largest share in the world, but resulting in only the 40th best health status among nations. Contemporary health care is arguably a largely ineffective, inequitable, counterproductive, and unsustainable industry carried on for the benefit of an unaccountable corporate-government-medical-research complex of vested interests.

Contemporary biomedicine has become marked by the arrogance and intransigence of mainstream biomedical research elites, excessive corporate profiteering through unsafe and ineffective "blockbuster" drugs and direct-to-consumer marketing (rather than true therapeutic breakthroughs), and the mirage of "biotech" cures. There has been substitution of hard-won medical knowledge and clinical judgment by distant and unaccountable insurance companies and government bureaucracies that results in withholding of care and health care rationing (ironically, that which had been the greatest fear under the "socialized medicine" of a single-payer system). For several decades, many have awaited the next "miracle" drug, biotech breakthrough, and, now, "information technology," and politicized, government-run "mandates" for solutions to our health care crisis. The new government-run health care system, at this writing, has proven only that it is the one entity even more dysfunctional than the current health care system itself. This book illustrates that often it is ancient knowledge and wisdom about healing that can, when adapted to new circumstances, provide truly innovative approaches to health problems.

In today's economy, the health care *crisis* seems to many practitioners and patients to be moving toward *collapse* as much as many courageous health professionals continue to shoulder the burdens to provide good medical care. Recent divisive partisan political efforts at health care "reform" do not represent true reform at all in terms of what we have discussed in this chapter. Many Americans may find themselves back on the medical frontier, where, fortunately, the natural healing and remedies once spurned are still abiding in the contemporary consumer movement labeled "complementary/alternative medicine."

A final point about alternative systems: Complementary and alternative medicine systems imply the importance of individuality and choice. In an era in which the active engagement of the individual in his or her own health is a paramount goal, the importance of individuality and choice could not be greater, although it has never been in greater peril. ∽

References

Light DW, Lexchin J, Darrow JJ: Institutional corruption of pharmaceuticals and the myth of safe and effective drugs, *J Law Med Ethics* 41(3):590–600, 2013.

Mayor DF, Micozzi MS, editors: *Energy medicine east and west: a natural history of qi*, London, 2011, Churchill Livingstone Elsevier.

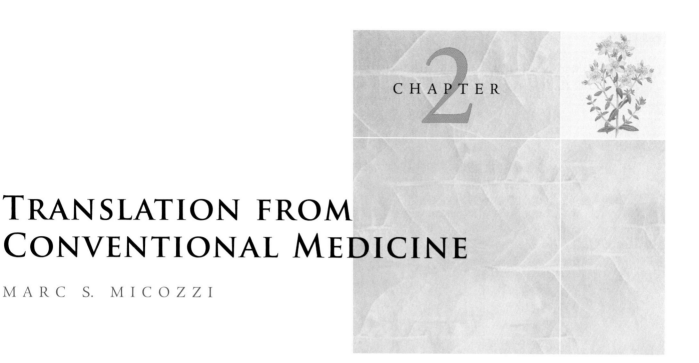

CHAPTER 2

TRANSLATION FROM CONVENTIONAL MEDICINE

MARC S. MICOZZI

What has been labeled "alternative/complementary medicine" in the United States is also a social phenomenon and consumer movement of significant dimensions. The term *complementary medicine* has been used interchangeably with *alternative medicine* and is a more accurate functional description of this social phenomenon, because most patients in the United States generally use "alternative medicine" as an *adjunct* to (not a replacement for) conventional medical care. Much of what we call "complementary and alternative medicine" in the United States, in fact, represents time-honored traditions of medical practice originating in other countries and other cultures or during earlier periods of European and American society as was presented at the end of the prior chapter. One of the most important distinctions we can make in studying and understanding CAM is to note the differences between two types of practices: (1) practices that are many years or centuries old and have a large body of practitioners and patients and a well-developed fund of clinical "wisdom" that is encoded into the belief system of a particular society or subgroup of people, and (2) practices that have been developed recently by one or a few practitioners in isolation from peers and without benefit of scientific testing and clinical studies (what may be appropriately called "unconventional therapy"). Practices in this second category can often be made to fit conceptually with the biomedical model but simply have not been tested using the standards of biomedical research and practice.

For example, with regard to the topics in this volume, CAM systems (alternatives) in the first category of time-tested traditions include the traditional medicine of China (with heterogeneous practice styles), manual therapies

(osteopathy, chiropractic, massage, and body work therapies), and naturopathy. Many time-tested traditions have in common, to a greater or lesser extent, aspects of mind–body medicine, a focus on nutrition and natural products, hands-on interaction between practitioner and patient, and an emphasis on listening to the patient. The five common characteristics of complementary and alternative medicine described in Chapter 1 are (1) a wellness orientation, (2) a reliance on self-healing, (3) an inference that bioenergetic mechanisms play a role, (4) the use of nutrition and natural products in a fundamental role, and (5) an emphasis on individuality.

For example, classical homeopathy stresses the importance of eliciting detailed symptoms and symptom complexes from the patient (and is not a system for placing patients into disease-based diagnostic categories). Thus, the practitioner must spend a great deal of time listening to the patient. The therapeutic benefits (and diagnostic value) of listening to the patient continue to be actively recognized among the "talk therapies" of contemporary mainstream medical practice in psychiatry and psychology, as well as general clinical practice as has been made explicit for some time now (Adler, 1997).

Because CAM therapies do not necessarily stress the assignment of patients to disease-based diagnostic categories, they are routinely prepared to deal with "functional" disorders and complaints (e.g., headache, pain, gastrointestinal dysfunction, menstrual dysfunction, other "subjective" symptoms) that do not carry a pathological diagnosis. Many CAM systems see these functional disorders as precursors of disease (rather than, for example, results of disease) and approach the clinical intervention on that basis.

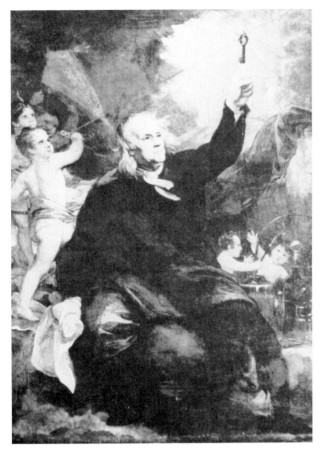

Figure 2-1 Poets, philosophers, and scientists of the late eighteenth and early nineteenth centuries were all interested in vitalism—finding the energy that animates life and the universe. Here Benjamin Franklin is shown in a heroic pose by Benjamin West figuratively "taming lightning." In fact, Franklin, like his contemporaries, was searching for insights into nature and human nature, not just exploring electricity in a contemporary utilitarian sense. Later, scientists thought that reductionist, materialist explanations substituted for the need for vitalist interpretations.

HOLISM AND VITALISM

Various CAM systems also refer to the importance of "energy" in the development of disorders and diseases and in their treatment and cure. Energy has a dynamic quality and is not measured in the usual ways that conventional medicine is accustomed to describing things, on the basis of materialist, reductionist biomedical mechanisms. The idea that whole, living systems and organisms have a "vital energy" that may not be present in nonliving entities or in parts or portions of an organism is an ancient concept among human cultures that is also reflected in European and U.S. intellectual traditions until the mid-nineteenth century (Figure 2-1).

CAM medical systems are sometimes considered vitalistic and holistic compared with allopathic medicine, which is considered materialistic and reductionistic (Table 2-1). Vitalism contends that there is an "energy" to living

TABLE 2-1 *Vitalism and Holism in Complementary Medicine*

Biomedicine	Complementary medicine
Reductionist	Holistic
Materialist	Vitalist

organisms that is nonmaterial. *Vitalism* is not an ecologic concept historically but posits non-naturalistic explanations for life. *Holism* is an ecological concept that the totality of biological phenomena in a living organism or ecological system cannot be reduced, observed, or measured at a level below that of the whole organism or system (Smuts, 1926). The term was first introduced by the South African naturalist and statesman Jan Smuts in the early twentieth century. Holism as an ecological concept is not consistent with the historic vitalist idea that living systems are somehow independent of nature. Holism was originally meant to be both antimechanistic and antivitalist.

While the term *holism* is relatively modern, the recognition in Western tradition that all things exist in relationship to a larger cosmic system dates back to Hippocrates, who said: "A physician without a knowledge of the cosmos should not call himself a physician. There is one common flow, one common breathing, all things are in sympathy." The cosmos spoken of here is not today's "pop" study of personality and the stars, which is far removed from its original purposes as used in ancient Greek, Chinese, and Indian cosmology and medicine, for example. These ancient cultures, living without the benefit of technology, were able to observe the heavens and detect relations among events on earth with what was happening in the universe.

Modern society, embedded and invested in technology, has led us away from the natural environment and the relations we as human organisms have with our own planet and the universe beyond. More importantly, it has also led us away from the "inner space" of our own body organism. Reconnecting with our inner spaces is something that Yoga and Qigong have to offer modern health and medicine, for example. In Chinese medicine, it is recognized that the microcosm (body) is a reflection of the macrocosm (universe), and the organ system is held in balance by the same powers that hold the cosmos in position. This concept is significant to physical health. It may not facilitate healing to take the part out of the context of its larger system, i.e., separating the cells from the tissues they form, the tissues from the organs they comprise, or the organs from the individual, that their functions are either helping or hindering. If all things exist in relationship, simply excising a problematic organ may or may not be the best solution. CAM endeavors to respect the relationship of the singular part to its whole. The word "heal" comes from the Old English word *Hal*, which means "whole."

VITALISM VS. HOLISM

Some interpretations of homeopathy, for example, rely on a vitalist mechanism while basing therapy on an essentially reductionist approach; that is, a whole organism's energetic mechanism is postulated to explain the effect elicited by minute doses of specific materia medica administered in little pills. Likewise, in Chinese medicine, the post-1949 traditional Chinese medicine style of practice veers toward a reductionist model while maintaining an essentially vitalist mechanism. Since 1978, the World Health Organization (WHO, 1998) has referred to traditional (cultural) medical systems as *holistic*, meaning:

> viewing humans in totality within a wide ecological spectrum, and emphasizing the view that ill health or disease is brought about by imbalance or disequilibrium of humans in the total ecological system and not only by the causative agent and pathogenic mechanism.

Historically, we might say that premodern medical systems could understand medicine only on the basis of observations of the whole organism, whose components were not well-known or understood. Modern reductionist biomedical science has allowed knowledge to be built on the basis of studying the individual, "de-vitalized" parts and pieces of the whole organism (e.g., tissue cells, DNA). A postmodern medicine might permit translation of the biomedical model back to the realm of the whole, vital organism. For example, new imaging technologies that permit observation of living cells for diagnostic and therapeutic purposes may provide one mechanism.

This view might consider that biomedicine has new technologies generally in the service of old, fixed ideas about health and healing, whereas CAM systems represent old technologies that may be interpreted in light of new ideas about health and healing.

Research has begun to be helpful in demonstrating the therapeutic benefit (or lack of benefit) of alternative medical practices that are not explainable on the basis of postulated mechanisms of action and that do not fit with the biomedical model. In this way, some regard such ideas as nonsense, or perhaps more precisely, "not sense." However, sense may be made of these ideas by considering a medical ecological or adaptational model.

MEDICAL ECOLOGY AND THE ADAPTATION MODEL

For medical traditions that have been encoded and carried as knowledge among different cultures for long periods, it is possible to study the adaptiveness and adaptive value of these practices. What benefits do these traditions confer on members of a society who follow certain health-related beliefs and practices? How do such practices help humans adapt to their circumstances? For cultural traditions that relate to medicine, anthropologists have now studied "ethnomedicine" for several decades (see Section VI).

Human physiology allows adaptation to occur, often instantaneously and insensibly, in response to environmental pressures over the *very short term* in each individual (homeostasis). Evolution allows adaptation to occur over the *very long term* in the population as a whole by altering gene frequencies that correspond to traits that have adaptive value to a changing environment. Operating in between the time scales of homeostasis and genetic adaptation, human culture is learned behavior that also has adaptive value. Culture is by definition learned behavior, which can be altered much faster than genetic evolution but much more slowly than individual homeostatic adjustments.

Among human populations, culture acts to fill this gap in time for adapting to the environment. Human cultural beliefs and behaviors surrounding health and medicine (ethnomedicine) are found to generally be rational, internally consistent responses that are adaptive to a given environment (Box 2-1).

At the end of the nineteenth century, European interpretations regarded traditional medical practices as myth, superstition, or magic (and sometimes madness), as illustrated in Sir James Frazer's *The Golden Bough* (1890). During the twentieth century, social scientists searched for the functional meanings and purposes of medically related traditions. European and North American social scientists

BOX 2-1 *Adaptation and Time Dimensions*

1. Individual adaptation
A. Homeostatic (seconds to months)
   For example, at high altitude (low partial pressure oxygen), increase respiratory rate in seconds; increase hematocrit and red blood cell count over weeks; "thicken" blood
B. Ontogenetic (during the growth period)
   For example, at high altitude, increase lung capacity during growth and development; over a lifetime
2. Population adaptation
A. Cultural
   Environmental determinism posits that environmental factors influence cultural practices (decades to centuries)
   For example, chewing of coca leaf at high altitude to prevent "thicker" blood from clotting
B. Genetic adaptation to environment
   Shifts in gene frequency (thousands to millions of years), such as hemoglobin polymorphisms, lactose tolerance, PTC taste sensitivity (ability to taste bitter compounds from plants)
C. Genetic adaption to cultural/agricultural practices
   With exposure to agriculture and animal domestication: gluten sensitivity, lactose tolerance/intolerance, "thrifty" gene, metabolic syndrome
   Cultural adaptions occur more quickly than genetic adaptions and can fill the gap in time for human populations, allowing them to adapt more rapidly and ultimately be more successful in their environments.

TABLE 2-2 *Representation of Traditional Health Systems*

Conceptual paradigm	Health system component	Methodology	Representation
"Social reality"	Health beliefs Health behaviors • Health practices, wellness maintenance • Care seeking, illness perceived — Structural-functional access — Cultural access	Informant interview/survey Participant observation	Cognitive Observational
"Scientific reality"	Health outcomes, disease defined	Technical evaluation: health and nutrition status indicators	Analytical

began describing the meanings of traditional medical practices in the 1920s. For example, if traditional societies, through plant domestication and agriculture, learn to obtain nutrients (foods) from the environment in which they live, they also learn to obtain medicines from their environment and to develop therapeutic techniques to provide medical care.

As previously stated, many contemporary CAM paradigms and practices derive from complex and sophisticated ancient and historical health systems and from indigenous cultures closely in touch with their natural and social environments. These health belief-behavior systems form part of the adaptation of these cultures to their respective environments, representing integral components of traditional societies (Micozzi, 1983). Health-related beliefs and behaviors that are widespread and persistent merit study to determine their adaptive value (Table 2-2).

To accept the validity of scientific investigation of "alternative/complementary" medical systems, one need only accept the possibility (or probability) of the adaptive value of human belief and behavior systems that are persistent and widespread. The adaptive value of human behavior is an important concept to both social and biological scientists. Whether human behavior is adaptive represents a persistent question in intellectual discourse. Some point to cultural practices that are widespread and that persist over generations as evidence of the adaptive value of such practices.

Although many hold out the symbolic power of beliefs and the transcendental value of ideas regardless of "adaptive" value, belief and behavior systems can often be demonstrated in a scientific sense to have associated outcomes relative to human health and disease. The British anthropologist–physician W.H.R. Rivers (1924) showed almost a century ago that traditional health systems are not magic or superstition but represent rational, ordered systems of knowledge and useful ways of understanding and interacting with the environment.

Bringing together social science and biomedical science in a more effective and integrated way requires rigorous application of the social sciences to the study of health and medicine. Social scientists often study health belief systems without adequately measuring health outcomes in a scientific sense, whereas biomedicine measures outcomes scientifically without being able to study the underlying belief systems. Social and cultural factors are amenable to study, but by techniques extrinsic to biomedical science. A conceptual paradigm may be considered to have reached the limits of explanation, or inquiry, when dependent variables can be measured but independent variables are unknown or immeasurable in the system of study.

This is one way I have interpreted some of the lessons of Thomas Kuhn's seminal work about scientific paradigms and conceptual and explanatory models, *The Structure of Scientific Revolutions* (Kuhn, 1973). (In fact, it was on the very day of my graduation from medical school that I met Dr. Kuhn on the train as he was traveling from his home in Princeton, NJ, to his sabbatical at Yale, in New Haven, CT, and had the opportunity to immediately further my postgraduate medical education, literally.)

If health outcomes are considered *dependent* variables, the explanatory limits of biomedical science become exceeded, because relevant *independent* variables are not made an explicit component of the explanatory model. A related issue is that an explanatory model may not be able to account for "how" a medical intervention actually "works" in terms of a mechanism of action (Chapters 3, 5).

For example, there are different ways of explaining how manual therapies work. Although their clinical applications and associated health outcomes have been accepted on the basis of biomechanical mechanisms, many manual therapy traditions invoke the manipulation of bioenergy as the mechanism.

BIOENERGETIC EXPLANATIONS FOR BODY WORK

First, all manual therapies imply that touching the patient in a particular manner is a primary means of therapy. Alternatively, the traditional view of the "laying on of hands" is to focus the attention of both practitioner and patient on the *intention* to heal and on the practitioner *undertaking to treat* the patient.

Manual therapies as CAM combine several approaches to healing traditions. Manual therapies can be seen to include North American historic traditions such as osteopathy and chiropractic and, more recently, "body work" (e.g., massage therapy, rolfing, Trager method, applied kinesiology, Feldenkrais method). Asian manual systems include Chinese tui na and more recently Japanese shiatsu. Techniques often viewed as manual therapy but more explicitly related to manipulation of bioenergy include the Asian systems of qigong (qi gong) and reiki and the North American technique of therapeutic touch.

The founder of *chiropractic,* Daniel David Palmer, was originally an "energy healer" or "magnetic healer" (following Franz Anton Mesmer), as was the founder of traditional *osteopathy,* Andrew Taylor Still. Both traditions were established within a few years and a few hundred miles of each other in the American Midwest frontier of the 1890s. In addition to embracing the concept of "vital energy," both Palmer and Still also rejected the use of drugs, which remained especially toxic during that period of history (Palmer, 1910; Still, 1902).

In this regard, Still and Palmer were actually supported by such mainstream medical figures as Sir William Osler and Dr. Oliver Wendell Holmes. In a famous statement to the Massachusetts Medical Society—publisher of the *New England Journal of Medicine*—in 1860, Holmes opined that "if the entire *materia medica* as currently practiced were sunk to the bottom of the sea, it would be all the better for humankind and all the worse for the fishes." However, chiropractic and traditional osteopathy went further by specifically identifying themselves as "drugless healing," which found many adherents, in reaction to the therapeutic excesses in mainstream medicine. After World War II, osteopathy was largely mainstreamed into modern medicine, which was partially driven by the chronic shortage of medical personnel in the U.S. military (who recruited D.O.s to supplement M.D.s), as well as the desire of osteopaths to participate in the full benefits of medical mainstream training and practice.

Therapeutic touch and *healing touch* are more recent developments, largely promulgated initially by two nurses in the United States, Dolores Krieger and Dora Kunz. Healing "touch" is notable in that the patient is not actually physi-cally touched. The technique therefore may be interpreted as a form of "energy healing" (perhaps the form most in practice in clinical settings in the United States) rather than manual therapy. The hands of the practitioner are thought to manipulate the flow of energy around the patient's body (Krieger, 1979; Kunz, 1991).

Other forms of hand-mediated healing include polarity therapy, Tibetan-Japanese reiki, Japanese *jin shin jyutsu,* external qigong, touch for health, reflexology, acupressure, and shiatsu massage.

Bioenergetic mechanisms are invoked to explain clinical observations of the efficacy of therapeutic touch. These concepts are difficult to translate into clinical medicine, which at the same time is recognizing that there is experimental reality beyond the realm of the contemporary biomedical paradigm (see Chapter 3).

AYURVEDA

Bioenergetic mechanisms have also been invoked in attempting to understand some aspects of Ayurveda, a traditional medicine of India (see Chapters 28 to 31). Traditionally, Ayurveda is not simply a medical system; rather, it is described as the "science of life" or *longevity* and relates more to what we would consider as a way of life or "lifestyle." A contemporary form of Ayurveda as provided by "Maharishi Ayurveda" represents itself as a revival of Ayurvedic traditions lost through centuries of foreign rule (Moslem/Mogul and European/British) in India (see Indian Medicine Table after ch 31), blended with "bioenergetic" and "quantum mechanical" interpretations of mechanism.

Empirically, Ayurveda makes use of correspondences among five cosmic elements of earth, air, fire, water, and space (similar to ancient Greek, Unani, and Persian concepts, as well as "humoral" Western medical systems extending into the nineteenth century). There are three constitutional body types based on the balance of three *doshas,* which represent these five elements as they occur in the human body (Table 2-3). The three primary body types

TABLE 2-3 *Characteristics of Three Constitutional Types in Ayurveda*

	Dosha		
	Vata	*Pitta*	*Kapha*
Somatotype (Sheldon)	Ectomorph	Mesomorph	Endomorph
Body type	Light, thin	Moderate	Solid, heavy
Skin type	Dry	Reddish	Oily, smooth
Personality	Anxious	Irritable	Tranquil, steady
Digestion	Irregular, constipation	Sharp	Slow
Activity	Quick	Medium	Slow, methodical
Season	Winter	Fall	Spring
Diseases	Hypertension	Inflammation	Sinusitis
	Arthritis	Inflammatory bowel disease	Respiratory diseases
	Rheumatism	Skin diseases	Asthma
	Cardiac arrhythmia	Heartburn	Obesity
	Insomnia	Peptic ulcer	Depression

(*prakriti*) represent an empirical system for describing predisposition to illness, proscribing against unhealthy behavior, and prescribing for treatment of disease. The three primary body types of *vata*, *pitta*, and *kapha* may be roughly translated to the Sheldon somatotypes of twentieth-century Western science describing body constitution as ectomorph, mesomorph, and endomorph. Ayurveda also demonstrates systematic correspondences among a number of cosmic elements, seasons, constitutions, personalities, diseases, and treatments.

The idea that body constitution predisposes to certain diseases is an old one. In biomedicine this idea now finds expression in the association of genetic factors with health and disease, a current preoccupation of contemporary biomedical science.

CHINESE MEDICINE

As with Ayurveda, we can also think of Chinese medicine as an empirical tradition of systematic correspondences making reference to five cosmic elements (one expression is in "five phases" approach) that dates back to about 3000 BC (Table 2-4). Although for comparative purposes Chinese medicine is often treated as a homogeneous monolithic structure, this view neglects the changing interpretations of basic paradigms offered by Chinese medicine through the ages and the coexisting plurality of differing opinions and ideas over thousands of years (Unschuld, 1985).

Likewise, this text uses the term *China's traditional medicine* or *traditional medicine of China*. The popular term "traditional Chinese medicine" (TCM) is a mid-twentieth-century invention, convention, or perhaps concoction that blends certain aspects of Chinese medicine with a scientific underpinning put into place by the Communist government of Mao Tse-tung beginning only in 1949 to provide basic health care to the Chinese population.

Much of what the Chinese medical practitioner does is thought to influence the flow or balance of the body's energy, called "qi." In one view, the Chinese concept of qi, which is translated as "energy," "bioenergy," or "vital energy" (if it actually translates to the Western concept of energy at all), has a metabolic quality. The Chinese character or pictogram for qi may be described as vapor or steam rising over rice (Figure 2-2). The term "rice" has a specific quality that we associate with the specific food, but it also has a generic meaning, "food" or "foodstuff." For example, the character "rice hall" is used to describe a restaurant in Chinese. The elusive meaning of qi may therefore be likened more to living metabolism than to the energy that we associate with electromagnetic radiation.

Energy or qi also has the dynamic qualities of "flow" and "balance." Because flow and balance are dynamic, they may be described in changing terms from one patient to the next, or in the same patient from one day to the next (again, without the use of static, fixed pathological diagnostic categories). Such concepts present great challenges in translation to the biomedical model.

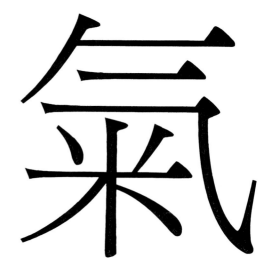

Figure 2-2 The Chinese character *qi,* described as vapor or steam rising over rice.

TABLE 2-4 *Correspondences of the Five Phases in Chinese Medicine*

Category	Wood	Fire	Earth	Metal	Water
Organ	Liver	Heart	Spleen	Lungs	Kidney
Bowel	Gallbladder	Small intestine	Stomach	Large intestine	Urinary bladder
Season	Spring	Summer	Late summer	Autumn	Winter
Time of day	Before sunrise	Forenoon	Afternoon	Late afternoon	Midnight
Climate	Wind	Heat	Damp	Dryness	Cold
Direction	East	South	Center	West	North
Development	Birth	Growth	Maturity	Withdrawal	Dormancy
Color	Cyan	Red	Yellow	White	Black
Taste	Sour	Bitter	Sweet	Pungent	Salty
Sense organ	Eyes	Tongue	Mouth	Nose	Ears
Odor	Goatish	Scorched	Fragrant	Raw fish	Putrid
Vocalization	Shouting	Laughing	Singing	Weeping	Sighing
Tissue	Sinews	Vessels	Flesh	Body hair	Bones

Acupuncture is a major modality for the manipulation of qi. Clinical observations of efficacy are increasing, and some biomedical explanations focus on the physiological effects of skin puncture and modulation of neurotransmitter substances. Some experiments indicate that the acupuncture needle has the same effect when it is merely held in place over the appropriate point in space (without puncturing the skin). If acupuncture needles operate by influencing the flow of energy, which is not limited by internal or external physical barriers, then puncturing the skin is not a necessary part of the mechanism of action. Perhaps pragmatic Chinese acupuncturists simply found a way to hold the needles in place by puncturing the skin when they were trying to influence more than two acupuncture points simultaneously (and had only two hands to hold the needles in position).

HOMEOPATHY

Homeopathy challenges several basic assumptions of allopathic medicine starting with the concept that "like cures like." (Here we reference the term *allopathic medicine* in reference to modern biomedicine, which is appropriate because it was actually the homeopaths who granted the term "allopathic" to the "regular" medicine of their day in the mid-nineteenth century). In homeopathy, a symptom should be seen as an attempt on the part of the body to correct itself, to fight disease, and to restore balance (homeostasis). For example, the case of fever may be seen as an adaptation to bacterial infection. Increased temperatures (above the normal body temperature) are observed to slow the rate of bacterial reproduction significantly (Figure 2-3). In this way, raising body temperature above normal is bacteriostatic and (as with many antibiotics) slows bacterial growth, which gives the immune system a chance to catch up and clear the infection.

Thus, the reason that homeopathy originally gave the name "allopathic" medicine to the "regular" medical mainstream approaches of the time (early nineteenth century) was because the medical focus is on the elimination or control of symptoms. In homeopathy, symptoms are everything, and describing them is the primary goal and guide to therapy. Of course, fully characterizing the symptoms of each individual involved listening to, and talking to, the patient—which is highly therapeutic in itself. The classic homeopath also included mental and psychological characteristics and "symptoms" in his profile, also providing an early form of "mind-body" medicine.

In classical homeopathic treatment, an empirical approach is taken by administering "provings" of substances (largely materia medica) in minute doses and observing whether the patient shows clinical improvement. This practice may also be considered reductionistic. Because many symptoms tend to improve over time, these provings cannot be considered controlled experiments, but the same observation may be applied to the administration of "cures" in other traditions as well.

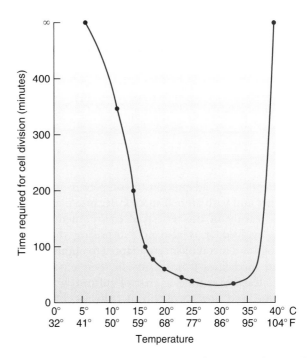

Figure 2-3 Relation between rate of cell division for *Bacillus mycoides* and temperature. (Data from *Encyclopaedia Britannica*, 1954 ed, s.v. "Bacteriology.")

NATUROPATHY AND WESTERN HERBALISM

Naturopathy is the most recent of alternative approaches to have developed as a complete system in North America (see Chapter 22). It emphasizes the healing power of nature and can also be understood in terms of the adaptational model. In practice, contemporary naturopathy is eclectic, consciously drawing on a number of models and systems (e.g., Chinese medicine, Ayurveda, homeopathy, manual therapies, Usani healing) in an effort to fit the patient profile and the clinical problem with appropriate medical systems and techniques. Because one of two central tenets is to establish "therapeutic order," naturopathy also provides an authentic approach to "integrative" medicine by matching the right treatment to the individual patient and complaint (Chapter 3). Naturopathy is well organized in several states in the West (notably Oregon, Washington, and Montana) and in New England, but may be practiced in a less formal fashion in other parts of the United States.

The use of nutrition, herbs, natural remedies, and other natural products is an important component of naturopathic medicine. Medical traditions around the world, from the most basic shamanistic approaches to healing to the highly complex and sophisticated systems of Chinese and Ayurvedic medicine, make use of medicinal plants in relation to their biological activity. Homeopathy (often included in the range of practice of naturopathic medicine) is also based largely on minute doses of materia medica.

From the standpoint of evolutionary biology, it is not surprising that plants develop biologically active

TABLE 2-5 *Medicinal Plant Constituent Actions*

Respiratory	Gastrointestinal	Neural
Expectorant	Emetic	Sedative
Antitussive	Antiemetic	Stimulant
Immunomodulative	Laxative	Cardiotonic
	Spasmolytic	Antidepressant

constituents as an adaptation to compete in nature with each other and with animal species. Because plants form a primary feature of the terrestrial environment in which humans evolved, it is also not surprising that human physiology and metabolism are adapted to obtaining nutrients and medicines from plants in their environments. Societies learn over time, as part of culture, which plants have value, and how to obtain or cultivate, harvest, and prepare them. Societies then encode and carry this empirical knowledge and behavior into their cultural traditions. In addition to each of the traditional medical settings for the use of medicinal plants, an eclectic system of herbal medicine has historically developed in the West, which can be referred to as "Western herbalism." Biologically active constituents of plants include carbohydrates, glycosides, tannins, lipids, volatile oils, resins, steroids, alkaloids, peptides, and enzymes.

Volatile oils form the primary basis of the practice of aromatherapy, or essential oils therapy. The active constituents have various physiological effects throughout the body (Table 2-5 and Box 2-2). Because biologically active constituents are present in combination in each medicinal plant, they are often observed to have synergistic effects. These synergistic effects have been useful, for example, in the application of crude extracts of medicinal plants to antibiotic-resistant bacterial infections and to chloroquine-resistant malaria. However, it is difficult to translate this approach to the active-ingredient model of reductionist biomedical research, as described in the next section.

COMPARATIVE GLOBAL PERSPECTIVES

Understanding complementary medical systems described here as "traditional" or "cultural" medicine in an ecological model, we can compare and contrast how they fit into their indigenous settings with how they are interpreted in the contemporary United States. In the U.S. health care system, we assume traditional herbal medicines to be of value only when their active principal or ingredient is known and can be purified for mass production. However, this "active ingredient" approach to medicinal plants and traditional medicine reflects a particular conceptual paradigm rather than a particular truth about how natural medicines may work.

On the basis of findings from U.S. biomedical plant-screening programs, therapeutic benefits are often observed

BOX 2-2 *Medicinal Plants as Adaptogens: Ginseng*

Another concept that is difficult to translate to biomedicine, and another category of medical plant constituent action, is that of *adaptogen*. An adaptogen has the interesting and nonpharmacological property of helping the body to adapt to whatever changes in environment may occur and to maintain homeostasis. Thus, it helps keep you warm if it is cold, or to stay cool if it is hot; stay awake when you need to be up, or sleep when it is time to retire; be alert when that is called for, or relax when it is time to restore your energy. This "tonic" property is not accounted for in Western pharmacology but is consistent with physiology, in which essentially the same metabolic "equipment" and mechanisms must adapt to constantly changing circumstances.

Ginseng is the prototype medicinal plant among adaptogens. There are Chinese ginseng, Siberian ginseng, and American ginseng. In a good illustration of the diffusion of Western herbalism, American ginseng was rapidly brought into the modern Chinese pharmacopeia when Chinese emigrants to the United States "discovered" it (there is that word again) and rapidly brought it into common use. American ginseng is highly prized, and it is "wild-crafted" today by American "sangers" in the Appalachian Mountains, who closely guard the secret of where and how to locate ginseng for gathering.

Today, other adaptogens are being found in Africa, such as *Sutherlandia frutescens*, or *kankerbos* (in South African Afrikaans).

to be limited. However, methodologies used in biomedicine often overlook the effects by which traditional medicines produce results because of a fixed and defined view of what constitutes therapeutic action. Although traditional health systems have acknowledged use in management of chronic, low-level conditions, they are assumed to be of no value in providing acute or emergency care. However, in some countries that have been held outside the Western global economy for extended periods (China, Vietnam, Nicaragua), traditional medicine is mandated and used effectively for trauma and major acute diseases. Historically, this necessity resulted from political and economic exclusion from other health care technologies. Much research already exists in other countries (often in languages other than English).

Traditional medicines are now being seen as valuable because they serve as sources of leads for new pharmaceuticals (so-called biodiversity prospecting), and the potential medical value of tropical rainforest species provides a basis for support to preserve and conserve regional biodiversity. However, this biodiversity prospecting assumption overlooks the role of traditional medical systems in addressing the needs of the people from whence come the medicinal plants and the knowledge about their appropriate use. The use of medicinal plants is not a botanical system, but a

TABLE 2-6 *Old Assumptions and New Perspectives on Complementary Medical Systems*

Old assumptions	New perspectives
"Primitive"	Holistic
Ineffective	Cost effective
Marginalized	Locally available
Extinct	Renewed
Should be regulated	Should be studied
Provides prospects for biomedicine	Valid in own right
Active ingredient model	Synergistic activity

system of human knowledge. If a medicinal plant grows in the forest, but no human is there, does it make a cure?

Old views had assumed the marginalization of traditional medical systems. A new perspective looks to them to provide complementary therapies and, in some cases, new solutions to our contemporary "health care crisis" (Table 2-6). Much of what is called complementary or alternative medicine in the United States represents primary care for 80% of the world's people (WHO, 1998). In this way, CAM may be considered to represent appropriate technology and affordable, sustainable medicine both for indigenous people, traditionally, and now for industrialized societies as well on a global basis (See also Ch 43).

References

Adler HM: The history of the present illness as treatment: who's listening, and why does it matter? *J Am Board Fam Med* 10:28, 1997.

Frazer JG: *The golden bough,* translated by TH Gaster, New York, 1959, New American Library. (originally published in 1890).

Krieger D: *The therapeutic touch: how to use your hands to help or to heal,* New York, 1979, Prentice-Hall.

Kuhn T: *The structure of scientific revolutions,* New Haven, CT, 1973, Yale University Press.

Kunz D: *The personal aura,* Wheaton, IL, 1991, Quest Books.

Micozzi MS: Anthropological study of health beliefs, behaviors and outcomes, *Hum Organ* 42:351, 1983.

Palmer DD: *Textbook of the science, art and philosophy of chiropractic,* Portland, OR, 1910, Portland Printing House.

Rivers WHR: *Medicine, magic and religion,* New York, 1924, Harcourt & Brace.

Smuts JC: *Holism and evolution,* New York, 1926, Macmillan.

Still AT: *Philosophy and mechanical principles of osteopathy,* Kansas City, MO, 1902, Hudson-Kimberly.

Unschuld P: *Medicine in China: a history of ideas,* Berkeley, 1985, University of California.

World Health Organization: *Traditional medicine,* Geneva, 1998, WHO Publications.

Suggested Readings

Hahnemann S: *Organon of medicine,* translated by W Boericke, ed 6, New Delhi, 1980, B Jain. (originally published in 1933).

Lust B: *Universal directory of naturopathy,* Butler, NJ, 1918, Lust.

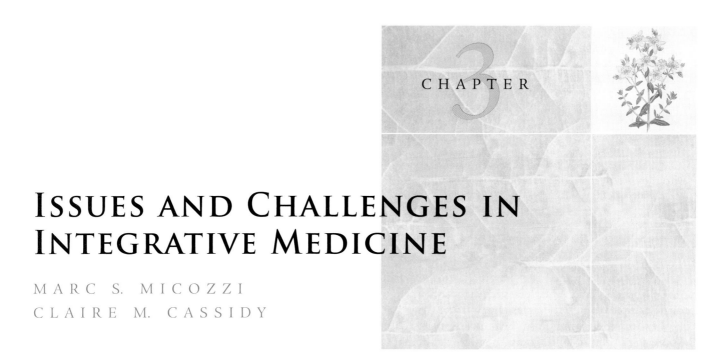

CHAPTER 3

ISSUES AND CHALLENGES IN INTEGRATIVE MEDICINE

MARC S. MICOZZI
CLAIRE M. CASSIDY

As discussed in Chapters 1 and 2, a major popular health movement of the twenty-first century is widespread interest in, and utilization of, what has been called "alternative," "complementary," or, often now, "integrative" medicine. The goal of this chapter is to explore the concept and problematics of "integration," especially the effort to "integrate" CAM practices into essentially biomedical venues.

With growing general recognition by the biomedical and scientific communities during the 1990s (such as the Chantilly conference and report, NIH Consensus Conferences, FDA decisions on classifying herbs and acupuncture needles; all discussed elsewhere in this text), there has been a corresponding movement among biomedical practitioners, administrators, academicians, and scientists to incorporate selected nonbiomedical modalities and techniques into their existing spheres of research, practice, and teaching. These movements are now causing the private sector, through institutional health systems and insurers, and the public sectors of state and federal governments, to invest more deeply and broadly in what is increasingly being labeled "integrative medicine" (Box 3-1).

Before going further, let us stop a moment to define our use of some words, and to examine the essential oddity of setting biomedicine off alone on a sort of pedestal raised above the very extensive plain containing all the other medical practices of the world.

Health care system: In this chapter and book we are concerned with *institutional* health care systems—that is, the economic, political, and legally mandated aspects of health care delivery at the national (or state, etc.) level that doesn't directly deliver health care, but attempts to answer questions about what care is appropriate and what can be afforded. Unless our scale is extremely local, such as a hospital or a single clinic, this level of organization is not concerned with the day-to-day delivery of medical care, apart from its institutional aspects, such as complying with HIPAA rules, or hiring properly licensed personnel. This institutional use of the phrase "health care system" is in contrast to the *cultural* concept of the health care system, which *is* concerned with delivery issues, and is discussed in depth in Chapter 5 (see Figure 5-1).

These two meanings are not truly separate in the sense that the concerns of the institutional system *reflect the explanatory model* that is dominant in a particular society or locale. In our society, biomedicine is the dominant Medicine, and has been for about a hundred years. Current assumptions of institutional health care systems accept the biomedical medical model as accurate and possibly sufficient, and assume that its dominance is normative and appropriate. In this way, all other medical systems become non-normative, *alternative,* perhaps, when one considers their independence and distinctive explanatory models, or potentially *complementary to biomedicine.*

Currently, some propose that there can be some sort of *integration* of selected aspects of these "others"—essentially always *into biomedicine.* This dominance issue markedly affects this book's title and topics: complementary and alternative medicine (CAM), and "integrative" medicine, because in both terminological cases, biomedicine continues to be set apart from other Medicines, in a manner as if it were the only valid Medicine. This issue is a sociological, cultural, and historical anomaly, discussed in Chapter 5, but relevant here because of the anxious territoriality that lies at the core of the labeling—and bleeds into the boundary-setting concerns of institutional health care systems.

Medicine: Medicine, with a capital M, refers to any medical practice, local or expanded, admired or not, that delivers "medical" or "health" care intended to protect or improve the health of individuals or the society, or to affect and improve the expression of symptoms or the outcome of illnesses. "Medical" care usually is used to refer to treating those already suffering malfunction; "health" care refers to efforts to prevent illness.

Health Care System: can refer either to a national or local level socioeconomic construct concerned with the costs and feasibilities of delivering medical and health education and care or to the cultural system that grows up around a medical explanatory model, and that permits the model to be actualized. The latter meaning is used in this chapter. Figure 5-1 shows that the socioeconomic meaning is a part of the larger cultural construct.

Biomedicine or Allopathy: is a highly technological and specialized Medicine that grew out of Greek roots, but gave up the ancient medical theory in favor of a materialist explanatory model, aiming to become more scientific, in the nineteenth and twentieth centuries. The primary practitioner is commonly called "a medical doctor" or "a physician"; affiliated specialties include nursing, psychotherapy, dentistry, and physical therapy/physiotherapy. This Medicine is socioeconomically and politically dominant in the Euro-American sphere, and has spread worldwide. The term "biomedicine" fronts its focus on biology and science; the term "allopathy" compares it with naturopathy, osteopathy, and homeopathy, for example. Either term, biomedicine or allopathy, is precise. Calling this Medicine by adjectives like regular, conventional, traditional, modern, scientific or the like is commonly encountered, but is not accurate or precise in this context. The reader is advised to keep these guidelines in mind regarding use of terminology.

Because biomedicine remains dominant and socioculturally normative, we may appropriately ask whence comes the pressure to invest in "integrative" medicine, or, more simply, to integrate some novel approaches into biomedicine? A large part of the answer is economic: people are voting for alternatives to biomedicine with their feet and their pocketbooks. In recent years, estimates indicate that the American public made more visits to alternative practitioners than to primary care biomedical physicians. Utilization of herbal remedies and dietary supplements is now supported by a multibillion-dollar industry in the United States and worldwide. Already a decade ago, in 2004, a report on complementary and alternative medicine (CAM) utilization by the U.S. National Center for Health Statistics, the largest and most methodologically sophisticated survey to that date, indicated that almost three-quarters of Americans had used CAM at some point in their lives and almost two-thirds had used CAM sometime in the prior year (Barnes et al, 2004). For some categories of patients, utilization of CAM is even higher, as with 80% or more of patients with cancer (Wootton & Sparber, 2003). These statistics also indicate that once a consumer starts using CAM, they continue using it.

Significantly, American consumers have paid for most of these products and services as out-of-pocket costs, receiving only limited, if any, insurance or tax benefits until recently (see later discussion in this chapter). It has also been estimated that the out-of-pocket amount spent by consumers for alternative care exceeds the out-of-pocket copayments and deductibles consumers make for health care covered by insurance. These observations are important when making assumptions, or debating the roles or even the need for, third-party payers in the provision of health care. A reality for health care professionals is that one last bastion of traditional fee-for-service medicine resides only among alternative and complementary medical practitioners. Ironically, a major motivation for the phenomenon of "integrative" medicine is to open the door to intrusion by third parties, such as insurance companies, and increasingly, the federal government. Such developments simply place more barriers between the practitioner and the patient.

Furthermore, the workforce supplying alternative, complementary, and integrative care is strikingly small compared with the current workforce of approximately 750,000 practicing physicians (see the section on Availability of Services).

NOMENCLATURE AND PHILOSOPHIES OF CARE

In trying to develop a nomenclature for CAM practices for descriptive purposes in the 1990s, the medical and scientific professions advanced various labels, such as "nontraditional," "unconventional," "unorthodox," "holistic," and "wholistic" (the latter two a revival from the 1960s). In the midst of the call for greater scientific evidence and objectivity, these labels had the characteristic of betraying cultural values, prejudices, and judgments about the validity and appropriateness of these practices. The more properly descriptive terminology of "alternative and complementary medicine" became generally accepted by the late 1990s.

Alternative, originally an American term, was meant to imply a systemic differentiation from the practice of biomedicine, such that a user might be clear about *which* Medicine they were using, and all Medicines could be seen as alternatives to one another. Such a *plural medical* situation is found in most countries worldwide. In contrast, in the post-WWII United States, biomedicine briefly achieved a near medical monopoly by the 1950s, but which has been steadily eroding since. Today, the United States has joined the rest of the world as a society that offers multiple medical choices to their citizens (medical pluralism).

Complementary grew out of European usage and nearly always implied that the CAM practices were functionally inferior to biomedicine, that is, that the non-biomedical practices might be used to enhance biomedicine, but the opposite would not be true. Nevertheless, this term remains popular as implying a degree of compatibility between biomedicine and other medical practices such that their use can be seen as an adjunct to, if not a replacement for, biomedicine.[1]

Integrative medicine, at its best, implies an active, conscious effort by the health professions and biomedical sciences to seek and sort out the evidence for and application of various complementary medical systems, modalities, and techniques for appropriate incorporation into the continuum of health care within the current parameters of the institutional health care system. Unfortunately, this meaning is rarely achieved in practice. Instead, as feared by many, "integration" has generally meant dominance by the mainstream biomedical model in terms of practice, accompanied by economic and professional constraints (Hunter et al, 2012).

A potentially irresolvable philosophical question relates to the intangible costs and benefits of integration within one limited medical system versus the continued existence of pluralism among healing choices for consumers. "Integration" is sometimes interpreted to mean improved standards of evidence, quality, appropriateness, and availability of care within the institutional health care system (largely biomedical). "Alternatives" imply greater choices to consumers for those willing and able to create their own menu of healing choices.

One view pivots on the limitations of the long-standing health care workforce situation (Micozzi, 1998), which may dictate that more appropriate care may be provided to more Americans through continued integration than with an uncoordinated landscape of different practices, each vying for primacy within as-yet incompletely defined, articulated, and accepted "evidence-based" scopes of practice. These considerations regarding "integration" may be overridden by current concerns about the economic crisis in health care, which may be seen as a sociocultural crisis brought about by pursuing a nineteenth-century paradigm about healing using expensive, invasive, twenty-first-century technologies (see Chapters 1 and 2). The existing health care infrastructure of biomedical clinics and hospitals may simply not be sustainable without major changes in character. These points should naturally lead to serious consideration about providing services in other types of health care facilities (Box 3-2).

Accordingly, in this new edition, we work with the realization that much of what we call CAM will not be

---

[1]Biomedicine has been increasingly politically and economically dominant in the United States since the late nineteenth century, and the United States became virtually a biomedical monoculture by the 1950s. The loss of such territorial dominance as CAM makes inroads creates anxiety accompanied by rejective behaviors, mild ("complementarity" concept) to extreme, and efforts to police medical professionals that in other settings might be accepted as colleagues. To see how acupuncture patients perceive and use their medical choices, see Cassidy (1998a, 1998b). For more discussion, see Chapter 5.

BOX 3-2 *The Nature Cure as a Remedy for Health Care*

- The U.S. health care system is in crisis and does not appear to be sustainable. Fortunately, alternative approaches to much of health and wellness are available.
- Presently, three-quarters of Americans use health services now labeled as "complementary and alternative medicine" (CAM) for health and wellness.
- Americans now pay for CAM services primarily out of pocket. These payments now exceed total out-of-pocket charges for all outpatient mainstream health services.
- CAM services in the United States are usually available only in an outpatient (ambulatory care) setting in private offices or health care facilities. This setting provides only limited potential for the full therapeutic benefits of CAM.
- Many people would benefit from the application of CAM therapies and protocols ("a cure") over successive days of treatment (residential care) outside of health care facilities in more healthful environments.
- CAM care can be provided in more healthful environments and at lower costs than in health care facilities while providing vastly enhanced levels of hospitality.*
- Resorts, natural springs, spas, and campgrounds are ideal settings for providing many CAM health and wellness services together with the benefits of a restful, stress-free, relaxing, and healthy environment.
- Historically in the United States, and in much of Europe and Asia today, CAM may be thought of as natural medicine, or "nature cures." There is a great deal of now largely forgotten historical evidence regarding the benefits of "nature cure" obtained during the late 1700s, 1800s, and early 1900s in the United States.
- The hidden or forgotten history of American medicine is highly relevant to fully understanding the potential benefits of CAM and natural healing today.
- There is a tremendous opportunity to integrate the historically proven benefits of "nature cure" with contemporary CAM therapies in natural settings.*

---

*Claire Cassidy in Chapter 5 comments to the effect that much of modern biomedicine can barely function in the absence of carefully controlled environments and perfectly sterile conditions.

effectively integrated into biomedical practice because it cannot be. That is, the concept and term CAM remains a largely undifferentiated amalgam of nonbiomedical practices (see Box 5-6), and much of CAM-as-presently-spoken-of is not actually focused on medical care, but rather on sickness prevention and wellness care, e.g., prayer, exercise, yoga, meditation, and the like. Such activities are really about about lifestyle and "self-care," and often take place in groups in the community or even the workplace (see Chapter 4). Admittedly, these "non-medical" activities may actually be the very ones easiest to introduce into biomedical venues such as hospitals, which can offer community or communal "space" if nothing else.

Much more difficult to integrate are modalities derived from global World Medicines such as Ayurveda, East Asian Medicine, Naturopathic Medicine, or chiropractic. Truly offering both wellness and medical care, and inherent "integration," these systems have their own explanatory models, which often do not mesh well with that of biomedicine. Further, they require extensive education and "integrative-willingness" to put into place in biomedical settings. There are twin dangers here. One is that a technique divorced from its medical model origins will be essayed by biomedical practitioners, with results that do not match those achieved by professional practitioners of that skill, and thus will be labeled "ineffective" and rejected (see below). The other danger is that a tertiary care setting such as a hospital will admit nonbiomedical practitioners to serve patients but will constrain their functions (and status) so intensively that the care cannot be given as intended.

The problem of **scale** (see Chapter 5) looms large here because only some of the CAM practices are small-scale and community-based; others represent complete medical systems and would require some deep changes in hospital and health care organization to put into place. In their "homes" of origin, they do have hospital settings and typically also use clinic settings, and they are not "community-based" in the way teaching yoga or mindfulness meditation would be.

Thus, the new and different resources that must be engaged in realistically achieving greater benefits from CAM, and realizing its full potential, do not reside in hospitals, or within biomedical practices, but outside and beyond what is called health care or medical practice per se. Approaches must be expanded to lifestyle, wellness, mind–body–spirit, wholeness, nature (air, water, sun), and world-view about health healing, which must be sought in the larger community and natural environment.

In today's biomedical practice, there comes a time when health care has done all that it can and patients are returned home to the community. In our system, the role of community and social workers has evolved to fill the transition back outside the health care setting, and to access the resources of the larger community. Social workers are learning about CAM approaches and can have an important new role in helping clients access the broader base of resources that applies to holistic health. We discuss this expanded approach in Chapter 4, the next chapter, which is a new chapter for this edition.

CAM PRACTICES

Many of the different physical aspects of the practices variously described as alternative, complementary, and integrative can be seen to exist on continua with biomedicine (Chapter 5) and are believed and increasingly shown to have measurable, physiological effects on the body. In this textbook, we have found it useful and instructive to arrange these techniques from "least invasive" to "most invasive"

(see Figure 5-3). Such an array also provides the beginnings of an approach to cost-effectiveness analyses in light of the general correlation between degree of invasiveness and costs, both the cost of providing the care and the cost of managing the known and accepted complications of that care. Such an approach is also well established as one of two fundamental principles, that of *therapeutic order,* in Naturopathic Medicine (Chapter 22), which represents an "eclectic," conscious, and authentic integration of CAM practices into a natural, holistic system of health.

To that end, true "health care reform" would devise a system by which the least expensive, least invasive therapeutic approach is provided first. Then, only as needed, would the patient be graduated to the more expensive, more invasive therapies. The situation in the United States has been almost the exact opposite for most patients, with the failures of invasive medical and surgical procedures often being bumped down into the hands of alternative practitioners for attempted remediation.

A case in point is low back pain (the most common cause of pain and disability in working Americans), surgery, and the sad phenomenon of "failed back" as an entirely new subspecialty of pain medicine (Chapter 19). The British National Collaborating Centre for Primary Care has developed a recommended sequence for dealing with chronic low back pain, which recommends precisely this layering of intensity of care (Savigny et al, 2009). The recommended sequence is exercise, OTC drugs, acupuncture, psychotherapy, chiropractic—all to be tried before X-rays or expensive tests such as MRIs. If, after 3 months, the patient "fails" all of these—and let us assume he or she is actively participating in recovery—then, only then, are "standard," more expensive and more invasive biomedical approaches to be applied.

One array for rationally ordering modalities is provided by the order: meditation, talk therapies, bioenergetic manipulation, massage, physical manipulation, insertion, ingestion, injection, and surgery. Alternative and complementary systems of practice are organized around the use of one or more of these modalities. For example, Chinese medicine uses bioenergy (qi), manipulation (tui na), moving meditation (qigong), insertion (acupuncture needles), and ingestion (herbs and foods) for medicinal purposes, approximating a more "complete" system of care. Chiropractic is traditionally limited to manipulative therapy, although many chiropractors incorporate acupuncture, herbal medicine, and nutrition into their individual practices.

Of course, individual practitioners within one system of care may incorporate other healing modalities that are traditionally outside that system of care (e.g., physician or chiropractor who incorporates acupuncture, acupuncturist who practices as a primary care provider and orders biomedical tests).

Some research suggests that individual techniques, when practiced in a manner that is removed from the traditional system of care (what may be called "formulary" or "protocol" approaches), can be effective, perhaps, as long as the medical issue is a simple one. For example, a patient might choose to consult a professional acupuncturist, perhaps someone trained for years in China and subsequently licensed to practice in the United States. Such a practitioner brings depth and width to her or his practice: besides offering acupuncture, she can offer herbal prescriptions, dietary counseling, meditative training, and manipulative therapy. For a relatively simple complaint—a swollen knee postsurgery, common cold, menstrual cramps—such an array of expertise may not be required, and the patient may get equal relief from an MD trained to deliver acupuncture needling in a six-week workshop. Noting that it costs less to train for six weeks than five years, one might be tempted to claim that the biomedical "integrated" approach is preferable, and might even better meet cultural expectations of how a medical encounter ought to go. Further, the fact that non-culturally based, formulary approaches "work" tells us that acupuncture needles must be tapping into some aspect of human physiology that may have been long set aside or been overlooked by mainstream biomedical approaches.

However, in a society in which complex medical situations are "sent back" to nonbiomedical practitioners, the non-formulary advanced expertise of the professional acupuncturist or Oriental Medical Doctor would likely be preferable. Further, studies show that patients report very good results and strongly prefer their professional acupuncture practitioners, in contrast to biomedical practitioners delivering acupuncture as formulary. When asked about the cultural embedding of their acupuncture care, these satisfied patients report seeking personal interaction with their practitioner, and "holism"; they often know little of the underlying East Asian medical model, points which do not seem to affect their ability to profit from acupuncture. This complex situation is evolving; those interested in the issue are encouraged to read, for example, Cassidy (1998a, 1998b), Cohen et al (2007), Frank & Stollberg (2004), Zhan (2009).

AVAILABILITY OF SERVICES

The availability of nonbiomedical practices is determined by (1) the existence, number, and location of practitioners trained (and licensed, where applicable) to provide these services and (2) access to these practitioners. In the world of the ordinary patient, access often begins with word of mouth, that is, a satisfied friend refers the patient to someone already tried. In the model of "integrative" medicine, access occurs through, in increasing order of complexity, clinics, hospitals, academic medical centers, institutional health care systems, and health insurance networks. Individual, traditional fee-for-service practices often thrive completely independently of the institutional health care system.

When considering "what works," we must take into account not only clinical effectiveness of the therapy, but whether the health care setting succeeds in actually delivering effective care—the interactional and managerial aspects of delivery. Patients are willing to pay for care with these attributes regardless of the role, or the absence, of third-party payers and health care rationers.

Although still much smaller in number relative to the mainstream biomedical workforce, the numbers of practitioners in the major professionalized CAM professions in the United States have been growing rapidly. So also have markers of public recognition and professionalization, such as school accreditation, state licensing, and the formation of professional organizations designed to support the Medicine. Manual and manipulative therapies are relatively well represented, with approximately 300,000 massage therapists and more than 54,000 licensed chiropractors. There are approximately half that number of osteopaths, with perhaps fewer than one-quarter of them maintaining any practice in traditional manual and manipulative therapy. Manipulative therapy is also relatively well regulated, with licensure for chiropractic in all 50 states and the District of Columbia and accreditation of graduate schools of chiropractic, whereas osteopathy has been fully subsumed under the credentialing processes of mainstream medicine.

In contrast, other fields of complementary medicine are sparsely represented. There are approximately 27,835 licensed professional acupuncturists in the United States (NCCAOM 2014), with licensure available in most states and the District of Columbia. In addition, there are approximately 5000 MD-acupuncturists. There are approximately 3000 homeopaths, most of them licensed physicians. There are approximately 7000 naturopaths, with licensure available in 17 states, in the northwestern United States, New England, and elsewhere, and six accredited graduate schools, primarily in the Northwest and Southwest.

Naturopathic Medicine includes the practice of what I (Micozzi) have called, from historic usage, an "eclectic" style of natural medicine and Western herbalism, drawing from herbal and many other Eastern and Western natural healing traditions of cultures worldwide. Hundreds of Ayurvedic practitioners may exist, with many following highly individuated practices and others ascribing to a tightly controlled Maharishi Ayurveda school of practice in North America.

In another tradition from India, thousands of yoga masters offer somewhat attenuated training in a variety of yoga, primarily designed as a meditative practice, intended to influence the physical body (*Hatha Yoga*). Although yoga has a meditative aspect (at least yoga done for health purposes), there is another tradition of Mindfulness Meditation, which is rapidly growing with thousands of meditation groups across the United States and worldwide. Energy healers now come from several organized schools of energy healing nationwide. The practice of energy healing is widespread among thousands of members of the U.S. nursing professions (Chapter 14), through healing touch and therapeutic touch, and among a number of physical therapists, who may also include such modalities as craniosacral therapy (Chapter 17).

MODELS OF INTEGRATION

There is a great deal of discussion about integrative medicine, from "integrating" CAM practices into individual clinics on a quasi-competitive basis, to providing access to CAM practitioners within academic or private hospital-based health networks and systems, to providing "discounts" or even partial coverage for CAM services under health insurance plans and alliances. Given the broad nature of the resources brought to bear, and the locations accessed in natural, holistic CAM medical systems, we should also consider at least theoretically what would be involved in integration at the scale of the entire, nationwide institutional health care system. Supposing that the national-level institutional health care system (or even the IHCS within a locality or a hospital group) chose to develop the concept of "integrative" medicine by supporting the creation of "integrative" clinics, what might be needed?

First, a philosophical issue: would such clinics always and inevitably be visualized as including biomedical practitioners, and functioning according to the biomedical and hospital management models? If so, it is likely that many CAM practitioners would simply continue as they are: in their own clinics and/or forming their own multimodel integrative clinics (e.g., chiropractic, massage therapy, acupuncture) that do not include biomedical practitioners. Assuming this problem could be resolved, "integrative" clinics need access to licensed CAM health care providers. CAM practitioners who accepted the challenge to work with biomedical practitioners would need to be convinced that there were significant advantages to linking up with them, and that the risks had been minimized. These very substantial risks include being treated as inferior and lesser than the biomedical practitioners, being paid less, being unable to treat freely, and having only "second-go" at incoming patients (common in clinics where all patients are required to "see the MD first").[2]

Another way to go about forming "integrative" clinics would be to train existing biomedical providers in one or more modalities of complementary care. It would make sense, at the same time, to train CAM practitioners in the basics of biomedical primary care. Handled well, such dual training could help both biomedical and CAM practitioners to understand the logic of the others' practice, and view each other as fellow medical professionals.

To support such an effort to develop "integrative" clinics, the institutional health care system may provide credibility, appropriate practice environments, and access to new clients for practitioners. Often the institutional health care system has opportunities to make capital investments in facilities required to provide care that are not available to individual practitioners. Sometimes the success of the integrative care clinic is based on attracting the individual practitioner's existing client base, whereas the individual practitioner comes to the health care system looking for new referrals. An important area for expansion of services is represented by appropriate referrals from within the health system host to their integrative clinics and inpatient services, if actually implemented as part of an "integrated" system.

If complementary medical services are added onto existing biomedical services (instead of selectively replacing them), they become a cost center rather than a cost-effective source of savings. In response to consumer demand, some managed care systems have offered access to a network of complementary care providers who have agreed to accept reduced rates. For example, one approach is to create a network of licensed "holistic" health providers, which offers an insurance rider to employers, unions, and associations for access to members at negotiated rates. These networks may be developed as part of corporate wellness programs, so that access to alternative providers becomes another employee benefit and factor for retention and recruitment of employees who seek these kinds of services.

Academic biomedical centers offer a further opportunity to develop the "integration" of clinical research and training together *with* the practice of integrative medicine. Presently, and unfortunately, many academic medical centers adopt an "arms-length" relationship with CAM with internally isolated efforts at research, or teaching, or practice, but only rarely all three, that are not at all functionally integrated themselves.

Integrative care has also been taken to imply the provision of various medical modalities under the supervision of a physician. To the extent that such physician-supervised centers function as full-service (or even fuller service) primary care biomedical facilities, there is fear that when primary care "gatekeepers" refer patients for complementary care, the patient may never come back to that biomedical provider. Such a result, were it to happen, might appropriately trip a re-examination of the referring clinic, the patient's complaint, and the validity of the feeling of loss. Follow-up might show that the patient has found a more effective form of care for her complaint, or a more welcoming environment, in which case, the referring clinic might wish to celebrate her success, and look to the management of their own clinic.

Within a health care system, an integrative medical practice may be managed as part of a primary care referral system for general hospital services. The national American Whole Health Network, based on a successful clinic in Chicago and intended to provide integrated medical services under physician supervision, was unable to receive adequate physician-patient referrals nationally and had to

---

[2]We won't even discuss the situation in which only the MDs get the parking spots! See Hunter et al (2012).

embark on costly direct-to-consumer marketing, ultimately going out of business. One response to the concern about physician referrals, developed by the late William Fair, Sr., of Memorial Sloan Kettering, were facilities for complementary care *not* supervised by a physician. This concept, initially developed as Synergy Health, opened in New York City in the late 1990s.

Another important direction in integrated medicine takes the provision of complementary care beyond the primary care provider and gatekeeper to the integration of appropriate complementary medical modalities into a medical specialty practice for the management of chronic diseases, for example, acupuncturists at pain clinics or in neurological rehabilitation centers. The initial primary care focus of integrated medicine is being supplemented by information on integrative medicine targeted to medical specialists such as orthopedic surgeons who create spine health centers. Significantly, there is now research and clinical protocols to support the use of safe and effective CAM therapies within the practices of many medical specialties: Neurology and pain management, cardiology, obstetrics–gynecology and women's health, and pediatrics are among the specialties for which textbooks have compiled such information. Churchill Livingstone's medical guides to complementary therapies includes, for example, the title *Complementary and Integrative Therapies for Cardiovascular Disease* (Frishman et al, 2005).

EFFECTIVENESS AND COST-EFFECTIVENESS

The establishment and expansion of the CAM research program at the National Institutes of Health (NIH), forced by leaders in the U.S. Congress, has increasingly emphasized clinical trials research to create a research database for evidence on the efficacy or lack of efficacy of available alternative medical modalities. Therefore the health care system has access to increasingly available, abundant, and credible data on efficacy. However, more practical understanding of the appropriateness and cost-effectiveness of care requires health care utilization research to better understand (1) patient motivation and satisfaction, (2) willingness to pay for care, (3) preference for one effective modality of care over another, (4) willingness to substitute care, (5) multidisciplinary guidelines for best practices in disease management, and (6) related types of analyses that can better inform health care decision makers, whether policy makers, administrators, or consumers. The Agency for Healthcare Research and Quality has worked within a very limited budget to provide important analyses on the effectiveness and cost-effectiveness of various modalities in the management of low back pain (Chapter 19), pharmaceuticals, surgery, spinal manual therapy, acupuncture, massage, and other therapies that are all available at various levels of accessibility, cost, and effectiveness.

The U.S. Health Resources and Services Administration, again with a tiny fraction of the NIH budget, has sponsored projects for development and dissemination of best practices, as well as an Internet-based distance learning network for applied aspects of the management and administration of integrative medical practice. Under the Health Insurance Portability and Accountability Act (HIPAA, originally the Kennedy–Kassebaum bill, developed by the Congressional Energy and Commerce Committee), the Centers for Medicare and Medicaid Services (CMS) was mandated to develop current practice terminology (CPT) codes for every therapy "in commerce," which implies that codes are to exist for CAM therapies currently in practice and for which consumers are paying. CMS contracts with the AMA to maintain and update the coding system, which AMA does through its Health Care Professions Advisory Committee (HCPAC). In 2003, one of the authors of this chapter (Micozzi) served on a panel to prepare testimony to CMS recommending that AMA add CAM practitioners to HCPAC so that such codes could be developed. Currently, there are codes, for example, for massage therapy, acupuncture, and chiropractic. These codes are providing a basis for expanded reimbursement of CAM by Medicare and Medicaid and serve as a precedent for other third-party payers. For improved effectiveness and cost savings to be realized by consumers, the health care system, and third-party payers, it is necessary to determine which therapeutic options can be appropriately and specifically provided to which patients in what order for cost-effective medical management.

REASONS WHY CAM MAY NOT WORK IN INTEGRATIVE PRACTICE

Over 20 years and five editions, this standard medical textbook has provided thousands of references and hundreds of pages of published scientific studies on the safety and efficacy of CAM. We have accordingly been able to move beyond the archaic arguments that CAM is not effective, or that it has not been proven to work, or even that "it cannot work," according to a particular scientific paradigm. Still, however—as is the case with all Medicines and medical interventions—we must confront the reality that a given CAM therapy may not work well, or work at all, for everyone, even if shown efficacious in clinical trials.

The concept of "working well" is usually taken to mean having a specific physiological balancing or healing effect. But, as is well known, medical care may also not "work well" if the delivery environment is unappealing. Thus, often, the better question is "Does it serve?" as in *does it serve patients such that they feel cared for and their symptoms are ameliorated?*

Let us consider some reasons why CAM interventions may sometimes not "work."

Incomplete or incorrect techniques taught in the absence of the comprehensive medical model of that CAM system. Some schools of CAM practice in the West have selectively adapted knowledge and practices without necessarily being aware of their historical embedding, or of what other models and interventions are available. An example of this trend is in the practice of the style of medicine called traditional Chinese medicine (TCM) (see Chapter 2). This style, developed after World War II on a biomedical model, specifically chose to exclude aspects of classical Chinese medicine, especially aspects concerned with emotions and spirit, both of which were defined as treatable by attention to the physical body alone (see Figure 5-4). TCM is the favored style in professional Chinese medical schools in the United States. Thus, it can be expected that those who *only* practice TCM will be unaware of and unable to provide a more comprehensive care, and may expect to have treatment failures. Fortunately, most schools, and postgraduate continuing education courses, help correct such limitations, expanding the practitioner's reach to draw upon more of the ancient knowledge actually available over centuries of Chinese medicine. This can help them deal with "difficult issues" (on which an entire classical treatise was written) or deal with second tier and third tier complicated cases. In short, limited training leaves some Oriental medical doctors (OMDs) open to limited success[3]; additional training allows them resort to further approaches. Awareness of this problem lies behind the rich continuing education offerings now available in the United States for professional acupuncture practitioners.

A related issue is the sometimes intentional "editing" of practices that may be considered too harsh or uncomfortable in the West. An example is the Maharishi Mahesh Yogi intentionally modifying traditional ancient Ayurvedic practices starting in the 1960s to make them more palatable and "friendly" to the West. Although this helped introduce the benefits of Ayurveda to the West, it left us with a less than fully potent set of practices (see Chapter 7). Similarly, some of the more strenuous and uncomfortable aspects of Yoga have been omitted in Western practice—while these omissions make Yoga more accessible as a practice, clearly it can limit its potency as a therapy (Chapter 21).

The Issue of "Trade Secrets." In addition to the issue of limited awareness of the totality of a medical model and its interventive procedures, there is the problem that most ethnomedical traditions include "trade secrets" (like clinical "pearls" of wisdom in the West) passed down orally within families or communities of healers. These "secrets" serve to make that community distinctive and potentially able to treat cases others can't help, thus earning more money or status. The more closely a Western-trained practitioner works with a traditionally trained practitioner of a Medicine, the more likely she is to gain the trust and perhaps be incorporated into depth-training in that practice, thus learning the clinical pearls of that tradition. This situation is much the same as what ideally happens when student physicians leave the classroom and begin to work directly under the guidance of a senior physician—they profit from the elder's extensive experience.

The potency of CAM in the West is also limited by being largely restricted to delivery on an outpatient basis. In chronic or traumatic situations—for example, poststroke, postamputation, postsurgery, chemotherapy—one or two treatments per week for 15 to 60 minutes cannot achieve the benefits of a residential care program (equivalent to "hospitalization") where all aspects of a patient's experience, including sleep, exercise, diet, and other healthful practices, are potentially addressed, in addition to delivering the specific therapy.[4] Going away and staying in residence at a resort-spa in the wilderness was one way historically of getting the benefits of an all-encompassing nature cure (see Chapter 1 and Box 3-2).

Individuality, both biological and cultural. Realistically, even the most lab-effective CAM practices may simply not work for patients taken as individuals. Although a focus on individualizing care is one of the idealized characteristics of CAM practices (Chapters 1 and 5), integrative medicine often makes the same "one size fits all" mistake of biomedicine. Rarely are objective efforts made to "screen" patients for appropriate therapy, and although "integrative" practitioners recognize and hold out the individuality of each patient, there is resistance to actually treating them as such in any disciplined, scientific way.

Some headway is being made. For example, this reality of individuality has been understood and accepted with hypnosis for decades. The Spiegel Hypnotic Susceptibility Scale (Chapter 10) is used to predict, based upon a simple statistical profile, who will benefit from hypnosis and who will not, on an objective scientific clinical basis. We now know that about 10% respond very well to hypnosis, another 10% are resistant, and everyone else falls somewhere on a continuum between.

For the past 20 years, whenever one of us (Micozzi) spoke to the CAM research community, he pointed out the need to develop similar "susceptibility scales," like that for hypnosis, for other CAM therapies as well, because their effectiveness generally falls along a continuum, rather than being an all-or-none phenomenon. Using psychometric analysis, Micozzi worked with a colleague, Michael Jawer, on the "personality boundary types" developed by Dr. Ernst Hartmann (d. 2013) at Tufts University, Boston, over 25 years. They have explored the predictive value of this "susceptibility scale" for many CAM modalities, including acupuncture, biofeedback, guided imagery, stress reduction, and meditation-yoga (see Chapters 9 and 10).

---

[3]This point applies equally to MDs trained in a single style of acupuncture care.

[4]Note that the typical biomedical hospital does not realistically address sleep, exercise, or diet among hospitalized patients: patients complain of noise and having their sleep interrupted, being restricted to bed or boring hall walking, and being offered diets of such low quality that it is sometimes barely recognizable as "food" and is certainly neither particularly nutritious nor healthful.

Without applying appropriate psychometric screening for patients, "integrative" medical practices cannot know which way to point their patients without engaging in time-consuming and costly "trial and error," and potentially failing altogether. Although there is a certain amount of "trial and error" in approaching optimal care for any patient, the potentially bewildering array of choices among CAM modalities (to both patient and "integrative" practitioner) mandates that a more disciplined approach to selecting appropriate therapies be taken than what is presently being offered.

PROBLEMS WITH INTEGRATIVE MEDICAL RESEARCH

Although it is important to realize that there can be misdirection in the use of CAM therapies, it is equally important to realize that much unnecessary confusion can also result from problems with the conduct of research on CAM modalities and techniques. There is a considerable literature on this issue (see Chapter 14 on Energy Medicine). In Chapter 24, we also provide a detailed discussion of research pitfalls in new assessments of herbal remedies that have already been in long-established historical use. Herbs (unlike many "hands-on" CAM therapies) can theoretically be studied effectively using a controlled clinical trial design identical to the same approach commonly used for drugs. Despite the appropriateness of this research methodology in theory, mainstream medical researchers nonetheless have mismanaged research design and reporting results in ways that have been highly counterproductive (see Appendix, Chapter 24).

GENERAL LIMITATIONS OF EVIDENCE-BASED MEDICINE AND MEDICAL RESEARCH

Beyond the problems particular to research on integrative medicine are concerns that have arisen regarding the so-called gold standard of any medical research in general, and the construction of any medical practice based only on so-called evidence-based medicine derived from that. There have been those (including a reviewer of this textbook!) who have taken the position—in direct opposition to historic, pragmatic uses of CAM as a basis for integrative medicine—that evidence-based medicine provides the only basis for integrative medicine, as well as for all of medical practice.

Multiple limitations of such an approach are dramatically illustrated by a recent book entitled, *Tarnished Gold: The Sickness of Evidence-Based Medicine*, by Drs. Steve Hickey and Hilary Roberts (Hickey & Roberts, 2011). In the tradition of Thomas Kuhn's ground-breaking *Structure of Scientific Revolutions* (Chapter 2), this new book provides important tools to help understand how statistical *data* become useful *information* (or not) in improving our understanding of nature and human biology and in guiding medical practice. Originally conceived as a post–World War II cost-saving strategy for England's socialist National Health Service (an early form of health care rationing), by the 1990s evidence-based medicine (EBM) was becoming the latest fashion in biomedical science.

In fact, the new statistical fashion of evidence-based medicine has simply become a cloak for establishing a sometimes false face of credibility and taking the "scientific high ground." This cloak is worn well by those statisticians who lack a working understanding of what my faculty advisor, Nobel Laureate Baruch Blumberg (1925–2011, to whom this edition is dedicated), liked to call "biological plausibility." It is also worn in an ill-fitting manner by physicians intimidated by elaborate uses of statistics. EBM has also become a kind of superficial marketing slogan for presumed respectability of costly big pharma and "big science" projects that increasingly crowd out other valid kinds of experimentation, observation, and research. This problem is painfully familiar to anyone providing or using natural medicine, nutritional medicine, complementary or alternative medicine, or integrative medicine. The human biological paradigm, model, or theory underlying any scientific approach and medical practice may differ, but it is important to *actually have one* in order to develop any sense of the plausibility for assigning a statistical association to having an actual role in the causation of health or disease.

Despite its high-blown claims of superiority, EBM typically sends practitioners to "cheat sheets," such as mindless lists of protocols/formularies, or the Hippocrates website, rather than paying attention to the specifics of the individual patient and actually using their education and training to *think* about what they are doing. For any medical practice, the biggest complaint about EBM is, most of all, that it eliminates *thinking* and thus makes any and all health practitioners into mere technicians. This approach can leave the patient in desperate straits.

"STATE-ISTICS"

Beyond the individual patient, when applied to public health and health policy, "State-istics" first turned a troubling corner with politicization and massive government intervention into the scientific process for "proving" that smoking is *the* cause of lung cancer during the 1970s–1980s. [One hundred years before, while Francis Galton (Charles Darwin's nephew) was working on statistical methods and observations, Otto von Bismarck in Germany was already encouraging the development of "vital statistics" as a measure of a nation's "war-fighting" capacity.] This unprecedented government intervention has set a different, more legalistic standard for how scientific *data* are translated into *information* about human biology to help guide public health and medical practice. This process leaves behind a lot of valid information about genetic and other risk factors and the fact that many nonsmokers get lung cancer. In fact, today there are 100,000 lung cancer victims who never smoked; and there are more former smokers than current smokers among lung cancer victims. So much for the government's single-minded smoking cessation and prevention research as the final solution for lung cancer.

The smoking and lung cancer precedent also helped create a role for government and industry bureaucrats in using statistics to force social agendas onto public health and medical practice. The diversity among patients and circumstances (a critical component of holistic, complementary or alternative, and integrative medical practices) is lost and replaced by arbitrary and illusory standards that in fact represent nothing (Hickey & Roberts, 2011).

We could consider the case of negligence regarding the need for vitamin D supplementation as an example of the seriously misdirected overall public health effort (see Chapters 15 and 26).

TRIALS ON TRIAL

The modern preoccupation with statistical manipulations forces every observation into an arbitrary placebo-controlled "gold standard" clinical trial—and now evidence-based medicine. This dark lens leaves physicians and scientists half-blind to critical observations from the daily realities of clinical practice, as well as to understanding basic biological sciences and how nature operates in the universe. Therefore, calling such approaches a "gold standard" in medical research is limiting and counterproductive and undermines true scientific innovation.

> Here are all our highly educated and intelligent MDs ostensibly trained in physiology who have *no* idea of the flow of anything at all, or of the linkages of all the body parts, etc. They can only think in nouns: you have asthma (pulmonologist); no, it's reflux (gastroenterologist); no, it's heart failure (cardiologist); no, it's a narrow return from the legs (well, the cardiologist says, he can't deal with blood vessels elsewhere in the body); no, it's allergies; no, it's ... and all this time the patient is suffering and the costs are rising. These are examples of people not thinking, not examples of using evidence-based medicine. ∾

It may all be summed up by Nobel Laureate (1908) Lord Ernest Rutherford, the discoverer of atomic theory, when he said a century ago, "If your result needs a statistician, then you should have done a better experiment."

SPECIFIC LIMITATIONS OF EVIDENCE-BASED MEDICINE

In sum, several specific issues hamper and limit the value of data and information gained from EBM and modern biomedical or CAM research in general:

- Because of the emphasis on reductionist research designs, immense amounts of information is lost about *individual* patients' health, and about the significance of the patient–practitioner interaction in the receipt of medical care.
- Research funding is heavily biased toward reductionist designs, and the asking of quantitative questions, to the detriment of answering "meaning" and "explanation" questions via qualitative research.
- The reductionist, hierarchical approach to what constitutes "evidence" markedly limits the kinds of research questions that are considered valid (see Chapter 1).
- Results are often withheld, or biased due to corporate ownership of data.
- Publication is biased such that only certain kinds of data get published due to decisions by researchers, authors, editors, and reviewers; these decisions are often fashion-based, and prejudicial to nonbiomedical medical models.
- The media are not free of fashion, and prefer "what sells," attitudes that also bias which published results get attention, and the kinds and degree of attention; all this affects popular perception without necessarily reflecting quality science.
- The medicalization of human biology whereby new "diseases" are continually being discovered, many of which are natural aspects of human life.
- Disreputable statistical analyses, including deliberate cheating, fraud, and misrepresentation in *in up to half* of the modern scientific literature due to academic careerist and funding pressures (Bauchner, 2013).

In October 2011, for example, the prestigious British journal *Nature* reported that published retractions had increased *ten times* over the past decade. In this view, EBM can be seen as a sort of "junk science" that misleads practitioners, researchers, politicians, government bureaucrats, journalists, and the public. EBM harms patients and suppresses true medical innovation and progress. In our opinion, patient-based rather than "evidence-based" medicine is a more productive approach—this point returns us to the earlier remark about asking "what serves." The average patient and physician may be less concerned with the considerations discussed above than they are with "good medicine" that they can "believe in" (Chapter 5), which is really the answer to "what serves."

To which might be added, as taught by my (Micozzi) mentor, medical school professor and U.S. Surgeon General C. Everett Koop (1915–2013, to whom this edition is also dedicated): "The least medicine that works is the best medicine." And, per Lord Rutherford, the fewer statistics needed to reach a conclusion, the better. Or perhaps it was best repeated by Mark Twain, who often quoted the British statesman Benjamin Disraeli: "There are three kinds of lies: lies, damned lies, and statistics."

SOLUTIONS FOR INTEGRATIVE PRACTICE

Reliance on the appropriate and safe use of CAM therapies, mind–body approaches, as well as food, nutrients, and herbs is a critical and fundamental component of integrative medical practices. To properly address these areas, more attention needs to be focused on biomedical education and public policy issues.

BIOMEDICAL EDUCATION

The issues considered thus far point to the clear need for improved biomedical education on dietary supplements, CAM therapies, and integrative medicine in biomedical schools, postgraduate biomedical training programs, and continuing biomedical education (CME) courses. CME programs are met with the challenge that current practitioners generally have had little to no exposure to these topic areas.

According to surveys conducted by the Center for Research in Medical Education and Health Care at Thomas Jefferson University, Philadelphia, the majority of today's biomedical students in all graduation years and in all current classes want more education in CAM and integrative medicine. The proportion has been increasing with each graduating year. Among biomedical school classes, the proportion is relatively high in the first year (when entering students carry the culture of the general population), declines somewhat in the second and third years (as students become socialized to the biomedical model and generally witness little reinforcement for the teaching of integrative medicine), and rises again in the fourth year (after students have been exposed to the problems and questions of patients).

The literature of integrative medicine is in the process of creation, with a need for both "basic science" and clinical texts, and journals in integrative medicine. Elsevier Health Sciences (subsuming the former C.V. Mosby of St. Louis, W.B. Saunders of Philadelphia, and Churchill Livingstone of Edinburgh and London) has developed many titles in complementary medicine, including medical guides to complementary and alternative medicine for which this text served as the foundation (www.elsevierhealth.com). A number of highly scientific and professional journals now exist to forefront CAM research, for example, *Journal of Complementary and Alternative Medicine* (founded by one of us, Micozzi; current executive editor, co-author Cassidy), *Complementary Therapies in Clinical Practice, Social Health and Illness,* and *Culture, Medicine and Psychiatry,* all of which reflect the whole field of CAM; there are also specialized journals as in chiropractic, Oriental medicine, and massage therapy.

Much curriculum and faculty development remains to be done in this area, and the traditional support of state and federal governments for medical education and training could help provide biomedical schools with the needed resources and incentives. Turning the other cheek, the same governmental agencies could choose to support improved medical education at CAM schools, particularly by offering cogent training in the medical model of biomedicine and some skills in primary care and patient communication (see Foreword to the third edition of this text

by former U.S. Surgeon General C. Everett Koop). In the interim, it is incumbent upon providers of health care services to help stimulate appropriate CME and in-service training for health professions staffs so that practitioners can be knowledgeable and helpful to their patients seeking guidance on the use of nutritional supplements, and integrative medicine, including developing skills in appropriate referral and patient assessment.

PUBLIC AND INSTITUTIONAL POLICY

State governments have developed a traditional role in regulating medical practice and in supporting medical education. The federal government has had a role in stimulating and supporting certain kinds of medical research, regulating medical products and devices, monitoring aspects of the public health, and helping fund health care infrastructure, and is now paying approximately one-third of the costs of health care in America. Policy makers at the state and federal levels should become more knowledgeable about the needs and opportunities relative to integrative medicine, which would represent true health care reform and cost savings.

REGULATION

Various health practitioners are regulated by an assembly of state boards and regulatory bodies that varies from state to state. Medical devices, including biophysical devices, which are employed in the application of various mind-body therapies are regulated by the FDA. A discussion of recent experiences with regulation of the acupuncture needle is provided in Chapter 29. Finally, herbal remedies and nutrients are classified and regulated as dietary supplements by the FDA under special legislation. Because dietary supplements are administered much like drugs are administered, there are theoretically certain similarities. However, unlike with pharmaceuticals, DSHEA (Dietary Supplement Health and Education Act) mandates that scientific information about health effects *cannot* be provided on the product label (or with the product as a product insert) for dietary supplements. Therefore, professionals and consumers must be educated in other ways about the appropriate use of dietary supplements.

PROFESSIONAL INFORMATION

Due to the increasing availability of credible third-party research on the efficacy of herbal and nutritional ingredients, as well as increasing recognition by the biomedical profession of the importance of dietary supplementation for optimal health, it is incumbent upon practitioners of integrative medicine to maintain a high standard of information and practice about herbal and nutritional ingredients. One approach to this requirement is to develop and maintain the capability for a clinic or hospital-based formulary of appropriate, effective, and high-quality sources of herbs and nutrients. Another approach is to integrate herbalists and nutritionists into staffing.

New information technologies are being brought online to provide distributors, consumers, and practitioners fair and accurate information about the appropriate use of dietary supplements.

The former Tai Sophia Institute in Laurel, Maryland, now the Maryland University of Integrative Health (www.muih.edu), the University of Exeter in the United Kingdom (www.ex.ac.uk), the University of Minnesota Center for Spirituality and Healing (www.csh.umn.edu), and other sources are all committed to developing accessible databases on dietary supplements and numerous other features for professional and patient reference in the practice of integrative medicine. (Websites accessed January 20, 2014.)

FEDERAL POLICY

While state governments have developed a traditional role in regulating medical practice and in supporting medical education, the federal government has had a role in stimulating and supporting certain kinds of medical research, regulating medical products and devices, monitoring the public health, and helping fund health care infrastructure, and is now paying approximately one-third of the costs of health care in America. Policy makers at the state and federal levels should become more knowledgeable about the needs and opportunities relative to integrative medicine, which would represent true health care reform and cost savings.

A bipartisan Congressional Caucus on Complementary and Alternative Medicine and Dietary Supplements was organized to help serve this purpose, co-chaired in the Senate by Tom Harkin (D-IA; retired January 2015), and Orrin Hatch (R-UT). In 2006, another House Caucus on Dietary Supplements was formed with Representatives Chris Cannon (R-UT) and Frank Pallone (D-NJ), as well as a continuing Caucus on Complementary and Alternative Medicine with Rep. Dan Burton (R-IN). Some professional groups had begun to work with members of these caucuses and other elected representatives to improve federal support for appropriate analyses and applied programs on dietary supplements, CAM, and integrative medicine. However, the effort to work with public policy leaders remains poorly organized and undermined by the desire of most "integrative medicine" programs, within their mainstream biomedical institutions, to maintain the status quo and not to "rock the boat" for higher priority, current federal funding support for mainstream education and research. With the final recognition of the overdue need for constraints on government overspending, the window of opportunity may well have been lost, and although the cost savings of appropriate CAM and integrative medicine would be huge, they may never be realized.

Although funding specifically for the National Center for Complementary and Alternative Medicine (NCCAM) research has increased each year since its creation was forced by Congress in 1992, it remains an insignificant percentage of medical research. It is also critical that other federal agencies charged with administering programs related to health resources and services, primary care, health professions training and workforce development, consumer education, health services research, and other areas direct their efforts to address the important challenges and opportunities offered by CAM and potentially integrative medicine. Integrative medicine can have an important role that requires further articulation in current congressional actions on medical liability insurance reform and the national patient safety and quality assurance initiative, not to mention the chimera of authentic health care reform.

Outside the government, private philanthropic support for CAM and integrative medicine has been paltry relative to mainstream medical causes and to the vast unrealized potential for improving medical practice, public health, and the health care economy. The burgeoning private, non-profit disease advocacy groups have generally been slow to recognize the potential of CAM, but instead tend to repeat the slogans formulated by the mainstream academic-industrial-biomedical complex for ever more public funding as the only measure of success—rather than focusing on true innovation.

Public support together with private innovation and respect for the art and science of the traditions of medical practice have been the hallmarks of medical advancement. All these must become part of the equation in order to make the case for effective integrative medicine.

References

Barnes PM, Powell-Griner E, McFann K, et al: Complementary and alternative medicine use among adults: United States, 2002, *Semin Integr Med* 2:54, 2004.

Bauchner H, Fontanarosa PB: Restoring confidence in the pharmaceutical industry, *JAMA* 309(6):607–609, 2013. doi: 10.1001/jama.2013.58.

Cassidy CM: Chinese Medicine users in the United States: Part I, Utilization, satisfaction, medical plurality, *J Altern Complement Med* 4(1):17–28, 1998a.

Cassidy CM: Chinese Medicine users in the United States: Part II: Preferred Aspects of Care, *J Altern Complement Med* 4(2):189–202, 1998b.

Cohen M, Ruggie M, Micozzi M: *The practice of integrative medicine: a legal and operational guide*, New York, 2007, Springer.

Frank R, Stollberg G: Medical acupuncture in Germany: patterns of consumerism among physicians and patients, *Sociol Health Illn* 26(3):351–372, 2004.

Frishman WH, Weintraub MI, Micozzi MS, editors: *Complementary and integrative therapies for cardiovascular disease*, St. Louis, 2005, Mosby Elsevier Health Sciences.

Hickey S, Roberts H: *Tarnished Gold: The Sickness of Evidence-Based Medicine*, Create Space, 2011.

Hunter J, Corcoran K, Phelps K, et al: The challenges of establishing an integrative medicine primary care clinic in Sydney, Australia, *J Altern Complemen Med* 18(11):1008–1013, 2012.

Micozzi MS: Complementary medicine: What is appropriate? Who will provide it?, *Ann Intern Med* 129:65, 1998.

NCCAOM (National Certification Commission for Acupuncture and Oriental Medicine): State Licensure Requirements, 2014. Available at: www.NCCAOM.org. Accessed 10 March 2014.

Savigny P, Juntze S, Watson P, et al: *Low back pain: early management of persistent non-specific low back pain*, London, 2009, National Collaborating Centre for Primary Care and Royal College of General Practitioners.

Wootton J, Sparber A: Surveys of complementary and alternative medicine usage: review of general population trends and specific populations, *Semin Integr Med* 1(1):1–16, 2003.

Zhan M: *Other-worldly: making Chinese medicine through transnational frames*, Durham NC, 2009, Duke University Press.

Suggested Readings

Astin JA: Why patients use alternative medicine: results of a national study, *JAMA* 279(19):1548, 1998.

Behnke K, Jensen GS, Graubaum HJ, et al: Hypericum perforatum versus fluoxetine in the treatment of mild to moderate depression, *Adv Ther* 19(1):43–52, 2002.

Cohen M, Ruggie M, Micozzi M: *A Legal and Operational Guide to Complementary and Integrative Medicine*, New York, 2007, Springer, p 202.

DeSmet PAGM: Herbal remedies, *N Engl J Med* 347:2046, 2002.

Druss BG, Rosenheck RA: Association between use of unconventional therapies and conventional medical services, *JAMA* 282(7):651, 1999.

Eisenberg DM, Davis RB, Ettner SL, et al: Trends in alternative medicine use in the United States, 1990–1997: results of a follow-up national survey, *JAMA* 280(18):1569, 1998.

Eisenberg DM, Kessler RC, Foster C, et al: Unconventional medicine in the United States: prevalence, costs, and patterns of use, *N Engl J Med* 328(4):246, 1993.

Fairfield KM, Fletcher RH: Vitamins for chronic disease prevention in adults: scientific evidence, *JAMA* 287:3116, 2002.

Fletcher RH, Fairfield KM: Vitamins for chronic disease prevention in adults: clinical applications, *JAMA* 287:3127, 2002.

Gruenwald J, Skrabal J: Kava ban highly questionable: a brief summary of the main scientific findings presented in the "In Depth Investigation on EU Member States Market Restrictions on Kava Products", *Semin Integr Med* 1(4):199, 2003.

Hatch O: *Square peg: confessions of a citizen senator*, New York, 2002, Basic Books, pp 81–95.

Kessler RC, Davis RB, Foster DF, et al: Long-term trends in the use of complementary and alternative medical therapies in the United States, *Ann Intern Med* 135(4):262, 2001.

Micozzi MS: *Complementary and integrative medicine in cancer care and prevention*, New York, 2007, Springer.

Shelton RC, Keller MB, Gelenberg A, et al: Randomized controlled trial of St. John's wort in major depression, *JAMA* 285(15):1978–1986, 2001.

Solomon PR, Adams F, Silver A: Gingko for memory enhancement: a randomized controlled trial, *JAMA* 288:835–840, 2002.

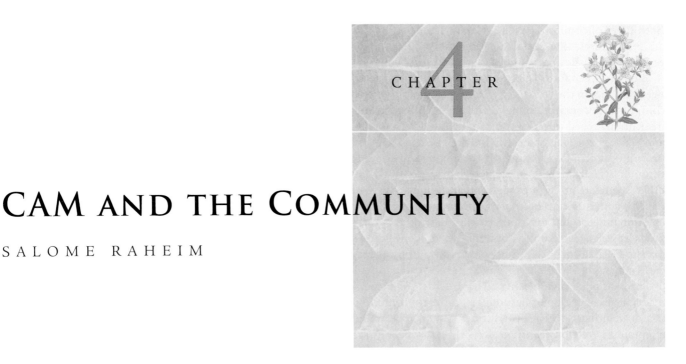

CHAPTER 4

CAM AND THE COMMUNITY

SALOME RAHEIM

Individual and population health are promoted or undermined by many factors that are largely rooted in the community. These factors are considered to be the social determinants of health—"the circumstances in which people are born, grow up, live, work and age, and the systems put in place to deal with illness" (Commission on Social Determinants of Health, 2008, p 3). Key social determinants of health include the quality and extent of access to food, education, health care, housing, transportation, and opportunities for income generation. Degrees of exposure to discrimination, crime, violence, and environmental toxins are also critically important (Wenger, 2012). By this definition, it is readily apparent that the vast majority of health factors and outcomes exist, occur, and are experienced entirely outside the "health care" system.

The World Health Organization (WHO) has identified general relationships among community-level factors and health outcomes:

- Higher income and social status are generally linked to better health. The greater the gap between the richest and poorest people, the greater overall differences in health.
- Low education levels are generally linked with poor health, more stress, higher blood pressure, and lower self-confidence.
- Clean air and water, healthy workplaces, safe houses, communities, and roads all contribute to good health.
- Employment contributes to good health, particularly for those who have more control over their working conditions.
- Greater support from families, friends, and communities is linked to better health.

- Access to (and use of) services that prevent and treat disease contributes to positive health outcomes (WHO 2013).

Most of what influences health happens *outside* of the biomedical health care system. What has been called "complementary and alternative medicine" (CAM), also theoretically considered as "holistic health," has been defined as ancillary to the dominant health care system (Chapters 3, 5). However, an ecological perspective, which includes social determinants of health, supports a much broader conceptualization that situates "holistic health" systems and practices within the broader context of community.

COMMUNITY, SOCIAL DETERMINANTS OF HEALTH, AND HEALTH OUTCOMES

Community may be understood in multiple ways. Two common conceptualizations are place-based and non–place-based communities. Neighborhoods, municipalities, and metropolitan areas are place-based or locality-based communities. They have distinctive geographic and political boundaries and contain a network of social groups and organizations, including families, as well as arts, business, civic, educational, governmental, health, human service, and religious groups and organizations (Netting et al, 2004; Weil, 2005). Non–place-based communities are "communities of interest" or "communities of identification" and are composed of people who share common characteristics and common identity, such as ethnicity, race, religion, lifestyle, ideology, or sexual orientation (Reed, 2005). Community commonality may also be based upon a significant physical characteristic or characteristics, such as hearing impairment (e.g., the deaf community).

35

Both types of communities are relevant to any effort that aims to address the social determinants of health and promote a holistic approach to health and well-being.

Biological, economic, emotional, intellectual, and social needs are met in the context of community. Locality-based communities contain within them the organizations and institutions relied upon to provide the tangible resources and services needed for health and well-being. They also provide opportunities for a sense of belonging and meaning through affiliation with civic, faith-based, political, and other membership groups and organizations. By their nature, communities of identification meet social and emotional needs and may meet intellectual and economic needs as well (Reed, 2005). Communities of identification may be situated within a locality-based community or may cross geographic boundaries to include regional, national, or international membership. The Internet and social media have created boundless opportunities for communities of identification to form, attract new members, and maintain interaction electronically.

Locality-based communities with abundant resources have greater capacity to meet members' needs and support the health and well-being of their members. Conversely, when communities experience major stressors, their capacity to promote health and well-being among members is compromised. These stressors may include economic decline, limited availability of nutritional foods, overcrowded or underperforming schools, poor housing stock, and high rates of unemployment, crime, violence, and/or pollution (Box 4-1). When persistent patterns of discrimination exist based on gender, racial or ethnic background, national origin, or other characteristics, affected groups may have less access to health-promoting circumstances even in well-resourced communities and are more seriously affected by the problems of stressed communities.

Despite U.S. affluence and the highest per capita spending on health care in the world, U.S. health outcomes are worse than those of most other wealthy nations (Murray et al, 2013). Heart disease, lung cancer, and other chronic diseases are the leading causes of death. Significant health disparities exist, which in many cases are associated with patterns of long-standing discrimination. U.S. Census Bureau data show that African Americans, American Indians/Alaska Natives, Asian Americans, Latinos/Hispanics, and Native Hawaiians/Pacific Islanders are less likely to have health insurance and are disproportionately affected by many chronic diseases and other poor health outcomes as compared to whites. It remains to be seen whether partisan political efforts at addressing this shortfall will actually have the benefits intended. With the exception of Asian Americans, each of these groups has a shorter life expectancy compared to white Americans. Examples of these disparities are noted below, as summarized by the U.S. Department of Health and Human Services Office of Minority Heath (2012):

- **African Americans**: The 2009 death rate was higher than whites for heart diseases, stroke, cancer, asthma,

BOX 4-1 *Example of Major Stressor to Community: Pollution*

Compared to affluent white communities, communities that are predominantly African American, Asian, and Latino and low-income communities are exposed to more hazardous air pollution (Pace, 2005; Katz, 2012). In these communities, studies have found higher concentrations of vanadium, nitrates, zinc, and fine particles—called PM2.5—that result from all types of combustion, including motor vehicles, power plants, and refineries (Dominici et al, 2006; U.S. Environmental Protection Agency 2013). These pollutants have been linked to asthma, cardiovascular and respiratory disease, low birth weight, and higher mortality rates (Bell & Dominici, 2008; Bell et al, 2007; Dominici et al, 2006).

For decades, grassroots organizations have advocated for local factories to reduce air-contaminating emissions. They have also worked to stop industrial waste plants and other high-polluting industries from locating near their communities (Chicago Tribune News, 1991). The People of Color Leadership Summit on the Environment is an exemplar of grassroots efforts to address these issues (Lee, 1991). To reduce the environmental causes of health disparities, community partnerships are critically important (Minkler et al, 2008).

influenza and pneumonia, diabetes, HIV/AIDS, and homicide.

- **American Indians/Alaska Natives**: The infant death rate is 60% higher than the rate for whites; they are twice as likely to have diabetes; the 2012 tuberculosis rate was 6.3 per 100,000, as compared to 0.8 for the white population.

- **Asian Americans**: In 2012, tuberculosis was 24 times more common among Asians, with a case rate of 18.9 per 100,000, as compared to 0.8 for the white population.

- **Latinos/Hispanics**: Higher rates of obesity than non-Hispanic whites; specifically, Puerto Ricans have a low birth weight rate that is twice that of non-Hispanic whites. Puerto Ricans suffer disproportionately from asthma, HIV/AIDS, and infant mortality. Mexican Americans suffer disproportionately from diabetes.

- **Native Hawaiians/Pacific Islanders**: The infant mortality rate (deaths per 1000 live births) for Native Hawaiians in 2002 was 9.6, higher than the rate for all Asian American/Pacific Islander groups combined (4.8) and for all of the population (7.0). The tuberculosis rate in 2012 was 15 times higher for Native Hawaiian/Pacific Islanders, with a case rate of 12.3 per 100,000, as compared to 0.8 for the white population.

The relations between community, the individual, and health are complex. Individual variables of income and education levels are linked to health outcomes, such as infant mortality, health during childhood (including childhood obesity), adult health (including diabetes and heart disease), and life expectancy. The 2013 Robert Wood Johnson Commission to Build a Healthier America Report explains:

> For each of these health indicators, people in the poorest or least educated groups have the worst health, but middle-class people also are less healthy than those who are better off. For example, 25-year-old college graduates can expect to live eight to nine years longer than those who have not completed high school—and two to four years longer than those who have attended but not graduated from college. (Braverman and Egerter, 2013, p 2)

Education level is positively correlated with income, and income is a major factor in individuals' and families' options, including options for where they can live, what they can eat, and how and where they can engage in physical activity. We also like to think that educating the public about health is a major factor in promoting health and preventing diseases. In turn, community level variables influence health directly, as well as individual health choices. According to the U.S. Department of Agriculture, more than 23 million people in America live in "food deserts"—urban neighborhoods and rural towns without ready access to fresh, healthy, and affordable food (Agriculture Marketing Service, 2013). These neighborhoods are more likely to have a higher density of fast-food restaurants, convenience stores, liquor stores, and ads for harmful substances, and less likely to have safe places to play and exercise (Braverman and Egerter, 2013). While eating healthy foods, hydration, exercise, and tobacco and substance abuse are individual choices that affect individual and population health, an ecological perspective makes clear that these choices are heavily influenced by the communities in which people live.

An ecological perspective also recognizes the reciprocal influence of individual behavior and the community. Not only does the community influence individual health and health behaviors, individuals shape the community and community health. Understanding this process of "reciprocal causation" is fundamental to developing and implementing strategies to improve individual, population, and community health (National Cancer Institute, 2005, p 11). Multiple points of intervention are required at the individual and community levels and include:

1. Increasing community capacity to provide health-promoting resources and services:
   - Creating needs-based programs that are more efficient and effective.
   - Removing barriers to healthy lifestyle choices.
2. Addressing the social determinants of health—addressing issues in the community context that negatively affect health.
3. Increasing access to existing resources and services for all community members.
4. Increasing individual members' knowledge and motivation to engage in health-promoting behaviors.

Despite CAM's commitment to "treat the whole person," when guided by the Western-centered value of individual-

ism, the person may still be viewed in a vacuum and the environmental context ignored. An ecological perspective that considers social determinants of health makes clear that health cannot be achieved through the narrowly focused interventions that are possible within biomedical health care systems, whether or not that health care system now includes additional CAM therapies under "integrative medicine." Instead, multiple systems are relevant and must be mobilized to effectively promote individual and population health.

CAM, SOCIAL WORK, AND COMMUNITY

By virtue of their core principles, "holistic" medical systems, such as Ayurveda and Chinese medicine, are ecological in their approach and address and incorporate the social determinants of health in diagnosis and treatment. Ancient Chinese medicine and many forms of traditional healing around the world explicitly involve the entire community in delivering "therapy," and the "patient" being treated is the community itself (see Sections V and VI). In Ayurveda, health is maintained or restored through creating harmony and integration of the social determinants of health, "including the biological, ecological, medical, psychological, sociocultural, spiritual and metaphysical factors" (Morandi et al, 2011, p 459). When these "alternative" systems and related practices are employed within a Western biomedical model, for example, in "integrative medicine," diagnosis and treatment are limited to the individual—and the community context remains beyond the boundaries of any "medicine."

The profession of social work operates beyond these boundaries of medicine, focuses on multiple systems, and is positioned to bridge the gap between the limits of medicine and the community level interventions that are required to promote health. Insofar as many of the approaches included with Ayurveda, Chinese medicine, "mind-body" medicine, and other healing traditions involve "lifestyle," they may be more effectively pursued and achieved by individuals and by groups outside the "health care" system and in the community.

A defining characteristic of the profession of social work is its ecological perspective. Social workers practice in a wide range of settings, including schools, hospitals, nursing homes, human service agencies, and community-based housing organizations. They engage in micro-level practice, which involves working directly with individuals and families in one-to-one and/or group work settings. They also work at the macro level, engaged in community organizing, policy advocacy, program development, and agency administration. What is common to the work done across settings and types of practice is a multisystemic, person-in-environment perspective.

As a profession that is historically grounded in community work and philosophically guided by an ecological perspective, social work's approach is inherently "holistic" and recognizes "the complexity of interactions between human beings and their environment, and the capacity of people both to be affected by and to alter the multiple influences upon them, including bio-psychosocial factors" (International Federation of Social Workers, 2013). Social work has a particular involvement with populations negatively impacted by the social determinants of health and that experience health disparities. The goal of social work intervention is to increase the "fit" between the individual and the environment, increase access to resources, and help individuals, families, and communities thrive. To accomplish these aims, social workers may engage in direct service provision, provide information and referral services, coordinate services, or advocate for client access to services.

Increasingly, social workers are incorporating CAM in their practices, working in or with integrative medicine settings, and bringing CAM to the community. Social workers are acting as sources of referral to CAM practitioners, providing services, establishing community programs, and advocating for access to services. In some cases, the focus of social work advocacy efforts is a community system or changing public policy so that clients will have access to the resources they need (Box 4-2). Some social workers are also advocating that training and practice in appropriate aspects of "CAM" be included in their spheres of work

within communities, such as group meditation, mindfulness, yoga, and other programs.

A considerable amount of these social work efforts are taking place outside of health care systems to address the needs of individuals, families, and communities, including among groups and communities that have been historically marginalized and/or who experience significant social, economic, and health disparities. When engaging in CAM modalities, a "bio-psycho-social-spiritual" approach is a useful orientation to keep in mind for the effectiveness of these therapies. Because of the dynamic interplay between the individual and the environment, imbalance in one area is likely to impact other areas of clients' lives and the community.

An intervention plan that addresses problems of daily living in tandem with treating a specific health condition may be essential to restore balance. For example, meditation has become a widely used intervention to reduce stress and related conditions, such as anxiety, high blood pressure, and heart disease (Chapter 10). If a client is living in unsafe housing, frequently witnesses neighborhood crime and violence, or is fearful of being victimized by crime in the community, a more comprehensive approach will be needed to support well-being than a mindfulness-based stress reduction–MBSR intervention can provide in isolation. Approaches like MBSR may be used to good effect in groups, such as schools or adult education, as well as targeted to individuals. However, support with problems of daily living may still be needed, which is the focus of micro-level social work practice.

COMPREHENSIVE APPROACHES: HEALTHY COMMUNITY INITIATIVES

When individual and community health are worked on at the same time, as part of a comprehensive strategy, success is more likely. Individual and population health can be improved through multisystem strategies, such as ones being used by organizations like Latino Health Access and the Lowell Community Health Centers (described below).

LATINO HEALTH ACCESS, SANTA ANA, CA

Latino Health Access is a nonprofit organization founded in 1993 in Santa Ana, California. The organization is located in the Station District area of Santa Clara, where the Latino population is 90.5%, the overall poverty rate for families is 29%, and the poverty rate for female-headed families with children under 18 years old is 47% (American FactFinder, 2011). Latino Health Access programs have emerged from the needs identified by community residents and aim to improve individual and community health through a wide range of strategies and programs, including health education, community organizing, community partnerships, and policy advocacy. Recognizing the role of cultural and linguistic competence in improving health outcomes, Latino Health Access trains community workers, called *promotoras* or *promotores*, to educate their

BOX 4-2 *Voice for HOPE*

Lori Strolin is a social worker and the vice president and cofounder of Voice for HOPE. The organization's mission is:

> To advance the well-being of humanity by ensuring that producers, practitioners, and consumers of natural healing and wellness services and products (including Complementary and Alternative Medicine) have meaningful participation in the development of public policy, through educating policy makers and the general public and promoting the rights of individual consumers and their families to information, access, redress and choice.

Voice for HOPE is an advocacy organization that trains individuals in communities across the United States to talk with congressional members and their staff about policy issues. The organization sponsors HOPE on the Hill, a lobbying event that occurs several times per year to advocate for national health reform to remove barriers and make CAM products and services more available and accessible to consumers. Voice for HOPE's goal is "to train Citizen Healers and organize HOPE Builders in each of the nation's 9500 congressional and state legislative districts as guides, helpers and information sources for policy makers."

Strolin uses an ecological approach to plan and lead these advocacy and training efforts.

Voice for HOPE, 2011 (U.S. Environmental Protection Agency, 2013).

own neighbors about diabetes, breast cancer, obesity, domestic violence, parenting, and other health-related issues. *Promotores* are employees and volunteers and may range from 6 to 76 years old. They interact with their neighbors in laundromats, churches, supermarkets, parking lots, apartments, streets, bus stops, living rooms, patios, schools, and other places. Residents and staff participate in group walks, exercise classes, and health education initiatives. They also engage in grass-roots fund raising and advocacy (Latino Health Access, 2012).

Latino Health Access obtained a $3.5 million state grant to build a park and community center in the "park-poorest area" of Orange County, where outdoor play areas are few:

> [The Station District area] is one example of many North County neighborhoods where children grow up with virtually no exposure to nature because of the absence of outdoor play areas. . . . The park is an important addition to the Station District area, which has less than a **half-acre of parkland** per 1,000 residents, according to the City Project, a Los Angeles-based nonprofit. South County cities like Irvine and Laguna Nigel have more than seven acres of parkland per 1,000 residents. (Wood, 2013, p 1)

Lowell Community Health Center

Located in Lowell, Massachusetts, the Lowell Community Health Center (LCHC) is an exemplar of a federally qualified health center that has taken a comprehensive, ecological approach to individual and community health with a population that experiences significant health disparities. Cambodian Americans represent 25% of the city of Lowell's population and 22% of the LCHC patient population (Grigg-Saito et al, 2010). Primary and secondary generational trauma is an important factor in health outcomes for this population and for provision of services. Cambodians experienced violence, torture, and starvation during the rule of the Khmer Rouge regime, and, subsequently, significant trauma and hardship in refugee camps. Consequently, culturally and linguistically competent, trauma-informed programs and services are essential to work effectively with Cambodian Americans (Marshall et al, 2005; Wong et al, 2006).

LCHC uses a "whole community model" in program planning and service delivery:

> This approach places physical-psychosocial-spiritual needs at its center and is based on relationship building to promote change and recognition of generational differences and the critical role of bilingual, bicultural community health workers. This model is attentive to individual and institutional barriers to care: language, health beliefs, and limited literacy, trust levels, and understanding of US health care. (Grigg-Saito et al, 2010, p 2027)

The whole community model requires comprehensive programming and a collaborative and coordinated approach to health and well-being. To implement this model, LCHC provides the following programs (Grigg-Saito et al, 2010; p 2026–2027):

- The Metta Health Center integrates Eastern and Western approaches for primary medical, mental health, and substance abuse care, with bilingual/bicultural staff and Buddhist monks as consultants.
- Cambodian Health Access Program provides education, support, and advocacy services on cardiovascular disease and diabetes. Interventions include outreach, peer support, stress management, case management, and media programs; uses a group disease self-management model; and integrates community health workers into clinical care.
- The Cambodian Youth Development Partnership was designed to reduce HIV transmission and substance abuse among Cambodian American youth through peer education and leadership and involving parents and community partners.
- Reaksmey Sangkhim provides an adult HIV/AIDS prevention and education program, using outreach, a culturally adapted curriculum, and local cable advertisements.
- The Refugee and Immigrant Safety and Empowerment Network focuses on supporting Cambodian domestic violence victims, working within a network of service providers.
- The Language Access System Improvement Team improves access to interpreter services for patients through in-house cultural competency training, signage, and patient input.

Evaluation of LCHC programs shows positive health outcomes, including improvements in patients' depression, diabetes, blood glucose levels, blood pressure, dietary habits, and medication compliance (Grigg-Saito et al, 2010). These data support the effectiveness of an ecological, culturally and linguistically competent approach, like the "whole community model" for advancing health and well-being.

SUMMARY AND CONCLUSION

Efforts to create sustainable improvement in individual and population health must be designed from an ecological perspective and rooted in the community. A truly holistic approach must view the person in the context of his or her environment. The full program and benefits of many CAM approaches and therapies cannot be realized within the boundaries of the present health care system whether delivered in a model of "integrative medicine" or otherwise (Chapter 3).

Further, restricting most CAM therapies to outpatient clinics in the present model of so-called integrative medicine denies the opportunity for the full potential of CAM with respect to health (Chapter 3). Training of health professionals in CAM is critical to expand the intellectual parameters of what is considered health and healing. Unlike social workers, most health care professionals do not work in the community settings where much of what the practice of CAM has to offer can be realized. A renewed partnership with social workers can help extend awareness and access to the whole range of CAM therapies and potentials in order to reach clients who spend only a small fraction of time in the health care system and spend the rest of their whole lives in their communities.

References

Agricultural Marketing Service: *Creating access to healthy, affordable food*, 2013, U.S. Department of Agriculture. http://www.ams.usda.gov/AMSv1.0/. Accessed January 13, 2014.

American FactFinder: *Community facts. 2011*, 2011, U.S. Census Bureau. http://factfinder2.census.gov/faces/nav/jsf/pages/index.xhtml. Accessed January 13, 2014.

Bell ML, Dominici F: Effect modification by community characteristics on the short-term effects of ozone exposure and mortality in 98 US communities, *Am J Epidemiol* 167(8):986–997, 2008.

Bell ML, Ebisu K, Belanger K: Ambient air pollution and low birth weight in Connecticut and Massachusetts, *Environ Health Persp* 115(7):1118, 2007.

Braverman P, Egerter S: *Overcoming obstacles to health in 2013 and beyond*, Princeton, NJ, 2013, Robert Wood Johnson Foundation Commission to Build a Healthier America. http://www.rwjf.org/en/about-rwjf/newsroom/features-and-articles/Commission.html.

Chicago Tribune News: *Minority groups protest pollution, plan to protect*, 1991, New York Times News Service. http://articles.chicagotribune.com/1991-10-25/news/9104060285_1_environmental-racism-contamination-minorities. Accessed January 13, 2014.

Commission on Social Determinants of Health: *Closing the gap in a generation: health equity through action on the social determinants of health. Final Report of the Commission on Social Determinants of Health*, Geneva, 2008, World Health Organization. http://www.who.int/social_determinants/en. Accessed January 13, 2014.

Dominici F, Peng RD, Bell M, et al: Fine particulate air pollution and hospital admission for cardiovascular and respiratory diseases, *JAMA* 295(10):1127–1134, 2006.

Grigg-Saito D, Toof R, Silka L, et al: Long-term development of a "whole community" best practice model to address health disparities in the Cambodian refugee and immigrant community of Lowell, Massachusetts, *Am J Public Health* 100(11):2026–2029, 2010.

International Federation of Social Workers (IFSW): Definition of social work, 2013. http://ifsw.org/policies/definition-of-social-work/. Accessed January 13, 2014.

Katz C: *Unequal exposures: People in poor, non-white neighborhoods breathe more hazardous particles. Environmental Health News*, Charlottesville, VA, 2012, Environmental Health Sciences. http://www.environmentalhealthnews.org/ehs/news/2012/unequal-exposures. Accessed January 13, 2014.

Latino Health Access, 2012. http://www.latinohealthaccess.net/. Accessed January 13, 2014.

Lee C: *Proceedings: The First National People of Color Environmental Leadership Summit*, New York, 1991, United Church of Christ.

Marshall GN, Schell TL, Elliott MN, et al: Mental health of Cambodian refugees 2 decades after resettlement in the United States, *JAMA* 294(5):571–579, 2005.

Minkler M, Vásquez VB, Tajik M, Petersen D: Promoting environmental justice through community-based participatory research: the role of community and partnership capacity, *Health Educ Behav* 35(1):119–137, 2008.

Morandi A, Tosto C, di Sarsina PR, Dalla Libera D: Salutogenesis and Ayurveda: indications for public health management, *EPMA J* 2(4):459–465, 2011.

Murray CJ, Abraham J, Ali MK, et al: The state of US health, 1990–2010: burden of diseases, injuries, and risk factors, *JAMA* 310(6):591–608, 2013.

National Cancer Institute: *Theory at a glance: A guide for health promotion practice*, ed 2, Washington, DC, 2005, U.S. Department of Health and Human Services, National Institutes of Health.

Netting FE, Kettner PM, McMurtry SL: *Social work and macro practice*, ed 3, Boston, 2004, Pearson.

Pace D: Minorities suffer most from industrial pollution. Environment, *NBC News* 2005. http://www.nbcnews.com/id/10452037/ns/us_news-environment/t/minorities-suffer-most-industrial-pollution/#.UjBTrDakprY. Accessed January 13, 2014.

Reed B: Theorizing in community practice: Essential tools. In Weil M, editor: *The handbook of community practice*, Thousand Oaks, CA, 2005, Sage, pp 84–102.

U.S. Department of Health and Human Services Office of Minority Heath: Data and statistics, 2012. http://minorityhealth.hhs.gov/templates/browse.aspx?lvl=1&lvlID=5.

U.S. Environmental Protection Agency: Fine particle (PM2.5) designations, 2013. http://www.epa.gov/pmdesignations/.

Voice for Hope, 2011. http://www.voiceforhope.org. Accessed April 27, 2014.

Weil M: Introduction: Contexts and challenges for 21st century communities. In Weil M, editor: *The handbook of community practice*, Thousand Oaks, CA, 2005, Sage.

Wenger M: *Place matters: Ensuring opportunities for good health for all: A summary of "Place Matters' community health equity reports*, Washington, DC, 2012, Joint Center for Political and Economic Studies. http://www.jointcenter.org/research/place-matters-ensuring-opportunities-for-good-health-for-all. Accessed January 13, 2014.

Wong EC, Marshall GN, Schell TL, et al: Barriers to mental health care utilization for US Cambodian refugees, *J Consult Clin Psych* 74(6):1116, 2006.

Wood T: *A welcome addition to OC's most park-poor neighborhood*, Santa Ana, CA, 2013, Voice of OC. http://www.voiceofoc.org/oc_central/santa_ana/article_471107c8-ce16-11e2-b480-001a4bcf887a.html. Accessed January 13, 2014.

World Health Organization (WHO): Health impact assessment: determinants of health, 2013. http://www.who.int/hia/evidence/doh/en/. Accessed January 13, 2014.

CHAPTER 5

SOCIAL AND CULTURAL FACTORS IN MEDICINE

CLAIRE M. CASSIDY

There are a great many health care systems in the world. All share the goals of alleviating the suffering of the sick, promoting health, and protecting the wider society from illness. All also offer answers to a series of fundamental questions about the body, life, death, and the doctor/healer relationship in health care.

Despite these universals, systems differ profoundly. They differ in degree of expansion into the world, so that some systems are practiced only locally, as among a single rainforest tribe, whereas others have spread to every corner of the globe. They differ in degree of technology, from systems that require virtually none to others that can barely function in the absence of electricity, computers, laboratories and perfect sanitation (see Box 3-2 in Chapter 3). Most importantly, these systems differ in their perceptions of the sick and well human body and in the ways in which they deliver health care. This topic is developed in this chapter.

Health care system similarities and differences have been systematically studied for more than a hundred years. As a result, we can now discuss both why so many systems exist and how differences among them matter. Basically, health care systems arise and persist because each one serves a need. Needs are similar everywhere, but the way needs are fulfilled is a matter of cultural interpretation. *Patients report satisfaction with care—no matter what kind—if that care is delivered in a manner that meshes with their cultural expectations.* Thus, the form that health care takes is first and fundamentally a matter of sociocultural interpretation: the "truth" that guides any health care system is *relative* and is *learned.*

> The form that health care takes is first and fundamentally a matter of sociocultural interpretation: the "truth" that guides any health care system is *relative* and is *learned.* ∾

This point, although implied by the very existence of numerous health care systems, surprises North Americans because, almost alone in the world, we have encouraged the belief that there is only one "best" health care approach. This belief is couched in language that argues for the primacy of scientific medicine, including the claim that only one Medicine—biomedicine or allopathy—is scientific (Boxes 5-1 and 5-2). As the voices of other types of practitioners gain strength, however, and as the world's cultural diversity increasingly bears in upon Americans, it becomes clear that most of what we know, even scientific fact, is culturally modeled. We remain unaware of this situation most of the time because our cultural assumptions are learned at an early age and are embedded within us to the point that we take them for granted. Only when these assumptions are challenged, as they will be by the material in this book, do we become aware of them. Once aware, we can choose either to expand our thinking or to defend the status quo.

This chapter offers an opportunity to expand thinking. It considers these questions:

1. What are the fundamental questions that health care systems try to answer?

BOX 5-1 *Definitions*

> *Medicine:* Medicine, with a capital M, refers to *any* medical practice, local or expanded, admired or not, that delivers "medical" or "health" care intended to protect or improve the health of the society or individuals. "Medical" care usually is used to refer to treating those already suffering malfunction; "health" care refers to efforts to prevent illness.
>
> *Health Care System:* can refer either to a national or local level socioeconomic construct concerned with the costs and feasibilities of delivering medical and health education and care (see Chapter 3) or to the cultural system that grows up around a medical explanatory model, and permits that model to be actualized. The latter meaning is used in this chapter. Figure 5-1 shows that the socioeconomic meaning is a part of the larger cultural construct.

BOX 5-2 *Definitions*

> *Biomedicine or Allopathy:* is a highly technological and specialized Medicine that grew out of Greek roots, but in the nineteenth and twentieth centuries gave up this medical model in favor of a materialist explanatory model, aiming to become more scientific. The primary practitioner is commonly called "a medical doctor" or "physician"; affiliated specialties include nursing, psychotherapy, dentistry, physical therapy/physiotherapy, and others. This Medicine is sociopolitically dominant in the Euro-American sphere, and has spread worldwide. The term "biomedicine" fronts its focus on biology and science; the term "allopathy" compares it with naturopathy, osteopathy, and homeopathy. Either term is acceptable; calling this Medicine by adjectives like "regular," "conventional," "traditional," "modern," "scientific" or the like is inaccurate and not recommended.
>
> *Humoral Medical Model:* this common model posits that there are "humors" (fluids), "elements," or "constitutions" that characterize individuals and help explain both the kinds of illnesses individuals get, and the kinds of diseases there are. Humoral models are guided by two principles: the selective use of opposites (treat hot with cool, for example), and the avoidance of extremes (avoid excessive cold, heat, damp, dry, wind). Humoral models derived from the classic Greeks were used in the West until the eighteenth century; today Ayurveda, East Asian Medicine, curanderismo, and other medical systems continue to find the humoral approach effective. For a brief summary, see Vejdemo (2010).

2. What kinds of medical models and health care systems grow out of their answers?
3. What are the similarities among systems?
4. What are the differences and what are the implications of the differences?

Before we begin, we need to be clear about our task. This chapter analyzes and compares medical systems, using concepts like relativity, explanatory model, and the concept of "system" itself. To make this material intellectually available to readers, it is helpful to establish some "ground rules." The first rule is *to use descriptive, neutral, inclusive—not judgmental—language*. This goal can be tricky! Many common formulations are in fact judgmental. Calling one Medicine "modern" implies that the others are outmoded. Actually, by definition, any practice extant today *is* "modern," in that it is contemporary, but in our society the concept of modernity has had such an overload of positivity that we prefer to apply it only to select admired actions. Again, calling one Medicine "conventional" (orthodox, scientific) implies that the others are unconventional, (unorthodox, unscientific). All these are judgmental adjectives, unnecessary, and misleading. So, the second rule we will follow is *to call each Medicine by its actual name*.

What we are talking about here is the problem of "the other." When we are deeply familiar with one way of being or thinking it is sometimes difficult to be open to other ideas. Here we wish to examine many "others" than the one Medicine (biomedicine, allopathy) to which most Western people have been socialized, and accept as "true." In this situation, learning of other Medicines can set off alarm bells, as in "how could anyone possibly believe something like that?" In teaching I have found it important to remind students that:

$$different \neq worse$$
$$description \neq criticism$$
$$analysis \neq criticism.$$

Here, we study different systems and we use specific neutral terms to examine them. Our goal is analysis, not criticism, which is the subject for a different kind of essay. Now let us examine the implications of the remark that "the 'truth' that guides any health care system is *relative* and *learned*."

> Physical symptoms are read narratively, contextually, and interpreted in cultural systems. A physician's diagnosis is a plot summary of a socially constructed pathophysiological sequence of events. The [breast] lump is there. It is a sign . . . a clue to a natural history that is unfolding. Science . . . explains it. . . . But the importance of that lump, the acts its discovery entails and what those acts will mean are social and cultural matters. (Montgomery, 2006, p 13)

RELATIVITY AND MODELS

A psychiatrist told me about a Mormon woman who came to him deeply distressed because 20 years and four children into her second marriage, she realized that she would be spending eternity with her first husband, a man who had died 6 months after their wedding. Mormon couples can be married both for this life and for "eternity," and she and her first husband had chosen to be linked in both ways. Now her first husband was a stranger to her, and she desperately wanted to spend the afterlife with her present husband and children. To his credit the psychiatrist realized that he could not help this patient. He called a Mormon colleague who quickly linked the patient with a bishop of the Mormon Church. In a single visit the bishop helped the woman straighten out her fears about the afterlife.

Why could the first psychiatrist not help the patient himself? Because he did not share her reality model. He could have denied her suffering, attempted to maneuver her into accepting his perception, or told her "not to be so silly." Instead, he took a logical and compassionate step and linked the sick woman with health care workers in her community who did share her reality model.

Consider another example. On a chilly wet day, a young woman laughingly pointed out her red tights and red boots, saying, "I always wear red on my feet on days like this, to keep me cooking from below up." What did she mean? Was she a bit crazy? Certainly, her remark did not make sense from within the biomedical model. But an acupuncturist would understand that the cold earthy element, water, can be warmed by the hot rising element, fire, and the symbolic color of fire is red. A similar interpretive pattern would be recognized by practitioners of Ayurveda, the traditional medicine of India (Chapter 30), or curanderismo, the folk medicine tradition of Mexico, Central America, and many Hispanic people in the United States (Chapter 39). It also survives in mainstream America when a mother boots up her kids on rainy days to keep them warm and to prevent colds.[1]

But perhaps people with such beliefs are irrational, or ignorant? A biomedical practitioner, writing in a women's popular magazine, comments: "Mothers may not believe this, but colds are not caused by standing in drafts, going without a hat, or getting feet wet. They occur when one sneezing, coughing child shares germs with another" (Sears, 1991).

Here you see two medical models in conflict: the mothers' humoral model (Box 5-2) and the physician's model in which he accepts the germ theory of disease as true. We can express it neutrally like that, but the biomedical writer could not: he has used a dismissive tone that implies that the mothers are stupid. Is his tone is likely to convince mothers of the truth of his remark?

These stories provide small illustrations of the statement that the form health care takes is first and fundamentally a matter of interpretation. The wide variety of lifeways shows that humans have found many different ways to answer the same life questions. We can enjoy these differences much as we enjoy a good conversation, or we can grapple with their meanings and implications. Those involved in delivering health care must grapple with these differences.

To grapple with meaning differences demands that readers, researchers, and medical practitioners stop twice. First is simply to *notice* that an idea or concept is disturbing—the point when the thinker can realize that she or he is experiencing conflict deriving from previous socialization and learning. Stopping to notice opens possibility. That possibility is to consider the internal logic of other medical explanatory models. Most health care systems are logical and rational systems of thought if the underlying assumptions are known. This does not mean that these assumptions are correct in some externally measurable way, only that they can be viewed as having been reached by the coherent use of reason (Snow, 1993). So, *second stop,* in analyzing medical systems, we want to identify their underlying premises, assumptions, and reality models, and this analysis will guide us toward understanding why they practice as they do.

That there are numerous cogent *models* of reality is often disturbing to people. In the West, battles have been fought and lives lost in defense of the ideal of a singular reality (Ames, 1993). Earlier in our history, the search for this reality ("truth") was mainly expressed in religious terms, but for more than 150 years, many have believed that science provides that singular reality. By this logic, health care practices that are not considered scientific are not trustworthy, and the path to acceptance demands "scientific research."

This situation helps explain why the preceding psychiatric example might be shrugged off. Laypeople are known to have beliefs, and clinicians must deal with them. But the point of this discussion is that *everyone has beliefs, and all* realities are constructed; the facts of science are as culturally contextualized as those of law, theology, or social manners. Scientific fact is only as stable as the logic that produced it and the systems that apply it.

Thus, science also experiences paradigm shifts, for example when a new technology permits new perceptions, and former "facts" fall by the wayside. Plasma physics operates by a different logic and perceives reality differently from Newtonian physics; population biology is quite a different kettle of fish from Linnaean systematic typology; and an ecological or holistic approach to gathering scientific knowledge is very different from a materialistic reductionistic one (Chapter 1).

> The point of this discussion is that *everyone has beliefs, and all* realities are constructed; the facts of science are as culturally contextualized as those of law, theology, or social manners. Scientific fact is only as stable as the logic that produced it and the systems that apply it. ❧

---

[1]That the remark makes sense within the logic of humoral models does not mean that practitioners would say that red boots "work," that is, that the boots themselves, or their color specifically, prevented the young woman from being invaded by cold damp. To determine whether an action is effective requires an entirely different level of analysis.

The curious thing about modular reality is that you are likely to find exactly what you expect. The observer is not separate from the observed (see discussion of the Heisenberg uncertainty principle in Chapter 1). Expectations are based on assumptions and the application of logic. When the assumptive base changes, so does the logic and, as a result, the appropriate response. Consider, for example, "strep throat." According to biomedicine the *Streptococcus* bacterium causes the sore throat. Logically, one could treat with antibiotics to destroy that bacterium. However, approximately 20% of the population carries this germ in their throats without developing an illness (Greenwood & Nunn, 1994). Only a minority of people who are exposed to the bacterium contract a sore throat. Thus, other factors must be involved; the presence of the bacterium, although necessary, is not sufficient.

Most "holistic" health care systems, such as homeopathy, Ayurveda, Tibetan, and East Asian medicine, understand this concept and focus more attention on the *other* factors—the host body reaction, the person with the condition, the environment—than on infectious microorganisms. Even the eighteenth and nineteenth century philosophy of Western medicine in France considered *le terrain*—the terrain or host factors—as critical to treating infection and emphasized strengthening the host response even before microbes were recognized as causing infections. Care is aimed at strengthening the person rather than destroying bacteria.

But surely, you might ask, people agree about such material body parts as the heart or blood? Not necessarily. For example, although everyone might agree that the heart is a pulsating organ located in the center of the chest, its energetic and spiritual capabilities are debated. Biomedical thinkers describe the heart as a pump, using a material and mechanical metaphor. Even biomedical physicians, however, once thought of the heart as the "seat of the soul," a memory our society revisits in many romantic songs. This idea still is active in East Asian medical thought, in which the physical heart beats while the energetic "Heart" fills the role of sovereign ruler: "Sovereign of being and pivot of life, the heart is the guarantor of the unity of a person's existence" (Larre & de la Vallee, 1995, p 174). In East Asian anatomy, the Heart even has a special "Protector," an organ unknown in biomedical anatomy.

Again, in biomedicine, blood is a living red substance that contains red and white cells and carries nutrients, enzymes, hormones, and oxygen; it is complex and constantly renews itself. It can be shared if genetically matched. In popular Jamaican thought, however, blood does not renew itself. Its purity (a social rather than medical concept) determines one's success in life (Sobo, 1993). Following this logic, many Jamaicans are loath to give or receive blood for transfusions. Resistance to donating blood (e.g., among Jehovah's Witnesses; Gohel et al, 2005; Ott & Cooley, 1977; Shan et al, 2002; Singelenberg, 1990) or to

receiving organ transplants (Lam & McCullough, 2000; O'Connor, 1995; Radecki & Jaccard, 1997; Shaheen et al, 2004; Tong et al, 2013) is common wherever people are guided by concepts of purity or believe the soul imbues all body parts.

CULTURAL RELATIVITY

For each of the preceding examples, a reader might ask, "Who is right?" This question is not useful because answers are judged "right" from within the logic of the model in use. "Rightness" also is modular or relative.

A truly useful question is, "How does this model *serve its users*?" To be able to ask this question, one must stand back from one's own beliefs and models and recognize them as constructed and not exclusively correct. To take this stance is to practice *cultural relativity*.

Cultural relativity is a technique for dealing with the many ways in which people explain themselves. It tells practitioners and researchers to remain in a fairly neutral, nonjudgmental stance, *knowing the values of people without adopting or rejecting them* (Kaplan, 1984; also see Salzman & Rice, 2010). From this position, clinicians, researchers, or students can observe their own perceptions and those of others and understand how these interpretations serve users' lives. They can avoid becoming mired in determining which method is true, because nothing is exclusively true when all realities are constructed.

On the other hand, ideas can be true in certain contexts or situations; that is, they make sense to their users. Therefore the observer must learn to synthesize his or her position with those of others, so as to design an effective response strategy. For example, if people think of penicillin as a cooling drug and therefore hesitate to use it to treat a "cold" illness such as pneumonia, the practitioner can neutralize the cold of penicillin by suggesting that the patient take the medicine along with a food perceived as "hot" (Harwood, 1977). This idea of balance also lies behind the multiple herbs ordinarily included in East Asian herbal prescriptions. Here, some herbs are included to address the symptoms, others to minimize side effects of the first set, and a final one or two, called *adaptogens*, are added to ensure that the previous herbs work well together (Chen & Chen, 2004). Compare this approach with the biomedical, which is guided by concepts of "purity" and "specificity" in creating pharmaceuticals and largely assumes that there *will be* side effects. Alternatively, as in the previous example of the Mormon woman, the clinician can refer a patient to a practitioner whose reality model more closely resembles that of the patient.

The practice of cultural relativity is pivotal to the study of medicine, because each system of medicine provides a different set of ideas about the body, disease, and medical reality. Readers will find it much easier to absorb and use this material if they can willingly—even playfully—step aside from their current beliefs and appreciations to let in new ones.

THE ISSUE OF SCALE

Cultural relativity is a technique to deal with difference. Scale is another that is often misunderstood or misused. Medical care can be studied or applied at many different levels or *scales of complexity* (Figure 5-1). Worldview is the largest and is discussed in the next section. The *system* comes next, and refers to all the ways in which a particular Medicine is understood and applied. Other concepts in Figure 5-1 indicate scalar levels *within* the system concept, *smaller in scale* than the system. A *modality* refers to the ways by which care is offered to the body-person. Biomedicine offers two main modalities: pharmacy and surgery. East Asian Medicine offers five: herbs, acupuncture, qigong, tui na massage, and dietary therapy. Other Medicines offer yet other modalities (Figure 5-2). Much smaller in scale than the modality is the *technique*; most modalities include multiple techniques. For example, pharmacy can be delivered via injection, transfusion, insertion, inhalation, cutaneously, and so on. Acupuncture can be delivered with long hair-thin needles (whole body), with short fat needles that remain in place for a time (ear), by electrical stimulation, by

vibration (light, sound), by touch, and by "sending qi" without actually touching the acupoint or patient.

In sum, a system is remarkably more complex and inclusive than a modality, which is in turn more complex and inclusive than a therapeutic technique. Similarly, a professionalized system is expanded further than a community-based system. Failure to understand such issues of scale can lead to confusion and can also result in invalid "data." For example, researchers attempting to survey use of non-biomedical practices often offer respondents lists of "alternative therapies" of completely different scales, as from garlic supplementation (a small-scale, single therapy a layperson can select from reading a popular magazine) to Ayurvedic medical care (a large-scale, professionalized urban health care system, the use of which demands a much higher level of decision-making). Often, items within the list are only peripherally about medical care, for example, listing as an alternative, prayer or exercise. Creating a list of such wildly different scalars cannot yield meaningful data; it is as pointless as comparing a volleyball to the entire Olympic Games, or an orange to a grocery chain.

This problem remains common in commentary about alternative and complementary medicine, because one system (biomedicine) has been set up as "standard," whereas everything else, of whatever scale of complexity, has been set aside into the "other" category (Box 5-3). This contrast habit itself is invalid and unscientific, and it is hoped that a wider view of medical care will eventually result in all medical systems being seen as alternatives to one another. Meanwhile, one must be careful of terms that lend themselves to scalar confusion. The single term *acupuncture* can refer to a system, a modality, or simply a needling technique. Which does a given writer or speaker mean? *Massage* can mean a single technique, or it can refer to a rapidly professionalizing and systematizing practice. Some people use the term *medicine* to refer exclusively to biomedicine; in this chapter, however, *Medicine* is a term that encompasses all the various ways in which people deliver health care.

In summary, it is most effective to refer to health care systems by their specific names and to distinguish clearly the scale at which one wants to speak or write.

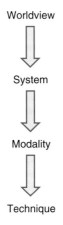

Figure 5-1 Scale of complexity in understanding health care.

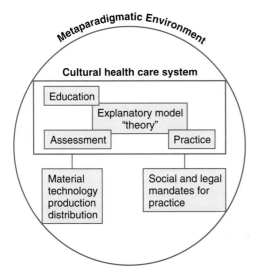

Figure 5-2 Cultural health care system.

BOX 5-3 *An Example of a Culturally Driven Scalar Error*

What is included under "CAM"?
> single supplements
  stand-alone techniques
    folk and tribal practices
      semi-professionalized practices
        World Medicines
          bioscientific practices not normative within biomedicine, e.g., nutrition

What is included under biomedicine?
> Biomedicine(!)

METAPARADIGMS

A metaparadigm is a conceptual model—a set of perceptions of how the world works—that imbues whole societies typically over a duration of hundreds of years. For our purposes two metaparadigms matter. They have many names. The one that is dominant in the Euro-American worldview is called the hierarchic, reductionist, materialist, categorical, Cartesian, or ontologic metaparadigm. It's more-or-less opposite is called the relational, processual, ecologic, holistic, or physiological metaparadigm. The easiest way to understand their characters and relations is to note that the reductionist is concerned with naming and states of being ... or *nouns*. It is characterized by *dichotomous thinking*—this or that, either/or, true or false, black or white—often with a judgmental element built in. Associated with this dichotomy are tendencies to competition, forcefulness, preferences for materialist explanations and an admiration for and celebration of technology and modernity (Cassidy, 1994; Kenner, 2002).

The processual or physiological is concerned with movement, flow and change ... *verbs*. It is characterized by *inclusive thinking*—e.g., both-and, body-person, body–mind-and-spirit. Although many people are intensely attached to one or the other position, here we use the concepts *descriptively* to better understand how medical systems work. We also remember that *sentences contain both nouns and verbs*—thus both serve usefully to help us "make sense" as we think and speak.

Biomedicine is an example of a preferentially reductionist system, though some specialties like family medicine, psychiatry, and psychoneuroimmunology, tend to be more inclusive in outlook. Biomedicine reflects reductionist patterns in (1) its concern for the expertise of the practitioner over that of the layperson or patient; (2) its tendency to magnify the importance of some specialties or diseases over others (cardiology over pediatrics, cancer over asthma); (3) its preference for specialist-delivered technological treatment modalities that cause obvious reactions in the physical body (surgery, pharmaceuticals); and (4) its focus on end-stage physical malfunction while largely ignoring "wellness" and less-developed "functional" conditions, and rejecting nonmaterial explanations of cause.

Biomedicine's materialist effort to segregate medicine from spirituality grew out of the secularist urge to embrace science late in the nineteenth century; this concept is artificial and is not shared by most of the world's health care systems. Indeed, most systems argue that the nonmaterial aspects of the body-person are as real and cogent as the material aspects and, further, that there is no true separation of these aspects:

> Sister Erma Allen once told me of having healed a small boy who had cut his head; she had silently said the (blood-stopping) verse over and over while at the same time applying ice to the wound. I asked how she knew that it was not the *ice* that had stopped the bleeding. After a pause she reprimanded me gently, "God sewed it with *His* needle, darlin'." (Snow, 1993)

Reductionist ideas lie behind scientific experiments in the randomized controlled clinical trial design: the goal is to study as *few* variables as possible; this approach is thought to provide the most accurate data about, for example, the utility of a pharmaceutical—but necessarily provides the least information about healing (see Chapter 3). In focusing on minimizing variables, it is common to limit the effects of opinion, expectation, and patient–practitioner interaction—which are often classed as troublesome "placebo" effects. In contrast, holistic researchers wish to work with "the whole picture"—and are not afraid of complexity, arguing that it characterizes real life, and the complex situation in which a patient interacts with a practitioner to receive medical care. Which is "right"? Remember: what we want to know is "what serves," because there is no absolute "right," only designs that are *appropriate or inappropriate to answer the question asked*.

Other Western health care systems, which literally originated in reaction to biomedicine (allopathy), include homeopathy, osteopathy, naturopathy, chiropractic, and Christian Science.[2] Others have been imported from Asia, such as East Asian medicine, Ayurveda, and Tibetan medicine. Most argue (not always convincingly) that their approaches to care are more egalitarian, less judgmental, and gentler than biomedicine. Several offer nonmaterialist explanations of cause and care. In making such arguments, these systems are calling on the *relational* (ecological, holistic, physiological) worldview. This worldview sees all things as connected in a network of relationships and considers how people, things, and energy interact and how these interactions affect the whole. Reflected into health care, this idea means that practitioners model health in terms of achieving balance (homeostasis), and patients are seen to have expertise different from that of the practitioner but expertise nonetheless. Thus, practitioner and patient form a partnership, and patients take some responsibility for their own care and development.

The fact that biomedicine prefers materialist explanations also implies that it does not deliver care to, or in, all parts of the body-person. This limitation is equally true for other systems. Each emphasizes a distinctive viewpoint (explanatory model) and develops expertise in only *some* of the potential areas of health care. For example, biomedicine has had great success in treating acute illness and trauma. Its control of technology allows for remarkable success in extending life[3] and in producing

---

[2]It should not be assumed that nonbiomedical is equivalent to holistic. Some nonbiomedical systems are reductionistic. Chiropractic and osteopathy originated in reductionistic explanatory models. Many faith-based healing systems also use reductionistic models.

[3]Not discussed here is public health, which uses bioscience findings to protect the health of populations, such as by providing clean water, sewerage systems, vaccine development and distribution, tracking and control of epidemics, and so on, largely outside the local sphere of biomedical care delivery. It is widely accepted that biomedicine's successes are built upon the enormous successes of population-level sanitation measures established since the mid-nineteenth century.

pharmaceuticals to address the physical and metabolic components of disease. Simultaneously, however, biomedicine is criticized for its relatively ineffective care of many chronic conditions and for repeated inefficiencies in human kindness and humane care, areas that easily escape the purview of its materialist model.[4]

Other systems, notably the so-called holistic systems, *integrate* human development into their usual care patterns. These systems also control technologies and techniques that address physical and metabolic functioning. Patients praise these systems for their care of chronic conditions and for their efforts to enhance wellness, which include weaning patients from excessive dependence on pharmaceuticals and even on health care specialists.

Two vital points emerge from this discussion and recur throughout this chapter:
1. No one medical system addresses the whole potential field of health care.
2. All medical systems address a considerable part of the field.

The logical corollaries are (1) no one system is always and singularly best for everything, and (2) systems overlap considerably in what they offer. There arises a temptation to argue that societies ought to achieve economies of scale by making sure that only the "best" approaches, by one definition or another, survive. Again, however, considering our discussion of cultural relativity, it is impossible to define "best" in a satisfactory manner. Logic demands that we determine who will be served well by which system and why (Box 5-4). We will return to this issue after discussing some of the important ways in which health care systems differ.

---

[4]For observations on the limits of reductionism, consider Engel (1992), Freedman (2010), Morris (2000), Velasquez-Manoff (2012).

BOX 5-4 *Review of Ground Rules*

· Use descriptive, neutral, inclusive language
· Call each Medicine by its own name
· Focus on analysis, not judgment
· Be aware of scale and use it appropriately
· When startled by information, stop and open to possibility
· Ask: how/who does this *serve?*

FUNDAMENTAL QUESTIONS HEALTH CARE SYSTEMS TRY TO ANSWER

We began by stating that among the universals are a set of questions that all health care or medical systems try to answer. These questions are summarized in Box 5-5.

We want to understand: *How does a medical practitioner know?* The first set of questions represent areas in which medical practitioners typically have answers to offer. The answers are offered in the form of a *medical explanatory model*, as in the first section of the equation:

PREMISES → Logic → Practice

The explanatory model (EM) is learned by apprenticeship, by schooling, and by a combination of the two, usually within a larger societal setting in which the relevant metaparadigm logic has already been learned. The learning of Medicine is then a form of specialization. It is also possible, of course, to shift paradigms. A traditional Dineh (Navajo) who chooses to become a biomedical physician can learn to think in reductionist terms but is likely to prove reflective (Alvord, 2003). A middle-class white American who decides to become a professional acupuncturist must typically make some special effort to learn to use the holistic paradigm.

We can then ask "What does a medical practitioner do?" and that moves us into examining the actions and technology of the medical practice.

In between is the logic: how premises are actualized in practice.

The next two sections discuss the larger construct, the cultural health care system, and develop the idea of the explanatory model.

CULTURAL CONCEPT OF THE HEALTH CARE SYSTEM

A cultural medical (or health care) system is a complex of beliefs, models, and linked activities that providers and users consider useful in bettering health or well-being and in relieving stress and disease. In Figure 5-2, note first that the health care system is itself embedded in a societal metaparadigm—this circumstance affects many components of the resulting system. Within the system, the explanatory model (EM) is embedded in the

BOX 5-5 *Medical Explanatory Models Offer Answers to Fundamental Questions*

How does a medical practitioner know?
What is a "body"? A "person?" A "body-person?"
What is a "live" body?
What is "health"? What is sickness ... or disease ... or
What causes sickness/disease/imbalance?   } imbalance?
What can be done about sickness/disease/imbalance?
What does a medical practitioner do?

middle—indeed, guides all the other parts of the system. Practitioners are educated (sub-box upper left) in the EM, and when that training is complete, focus on the sub-box labeled Practice, delivering care that reflects the EM. All systems also assess the success of their care (sub-box lower left). Practitioners observe "what works," keeping track within their personal practice, testing within practice, and learning from others. Eventually, more formal methods of assessment grew up—scientific experiments to see if particular interventions "work" or "work better" than a comparison case. In short, as the medical system becomes more expanded, professionalized and "scientific," assessment and evaluation tends to move away from the practitioner and into the hands of "research specialists."

At the bottom of Figure 5-2 are two other important boxes. On the left is a sub-box that indicates that the technology necessary to perform the Medicine must be produced. In small-scale settings, it may be the practitioner herself who gathers and prepares the herbs, creates the sand painting, or makes the drum. But in large-scale urban Medicines, a host of producers, often corporate in size, not only build equipment and produce medicinal capsules, but also advertise, sell, and distribute at a high level of economic and regulatory complexity. Meanwhile, societies also determine *who* may practice medicine (right lower subbox). In small-scale societies we may say one is chosen by divination or accolade after sufficient training and demonstration of competence (see Section 6). As the scale enlarges, and as the Medicine becomes more professionalized, legal and formal economic controls begin to act: for example, practitioners may be tested by exam, licensed by the state, and perhaps also board-certified by members of their own profession.

The terms *professionalized systems* and *community-based systems* distinguish between systems that serve large, heterogeneous patient populations and those smaller, more localized systems that serve culturally homogeneous populations.

A professionalized system tends to be found in urban settings, is taught in schools with the aid of written texts, and demands formal, usually legal, criteria for practice (Foster & Anderson, 1978; Shahjahan, 2004). Students enter the system by choice and are approved by entrance examinations. They become practitioners upon completing a designated plan of study, passing more examinations, and often being licensed by the state or nation. Health care typically is delivered on a one-practitioner-to-one-patient basis in locales that have been set aside for this purpose, such as offices, clinics, and hospitals. Practitioners form membership organizations dedicated to policing their respective specialties and practitioners, and presenting them in a positive light to outsiders. The dominant health care systems of modern nations are always professionalized systems. Examples include Ayurveda, biomedicine, chiropractic, East Asian medicine, homeopathy, osteopathy, and Unani (the traditional system used in Pakistan and neighboring Muslim nations, and in Nepal).

Community-based systems, also known as *folk* or *tribal* systems, are less expanded than professionalized systems, although they may have equally complex explanatory models and equally lengthy histories. These systems are found in both urban and rural settings, and training is often by apprenticeship. People enter training sometimes by inheritance, sometimes by receiving a call from the unseen world, indicating that he or she has the special capacity necessary to become a healer. Training ends when the teacher considers the student ready to practice. Rather than taking written examinations, students are tested by practicing medicine under guidance; essentially the community itself determines whether a student is "good enough." Care is often offered in people's homes, and community-based healers often practice on a part-time basis. Some folk healers form professional associations, with the same goals as professionalized doctors. Examples of community-based systems include Alcoholics Anonymous and similar urban self-help groups (Chapter 4), curanderismo (among the most expanded of folk systems), rootwork (an African-derived system used by some African Americans), and traditional health care in Native American and Euro-American rural groups (Box 5-6).

A third type of system is often called "popular" health care. Popular health care is not organized systematically; rather, it consists of simple techniques associated with the care of particular conditions. Examples familiar in the United States include using cranberry juice for bladder infections, Echinacea tea or chicken soup for colds, and hot toddies for sore throats. In biomedically dominant regions, much of what is published in general-reader magazines, on the Internet, or discussed on talk shows is popular medicine, and is typically presented using biomedical terminology; it is often simplified biomedicine. Where biomedicine is an imported model, popular medicine reflects the historical ideas of the locality. For example, in China, popular medicine is often simplified classical Chinese medicine.

Distinctions of complexity among health care systems are not absolute. For example, most professionalized systems continue to insist on considerable hands-on training, similar to apprenticeships. Some folk systems, especially urbanized ones (e.g., Alcoholic Anonymous), train practitioners in schools and do not expect students to have received an avocational "call" to practice; these practitioners often earn their living through full-time health care work.

This discussion makes it clear that a health care *system* is complex and multilayered. Even simple systems, such as those limited in scope to one ethnic group, or one therapeutic technique like reiki, are difficult for one person to master or describe. Larger systems are correspondingly more complex, encompassing a wide range of viewpoints, numerous subspecialties, and distinctive styles of practice. Biomedicine includes specialties ranging from the intensely material practice of surgery to the much more relational specialties of family medicine and psychiatry. Biomedical

BOX 5-6 *Classic Sources Describing Community-Based Systems in North America*

American folk medicine (Hand, 1976)

An epidemic of absence: a new way of understanding allergies and autoimmune diseases (Velasquez-Manoff, 2012)

Becoming a Diné Navajo medicine man (Benally, 2011)

Big doctoring in America: profiles in primary care (Mullan, 2002)

Biomedicine examined (Lock & Gordon, 1988)

Black Elk: the sacred ways of a Lakota (Black Elk & Lyon, 1990)

Cave and cosmos: shamanic encounters with another reality (Harner, 2013)

Chinese medicine users in the United States, Part 2: Preferred aspects of care (Cassidy, 1998b)

Concepts of health: illness and disease, a comparative perspective (Currer & Stacey, 1986)

Cry of the eagle: encounters with a Cree healer (Young et al, 1989)

Culture, health and illness (Helman, 2007)

Curanderismo: Mexican-American folk healing (Trotter & Chavira, 1997)

Differences in medicine: unraveling practices, techniques and bodies (Berg & Mol, 1998)

Energy medicine, East and West: a natural history of qi (Mayor & Micozzi, 2011)

Ethnic medicine in the Southwest (Spicer, 1979)

Feeling the qi: emergent bodies and disclosive fields in American appropriations of acupuncture (Emad, 1998 [dissertation])

Healing by hand: a cross-cultural primer for manual therapies (Oths, 2004)

Healing traditions: alternative medicine and the health professions (O'Connor, 1995)

Healing Ways: Navajo health care in the twentieth century (Davies, 2001)

Herbal and magical medicine: traditional healing today (Kirkland et al, 1992)

How doctors think: clinical judgment and the practice of medicine (Montgomery, 2006)

"I choose life": contemporary medicine and religious practices in the Navajo world (Schwartz, 2008)

Indigenous theories of contagious disease (Green, 1999)

Knowledge, power and practice: the anthropology of medicine in everyday life (Lindenbaum & Lock, 1993)

Masters of the ordinary: integrating personal experience and vernacular knowledge in Alcoholics Anonymous (Scott, 1993 [dissertation])

Meaning, medicine and the "placebo effect" (Moerman, 2002)

Medicine as culture, illness, disease and the body in Western societies (Lupton, 2003)

Narrative and cultural construction of illness and healing (Mattingly & Garro 2000)

9000 needles [documentary film] (Dearth, 2011)

Practicing acupuncture in an in-patient setting [dissertation] (Kielczynska, 2012)

Powwowing in Union County: a study of Pennsylvania German folk medicine in context (Reimansnyder, 1989)

Ritual healing in suburban America (McGuire, 1994)

Spirit Talkers, North American Indian Medicine Powers (Lyon, 2012)

Susto: a folk illness (Rubel et al, 1984)

The Cuban Chinese medical revolution. (Lo & Renton, 2012)

The expressiveness of the body, and the divergence of Greek and Chinese medicine (Kuriyama, 2002)

The hands feel it: healing and spiritual presence among a Northern Alaskan people (Turner, 1996)

This other kind of doctors: traditional medical systems in black neighborhoods in Austin, TX (Terrell, 1990)

The world we used to live in: remembering the powers of the medicine men (Deloria, 2006)

Walkin' over medicine (Snow, 1993)

Walking Thunder, Diné medicine woman (Walking Thunder & Nickerson, 2001)

What does it mean to practice an energy medicine? (Cassidy, 2011)

What I learned in medical school: personal stories of young doctors (Takakuwa et al, 2004)

What is medicine? Western and Eastern approaches to healing (Unschuld, 2009)

Wolfkiller: wisdom from a nineteenth century Navajo shepherd (Wetherill & Leake, 2007)

---

complexity is compounded by the fact that it is practiced rather differently in different countries:

Even the best simultaneous translator is going to have trouble dealing with the fact that *peptic ulcer* and *bronchitis* do not mean the same things in Britain that they do in the United States; that the U.S. *appendectomy* becomes the British *appendicectomy*; that the French tendency to exaggerate means there are never headaches in France, only migraines, and that the French often refer to real migraines as "liver crises"; that the German language has no word for chest pain, forcing the German patient to talk of heart pain, and that when a German doctor says "cardiac insufficiency" he may simply mean that the patient is tired. . . . How can [bio]medicine, which is commonly supposed to be a science, be so different in four countries whose peoples are so similar genetically? The answer is that while

[bio]medicine benefits from a certain amount of scientific input, culture intervenes at every step of the way (Payer, 1988).

This complexity is equally true of East Asian medicine, which embraces many *styles,* including traditional Chinese medicine (TCM), Worsley Five Element style, Matsumoto style, French energetic, numerous Japanese and Korean styles, and more (see Chapter 35). Like biomedicine, it too is practiced differently in different countries (Scheid & MacPherson, 2012); increasingly, practitioners are also specializing, for example, in gynecology, or in pain care. Even community-based or folk systems may have different specialties. Lakota (Sioux) people distinguish medicine men and women who emphasize herbal treatment from holy men and women who practice shamanically (Hultkrantz,

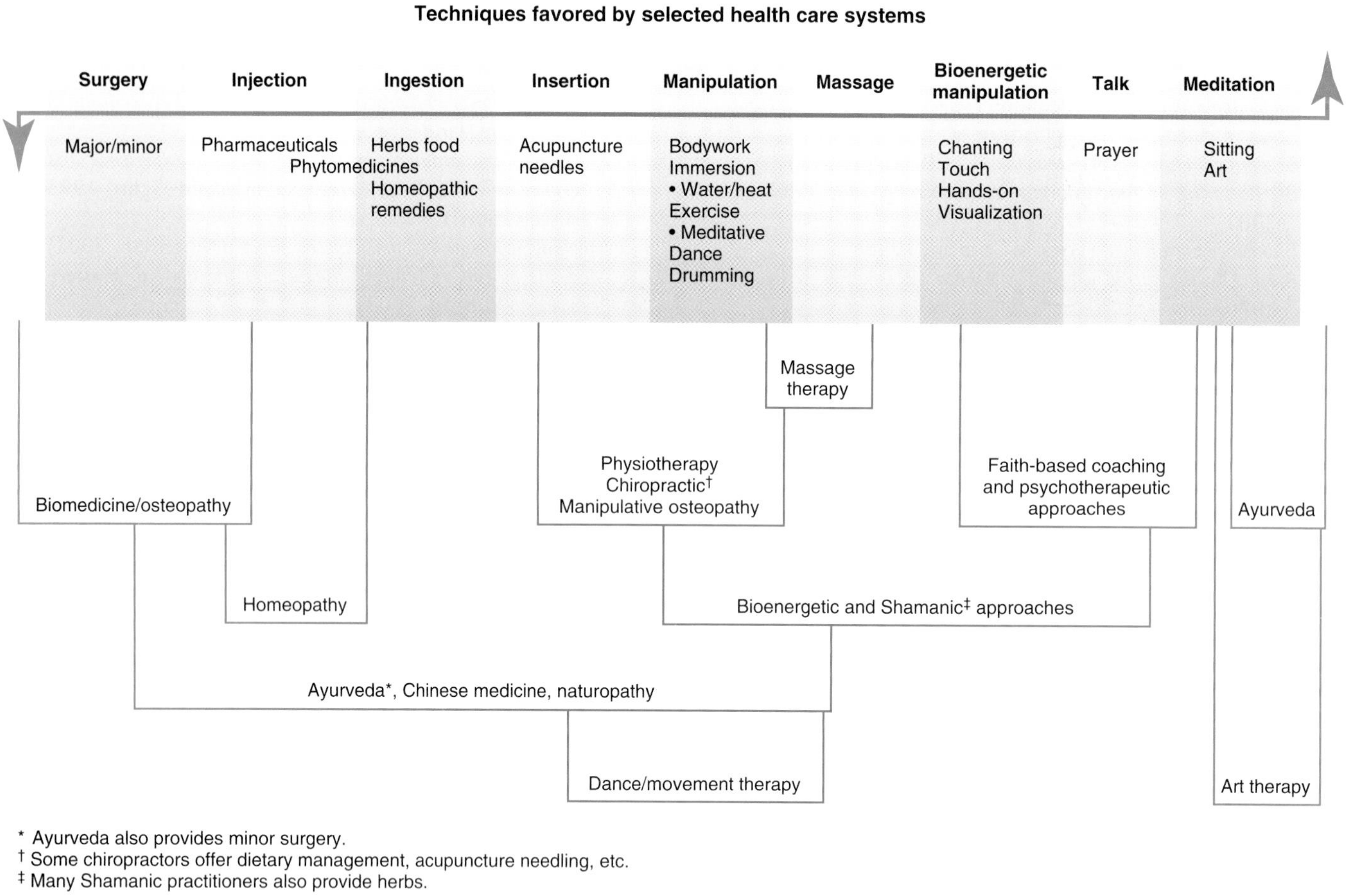

Techniques favored by selected health care systems

Surgery	Injection	Ingestion	Insertion	Manipulation	Massage	Bioenergetic manipulation	Talk	Meditation
Major/minor	Pharmaceuticals Phytomedicines Homeopathic remedies	Herbs food	Acupuncture needles	Bodywork Immersion • Water/heat Exercise • Meditative Dance Drumming		Chanting Touch Hands-on Visualization	Prayer	Sitting Art

Massage therapy

Physiotherapy
Chiropractic[†]
Manipulative osteopathy

Faith-based coaching and psychotherapeutic approaches

Biomedicine/osteopathy

Ayurveda

Homeopathy

Bioenergetic and Shamanic[‡] approaches

Ayurveda*, Chinese medicine, naturopathy

Dance/movement therapy

Art therapy

* Ayurveda also provides minor surgery.
† Some chiropractors offer dietary management, acupuncture needling, etc.
‡ Many Shamanic practitioners also provide herbs.

Figure 5-3 Relative physical invasiveness of selected therapeutic techniques, from most invasive (left) to least invasive (right).

1985). The Dineh (Navajo) recognize three types of diagnosticians, plus Singers who work with ritual, herbs, and the psychosocial body to deliver health care (Benally, 2011; Davies, 2001; Lyon, 2012; Morgan, 1977; Schwartz, 2008; Walking Thunder & Nickerson, 2001). Biomedicine is famous for its numerous *specialties*, and other health care systems also offer specializations.

On a much smaller scale than the system or the style is the *technique*. A technique is comparatively simple; it might be a single therapy and often can be practiced without being linked to an explanatory model, detailed training, or professional oversight. Some practitioners specialize in offering single therapies, such as bee-sting injections, colonic irrigations, biofeedback, specific dietary supplements, or Swedish massage; within biomedicine single-skill *phlebotomists* are technicians who draw blood for laboratory tests.

Single-therapy practitioners can provide *symptomatic relief* to their patients, but they cannot provide *systematic care*, that is, care guided by a well-developed model of how the body-person works, how the malfunction arose, and how intervention can help.

MODALITIES OF HEALTH CARE

Whatever the other aspects of their character, all health care practices care for people. To do so, they offer a variety of complex sets of interventions, or *modalities*, such as surgery, injection or ingestion of pharmaceuticals, use of biologicals or botanicals, needling, dietary management, manipulation, bodywork, meditative exercises, dancing, music therapy, art therapy, water and heat treatments, bioenergetic manipulation, talk therapy, shamanic journeying, sitting meditation, and prayer.

Figure 5-3 sorts selected modalities along a line from intensely to lightly physically invasive. This spectrum corresponds roughly with a movement from materialist to nonmaterialist views of the body-person. The more invasive modalities enter the physical body by cutting, pricking, insertion, or ingestion. Less invasive techniques involve touching the surface of the body. Even softer modalities access energetic or spiritual levels of the body without touching the skin. Among techniques that break into the body there are differing degrees of intensity: replacing a hip is more intrusive than removing a cataract. Pharmaceutical drugs generally are more toxic than phytomedicines (semi-purified plant medicines), which are in turn more forceful than herbs. However, forcefulness does not connote effectiveness. Mild and gentle modalities can be equally effective.

Actual health care systems employ several modalities and can be roughly mapped with regions of the line in the figure, which provides further evidence that each system

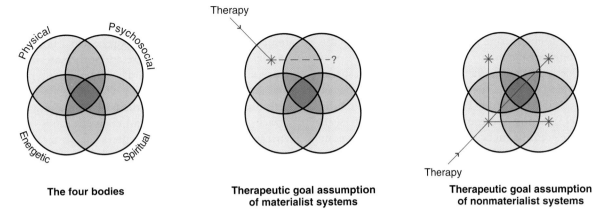

The four bodies

Therapeutic goal assumption of materialist systems

Therapeutic goal assumption of nonmaterialist systems

Figure 5-4 The four bodies addressed by health care.

emphasizes certain parts, but not the entire spectrum, of health care options.

For example, a community-based system such as curanderismo uses bodywork, dietary manipulation, herbs, first-aid techniques, and shamanic techniques to treat a wide range of physical, psychosocial, and spiritual malfunctions (Rubel et al, 1984; Spicer, 1979; Trotter & Chavira, 1997). Ayurveda offers surgery, a variety of water treatments from purges to baths, numerous biological and herbal remedies, bodywork, dietary management, and both sitting and moving forms of meditation (Krishan, 2003; Morrison, 1995). Biomedicine is unusual in focusing at the left of the line in Figure 5-3, the most invasive region, but associated practitioners such as physical therapists, nurses, and psychotherapists use modalities farther to the right along the line.

EXPLANATORY MODELS

We have completed our introduction to the cultural health care system, and can now examine the aspect that guides all the rest, and provides answers to fundamental questions including the preferred relationship between patients and practitioner: the *explanatory model* (EM).

> *The truth. . . . is that . . . there are no fixed and unmistakable signs. . . . Changes and features that speak eloquently to experts in one culture can thus seem mute and insignificant, and pass unnoticed, in another. [Ancient] Greek pulse takers ignored the local variations that their counterparts in China found so richly telling; Chinese doctors saw nothing of muscular anatomy. (Kuriyama, 2002, p 272)*
> *. . . both traditions [early Chinese and Greek Medicines] were based on certain realities of morphology, physiology and pathologic types. Yet the way these were seen, and that they were seen at all, and the way they were interpreted and used as a call to action for the prevention and therapy of illness, was laid down for scientists and physicians by social reality, not by nature. (Unschuld, 2009, p 65)* ❧

CONCEPTS OF THE BODY-PERSON

There is not one human body, not one anatomy, not one physiology, but many. To understand any system, we must understand its concept of body. Figure 5-4 depicts the body-person as four intersecting circles. The figure is simplified, because even within each of the circles, there are many ways in which systems can phrase their material, energetic, spiritual, or social perceptions of the body-person.

The biomedical model of the body-person focuses on the physical body, specifically the structure of its tissues and the movement and transformation of chemicals within and between cells. Classic chiropractic and osteopathic models of the body are also materialistic, emphasizing connections and communications between bones, nerves, and muscles and the rest of the physical body. In the twenty-first century osteopathic medicine is legally recognized as equivalent to biomedicine with only a minority of practitioners maintaining the manipulative tradition (Johnson & Kurtz, 2001). Chiropractic maintains its independence, and offers distinct styles of practice, some of which employ an "energy" model to help explain changes (Mootz & Phillips, 1997). Note that such primarily materialist systems "enter" the body through the physical route and commonly view this aspect as the goal of treatment, only hesitantly accepting that the psychosocial being may also be affected.

Other medical systems focus initial care on other aspects of the body-person and characteristically assume that care will redound on all parts. Several systems begin with "energy," and much current research aims to develop this concept (MacPherson et al, 2007; Mayor & Micozzi, 2011; Oschman, 2003; Scheid & MacPherson, 2012; Stux et al, 2001). Existing systems use traditional language; for example, homeopathy views the physical body as having three significant layers and the body-person as having three distinct aspects (Vithoulkas, 1980), each imbued with *vital spirit* or *vital energy*. Acupuncture analyzes the physical body in terms of the flow of energy through *channels*, or *meridians*, that do not directly correlate with known anatomical entities. The energy that flows through and animates the material body is called *qi* (*ch'i, ki*)[5] and closely resembles the homeopathic concept of vital spirit or the Ayurvedic concept of *prana*.

Biofield or bioenergetic therapies intervene in aspects sometimes referred to as energy whorls, emanations, or auras, and specialists identify them somewhat differently. Wirkus (1993), using bioscience terminology, refers to the thermal, electromagnetic, and acoustic fields. Brennan (1988), using esoteric science terminology, labels these three as the etheric, astral, and mental bodies. Bruyere (1994) focuses on chakras.

Spiritual and shamanic healers also work with nonmaterial and normally invisible bodies. Most believe that these spiritual forces imbue the physical body, although some say they extend beyond it, and some say that parts can travel (as during sleep), be removed (by exorcism), or get lost (Eliade, 1964; Harner, 2013; Ingerman, 1991, 1994; Targ et al, 1999).

Psychotherapists typically begin work with the psychosocial body, that is, the "person" who lives within the other bodies and interacts with the world outside. Terms for this aspect include *mind* and *emotions*, as well as technical terms that each subspecialty uses to showcase its particular explanatory model.

The several bodies are not separate: only one body-person stands before the practitioner seeking help. But who can say where the physical body, with its ongoing chemical and electrical changes, merges into the energetic body and where the latter extends into the spiritual body? All are immersed in the psychosocial body. For what a person believes greatly affects how he or she will respond to illness and to treatment or what he or she will deliver in the way of health care.

But how can just a thought do any harm? I asked. He seemed surprised that I did not realize that a thought could have much power, even though it was unexpressed. "*A thought, whether spoken or not, is a real thing,*" he explained. "Don't you know that if someone is very ill and the medicine man is trying to cure him, there must not be anyone around whose thought are working against the medicine man? No one must say or think anything but good. No one must think that the patient will not recover. If someone among us does not have faith, the work is all lost. We must all believe that our prayers will be answered and that all will be peace. (Wetherill & Leake, 2007, p xvi; emphasis added.)

See the section on nocebo effect in Chapter 9.

---

[5]Qi equated to "energy" troubles many. Traditional sources often speak of "breath," not energy. However, the "translation" of qi as "energy" has become so popular in Western countries that many no longer question it (see Mayor & Micozzi, 2011).

With the exception of heavily materialist models that perceive themselves as treating the physical body and only reluctantly acknowledge the psychosocial body, all health care systems argue that there are both material and non-material aspects to the body, and that intervention in one area will affect all others. Thus, when a professional acupuncturist needles a patient who is having an asthma attack, he or she enters the energetic body and moves energy. The acupuncturist expects the physical, psychosocial, and spiritual bodies to respond as well: the bronchial tubes will dilate, and pain, anxiety, and fear will dissipate. These changes are not thought to be coincidental; according to this system's explanatory model, all the aspects of the body can work at ease when energy flows smoothly. Similarly, a shamanic practitioner offers healing first through the spiritual body, but assumes that harmoniousness will result in improved function in all bodily aspects. Gathering scientific evidence for bodily interrelatedness is the subject of the field of psychoneuroimmunology (Ader et al, 2008; Martin, 1999; Moss et al, 2002; Wisnesky & Anderson, 2009).

CONCEPTS OF SICKNESS, DISEASE, AND IMBALANCE

Although often used generically, the terms *sickness* and *illness* formally refer to an experience of discomfort or malfunction. *Disease* and *imbalance*, however, are abstracted concepts. Thus a person has an illness or sickness, and a practitioner *assigns meaning* to this experience by diagnosing and explaining what has happened. The answers provided by the practitioner are guided by the explanatory model of his or her health care system. Cultural learning also guides the expression of the patient's illness and the practitioner's diagnostic values (Dimou, 1995; Hallenback, 2006; Nilchaikovit et al, 1993; Schouten & Meeuwesen, 2006), so much so that even the pain people feel and report is related to such learned aspects of being as gender and ethnicity (Bachiocco et al, 2002; Bates, 1996; Bates et al, 1995; Emad, 1994); and even the preferred means of suicide reflects ethnicity (Bhui et al, 2012; Micozzi, 2014; Tuck et al, 2011).

A system's preferred malfunction concept is closely linked to its perception of the body-person, particularly whether a system tends to perceive cause as primarily *external* or *internal* (Cassidy, 1982, 1995; Fabrega, 1974; Foster & Anderson, 1978; Helman, 2000; Kleinman, 1980; Lindenbaum & Lock, 1993; Mattingly & Garro, 2000; Murdock, 1980). Most health care systems accept that both occur, although most also prefer to emphasize either the invader or the responding organism. External models argue that malfunctions attack from *outside* the body-person, invading and destroying. Internal models argue that something must first go wrong *internally*, which allows outer influences to penetrate where they previously could not. These conceptual differences affect each system's view of patient and practitioner. External theorists see the patient as passive and the practitioner as authority, whereas internal ideology interprets the patient as responsible and the practitioner as partner to that responsibility. Notice again the interplay between EM and metaparadigm: external cause theorists tend to prefer reductionism, whereas internal cause theorists often speak from the holistic position.

DISEASE

The concept of *disease* is preferred by external models. In this view the body-person is relatively passive, whereas the surrounding environment teams with danger. Body-persons are thought to respond similarly to the same invaders; that is, one person with mumps, leukemia, or pneumonia experiences it much as others do. If people are similar and the environment is dangerous, it is logical to emphasize the actions of the invader, and to find that every different type of invader creates a different disease. These externalizing reductionist assumptive patterns lead to the naming of many different diseases, and a major function of practitioners is to distinguish among them (*diagnose* disease). Their second job is to remove, destroy, or immobilize invaders, and thereby cure the patient.

This model, consistent with the late-nineteenth-century "germ theory" of disease, has long been preferred by biomedicine and has yielded familiar metaphors (Montgomery, 2006; Sontag, 1977). Tumor cells and microorganisms that have been awaiting their chance in "reservoirs" invade human "victims." The body "wages war," and surgeons and physicians are "warriors in white," "battling" the invaders.[6] Diseases that fit this classic model have distinctive symptoms and signs, have single causes, and respond to specific therapies. Treatment results in cure. To emphasize the separation of ailment from patient, the former often are called disease *entities*.

Despite the power and familiarity of this model, only a minority of the "disease entities" defined by biomedicine fit the invasion model. Chronic, degenerative, and stress-related disorders frustrate the system because they do not have specifiable boundaries, single causes, "cures," or predictable outcomes of "entities." These disorders force biomedicine to consider explanations that fall outside the usual framework: (1) the body-person is not passive but plays some part in the genesis of disease; (2) many (often unspecifiable) factors must interact before disease arises; (3) some of these factors might be psychosocial; and (4) the practitioner's role is less to prescribe than to educate. The area of biomedicine that best reflects this opening state of mind is that of "lifestyle" diseases, or conditions that arise from and can be ameliorated by changes in how people behave and believe (Ornish, 1998). Interestingly, even this door has not opened too widely; most lifestyle discussions still focus on ameliorative factors that address

the physical body, such as diet and exercise. Biomedical practitioners who recommend acupuncture, visualization, or meditation are likely to consider themselves "avant-garde," or perhaps say they are practicing "integratively" (see Chapter 3).

As noted, chiropractic and osteopathy share biomedicine's primarily material and mechanistic view of disease, although these systems focus on the spine and nerves rather than cells and chemicals. Patient instructions also tend to take a physical form, such as changes in diet and exercise.

IMBALANCE

Many health care systems stress internal models of disorder and emphasize *imbalance* rather than disease. Their therapeutic goal is to return the person to a state of balance. These systems often name conditions according to their process within the person. For example, in East Asian medicine, *rising Liver fire* describes a person's condition momentarily or repeatedly, but it is not a freestanding and categorical concept such as the biomedical disease entity *migraine headache*.

Balance can be perturbed by external invaders or by interruptions in the smooth working of the internal milieu. External causes, however, rarely harm a body-person who is in balance. Health care therefore tends to the self-protective abilities of the body-person, maintaining and strengthening them. This approach is not curing but healing; the practitioner's goal is less to "battle" the invader[7] or "fix" the patient but rather to prune, weed, and plant, like an ecological system within the patient, enabling the person to grow a vibrant internal "garden" in which all aspects of his or her body-person function harmoniously despite the vagaries of the external environment (Beinfield & Korngold, 1991).

Treatment within internal-cause systems is individualistic, because the logic of this model is such that each person is considered to have a unique history and constitution that affect how he or she will respond to the myriad circumstances of life. The practitioner examines the current condition of the patient, relates it to the patient's social and medical history, and then selects therapy on the basis of the entire assessment.

Although diet, exercise, rest, and other physical interventions are prescribed, these "treatments" are usually offered in formats that also address the spiritual and energetic bodies. For example, exercises such as yoga, t'ai chi, or qi gong offer movement, energy balancing, energy storage, and meditation simultaneously. A patient might be advised to develop his or her spiritual and emotional body through creative activities such as art, dance, and chanting, or may

---

[6]Similar metaphors are used to describe the need for exorcism: invasion by an evil entity demands a spiritual battle to defeat it. Faith-based systems that use exorcism therapeutically also use external models of disease causation.

[7]Classical Chinese medicine did often use "battle" metaphors to discuss disorder, and had a well-developed model of invasion/infection. The emphasis on "holism" and metaphors of "gardening" is popular among professional acupuncturists in English-speaking countries who emphasize "holism" and "patient-centered care."

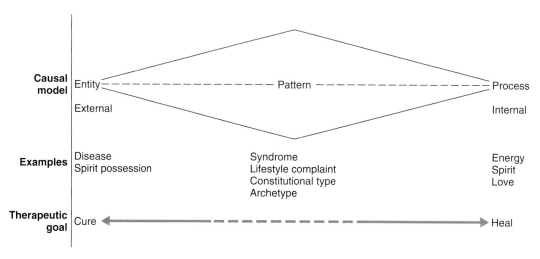

Figure 5-5 Three major approaches to interpreting symptoms.

be encouraged to minimize vulnerability to psychic attack by meditation, shamanic journeying, or prayer. Diet counseling may include attention not only to nutrient content but also to seasonal, constitutional, and essential (as opposed to literal) temperature appropriateness (see Chapter 30).

CONSTITUTIONAL TYPES

The disease entity and imbalance models represent ideals. Practitioners know that neither model works all the time. Thus, biomedicine recognizes as *syndromes* those conditions with multiple linked causes, not all of which can be specified. Similarly, internal-cause systems know that individuality is not absolute, because people do present commonalities or patterned responses to similar challenges.

Many health care systems have developed sophisticated models to link certain constitutional types with the probability of the development of particular illnesses. In the European, Mediterranean and Middle Eastern system that preceded biomedicine, persons were categorized as melancholic, phlegmatic, sanguine, or choleric. Although current biomedical practitioners may view these concepts with an indulgent smile, the underlying idea is by no means absent in modern biomedicine. In the mid-twentieth century, biomedical scientists attempted to link physical and psychosocial diseases with the endomorphic, mesomorphic, and ectomorphic types (Sheldon et al, 1949). At present there also remains much interest in type A or C personalities, which are said to be linked to heart disease (Friedman, 1996), and other types possibly linked to cancer. A popular diet that has been "debunked" attempts to relate blood type to diet (Adamo, 1996). Constitutional typologies are well developed in the Ayurvedic system (the *doshas* of *pitta*, *vata*, and *kapha*) and in some styles of East Asian medicine (the five elements of wood, fire, earth, metal, water). The old European categories survive in the hot–cold systems of Latin America (Chapters 38, 39) and the Philippines (Chapter 40). Meanwhile, psychometric evaluations such

as the Spiegel Hypnotic Susceptibility Scales, and the development of Hartmann's Personality Boundary Types by Micozzi and Jawer, have been quite useful in matching the individual patient to the appropriate CAM therapies (see Chapter 10), which remains a major challenge for so-called integrative medicine (see Chapter 3).

Figure 5-5 summarizes the data of this section in a linear model. The "categorical disease entities" model forms one extreme on one end of a continuum, with the "process-related imbalance" model at the other end. At the midpoint are patterned responses, including constitutional types. At the end featuring diseases, the individual person essentially has been deleted from the argument ("One person suffers much like others, so focus on identifying the disease"), whereas at the other extreme the person is the final focus and arbiter of interpretation ("In this individual these symptoms mean *x,* which I know from experience of him/her. . . . They may mean *y* in another individual"). In the middle are positions that share both interpretive energies ("Certain characteristics make it more likely that he or she will experience these symptoms, so perhaps I can reduce my diagnostic chore").

COMMUNICATION ISSUES

Biomedical disease entity names have become standard vocabulary, but these diseases (not the symptoms) are "real" only to people who use the biomedical model. Practitioners of other systems may use these terms out of familiarity to communicate with patients or with fund granting agencies or to complete insurance claim forms, but within their own systems of health care, such labels have little cogency. Acupuncturists, for example, treat what their patients and referring physicians call "depression," but the concept does not exist in East Asian medicine. Research has shown that in samples of people with the biomedical diagnosis of depression, Chinese medical practitioners can recognize at least five different, distinct energetic imbalance conditions (Schnyer, 2002; Schnyer & Allen, 2001). The significant point is that two patients with the same biomedical diagnosis might appropriately receive different diagnoses *and therapies* from an East Asian medicine practitioner.

As it happens, this example directly addresses a problem within biomedicine: practitioners often can't distinguish which patients will respond to which anti-depression drug treatments. Weeks may be spent trying to identify an effective pill—if ever. What if each depressed patient were assessed in East Asian medical terms? By linking symptoms as perceived by EAM with those known to characterize the drugs, perhaps a patient could more quickly receive a suitable pharmaceutical or herbal prescription. This kind of "technology transfer" would be an example of pragmatic and true medical integration. Will we "get there" someday?

Because each system defines disorder differently, practitioners and scientists must be careful in their use of biomedical terminology, not assuming that it is sufficient. It is better to describe symptoms and then affix a biomedical label (if appropriate) while clearly stating that the biomedical label may not reflect the way of knowing of another system. This approach can serve because symptoms are widely recognized; but it is the *interpretations* that differ. By focusing on symptoms, the malfunction labels of the other systems might begin to take on the kind of reality that now is owned only by the biomedical labels. The medical conversation would become more accurate and broader.

CONCEPTS OF DEEP CAUSE

External and internal causative factors mentioned so far can be understood as proximate causes of malfunction. With the issue of deep cause, we contemplate why *this* person at *this* time or in *this* place has become ill in *this* way. We want to consider sociocultural answers, not epidemiological ones. We explore the issue first by returning to our discussion of the body-person and considering the developmental nature of illness, and second by considering the intentional component of illness.

DEVELOPMENTAL NATURE OF ILLNESS

An ancient "chicken-and-egg" philosophical argument questions whether the physical body comes first, giving rise to nonmaterial constructs such as emotions and mind, or whether mind (spirit, soul) comes first and animates the physical body. Materialist models prefer the first argument, whereas nonmaterialist models favor the second.

This choice affects both the theory and the politics of health care. If one accepts as real only what one can see, hear, or measure with machines, delivering care to the nonmaterial bodies seems, at the least, puzzling, and quite possibly, ridiculous. Efforts to test nonmaterialist systems include designing machinery to "prove" that the claimed bodies exist, such as using electrical point locators to find acupuncture points and meridians or Kirlian photography to find auras (Chapters 14, 15). Materialists suspect nonmaterialist practitioners of misleading their patients or achieving effects primarily by activating the placebo response (Chapter 9). Cynics also argue that nonmaterialist practitioners have their greatest successes in the care of functional, or psychosomatic, diseases. Such diseases are disvalued in materialist systems precisely because they lack specific material signs such as germs, malfunctioning genes, tumor cells, abnormal metabolic values, broken bones, or other "pathologies." Materialists suspect that those who suffer functional conditions are not really sick.

Nonmaterialist thinkers consider malfunction in the nonmaterial aspects of the body to be as real as physical malfunction. All patient complaints signal true distress and suffering; the diagnostic task is not with triaging between the real and the imaginary, but with identifying what aspect of the person will respond most efficaciously to treatment, and to rationally alleviate suffering (Chapter 1).

Many such systems use a developmental model of malfunction, in which sickness starts in the nonmaterial bodies and ultimately becomes expressed in the physical body only later. They fault materialist systems for paying attention only to end-stage (i.e., physical) malfunction and failing to treat conditions *before* they become entrenched. They further argue that a focus on the material level alone provides only symptomatic relief and ignores deep cause, allowing underlying causes and malfunctions to remain unaddressed. Nonmaterialist systems assume that care can modify all parts of the body-person. Some also claim that as persons heal, they cycle backward through layers of long-buried symptoms until finally they express the oldest symptoms, release them, and are well. This pattern is called the "law of cure."

For example, a child might experience a spiritual trauma from loss of intimacy (Jarrett, 1998) such as parental divorce. Afterward this child has eczema. Later still the child has allergies and asthma. Untreated, the original spiritual wound or deep cause has been magnified and becomes overt and disabling. Appropriate treatment of the asthma not only will relieve wheezing but also might instigate a recrudescence of eczema and grief until the original spiritual wound is healed.

By the logic of internal-cause systems, it is advantageous (as well as cost effective) to treat complaints before malfunction is manifested physically. Nonmaterial complaints are real because any suffering affects the whole body-person, and potentially, the whole community.

Systems that use only nonmaterial therapies, such as bioenergetic healing, psychotherapy, and shamanism, focus care on the nonmaterial aspects of the person and expect that the physical body will respond. However, many systems use a combination of material and nonmaterial therapeutic modalities. The techniques themselves often have a layered character. For example, acupuncture points have multiple functions and in combination have predictable and specific physical, spiritual, and emotional effects (Ross, 1995). The same is true of herbal remedies and some forms of bodywork. Nonmaterialist models also view the person as having an active role in creating and treating his or her own condition. The role of practitioner is reformulated from authority to facilitator, from the one who does the curing to the one who helps persons heal themselves. As treatment is administered, such practitioners encourage patients to consider what attitudes of mind or spirit may have played a part in their illness and to explore new, life-enhancing ways of believing and behaving—wellness training. The goals of nonmaterialist health care are to care for the nonsomatic aspects of the patient so completely that the somatic aspect rarely suffers or surfaces.

> AKT, a professional acupuncturist, explains:
> [Acupuncture is] this ancient process of using needles ... to affect the vitality of another human being in a way that **helps that person become more in a homeostatic state, or more who they're meant to be.** Basically all that an acupuncturist is trying to do is to help the parson show up in the best possible well-being. ... What I would like to do best is to be so present to someone that I get out of the way, and ... understand that they are already whole, and [what] I am doing is providing a space for them finding their own wholeness. (Cassidy, 2011, p 171; emphasis added)

Unfortunately, in the hands of some practitioners the focus on patient responsibility becomes excessive, and patients feel guilt about their sickness. The materialist emphasis on the patient as the victim of disease can be equally harmful, resulting in patients who feel helpless to change themselves or learn and implement health-enhancing behaviors.

INTENTIONAL COMPONENT OF ILLNESS

Whereas practitioners discuss proximate and deep causes of sickness, medical social scientists recognize another cross-cutting domain of causality and contrast, called the *naturalistic* and *personalistic* explanatory approaches. According to the *naturalistic* approach, the causes of sickness are found in the natural world and lack intention; they cause malfunction by unintentionally ending up in the wrong place or by causing damage as they go about their own lifeways. Illness is considered a normal experience of life, natural and inevitable. The *personalistic* approach, in contrast, maintains that some form of intention is present, and sickness is an unnatural result of one's own misbehavior or of attracting the attention of the wrong entities (Foster & Anderson, 1978).

When a person says he or she has lung cancer and attributes it to 30 years of two-pack per day cigarette smoking, the person speaks in a naturalistic mode. However, if the person complains of having been inveigled into smoking or declares that this habit is an expression of weak character, the person is moving in a personalistic direction. If

people attribute their cancer to the corrective or punitive actions of a spiritual entity such as God, they speak fully in the personalistic mode (Chapter 11).

These tendencies coexist in most health care systems, although one or the other usually is emphasized. Professionalized health care systems generally prefer naturalistic explanations such as microorganisms, malformations, toxins, age-related degeneration, winds, hot and cold, or damp and dry. Within these systems, however, some practitioners recognize, even specialize in, the personalistic approach. In biomedicine, psychiatry and psychology emphasize this structure, usually attributing malfunction to troubles in the psychosocial body rather than in the spiritual or energetic bodies. In other major systems, practitioners deal with expressions of self-distrust or the results of psychic attacks in much the same way as they deal with physical conditions.

Faith-based systems are primarily personalistic in approach. They ask patients to confess ways in which they have angered God, who may have retaliated by sending disease. Some also recognize invasion by evil spiritual entities and offer exorcism as a treatment. Prayer is offered to alleviate pain and prevent sickness. Some faith-based systems also practice the "laying on of hands."

> But she seems to be an intelligent woman," one family practitioner kept repeating as he told me of the woman who had refused the surgical removal of uterine fibroids. What he viewed as a completely medical (and secular) situation his patient took to be a tangible sign of divine displeasure. God would heal her if it would be his will; no scalpels necessary (Snow, 1993).

Shamanic systems combine naturalistic and personalistic approaches. Natural events, such as experiencing a severe emotional or physical shock, may cause parts of the soul to be lost. The shaman recognizes the situation from the symptoms and takes a spiritual journey to retrieve and return the soul parts, thus reintegrating the body-person. Again, a person with an insufficient degree of psychic protection may be psychically attacked by someone else, either purposefully, during an argument, or even by being looked at with envious eyes (the "evil eye"—see Chapter 34). The shaman's task is to heal the psychospiritual wound and then help the patient to develop stronger personal protective skills. Shamans also serve communities by mediating arguments, changing weather, and treating physical illness with herbs and psychospiritual support (Box 5-6 provides sources).

Notice that the naturalistic-personalistic frame cuts across the materialist-nonmaterialist frame. Naturalistic explanations often deal with causes that are nonmaterial, such as temperature changes or wind invasions. Similarly, personalistic explanations can be materialist; some people see, hear, or feel entities such as ghosts and spirits, and material objects such as hair and fingernails store aspects of soul and thus can be used to heal or harm. Most importantly, however, even when the system

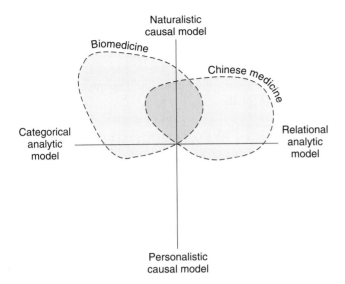

Figure 5-6 A cognitive map for health care systems.

and practitioner prefer naturalistic explanations, patients regularly demand to know, "Why me, Lord?" and offer answers couched in the personalistic framework. We use such perceptions again in developing the model in Figure 5-6.

CONCEPTS OF THE PRACTITIONER–PATIENT RELATIONSHIP

The EM also offers guidance on how the practitioner is to relate to the patient. It is essentially an issue of the balance between attention to doctor–patient *interaction*, and attention to *intervention*. If a system emphasizes diagnosis and material intervention—prescribing pills, for example—the tendency to interaction is correspondingly less, and may even be frowned upon to the extent that the practitioner is defined as "expert" in a hierarchical relationship to "patient." In those systems that argue that the "whole" matters, especially where diagnosis and treatment are "hands-on" (e.g., acupuncture, massage therapy), the practitioner's interaction with the patient (or client) is likely to be more intense, closer, "warmer." A study of American acupuncture patients' assessment of their care (Cassidy, 1998a) found that when respondents were asked to choose the best word to describe their relationship to their practitioner—for example, teacher, boss, doctor, guide, friend—the majority chose "friend."[8] However, although the EM does offer a degree of guidance on this issue, this guidance is cut across (and may be extinguished) by issues of personal tendency ("cool" vs "warm" personalities), locale of care delivery, and habit. Holistic practitioners working in a reductionist environment, such as a hospital,

may have to restrain their interpersonal warmth to fit the local culture (Kielczynska, 2012). Practitioners working in a community-based medical system, such as a Navajo Sing, "perform" in front of an audience and must also meet the expectations of the locale (Chapters 13, 37).

Additionally, systems that prefer external causative models characteristically view the body-person as passive, a victim, and, logically enough, interpret the practitioner as active, the one who cures. By contrast, systems that prefer internal causative models view the body-person as active and as already capable of healing. The practitioner's task is to facilitate the discovery of this capacity and develop it. The patient in this model has life expertise, and the practitioner must use medical expertise in *partnership* with the patient.

The personality of some patients is passive regardless of what is asked of them, and others always demand a say in their care. The biomedical literature discusses this issue under the rubrics of external locus and internal locus of control (Carlson et al, 2009). However, this chapter makes the point that not only practitioners or patients, but entire systems are modeled to emphasize one or the other style of care giving. Systems that want patients to be passive find and label active patients as frustrating, irritating, and intrusive, even "noncompliant." Systems that want patients to be active find and label passive patients as unresponsive, helpless, and in denial, or again, noncompliant.

A lucid practitioner might be able to match his or her style to the patient's needs, providing either authoritarian or relational (patient-centered) care to fit the situation. However, practitioners also have preferences and personal styles that cannot be modified easily. Health professions students are likely to select health care practices and specialties that fit their own personalities and personal styles.

MAKING SENSE OF ALL THE VARIABILITY

The chapter began with the statement that health care systems vary in many ways and that the variety can be analyzed with the help of conceptual models. Now we must ask, "How can this information be applied in a world in which patients use many health care systems and modalities ('medical pluralism'), and practitioners are advised to understand and sympathize with them?" See the case example below.

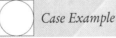

Case Example

August 2013: An educated rural white woman tells a medical use story.

I was seventy when I fractured my left hip and femur. [After hospital care] there was little I could do except keep flexible and walk and exercise for the first year. The left leg was healing 1.25″ short. The physical therapist said the doctors would insert a longer rod

---

[8]Professional acupuncturists working in English-speaking countries offer good examples of holism in practice. Patients of MD-acupuncturists, as in Germany, do not report equivalent levels of warmth or effectiveness, another indication of the difference a metaparadigm can make (Frank & Stollberg, 2004).

after a year. It was then [that] I sought the aid of a shaman. The right leg at that time was angry from bearing the weight of the whole body for so long. I was angry at the doctors for measuring incorrectly. The shaman released all the anger. I sought the aid of a chiropractor and massage therapist. The chiropractor gained an inch and told me I would lose it soon, and to come back. I have been working with the massage therapist, who is also a Tibetan doctor. He gains the 1.25″ which I am able to maintain for about 10 days, walking with very little limp. I then return for another treatment.

This case example shows a woman in deep communication with her own body, certain her leg will learn to stay extended, effectively using health care options available in her mountain valleys, avoiding costly and painful secondary biomedical care, and satisfied with her choices and progress. It also shows the potential of offering citizens multiple medical care options in a world that recognizes that "other" Medicines have much to offer.

This section explores this issue by discussing an example that compares biomedicine and East Asian medicine. I have developed a conceptual map that allows any system to be rapidly compared with another (Figure 5-6). The chapter concludes by summarizing what makes biomedicine actually quite unusual, yet allowing it to remain convinced that it is normative.

COMPARISON OF CARE IN TWO MEDICAL SYSTEMS

As discussed, biomedicine prefers reductionistic, categorical explanatory models, whereas East Asian medicine (Chinese, Oriental) prefers relational, process-oriented explanatory models (Beinfield & Korngold, 1991, Cassidy, 2002, 2010, 2011; Kaptchuk, 1983; Lock & Gordon, 1988; Mayor & Micozzi, 2011; Scheid & MacPherson, 2012; Stein, 1990). Both are heterogeneous systems, so relational tendencies can be found in biomedicine, and categorical tendencies exist in East Asian medicine. How different do these preferences really make these two systems?

SIMILARITIES BETWEEN BIOMEDICINE AND EAST ASIAN MEDICINE

1. Both aim to provide comprehensive health care, which includes health-enhancing, preventive, reproductive, acute and chronic illness, and trauma care.
2. Both prefer to deliver care in specific locales such as clinics or hospitals and in practitioner-to-patient dyads; group-based and home- or community-based practices are viewed as possible but nonmodal.
3. Both prefer naturalistic explanations of malfunction, arguing that impersonal forces are the main sources of ill health. However, if sometimes reluctantly, both also recognize that personalistic explanations sometimes make sense.
4. Both subsume a wide range of practices or specialties. Although specialties within internal medicine represent the intensively reductionist naturalistic components of biomedicine, psychiatry (particularly psychoanalysis) veers toward personalistic explanatory models, and immunotherapy, clinical ecology, and approaches empha-

sizing lifestyle intervention have a relational flavor. Again, although some styles of acupuncture practice aim to be primarily relational and holistic in outlook, the post-1949 TCM style (see Chapters 3, 28) veers toward the reductionist model and borrows many ideas from biomedicine.

DIFFERENCES BETWEEN BIOMEDICINE AND EAST ASIAN MEDICINE

1. Biomedicine focuses on trauma, acute illness, and end-stage chronic disease intervention. Although prevention is discussed as part of biomedical care, wellness is not a core concept. East Asian medicine emphasizes wellness and preventive care, and treats chronic and acute illness conditions, but avoids surgery.
2. Biomedicine emphasizes materialist explanations, whereas East Asian medicine emphasizes nonmaterialist explanations based on a distinctive concept of qi (ch'i, vital energy) flow. Their views of anatomy and physiology and their favored bodily metaphors are distinctly different (Beinfield & Korngold, 1991; Kuriyama, 2002; Unschuld, 2009).
3. Biomedicine emphasizes the physical body as the locus for intervention, recognizes but remains uncomfortable with the concept of the psychosocial body, and largely denies the existence of the energetic and spiritual bodies. By contrast, East Asian medicine uses the energetic body as the first locus for intervention and assumes that interventions at that level will redound on all the other bodies, including the physical.
4. Biomedicine sees humans as biologically similar; therefore, diseases will present similarly and can be treated similarly, for example, by prespecified standard protocols. East Asian medicine sees each human as unique and assumes that even if symptoms appear to be similar, the deep cause might be dissimilar; thus, care should be delivered individualistically.
5. Biomedicine has defined an immense universe of distinct disease "entities," assumes they will each and all present similarly in most people, focuses much energy on disease diagnosis and classification, and defines success only as cure. Controlling or palliating symptoms is considered a lesser success, and death (while fully inevitable at some point) is commonly thought of as failure. East Asian medicine focuses on the flow of energy within the body and between the patient and the cosmos. Ill health arises when this flow is disrupted or impeded or when there is insufficient energy. Because this disorder can happen in many ways, the practitioner also spends much time diagnosing by assessing the character of the flow, hearing the patient's story, and listening in on the energetic body (e.g., by taking the pulses). Imbalance is viewed as commonplace and natural, and there is little to cure; instead the practitioner hopes to maintain or improve the coherence of the body-person, that is, heal the person. Death is also

deemed natural; the dying patient can use acupuncture to ease pain and to achieve a final energetic balance.

CONCEPTUAL MAPPING OF HEALTH CARE SYSTEMS

It is possible to map differences among health care systems to allow these similarities and differences to be rapidly grasped and applied. Figure 5-6 shows a matrix with the categorical (reductionist) versus relational (process-related) worldview represented on the horizontal axis and the naturalistic to personalistic causal model on the vertical axis. Using this diagram, we can—hypothetically—locate virtually any system of health care in such a way as to compare it rapidly with any other system. Knowing more about the terrain of systematic health care differences makes it easier to understand and use the insights from other systems of health care. Practitioners can use such information to design research, to make themselves and their patients aware of their own prejudices, and to listen more openly to the users of different health care systems.

Figure 5-6 maps only the two systems cited in our example; readers are encouraged to map others as they learn about them in this text. Note, however, that each of the two systems mapped covers a wide area. Biomedicine, although clearly within the realm of categorical naturalistic thinking, spills over the horizontal line into personalistic models (psychology, psychiatry) and over the vertical line into relational territory (family practice, psychoneuroimmunology, lifestyle approaches). In fact, biomedical practice overlaps the East Asian medicine outline at the center of the figure.

The map also shows that in terms of preferred worldview, East Asian medicine is opposite that of biomedicine. On the other hand, it is similar to biomedicine in its general preference for naturalistic causal explanations. These twin characteristics map East Asian medicine into the upper right quadrant. Note again, however, the wide range of practice under the umbrella of East Asian medicine. The more symptomatic and categorical styles of practice map left toward the reductionistic quadrant, and the traditional shamanistic components of East Asian medicine map below the horizontal line.

This map reminds us that no single health care system serves the whole field, and that systems differ but also share similarities.

WHY BIOMEDICINE FINDS OTHER SYSTEMS UNCONVENTIONAL

Although not drawn onto the map, the other health care systems tend to cluster more centrally or to the right of the center on both sides of the horizontal axis. Thus the mapping exercise also provides a visual clue as to why biomedicine, from its perch in the upper left quadrant, might find the other systems unconventional. They are nonmodal when judged from biomedicine's position. However, biomedicine is equally unconventional when viewed from the position of most systems. From a worldwide viewpoint, biomedicine is unusual, or not conventional, in the following ways:

1. Its intense, almost exclusive attachment to materialist interpretive models.
2. Its focus on the physical body, almost to the exclusion of other possibilities.
3. Its focus on the disease "entity," often to the exclusion of the person or "host.'
4. Its vast development of disease types and typology.
5. Its highly technological healthcare delivery system.
6. The extreme invasiveness of even first-resort care modalities.
7. Its emphasis on acute disease, trauma, and end-stage malfunction
8. Its relative lack of focus on prevention, "functional disorders," or wellness.
9. Its high cost.

Despite these oddities, biomedicine considers itself conventional and other systems "alternative." How did this situation come about, and why is it not surprising to most Western urban people? Furthermore, why is it difficult for people to consider biomedicine as just one more alternative?

> Biomedicine's faith in science as the unmediated discovery of reality means that biomedicine is not self-reflective. Meanwhile, complementary and alternative medicine, faced with the power imbalance between the two regimes, is inspired to wrestle with important questions about the nature of skill, the constitution of evidence, the role of autonomy in standardized practice, and the challenges of "integration" in a range of circumstances.... Above all complementary and alternative medicine must seek out and defend appropriate research methodologies for questions that biomedicine for the most part neglects, even fails to recognize. (Montgomery, 2012, p 229)

Health care is not free of culture, economic interests, or politics. In the United States, we are accustomed to thinking of biomedicine as the best system because it has become the most expanded, being practiced in every country in the world, although East Asian medicine, chiropractic and homeopathy are close seconds. Biomedicine also has the largest educational, legal, and economic mandate. Finally, its explanatory model closely fits the dominant European and North American worldview, or metaparadigm: categorical and reductionist.

As part of the expression of this worldview, many state that biomedicine is the most scientific system. This argument is controversial and must be examined carefully.

Science is a particular method for gathering information and constructing knowledge. In contrast to other systems—such as theology, which allows for revelation, and law, which allows for precedence ("common law")—science demands that information be sought in the natural world and that interpretations be tested for accuracy. This approach is extremely unusual: it means that a person's opinion or mere observation and consequent certitude are not enough to make the person's position acceptable to scientists. Instead, the person must show that he or she has gathered data systematically and accounted for potential biases, then must submit his or her interpretations to others for examination and retesting. Furthermore, the researcher is enjoined to be a relativist; that is, not to become enamored of his or her interpretations but to hold them always as *models* of reality or approximations. This approach provides remarkable training in humbleness, but to be frank, not many researchers achieve it.

ROLE OF SCIENCE

Euro-American society in particular has developed science to be *the* believable knowledge method, the knowledge orthodoxy since the late nineteenth century. The determination with which Westerners cling to their cultural preference concerning the power of science approaches a religious fervor (Chapter 34). Biomedicine gradually took on the cloak of this scientism with the rise of clinical medicine in the mid-nineteenth century, moving toward a laboratory-based experimental model by the late nineteenth century. Although the laboratory experiment is only one narrow way to gather valid data by use of the scientific method, this approach became accepted as *the* "scientific" approach. By the early twentieth century, American biomedicine had already contrasted itself to other systems by claiming to be experimental and thus uniquely scientific (Chapter 22). Given that the other major systems are historically not experimental—they depend on well-developed clinical observation skills and empirical experience guided by their explanatory models—it becomes clear why a system that perceives itself as scientific can consider "nonscientific" (by this definition) systems as inferior *in our cultural milieu*.

The biomedical model assumes diseases to be fully accountable by deviations from the norm of measurable biologic (somatic) variables. It leaves no room within its framework for the social, psychological, and behavioral dimensions of illness. The biomedical model has thus become a cultural imperative, its limitations easily overlooked. In brief, it has now acquired the status of dogma. In science, a model is revised or abandoned when it fails to account adequately for all the data. A dogma, on the other hand, requires that discrepant data be forced to fit the model or be excluded (Engel, 1977).

So, is biomedicine really scientific if judged from the perspective of science rather than cultural preference? Does biomedicine function as a "science" or a "dogma," or both? Though difficult to measure accurately, estimates suggest that only about 30% of what biomedicine performs has been tested adequately (Altman, 1994; American Iatrogenic Association, n.d.; Andersen, 1990). (Such observa-

tions were routinely reported by the U.S. Congressional Office of Technology Assessment during the 1970s and 1980s; the office was closed in 1995. A partial replacement is the U.S. Preventive Services Taskforce.) Fully 70% of practice uses only the same well-developed clinical observation skills and experience guided by the explanatory model that powers the other health care systems, and is not based on clinical trials evidence.

Those who can stand back dispassionately—that is, those who really do think like scientists and not dogmatists—understand that a great deal of the argument over which systems are modal and "normative, or alternative, is really an argument over cultural turf. As such, victory in this argument serves the usual economic and political purposes of maintaining power by insisting on the virtue of one's own values, often by attacking the perceptions of one's rivals. But these are political and economic, not scientific, actions.

HEALTH CARE AS A MATTER OF CULTURAL MODELING

That health care is a matter of cultural modeling rather than scientific truth is important to practitioners whose rational goals are to relieve suffering. It also is important to those who want to be scientific in their thoughts and choices. Differences must be addressed. So, pragmatically, we end by asking, "Who do the differences serve?" and "How do the differences serve?"

USERS OF ALTERNATIVE MEDICINE

Demand for nonbiomedical health care in Europe and North America is at a peak that has not been seen for about 125 years. Surveys of users of alternative or integrative medicine tell similar stories. People want to feel cared for, and do not appreciate biomedicine's (a) emphasis on laboratory medicine, (b) factoring of the individual person out of the diagnostic and treatment equation, (c) invasive treatments associated with high levels of painful and debilitating side effects,[9] (d) rushed and stingy delivery and rationing of care, and (e) immensely high and ever-rising costs. All these factors connote an "uncaring" health care system, making biomedicine increasingly unattractive to increasing numbers of people. Meanwhile this is the kind of care that is now being mandated by the federal government.

Who are these people? Surveys in the late twentieth century indicated that the users of the major nonbiomedical systems were mainly urban, female, and well educated, with middle to high incomes (Cassidy, 1998a; Cassileth et al, 1984; Eisenberg et al, 1993, 1998; McGuire, 1994); today CAM is used by *all* demographic groups. Original

---

[9]Approximately 20% of illnesses that lead to hospitalization are iatrogenic, that is, caused by the biomedical care itself (Greenwood & Nunn, 1994). Iatrogenesis is thought to be the third leading cause of death in the United States (Anonymous, 2013; also see Permpongkosol, 2011).

users—"early adopters"—were in excellent positions to judge the quality of the care they received from the variety of practitioners that they consulted, and they passed on their success stories by "word of mouth" because there was no other way of doing so within the dominant health care system of biomedicine. This point matters, because mainstream practitioners and researchers often attacked nonbiomedical health care by saying that the consumers were being misled, either purposefully by the practitioners or by their own desires, distress, and ignorance.

Such defensive, politically motivated arguments are increasingly weakened by the following facts:

1. Studies show that where health care is obviously pluralistic, laypeople are astute at matching systems with complaints (Cassidy, 1998a; Scheid & MacPherson, 2012; Young, 1981).

2. On the whole, patients report satisfaction with alternative health care (Alraek & Baerheim, 2001; Baarts & Pedersen, 2009; Cassidy, 1998b; Coulter et al, 2002; Emad, 1994; Gaumer, 2006; Gould et al, 2001; Hendrickson, 2001; Hughes, 2009; O'Connor, 1995; Paterson & Britten, 2003; Paterson & Britten, 2004; Workshop on Alternative Medicine, 1994; also see Dearth, 2011, a documentary film entitled *9000 Needles*).

3. Rapidly accumulating results of scientific research on alternative treatments show that they are often as effective or more effective, more cost-effective, and/or safer, than biomedical treatments for identical conditions, or that they provide valuable complementary effects when biomedicine is in use (Benor, 1993; Byrd, 1988; Carlston, 2003; Cassidy, 2002; Corbett et al, 2013, Dossey, 1997, Edzard et al, 2001; Hertzman-Miller et al, 2002; Jacobs et al, 1994; Jobst, 1995, 2004; O'Connor, 1995; Reilly et al, 1994; Savigny et al, 2009; see also articles in *Journal of Alternative and Complementary Medicine, Alternative Therapies*, and other journals on PUBMED (www.ncbi.nlm.nih.gov/pubmed), and NICE (www.nice.org.uk); and see reports of the National Institutes of Health, Center for Complementary and Alternative Medicine, http://nccam.nih.gov (websites accessed January 27, 2014).

4. Methodological skills for analyzing systems that differ deeply from biomedicine are developing rapidly beyond the myth of so-called evidence-based medicine (see Chapter 3; Cassidy & Thomas, 2012; Cassidy, 1995; Edzard et al, 2001; Grimes, 2003; Jonas et al, 2003; MacPherson et al, 2007; Paterson & Schnyer, 2012; Scheid & MacPherson, 2012; Verhoef et al, 2005; Wisnesky & Anderson, 2009).

CONSTITUENCY FOR ALTERNATIVE MEDICINE

Current biomedical discussion on the best use of nonbiomedical alternatives focuses either on annexing ("integrating") particular techniques (in the process, discarding the systemic embedding of the techniques within their native explanatory models) or on using the alternatives adjunc-

tively (e.g., recommending acupuncture as adjunctive therapy to minimize the side effects of chemotherapy). This approach to "integrative medicine" is analogous to building a separate annex in back of a building, not redesigning the building. Readers are now prepared to interpret these "integrative" approaches as expressions of a biomedical perspective that claims its health care reality is superior to all others.

Of course, the situation looks a little different from the viewpoints of alternative practitioners, as well as from the perspective of potential patients, many of whom are happy that "modern" health care provides a menu of alternatives from which to choose (Montgomery, 2012, p 229), and that alternative care is still available outside of "integrative medicine" facilities and practices. At times, for example, Chinese medical practitioners might want to use biomedicine adjunctively, and some biomedical diagnostic techniques are well integrated into nonbiomedical systems of health care. In the United States, some states (e.g., New Mexico, Florida) license professional acupuncturists as primary care providers. Thus they must master many concepts and techniques from biomedicine, "integrating" them into their East Asian medical practice, and can treat patients much as a family practitioner might. Increasingly, practitioners develop clinics that offer a range of medical practices, sometimes but not always including biomedical physicians. Physicians who initiate or choose to work within such a clinic often define themselves as "integrative" practitioners, and typically have extended their biomedical training to include knowledge of nonbiomedical modalities, which may be all over the scalar map, such as herbal therapy, enzyme therapy, or acupuncture.

Indeed, many would benefit if the U.S. health care system were organized so that several alternatives were widely available, had adequate staffing, and people learned about them from childhood (Box 5-7).

Note that this discussion assumes that there is space (and resources) for all forms of health care. This choice *should* be true in a democratic society, and it *is* true in the

BOX 5-7 *Beneficiaries of Widely Available Alternative (or Integrative) Health Care Systems in the United States*

- Those who have a high need for affiliation and who therefore want a relational style of health care
- Those who want to alleviate symptoms gently or with fewer side effects
- Those who will not take "hopeless" for an answer
- Those who want to prevent disease or enhance wellness
- Those who interpret the body-person as having more than a physical aspect and who want to be able to address the energetic, psychosocial, and spiritual bodies when receiving or delivering health care
- Those who are concerned with the end-stage focus and invasiveness of typical biomedical care

sense that all the systems already exist and serve people. While NIH, for example, remains focused on conducting ever more controlled clinical trials, another contemporary and more productive drive behind current research is to discover what services each system can provide and to compare their effectiveness in providing these services (Corbett et al, 2013; Savigny et al, 2009). Further work remains to be done on matching each individual patient to the treatment(s) that will work best for them (Chapter 10). This direction will fail if it is expressed solely in terms of conditions or complaints, which is only half the equation. The other half consists of the people who are to receive the care. There always will be a range of desires and needs; some patients will always expect and prefer care that is technological, "sterile," and has rapid overt effects, whereas others will always prefer care that is relational, gentle, and virtually contemplative.

It may be anticipated that the world's people will continue to become more skilled at using all our health care resources and options, to make it possible for everyone—practitioners and patients, funders, payers and policy makers—to know enough about their options to triage care successfully in a manner that maximizes patient satisfaction and health while minimizing suffering, iatrogenic diseases, and costs, and optimally improving quality of life.

It remains for you to consider your own goals for practice. Where do you fall on the various continua discussed in this chapter? Are you satisfied with the care that you deliver, or would you like to modify some rough spots? How can the existing range of medical options help you do so? How can developing your skill and referral base in alternatives to your own medicine aid your current or future patients, and in your current and future practice? Are you prepared to recognize as fellow professionals people trained in a different Medicine? Are you ready to refer patients out to them when you sense it would be beneficial?

SUMMARY AND CONCLUSIONS

This chapter introduces concepts that are fundamental to understanding values and issues in the practice of health care and provides a sociocultural context and models that will be useful in understanding the practices described in subsequent chapters.

Some take-away messages include: Health care is fundamentally a matter of sociocultural interpretation. Health care systems differ in important ways and no one system provides all the answers, or even the best answers, for all users or circumstances. Differences among systems are not random but are driven and logically organized by underlying assumptive patterns that are revealed in explanatory models, therapeutic modalities, and styles of practice.

These differences are *not* unbridgeable; the concepts developed in this chapter and textbook should allow most practitioners and researchers to approach even strange ideas with new appreciation, as well as provide them with tools that allow for better communication and under-standing. After all, the deepest and most common goal of all health care systems is to relieve pain and alleviate suffering—let us share the space.

Acknowledgments

Special thanks to Haig Ignatius, MD, MAc (1927–2004) and Marc Micozzi, MD, PhD, for their generous readings of the original chapter in its draft stages. Warm thanks to Sonya Pritzger, PhD, LAc, for her insightful reading of this version, and to Marc Micozzi and Carole O'Leary for their continuing attention to this chapter and its implications. As always, much thanks to many colleagues whose deep thinking about medical philosophical and practice issues guides and sustains my own explorations. And to my husband and daughter, always, your love and support are most precious.

References

Adamo PJ: *Eat right for your type*, New York, 1996, Putnam.

Ader R, Felten DL, Cohen N: *Psychoneuroimmunology*, ed 4, 2 volumes, 2008, Academic Press.

Alraek T, Baerheim A: "An empty and happy feeling in the bladder …": health changes experienced by women after acupuncture for recurrent cystitis, *Complement Thera Med* 9:219–223, 2001.

Altman D: The scandal of poor medical research, *BMJ* 308:283, 1994.

Alvord LA: Medicine: Navajo, 2003. http://www.cradleboard.org/cnat/resource/navajo.htm. Accessed January 27, 2014.

American Iatrogenic Association: Home page, n.d., Available at http://www.iatrogenic.org. Accessed January 27, 2014.

Ames R: *Sun-Tzu: the art of warfare*, New York, 1993, Ballantine Books.

Andersen B: *Methodological errors in medical research*, Oxford, 1990, Blackwell.

Anonymous: Iatrogenesis. http//en.wikipedia.org/wiki/iatrogenesis. Accessed February 3, 2014.

Baarts C, Pedersen IK: Derivative benefits: exploring the body through complementary and alternative medicine, *Sociol Health Illn* 31(5):719–733, 2009.

Bachiocco V, Tiengo M, Credico C: The pain locus of control orientation in a health sample of the Italian population: sociodemographic modulating factors, *J Cultur Divers* 9(2):55, 2002.

Bates MS: *Biocultural dimensions of chronic pain: implications for treatment of multi-ethnic populations*, Plattsburgh, 1996, State University of New York Press.

Bates MS, Rankin-Hill L, Sanchez-Ayendez M, et al: A cross-cultural comparison of adaptation to chronic pain among Anglo-Americans and native Puerto Ricans, *Med Anthropol* 16(2):141, 1995.

Beinfield H, Korngold E: *Between heaven and earth: a guide to Chinese medicine*, New York, 1991, Ballantine Books.

Benally C: Explore: Becoming a Diné Navajo medicine man, 2011. http://explore.org/#!/videos/player/becoming-a-dine-navajo-medicine-man. Accessed February 3, 2014.

Benor D: *Healing research: holistic energy medicine and spirituality*, Munich, 1993, Helix Verlag.

Berg M, Mol A, editors: *Differences in medicine, unraveling practices, techniques, and bodies*, Durham NC, 1998, Duke University Press.

Bhui KS, Dinos S, McKenzie K: Ethnicity and its influence on suicide rates and risk, *Ethn Health* 17(1–2):141–148, 2012.

Black Elk W, Lyon WS: *Black Elk: the sacred ways of a Lakota*, San Francisco, 1990, Harper & Row.

Brennan B: *Hands of light: a guide to healing through the human energy field*, Toronto, 1988, Bantam Books.

Bruyere R: *Wheels of light: chakras, auras and the healing energy of the body*, New York, 1994, Fireside Books.

Byrd RC: Positive therapeutic effects of intercessory prayer in a coronary care unit population, *South Med J* 81:826, 1988.

Carlson NR, Buskist W, Heth CD, Schmaltz R: *Psychology: the science of behaviour*, Canadian ed 4, Toronto ON, 2009, Pearson Education Canada.

Carlston M: *Classical homeopathy*, Edinburgh, 2003, Churchill Livingstone.

Cassidy CM: Protein-energy malnutrition as a culture-bound syndrome, *Cult Med Psychiatry* 6:325, 1982.

Cassidy CM: Unraveling the ball of string: reality, paradigms, and the study of alternative medicine, *Adv J Mind-Body Health* 10:3, 1994.

Cassidy CM: Social science theory and methods in the study of alternative and complementary medicine, *J Altern Complement Med* 1:19, 1995.

Cassidy CM: Chinese medicine users in the United States. I. Utilization, satisfaction, medical plurality, *J Altern Complement Med* 4(1):17–28, 1998a.

Cassidy CM: Chinese medicine users in the United States. II. Preferred aspects of care, *J Altern Complement Med* 4(2):89–202, 1998b.

Cassidy CM, editor: *Contemporary Chinese medicine and acupuncture*, Edinburgh, 2002, Churchill Livingstone.

Cassidy CM: How acupuncture is actually practised, and why this matters to clinical research design, *EJOM* 6(4):20–25, 2010.

Cassidy CM: What does it mean to practice an energy medicine? In Micozzi M, Mayor D, editors: *Energy medicine East and West, a natural history of qi*, 2011, pp 165–184. Chapter 13.

Cassidy C, Thomas K: Patient pattern of use and experience of acupuncture. In Scheid V, MacPherson H, editors: *Integrating East Asian medicine into contemporary healthcare*, Edinburgh, 2012, Churchill-Livingstone Elsevier, pp 37–56. Chapter 3.

Cassileth B, Lusk E, Strouse R, et al: Contemporary unorthodox treatments in cancer medicine: a study of patients, treatments and practitioners, *Ann Intern Med* 101:105, 1984.

Chen JK, Chen TT: *Chinese medical herbology and pharmacology*, City of Industry CA, 2004, Art of Medicine Press.

Corbett MS, Rice SJC, Madurasinghe V, et al: Acupuncture and other physical treatments for the relief of pain due to osteoarthritis of the knee: network meta-analysis, *Osteoarthritis Cartilage* 21:1290–1298, 2013.

Coulter ID, Hurwitz EL, Adams AH, et al: Patients using chiropractors in North America: who are they and why are they in chiropractic care? *Spine* 27(3):291–297, 2002.

Currer C, Stacey M: *Concepts of health, illness and disease, a comparative perspective*, 1986, Berg. 3PL.

Davies W: *Healing ways: Navajo health care in the twentieth century*, Albuquerque, 2001, University of New Mexico Press.

Dearth D: *9000 needles* [documentary film], 2011. http://www.acupunctureinlondon.com/2011/06/9000-needles-documentary-film-familys.html. Accessed January 27, 2014.

Deloria V: *The world we used to live in: remembering the powers of the medicine men*, Golden CO, 2006, Fulcrum Group.

Dimou N: Illness and culture: learning differences, *Patient Educ Couns* 26(1–3):153–157, 1995.

Dossey L: *Prayer is good medicine: how to reap the healing benefits of prayer*, San Francisco, 1997, Harper San Francisco.

Edzard M, Ernst D, Pittler M, et al: *Desktop guide to complementary and alternative medicine: an evidence-based approach*, St Louis, 2001, Mosby.

Eisenberg D, Davis RB, Ettner S, et al: Trends in alternative medicine use in the United States, 1990–1997: results of a follow-up survey, *JAMA* 280:1569, 1998.

Eisenberg D, Kessler R, Foster C, et al: Unconventional medicine in the United States, *N Engl J Med* 328:246, 1993.

Eliade M: *Shamanism: archaic techniques of ecstasy*, Princeton, NJ, 1964, Princeton University Press.

Emad M: Does acupuncture hurt? Ethnographic evidence of shifts in psychobiological experiences of pain, *Proc Soc Acupunct Res* 2:129, 1994.

Emad M: *Feeling the qi: emergent bodies and disclosive fields in American appropriations of acupuncture*, doctoral dissertation, Houston, 1998, Rice University.

Engel GL: The need for a new medical model challenge for biomedicine, *Science* 196(4286):129, 1977.

Engel GL: How much longer must medicine's science be bound by a seventeenth century world view? *Psychother Psychosom* 57(1–2):3–16, 1992.

Fabrega H: *Disease and social behavior: an interdisciplinary perspective*, Cambridge, Mass, 1974, MIT Press.

Foster G, Anderson B: *Medical anthropology*, New York, 1978, John Wiley & Sons.

Frank R, Stollberg G: Medical acupuncture in Germany: patterns of consumerism among physicians and patients, *Sociol Health Illn* 26(3):351–372, 2004.

Freedman DH: Lies, damned lies, and medical science. www.theatlantic.com/magazine/archive/2010/11/lies…lies/308269. Accessed January 27, 2014.

Friedman M: *Type A behavior: its diagnosis and treatment*, New York, 1996, Plenum Press (Kluwer Academic Press).

Gaumer G: Factors associated with patient satisfaction with chiropractic care: survey and review of the literature, *J Manipulative Physiol Ther* 29(6):455–462, 2006.

Gohel MS, Bulbulia RA, Slim FJ, et al: How to approach major surgery where patients refuse blood transfusion (including Jehovah's Witnesses), *Ann R Coll Surg Engl* 87(1):3–14, 2005.

Gould A, MacPherson H: Patient perspectives on outcomes after treatment with acupuncture, *J Altern Complement Med* 7(3):261–268, 2001.

Green EC: *Indigenous theories of contagious disease*, Walnut Creek CA, 1999, Altamira Press.

Greenwood M, Nunn P: *Paradox and healing: medicine, mythology and transformation*, ed 3, Victoria, BC, 1994, Paradox.

Grimes D: Identifying worthy medical research, *Network* 23(1): 2003.

Hallenback J: High context illness and dying in a low context medical world, *Am J Hosp Palliat Care* 23(2):113–118, 2006.

Hand WD, editor: *American folk medicine: a symposium*, Berkeley, 1976, University of California Press.

Harner MJ: *Cave and cosmos: shamanic encounters with another reality*, Berkeley CA, 2013, North Atlantic Books.

Harwood A: The hot-cold theory of disease: implications for treatment of Puerto Rican patients, *JAMA* 216:1153, 1977.

Helman CG: *Culture, health and illness*, ed 4, London, 2000, Arnold.

Helman CG: *Culture, health and illness*, ed 5, London, 2007, HodderArnold.

Hendrickson M: Clinical outcomes and patient perceptions of acupuncture and/or massage therapies in HIV-infected individuals, *AIDS Care* 13(6):743-748, 2001.

Hertzman-Miller RP, Morgenstern H, Hurwitz HL, et al: Comparing the satisfaction of low back pain patients randomized to receive medical or chiropractic care: results from the UCLA low-back pain study, *Am J Public Health* 92(10):1628-1633, 2002.

Hughes JG: "When I first started going I was going in on my knees, but I came out and I was skipping": Exploring rheumatoid arthritis patients' perceptions of receiving treatment with acupuncture, *Complement Ther Med* 17:269-273, 2009.

Hultkrantz A: The shaman and the medicine man, *Soc Sci Med* 20:511, 1985.

Ingerman S: *Soul retrieval: mending the fragmented self*, San Francisco, 1991, HarperCollins.

Ingerman S: *Welcome home: following your soul's journey home*, San Francisco, 1994, Harper San Francisco.

Jacobs J, Jimenez LM, Gloyd SS, et al: Treatment of acute childhood diarrhea with homeopathic medicine: a randomized clinical trial in Nicaragua, *Pediatrics* 93(5):719, 1994.

Jarrett L: *Nourishing destiny: the inner tradition of Chinese medicine*, Stockbridge, Mass, 1998, Spirit Path Press.

Jobst KA: A critical analysis of acupuncture in pulmonary disease: efficacy and safety of the acupuncture needle, *J Altern Complement Med* 1:57, 1995.

Jobst KA: Energy medicine: science and healing from bioelectromagnetics to the medicine of light, *J Altern Complement Med* 10(1):1, 2004.

Jonas W, Crawford C, editors: *Healing, intention and energy medicine: science, research methods, and clinical implications*, Edinburgh, 2003, Churchill Livingstone.

Johnson SM, Kurtz ME: "Diminished use of osteopathic manipulative treatment and its impact on the uniqueness of the osteopathic profession", *Acad Med* 76(8):821-828, 2001.

Kaplan A: Philosophy of science in anthropology, *Annu Rev Anthropol* 13:25, 1984.

Kaptchuk T: *The web that has no weaver: understanding Chinese medicine*, New York, 1983, Congdon & Weed.

Kenner D: Putting it all together: practicing Oriental medicine. In Cassidy CM, editor: *Contemporary Chinese medicine and acupuncture*, Edinburgh, 2002, Churchill Livingstone.

Kielczynska BB: *Practicing acupuncture in an in-patient setting: a phenomenologic study*, 2012, Drew University. Dissertation.

Kirkland J, Mathews HF, Sullivan CW III, et al, editors: *Herbal and magical medicine: traditional healing today*, Durham, NC, 1992, Duke University Press.

Kleinman A: *Patients and healers in the context of culture*, Berkeley, 1980, University of California Press.

Krishan S: *Essential Ayurveda: what it is and what it can do for you*, Novato, CA, 2003, New World Library.

Kuriyama S: *The expressiveness of the body, and the divergence of Greek and Chinese medicine*, NY, 2002, Zone Books.

Lam WA, McCullough LB: Influence of religious and spiritual values on the willingness of Chinese–Americans to donate organs for transplantation, *Clin Transplant* 14:449-456, 2000.

Larre C, de la Vallee ER: *Rooted in spirit: the heart of Chinese medicine*, Barrytown, NY, 1995, Station Hill Press.

Lindenbaum S, Lock M: *Knowledge, power and practice: the anthropology of medicine and everyday life*, Berkeley, 1993, University of California Press.

Lo V, Renton A: The Cuban Chinese medical revolution. In Scheid V, MacPherson H, editors: *Integrating East Asian medicine into contemporary healthcare*, Edinburgh, 2012, Churchill Livingstone Elsevier, pp 213-228. Chapter 13.

Lock M, Gordon DR, editors: *Biomedicine examined*, Dordrecht, The Netherlands, 1988, Kluwer.

Lupton D: *Medicine as culture: illness, disease and the body in Western societies*, ed 2, Thousand Oaks CA, 2003, Sage Publications.

Lyon WS: *Spirit Talkers: North American Indian Medicine Powers*, Kansas City MO, 2012, Prayer Efficacy Publishing.

Martin P: *The healing mind: the vital links between brain and behavior, immunity and disease*, New York, 1999, St Martin's Griffin.

Mattingly C, Garro L: *Narrative and the cultural construction of illness and healing*, Berkeley, 2000, University of California Press.

MacPherson H, Hammerschlag R, Lewith G, Schnyer R: *Acupuncture research, strategies for establishing an evidence base*, Edinburgh, 2007, Churchill Livingstone Elsevier.

Mayor D, Micozzi MS, editors: *Energy medicine, East and West: a natural history of qi*, Edinburgh, 2011, Churchill Livingstone Elsevier.

McGuire MB: *Ritual healing in suburban America*, New Brunswick, NJ, 1994, Rutgers University Press.

Micozzi MS: "Medical-legal investigation of death," In Rubin E, Strayer D, editors: *Rubin's textbook of pathology*, Philadelphia, 2014, Wolters Kluwer/Raven Lippincott. (in press).

Moerman DE: *Meaning, medicine and the 'placebo effect'*, 2002, Cambridge University Press.

Montgomery K: *How doctors think: clinical judgment and the practice of medicine*, 2006, Oxford University Press.

Montgomery K: Redescribing biomedicine: toward the integration of East Asian medicine into contemporary healthcare. In Scheid V, MacPherson H, editors: *Integrating East Asian medicine into contemporary healthcare*, Edinburgh, 2012, Churchill Livingstone Elsevier, pp 229-234. Chapter 14.

Mootz RD, Phillips RB: "Chiropractic belief systems". In Cherkin DC, Mootz RD, editors: *Chiropractic in the United States: training, practice, and research*, Rockville, MD, 1997, Agency for Health Care Policy and Research, pp 9-16.

Morgan W: Navajo treatment of sickness; Diagnosticians. In Landy D, editor: *Culture, disease and healing: studies in medical anthropology*, New York, 1977, Macmillan, p 163. (originally published in 1931).

Morris DB: How to speak postmodern: medicine, illness, and cultural change, *Hastings Cent Rep* 30(6):7-16, 2000.

Morrison J: *Book of Ayurveda: a holistic approach to health and longevity*, New York, 1995, Fireside.

Moss D, McGrady A, Davies T, et al: *Handbook of mind-body medicine for primary care*, Thousand Oaks CA, 2002, Sage.

Mullan F: *Big doctoring in America: profiles in primary care*, Berkeley and Los Angeles CA, 2002, University of California Press.

Murdock GP: *Theories of illness: a world survey*, Pittsburgh, 1980, University of Pittsburgh Press.

Nilchaikovit T, HIll JM, Holland JC: The effects of culture on illness behavior and medical care. Asian and American differences, *Gen Hosp Psychiatry* 15(1):41-50, 1993.

O'Connor BB: Hmong cultural values, biomedicine and chronic liver disease. In *Healing traditions, alternative medicine and the health professions*, Philadelphia, 1995, University of Pennsylvania Press.

Ontario Consultants on Religious Tolerance: Jehovah's Witnesses, n.d., Available at http://www.religioustolerance.org. Accessed January 27, 2014.

Ornish D, Scherwitz LW, Billings JH, et al: Intensive lifestyle changes for reversal of coronary heart disease, *JAMA* 280:2001–2007, 1998.

Oschman J: *Energy medicine in therapeutics and human performance,* Philadelphia, 2003, Butterworth-Heinemann.

Oths K: *Healing by hand: a cross-cultural primer for manual therapies,* Walnut Creek CA, 2004, Alta Mira Press.

Ott DA, Cooley DA: Cardiovascular surgery in Jehovah's Witnesses: report of 542 operations without blood transfusion, *JAMA* 238(12):1256–1258, 1977.

Paterson C, Britten N: Acupuncture for people with chronic illness: combining qualitative and quantitative outcome assessment, *J Altern Complement Med* 9(5):671–681, 2003.

Patterson C, Britten N: Acupuncture as a complex intervention: a holistic model, *J Altern Complemen Med* 10(5):791–801, 2004.

Paterson C, Schnyer R: Measuring patient-centred outcomes. In Scheid V, MacPherson H, editors: *Integrating East Asian medicine into contemporary healthcare,* Edinburgh, 2012, Churchill Livingstone Elsevier, pp 77–93. Chapter 5.

Payer L: *Medicine and culture: varieties of treatment in the United States, England, West Germany, and France,* New York, 1988, Penguin.

Permpongkosol S: Iatrogenic disease in the elderly: risk factors, consequences, and prevention, *Clin Interv Aging* 6:77–82, 2011.

Radecki CM, Jaccard J: Psychological aspects of organ donation: a critical review and synthesis of individual and next-of-kin donation decisions, *Health Psychol* 16(2):183–195, 1997.

Reilly D, Taylor MA, Bettie N, et al: Is evidence for homeopathy reproducible? *Lancet* 344(8937):1601, 1994.

Reimansnyder BL: *Powwowing in Union County: a study of Pennsylvania German folk medicine in context,* New York, 1989, AMS Press.

Ross J: *Acupuncture point combinations: the key to clinical success,* Edinburgh, 1995, Churchill Livingstone.

Rubel A, O'Nell CW, Ardon RC: *Susto: a folk illness,* Berkeley, 1984, University of California Press.

Salzman PC, Rice PC: *Thinking anthropologically: a practical guide for students,* ed 3, 2010, Pearson.

Savigny P, Juntze S, Watson P, et al: *Low back pain: early management of persistent non-specific low back pain,* London, 2009, National Collaborating Centre for Primary Care and Royal College of General Practitioners.

Scheid V, MacPherson H, editors: *Integrating East Asian medicine in contemporary healthcare,* Edinburgh, 2012, Churchill Livingstone Elsevier.

Schouten BC, Meeuwesen L: Cultural differences in medical communication: a review of the literature, *Patient Educ Couns* 64 (1–3):21–34, 2006.

Schnyer R: Acupuncture in depression and mental illness. In Cassidy CM, editor: *Contemporary Chinese medicine and acupuncture,* Edinburgh, 2002, Churchill Livingstone.

Schnyer R, Allen J: *Acupuncture in the treatment of depression: a manual for practice and research,* Edinburgh, 2001, Churchill Livingstone.

Schwartz MT I: *Choose life: contemporary medicine and religious practices in the Navajo world,* Norman, 2008, University of Oklahoma Press.

Scott AW: *Masters of the ordinary: integrating personal experience and vernacular knowledge in Alcoholics Anonymous,* doctoral dissertation, Ann Arbor MI, 1993, Michigan Microfilms.

Sears: Sick enough to stay home? *Redbook* 1991.

Shaheen FA, Al-Jondeby M, Kurpad R, Al-Khader AA: Social and cultural issues in organ transplantation in Islamic countries. transplantation, *Ann Transplant* 9(2):11–13, 2004.

Shahjahan R: Standards of education, regulation, and market control: perspectives on complementary and alternative medicine in Ontario, Canada, *J Altern Complement Med* 10:409, 2004.

Shan H, Wang JX, Ren FR, et al: Blood banking in China, *The Lancet* 360(9347):1770–1775, 2002.

Sheldon WH, Hartl EM, McDermott E: *Varieties of delinquent youth: an introduction to constitutional psychiatry,* New York, 1949, Harper & Brothers.

Singelenberg R: The blood transfusion taboo of Jehovah's Witnesses: origin, development and function of a controversial doctrine, *Soc Sci Med* 31(4):515–523, 1990.

Snow LF: *Walkin" over medicine,* Boulder CO, 1993, Westview Press.

Sobo EJ: *One blood: the Jamaican body,* Albany, 1993, State University of New York Press.

Sontag S: *Illness as metaphor,* New York, 1977, Farrar, Straus & Giroux.

Spicer EH, editor: *Ethnic medicine in the southwest,* Tucson, 1979, University of Arizona Press.

Stein HF: *American medicine as culture,* Boulder Co, 1990, Westview Press.

Stux G, Hammerschlag R, editors: *Clinical acupuncture: scientific basis,* Berlin, 2001, Springer.

Takakuwa K, Rubashkin N, Herzig K, editors: *What I learned in medical school: personal stories of young doctors,* 2004, University of California Press.

Targ R, Katra J: *Miracles of mind: exploring nonlocal consciousness and spiritual healing,* Novato CA, 1999, New World Library.

Terrell SJ: *This other kind of doctors: traditional medical systems in black neighborhoods in Austin TX,* New York, 1990, AMS Press.

Tong A, Chapman JR, Wong G, et al: Public awareness and attitudes to living organ donation: systematic review and integrative synthesis, *Transplantation* 96(5):429–437, 2013.

Trotter R, Chavira JA: *Curanderismo: Mexican-American folk healing,* Atlanta, 1997, University of Georgia Press.

Tuck A, Bhui K, Nanchahal K, McKenzie K: Suicide by burning in South Asian origin population in England and Wales: a secondary analysis of a national data set, *BMJ Open* 1(2):e000326, 2011.

Turner E: *The hands feel it: healing and spirit presence among a northern Alaskan people,* DeKalb, 1996, University of Northern Illinois Press.

Unschuld PU: *What is medicine? Western and Eastern approaches to healing,* 2009, University of California Press.

Vejdemo S: Linguistics of temperature, 2010. http://temperature.ling.su.se/index.php/Vejdemo. Accessed February 3, 2014.

Velasquez-Manoff M: *An epidemic of absence: a new way of understanding allergies and autoimmune diseases,* New York, 2012, Scribner.

Verhoef MJ, Lewith G, Ritenbaugh C, et al: Complementary and alternative medicine whole systems research: beyond identification of inadequacies of the RCT, *Complement Ther Med* 13(3):206–212, 2005.

Vithoulkas G: *The science of homeopathy,* New York, 1980, Grove Press.

Walking Thunder, Nickerson KL: *Walking Thunder: Diné medicine woman,* 2001, Ringing Books Press.

Wetherill LW, Leake H: *Wolfkiller: wisdom from a nineteenth century Navajo shepherd*, Layton Utah, 2007, Gibbs Smith, Publisher.

Wirkus M: School of bioenergy, the healing art, *Newslett Int Soc Study Subtle Energies Energy Balance* 4(2):8, 1993.

Wisnesky L, Anderson L: *The scientific basis of integrative medicine*, Boca Raton FL, 2009, CRC Press.

Workshop on Alternative Medicine: *Alternative medicine: expanding medical horizons, Chantilly, Va.*, Report to the National Institutes of Health on Alternative Medical Systems and Practices in the United States, NIH Pub No 94-066, Washington, DC, 1994, US Government Printing Office.

Young D, Ingram G, Swartz L: *Cry of the eagle: encounters with a Cree healer*, Toronto, 1989, University of Toronto Press.

Young JC: *Medical choice in a Mexican village*, New Brunswick, NJ, 1981, Rutgers University Press.

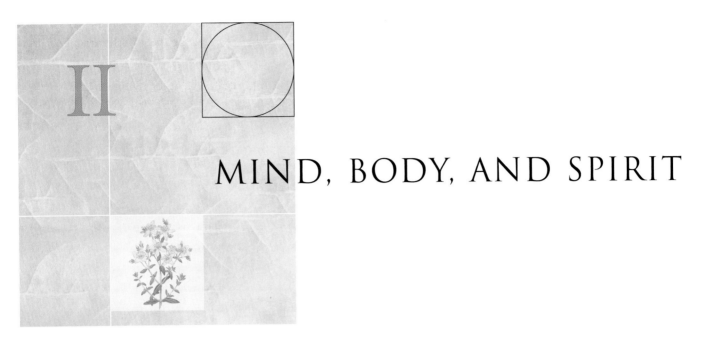

MIND, BODY, AND SPIRIT

Most forms of complementary and alternative medicine can be seen to draw, at least partially or even almost exclusively, on a "mind–body" connection. The complementary medical approaches described in this section explicitly make use of physiological mechanisms by which mental states are reflected in direct biological responses. Likewise, although vital energy, or "bioenergy," is invoked in many complementary modalities and alternative medicine therapies, energy medicine itself uses this energetic property as the sole means and primary mode of cure.

Historically, virtually all phases of Western societies have considered the mind–body-spiritual connection to have an important role in health and healing—extending all the way, literally, to "mind over matter," or mind cure, variations of which remain in practice to this day. Such approaches posit an energy that animates life not subject to explanations that govern inanimate matter. The first chapter in this section reviews this question of "vitalism" from ancient times to the twenty-first century. Ultimately, mind and energy may be reflected in the "consciousness" approach of many complementary and alternative medicine forms of traditional healing.

CHAPTER 6

VITALISM

DAVID F. MAYOR

The basic metaphors of vitalism are present for all of us. Whether they originate in our genes or in our inner, intrauterine, or early life experience; are intellectually molded later on by our sociocultural environments; or are part of our individual energy or thought fields, they are there whether we like it or not. Whether we consider ourselves cool rationalists or hot-blooded intuitives, vitalism remains a pervasive influence. It is sustained in the writing of influential Romantic authors such as Percy Bysshe Shelley (1792-1822), his wife Mary Wollstonecraft Shelley (1797-1851), and Honoré de Balzac, as well as by post-Romantics such as Gustav Meyrink (1868–1932) and D.H. Lawrence (e.g., in *Women in Love*, with its ubiquitous flows of *kundalini*-like "fierce electric energy"). It is difficult even now to find a novel that, in some form or other, does not make use of the language of vitalism, whether consciously or unconsciously.

Folk (medical) traditions from around the world also lay stress on the flow, transmission, and balance of life energies, as for instance in the positive or negative *vibraciones* of *curanderismo* (see Chapter 39). As can be seen from the ubiquity of various forms of vitalism in the many CAM practices discussed in this text, its multivalent possibilities have made it endlessly attractive. Its very imprecision allows for enormous flexibility and adaptability, explanatory models morph and coalesce, and there are

so many strands to its history that it is now probably impossible to disentangle. However, some aspects of vitalism do appear consistently across the various modalities of CAM, more or less in the order shown in Figure 6-1 (a more detailed schema can be found in Mayor & Micozzi [2011]).

In conventional medicine it is sometimes too easy for a person to become a thing, an object, an irrelevant spectator, overwhelmed by a mechanical world of technology, tests, and surgery in which stress may adversely affect self-healing. The vitalist perspective, on the other hand, aligns itself with coherent, life-affirming principles. The vitalist universe is not random, detached, or mindless; it is benign, coherent, and hospitable. Instead of a medicine whose central issues can seem coldly mechanical and buried in inaccessible molecular biology, vitalism instinctively invites a person to experience a unifying, transcendent, and reassuring ontological presence. Whatever the outcome of scientific investigations of vitalist medical traditions, and despite ongoing vociferous protests from pseudo-scientist "quackbusters," vitalism's attractiveness for practitioners and patients is likely to remain a growing presence in health care, provided we can give it the necessary time in our own new and accelerating "axial age." As such, it is part of an increasing awareness of ecology as central to our very survival on this small planet.

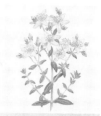

CHAPTER 7

Mind–Body Thought and Practice: Great Britain to Early and Late America

DONALD MCCOWN

MARC S. MICOZZI

Contemplative practice regarding what are now called mind–body approaches dates back to British colonial and early American history and has continued until its resurgence in late, or "postmodern," America. This thinking and practice did not, of course, originate from early physiological or medical studies nor from the current recognition of psychoneuroimmunology in medical science (the topic of the next chapter in this section). Like much of complementary and alternative medicine, it arose in the popular consciousness from nonmedically related cultural and spiritual movements based on experiential and existential (not experimental) thinking, studies, and philosophies. Therefore, as introduced in Chapter 3 and discussed in chapter 5, most of its substance resides outside of what we typically consider medical practice or health care—and our discussion in this chapter takes us well outside the traditional boundaries of medical discourse.

FROM GREAT BRITAIN TO EARLY AND LATE AMERICA

It is possible to trace a European intellectual connection to Asian spiritual thought and practice as early as the ancient Greek histories of Herodotus, Alexander the Great's Indian campaign in 327 to 325 BC (Hodder, 1993), or Petrarch's mention of Hindu ascetics in his *Life of Solitude,* written 1345–1347 (Versluis, 1993). A more substantive start, however, would be 1784, which marks the founding by British scholars and magistrates of the Asiatic Society of Bengal, from which quickly flowed first translations of

Hindu scriptures directly from Sanskrit texts into English. Sir William Jones was the preeminent member of the group. His tireless work included translations of Kalidasa's *Sakuntala* (1789), Jayadeva's *Gitagovinda* (1792), and the influential *Institutes of Hindu Law* (1794). His early tutor in Sanskrit, Charles Wilkins, holds the distinction of making the first translation of the *Bhagavad Gita* (1785). In 1788, the group founded a journal, *Asiatik Researches,* that was widely circulated among the intelligentsia, including the future second U.S. president John Adams, an enthusiastic subscriber (Hodder, 1993; Versluis, 1993). An effect of this flow of scholarly and objective information about Indian culture and religion was the beginning of a profound shift in Western views of the East—"from the earlier presupposition of the East as barbarous and despotic, 'Oriental despotism,' to a vision of an exotic and highly civilized world in its own right" (Versluis, 1993, p 18).

The new language, ideas, images, and narratives embedded in such texts immediately touched something in poets, philosophers, and artists, particularly in England and Germany—powerful influences on the development of American culture. In England, the Romantics embraced all things "Oriental" as a celebration of the irrational and exotic. Their use of the scriptures, stories, lyrics, and images becoming ever more available to them from Hinduism, Buddhism, Confucianism, and Islam was not discrete, but rather an amalgam. Their drive was not for a practical use of these new elements of discourse in expressing some tacit knowledge heretofore inexpressible; to the contrary, as Versluis (1993) notes, "their Orientalism was not serious but rather a matter of exotic settings for poems" (p 29). The confounding of international relations by "Orientalism" (Said, 1978) was a serious consequence.

Johann Gottfreid von Herder, Johann Wolfgang von Goethe, and the Romantics who followed them in Germany found "Oriental" thought a refreshing alternative to the stifling rationality (and then nationality) of their time. Yet, again, their usage of the new raw material that became available was not entirely pragmatic. Their philosophical and poetic insights *could* have been expressed in the preexisting discourse of Christian mysticism, Neo-Platonism, and Hermeticism and the charismatic movement. What the use of Oriental religious discourse by a poet of spiritual power such as Novalis (Freidrich von Hardenberg) did do was to suggest that the full range of Eastern and Western religious expression pointed to a Transcendent (with a capital T) reality, and that all—*in essence*—offered truth (Versluis, 1993). It is this last point that brings us to America, to the Transcendentalists, and, at last, to the pragmatic use of the Eastern discourses to better understand and express a personal tacit knowledge.

AMERICAN BEGINNINGS

In writers such as Ralph Waldo Emerson and Henry David Thoreau, and in the utopian vision of the Transcendentalist Old Concord Farm and other communities, the influence of Eastern thought is evident (Brooks, 1936; Hodder, 1993; Versluis, 1993). Through the *Dial,* the journal that did much to shape American Transcendentalism, they brought out translations of Hindu, Buddhist, and Confucian texts, and of the Sufi poets, such as Hafiz, Rumi, and Saadi. In these "transcendentalations" a new, rich brew began to find ways to give voice to tacit experience.

It is possible to see both Emerson and Thoreau as natural (and learned) contemplatives whose entwined and inter-twined literary and spiritual lives reflect experiences that required a larger discourse than the West provided for more explicit understanding and more elaborated communication.

EMERSON'S IMMERSION

Emerson's early (1836) essay "Nature," written before his deep engagement with Eastern thought, contains a description of such an experience:

> Crossing a bare common, in snow puddles, at twilight, under a clouded sky, without having in my thoughts any occurrence of special good fortune, I have enjoyed a perfect exhilaration. Almost I fear I think how glad I am. In the woods, too, a man casts off his years, as the snake his slough, and at what period so ever of life is always a child. In the woods, is perpetual youth. Within these plantations of God, a decorum and a sanctity reign, a perennial festival is dressed, and the guest sees not how he should tire of them in a thousand years. In the woods, we return to reason and faith. There I feel that nothing can befall me in

life,—no disgrace, no calamity, (leaving me my eyes,) which nature cannot repair. Standing on the bare ground,—my head bathed by the blithe air, and uplifted into infinite space,—all mean egotism vanishes. I become a transparent eye-ball. I am nothing. I see all. The currents of the Universal Being circulate through me; I am part or particle of God.

As Emerson began reading the amalgam of Oriental writings in earnest, which consumed him for the rest of his life, his enterprise became the essentialization (distillation) and integration of the insights that supported his experience and vision on both a personal and a cultural scale. Versluis notes that, "For Emerson . . . the significance of Asian religions—of all human history—consists of assimilation into the present, into this individual here and now" (1993, p 63). He was reading and feeling and thinking his way toward a universal, literally Unitarian religion. (Imagine if the early New England settlers had not provided "commons" as the centerpieces of their settlements, as spiritual practices evolved from Puritanism to Congregationalism to Unitarianism and Universalism.)

LOOKING THROUGH THOREAU

It seems Thoreau had a different enterprise underway, using the same raw materials. Whereas Emerson was grappling with universals and theory to make sense of the larger world, Thoreau was intent that particulars and practice would make sense of his *own* world. Though he had only the translated texts to guide him, he did more than just *imagine* himself as an Eastern contemplative practitioner. He wrote to his friend H.G.O. Blake in 1849, "rude and careless as I am, I would fain practice the yoga faithfully. . . . To some extent, and at rare intervals, even I am a yogin" (quoted in Hodder, 1993, p 412). Thoreau offers descriptions of his experience, such as this from the "Sounds" chapter of *Walden:*

> I did not read books that first summer; I hoed beans. Nay, I often did better than this. There were times when I could not afford to sacrifice the bloom of the present moment to any work, whether of the head or hands. I love a broad margin to my life. Sometimes, in a summer morning, having taken my accustomed bath, I sat in my sunny doorway from sunrise till noon, rapt in a revery, amidst the pines and hickories and sumachs, in undisturbed solitude and stillness, while the birds sang around or flitted noiseless through the house, until by the sun falling in at my west window, or the noise of some traveller's wagon on the distant highway, I was reminded of the lapse of time. I grew in those seasons like corn in the night, and they were for me far better than any work of my hands would have been. They were not time subtracted from my life, but so much over and above my usual allowance. I realized what the Orientals mean by contemplation and the forsaking of works.

Like Emerson, Thoreau read the "Orientals" back into his own experiences, to help express that which was otherwise inexpressible without them. A journal entry from

1851 states, "Like some other preachers—I have added my texts—(derived) from the Chinese and Hindoo scriptures—long after my discourse was written" (quoted in Hodder, 1993, p 434). That original inarticulate discourse of ecstasy in nature was capable of transformation with the insights he found in the translations of Jones and Wilkins. It was the here-and-now value of the new language, images, and stories that counted. An emphasis on the moment-to-moment particulars of nature and his own experience was the central concern of his later life. He became, in his own words, a "self-appointed inspector of snowstorms and rainstorms," which is, perhaps, as cogent a description of an alternative practice as any from the Eastern traditions.

OPENING TO EAST ASIA

Although India and, particularly, Hindu thought had taken the primary place in the discussion so far, America's engagement with the East by the middle of the nineteenth century also included East Asian culture, with Chinese, Korean, and Japanese arts, literature, and religion—including the Buddhism of these areas—shaping the intellectual direction of an emerging American modernism. For example, the work of Ernest Fenollosa, American scholar of East Asian art and literature, and convert to Tendai Buddhism, brought this spirit into wider intellectual discourse (Bevis, 1988; Brooks, 1962). Fenollosa represents a more specific, scholarly, but no less engaged, use of the East by an American. A few lines from Fenollosa's poem "East and West," his Phi Beta Kappa address at Harvard in 1892, reflect a growing need of Western thought for contemplative space. Addressing a Japanese mentor, Fenollosa says, "I've flown from my West / Like a desolate bird from a broken nest / To learn thy secret of joy and rest" (quoted in Brooks, 1962, p 50).

At Fenollosa's death, his widow gave his unpublished studies of the Chinese written language and notebooks of translations from the classical Chinese poet Li Po to the influential American poet Ezra Pound, for whom a whole new world opened. Pound's Chinese translations drawn from Fenollosa's work radically transformed the art of the time. Indeed, Pound had arguably the most powerful influence of any single poet in shaping the poetry, not only of his modernist contemporaries, but of the generation that would come to maturity in the middle of the twentieth century.

Although Pound's use of Eastern influences was mainly stylistic, a very different sort of poet, Wallace Stevens, used his own encounter with the East—studying Buddhist texts and translating Chinese poetry with his friend the scholar poet Witter Bynner—to better understand and express his tacit experience (Bevis, 1988). Perhaps "The Snow Man," an early poem (written in 1908 and first published in 1921), suggests this (Stevens, 1971, p 54).

One can also cite a description of an alternative, meditative stance, using an image from the poet's Connecticut landscape, and rhetoric from his East Asian studies,

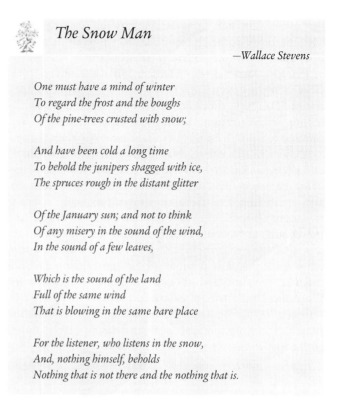

The Snow Man
—Wallace Stevens

One must have a mind of winter
To regard the frost and the boughs
Of the pine-trees crusted with snow;

And have been cold a long time
To behold the junipers shagged with ice,
The spruces rough in the distant glitter

Of the January sun; and not to think
Of any misery in the sound of the wind,
In the sound of a few leaves,

Which is the sound of the land
Full of the same wind
That is blowing in the same bare place

For the listener, who listens in the snow,
And, nothing himself, beholds
Nothing that is not there and the nothing that is.

perhaps. Yet it is possible that this is *also* an articulation of personal experience. Stevens did not study meditation formally, but, like Thoreau, he was a prodigious walker. In any season or weather, a perambulation of 15 miles or so—in a business suit—was a common prelude to writing (Bevis 1988). This practice is neatly captured in a few lines from "Notes for a Supreme Fiction": "Perhaps / The truth depends on a walk around a lake, // A composing as the body tires, a stop / To see hepatica, a stop to watch / A definition growing certain and // A wait within that certainty, a rest / In the swags of pine trees bordering the lake" (Stevens, 1971, p 212).

A transparent eyeball. An inspector of snowstorms. A mind of winter. These are powerful metaphors to describe experiences that sought and found elaboration through encounters with Eastern thought. For these individual authors, there was a willingness to use whatever comes to hand—from whatever culture or tradition suggests itself or is available—to understand what is happening in the here and now. This stance also reflects a perennial American pragmatism, which endures today in much of the discourse of complementary, alternative and "integrative" medicine: Hatha Yoga mixes with Buddhist meditation, whereas Sufi poetry and Native American stories illuminate teaching points, and the expressive language of the Christian and Jewish contemplative traditions hovers in the background.

BUDDHISM AND BIASES

In the same early time frame, a more specific connection to Buddhism began developing, as well. Of the major traditions in the Oriental matrix, Buddhism appears to have been the least understood and the most scorned during the earlier part of the nineteenth century. Reasons include Christian defensiveness and hostile reporting from the mission field; a portrayal of Buddhist doctrines as atheistic, nihilistic, passive, and pessimistic; and even the contagious anti-Buddhist biases of the Hindu scholars themselves who taught Sanskrit to the English translators of the Asiatic Society of Bengal (Tweed, 1992; Versluis, 1993). The "opening" of Japan to the United States in the 1850s commencing with Commodore Matthew Perry's visit, and China, and then subsequent travels, study, and writing of American artists, scholars, and sophisticates, including Ernest Fenollosa, Henry Adams (great-grandson of the aforementioned John Adams), John LaFarge, and Lafcadio Hearn (all had direct contact with Buddhism) did much to increase interest and sympathy for Buddhism. Then, the 1879 publication of *The Light of Asia*, Edwin Arnold's poetic retelling of the life of the Buddha, drawing parallels with the life of Jesus, turned interest into enthusiasm. Sales estimates of between 500,000 and a million copies put it at a level of popularity matching that of, say, *Huckleberry Finn* (Tweed, 1992) by Mark Twain or the number one bestseller of that time, *Ben Hur*, by retired Civil War general and adventurer Lew Wallace.

Buddhism became a new possibility for those at the bare edge of the culture who intuited the tidal shift of Christian believing that Matthew Arnold had poignantly articulated in the final stanzas of "Dover Beach" in 1867.

Dover Beach

The Sea of Faith
Was once, too, at the full, and round earth's shore
Lay like the folds of a bright girdle furled.
But now I only hear
Its melancholy, long, withdrawing roar,
Retreating, to the breath
Of the night-wind, down the vast edges drear
And naked shingles of the world

Ah, love, let us be true
To one another! for the world, which seems
To lie before us like a land of dreams,
So various, so beautiful, so new,
Hath really neither joy, nor love, nor light,
Nor certitude, nor peace, nor help for pain;
And we are here as on a darkling plain
Swept with confused alarms of struggle and flight,
Where ignorant armies clash by night.

And for some, Buddhist belief became a formal identity. Madame Olga Blavatsky and Henry Steele Olcott,

founders of the Theosophical Society (and the alternative practice of Theosophical Medicine), were long engaged with Buddhism. In Ceylon in 1880, they made ritual vows in a Theravada temple to live by the five precepts and take refuge in the Buddha, the teachings, and the community. The most powerful single event, however, was the face-to-face encounter with Buddhist masters afforded by the Parliament of World Religions, particularly the Theravadin Anagarika Dharmapala and the Rinzai Zen Master Soyen Shaku. Both of these teachers continued to raise interest in Buddhism through subsequent visits. In fact, Soyen Shaku bears significant responsibility for the popularization of Buddhism through to the present day. The vision of Buddhism that he presented fit perfectly with the early modern scientific and moral outlooks. The themes he presented—"an embrace of science combined with the promise of something beyond it, and a universal reality in which different religions and individuals participate, but which Buddhism embodies most perfectly" (McMahan, 2002, p 220)—still resonate today. (These themes resonate, for example, with contemporary attempts at reconciliation of ancient, traditional Ayurvedic precepts with quantum mechanics and fundamental particle physics in the re-formulations *of Maharishi Ayurveda*.) Soyen Shaku also had a "second-generation" impact through the 1950s and 1960s, as he encouraged his student and translator for the Parliament visit, the articulate Zen scholar D.T. Suzuki, to maintain a dialogue with the West through visits and writing (McMahan, 2002; Tweed, 1992).

It is important to note that the character of Buddhist "believing" during this period was an engagement with philosophy and doctrine, a search for a replacement for the Judeo-Christian belief system that some felt was no longer sustaining, as with Matthew Arnold's dark vision. Consider that two other Buddhist "bestsellers" besides Arnold's *Light of Asia* were Olcott's *Buddhist Catechism* and Paul Carus's *Gospel of Buddha*, whose titles even reflect a Christian, belief-oriented approach to Buddhism.

In the best Evangelical Protestant tradition comes the story of the first "Buddhist conversion" in America. In Chicago in 1893, Dharmapala was speaking on Buddhism and Theosophy to an overflow crowd in a large auditorium. At the end of the talk, Charles Strauss, a prominent German Swiss-American businessman of Jewish background, stood up from his seat in the audience and walked deliberately to the front. One can imagine the hush and expectancy. As planned in advance, he then—to use an Evangelical Protestant phrase—"accepted" Buddhism, repeating the refuge vows for all to hear (Obadia, 2002; Tweed, 1992).

Belief versus Practice

The connection of most of the 2000 or 3000 Euro-American Buddhists and the tens of thousands of sympathizers at this time (Tweed, 1992) was, with a few exceptions, intellectual. The popular appeal of Buddhism was as a form of

BOX 7-1 *Three Buddhisms in America*

It is important to note that the narrative that shapes the discourse of alternative medical professionals today sidelines the story of ethnic Asian Buddhism in America. Religion scholar Richard Hughes Seager (2002) describes three Buddhisms in America:

1. Old-line Asian American Buddhism, with institutions dating back to the nineteenth century.
2. Euro-American or convert Buddhism, centered in the Westernized forms of Buddhism—often generically parsed as Zen, Tibetan, and Theravada (or Vipassana or Insight), which are centered on meditation practice; and Soka Gakkai International, an American branch of a Japanese group, which, with a rich mix of Asian Americans, Euro-Americans, and substantial numbers of African Americans and Latino Americans, is the most culturally diverse group and is centered on chanting practice rather than meditation.
3. New immigrant or ethnic Buddhism, which is most easily parsed by country of origin.

belief, not as a form of spiritual *practice*. According to Tweed (1992), the fascination with Buddhist believing reached a high-water mark around 1907 and declined precipitously thereafter. A small nucleus of Euro-Americans interested in the academic or personal study of Buddhism maintained organizations and specialized publishing, but few Asian teachers stayed in the United States, and impetus for growth was lost. Dharmapala, in 1921, wrote in a letter to an American supporter, "At one time there was some kind of activity in certain parts of the U.S. where some people took interest in Buddhism, but I see none of that now" (in Tweed, 1992, p 157). Charges by the status quo religious and cultural powers that Buddhism was passive and pessimistic—terrible sins in a culture fueling itself on action and optimism—drowned dissenting Buddhist voices (Box 7-1).

Perhaps it was the separation of philosophy and doctrine, separate from practice, that led to what might be considered a "scientific," rather than a purely theological approach to Buddhism. The "scientific Buddha" is presented in two books by religion scholar, Donald Lopez (*Buddhism and Science: A Guide for the Perplexed*, and *The Scientific Buddha*). Lopez locates the birth of the scientific Buddha right in this wheelhouse of the mid-nineteenth century. The new science (of Darwinian biology) had taken away a traditional way of understanding the world, and Buddhism, presenting itself as scientific, offered a new way of understanding.

Taking a "scientific" approach to cultural and religious beliefs and practices that relate to health and medicine (but are not delimited by them) and more broadly to lifestyle, avocation, and spiritual orientation, continues to present challenges to the contemporary Western medical approach of "integrative medicine" (see Chapter 3).

MEDITATION COMES TO THE MASSES

In the aftermath of World War II, the applications of Eastern thought to Western experience developed a more powerful momentum. Western soldiers and sailors, many drawn from professional life into active duty, were exposed in great numbers to Asian cultures, from India, Burma, and China. In Japan, physicians, scientists, and artists and intellectuals who held posts in the occupation forces under Gen. Douglas MacArthur were exposed to a culture that included the aesthetic, philosophical, and spiritual manifestations of Japanese Buddhism, particularly its Zen varieties. Some stayed to study, and East-West dialogues that had been suspended were resumed, such as with D.T. Suzuki and Shinichi Hisamatsu. Most important for the discourse of mind–body medicine and psychotherapy, American military psychiatrists were exposed to Japanese psychotherapy, particularly that developed by Shoma Morita, which is based on a paradox that had enormous repercussions in Western practice. Instead of attacking symptoms as in Western approaches, Morita asked his patients to allow themselves to turn *toward* their symptoms (consistent with other alternative medical approaches) and fully experience them, to know them as they are (Dryden & Still, 2006; Morita, [1928] 1998).

Morita therapy was of interest and intellectually available to those Westerners in Japan for two powerful reasons. First, it is a highly effective treatment for what Western practitioners would identify as postwar anxiety-based disorders; reports of rates of cure or improvement of more than 90% were common (Morita, [1928] 1998; Reynolds, 1993). Morita developed a diagnostic category of *shinkeishitsu* for the disorders he targeted, which he describes as anxiety disorders with hypochondriasis (Morita, [1928] 1998). Second, Morita did not develop his work in cultural isolation. Working contemporaneously and internationally with French neurologist Charcot, American psychologist William James, Austrian psychiatrist Sigmund Freud, and Swiss psychotherapist Carl Gustav Jung, Morita read, referenced, and critiqued Western developments. He was particularly interested in the therapies that paralleled his own in certain ways, such as Freud's psychoanalysis, Philadelphia neurologist S. Weir Mitchell's nineteenth-century rest therapy (also rest cure, West cure, and nature cure—famously undertaken by a young Teddy Roosevelt), Otto Binswanger's life normalization therapy, and Paul DuBois's persuasion therapy (LeVine, 1998). It all integrated East and West—but from an *Eastern* perspective.

The entire regimen of Morita therapy, a four-stage, intensive, residential treatment has rarely been used in the United States, as is often the case with such therapies (see Chapter 3). David Reynolds (1980, 1993) adapted it and other Japanese therapies for the West and two of its basic insights had immediate and continuing effects. The first is the seeming paradox of turning toward rather than away from symptoms for relief. The second is the insistence on the nondualistic nature, or the unity, of the body and mind. Although the influence of Zen is easily seen in his therapy, Morita did not wish to promote a direct religious association, fearing that the treatment might be seen as somehow less serious, exacting, and effective (LeVine, 1998). Paradoxically, perhaps, it was the Zen connection that actually drew the interest of the Westerners.

Morita Therapy: Mushoju-shin and the Stages of Treatment

In the nutshell version of Morita therapy, the Zen term *mushoju-shin* points to the end, or the beginning. It describes a healthy attention. In Morita's ([1928] 1998) metaphor, it is the attention you have when you are reading while standing on the train. You must balance, hold the book, read, remember the next station, and be aware of others. That is, you cannot focus on any one thing too tightly. You must be willing to be unstable, to be open to whatever happens, and to be able to respond and change freely. In short, you are not "self" focused; rather, mind–body–environment are one. "This is the place from where my special therapy begins" (p. 31), says Morita. It is also the place that Morita therapists are required to inhabit as they work. ✎

First Stage: Isolation and Rest (5 to 7 Days)

Disposition: After careful assessment to ensure safety, patients are isolated and asked to remain in a lying down posture, except to use the bathroom.

Instructions: Experience the anxieties and illusions that arise; let them run their course, without trying to change or stop them.

Purpose: There is a Zen saying that if you try to eliminate a wave with another wave, all you get is more waves, more confusion. This becomes clear.

Second Stage: Light Occupational Work (5 to 7 Days)

Disposition: Isolation is maintained; there is no conversation or distractions. Sleep is restricted to seven or eight hours a night. Patients must be working during the day, and may not return to the room to rest.

Instructions: Move gently into mental and physical activity again, tidying the yard by picking up sticks and leaves, and moving into more effortful activities over time. Allow physical and mental discomfort to be just as it is.

Purpose: Break down the "feeling-centered attitude" by de-emphasizing judgments of comfort and discomfort and promoting spontaneous activity of mind and body.

Third Stage: Intensive Occupational Work (5 to 7 days)

Disposition: Same as in stage two.

Instructions: Patients are assigned more strenuous labor, such as chopping wood and digging holes, and are encouraged to do art or craft projects that please them and to be spontaneous.

Purpose: Learn to be patient and to endure work, build self-confidence, and own their subjective experiences.

Fourth Stage: Preparation for Daily Living (5 to 7 days)

Disposition: Patients may interact purposefully with others but not to speak of their own experience, and may leave the hospital grounds for errands.

Instructions: The work and activities are not chosen by the patient.

Purpose: Learn to adjust to changes in circumstances; to not be attached to personal preferences. Prepare for return to the natural rhythms of living.

MEDITATIVE THOUGHT IN POST-WWII AMERICA: FROM A TO ZEN

Zen had a double-barreled influence in America, particularly in the postwar "Zen boom" years of the 1950s and 1960s, touching both the intellectual community and the popular culture. With the first barrel, it had significant impact on the serious discourse of scholars, professionals, artists, and Western religious thinkers. One person was so profoundly influential in conveying the spirit of Zen that he epitomizes this impact: D.T. Suzuki. As a young man, you will remember, Suzuki had played a role in the Buddhist enthusiasm of the 1890s and 1900s as translator for Soyen Shaku. Suzuki had then lived for a time in the United States, working for Open Court, a publishing company specializing in Eastern thought, and had married an American woman. After the war, Suzuki returned to the West, where he continued to write books of both scholarly and popular interest on Zen and Pure Land Buddhism, traveled and lectured extensively in the United States and Europe, maintained a voluminous correspondence, and affected an incredibly varied range of thinkers. Three short examples involving Thomas Merton, John Cage, and Eric Fromm give a glimpse into the wide-ranging effects of Suzuki's Zen on intellectual discourse.

The Trappist monk Thomas Merton was greatly influenced by Suzuki's work—which he had first known in the 1930s before entering the monastery. An engagement with Eastern religious and aesthetic thought—particularly Zen, and particularly through Suzuki's work—shaped Merton's conception and practice of contemplative prayer, which has had a powerful influence on Christian spiritual practice to the present day (e.g., Merton, 1968; Pennington, 1980). Merton began a correspondence with Suzuki in 1959, asking him to write a preface for a book of translations of the sayings of the "Desert Fathers." Merton's superiors felt such collaboration in print was "inappropriate," yet in practice, they encouraged Merton to continue the dialogue with Suzuki, once telling him, "Do it, but don't preach it" (Mott, 1984, p 326). This *practice without preaching* stance represented a reversal of the earlier Buddhist fusion of *belief without practice*. The dialogue did indeed continue, with each endeavoring to explore and understand Christianity and Zen from their own perspectives. The relationship meant so much to Merton that, although his vocation had kept him cloistered in the Monastery of Gethsemane in Kentucky from 1941, he sought and gained permission from his abbot to meet Suzuki in New York City in 1964, Merton's first travel in 23 years (Merton, 1968; Mott, 1984; Pennington, 1980). Suzuki summed up the burden of their two long talks this way: "The most important thing is Love" (Mott, 1984, p 399).

The composer John Cage, who was deeply influenced by Hindu, Buddhist, and Daoist philosophy and practice, regularly attended Suzuki's lectures at Columbia University in the 1950s. His statement that in choosing to study with Suzuki he was choosing the elite—"I've always gone—insofar as I could—to the president of the company" (Duckworth, 1999, p 21)—suggests the value of Suzuki's thought to him and to much of the *avant garde*. The Zen influence on Cage's work is captured in his conception of his compositions as "purposeless play" that is "not an attempt to bring order out of chaos, nor to suggest improvements in creation, but simply to wake up to the very life we are living, which is so excellent once one gets one's mind and desires out of the way and lets it act of its own accord" (Cage, 1966, p 12). Suzuki's expansive sense of play is reported by Cage in an anecdote: "An American lady said, 'How is it, Dr. Suzuki? We spend the evening asking you questions and nothing is decided.' Dr. Suzuki smiled and said, 'That's why I love philosophy: no one wins'" (Cage 1966, p 40).

THE BIRTH OF "WELLNESS"

The psychoanalyst Erich Fromm (author of *Escape from Freedom,* about the attraction of fascism before and during World War II) was one of many in the psychoanalytic community of the time to be drawn to Zen and Suzuki's exposition of it. At a conference held in Mexico in 1957 entitled "Zen Buddhism and Psychoanalysis" and attended by about 50 psychoanalytically inclined psychiatrists and psychologists, Suzuki was a featured speaker and engaged in dialogue particularly with Fromm and the religion scholar Richard DeMartino. A book of the lectures was published after the conference (Fromm et al, 1960). Fromm suggests that psychoanalysis and Zen both offer an answer to the suffering of contemporary people: "The alienation from oneself, from one's fellow man, and from nature; the awareness that life runs out of one's hand like sand, and that one will die without having lived; that one lives in the midst of plenty and yet is joyless" (p 86). The answer, then, would not be a cure that removes symptoms, but rather *"the presence of well being"* (p 86; Fromm's italics).

Fromm defines *well being* as:

> to be fully born, to become what one potentially is; it means to have the full capacity for joy and for sadness or, to put it still differently, to awake from the half-slumber the average man lives in, and to be fully awake. If it is all that, it means also to be creative; that is, to react and respond to myself, to others, to everything that exists. (p 90)

This definition takes us well beyond the bounds of what would traditionally be considered the province of medical practice, or the "health care system," although the old psychoanalysis and the "new" mind–body approaches addressed in this section also take us there.

For Fromm, the work was not just to bring the unconscious into consciousness, as Freud suggested, but rather to heal the rift between the two. What was most intriguing for Fromm in the possibilities Zen offered for such a project was *koan* practice—the use of paradoxical or nonrational questions, statements, and stories to back the student's ego-bound intellect against a wall, until the only way out is through. This process of amplifying the root contradiction of ego-consciousness, leading to its overturning—*satori,* or enlightenment—was the subject of DeMartino's contribution to the conference and book. Fromm drew a parallel between this process and the work of the analyst, suggesting that the analyst should not so much interpret and explain, but rather should:

> take away one rationalization after another, one crutch after another, until the patient cannot *escape* any longer, and instead breaks through the fictions which fill his mind and experiences reality—that is, becomes conscious of something he was not conscious of *before.* (p 126)

Love, play, and well-being: it was not just Suzuki's erudition that attracted so many, it was his embodiment of what he taught. Alan Watts, the scholar-entertainer to whom we shall turn next, who got to know Suzuki at the Buddhist Lodge in London in the 1920s, described him as "about the most gentle and enlightened person I have ever known; for he combined the most complex learning with utter simplicity. He was versed in Japanese, English, Chinese, Sanskrit, Tibetan, French, Pali, and German, but while attending a meeting at the Buddhist Lodge he would play with a kitten, looking right into its Buddha nature" (Watts, 1972). Suzuki should have a few words here on his own way of being, and what he wished to communicate to others:

> We cannot all be expected to be scientists, but we are so constituted by nature that we can all be artists—not, indeed, artists of special kinds, such as painters, sculptors, musicians, poets, etc., but artists of life. This profession, "artist of life" may sound new and quite odd, but in point of fact, we are all born artists of life and, not knowing it, most of us fail to be so and the result is that we make a mess of our lives, asking, "What is the meaning of life?" "Are we not facing blank nothingness?" "After living seventy-eight, or even ninety years, where do we go? Nobody knows," etc.,

etc. I am told that most modern men and women are neurotic on this account. But the Zen-man can tell them that they have all forgotten that they are born artists, creative artists of life, and that as soon as they realize this fact and truth they will all be cured of neurosis or psychosis or whatever name they have for their trouble. (Fromm et al, 1960, p 15)

Certainly, such a vision of unfettered creativity and immediate relief from the pains of living would be resonant in postwar American culture.

It should be noted, however, that in the 1950s and 1960s, despite his tremendous stature, Suzuki was also criticized—accused by the ivory tower, *academic* Buddhist community of being a reductionist "popularizer" of Zen and also dismissed by the *practice* community as one who did not sit in meditation with enough discipline and regularity. On the one hand, these may be valid charges, yet on the other, they may be the significant reasons for Suzuki's influence. This was a time when Western intellectuals were in search of new rhetoric and new philosophy to help express and ground their shifting experiences and intuitions; for many, it was a time of wide-ranging dialogue, of exploring possibilities, of framing a debate, rather than a time of grounding, of digging in, of focus on details. Indeed, the charges might simply be moot, when Suzuki's enterprise is cast in the mode of his teacher Soyen Shaku, or even the mode of Ralph Waldo Emerson, of attempting to universalize spiritual experience. In his dialogue with Christian mysticism, for example, Suzuki (1957) found it possible that "Christian experiences are not after all different from those of the Buddhist" (p 8).

A 60s WATTS LIGHT

Just as Suzuki epitomized the intellectual reach of the Zen boom, it may be possible to capture the more popular facets of the time and continue the story through the 1960s by focusing on a single character: the transplanted Englishman Alan Watts. Watts's eccentric career as a scholar-entertainer travels a ragged "arc" from the 1930s to the early 1970s, along the way touching most of the important figures and movements in the meeting of Eastern and Western religious thought and practice, particularly as they offered insights that could be used in psychotherapy. The arc described here is drawn with the help of his autobiography, *In My Own Way* (1972), whose punning title suggests the paradox of sustaining a powerful public self to earn a living while simultaneously discussing the dissolution of the ego, and Monica Furlong's feet-of-clay biography, whose original title, *Genuine Fake* (1986), carries an ambiguous truth.

An intellectually precocious and sensitive religious seeker, Watts spent his early years at King's School, Canterbury, which is next to the ancient cathedral. There, the history-steeped atmosphere and rich liturgical expression cast a spell and created a love of ritual that never left him. In his adolescent years at the school, he developed an interest in Buddhism, which he was able to defend on a very high level in debates with faculty. He wrote to Christmas Humphries, the great promoter of Buddhism and Theosophy, and the founder of the Buddhist Lodge in London, who assumed the letters were from a faculty member. When they finally met, Humphries became a mentor, providing guidance for reading and practice, and connecting Watts to other Asian scholars, including D.T. Suzuki. By 1935, having foregone an Oxford University scholarship to study what appealed to him, Watts published his first book, written at age 19, *The Spirit of Zen,* which was almost a guidebook to the densities of Suzuki's *Essays on Zen.* As Watts's studies expanded, he came to read and write Chinese at a scholarly level, and he read deeply in Daoism, as well as Vedanta, Christian mysticism, and Jung's psychology.

Through the Buddhist Lodge, he met a mother and her adolescent daughter, Ruth Fuller Everett and Eleanor. Ruth had been a member of the "ashram-cum-zoo," as Watts called it, of Pierre Bernard—known as "Oom the Magnificent"—who catered to New York society ladies by teaching Hatha Yoga and Tantrism. Through that association, Ruth learned of Zen Buddhism and, taking Eleanor as a traveling companion, set off for Japan. The two became the first Western women to sit in meditation in a Zen monastery. Years later, Ruth married a Zen teacher and eventually became a teacher herself. Watts and Eleanor courted, in a way, and attended meditation sessions together.

Watts's "practice" at the time was simply to be *in the present moment,* learned from the independent spiritual teachers J. Krishnamurti (who called it "choiceless awareness") and G.I. Gurdjieff (who called it "constant self-remembering"). He was becoming frustrated with his inability to concentrate on the present and discussed this with Eleanor on their walk home from a session at the Buddhist Lodge. Eleanor said, "Why try to concentrate on it? What else is there to be aware of? Your memories are all in the present, just as much as the trees over there. Your thoughts about the future are also in the present, and anyhow I just love to think about the future. The present is just a constant flow, like the Tao, and there's simply no way of getting out of it" (Watts, 1972, p 152–153). That was *it.* He came to think of this stance as his true way of life and continued to practice in this way in various guises throughout his lifetime.

The couple married and moved to the United States, just ahead of the war in Europe. After all his resistance and protest, at this point in his development Watts felt drawn to try to fit himself into a vocation that made sense in the West. With his rich Anglican background, the logical choice was the priesthood of the Episcopal Church. Although he had no undergraduate degree, Watts proved the depth of his learning and entered Seabury-Western Seminary in Chicago for a two-year course of study. In his second year, his standing was so far advanced that he was excused from classes and undertook expansive theological reading in personal tutorials. His research resulted in the book *Behold the Spirit,* which brought insights from the

Eastern religions into profound dialogue with a Christianity he painted as in need of refreshment. Reviewers in and outside the church greeted it warmly. Ordained, he was made chaplain of Northwestern University, where his feeling for ritual, his skills as a speaker, and his ability to throw a great party brought quick success. Yet tensions in his growing family and his own tendency for excess ended his career; the church in 1950 did not take affairs and divorce lightly.

With a new wife and no job, Watts's prospects were indeed uncertain as he began work on a new book, *The Wisdom of Insecurity* (1951). An influential friend, mythologist Joseph Campbell, managed to get Watts a grant from the Bollingen Foundation, funded by one of C.G. Jung's wealthy patients, to support research on myth, psychology, and Oriental philosophy. The book, fueled perhaps by the indigence and indignities of his situation, brought him to the directness and clarity of expression that characterize his work from then on. Here is a description of working with pain by trusting that the mind "has give and can absorb shocks like water or a cushion" (p 96):

> How does the mind absorb suffering? It discovers that resistance and escape—the "I" process—is a false move. The pain is inescapable, and resistance as a defense only makes it worse; the whole system is jarred by the shock. Seeing the impossibility of this course, it must act according to its nature—remain stable and absorb.
>
> . . . Seeing that there is no escape from the pain, the mind yields to it, absorbs it, and becomes conscious of just pain without any "I" feeling it or resisting it. It experiences pain in the same complete, unselfconscious way in which it experiences pleasure. Pain is the nature of this present moment, and I can only live in this moment.
>
> . . . This, however, is not an experiment to be held in reserve, as a trick, for moments of crisis. . . . This is not a psychological or spiritual discipline for self-improvement. It is simply being aware of this present experience, and realizing that you can neither define it nor divide yourself from it. There is no rule but "Look!"(Watts, 1951, pp 97–99)

In no time, Watts landed on his feet, invited into a position at the founding of the American Academy of Asian Studies in San Francisco, a precursor of today's California Institute of Integral Studies. He also landed in creative ferment. Instead of business people and diplomatic and government officials learning Asian languages and culture that had been the students anticipated, the academy drew artists, poets, and religious and philosophical thinkers open to the kind of exploration for which Watts and his faculty colleagues had prepared their whole lives. Students included the Beat poet Gary Snyder, with whom Watts struck up a deep friendship; Michael Murphy and Richard Price, who would found *Esalen Institute;* and Locke McCorkle, who would become a force in *est* (Erhard Seminars Training).

As Watts added administrative duties to his teaching, he brought in a wide range of guest lecturers: old friends such as D.T. Suzuki; his ex-mother-in-law, Ruth Fuller Sasaki,

who spoke on Zen *koan* practice; Pali scholar G.P. Malalasekera; Theravada Buddhist monks Pannananda and Dharmawara; and the Zen master Asahina Sogen. As the academy found its place in the community, local connections were made with Chinese and Japanese Buddhists. Through the academy, the Zen master Shunryu Suzuki came to understand the need for a Western Zen institution, later creating the San Francisco Zen Center. Watts himself spoke and gave workshops up and down the West Coast and began a relationship with the Berkeley radio station KPFA, the first community-funded station in the United States, broadcasting regularly and appearing as well on the educational public television station KQED. He was stirring what was fermenting and that would soon distill itself as a kind of renaissance.

AND THE BEAT GOES ON

The core of the Beat writers coalesced for a moment in 1956 in San Francisco, and Jack Kerouac captured it in his novel *The Dharma Bums* (1958). Its central character is the poet and Zen student Japhy Ryder (Gary Snyder), whom the narrator Ray Smith (Kerouac) idolizes for his "Zen lunatic" lifestyle, combining Zen discipline and aesthetics with freewheeling sensuality. One scene in the novel recounts the Six Gallery poetry reading, at which Snyder, Philip Whalen, Michael McClure, and Philip Lamantia read, and Allen Ginsberg's incantation of *Howl* did, indeed, scream for a generation about the agonies of 1950s fear and conformity (and fear of conformity, and conformity as a form of dealing with fear). *The Dharma Bums,* coming fast on the heels of Kerouac's bestselling *On the Road* (1957), drew a huge readership of the young and aspiring hip, who saw in Ryder/Snyder a new template for living, a chance to go beyond the confines of suburban expectations. This work helped fuel the Zen boom from the popular culture side, prompting complaints from the Western Zen community of practitioners and academics about the authenticity of the Beats' Buddhism. Both the popular and elite outlooks drew a chastening commentary from Watts in his essay "Beat Zen, Square Zen, and Zen" ([1958] 1960), as he showed that their differences arose from the same fundamental background and impulse:

> The Westerner who is attracted to Zen and who would understand it deeply must have one indispensable qualification: he must understand his own culture so thoroughly that he is no longer swayed by its premises unconsciously. He must really have come to terms with the Lord God Jehovah and with his Hebrew-Christian conscience so that he can take it or leave it without fear or rebellion. He must be free of the itch to justify himself. Lacking this, his Zen will be either "beat" or "square," either a revolt from the culture and social order or a new form of stuffiness and respectability. For Zen is above all the liberation of the mind from conventional thought, and this is something utterly different from rebellion against convention, on the one hand, or adapting to foreign conventions, on the other. (p 90)

Watts, already a friend and admirer of Snyder, whom he exempted from his criticisms due to Snyder's level of Zen scholarship and practice, soon came to count the rest of the Beats as friends and accepted many of them as "serious artists and disciplined yogis" (Watts, 1972, p 358). He had connections to many seemingly disparate worlds. There were old guard spiritual seekers, like his expatriate British friend Aldous Huxley (*Brave New World*); members of the highest circles of art, music, and literature; Asian meditation teachers from many different traditions and cultures; psychotherapists of every stripe; and the old guard bohemians, the Beats, and the students. All of whom, as the 1960s began, would come together to create a culture into which Watts was not fitted, but had built.

A catalyst of the new culture in the revolutionary 1960s was the beginning of experimentation with lysergic acid diethylamide (LSD) and other psychedelic drugs in the 1950s, and the publicity surrounding it. Aldous Huxley's descriptions of his experiences in *The Doors of Perception* (1954) were illuminating, but for Watts, it was about embodiment—that his once ascetic and severe "Manichean" friend had been transformed into a more sensuous and warm man made the promise real. Watts's own controlled experiments, in which he found his learning and understanding of the world's mystical traditions and meditative practices extremely helpful, resulted in powerful experiences, followed (inevitably) by enthusiastic essays and broadcasts, as well as by a book, *Joyous Cosmology: Adventures in the Chemistry of Consciousness* (1962).

Watts's position as a proponent of these drugs for experienced, disciplined explorers of consciousness helped fan an interest—the more so when Watts coincidentally was given a two-year fellowship at Harvard just as Timothy Leary and Richard Alpert (later Ram Das) were beginning their engagement with psychedelics there. The spread of psychedelics beyond the specialists added a key facet to what Roszak in 1969 dubbed the "counterculture":

> It strikes me as obvious beyond dispute, that the interests of our college-age and adolescent young in the psychology of alienation, oriental mysticism, psychedelic drugs, and communitarian experiments comprise a cultural constellation that radically diverges from values and assumptions that have been in the mainstream of our society since at least the Scientific Revolution of the seventeenth century. (quoted in Furlong, 1986, p 143)

ZEN, BEAT AND BOOM

Just as the 1950s Zen boom can be captured in the Fromm-Suzuki meeting in Mexico in 1957, the 1960s can, perhaps, be captured in a meeting ten years later—admittedly much larger—the "Human Be-In" at the polo field in Golden Gate Park, San Francisco, in 1967. A procession led by Snyder, Ginsberg, and Watts, among others, circumambulated the field as in a Hindu or Buddhist rite to open the day. Tens of thousands found their way there, dressed in colorful finery, raising banners, "dropping acid," listening to the Grateful Dead, Jefferson Airplane, and Quicksilver Messenger Service, and "digging" the mix of the crowd—Timothy Leary and Richard Alpert, political radical Jerry Rubin, Zen master Shunryu Suzuki, and activist-comedian Dick Gregory suggest the organizers' intention to unify "love and activism." The be-in became a model for gatherings around the United States and the world. The color, light, and promise of the day were slickly captured by Paul Kantner of Jefferson Airplane in "Won't You Try / Saturday Afternoon" (Kantner 1967). The soaring harmonies and instrumental arrangement convey a fuller experience.

And another shift had already begun. At the leading edge of cultural change, seekers had learned what was to be learned from psychedelic experience and were turning toward the practice of meditation. As Watts (1972) put it in his unique blend of the pontifical and the plain, "When one has received the message, one hangs up the phone" (p 402). Where an infrastructure for teaching and practice of Zen Buddhism already existed, such as in San Francisco, seekers turned in that direction, following Watts and Snyder. Another infrastructure had also been building, since 1959, using a mass marketing model to encompass much of the Western world: the Maharishi Mahesh Yogi's Transcendental Meditation (TM). This was an adaptation of Hindu mantra meditation for Western practitioners, in which the meditator brought the mind to a single pointed focus by repeating a word or phrase—in TM, the mantra was secret, potently exotic, and "specially chosen" for the meditator (Johnston, 1988; Mahesh, Yogi 1968). The Beatles, among many other celebrities, discovered (or were "recruited" into) TM in 1967, which not coincidentally brought it to prominence on the world stage. (When the Beatles invited one of the Hindu yogis to visit London, he responded, "London? I am London.") The connection seemed direct.

Perhaps the psychedelic experience linked more directly to Hindu meditation than to Zen, as well. Watts (1972) describes this view from his own experience:

> LSD had brought me into an undeniably mystical state of consciousness. But oddly, considering my absorption in Zen at the time, the flavor of these experiences was Hindu rather than Chinese. Somehow the atmosphere of Hindu mythology slid into them, suggesting at the same time that Hindu philosophy was a local form of a sort of undercover wisdom, inconceivably ancient, which everyone knows at the back of his mind but will not admit. (p 399)

TM was able aggressively to take advantage of the publicity available to it. In 1965, there were 350 TM meditators in the United States, and by 1968, there were 26,000; by 1972, there were 380,000; and by 1976, there were 826,000. (Later, Deepak Chopra was able to vault onto the *New York Times* bestseller list with appropriated ancient Ayurvedic wisdom by asking each of the TM meditators to buy 10 copies of his first book during one week.)

The TM marketing strategy targeted specific populations, giving the practice and its benefits a spiritual spin, a political change spin, or a pragmatic self-help spin depending on the target. The pragmatic approach, designed to reach the middle-class, middle-management heart of the market, was given impetus through scientific research into TM's physical and psychological outcomes (e.g., Seeman et al, 1972; Wallace, 1970), which subsequently captured the attention of the medical establishment. The result was development of and research on medicalized versions, such as the relaxation response (Benson, 1975) and clinical standardized meditation (Carrington, 1998) (see Chapter 10). The factors at work here—translation into Western language and settings, popular recognition, adoption within scientific research in powerful institutions, and the use of sophisticated marketing and public relations techniques—represent a model for success in the building of new social movements (Johnston, 1988).

On both the substantive and popular levels, then, the market for Eastern and Eastern-inflected spiritual practices grew steadily. Looking from 1972 back to himself in 1960, Watts provides perspective on this growth:

> In my work of interpreting Oriental ways to the West I was pressing a button in expectation of a buzz, but instead there was an explosion. Others, of course, were pressing buttons on the same circuit, but I could not have believed—even in 1960—that [there would be] a national television program on yoga, that numerous colleges would be giving courses on meditation and Oriental philosophy for undergraduates, that this country would be supporting thriving Zen monasteries and Hindu *ashrams,* that the *I Ching* would be selling in hundreds of thousands, and that—wonder of wonders—sections of the Episcopal church would be consulting me about contemplative retreats and the use of mantras in liturgy. (1972, p 359)

At the turn of the decade of the 1960s, through political dislocations, waves of immigration, and economic opportunism, new teachers from many of the Eastern traditions became available to offer instruction in the West. At the same time, Westerners of the post–World War II cohort who studied in the East, or with Eastern teachers in the West, began to find their own approaches and voices for teaching as well.

The decade of the 1970s was a time of institution building on an unprecedented scale, a time in which, for example, Buddhism in America took its essential shape. Watts only flashed on this institutionalization, only saw this promised land from afar. He died in 1973, at age 58, of a heart attack. His health had been in decline for some time, due to overwork and problems with alcohol. And in that, his example was again prophetic—foreshadowing the revelations in the 1980s of many spiritual teachers' feet of clay.

GOING A LONG WAY TO FIND WHAT WAS LEFT AT HOME

The injunctions to relieve suffering and to live a more integrated, creative life by paying attention to what is arising in the present moment and turning toward discomfort—mindfulness (Figure 7-1) and acceptance—are also easily

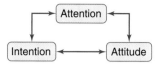

Figure 7-1 Three axioms of mindfulness: attention, attitude and intention. **Defining mindfulness:** With all the history of this chapter as background, Jon Kabat-Zinn, developer of Mindfulness-Based Stress Reduction (MBSR), a highly researched and extremely popular intervention in medicine and mental health care, offhandedly defined mindfulness as "paying attention in a particular way: on purpose, in the present moment, and non-judgmentally" (McCown et al 2009, Kabat-Zinn, 1994, p 4). The scientific community, as it continues to wrestle with defining and operationalizing mindfulness for research, is influenced by this basic tripartite structure. An influential proposed definition uses three axioms of mindfulness—Intention, Attention, and Attitude (IAA). These three are not engaged in any order or sequence; rather, they are engaged simultaneously in the process of mindfulness, as shown above (Shapiro et al, 2006). (From McCown D, Micozzi M, 2012, *New world mindfulness: from the founding fathers, Emerson and Thoreau to your daily practice,* Rochester, VT: Healing Arts Press/Inner Traditions, with permission.)

located within the three Abrahamic religions, the ones closest to home. But the encrustation of tradition and the carelessness of familiarity hide them quite well.

In Judaism, there is the marvelous text from Ecclesiastes (3:1–8), given here in the King James Version, which may ring in your ears to the tune "To everything, turn, turn, turn" and the motion of the chorus of the song by Pete Seeger.

> To every thing there is a season, and a time to every purpose under the heaven: a time to be born, and a time to die; a time to plant, and a time to pluck up that which is planted; a time to kill, and a time to heal; a time to break down, and a time to build up; a time to weep, and a time to laugh; a time to mourn, and a time to dance; a time to cast away stones, and a time to gather stones together; a time to embrace, and a time to refrain from embracing; a time to get, and a time to lose; a time to keep, and a time to cast away; a time to rend, and a time to sew; a time to keep silence, and a time to speak; a time to love, and a time to hate; a time of war, and a time of peace.

There is also the tradition that everything should be blessed. Indeed, when one hears good news the blessing traditionally said is, "Blessed are you G-d, Sovereign of the Universe (who is) good and does good." On hearing bad news such as the death of a friend or relative one says, "Blessed are you G-d, Sovereign of the Universe, true judge." Such blessings acknowledge G-d as the source of everything, good or bad (Kravitz, 2008). In Christianity, the natural mode for many is to do for others, to focus outward. This "Letter to a Christian Lady" from C.G. Jung (who had carved over the doorway of his home in Zurich, "summoned or unsummoned, G-d will be there"), which was made into a text for speaking by Jean Vanier (2005, pp 63–64), is a refreshing corrective:

> I admire Christians,
> because when you see someone who is hungry or thirsty,
> You see Jesus.
> When you welcome a stranger, someone who is "strange,"
> you welcome Jesus.
> When you clothe someone who is naked, you clothe Jesus.
> What I do not understand, however,
> is that Christians never seem to recognize Jesus
> in their own poverty.
> You always want to do good to the poor outside you
> and at the same time you deny the poor person
> living inside you.
> Why can't you see Jesus in your own poverty,
> in your own hunger and thirst?
> In all that is "strange" inside you:
> in the violence and the anguish that are beyond your control!
> You are called to welcome all this, not to *deny* its existence,
> but to accept that it is there and to met Jesus *there*.

The Christian contemplative teacher Richard Rohr (1999) suggests that, for him, Jesus' refusal of the drugged wine as he hung on the cross is a model of a radical acceptance of what is happening in the moment (Box 7-2).

Growth and definition of Buddhism in America occurred as a great variety of teaching and practice became available that more palatable. The turn away from psychedelic culture to more disciplined and thoughtful practice began as the 1960s waned. There was a range of Eastern and Western teachers in Hindu, Buddhist, Sufi, and the independent and occult traditions. There were new takes on Western traditions such as the Jesus People or "Jesus Freak" manifestation of Christianity, and the resurgence of interest in the mysticism of Kabbalah in Judaism. Yet, in tracing the discourse of mindfulness, by far the most influential tradition was Buddhism. This turn-of-the-decade moment is a fruitful place to focus, as all of the elements at play today came into view.

A TIME FOR GROWTH

This was a time of growth. For example, the San Francisco Zen Center, which had been started for Western students under the teaching of Shunryu Suzuki Roshi in 1961, expanded in 1967 to include a country retreat center at Tassajara Hot Springs, for which more than a thousand people had contributed money; and by 1969, the center had moved to larger quarters in the city and had established a series of satellite locations. The Zen presence was the most well established in the United States, whereas Tibetan and Theravada-derived teaching and practice infrastructures were in earlier developmental stages. It is

BOX 7-2 *Rumination by Sufi Poet Rumi*

The Sufi poet Rumi makes the injunction for acceptance come alive in "The Guest House," a poem translated by Coleman Barks (1995, p 109), which has become a very common teaching:

This being human is a guest house.
Every morning a new arrival.

A joy, a depression, a meanness,
some momentary awareness comes
as an unexpected visitor.

Welcome and entertain them all!
Even if they are a crowd of sorrows,
who violently sweep your house
empty of its furniture,
still, treat each guest honorably.
He may be clearing you out
for some new delight.

The dark thought, the shame, the malice,
meet them at the door laughing and invite them in.

Be grateful for whatever comes,
because each has been sent
as a guide from beyond.

For further exploration of Sufism and healing, see Chapter 33.

these three traditions, generalized, that represent the shape that Buddhism in America has taken. There were again three different types of Buddhism in America as there had been one hundred years before.

However, the task of characterizing and defining something that could be called *American Buddhism* is an enormous task, because it requires the parsing of, at a minimum, two phenomena under that title. Prebish (1999) suggests that identifying two divisions approximating "Asian immigrant Buddhism" and "American convert Buddhism" can be informative; it should be noted, however, that there is considerable disagreement among researchers about how and if such distinctions can be made. For our purposes it might reasonably be said that the former group is more interested in preserving religious and community traditions, whereas the latter is more interested in transforming religious traditions for an elite population.

American convert Buddhism is not a mass movement, but is the preserve of an elite. It is also an extremely important factor in the development of the popularity of alternative medicine. The group is highly educated, economically advantaged, politically and socially liberal, and overwhelmingly of European descent. This was also true of the crowd at the World Parliament of Religions in 1893, as it was of the students and intellectuals who made the shift from psychedelic experience to meditative experience. And it is now true of the medical, mental health care, and other professionals exploring the roots of alternative medicine. Indeed, there is a continuity not just of types, but of persons (Coleman, 2001; Nattier, 1998).

The signal characteristic of the American converts is a focus on meditation, almost to the exclusion of other forms of Buddhist practice and expression (Prebish, 1999). It is not surprising, then, that the expressions of world Buddhism they have "imported" for their use (as Nattier, 1998, would characterize it) are the meditation-rich Zen, Tibetan, and Theravada-derived traditions. A quick overview of the development and essential practice of each in the United States may be of value.

BOOMS AND ECHOES

Zen was the first wave and the "boom" of Buddhism in America. In keeping with the elite nature of American interest, the highly aristocratic Rinzai sect, represented by Soyen Shaku and D.T. Suzuki, was influential until the 1960s. Rinzai emphasizes *koan* practice leading to *satori* or kensho—concentrating on a paradoxical question or story to heighten intensity and anxiety (suspense) until a breakthrough occurs. This technique is central in the dialogues of D.T. Suzuki, Fromm, and DeMartino, for example. In the 1960s, however, the more popular Soto Zen sect began to reach beyond the Japanese American communities to American converts. Two of the most important figures in this shift and in the development of Buddhism in America, are from this community: Shunryu Suzuki and Taizan Maezumi. Maezumi Roshi founded the Zen Center of Los Angeles in 1967 to reach Western students. He was in the Harada-Yasutani lineage, which includes *koan* practice and significant intensity and push for enlightenment.

Two Western teachers were also part of this lineage and began their teachings at this same period: Robert Aitken founded the Diamond Sangha in Hawaii in 1959, and Philip Kapleau founded the Rochester Zen Center in 1966. Shunryu Suzuki Roshi of the San Francisco Zen Center was of a more traditional Soto lineage and presented an approach that must have clashed with what most of his students would have read or known about Zen. His focus was not on enlightenment but on what he presented as the heart of the matter, just sitting. That is, "Our *zazen* is just to be ourselves. We should not expect anything—just be ourselves and continue this practice forever" (quoted in Coleman, 2001, p 71). Zen in its original Chinese form, Chan, as well as Korean (Son) and Vietnamese (Thien) forms, arrived much later in the United States. Yet, teachers such as the Korean Seung Sahn and the Vietnamese Thich Nhat Hahn have had significant influences on Buddhism in America—particularly the genuine witness of "engaged Buddhism" advocate Thich Nhat Hahn, who was nominated for the Nobel Peace Prize by Martin Luther King, Jr., for his peace work during the Vietnam War, 1965-1975.

THE OTHERS

The foundational teachers mentioned here had authorized others to carry on their lineages of teaching. These others often went on to found their own centers. Some have hewn closely to their teachers' approaches, whereas others have continued to make adaptations to bring Zen to more Americans. To suggest the flavor of this process, in the Maezumi line, John Daido Loori founded Zen Mountain Monastery in Mount Tremper, New York, keeping more toward traditional monastic training, yet creating a highly advanced computer-based communications and marketing infrastructure. Bernard Glassman Roshi, Maezumi's heir, extended not simply Zen training, but a deeply felt social engagement, from highly successful initiatives to bring education and employment opportunities to the homeless in Yonkers, New York, to the founding of the Zen Peacemaker Order (Prebish, 1999; Queen, 2002). In Kapleau's line, Toni Packer, who had been his successor in Rochester, New York, became disillusioned by the traditional hierarchy and protocols and left that all behind to form an independent center with a Zen spirit all but devoid of the tradition—including that of lineage (Coleman, 2001; McMahan, 2002).

TYPICAL ZEN

If it were possible to characterize "typical" Zen practice, one might see most of the following four practices (Coleman, 2001; Prebish, 1999): (1) protocols for meeting teachers and entering and leaving meditation halls, including bowing; (2) chanting, often in the original Asian language; (3) ceremonial marking of changes in status, anniversaries of events, and the like; and (4) a meditative engagement with manual work around the center. Also central to Zen is the sitting practice, *zazen,* in which the adherence to correct physical posture is considered extremely important. Initial instruction may be to count one's breaths—say, to 10—and, when the attention has wandered, just to notice that it has happened and begin the count again. When capacity for concentration has grown, one may begin *shikantaza,* "just sitting" with full awareness, without directing the mind (Coleman, 2001; Suzuki, 1970). Retreats, or *sesshins,* are intensely focused on sitting meditation, with short periods of walking meditation in between; retreats are rarely longer than seven days.

SEVEN YEARS IN TIBET

Tibetan teachers began to leave Tibet in response to the Chinese repression in the 1950s that killed or drove more than a third of the population into exile. Buddhism's central role in the culture made teachers and monastics a major target. Although a few scholars had come to the United States in the 1950s—notably Geshe Wangal, Robert Thurman's first teacher—it was not until 1969 that Tibetan teachers reached out seriously to American students. Tarthang Tulku established the Tibetan Nyingma Meditation Center in Berkeley. The basic approach was very traditional, with students asked to undertake hundreds of thousands of prostrations, vows, and visualizations before meditation instruction is given. Tarthang Tulku created the Human Development Training Program to teach Buddhist psychology and meditation techniques to a professional health care and mental health care audience, and created as well the Nyingma Institute to support Buddhist education and study. In 1971, Kalu Rinpoche, who had been asked by the Dalai Lama to teach in North America, came first to Vancouver to start a center and later created a center in Woodstock, New York (Coleman, 2001; Seager, 2002).

Chogyam Trungpa, who had escaped from Tibet to India in 1959, came to the West to study at Oxford University; during the years he spent in the United Kingdom, he moved away from the traditional monastic teaching role and eventually gave up his vows. In 1970, as a lay teacher, he came to the United States, where he had an instant effect. He had arrived after the "boom," after the Beats, but the term "Beat Zen" described him better than any type of Zen master. Allen Ginsberg became a student, and many of the original Beat contingent taught at the Naropa Institute (now Naropa University) in Boulder, Colorado, which Trungpa founded. The appeal to the counterculture was swift and far reaching. In a very short time, he created a thoroughgoing infrastructure, including a network of practice centers (now worldwide) and developed a "secular path" called "*Shambhala* Training," to make the benefits of meditation practice and Buddhist psychological insights more available. Trungpa's approach to teaching was not the traditional one, but an amalgam that included much that he had learned from his Oxford education in comparative religion as well as wide-ranging exposure to Western psychology, which flavor finds its way into the new translations offered by Shambhala Publications. He not only powerfully shaped Tibetan Buddhism in the West, he offered spiritual perceptions that had a much wider reach—particularly the idea of "spiritual materialism," which he defined in this way: "The problem is that ego can convert anything to its own use, even spirituality. Ego is constantly attempting to acquire and apply the teachings of spirituality for its own benefit" (Trungpa, 1973).

Tibetan Buddhist practice in America is richly varied; characterizing it in a paragraph is a hopeless challenge. It is the most exotic and sensual of the three traditions under consideration. The iconography and rituals are complex; the teachers are often Tibetan, rather than Westerners as is common in the other traditions. There is considerable emphasis on textual study. The ritual relationship of student to teachers is hierarchical and devotional. Many of the difficult issues of "belief" that are subdued in the other traditions are right at the surface in Tibetan doctrine and practice—karma, rebirth, realms of supernatural beings. And the practices themselves are guarded, only revealed by initiation, face to face with an authorized teacher. Vajrayana or tantric practice, roughly conceived, includes visualization by the meditator of himself or herself with the attributes of a particular enlightened being. Less traditional teachers work differently.

Trungpa began his students with sitting meditation much like that of his friend Shunryu Suzuki. The *dzogchen* teachers have an approach that seems easily accessible to Western students, a formless meditation akin to *shikantaza* in Zen. Within the tradition, this approach is considered a high teaching, available only after years of preparation. In the West, however, it is offered differently. Lama Surya Das, a Westerner, explains: "One surprise is that people are a lot more prepared than one thinks. Westerners are sophisticated psychologically, but illiterate nomads (as in Tibet) are not" (quoted in Coleman, 2001, p 109). Retreats in the Tibetan tradition may be adapted for Americans as daylong or weeks long, or as more traditional lengths such as three months or three years.

HISTORICAL BUDDHA MAKES A COMEBACK

Vipassana meditation is the latest tradition to flower in North America. It is drawn from Theravada Buddhist practice, the tradition most directly connected to the historical Buddha, and perhaps the most conservative. Theravada was an early and profound influence on the development of Buddhism in the United Kingdom and Europe, dating back to the nineteenth century, through colonial connections. In the United States, the connection eventually came much later, in the Buddhist Vihara Society of Washington, DC, founded in 1966, with teachers Dickwela Piyananda and Henepola Gunaratana. Also, young Americans in the Peace Corps, serving in Vietnam, or traveling in southern Asia in the 1960s came into contact with Theravada teachers, such as Mahasi Sayadaw, S.N. Goenka, and U Ba Khin.

The influential Vipassana or Insight movement in the United States can be said to have begun when two of those young Americans, Joseph Goldstein and Jack Kornfield, came together to teach Vipassana at Chogyam Trungpa's request at Naropa Institute in 1974. Their connection, which also included Goldstein's friend Sharon Salzberg, another of the travelers to become a teacher, deepened. In 1975, under their leadership, the Insight Meditation Society (IMS) was founded, in rural Barre, Massachusetts. IMS grew quickly into a major retreat center, as the Insight approach found broad appeal. In 1984, Jack Kornfield left IMS for California to found Spirit Rock Meditation Center, which quickly became a second wing in American Vipassana practice (Coleman, 2001; Fronsdal, 2002; Prebish, 1999).

NEW INSIGHT

The Insight movement is the most egalitarian and least historically conditioned of the three traditions under consideration. Ritual, ceremony, and hierarchy are deemphasized, and meditation is of central importance. In contrast to Zen orderliness and Tibetan richness, there is ordinariness and a very American democratic, individualistic atmosphere. Students and teachers alike wear casual clothes and are known by first names. Teachers are less authority figures than they are "spiritual friends," and language is more psychological than specifically Buddhist. Vipassana is highly psychologized; in fact, many, if not a majority, of Vipassana teachers in the Insight movement are trained psychotherapists.

Meditation practice commonly includes two forms, concentration on the breath and open awareness (insight) of whatever is arising in the moment. Practices for cultivating loving kindness, as well as compassion, sympathetic joy, and equanimity, are also a part of training. Retreats are commonly 10 days in length, with long days of intense practice in silence. A typical schedule would find retreatants rising at 5:00 in the morning and moving through periods of sitting and walking (walking periods are as long as sitting periods, in contrast to the short breaks in Zen) with breaks for meals, until 10:00 in the evening (Coleman, 2001; Fronsdal, 2002; Prebish, 1999).

Perhaps most important for the discourse is not the differences in these three current traditions, but rather the essential similarities. Stephen Batchelor (1994) neatly summarizes:

> The distinctive goal of any Buddhist contemplative tradition is a state in which inner calm (*samatha*) is *unified* with insight (*vipassana*). Over the centuries, each tradition has developed its own methods for actualizing this state. And it is in these methods that the traditions differ, *not* in their end objective of unified calm and insight.

THE OTHER SHOES DROP

If the 1960s and 1970s were the period of foundation and growth, the 1980s and 1990s could be seen as the painful passage to maturity. In the many Buddhist centers around the United States, large but intimate communities had grown up, often with charismatic leaders. In most instances, the sharp discipline of Asian monastic practice, with celibacy and renunciation at its core, had been replaced by more casual, worldly, "extended family" types of community. As Suzuki Roshi told the San Francisco Zen Center, and Downing (2001) construed as a warning, "You are not monks, and you are not lay people" (p 70). There was no map, as communities sought ways forward. Perhaps the scandals around sexuality, alcohol, finances, and power that began to plague these institutions could not have been avoided and were necessary in catalyzing change. By 1988, Jack Kornfield could write, "Already upheavals over teacher behavior and abuse have occurred at dozens (if not the majority) of the major Buddhist and Hindu centers in America" (quoted in Bell, 2002). None of the three traditions was spared. A précis of a scandal from each will help illustrate the commonality of the problems and the importance of their aftermaths and resolutions.

HALF-BAKED HORRORS

At the San Francisco Zen Center, Suzuki Roshi appointed Richard Baker his successor, not just as abbot but as principal authority over the entire enterprise, which included associated meditation centers and successful businesses such as the Tassajara Bakery and Greens Restaurant. Following Suzuki's death in 1971, Baker held a tight rein over the institution, with little input from board members or other authorized teachers. In 1983, the board called a meeting, and the outcome was Baker's taking a leave of absence. This action was precipitated by an incident in which it became obvious that Baker, married himself, was having a sexual relationship with a married female student—indeed, the wife of a friend and benefactor. This kind of abuse was not an unprecedented situation; Baker had amassed a considerable history of infidelities with students.

There was more: in a community in which the residents willingly worked long hours for low wages, Baker spent more than $200,000 in a year (in the 1970s), drove a BMW, and had his personal spaces impeccably furnished with antiques and artwork. Further, Baker had surrounded himself with an inner circle of "courtiers" and failed to treat other senior members who had been ordained by Suzuki Roshi as valued peers. The most painful thing for the community was Baker's reaction: he did not comprehend that he had done anything wrong. More than 10 years after "the apocalypse," as it came to be known, he stated, "It is as hard to say what I have learned as it is to say what happened" (quoted in Bell, 2002, p 236; Downing, 2001).

"WISDOM" IN EXCESS

In Chogyam Trungpa Rinpoche's organization, excess was framed as "crazy wisdom" and accepted by many; in fact, failure to accept it was characterized as failure to understand the teaching. Trungpa's sexual liaisons with female students, his destructive meddling in students' lives and relationships, his drunkenness, and his aggressive, even violent outbursts were all well known. He was both open and unapologetic about his behavior (Bell, 2002; Clark, 1980; Coleman, 2001). Trungpa chose a Westerner, Osel Tendzin, as his heir. When Trungpa died in 1987, Tendzin became what amounted to supreme ruler of the enterprise, holding untouchable spiritual and executive power. In 1988, it was revealed to members that Tendzin had tested positive for human immunodeficiency virus (HIV) and that, although he was aware of his condition, he had continued to have unprotected sex with both male and female members. Not only had Tendzin known of his condition, but board members had known as well and had kept silent (Bell, 2002; Coleman, 2001). Tendzin, at the urging of a senior Tibetan teacher, went into retreat and died soon after.

RETREAT TRICKS AND TREATS

At the end of an IMS retreat taught by an Asian Theravada teacher, Anagarika Munindra, a woman came forward to say that she had had sex with the teacher—*during* the retreat. The woman had been psychologically troubled, and this incident had traumatized her further. The IMS guiding teachers were divided as to how to handle the situation—how much to reveal publicly, and how to deal with Munindra, who had already returned to India. Kornfield pushed for complete disclosure and an immediate confronting of Munindra. As he put it, "If parts of one's life are quite unexamined—which was true for all of us—and something like this comes up about a revered teacher, it throws everything you've been doing for years into doubt. It's threatening to the whole scene" (quoted in Schwartz, 1995, p 334). Eventually, Kornfield was sent by the board to India to speak directly with Munindra, who agreed to apologize to the community.

Aftermath

In the aftermath and resolution of all of these incidents, American Buddhism lost its idealized self-image and came to the maturity it carries now. In this process, common themes and practices arose. Leadership power moved away from the charismatic models and was rationalized and distributed more widely, with checks and balances, and boards accountable for oversight. Ethics were addressed formally with statements and policies. The model of teacher–student interaction was scrutinized, and methods for diluting intensity were developed and instituted, as much as possible. Of course, the teacher–student relationship remains the most difficult to manage, because meditation training carries the teacher–student dyad into areas of friendship, intimacy and power differential analogous to those in psychotherapy.

Universal Discourse

A universalizing and secularizing discourse draws together four themes. The first theme is the need for an expanded vocabulary of words, images, and ideas with which to express tacit experience. As more experience comes into shared language—verbal or nonverbal—the possibilities for teaching expand. The second theme is the drive for universalizing the experiences and language surrounding them. This theme may emerge in explicitly spiritual language, as with Emerson or D.T. Suzuki, or in more secular language, as in the current mindfulness-based interventions. The third theme, more specific, is the discovery or rediscovery of the principle of turning *toward* suffering and taking on the attitude of acceptance. This universal insight is both spiritual and psychological in nature, and suggests that such a distinction is of little expressive value. As the verbal and nonverbal discourse of mindfulness continues to expand, universalize, and secularize, the potentials for teaching expand as well. But this is only possible if the fourth theme is considered: the fact that this discourse is predominantly a product of an elite social group, with significant socioeconomic advantages and a level of education that is "right off the charts" (Coleman, 2001, p 193). As professionals and members of an elite, we teach from our own experience and give voice to it in language that may reflect that elite position. Therefore, we must continually be sensitive to, and learn from, the language of our clients, patients, and students.

One window into the possibilities of expanding discourse is suggested in the work of the postmodern theologian Don Cupitt (1999), who undertook an exercise in "ordinary language" theology. He collected and analyzed more than 150 idiomatic expressions in English that use the term *life*. His hypothesis was that these idioms have arisen as the overall population's reaction to the shifts in religion or spirituality from the mid-nineteenth century onward—the era of the development of the East–West discourse under consideration. He suggests that for a great many people, *life* has become the privileged religious object. Consider, for example, the switch since the mid-twentieth century from funerals oriented toward the deceased's place in the hereafter to a "celebration of the life of" the deceased. It might be said of the deceased that "she loved life." Phrases like "the sanctity of life," "the value of life," "the quality of life," "pro-life," have all become current since the 1950s; in fact, in health care, there are scales to measure "quality of life." And then there is the imperative phrase "Get a life!" that became so popular in the 1990s. What are its implications as a spiritual phrase?

The usual rhetoric about spirituality and religion in contemporary Western culture is that it has been *secularized*. Cupitt suggests just the reverse, that ordinary life has been *sacralized*. We can trace the roots of this shift back again to its mid-nineteenth century roots: Thoreau recorded this new attitude in *Walden,* as he went to the woods to "live deliberately," as he put it. Says Cupitt (1999):

> It is clear straightaway that Thoreau is not going to live in the wilderness for any of the Old World's traditional reasons. He's not going into the desert like Elijah or Muhammad to listen out for the voice of God; he's not going like Jesus or Anthony to be tempted of the devil; and he's not going, like Wittgenstein or Kerouac, in order to seek relief for his own troubled psychology. He's going to try to find out for himself what it is to be a human being with a life to live. (p 21)

This attitude is of considerable importance. For example, a poem such as Mary Oliver's "The Summer Day," with the last lines "Tell me, what is it you plan to do / With your one wild and precious life?" dropped into the silence of a meditation class creates a sacred space and a sacred pause for reflection. It is secular liturgy.

Another Window

Another window into the further possibilities is suggested by the sociologist of religion Robert Wuthnow. In *After Heaven: Spirituality in America since the 1950s* (1998), he maps out three approaches to spirituality that may suggest language, images, metaphors, and assumptions that connect contemporary Americans to alternative practices. The approaches he names follow the arc of the narrative of this chapter: the traditional *spirituality of dwelling,* the contemporary *spirituality of seeking*, and the emerging *spirituality of practice*.

Dwelling spirituality dominates in settled times in history, when it is possible to create stable institutions and communities, when sacred spaces for worship can be *inhabited*. The metaphor of this spirituality is a *place*. In the narrative we've been following, the hundred years from mid-nineteenth to mid-twentieth century were dwelling times. In America, the overwhelming majority of the population identified with Jewish or Christian tradition. Towns were small, church buildings and synagogues were central, often "commons" occupied the center of town, and one—and one's entire family—simply *belonged*. Lives were spent from infancy to funeral participating within a community, a place. The few at the end of the nineteenth century who saw and felt Matthew Arnold's ("Dover Beach") "withdrawal of the tide of the sea of faith"—the first Buddhists—were anomalous harbingers.

Seeking spirituality dominates in unsettled times, when meaning must be negotiated, and all that is on offer may be explored. Wuthnow notes that a major shift was beginning in the post-WWII America of the 1950s, as the culture became more fluid, complex, and threatening to individual identities. The opening to new possibilities from the East, and from the culture of recovery and self-help, brought new products, programs and perspectives into the spiritual marketplace. The seeking of the 1960s and 1970s was pervasive, and continues today, as the market becomes even more fragmented and the culture more unstable.

THE METAPHOR FOR SEEKING SPIRITUALITY IS A JOURNEY

Practice spirituality is the new bright edge in the culture. In a profound way, it integrates both dwelling and seeking. It requires setting aside a sacred space-time for the practice, yet that space-time is potentially fluid. Further, practice spirituality begins to reconcile or mediate the split between dwelling and seeking. Practice encourages both discipline and wide-ranging exploration, and can be undertaken either dwelling within the shelter of an organization and community, or pursued and sought independently. There is not a metaphor for practice, but rather an impulse and attitude to "live deliberately," as first Thoreau and now Cupitt suggest.

It is here, now, in this emerging moment, that alternative medical approaches are growing and evolving with a democratic and ethical view of spiritual teacher–student relations, a secular spirituality of life, and a drive for the paradoxical fluidity and stability of spiritual practice. We have had nearly one-quarter millennium of evolving East-West discourse behind and within alternative thought and practice. We may finally be ready to reap the rewards by a radical reorganization of our ideas and approaches to health care in America.

This chapter has explored the historical, social and cultural "equipment" we have for engaging in mind–body thought and practice. The next chapter presents the growing scientific evidence for all the anatomical, biochemical and physiological connections between the brain and the body, and an expansion of what can be considered as "mind" for purposes of health and healing.

References

Barks C: *The essential Rumi*, San Francisco, 1995, Harper.

Batchelor S: *The awakening of the West*, Berkeley, CA, 1994, Parallax.

Bell S: Scandals in emerging Western Buddhism. In Prebish CS, Baumann M, editors: *Westward dharma: Buddhism beyond Asia*, Berkeley, CA, 2002, University of California Press.

Benson H: *The relaxation response*, New York, 1975, Morrow.

Bevis WW: *Mind of winter: Wallace Stevens, meditation, and literature*, Pittsburgh, 1988, University of Pittsburgh Press.

Brooks VW: *The flowering of New England, 1815–1865*, New York, 1936, EP Dutton.

Brooks VW: *Fenollosa and his circle, with other essays in biography*, New York, 1962, EP Dutton.

Cage J: *Silence: lectures and writings*, Cambridge, MA, 1966, MIT Press.

Carrington P: *The book of meditation: the complete guide to modern meditation*, Boston, 1998, Element. (rev ed of *Freedom in meditation*, East Millstone, NJ, 1975, Pace Educational Systems).

Clark T: *The great Naropa poetry wars*, Santa Barbara, CA, 1980, Cadmus Editions.

Coleman W: *The new Buddhism: the Western transformation of an ancient tradition*, New York, 2001, Oxford University Press.

Cupitt D: *The new religion of life in everyday speech*, London, 1999, SCM Press.

Downing M: *Shoes outside the door: desire, devotion, and excess at San Francisco Zen Center*, Washington, DC, 2001, Counterpoint.

Dryden W, Still A: Historical aspects of mindfulness and self-acceptance in psychotherapy, *J Ration Emot Cogn Behav Ther* 24(1):3, 2006.

Duckworth W: *Talking Music: conversations with John Cage, Philip Glass, Laurie Anderson, and five generations of American experimental composers*, Cambridge, Mass, 1999, Da Capo Press.

Fromm E, Suzuki DT, DeMartino R: *Zen Buddhism and psychoanalysis*, New York, 1960, Harper & Row.

Fronsdal G: Virtues without rules: ethics in the Insight Meditation movement. In Prebish CS, Baumann M, editors: *Westward dharma: Buddhism beyond Asia*, Berkeley, CA, 2002, University of California Press.

Furlong M: *Genuine fake: a biography of Alan Watts*, London, 1986, Heinemann.

Hodder AD: "Ex Oriente Lux": Thoreau's ecstasies and the Hindu texts, *Harv Theol Rev* 86(4):403, 1993.

Johnston H: The marketing social movement: a case study of the rapid growth of TM. In Richardson JT, editor: *Money and power in the new religions*, Lewiston, NY, 1988, Edwin Mellen Press.

Kabat-Zinn J: *Wherever you go, there you are*, New York, 1994, Hyperion.

Kantner P: Won't you try/Saturday afternoon. On Jefferson Airplane: *After bathing at Baxter's* [LP], New York, 1967, RCA Victor.

Kravitz Y: Personal communication August 8, 2008.

Levine P: Introduction to *Morita therapy and the true nature of anxiety based disorders (Shinkeishitsu)* (1928), translated by

Akihisa Kondo, Albany, NY, 1998, State University of New York Press.

Mahesh Yogi M: *Transcendental meditation*, New York, 1968, New American Library.

McCown DM, Micozzi MS: *New world mindfulness: from the founding fathers, Emerson and Thoreau to your daily practice*, Rochester, VT, 2012, Healing Arts Press/Inner Traditions.

McCown DM, Reibel D, Micozzi MS: *Teaching mindfulness*, New York, 2009, Springer.

McMahan DL: Repackaging Zen for the West. In Prebish CS, Baumann M, editors: *Westward dharma: Buddhism beyond Asia*, Berkeley, Calif, 2002, University of California Press.

Merton T: *Zen and the birds of appetite*, New York, 1968, New Directions.

Morita S: *Morita therapy and the true nature of anxiety based disorders (Shinkeishitsu) (1928)*, translated by Akihisa Kondo, Albany, NY, 1998, State University of New York Press.

Mott M: *The seven mountains of Thomas Merton*, Boston, 1984, Houghton Mifflin.

Nattier J: Who is a Buddhist? Charting the landscape of Buddhist America. In Prebish CS, Tanaka KK, editors: *The faces of Buddhism in America*, Berkeley, CA, 1998, University of California Press.

Obadia L: Buddha in the Promised Land: outlines of the Buddhist settlement in Israel. In Prebish CS, Baumann M, editors: *Westward dharma: Buddhism beyond Asia*, Berkeley, CA, 2002, University of California Press.

Pennington MB: *Centering prayer: renewing an ancient Christian prayer tradition*, New York, 1980, Image Books.

Prebish CS: *Luminous passage: the practice and study of Buddhism in America*, Berkeley, CA, 1999, University of California Press.

Queen CS: Engaged Buddhism: agnosticism, interdependence, globalization. In Prebish CS, Baumann M, editors: *Westward dharma: Buddhism beyond Asia*, Berkeley, CA, 2002, University of California Press.

Reynolds DK: *The quiet therapies: Japanese pathways to personal growth*, Honolulu, 1980, University of Hawaii Press.

Reynolds DK: *Plunging through the clouds: constructive living currents*, Albany, 1993, State University of New York Press.

Rohr R: *Everything belongs: the gift of contemplative prayer*, New York, 1999, Crossroad.

Said EW: *Orientalism*, New York, 1978, Pantheon Books.

Schwartz T: *What really matters: searching for wisdom in America*, New York, 1995, Bantam Books.

Seager RH: American Buddhism in the making. In Prebish CS, Baumann M, editors: *Westward dharma: Buddhism beyond Asia*, Berkeley, CA, 2002, University of California Press.

Seeman W, Nidich S, Banta T: Influence of Transcendental Meditation on a measure of self-actualization, *J Couns Psychol* 19: 184, 1972.

Shapiro S, Carlson L, Astin J, Freedman B: Mechanisms of mindfulness, *J Clin Psychol* 62(3):373–386, 2006.

Stevens W: *The palm at the end of the mind; selected poems and a play*, New York, 1971, Alfred A Knopf.

Suzuki DT: *Mysticism: Christian and Buddhist*, New York, 1957, Harper & Brothers.

Suzuki S: *Zen mind, beginner's mind*, New York, 1970, Weatherhill.

Trungpa C: *Cutting through spiritual materialism*, Berkeley, CA, 1973, Shambhala.

Tweed T: *The American encounter with Buddhism, 1844–1912: Victorian culture and the limits of dissent*, Bloomington, 1992, Indiana University Press.

Vanier J: *Befriending the stranger*, Grand Rapids, MI, 2005, Eerdmans.

Versluis A: *American Transcendentalism and Asian religions*, New York, 1993, Oxford University Press.

Wallace RK: Physiological effects of Transcendental Meditation, *Science* 167:1751, 1970.

Watts A: *The wisdom of insecurity*, New York, 1951, Pantheon Books.

Watts A: *This is it: and other essays on Zen and spiritual experience*, New York, 1960, Pantheon Books.

Watts A: *Joyous cosmology: adventures in the chemistry of consciousness*, New York, 1962, Pantheon Books.

Watts A: *In my own way, an autobiography*, New York, 1972, Vintage Books.

Wuthnow R: *After heaven: spirituality in America since the 1950s*, Berkeley, CA, 1998, University of California Press.

Suggested Readings

Baer R: *Mindfulness-based treatment approaches: clinician's guide to evidence base and applications*, Boston, 2006, Elsevier/Academic Press.

Didonna F: *Clinical handbook of mindfulness*, New York, 2009, Springer.

Hayes SC, Follette VM, Linehan MM: *Mindfulness and acceptance: expanding the cognitive-behavioral tradition*, New York, 2004, Guilford.

Metcalf FA: The encounter of Buddhism and psychology. In Prebish CS, Baumann M, editors: *Westward dharma: Buddhism beyond Asia*, Berkeley, CA, 2002, University of California Press.

Polanyi M: *The tacit dimension*, Garden City, NY, 1966, Doubleday.

Resources for Teaching Mindfulness: *Cross-cultural and International Handbook*, New York, 2015, Springer.

Watts A: *Psychotherapy East and West*, New York, 1961, Pantheon.

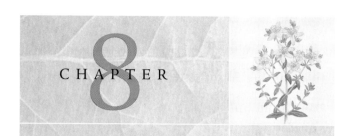

CHAPTER 8

NEUROHUMORAL PHYSIOLOGY AND PSYCHONEUROIMMUNOLOGY

HAKIMA AMRI

MARC S. MICOZZI

NEUROHUMORAL MECHANISMS

The autonomic nervous system (ANS) maintains homeostasis by a series of humoral and nervous system interactions that continually occur on a subconscious, involuntary level. The ANS sends nervous impulses to all parts of the body as directed by the integration of several complex biofeedback mechanisms.

The information from these biofeedback loops is integrated in the central nervous system (CNS), and appropriate neural directives are passed along to the organs of respiration, circulation, digestion, excretion, and reproduction via the ANS.

Thus the body is maintained in a state of dynamic equilibrium, continually responsive to stimuli from internally monitored systems and environmental influences. These mechanisms are a major component of the ability of the human organism to adapt to instantaneous and short-term changes in the environment, as part of a continuum of adaptive responses (see Chapter 2).

DIVISIONS OF THE AUTONOMIC NERVOUS SYSTEM

The functional anatomy of the ANS has important implications for therapeutics (Table 8-1). The division of the system into two major parts—sympathetic and parasympathetic—provides a series of checks and balances to regulate body functions. This division enables an ongoing dialogue between the two parts to maintain dynamic equilibrium. The opposition of two vital forces may be likened to the Asian concept of the yin and the yang, in which the interaction of these opposing forces maintains the balance and harmony of humans and the

universe (see Chapters 1 and 2). Accordingly, each of the two forces may take on some characteristics of the other. An analogy lies in the sympathetic and parasympathetic divisions of the nervous system, which are antagonistic, with a few notable exceptions. Coronary and pulmonary blood vessels are dilated by both divisions of the ANS, whereas the vessels supplying blood to skeletal muscles may be dilated by the sympathetic system in exercise or by the postganglionic parasympathetic neurotransmitter at rest. These versatile exceptions have significance for the relaxation response and mind–body therapies (Chapter 10).

The unique short-term and long-term adaptability of the human organism to environmental stimuli is facilitated by the actions of the ANS. The so-called fight-flight or defense-alarm responses are promulgated by the *sympathetic nervous system,* which raises blood oxygenation and pressure, regulates blood flow to the musculoskeletal system for activity and to the skin for thermal regulation, and causes retention of fluids and electrolytes in a state of arousal. These acute physiological responses are adaptive in the short term and allow long-term survival of the human organism.

The "relaxation response" is mediated by the dynamic opponent of the sympathetic system—the parasympathetic system. The *parasympathetic nervous system* directs the normative functions of the organism, allowing development of an ongoing state of well-being and physiological equilibrium. The maintenance of vegetative functions has facilitated human development and cultural evolution. The ability to relax has allowed humans to reserve some portion of physical and mental energy for the pursuit of activities peripheral to primary survival. This ability has given

TABLE 8-1 *Sympathetic and Parasympathetic Divisions of the Autonomic Nervous System*

	Sympathetic	Parasympathetic
Synonym	Adrenergic	Cholinergic
Preganglionic fiber	Short	Long
Neurohumoral agent[a]	Acetylcholine	Acetylcholine
Ganglion location	Paravertebral	End organ
Postganglionic fiber	Long	Short
Neurohumoral agent[a]	Norepinephrine	Acetylcholine
Extra-autonomic sites	Adrenal medulla	Neuromuscular junction
Evolutionary role	Fight-flight/defense-alarm	Relaxation response, vegetative functions
Activators	Multiple	Specific
Blockers	Diffuse, nonspecific	Selective, cholinesterase
Degradative enzymes	Monoamine oxidase, methyltransferase	

[a]These compounds are referred to as neurohumoral agents because they are present both in the general circulation and within nervous tissue. They are neurotransmitters because they manifest their activity across presynaptic or postsynaptic junctions during transmission of nerve impulses.

humans their unique cultural attributes, which enables each individual to express their inclination for creativity. The selective responsiveness of the ANS has enabled humans, both as individuals and as a species, to make the successful adaptation to the environment that has characterized human evolution.

The anatomical divisions corresponding to the functional autonomy of the sympathetic and parasympathetic nervous system can be traced along the length of the brain and spinal column (Figure 8-1). The ANS begins with cranial nerve X, the vagus, a single bundle of parasympathetic nerves that originates from the brainstem and courses throughout the body. Cranial nerves III, VII, and IX also send some parasympathetic fibers to the eyes, nose, and salivary glands. *Vagus* means "wanderer" in Latin, and no other nerve interfaces at so many diverse points along the functional anatomy. Passing down along the spinal cord, the cervical, thoracic, and lumbar divisions send sympathetic nerves throughout the body. Finally, the sacral divisions of the spinal cord send a few parasympathetic nerves to the lower regions of the body (Figure 8-1).

SEGMENTS AND SYNAPSES OF THE AUTONOMIC NERVES

Each nerve of the ANS has two longitudinal divisions or segments as it passes from the CNS to the end organs. The initial, or *preganglionic*, nerve fiber originates in the CNS and terminates in a nerve ganglion. Here it synapses with a new continuation—the postganglionic nerve fiber. This *postganglionic* fiber originates in the ganglion and terminates at a site of action. Autonomic nerve impulses travel in a continuum along the preganglionic fiber, through the synapse, and onto the postganglionic fiber to the site of action. In the sympathetic division, the preganglionic fibers are short and end in nearby ganglia, which occur in chains along the thoracic and lumbar vertebrae. From

there, the postganglionic fibers travel to the diverse sites of action. In the parasympathetic system the preganglionic fibers are long and travel into ganglia located near end organs. From there, postganglionic fibers traverse a short distance to the sites of action.

The occurrence of *synapses* in the ganglia between the preganglionic and postganglionic fibers is important to therapy. Local anesthetics affect nerve conduction in the nerve fiber. Otherwise, these nerve impulses may be influenced by activities at the synaptic junction site. The *interactions that occur in the synapse are a microcosm of neurophysiology* and serve to distinguish the sympathetic system functionally from the parasympathetic system. These distinctions are utilized extensively in pharmacological, and inherently recognized in ethnopharmacalogical, and herbal therapies (Chapter 24).

Each of these systems makes use of characteristic endogenous neurohumoral agents for the unique transmission of nervous impulses throughout the body. The preganglionic fibers of both divisions use *acetylcholine* as the neurotransmitter across the synapse. The postganglionic parasympathetic transmitter is also acetylcholine, but the sympathetic transmitter is *norepinephrine (noradrenalin)*. The exclusive postganglionic use of acetylcholine as the parasympathetic and norepinephrine as the sympathetic neurotransmitter holds throughout the ANS, except in the case of sweating of the palms, soles, and axilla, where the autonomic innervation is adrenergic but the neurotransmitter is acetylcholine. These neurohumoral compounds used in the transmission of impulses across the synaptic junction are distinct chemical entities that tend to accumulate at their sites of release. Such a circumstance would limit the effectiveness of the ANS in providing sensitive, instantaneous regulation of body systems. Thus the synaptic sites maintain extensive and sophisticated mechanisms for the reuptake and degradation of released neurohumoral transmitters, and the synaptic junctions are kept

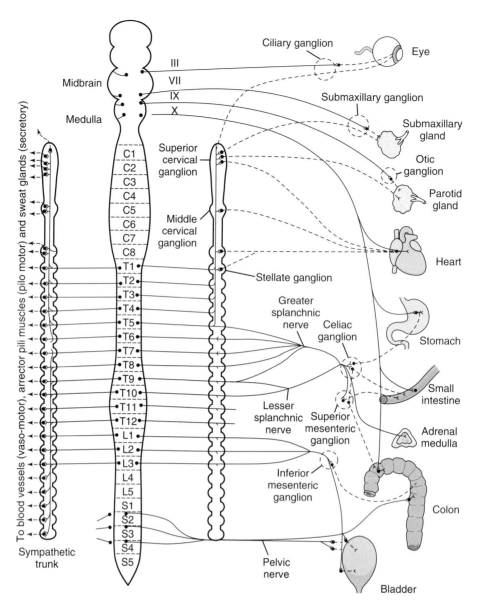

Figure 8-1 Autonomic nervous system and cranial nerves. (From Williams PL: *Gray's anatomy,* Edinburgh, 1995, Churchill Livingstone.)

clear of accumulated active compounds on an ongoing basis.

Specific enzymes degrade norepinephrine in the sympathetic postganglionic synapses, as well as their metabolic products. The concentration of these metabolites may be increased in certain pathological conditions and detected by analytical chemical techniques.

The enzyme responsible for the breakdown of acetylcholine in the postganglionic parasympathetic synapse is *acetylcholinesterase.* Although acetylcholine itself cannot practically be administered even when its properties are desired, a "functional dose" may be given through inhibition of its breakdown by cholinesterase. Thus, anticholinesterases form the basis for parasympathetic nervous stimulation in clinical therapeutics.

A phenomenon known as *denervation hypersensitivity* greatly depends on this system of reuptake and degrada-

tion. When the autonomic innervation to an organ is anatomically interrupted (denervation), the postganglionic synaptic site loses its induced degradative enzymes, and the synaptic receptor becomes extremely sensitive (hypersensitive) to the neurohumoral agent. Thus any amount of the original neurohumoral agent introduced into the site by the circulation, through administration or otherwise, will have a magnified effect because the activity will not be mitigated by action of its appropriate degradative mechanism.

PATHOPHYSIOLOGICAL AND THERAPEUTIC SIGNIFICANCE

The functional divisions of the ANS have great pathophysiological and therapeutic significance. For example, the entire gastrointestinal (GI) tract is extensively innervated by nerve fibers from both the sympathetic and the parasympathetic divisions. In fact, there are more neuropeptides present in the long GI tract than there is in the CNS itself—perhaps leading to the truth of the colloquial expression of a "gut feeling" (Chapters 9, 10).

As previously discussed, the parasympathetic ganglia, where preganglionic fibers synapse with postganglionic fibers, are located near the sites of action in end organs. In the case of the GI tract, the parasympathetic ganglia lie in two areas of the esophageal, gastric, intestinal, and colonic walls: the Auerbach myenteric plexus and Meissner submucosal plexus. These ganglia may be congenitally absent, as in Hirschsprung disease, or destroyed by a number of pathogenic agents. The resultant disease depends on the location of the deficiency or insult along the GI tract.

With destruction of the parasympathetic ganglia, there is prolonged, unopposed sympathetic stimulation. The characteristic effect is for the diseased segment to become constricted, with impaired motility and loss of peristaltic action. The segment of the GI tract proximal to the constriction lesion becomes extensively dilated as a pathological response to the event.

Achalasia of the esophagus, where a local area of constriction leads to proximal dilation of the esophagus that must be surgically corrected, is such a condition (Nemir & Micozzi, 1977). It has been thought that achalasia is caused by degenerative disease of the parasympathetic vagus nerve, which innervates this area.

Pyloric stenosis of the gastric outlet is a similar condition. A ganglionic megacolon, or Hirschsprung disease, is caused by a congenital lack of parasympathetic ganglion cells in the intestinal tract.

Chagas disease, or South American trypanosomiasis, caused by the parasitic organism *Trypanosoma cruzi*, may be associated with both megaesophagus and megacolon resulting from the toxic degeneration of the intraluminal nerve plexus through *T. cruzi* infection. On the other hand, selective loss of sympathetic activity occurs in Horner syndrome, with the characteristic triad of ptosis, miosis, and anhydrosis (lid lag, pupillary constriction, and loss of sweating). Horner syndrome occurs with injury to the cervical sympathetic trunk and unopposed parasympathetic innervation.

No autonomic therapeutic agent has been developed for the effective treatment of disorders such as Horner syndrome or irreversible disorders of the GI tract. However, autonomic agents to treat diseases of the circulatory and respiratory systems are common therapies in medicine. These same neurohumoral mechanisms involved in medical therapeutics may also be recruited in a nonpharmacological manner by many of the "mind-body" techniques of complementary, integrative, and alternative medicine (Chapter 10). The presence of these and other physiologic connections, pathways, and feedback loops among "mind" and "body" are outlined in Figure 8-2. These connections and pathways are being investigated by the field of psychoneuroimnunology (PNI) and will be discussed in the next section of this chapter, and the follow-

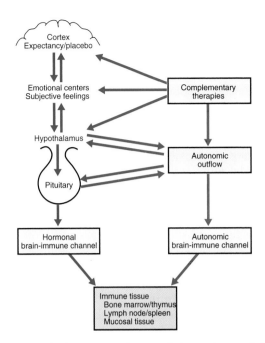

Figure 8-2 Brain–immune pathways of alternative medicine.

ing chapters. PNI demonstrates how thoughts, emotional states and states of consciousness can be translated into physiologic, nervous, humoral and immune responses in the body.

PSYCHONEUROIMMUNOLOGY

The Romans' view of *mens sanum in corpore sano,* "a sound mind in a sound body," as well as the Greek physician Galen's observation that women suffering from depression had a predisposition toward developing breast cancer, reflected the early recognition of mind–body interactions and their significance in health and disease. Understanding the connections and functioning of the mind has been the subject of discussions from the ancient era and transcended the Renaissance to modern times. Even today, scientists are still debating the "primitive mechanisms of trauma" (Baldwin, 2013).

This debate is witnessed by the philosophical writings of Pythagoras that "the brain served as the organ of the mind and the temple of the soul," (Chapter 1) and Anaximander, another Greek philosopher, that "mind gives body a life force" (Cassano, 1996). The European Renaissance was marked by the work of Leonardo da Vinci and Michelangelo. Da Vinci was interested in answering the question of how the brain processes sensory inputs; Michelangelo, an expert in anatomy, painted detailed structures of the human brain. René Descartes, a post-Renaissance philosopher, declared the connection between the body and the soul to be located in the pineal gland (Lokhorst & Kaitaro, 2001), while today he is also accused of being the responsible party for having separated the mind from the body for purposes of medical study and theory.

The development of electrochemistry in the eighteenth and nineteenth centuries led to the identification of different gases and their role in maintaining life through respiration, which also made the lungs the new indispensable organ to be seriously considered. It is basically what Hippocrates and Avicenna (Ibn Sina) called the "air element" that distributes the spirits (oxygen) inside the body (Tercier, 2005; Abu-Asab et al, 2013). The importance of breathing and the breath (as inspiration, literally) started then to occupy the discussion about what animates vital, living beings (Chapter 6). The twentieth century was marked by rapid technological developments, especially imaging, in which the functional brain is visualized and its metabolites measured. A similar trend is currently being followed in the twenty-first century.

It was not until studies in the 1950s and 1960s verified the impact of stress on overall health that mind–body connection research started to become a focus of attention. Motivated by advances in aviation and manned exploration of outer space during the late 1950s and 1960s, investigators attempted to better describe the interactions among mind and body as a result of stress exposure. The early work of Rasmussen et al (1957) showed that animals exposed to stress had increased susceptibility to infection. George Engel's view that genetics is not the only cause of poor health and that social and psychological factors have a direct impact on all biological processes further expanded this model during the new era of "holistic medicine" which became identified as "psychoneuroimmunology," or PNI (Engel, 1977; Lutgendorf & Costanzo, 2003).

Subsequent research strongly suggested that the higher cognitive and limbic emotional centers are capable of regulating virtually all aspects of the *immune system* as well and therefore play a significant role in health and disease (Ader, 1991; Blalock, 1994; Reichlin, 1993). The pioneering work of Besedovsky et al (1975) revealed the role of hormones and cytokines in modulating both brain and immune functions (Besedovsky et al, 1975). The Institute of Medicine issued reports in 1982, and again in 2001, on health and behavior with a special focus on understanding the role and interactions of the biological, behavioral, and social factors in health and disease, which signaled that it had become acceptable (and thus fundable) to begin investigating the role of these factors in medical research.

AUTONOMIC AND NEUROENDOCRINE PROCESSES

Autonomic and neuroendocrine processes are included among the mind–body pathways of communication (Figure 8-2). The ANS also innervates the bone marrow, thymus, spleen, and mucosal surfaces, the areas where immune cells develop, mature, and encounter foreign proteins (Felten et al, 1992). This innervation involves sympathetic, parasympathetic, and nonadrenergic noncholinergic fibers. As presented earlier (see Figure 8-1), signal transmission through ANS nerve synapses occurs through epinephrine, norepinephrine, acetylcholine, and neuropeptides. These chemical messengers also exert tissue-specific inflammatory or anti-inflammatory effects on immune target tissues, and nerves and inflammatory cells mutually influence each other in a time-dependent manner (Watkins, 1995).

Development and aging of the immune system and the ANS appear to be closely related (Ackerman et al, 1989; Bellinger et al, 1988). Levels of natural killer (NK) cells, first identified by Dr. Jerry Thornthwaite and now considered to be the first line of immune defense against viral infections, were found to be dramatically reduced in individuals exposed to chronic life stress as well as in those with major depression. The levels of NK cells returned to normal levels after the depression episodes subsided (Irwin & Miller, 2007). Studying 245 patients who had depression and were stratified by smoking habits, Jung and Irwin (1999) noted that the combination of depression and smoking caused a more pronounced decline in levels of NK cells than depression or smoking alone.

Several studies published in the past 30 years have clearly demonstrated that behavior affects immunity and have deciphered neuroimmune pathways governing the observed effects. The neuroimmune system also affects behavior, functioning as a bidirectional highway of communications involving neuropeptides and cytokines. It has been hypothesized that altered cytokine profiles, including levels of interleukin-1 (IL-1), IL-6, and tumor necrosis factor, might contribute to symptoms of depression, such as insomnia and fatigue (Irwin & Miller, 2007).

Recent studies have confirmed the connection between IL-6 and tumor necrosis alpha (TNF-α) in melancholic and atypical major depression. Whereas IL-6 was significantly elevated in patients with melancholic major depression, and not in those with atypical major depression, TNF-α was decreased in both groups when all were compared to healthy controls (Dunjic-Kostic et al, 2013). Furthermore, two immunomodulatory growth factors—IL-7 (a regulator of T cells homeostasis) and granulocyte-colony stimulating factor (G-CSF)—were measured in patients suffering major depressive disorder. These patients exhibited lower levels of IL-7 but no change in G-CSF. This observation indicates the close involvement of the immune system in these neuropsychological disorders (Lehto & Huotari, 2010).

MOLECULES OF EMOTION

The neuroendocrine pathway constitutes the second indirect communication channel involving the hormonal regulation of immune cell function. Immune cells have surface receptors for endorphins, enkephalins, and the various hormones, such as growth hormone, thyroid-stimulating hormone, sex hormone-releasing hormones, vasopressin, and prolactin (Blalock, 1994; Felten et al, 1992). The release of many of these hormones is intimately related to thoughts feelings, and emotions, and has a profound effect on immune system function (Jawer & Micozzi, 2009, 2012; Chapters 9, 10).

These "molecules of emotion" therefore govern the immune response through the endocrine system, leading to either suppression or enhancement (Pert et al, 1998). The neuroendocrine peptide corticotropin-releasing hormone (CRH) received special attention, especially after it was found that depressed patients had elevated central CRH levels as measured in the cerebrospinal fluid. Furthermore, acute administration of CRH centrally caused dramatic reduction in innate and cellular immune responses in animal models (Irwin et al, 1987, 1989; Strausbaugh & Irwin, 1992). These studies showed that the central action of this neuropeptide could affect the peripheral immune response. CRH is considered as the major neuroimmunoendocrine integrator. Thorough updates on the scientific research in this field are provided in reviews by Weschenfelder and Sander (2012) and Lang and Borgwardt (2013).

As thoughts, feelings, emotions, and perceptions alter immunity (Watkins, 1995), complementary therapies targeted at these areas should affect health and elicit positive changes in pathological conditions (Watkins, 1994).

Epilepsy illustrates the effect of the mind on the brain. Epileptic seizures can be triggered by stressful events (Fenwick, 1998), and negative emotions exacerbate the condition. A potential mechanism is the activation of the cytokine network (Hulkkonen et al, 2004), which corresponds to seizure activity, but whether it is cause or effect remains unclear.

The reverse scenario is reflected in a long-term study involving healthy World War II veterans who were asked to write about their war experiences and themselves. The essays were rated on a scale ranging from extreme optimism to extreme pessimism. When the study participants reached the age of 45, health status positively correlated with optimistic scoring at the beginning of the study (Peterson & Bossio, 1993). Recently, a new approach using multiplex immunoassay was applied to assess the relationship of 11 T-cell cytokines and chemokines to behavior. Mommersteeg et al (2008) investigated whether cytokine and chemokine profiles correlated to hostility in 304 healthy Dutch military males before deployment. In addition to finding that hostility was related to various clusters of proinflammatory and anti-inflammatory cytokines and chemokines and to potential risk factors including age, body mass index, smoking, drinking, previous deployment, early life trauma, and depression, the authors found that "hostility was significantly related to decreased IL-6/chemokine secretion and increased proinflammatory and anti-inflammatory cytokines" (Mommersteeg et al, 2008).

EVIDENCE FOR PSYCHONEUROIMMUNOLOGICAL MEDIATION OF THE EFFECTS OF COMPLEMENTARY AND ALTERNATIVE THERAPIES

The use of PNI-mediated techniques has dramatically increased in the United States. According to a recent survey, one in five adults reported using one or more mind–body therapies during the previous year (Wolsko et al, 2004). Relaxation techniques, guided imagery, hypnosis, and biofeedback are the most frequently used modalities. Patients sought these PNI-related techniques for treatment of chronic diseases such as anxiety (34%), depression (27 %), headaches (19%), back or neck pain (18%), heart problems or chest pain (18%), arthritis (15%), digestive disorders (13%), and fatigue (12%).

The authors estimated that the absolute numbers of patients using the modalities listed were as follows: for back and neck pain, 11.2 million; for anxiety, 6.3 million; and for fatigue, 6.8 million. Between 29% and 55% of patients found these therapies "very helpful" for their respective health condition. A recent study on the prevalence of complementary and alternative medicine (CAM) use in the military population showed that 37% of the 1305 individuals in a random sample of active duty and Reserve and National Guard members contacted between December 2000 and July 2002 had used at least one CAM modality in the previous year (Smith et al, 2007). A recent survey showed that CAM use was more prevalent in the military population (45%) as compared to the surveys conducted on civilians (36% to 38%) during the 2000 U.S. census (Goertz & Marriott, 2013).

What is the evidence that complementary, integrative, and alternative therapies work through the previously outlined mind–body pathways? (See Figure 8-2.) To date, few studies have actually investigated the *mechanism of action* of these therapies. Some data suggest that the activity of the ANS may be altered by chiropractic intervention (Beal, 1985; Bouhuys, 1963), hypnosis (DeBenedittis et al, 1994; Neild & Cameron, 1985), conditioning (Hatch et al, 1990), and acupuncture (Han et al, 1980; Jian, 1985). Other studies have indicated that the benefit derived from acupuncture (Kasahara et al, 1992) and spinal manipulation (Vernon et al, 1986) might be mediated through endorphin release.

Acupuncture

Several studies demonstrate that acupuncture-induced analgesia is blocked by naloxone, an opioid antagonist, which indicates that an opioidergic mechanism mediates the acupuncture analgesic response (Mayer et al, 1977; Sjolund & Eriksson, 1979). In electroacupuncture, electrical pulses are applied via acupuncture needles. Opioid and nonopioid pathways govern the antinociceptive effect induced by electroacupuncture. However, the PNI-mediated mechanism in electroacupuncture occurs at the level of neuronal nitric oxide synthase, nitric oxide expression and synthesis in the brain, and the therapeutic response induced by acupoint ST36 (Ma, 2004).

Another hypothesis on the mechanism of acupuncture involving neutrophins and cytokines has been postulated (Kavoussi & Ross, 2007). The beneficial effects of acupuncture on inflammatory pain, as well as neurodegenerative and psychiatric diseases, could indeed be mediated by nerve growth factor, brain-derived neurotrophic factor, neurotrophin 3, or neurotrophin 4/5, as well as by IL-1,

IL-2, IL-6, TNF-α, and transforming growth factor β. The dynamic crosstalk between the central and peripheral nervous systems could shed light on the mechanism of acupuncture (Du, 2008).

Acupuncture has also been used to relieve stress and anxiety, which are known to affect the immune response. In a study investigating the effects of acupuncture in women with anxiety, Arranz et al (2007) tested several immune functions: adherence, chemotaxis, phagocytosis, basal and stimulated superoxide anion levels, lymphocyte proliferation in response to phytohemagglutinin A, and NK activity of leukocytes (neutrophils and lymphocytes). Ten 30-minute sessions of manual acupuncture using 19 acupoints were administered to 34 women aged 34 to 60 years with anxiety, as assessed by the Beck Anxiety Inventory, and 20 healthy controls. The investigators found that the most positive effects of acupuncture on the immune parameters appear 72 hours after a single session and persist for 1 month after the full treatment regimen. The abnormal immune profiles of women with anxiety were normalized and the immune functions significantly enhanced by acupuncture (Arranz et al, 2007).

Using state-of-the-art technology (e.g., two-dimensional electrophoresis-based proteomics) and an animal model for neuropathic pain, Sung et al (2004) detected 36 proteins that were differentially expressed in the brains of injured animals compared with control subjects. Most interestingly, normal levels of these proteins were restored after the injured animals were treated with electroacupuncture. Of these proteins, 21 have been characterized as playing a role in inflammation, enzyme metabolism, and signal transduction, and this study undoubtedly will elucidate other pathways triggered by acupuncture (Sung et al, 2004).

The effectiveness of acupuncture across the trauma spectrum was assessed in a systematic review of reviews available in the searchable databases. Out of 1480 citations, 52 high-quality systematic reviews or meta-analyses were analyzed and showed effectiveness of acupuncture for treating headaches. However, less evidence was reported for anxiety, sleep problems, depression, and chronic pain (Lee et al, 2012).

Meditation

A growing body of evidence suggests that *meditation* alleviates anxiety, fosters a positive attitude, and improves the immune response. A meditation training program known as "mindfulness-based stress reduction" (MBSR), developed by Jon Kabat-Zinn in the late 1970s, yielded increased left frontal lobe activation in response to both negative and positive emotion induction. When vaccinated after intervention, the meditation group experienced a significantly increased rise in antibody titers. The correlation between the shift toward left-sided brain activation and the elevated immune response demonstrates the relationship between the PNI system and meditation (Davidson et al, 2003). Similarly, cancer outpatients using the same MBSR technique experienced improved mood, which correlated with a more favorable hormone profile with regard to melatonin, cortisol, dehydroepiandrosterone sulfate (DHEA-S), and the cortisol/DHEA-S ratio, as well as an enhanced immune response (Carlson et al, 2004).

The quasi-experimental study carried out by Robinson et al (2003) using an 8-week structured MBSR intervention in patients with human immunodeficiency virus (HIV) infection showed that NK cell activity and numbers increased significantly in the MBSR group compared with the control subjects. In a more recent single-blind randomized controlled trial, Creswell et al (2009) assessed the efficacy of an 8-week MBSR meditation program compared with a 1-day control seminar on CD4[+] T-lymphocyte counts in HIV-positive adults suffering from stress. Participants in the 1-day control seminar had reduced CD4[+] T-lymphocyte counts, whereas counts among participants in the 8-week MBSR program were unchanged from baseline to postintervention. Another study also found an indication that mindfulness meditation training can buffer CD4[+] T-lymphocyte declines in adults infected with HIV-1.

Beneficial effects of MBSR have also been reported among cancer patients. Quality of life, mood, endocrine, immune, and autonomic parameters have been assessed in patients with early stage breast and prostate cancer enrolled in an MBSR program. In this study the authors carried out preintervention and postintervention as well as 6- and 12-month follow-up measurements of the psychobehavioral and physiological parameters. They found significant general improvements in stress symptoms, which were preserved through the follow-up periods. In addition to a steady decrease in salivary cortisol level throughout the follow-up period, improvements in immune patterns were also maintained as shown by a decrease in the proinflammatory T helper cell type 1 cytokines. Reductions in heart rate and systolic blood pressure were positively correlated with improvements in self-reported stress symptoms. This pilot study data clearly showed the longer-term effects of MBSR on a range of potentially important psychoimmunophysiological biomarkers (Carlson et al, 2007).

Another study enrolled women who had been recently diagnosed with early stage breast cancer and were not currently receiving chemotherapy into an MBSR program. Compared with the levels before MBSR intervention, postintervention and 4-week follow-up assessments in the MBSR group showed an increase in peripheral blood mononuclear NK cell activity and cytokine production accompanied by a decrease in IL-4, IL-6, and IL-10 production, whereas the non-MBSR control group showed reduced NK cell activity and interferon-γ levels and increased IL-4, IL-6, and IL-10 production. Furthermore, the MBSR-intervention group demonstrated reduced cortisol levels, improved quality of life, and improved coping effectiveness (Witek-Janusek et al, 2008). Similar results were found in women who completed breast cancer treatment and participated in MBSR sessions; changes in their cortisol awakening response were recorded in favor of improved self-reported stress, reduced depressive symptomatology, and medical symptoms (Matousek et al, 2011).

Relaxation Therapy

Among the other mind–body programs is the one developed by Herbert Benson, MD, in the 1970s, in which he emphasized the *relaxation response*. A large body of evidence has been developed showing its beneficial effects on a wide array of diseases and disorders, and it is only recently that a special interest in its *mechanism(s) of action* has been developed. Building upon newly developed hypotheses that nitric oxide plays a role in the immune response and in stress-related diseases (Tripathi, 2007), an association between oxygen consumption, through breathing exercises, and nitric oxide production has been elucidated (Dusek et al, 2006).

Furthermore, the new technological approaches of high-throughput genomic analyses have been applied to mechanistic investigations of the relaxation response. Thus, genomic counterstress alterations induced by the relaxation response have been detected using whole blood transcriptional profiles. Genomic profiles were compared in 19 long-term practitioners of relaxation, 20 novice individuals who completed an 8-week relaxation program, and 19 healthy controls. Over 2200 genes in the long-term practitioners and 1561 genes in the novice group were differentially expressed compared with the control group. Among these genes, the long-term practitioners and novices shared 433 genes. The gene analysis revealed changes in gene expression related to cellular metabolism, oxidative phosphorylation, and production of reactive oxygen species and regulation of oxidative stress, especially among the relaxation response practitioners (Dusek et al, 2008).

Using a similar clinical design of long-term meditators and novices, the same team showed that one session of relaxation altered the transcriptome as measured in peripheral blood before and right after (15 minutes) eliciting a relaxtion response in comparison to the active control group, using health education. They founds that "RR practice enhanced expression of genes associated with energy metabolism, mitochondrial function, insulin secretion and telomere maintenance, and reduced expression of genes linked to inflammatory response and stress-related pathways concluding that mitochondrial resiliency might also be promoted by RR-induced downregulation of NF-κB-associated upstream and downstream targets that mitigates stress" (Bhasin et al, 2013).

T'ai chi

T'ai chi is a Chinese martial art that emphasizes meditative aerobic activity and relaxation. Its practice in the West is witnessing great development. Several studies using t'ai chi as intervention in subjects who either had their immune response clinically challenged or had immune-related diseases have been published. In a prospective randomized controlled trial, 112 healthy adults were vaccinated with Varivax® (attenuated varicella-zoster virus) and divided into either t'ai chi or health education groups. The t'ai chi group showed a significant improvement in scores on the Short-Form Health Survey (SF-36); in addition, the cell-mediated immune response to the vaccine was not only higher but also increased at a higher rate than in the control group (Irwin et al, 2007).

Another randomized clinical trial tested whether t'ai chi could improve immune function and psychosocial functioning in 252 individuals infected with HIV compared with a wait-listed control group. Although only modest effects were observed on the psychosocial test results, a significant increase in the lymphocyte proliferation function was found. The investigators concluded that t'ai chi could be considered to be an effective alternative intervention in patients with immune-mediated diseases (McCain et al, 2008).

In a recent systematic review and meta-analysis, the authors compiled 37 randomized controlled trials and 5 quasi-experimental trials from English-language and Chinese studies that used t'ai chi for depression, anxiety, and psychological well-being. They found that t'ai chi had beneficial effects on a range of well-being methods (Wang et al, 2013).

Yoga

Yoga has become a popular practice in Western culture (see Chapter 21). Based on the development and balance of psychophysical energies, yoga has proven to be beneficial in pulmonary and cardiovascular conditions, including asthma, chronic bronchitis, and hypertension (Raub, 2002). A study investigating the effects of yoga and meditation on psychological profile, cardiopulmonary performance, and melatonin secretion, demonstrated increased well-being, improved performance, and elevated plasma melatonin levels (Harinath et al, 2004).

Yoga has been administered as adjuvant therapy in treatment of other health conditions, in addition to the afore-mentioned disorders. Premenstrual syndrome is considered to be a stress-related psychoneuroendocrine disorder for which the numerous available treatments have not brought satisfactory relief. Fifty healthy women of reproductive age were assigned either to a Hatha Yoga group performing a 61-point relaxation exercise or to a no intervention control group. Several physiological parameters (heart rate, systolic and diastolic blood pressure, electromyographic activity, electrodermal galvanic activity, respiratory rate, and peripheral temperature) were measured. After 10 minutes of Hatha Yoga practice, values of all parameters declined significantly except that temperature increased, which suggests a reduction in sympathetic activity and basal sympathetic tone. Thus, Hatha Yoga could be used as an adjuvant to other medical treatment in alleviating premenstrual syndrome symptoms (Dvivedi et al, 2008).

Psychological outcomes, perceived stress, anxiety, and depression levels as well as radiation-induced DNA damage were assessed in 68 breast cancer patients undergoing radiotherapy and enrolled in an integrated yoga program. The psychological outcomes were significantly improved in the yoga group, but only a slight decrease in DNA damage was seen compared with the no intervention group (Banerjee et al, 2007).

In another study, 98 outpatients with stage II or III breast cancer were assigned to either yoga or supportive therapy. Data were analyzed only for those who underwent surgery followed by radiotherapy and chemotherapy. Subjects were assessed using the State Trait Anxiety Inventory (STAI) before and after 60 minutes of daily yoga sessions. Results showed a general decrease in self-reported STAI scores in the yoga group and a positive correlation of these scores with distress during conventional treatment intervals (Rao et al, 2009).

Looking into the neuroendocrine mechanisms underlying the effect of yoga, Madanmohan et al (2002) approached the question of whether yoga modulates the stress physiological response from a different angle. They used the cold pressor test to trigger a stress response in 10 healthy subjects who were taught shavasan practice. They measured the respiratory rate interval variation, deep breathing difference, and heart rate, blood pressure, and rate-pressure-product response to cold pressor test before and immediately after a yoga session. A significant increase in deep breathing difference and a close to significant increase in respiratory rate interval variation were observed, which indicate improved parasympathetic activity. Values of the other parameters mirroring sympathetic activity were blunted, which suggests that yoga practice helps reduce the sympathetic load on the heart (Madanmohan et al, 2002).

Biochemical and genomic approaches have also been undertaken to understand the action mechanisms underlying the stress reduction effects of *Sudarshan Kriya* Yoga. Whole blood drawn from 42 healthy subjects was used to measure glutathione peroxidase levels, and red blood cell lysate was used for superoxide dismutase activity assay as well as to estimate glutathione levels. White blood cells were separated and processed for gene expression. The results showed a better immune status and antioxidant profile both at the enzyme activity and at the RNA level in the yoga intervention group. A prolonged lymphocyte life span supported by the upregulation of antiapoptotic and survival genes was also observed. All together, these results suggest that *Sudarshan Kriya* Yoga has beneficial effects on immunity, cell death, and stress regulation through transcriptional pathways (Sharma et al, 2008).

In a systematic review assessing the existing evidence for yoga practice in neuropsychiatric disorders, the authors reported different grades of evidence. From the 124 trials collected, only 16 met the set-forth criteria. Among those, four randomized controlled trials showed benefits of yoga for depression and three for schizophrenia (as adjunct to drugs), two for attention deficit hyperactivity disorder in children, all with a grade B evidence;

however, only grade C evidence was recorded for the benefit of yoga on sleep disturbances in two randomized controlled trials (Balasubramaniam et al, 2013). There is insufficient evidence showing other aspects of yoga benefits such as comparative effectiveness, molecular mechanisms, and population diversity.

PLACEBO EFFECT AND PSYCHONEUROIMMUNOLOGY

A *placebo* is an inert substance or a control method used to evaluate the psychological and physiological effects of a new drug or procedure. The response to the placebo should not exceed that to the experimental drug or method, which would otherwise be considered ineffective. The placebo response had been seen as unpredictable and unreliable, and mediated by nonspecific mechanisms that were once dismissed as immeasurable and irrelevant (Chapter 9).

How does the psychoneuroimmunological complex relate to the placebo effect? It has been argued that every therapeutic intervention—whether complementary, integrative, and alternative medicine, or allopathic medicine—involves a placebo effect (Figure 8-3). Most allopathic physicians had considered it unethical or even deceitful to actively encourage a placebo response. However, in a survey of 1200 practicing internists and rheumatologists in the United States that inquired about behaviors and attitudes regarding the use of placebo treatments, among those who responded ($n = 679$), half reported prescribing placebo treatments on a regular basis within the previous year in the form of saline, sugar pills, over-the-counter analgesics, and vitamins. Most physicians describe these substances to their patients as potentially beneficial or as a treatment not typically used for the patient's condition, and most physicians believe this practice to be common and ethically allowable (de la Rochefordière et al, 1996).

PNI research demonstrates that an expectation of recovery can alter subjective feelings of well-being and result in ANS activation and pituitary hormone production. Thus, specific verifiable pathways have been identified by which expectation can alter immunity. However, expectation

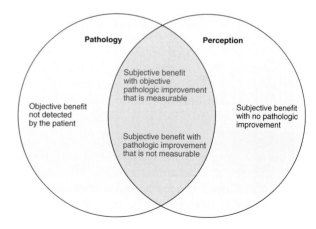

Figure 8-3 Overlap of objective and subjective therapeutic benefits.

likely has different effects in different individuals, producing large shifts in autonomic balance and hormonal output in some and negligible changes in others, which explains the unpredictability of the placebo response. Together with the idea that complementary therapies affect merely "subjective" measures of disease activity, these observations have formed some of the planks in the platform on which allopathic physicians argue that complementary practices are fundamentally flawed and of limited benefit.

Although fallacious, defeatist, and ultimately counterproductive, these arguments persist. The expectation of recovery that promotes a placebo response is separate from any subjective improvement and, incidentally, is also different from hope. It is possible to feel subjectively better without expecting a full recovery. Similarly, it is possible to expect recovery without feeling better at all (Figure 8-3). Complementary therapies cannot be dismissed as mere placebos, and it is becoming increasingly obvious that they produce substantial subjective and objective clinical benefits unrelated to the placebo effect per se.

Individuals differ in their responsiveness to the various activation stimuli, whether expectancy, subjective sensations, or complementary therapies. This individuality would explain why complementary therapies that are supposedly mediated by placebo mechanisms, as in allopathic arguments, could outperform placebos in a double-blind trial. It would also explain the need to combine a number of complementary approaches to ensure that these pathways are optimally activated (see Chapter 10).

There is a growing body of scientific literature published since 2006 from psychoneurologists and neuroscientists addressing the specific issues of placebo and *nocebo*, which is the worsening of symptoms due to a nonspecific response, and their potential biological mechanisms. According to Eccles (2007), the placebo response in clinical medicine could be compared to a component of an allergy treatment that possesses "nonspecific effects" (e.g., natural recovery) and a "true placebo effect" represented as the psychological therapeutic effect of the treatment.

Intrinsic positive belief in the efficacy of the treatment characterizes the true placebo effect, which can be enhanced by extrinsic factors such as the interaction with physician. Negative belief, however, can engender a nocebo effect that may elucidate some psychogenic diseases (Eccles, 2007). To examine placebo and nocebo symptoms, college students were recruited into what appeared to be a clinical trial evaluating the effectiveness of an herbal supplement on cognitive performance. Subjects received either an herbal supplement or a placebo (both were placebo inactive pills) and a list of positive and adverse effects. Most participants reported symptoms, and those who believed they were ingesting the herbal supplement reported significantly more symptoms than those who thought they were taking a placebo. In this case the belief may exacerbate the placebo response (Link et al, 2006). Further discussion of placebo and nocebo is provided in Chapters 9 and 10.

SUMMARY

The medical and scientific communities are showing growing interest in the neurohumoral mechanisms underlying PNI responses to complementary therapies.

The latest research in the biomedical sciences and the social/behavorial sciences is beginning to demonstrate mechanisms of action by which CAM therapies exert their benefits. The studies published to date have been carried out with relatively small groups of subjects and reflect conventional study criteria and design. Although complementary medicine research currently follows the conventional scientific approach in attempt to satisfy critics, evaluation of the efficacy of various complementary, integrative, and alternative modalities may require the development of additional methodologies based on a new paradigm to overcome foreseeable limitations.

It is noteworthy that the criticism of alternative and integrative therapies as being placebos has moved basic and clinical scientists to question the placebo and nocebo response itself. There is a call to expand the thinking beyond the "expectation and brain reward circuitry" or Pavlovian conditioning to include other pathways and mechanisms that reflect the psychoneuroimmunoendocrine paradigm. This theoretical framework needs to be redefined, and methodological as well as ethical paradigms should be developed to elucidate the placebo/nocebo response.

References

Abu-Asab M, Amri H, Micozzi MS: *Avicenna's medicine: a new translation of the 11th-century canon with practical applications for integrative medicine,* 2013, Healing Arts Press.

Ackerman KD, Felten SY, Dijkstra CD, et al: Parallel development of noradrenergic innervation and cellular compartmentation in the rat spleen, *Exp Neurol* 103(3):239–255, 1989.

Ader R, editor: *Psychoneuroimmunology,* 1991, Academic Press.

Arranz L, Guayerbas N, Siboni L, De la Fuente M: Effect of acupuncture treatment on the immune function impairment found in anxious women, *Am J Chin Med* 35(1):35–51, 2007.

Balasubramaniam M, Telles S, Doraiswamy PM: Yoga on our minds: a systematic review of yoga for neuropsychiatric disorders, *Front Psychiatry* 3:117, 2013.

Baldwin DV: Primitive mechanisms of trauma response: an evolutionary perspective on trauma-related disorders, *Neurosci Biobehav Rev* 37(8):1549–1566, 2013.

Banerjee B, Vadiraj HS, Ram A, et al: Effects of an integrated yoga program in modulating psychological stress and radiation-induced genotoxic stress in breast cancer patients undergoing radiotherapy, *Integr Cancer Ther* 6(3):242–250, 2007.

Bhasin MK, Dusek JA, Chang BH, et al: Relaxation response induces temporal transcriptome changes in energy metabolism, insulin secretion and inflammatory pathways, *PLoS ONE* 8(5):e62817, 2013.

Beal MC: Viscerosomatic reflexes: a review, *J Am Osteopath Assoc* 85(12):786–801, 1985.

Bellinger DL, Felten SY, Felten DL: Maintenance of noradrenergic sympathetic innervation in the involuted thymus of the aged Fischer 344 rat, *Brain Behav Immun* 2(2):133–150, 1988.

Besedovsky H, Sorkin E, Keller M, Müller J: Changes in blood hormone levels during the immune response, *Proc Soc Exp Biol Med* 150(2):466–470, 1975.

Blalock JE: The immune system: our sixth sense, *The Immunologist* 2:8–15, 1994.

Bouhuys A: Effect of posture in experimental asthma in man, *Am J Med* 34:470–476, 1963.

Carlson LE, Speca M, Faris P, Patel KD: One year pre-post intervention follow-up of psychological, immune, endocrine and blood pressure outcomes of mindfulness-based stress reduction (MBSR) in breast and prostate cancer outpatients, *Brain Behav Immun* 21(8):1038–1049, 2007.

Carlson LE, Speca M, Patel KD, Goodey E: Mindfulness-based stress reduction in relation to quality of life, mood, symptoms of stress and levels of cortisol, dehydroepiandrosterone sulfate (DHEAS) and melatonin in breast and prostate cancer outpatients, *Psychoneuroendocrinology* 29(4):448–474, 2004.

Cassano D: Neurology and the soul: from the origins until 1500, *J Hist Neurosci* 5(2):152–161, 1996.

Creswell JD, Myers HF, Cole SW, Irwin MR: Mindfulness meditation training effects on CD4+ T lymphocytes in HIV-1 infected adults: A small randomized controlled trial, *Brain Behav Immun* 23(2):184–188, 2009.

Davidson RJ, Kabat-Zinn J, Schumacher J, et al: Alterations in brain and immune function produced by mindfulness meditation, *Psychosom Med* 65(4):564–570, 2003.

de la Rochefordière A, Mouret-Fourme E, Asselain B, et al: Metachronous contralateral breast cancer as first event of relapse, *Int J Radiat Oncol Biol Phys* 36(3):615–621, 1996.

DeBeneditttis G, Cigada M, Bianchi A, et al: Autonomic changes during hypnosis: a heart rate variability power spectrum analysis as a marker of sympatho-vagal balance, *Int J Clin Exp Hypn* 42(2):140–152, 1994.

Du J: [The messengers from peripheral nervous system to central nervous system: involvement of neurotrophins and cytokines in the mechanisms of acupuncture], *Zhen Ci Yan Jiu* 33(1):37–40, 2008.

Dunjic-Kostic B, Ivkovic M, Radonjic NV, et al: Melancholic and atypical major depression–connection between cytokines, psychopathology and treatment, *Prog Neuropsychopharmacol Biol Psychiatry* 43:1–6, 2013.

Dusek JA, Chang BH, Zaki J, et al: Association between oxygen consumption and nitric oxide production during the relaxation response, *Med Sci Monit* 12(1):CR1–CR10, 2006.

Dusek JA, Otu HH, Wohlhueter AL, et al: Genomic counter-stress changes induced by the relaxation response, *PLoS ONE* 3(7):e2576, 2008.

Dvivedi J, Dvivedi S, Mahajan KK, et al: Effect of '61-points relaxation technique' on stress parameters in premenstrual syndrome, *Indian J Physiol Pharmacol* 52(1):69–76, 2008.

Eccles R: The power of the placebo, *Curr Allergy Asthma Rep* 7(2):100–104, 2007.

Engel GL: The need for a new medical model: a challenge for biomedicine, *Science* 196(4286):129–136, 1977.

Felten DL, Felten SY, Bellinger DL, Lorton D: Noradrenergic and peptidergic innervation of secondary lymphoid organs: role in experimental rheumatoid arthritis, *Eur J Clin Invest* 22(Suppl 1):37–41, 1992.

Fenwick PB: Self-generation of seizures by an action of mind, *Adv Neurol* 75:87–92, 1998.

Han JS, Tang J, Ren MF, et al: Central neurotransmitters and acupuncture analgesia, *Am J Chin Med* 8(4):331–348, 1980.

Harinath K, Malhotra AS, Pal K, et al: Effects of Hatha yoga and Omkar meditation on cardiorespiratory performance, psychologic profile, and melatonin secretion, *J Altern Complement Med* 10(2):261–268, 2004.

Hatch JP, Borcherding S, Norris LK: Cardiopulmonary adjustments during operant heart rate control, *Psychophysiology* 27(6):641–648, 1990.

Hulkkonen J, Koskikallio E, Rainesalo S, et al: The balance of inhibitory and excitatory cytokines is differently regulated in vivo and in vitro among therapy resistant epilepsy patients, *Epilepsy Res* 59(2–3):199–205, 2004.

Goertz C, Marriott BP: Military report more complementary and alternative medicine use than civilians, *J Altern Complement Med* 19(6):509–517, 2013.

Irwin M, Daniels M, Smith TL, et al: Impaired natural killer cell activity during bereavement, *Brain Behav Immun* 1(1):98–104, 1987.

Irwin M, Jones L, Britton K, Hauger RL: Central corticotropin releasing factor reduces natural cytotoxicity. Time course of action, *Neuropsychopharmacology* 2(4):281–284, 1989.

Irwin MR, Miller AH: Depressive disorders and immunity: 20 years of progress and discovery, *Brain Behav Immun* 21(4):374–383, 2007.

Irwin MR, Olmstead R, Oxman MN: Augmenting immune responses to varicella zoster virus in older adults: a randomized, controlled trial of Tai Chi, *J Am Geriatr Soc* 55(4):511–517, 2007.

Jawer MA, Micozzi MS: *Spiritual Anatomy of Emotion*, Rochester VT, 2009, Inner Traditions/Healing Arts Press.

Jawer MA, Micozzi MS: *Your Emotional Type*, Rochester VT, 2012, Inner Traditions/Healing Arts Press.

Jian M: Influence of adrenergic antagonist and naloxone on the anti-allergic shock effect of electro-acupuncture in mice, *Acupunct Electrother Res* 10(3):163–167, 1985.

Jung W, Irwin M: Reduction of natural killer cytotoxic activity in major depression: interaction between depression and cigarette smoking, *Psychosom Med* 61(3):263–270, 1999.

Kasahara T, Wu Y, Sakurai Y, Oguchi K: Suppressive effect of acupuncture on delayed type hypersensitivity to trinitrochlorobenzene and involvement of opiate receptors, *Int J Immunopharmacol* 14(4):661–665, 1992.

Kavoussi B, Ross BE: The neuroimmune basis of anti-inflammatory acupuncture, *Integr Cancer Ther* 6(3):251–257, 2007.

Lang UE, Borgwardt S: Molecular mechanisms of depression: perspectives on new treatment strategies, *Cell Physiol Biochem* 31:761–777, 2013.

Lee C, Crawford C, Wallerstedt D, et al: The effectiveness of acupuncture research across components of the trauma spectrum response (tsr): a systematic review of reviews, *Syst Rev* 15(1):46, 2012.

Lehto SM, Huotari A: Serum IL-7 and G-CSF in major depressive disorder, *Prog Neuropsychopharmacol Biol Psychiatry* 34(6):846–851, 2010.

Link J, Haggard R, Kelly K, Forrer D: Placebo/nocebo symptom reporting in a sham herbal supplement trial, *Eval Health Prof* 29(4):394–406, 2006.

Lokhorst GJ, Kaitaro TT: The originality of Descartes' theory about the pineal gland, *J Hist Neurosci* 10(1):6–18, 2001.

Lutgendorf SK, Costanzo ES: Psychoneuroimmunology and health psychology: an integrative model, *Brain Behav Immun* 17(4):225–232, 2003.

Ma SX: Neurobiology of acupuncture: toward CAM, *Evid Based Complement Alternat Med* 1(1):41–47, 2004.

Madanmohan, Udupa K, Bhavanani AB, et al: Modulation of cold pressor-induced stress by shavasan in normal adult volunteers, *Indian J Physiol Pharmacol* 46(3):307–312, 2002.

Mayer DJ, Price DD, Rafii A: Antagonism of acupuncture analgesia in man by the narcotic antagonist naloxone, *Brain Res* 121(2):368–372, 1977.

Matousek RH, Pruessner JC, Dobkin PL: Changes in the cortisol awakening response (CAR) following participation in mindfulness-based stress reduction in women who completed treatment for breast cancer, *Complement Ther Clin Pract* 17(2): 65–70, 2011.

McCain NL, Gray DP, Elswick RK, et al: A randomized clinical trial of alternative stress management interventions in persons with HIV infection, *J Consult Clin Psychol* 76(3):431–441, 2008.

Mommersteeg PM, Vermetten E, Kavelaars A, et al: Hostility is related to clusters of T-cell cytokines and chemokines in healthy men, *Psychoneuroendocrinology* 33(8):1041–1050, 2008.

Neild JE, Cameron IR: Bronchoconstriction in response to suggestion: its prevention by an inhaled anticholinergic agent, *Br Med J (Clin Res Ed)* 290(6469):674, 1985.

Nemir P, Micozzi MS: Combined aneurysmal and occlusive arterial disease, *Circulation* 56(3):169–170, 1977.

Pert CB, Dreher HE, Ruff MR: The psychosomatic network: foundations of mind-body medicine, *Altern Ther Health Med* 4(4):30–41, 1998.

Peterson C, Bossio L: *Healthy Attitudes: Optimism, Hope, and Control*, Yonkers, NY, 1993, Consumer Reports Books.

Rao MR, Raghuram N, Nagendra HR, et al: Anxiolytic effects of a yoga program in early breast cancer patients undergoing conventional treatment: a randomized controlled trial, *Complement Ther Med* 17(1):1–8, 2009.

Rasmussen AF Jr, Marsh JT, Brill NQ: Increased susceptibility to herpes simplex in mice subjected to avoidance-learning stress or restraint, *Proc Soc Exp Biol Med* 96(1):183–189, 1957.

Raub JA: Psychophysiologic effects of Hatha Yoga on musculoskeletal and cardiopulmonary function: a literature review, *J Altern Complement Med* 8(6):797–812, 2002.

Reichlin S: Neuroendocrine-immune interactions, *N Engl J Med* 329(17):1246–1253, 1993.

Robinson FP, Mathews HL, Witek-Janusek L: Psycho-endocrine-immune response to mindfulness-based stress reduction in individuals infected with the human immunodeficiency virus: a quasiexperimental study, *J Altern Complement Med* 9(5):683–694, 2003.

Sharma H, Datta P, Singh A, et al: Gene expression profiling in practitioners of Sudarshan Kriya, *J Psychosom Res* 64(2):213–218, 2008.

Sjolund BH, Eriksson MB: The influence of naloxone on analgesia produced by peripheral conditioning stimulation, *Brain Res* 173(2):295–301, 1979.

Smith TC, Ryan MA, Smith B, et al: Complementary and alternative medicine use among US Navy and Marine Corps personnel, *BMC Complement Altern Med* 7:16, 2007.

Strausbaugh H, Irwin M: Central corticotropin-releasing hormone reduces cellular immunity, *Brain Behav Immun* 6(1): 11–17, 1992.

Sung HJ, Kim YS, Kim IS, et al: Proteomic analysis of differential protein expression in neuropathic pain and electroacupuncture treatment models, *Proteomics* 4(9):2805–2813, 2004.

Tercier J: *The contemporary deathbed: the ultimate rush*, Basingstoke, 2005, Palgrave Macmillan.

Tripathi P: Nitric oxide and immune response, *Indian J Biochem Biophys* 44(5):310–319, 2007.

Vernon HT, Dhami MS, Howley TP, Annett R: Spinal manipulation and beta-endorphin: a controlled study of the effect of a spinal manipulation on plasma beta-endorphin levels in normal males, *J Manipulative Physiol Ther* 9(2):115–123, 1986.

Wang F, Lee EK, Wu T, et al: The effects of tai chi on depression, anxiety, and psychological well-being: a systematic review and meta-analysis, *Int J Behav Med* September 28, 2013. [Epub ahead of print].

Watkins AD: Hierarchical cortical control of neuroimmunomodulatory pathways, *Neuropathol Appl Neurobiol* 20(5):423–431, 1994.

Watkins AD: Perceptions, emotions and immunity: an integrated homeostatic network, *QJM* 88(4):283–294, 1995.

Weschenfelder J, Sander C: The influence of cytokines on wakefulness regulation: clinical relevance, mechanisms and methodological problems, *Psychiatr Danub* 24(2):112–126, 2012.

Witek-Janusek L, Albuquerque K, Chroniak KR, et al: Effect of mindfulness based stress reduction on immune function, quality of life and coping in women newly diagnosed with early stage breast cancer, *Brain Behav Immun* 22(6):969–981, 2008.

Wolsko PM, Eisenberg DM, Davis RB, Phillips RS: Use of mind-body medical therapies, *J Gen Intern Med* 19(1):43–50, 2004.

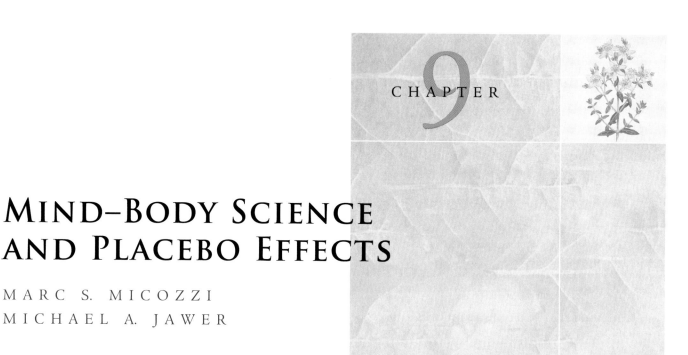

CHAPTER 9

MIND–BODY SCIENCE AND PLACEBO EFFECTS

MARC S. MICOZZI
MICHAEL A. JAWER

ealing, like life itself, can often be mysterious. The essence of the universe, including the universe of mind and body, remains challenging to explain or comprehend. The void inside every atom is pulsating with information, or perhaps unseen consciousness or intelligence. Molecular biologists and geneticists locate this information or intelligence within DNA, primarily for the sake of convenience. Life unfolds as DNA imparts its coded intelligence into a sequence in which energy and information are interchanged for the purpose of building life from matter—based on an ontogenetic blueprint by which cells develop into organisms along phylogenetic lines.

The view of reality ushered in by quantum physics made it possible to manipulate the invisible intelligence that underlies the visible world. Albert Einstein taught that the physical body, as with all material objects, is like an illusion, and trying to manipulate it can be like grasping the shadow and missing the substance. The subatomic world, while unseen, is nonetheless real. Similarly, if we are willing to explore the immense creative power that lies within the mind, we can access unseen dimensions of the body (see Chapter 14).

HISTORICAL OVERVIEW

While mainstream medicine has awakened to the inherent power of the mind, some of the earliest records of certain mind–body techniques arose in Babylonia and Sumer well before the rise of experimental science. In the third century BC, Hippocrates was well versed in the art of mental healing. A serpent coiled around a staff is the Hippocratic symbol historically used to portray the medical and healing professions. Other history reveals that the coiled serpent also can symbolize the healing energy possessed within each body, lying dormant at the base of the spine (as literally in Kundalini Yoga), with the staff representing life itself. Some Asian philosophy posits that when the serpent is unleashed, healing energy spirals up the spine and out the forehead. This energy, said to be mental in nature, can then be used to heal the physical body (see Chapter 21).

Most ancient and indigenous medical systems make use of the extraordinary interconnectedness of the mind and body. Native American, Asian Indian, and other cultures believe their members to be in contact with natural healing forces through their dreams, visions, and mystical experiences (see Sections V and VI).

The ancient Greeks were known for their healing temples. These centers existed for more than 800 years and endured until the rise of the Christian era. Patients would travel long distances to experience one of these Aesculapian healing temples. The first step in seeking a cure was to create inner cleanliness by taking a purifying bath. Patients then were put on a special diet or fast. They would attend one of the great dramas of Euripides or Sophocles, observing the tensions and movements of life. Later, they were taken to visit one of the shrines, where healers used imagery to visualize the affected part of the body. During sleep the priests entered the patients' rooms and touched the diseased parts. Thereafter, patients would dream and were said to awaken healed.

Philippus Aureolus Theophrastus Bombastus von Hohenheim, known as Paracelsus, was a sixteenth-century Renaissance physician. Often considered the father of modern drug therapy and scientific medicine, he opposed the idea of separating the mind from the healing processes of the body. Along with his esteemed medical theories, he held that imagination and faith were the cause of healing power:

> Humans have a visible and an invisible workshop. The visible one is the body and the invisible one is the imagination of the mind. The spirit is the master, imagination the tool, and the body the plastic material. The power of the imagination is the great factor in medicine. It may produce diseases in humans and it may cure them. Ills of the body may be cured by physical remedies or by the power of spirit acting through the soul.

Paracelsus also believed that physicians could heal by tapping the spiritual power of God. He believed that dreams gave humans clairvoyance and the ability to diagnose illness from long distances.

The philosophies of all these cultures held a common belief in a spiritual center that resides within each human being. They believed in spirit over matter, mind over body. In contrast, modern allopathic medicine has regarded these connections as nonscientific and of secondary, if any, importance. Scientific healing, in the form of drug therapy and surgery, has grown to become the dominant Western form of treatment. Since the early 1900s, however, many medical scientists began to reinvestigate the role the mind plays in healing. In critical situations, physicians have been known to say, "We have done all we can do—it is in God's hands now," or "It depends on the patient's will to live."

Physicians often witness miraculous recoveries unexplainable by a strictly scientific understanding. Labeling a recovery as a "spontaneous remission" is the commonplace term to describe a healing that cannot be explained by conventional medical standards. Physicians have also long recognized the effectiveness of placebos, substances with no known pharmacological action or benefit. In some cases, placebos can be as much as 70% effective in the treatment of illness, thereby proving the theory that a patient's therapeutic expectation is a strong contributing factor to healing.

EVOLUTION IN UNDERSTANDING

During the past four decades, the scientific community has made great strides in exploring the mind's capacity to affect the body. This movement has received its impetus from several sources. The rise in the incidence of chronic illness over the past few decades and the rapidly increasing costs and dangers of conventional treatment have set the stage for deeper exploration of mind–body therapies. These therapies show great promise for mobilizing the body's inherent power to heal itself.

Recent studies, for instance, are deepening our understanding of the effects of stress on the body. Convincing evidence supports the premise that the immune system, along with other organs and systems in the body, can be powerfully influenced by the mind (a scientific concept known as psychoneuroimmunology [Box 9-1], mentioned again later in this chapter, and discussed in Chapter 8). These research efforts and clinical experiments suggest that any separation between mind and body, long taken for granted in Western philosophy, is difficult to identify or quantify. This challenge is part of a new approach to medical science: proving that the mind—including our thoughts, memories, and emotions—has a significant impact on the body's health.

BOX 9-1 *Mind and Immunity*

Psychoneuroimmunology, a term coined by the late Robert Ader, an experimental psychologist at the University of Rochester, was first introduced to the scientific community in 1981. Ader had previously conducted laboratory experiments showing that the immune system could be conditioned and therefore did not operate autonomously, but was actually under the influence of the brain (see Chapter 8).

In subsequent research, Ader and Nicholas Cohen showed that the immune system can be trained, or conditioned, to respond to a neutral stimulus (placebo). They found that the administration of an immune-suppressing drug and placebo together conditioned the immune system to respond to the placebo alone after the drug was discontinued. They also found that by alternating the administration of real medication and placebo, thus conditioning the body's physiological response to the placebo, the beneficial effects of a drug can be increased and the side effects of drug dependence could be decreased (see Chapter 8).

Considering the brief time that psychoneuroimmunology has existed as an accepted field of research, a great amount of data has been collected in support of the idea that homeostatic mechanisms are the product of an integrated system of defenses of which the immune system is a critical component. Now that we know that neuropeptides and their receptors are simultaneously present in the nervous system, the digestive system, and the immune system, it is not surprising to learn that immunological reactivity can be influenced by stressful life experiences.

Research and clinical observations continue to shed light on the mechanisms by which the power of the mind is manifest. How else can an individual's attitudes or the anticipation of a physical effect actually bring about bodily change? How can such knowledge be used to enhance medical treatment or promote good health? What is the mechanism that underlies spontaneous remission (which is known to occur in supposedly "incurable" cancer more often than any other disease)? Mind–body practitioners and medical researchers are answering many questions regarding the clinical, scientific, and ethical dimensions of placebo and the placebo effect.

For patients, this new synthesis has very practical significance. It suggests that by paying attention to and exerting influence over mental and emotional states, they may actually contribute to prevention of, recovery from, and management of disease. The conscious participation of the patient in the process of healing not only offers new insights but also raises new questions about the nature of consciousness.

A fundamental tenet of mind–body medicine is the concept of *treating the whole person.* Another significant tenet is that people can be active participants in their own health care and may be able to prevent disease or shorten its course by taking steps to manage their own mental and emotional processes.

Medical researchers are beginning to rediscover techniques that other cultures have historically used in their healing systems, such as meditation, hypnosis, and imagery.

Grounded in ancient philosophy, these interventions are capable of stimulating the mind's capacity to affect the body. Experimentation has given practitioners the opportunity to offer nontoxic, noninvasive therapies while examining the specific links between mental and emotional processes and autonomic, immune, and nervous system functioning. While no serious practitioner can promise that people can completely cure themselves of disease solely by adjusting their mental attitudes, mind–body approaches can be used to reduce the severity and frequency of biological symptoms and can potentially help strengthen the body's resistance to disease.

The techniques of mind–body medicine are reasonably well accepted for treating certain chronic and difficult-to-treat medical conditions, from pain syndromes to hypertension. In well-designed studies, relaxation, guided imagery, biofeedback, hypnosis, and related strategies have been proven effective and highly practicable. For example, in a meta-analysis encompassing 191 studies and more than 8600 patients, psychosocial–behavioral interventions showed reliable, moderate effects in improving recovery, reducing pain, and decreasing psychological distress (see Chapter 10).

Mainstream medical institutions are beginning to take steps toward implementing these approaches within departments of psychology, psychiatry, oncology, neurology, and rehabilitation. Mind–body departments have been established in medical schools and hospitals worldwide. More impressively, both conventional and holistic professionals are beginning to incorporate these approaches into their professional practices, as well as their own personal regimens for greater health and wellness. Interestingly, the professions of psychiatry and psychology have, by and large, been more reluctant to adopt mind–body therapies than have integrative physicians.

This chapter discusses the research evidence that supports mind–body approaches, describes the more widely used and accepted techniques, and summarizes results from some of the most effective interventions. Beyond demonstrating dramatic results in many cases, such mind–body approaches amount to a basis for a new perspective for medicine and healing. From this perspective, it becomes evident that every interaction between physician and patient has the potential to affect the mind and, in turn, the body of the patient.

ROLE OF CONSCIOUSNESS

PRIOR DISMISSAL OF THE MIND

Although ancient healers, mystics, and physicians believed in the power of the human mind, Western science began to question such matters by the mid-1800s. The prevailing philosophy until that time was that the patient's inner life and social being were vital components of all diagnosis and treatment. Medicine, it was understood, should take into account not only biological but also behavioral, psychological, and spiritual factors.

These models and methods began to fade by the end of the nineteenth century, however, and an individualized, patient-specific model of treatment gave way to a disease-specific model. During the rise of this era of experimental, materialist, and reductionist science, four leading German physiologists (Hermann von Helmholtz, Carl Ludwig, Emil du Bois–Reymond, and Ernst Wilhelm von Brücke) pledged themselves to account for all bodily processes in purely physical terms. They considered that any reported connection between mental states and bodily functions were biased, subjective, nonmeasurable, and scientifically unreliable (Figure 9-1). More than 15,000 American physicians traveled to Germany to study the fascinating laboratory experimentations being introduced at that time. These innovative breakthroughs were in direct contrast with the styles of medicine that had been practiced for centuries. It was believed that proper research could be conducted only in laboratories on isolated constituents—microorganisms, components of blood and urine, tissue, and organs—with

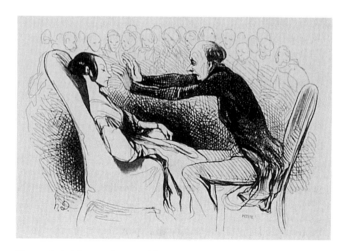

Figure 9-1 Mesmerism and hypnotism were the object of satire and a number of caricatures during the nineteenth century. (Courtesy Bibliothèque Interuniversitaire de Médecine, Paris.)

the focus on devising remedies that would apply universally to all patients. This approach has put contemporary medicine in the position of having to relearn the scientific basis of something it had actually known about for centuries: that beliefs, thoughts, and feelings affect physiology (see Chapter 8).

POWER OF PLACEBO

The word *placebo* is Latin for "I shall please." Its roots in colloquial speech implying "false consolation" date back to the twelfth century (Stefano et al, 2001). This concept is well illustrated by an anecdote concerning Sir William Osler (1849-1919). One of North America and England's busiest and most famous physicians, Osler brought new light to the power of placebo near the turn of the twentieth century. He once made a house call to a dying boy who had been unresponsive to any previous treatments. Osler appeared at the boy's bedside dressed in magnificent scarlet academic robes. After a brief examination, Osler sat down at the boy's bedside, peeled a peach, sugared it, and cut it into pieces. He then fed it, bit by bit, with a fork to the entranced patient, telling him that it was a most special fruit and that if he ate it, he would not be sick. (Perhaps Osler had read the account of "*Hanuman, the White Monkey, Eating the Magic Peach*" from the Sanskrit creation epic, *The Ramayana*.)

Osler confided to the boy's father that his son's chances for survival were slim. He continued to visit the boy daily for more than a month, always dressed in his majestic scarlet robes and offering the boy nourishment with his own two hands. This dramatic presentation inspired belief well beyond laboratory science and helped catalyze the boy's unexpected and complete recovery (what we would now term a spontaneous remission).

Eloquently summing up the placebo's power, Osler (1953) wrote the following:

> Faith in the gods or saints cures one, faith in little pills another, hypnotic suggestion a third, faith in a plain common doctor a fourth.... The faith with which we work ... has its limitations [but] such as we find it, faith is the most precious commodity, without which we should be very badly off.

EARLY PLACEBO STUDIES

During World War II the anesthesiologist Henry Beecher noted with surprise, as he examined men with serious shrapnel wounds at Anzio beach, that many of them refused morphine for pain. This behavior was something that he almost never saw in Boston when he tended to patients with far less serious wounds in the aftermath of surgery. How could such a phenomenon be explained? Under conditions that produce extreme stress or fear, higher emotional centers in the brain can activate a descending system that suppresses incoming pain signals. This descending analgesic system utilizes the body's own endogenous opiate-like neurotransmitters, the endor-

phins. The threshold for activation of descending analgesia by stress is high; otherwise pain would lose its survival value. But the nervous system appears to be organized so that in circumstances that produce the greatest stress or fear—for example, pursuit by a predator or mortal combat, circumstances in which the survival value of running or fighting far outweighs the risk of using already damaged limbs—pain can be completely suppressed (see Chapter 8).

Among early placebo studies are those conducted by Dr. Ronald Katz, Chairman of the Department of Anesthesiology at the University of California at Los Angeles School of Medicine. Katz reported a series of observations involving patients who were informed that headaches were a complication of spinal anesthesia. At the last minute the patients were told that the choice of anesthesia had been changed from spinal to general. Despite the change, all the patients experienced the symptoms associated with spinal anesthesia (see Chapter 8).

Dr. J.W.L. Fielding conducted a study at the Department of Surgery at the Queen Elizabeth Hospital in Birmingham, England, that similarly investigated the role of expectation. In compliance with informed consent procedures, 411 patients were told that they could expect to lose hair as a result of the chemotherapy being administered. Thirty percent of the patients unknowingly received placebos instead of chemotherapy and experienced hair loss even though the pills they had taken contained no medication.

THE PLACEBO EFFECT

Drawing on the well-established mind-body connection, a psychophysiological effect that is also a potent and versatile therapeutic tool is called the "placebo effect." A placebo is an inert substance (e.g., sugar pill or saline injection) or a sham physical/electrical manipulation believed to have no material (chemical, electrical, or physical) effect on the patient. Nonetheless, powerful chemical, electromagnetic, and physical transformations are often observed after patients' exposure to placebos. For example, placebos have been used to "switch on" and "switch off" serious breathing difficulties associated with asthma. A mind-body dimension to this medical problem is further suggested by the occurrence of psychogenic asthma, and by the effectiveness of acupuncture as a treatment (see Chapter 29)—for which conventional Western medicine has no explanations for a mechanism of action.

The potential of the placebo effect ranges from the simple, benign properties of a sugar pill to sham surgical procedures that were once performed where nothing was actually done to benefit the patients, who nonetheless reported "feeling better" after the operation. Even in cases of open-heart surgery, Nobel laureate (1985) Bernard Lown's lifelong research has forcefully questioned the ultimate benefits in terms of morbidity and mortality. One of us (MSM) has suspected, since "scrubbing in" on many open-heart surgeries during the 1970s, that there is a strong placebo component to the procedure. After all, it is difficult to exceed the "miraculous" effects of stopping the heart, working inside the chest, and then starting the heart again, effectively bringing the patient back to life.

Placebos have demonstrated remarkable potency in relieving intractable symptoms (pain, depression, anxiety, and so on), alleviating signs associated with a wide variety of illnesses (involving virtually every part of the body), shortening recovery time from invasive medical procedures and even reducing mortality. Objective and measurable physiologic functions that generally elude conscious control (e.g., concentrations of hormones, immunological markers, and neurotransmitters, as well as electrical activity of the heart) have been changed following participation in the placebo arms of research studies (Box 9-2).

Because these health effects are not the result of a potent drug or a powerfully precise surgical procedure, what explanations are possible? This chapter investigates possible explanations and delineates issues related to the use of placebos and the mobilization of inner, self-healing abilities.

EVOLUTION OF THE ART

A clear distinction should be made between questionable "placebo interventions" and the beneficial placebo effect. When applied in modern clinical practice, the former often

represent deceptive practices that harm rather than benefit patients. Frequently, the use of placebos is simply not consistent with good science or ethical professional practice. (This shortcoming will be addressed more fully later in this chapter.)

In contrast, the placebo effect is a desirable outgrowth of a skilled application of the ancient art of healing, regardless of the medical discipline or the setting where care is provided. Clinicians should always consider the benefits of this art form when providing care, and to help patients access and mobilize their own self-healing capabilities.

Technically, a placebo is an intervention designed to simulate medical therapy, but that is not believed by the investigator or clinician to actually be beneficial. Placebos are understood to produce an effect in patients resulting from implicit or explicit intent and not from any physical or chemical properties of the intervention. Placebos often take the form of sugar pills, saline injections, miniscule doses of drugs, or sham procedures designed to be void of any known therapeutic value (Bok, 1974).

Placebos are known to mimic the action of a wide variety of drugs, even exhibiting measurable drug-like properties (Fine et al, 1994). When given intravenously, a placebo begins to work in 15 to 60 minutes, with a peak effect over the next 15 to 45 minutes and an overall action that can last several hours or days. Pills or injections have

---

BOX 9-2 *Nature's Pain Killers*

Although it has sometimes confounded as much as clarified, the mechanisms of pain and the placebo effect have provided fascinating clues to investigators of the mind–body healing response. In one landmark study in 1978, dental patients experiencing the aftereffects of an extracted tooth were given a sugar pill and told it was a powerful painkiller. They reported significant pain relief. Experimenters then added another agent: along with the placebo, a separate group of dental patients were given a chemical known to block the action of the brain's own endorphins. The second group experienced significantly less pain reduction than the first group (Levine et al, 1978).

Here was a study that indicated a specific mechanism for placebo—endorphins—without which the "magical" effect would not have occurred. These studies and many similar ones led scientists to believe that endorphins mediate much of the mind–body effect, whether that effect is activated by placebo, hypnosis, meditation, dissociation, or any other process or agent.

There are many mind–body routes, with many mechanisms to create similar effects. Therefore, different states of mind may affect the body along different pathways, or the same substances may have multiple systemic influences. Pain relief, it is now understood, may also stimulate immune function because pain-relieving endorphins are key messenger molecules that also "talk" to the immune system.

The late Candace Pert, co-discoverer of endorphins at Johns Hopkins University the 1970s, made some startling revelations regarding the existence of neuropeptide receptors throughout the entire body. Pert found that the endocrine system, the digestive system, and even the immune system incorporate these "messenger" molecules. The implication is that neuropeptide molecules are involved in a psychosomatic communication network and that the biochemistry of emotion could be mediating the transmittal of information flowing throughout the body. Pert maintains that emotions are the bridge between the mental and the physical, which makes them prime candidates for a variety of links between thought and healing.

The natural conclusion emerging from such research is that expectation or belief affects biology. The emotional responses of individuals to the world around them—hopes and joys, fears and anguish—have a potential effect on the physical body. This understanding is fundamental to the treatment of illness. However, it does not imply that conventional medical treatment should be wholly supplanted by mind–body approaches. The most effective and comprehensive strategy of treatment should be *expanded* to include the awareness of emotional and psychological factors in concert.

an onset, peak, and duration of action the same as the drug for which they are substituting (Wall, 1992). Dose-response effects have been demonstrated. For example, two capsules work measurably better than one and injections are more potent than pills. Larger pills or capsules (especially the color brown or purple) typically work better than smaller ones—with the exception of very small bright red or yellow pills, which have been shown to be most effective (Turner et al, 1994).

RANGE OF EFFECTS

The variety of disorders that improve with placebos is quite extensive (Beecher, 1955; Benson & Epstein, 1975; Blanchard et al, 1990; Cobb et al, 1959; Gowdy, 1983; Lavin, 1991; LeVasseur & Helme, 1991). Placebos have successfully treated stomach ulcers, hypertension, bedsores, and herpes infections, and have even been shown to have profound benefits for some people with incurable cancer (Brody, 1980; LeVasseur & Helme, 1991; Tsolka et al, 1992). Placebos have been used to control physical symptoms associated with angina pectoris, headache, rheumatoid and degenerative arthritis, temporomandibular joint disorder, reflex sympathetic dystrophy, asthma, and even the common cold (Beecher, 1955; Benson & Epstein, 1975; Blanchard et al, 1990). Placebos are also useful in controlling emotionally mediated conditions such as anxiety, depression, insomnia, and premenstrual tension (Gowdy, 1983; Lavin, 1991).

At Harvard Medical School in 1955, Dr. Henry Beecher conducted a landmark analysis that summarized reports from over 1000 patients with different types of pain. Thirty-five percent of patients gained satisfactory relief from placebos, even patients with severe postoperative pain (Beecher, 1955). Other investigators administering placebos have reported a reduction in edema, blood pressure, gastric acid, and serum cholesterol levels, as well as improved blood counts and electrolyte and hormonal balances (Gowdy, 1983). Favorable electrocardiographic changes were noted in heart disease patients following a placebo intervention (Cobb et al, 1959).

THE SYMBOLISM BEHIND THE PLACEBO

The placebo effect is a measurable and, indeed, desirable consequence of the symbolism implicit in therapeutic treatment (i.e., the fact and intention of undertaking therapy, rather than any direct influence on the physical or chemical structure or function of the body). Physical and chemical changes, however, do occur. These changes may result from the presence or influence of a caring person (Diers, 1972), or what is termed the "healer effect." Particularly in a culture accustomed to all the latest advancements in medical technology (see Chapter 5), the healing intent manifest in novel, high-tech techniques can be especially effective at eliciting a placebo effect (Meehan, 1993; Turner et al, 1994; Wall, 1992), especially to the extent that patients are encouraged to avail themselves of the newest opera-

tions, latest drugs, and most sophisticated technologies. Upon introduction of an innovative treatment, 70% of patients will have a good or excellent response for several years, until that treatment becomes discredited or superseded in favor of a still newer technology that will go on to elicit that same effect (Murray, 1987).

SURGICAL PLACEBO

Surgery often has a strong placebo effect related to the confidence-instilling attitude of the surgeon. As one of us (MSM) was taught by the internationally recognized hypnotherapist Martine Orne, MD, regardless of one's general view of medicine or surgery, the night before the operation every patient always has the best surgeon in the world. This may involve an aspect of self-hypnosis (see Chapter 10).

The 1950s saw two famous, double-blind randomized trials of internal mammary artery ligation surgery for the treatment of angina pectoris due to insufficiency of blood flow to the heart muscle. The idea was that blood from the interior chest wall would be shunted toward the coronary arteries, improving blood flow (or not, in the case of false ligation). These studies showed a marked improvement in angina from skin incision alone, with benefits such as reduced pain, fewer medications required, and improved electrocardiogram tracings lasting at least 6 months (Cobb et al, 1959). Other sham surgical procedures for temporomandibular joint disease and disabling back pain have been demonstrated to be as effective as the standard surgical procedures (Tsolka et al, 1992, Turner et al, 1994).

These were rare examples of the so-called gold standard of clinical trials (see Chapter 3) being rigorously applied to a surgical procedure. For obvious reasons, the majority of surgical procedures are never subjected to controlled clinical trials, which may be why so many are ultimately discarded. It also helps account for the observation, by the former US Congressional Office of Technology Assessment in the 1970s and 1980s, that 70% to 80% of surgical procedures had no scientific evidence to support their use (see Chapter 3). (This office was later disbanded, perhaps because of its findings.) In the case of back surgery, we now know that the vast majority of low back pain improves with conservative measures of spinal manual therapy, physical therapy, massage, or acupuncture (see Chapter 19). (Far too many back surgeries result in the intractable pain of "failed back syndrome," spawning an entire new subspecialty of medicine to treat it, as well as the fact that in certain states, it is almost impossible for surgeons to obtain malpractice insurance for performing back surgery.)

DRUG BENEFITS

In Beecher's 1955 paper, he estimated that 50% of the therapeutic benefit of any drug administered is related to the placebo effect. Considerable variation was noted among studies regarding the percentage of patients who benefited from the placebo effect. On average, 35% of patients experienced placebo effects; however, response rates ranged from 15% to 80% in the various studies considered (Beecher, 1955). Beecher noted that more confident, enthusiastic physicians seemed to have better results, accounting for at least part of this discrepancy. Of course, at the other end of the spectrum, medical science has learned that a downcast, doom-saying, negative practitioner can elicit an opposite effect (the "nocebo effect").

Nocebos

Despite all their potential benefits, drugs or surgical procedures can actually exert a powerfully negative nocebo effect that can increase pain and suffering, or worsen disease based on the belief that these undesired outcomes will occur. We often hear in "direct-to-consumer" marketing of pharmaceuticals that "the occurrence of side effects is similar to that of sugar pills." What goes unsaid is that mild side effects are experienced by 20% to 30% of patients receiving placebos, including edema, pain, diarrhea, nausea, palpitations, urticaria, and rashes (Wolf & Pinsky, 1954). The rate of nocebo responses can also vary considerably. One sham treatment (a nonexistent "electric current" applied to the scalp) produced headaches in 70% of healthy subjects (Turner et al, 1994).

Harmful effects attributed to negative beliefs about a treatment include dizziness, depression, insomnia, drowsiness, vomiting, numbness, hallucinations, or addiction (Lasagna, 1986; Lavin, 1991; Turner et al, 1994; Wolf & Pinsky, 1954). In other patients, symptoms can worsen because the placebo failed to treat what is wrong with them. Nearly one-quarter of patients in one study believed that they were permanently disabled and destined to live with greater intensity of pain because they happened to participate in the placebo arm of a study (Turner et al, 1994).

The nocebo effect has been linked to untimely deaths (e.g., in cases in which people seemingly "will" themselves to die under certain circumstances). Anecdotes have been widely published about physicians or clergy proceeding with end-of-life care, or administering extreme unction rites (literally the final anointing with oil) to the wrong patient. The anointed patient subsequently dies, whereas the intended recipient survives for a prolonged period. Data linking the nocebo effect to death comes from the multi-decade Framingham Study, which showed a nearly fourfold greater rate of death from heart attacks among women who believed they would die from heart disease, even after controlling for all putative risk factors such as smoking, cholesterol levels, and high blood pressure (Eaker et al, 1992).

The nocebo effect may represent a major public health problem, with pain, infectious diseases, and stress-related and autoimmune disorders all theoretically linked by related physiological mechanisms (Stefano et al, 2001; see also Chapter 8). Hahn (1997), an anthropologist and epidemiologist, expressed concern about the rampant media coverage of health-related problems that are often poorly interpreted or understood. Sociogenic (also called psychogenic) illnesses, mass hysteria, or "assembly line" hysteria may result from nocebo effects in the general public.

When the movie *Outbreak*—about a rare African virus rapidly transmitted via a monkey bite in the jungle to large urban populations—came out in the early 1990s, it elicited a degree of public hysteria. One of us (MSM) was interviewed by host John Tesh for the popular TV show *Entertainment Tonight*. He asked whether such an epidemic or pandemic could really occur in the United States as depicted in the movie. I suggested that rather than let our imaginations run rampant, we could witness what a real "outbreak" looks like with the annual influenza pandemic—which only once in a hundred years (the 1918–1919 Spanish flu pandemic) produced results anywhere near what was depicted.

Hahn postulates that the nocebo phenomenon may account for a significant proportion and a substantial variety of pathologies currently experienced around the world (Hahn, 1997). Support for this hypothesis is provided by several cases where outbreaks of disorders is more closely aligned with the beliefs of the sufferers rather than with any known medical condition or diagnosis. (Münchausen syndrome and Münchausen syndrome by proxy are related disorders in which the afflicted person imagines symptoms in oneself or one's child.) One might consider an element of self-hypnosis, or autosuggestion, given that the persons afflicted do not manifest the actual behavior of the disease but what they *think* it behaves like (see Chapter 10). Hahn (1997) and Gladwell (2000) also point out a convincing link between media coverage of suicides and an increase in both suicides and motor vehicle fatality rates. Of course, the media generally does not give much attention to suicides versus homicides, although suicides generally occur at about the twice the rate of homicides in the average jurisdiction (Micozzi, 2015), except in the case of mass suicide, such as at Jonestown, Guyana, in 1978.

Hahn concludes that, until we learn more about the nocebo effect, it may be healthier for society if the media were to err on the side of optimism when reporting messages about health, and to err on the side of caution when reporting suspected causes of disease. However, the media watchword has long been "If it bleeds, it leads," and since Hahn's report there has been a proliferation of pessimistic TV programs and sensational newspaper and Internet stories that play up the seemingly "catastrophic" consequences of exposure to relatively innocuous agents in the environment.

The Power of Intent

The power of the placebo effect may reside among all therapies based on the quality of the provider–patient interaction. As a health care practitioner, consider the potential benefit of spending a few minutes of your encounters helping the patient develop confidence in you and the treatment, fostering a sense of hope and developing trust. In past generations, when medical technology did not have as much to offer, beneficial intention was always a potent resource available to the healer. Research suggests that the quality of the patient–provider interaction can have either a therapeutic or toxic effect on the patient. Caring interactions may well mobilize the comforting and self-healing potential within individuals (Diers, 1972). In Chapters 3 and 24, we present the results of a Harvard study on clinical depression, in which neither a potent new selective serotonin reuptake inhibitor antidepressant nor a historically proven herbal remedy showed any benefit over placebo. However, the "placebo control" included many hours of intensive interaction with highly skilled mental health professionals. The patients who benefited were doubtless influenced not only by the skill but the healing *intent* of the providers.

Placebo effects are shown to be strongest when the provider is friendly, warm, concerned, sympathetic, empathetic, prestigious, thorough, and competent (Alagaratnam, 1981; Hojat et al, 2003; Seeley, 1990). In addition to the patient's belief in the professional's abilities, the practitioner's explanation of the diagnosis (Thomas, 1987) and his or her own manifest belief in the treatment being offered (Graceley et al, 1985) is important. Thus, rapport with the patient, confidence in the diagnosis, enthusiasm for the treatment, and the patient's own receptive attitude are all likely to enhance the effectiveness of an intervention.

MORE ON PATIENT EXPECTATIONS

The role of patient expectations was demonstrated in a remarkable study of individuals with asthma. These subjects were given two different inhalers. The first inhaler, they were told, contained an allergen that would aggravate their asthma symptoms in order to test a powerful new form of therapy that was being evaluated through the second inhaler. Inhaling two puffs from the first inhaler resulted, for nearly half the patients, in an increase in airway obstruction and reduced air volume measures. Then the second inhaler was administered, causing the airways to open up and improve objective measures of effective breathing. In fact, both inhalers contained the same concentration of only salt water (Benson & Epstein, 1975).

Evans (1974) calculated the pain-relieving potency of placebos to be equivalent to approximately 5 mg of morphine when patients thought they had received a standard 10 mg dose morphine, but the effect dropped to the pain-relieving potency of just 1 mg of morphine when the patients thought they had received aspirin (which itself had the potency of 2 mg morphine).

PROVIDER EXPECTATION

As noted earlier, provider expectations form another key ingredient of the placebo effect. In a multicenter trial of a new antihypertensive agent, investigators at one research site were highly enthusiastic about the safety and superior efficacy of a new drug that had apparently brought about substantial reductions in blood pressure. When discussing their results with other researchers, it became apparent that the drug was no better than placebos used in the other research settings. The researchers' enthusiasm for the new drug then waned, but they agreed to complete the study. Both the experimental and placebo groups then went on to experience a marked and sustained elevation in blood pressure (Graceley et al, 1985).

The way that clinicians communicate their expectations to patients is another important component of the placebo effect. Thomas (1987) randomly selected patients who reported symptoms, but displayed no signs of disease. He found that, by giving the patient a diagnosis and telling him or her that they would get better in a few days, twice as many patients "recovered" than those who were informed of the physician's uncertainty about their illness.

Kong et al (2013), examining subjects' tolerance to pain, found that response to a placebo depends on diverse factors, including the way the treatment was administered, environmental cues, and learning based on verbal suggestions—in other words, that the placebo effect turns on the interaction of the given patient and the given practitioner in a given circumstance.

Spiegel (1997) states, "The placebo effect can occur when conditions are optimal for hope, faith, trust and love." Similarly, Lasagna (1986) found that placebo effects tend to occur in patients who have an affirming, cooperative attitude. (Ironically, these are the patients least likely to receive placebos [Goodwin et al, 1979].)

PATIENT CHARACTERISTICS

A full reckoning of the placebo effect must account for the fact that not even the most confident, enthusiastic practitioner will activate the same response in all patients. Spiegel (1997) has proposed that the patient's level of "suggestibility" is an important factor in placebo responsiveness. The degree of suggestibility is measurable by techniques used to evaluate "hypnotizability" (i.e., the Spiegel Hypnotic Susceptibility Scales; see Chapters 3 and 10). Hypnotic susceptibility varies among the general population along a bell-shaped curve. Some people can be easily hypnotized, others not at all (see www.hypnosisandsuggestion.org/measurement.html for more detail regarding how hypnosis is measured).

Examining the phenomenon more broadly, Ernest Hartmann, of Tufts University, has found evidence that "thin boundary" people (i.e., individuals who are extremely sensitive, open, or vulnerable) are more suggestible as well as hypnotizable (Hartmann, 1991). If the placebo effect is mediated by similar traits (openness, trust, sensitivity), we could reasonably suppose that thin boundary people will derive more benefit from placebos than "thick boundary" people (i.e., those who are hard-headed, rigid, or skeptical). (Hartmann's Boundary Questionnaire, which has been in use since the late 1980s, is a psychometric tool that assesses boundary type and, by extension, the likelihood of a person manifesting the placebo effect [Hartmann, 1991; see Chapter 10].)

Furthermore, a person's ability to dissociate his or her thoughts from bodily awareness, as well as the ability to focus intensively on an idea, subject matter, or instruction ("absorption," a concept elucidated by Tellegen & Atkinson [1974]), are thought to be important traits of people who readily experience placebo effects. The Dissociative Experiences Scale (Colin A. Ross Institute for Psychological Trauma, www.rossinst.com/dissociative_experiences_scale.html) and Tellegen Absorption Scale are measurement approaches used to document variability among individuals in these respects.

Theoretically, such psychometric approaches can be used to gauge susceptibility to *any* disorder or therapy, and may be especially useful where Western medicine struggles to understand the cause(s) of the disorder and the mechanism of action of therapies—especially when the given illness appears to have a strong mind–body component.

CONDITIONED RESPONSES

In addition to the role of expectations, prior experiences can set the stage for a conditioned response to play a part in the placebo effect. One familiar example involves college students who have been known to go to social gatherings, consume alcohol, and show signs of intoxication. Anecdotally, an annual lesson at one school of pharmacy involves a holiday party where word gets out that the punch is "spiked" with a high potency, colorless, tasteless form of alcohol. Some students attending this party become visibly intoxicated, whereas others feel woozy and sick. At the end of the party, however, the students are assured that there was no alcohol in the punch. Invariably, the signs of intoxication diminish rapidly.

Similarly, in a double-blind crossover study using a potent narcotic agent in one arm of the study, patients who got the active ingredient first demonstrated a stronger effect than those who received the placebo first. In the second phase of the study, the patients who never received any active ingredient were the only group not to elicit a placebo effect (Amanzio et al, 2001).

Several animal-based research studies also point toward operant conditioning being a significant mechanism in the placebo effect. Rats (like some college students) have demonstrated hyperactive, intoxicated behavior in response to sugar water after first being conditioned with amphetamines. The rats that were not previously conditioned did not demonstrate these behavioral changes. This conditioned response hypothesis has some support in humans as well.

OTHER POSSIBLE FACTORS

Although the role of expectations and conditioning has strong research support, there is a vast range of other possible explanations for placebo/nocebo effects. In light of homeostasis and the tendency of the physiology to correct or balance itself, many conditions simply improve on their own (at least prior to the onset of irreversible pathologic changes).

At one end of the spectrum is the popular idea that the placebo effect is simply the "tincture of time," explainable by natural healing processes for acute illnesses or injuries, and a "regression to the mean" for chronic ailments.

At the other end of the spectrum is a claim that universal healing energies are tapped and directed to the patient through the healer's compassion and intent to help. Early work by Donna Diers (1972) and more recent research supporting the benefits of therapeutic touch are marshaled as support for this latter perspective (see Chapters 14 and 17).

Evidence from the field of psychoneuroimmunology (see Chapter 8) indicates that particular thought patterns are capable of activating psychophysiological, self-regulatory mechanisms that mobilize hormones, neurotransmitters, and components of the immune system. One important line of research supports a link between an optimistic belief in one's own abilities ("self-sufficiency") and health benefits. In separate research studies, people with stronger self-efficacy beliefs were found to have higher levels of endorphins (natural pain relievers) (Bandura et al, 1987). In contrast, people who had belief patterns associated with learned helplessness had suppressed levels of beta endorphin (Tejedor-Real et al, 1995) and (perhaps as a nocebo response) reported more pain and depression. Similarly, Bandura et al (1987) determined that a pain-relieving placebo effect was mediated by at least two different mechanisms. The first mechanism was attributable to higher self-efficacy beliefs that raised patients' pain thresholds. In the second mechanism, as cognitive control over pain diminished, the body's production and release of endorphins was found to increase pain tolerance (Bandura et al, 1987).

Further support for a biobehavioral link between the placebo effect and the body's production of endorphins is provided by two studies that found, on the one hand, elevated endorphin levels correlated to placebo responses and, on the other, that the morphine antidote naloxone could reverse this beneficial placebo effect (Levine et al, 1978; Lipmann et al, 1990).

Strong physiological similarities have been established between the placebo effect and the "relaxation response" (see Chapter 10). Both involve activation of natural endogenous antibacterial and antinociceptive peptides, while suppressing potentially harmful inducible catecholamines and cytokines (Stefano et al, 2001). Most recently, Benson et al (2013) have demonstrated the ability of measured relaxation to influence the expression of several genes that could account for the role and mechanism of these endogenous biochemicals.

It is possible to conclude, through decades of research in addition to emerging functional MRI imaging evidence (see Chapter 8), that a remarkable number of stress-related conditions are amenable to the placebo effect, thus supporting the explanatory relevance of psychoneuroimmunology.

PLACEBOS IN RESEARCH

The placebo effect raises interesting and important larger questions for science and epistemology within the health professions and healing arts. Is it possible to truly know a patient or demonstrate the actual effectiveness of medical interventions given the existence of the placebo effect? Does the use of placebos in clinical research indicate that modern medicine ultimately values the power of drugs over interpersonal knowledge and healing intention? It is arguable that progress in the healing arts and sciences is not being accelerated but stifled by the current methods of inquiry (see Chapter 3).

Experimental design is considered to be the only method to generate evidence that can establish a cause–effect relationship (see Chapters 3 and 5). However, the use of placebos is not required for this methodology; their use, in fact, may confound the interpretation of findings from studies using this esteemed, "gold standard" design (Chiodo et al, 2000; Enserink, 2000; Krishnan, 2000). Experiments are often designed to include a control group that receives no intervention; by the same token, it is clear that giving a placebo is not the same as simply doing nothing.

Soon after the standardization of randomized clinical trial methodology in the late 1940s, it became evident that the magnitude of placebo effects often encountered (yielding both false-positive and false-negative results) invalidated the findings of even well-designed studies. Investigators were left wondering whether the outcomes resulted from *specific* treatment effects being studied or from nonspecific placebo effects. Despite these well-established limitations, the randomized clinical trial remains for many researchers the ultimate standard among research methodologies.

Given that the placebo effect is such a potent confounding variable, it is arguable that placebos are not really required to conduct experimental research. General consensus counters that randomized clinical trials are best when a "double-blind" method is used. Double-blind means that neither the investigator nor patient is aware of whether they are receiving the active or placebo treatment. Many randomized clinical trials, however, cannot truly be double-blind because either the investigator and/or patient is unavoidably aware of which treatment is being used. The more potent the drug being tested, or the stronger the side effect burden, the more likely it is that the study cannot truly be blind. Animal and human studies have shown inherent weaknesses in these types of studies, which essentially become "single-blind" (Enserink, 2000; Wall, 1992) and blur the ability to distinguish treatment effects from placebo effects.

Another criticism of randomized clinical trials relates to their being focused on only a small, artificial part of the patient experience, separate from the whole person and his or her social/environmental interactions in everyday life. In this context, it is easy to miss the actual cause–effect relationships affecting the phenomenon being studied. In the evolving debate within the health sciences, there is some support for mixing research methods to obtain a richer, more insightful, and more realistic perspective. The standard FDA drug approval process leaves many unhappy surprises as to all the real effects of drugs until they enter the public realm and are subjected to "post-marketing surveillance."

Although considerable value for evidence-based medicine remains, a call has arisen to look beyond disease-specific outcomes to include Patient Oriented Evidence that Matters (POEMs). By including data that relate to subjects' perceptions of their conditions and the interventions (e.g., patient satisfaction or improved quality of life), a more comprehensive understanding is likely to be gained and the healing process itself is likely to be enhanced (Ganiats, 2000).

In addition, research can be strengthened if it is independently evaluated by investigators who are not intervening or collecting the data (Wall, 1992). When a control treatment group is used, it should be as similar as possible to the active treatment group to create similar expectations. Patients in both groups should have the same frequency of contact and quality of support by the investigator (Geden, 1984). A completely untreated group controls for effects due to the passage of time, but not for effects stemming from patient expectations. Many investigations that include a control group, therefore, also include a standard treatment group, or simply compare the experimental group to the standard treatments with established efficacy.

Another method of double-blind study to overcome some of the problems inherent in the use of placebos uses patients as their own controls. One simple example is the crossover design, or "before and after" study. This method is a randomized clinical trial designed specifically for individual patients. The patient consents to try a random sequence of treatment trials. Some treatments are believed to be "active," others are not (subtherapeutic doses of active medications may be used rather than a placebo). Both the patient and the researcher are blind as to whether the treatment is active or not. Results are observed until a clear difference (or lack of difference) is noted between the treatment groups (Enserink, 2000). This methodology may be "un-blinded" by perceptible effects (whether desirable or adverse) of the active treatments, and because this method does not account for the effects of time during the lengthy trials that require "washout" periods in between treatments to prevent the carryover effects of drugs, nutrients, or metabolites.

Amanzio et al (2001) have described an approach that controls for the placebo effect in multiple ways. First, the use of open versus hidden administrations controls for patient expectations (hidden administrations are less effective). Second, the use of reversal agents (e.g., the morphine antidote naloxone) controls for biobehavioral aspects of the placebo response. Lastly, a completely untreated group is used to control for the nonspecific effects of the passage of time. While Amanzio's is more comprehensive than previous methodologies, factors such as the effects of conditioning and individual and interpersonal variables cannot be controlled.

In addition to methodological concerns, the use of placebos in research raises *ethical* concerns. Tesh (1983) discussed the conundrum of a science–ethics dualism where researchers may become aware of ethical problems related to their research but, if they should break their code of silence, they will be discredited as subjective and "unscientific." A prime example was the Tuskegee Syphilis Experiment begun during the 1920s. Six hundred poor black men (399 who had previously contracted syphilis before the study began, and 201 without the disease) were not told they had syphilis, or that some were being treated only with placebos. They received a hot meal once a year (so doctors could perform a physical examination and obtain a blood sample), with burial money paid upon death, in exchange for the US Public Health Service to follow how long it takes untreated syphilis to result in death. Dozens of nurses, hundreds of researchers, and an estimated 100,000 practicing physicians were aware of the study but did not try to stop it for 40 years until 1972, when the Associated Press broke the story (Jones, 1993).

A more contemporary concern is reflected in the Stockholm Declaration that researchers should not administer solely treatments they do not believe are efficacious (see Chapters 3, 24). Of course, clinical studies of cancer treatment are conducted by giving patients new treatments together with standard treatments; nobody with cancer is given only placebo.

CLINICAL PRACTICE

The use of placebos in medical practice preceded their use in medical research. In the early 1800s, Samuel Hahnemann in Germany was developing homeopathic medicines that were more than 99.9% inert (Tesh, 1983), and Thomas Jefferson was reporting the use of bread pills or colored water by the most successful physicians of the day. Jefferson called this practice a "pious fraud," as it was actually less harmful than the then-standard treatments, which included purging, puncturing, cupping, leeching, and the use of poisons (such as snake oil), lizard's blood, crocodile dung, and fox lungs. Within 50 years—despite the ethical issues involved—40% of treatments prescribed had become placebos (Brody, 1980). Mary Baker Eddy, founder of Christian Science (see Chapter 6) consciously deceived patients who insisted on drug treatments by administering unmedicated pellets to them (Kaufman, 1971). Given the toxicity of many of the standard medicines of the 1800s, many forms of "drugless healing" arose and thrived (initially on the American frontier). Physicians and patients who were often repelled by the regular treatments were attracted to the newly arising approaches (see Section IV).

Some clinicians today still administer placebos, either to patients whose motives are questioned or because they

believe (correctly or not) that the benefits of placebos outweigh the harms of available active treatments. Kleinman et al (1994) described the type of patients that are most likely to be prescribed placebos. These patients may be perceived as seeking drugs for abusive rather than therapeutic reasons. Typically the patients have a long and unusual medical diagnosis, or get worse instead of better during regular treatment. Patients who are given placebos are more likely to have difficulties with interpersonal relationships, especially with the medical team providing care. Physicians will also administer placebos for subjective symptoms, such as pain, because they mistakenly believe the treatment will be useful in distinguishing between organic and functional conditions, or to prove that a patient is malingering, exaggerating symptoms for secondary gain, has some undiagnosed psychiatric disorder, or has Münchausen syndrome. It is ironic that placebos are used by health professionals who do not believe patients are being honest, because the integrity of the deceptive health professional is then open to question.

It is medically narrow-minded to consider that all placebo responders had nothing wrong with them in the first place. This is especially so given the extensive evidence presented in this chapter that many patients respond to empathetic and confident practitioners, and that other patients are prone to a strong placebo response based on factors including suggestibility, absorption, and thin boundaries. However, there are still reports in the literature that some professionals interpret the effectiveness of placebos as evidence discrediting the patient's report of discomfort (Verdugo et al, 1994). Especially in the area of pain management, most specialists agree that *absence of evidence is not evidence of absence*, meaning that pain is real, even if the magnetic resonance image does not reveal an anatomical abnormality.

LEGAL AND ETHICAL ISSUES

The unconsented use of placebos raises clinical concerns and jeopardizes patient trust; it also damages the reputation of a profession that permits such deception. Whereas some professionals argue that the beneficial outcomes of placebos justify their use, others consider this justification to be misguided and potentially dangerous (Elander, 1991). Failure to believe what a patient is reporting risks decreased vigilance, a missed diagnosis, worsening of symptoms, or even death or disability from failure to treat a treatable condition.

The current use of placebos in clinical practice seems to depend on a physician's right to exercise therapeutic privilege overriding a patient's right to informed consent. Clinical practice guidelines established by the Agency for Health Care Policy and Research (1994), the American Society of Pain Management Nurses, and the American Pain Society (1992) clearly state that the clinical use of placebos is potentially harmful, represents substandard care, and is morally wrong. Most professional codes of ethics similarly support the notion that placebo use is unacceptable.

Professionals are expected to tell the truth and protect patients from substandard care, unethical practices, misrepresentation, or threats to the patients' right to self-determination.

The concealed use of placebos carries the risk of liability for fraud, malpractice, breach of contract, and the violation of informed consent requirements (Fox, 1994). Attorneys from different parts of the country have concurred that placebos violate informed consent and their use constitutes both medical negligence and deception that no court would excuse (Fox, 1994). This presumption has proven correct in many cases (e.g., when a court awarded $15 million to the estate of Henry James, a 71-year-old bone cancer patient, who had been given placebos instead of opiates for pain) (Brider, 1991).

A less obvious (though not insignificant) concern is that prescribing a placebo, when no effective medication exists, only reinforces the attitude that drugs are the only way to treat illness and human suffering. It also raises expectations that relief of disease or pain is as simple as swallowing a pill—shifting the burden of responsibility for healing away from the patient and the health care provider, who might otherwise identify behaviors or treatments that could prove constructive.

PLACEBO AND COMPLEMENTARY/ ALTERNATIVE MEDICINE

The last 25 years have seen a resurgence of interest in a variety of neglected or marginalized mind–body healing techniques. Although this could easily be viewed as a renaissance of the art of healing, skeptics of complementary and alternative medicine (e.g., acupuncture, mindfulness meditation, homeopathy, and so on) maintain that all these approaches represent nothing more than the placebo effect (Freedman, 2001). Given the flaws cited earlier with even well-designed research, however, it can be shown that a major portion of the benefit of modern therapeutics itself is *also* derived from the placebo effect. This circumstance is especially true given how technological advances (including medical technology) have fueled the expectations of the public (see Chapters 3 and 5).

There is strong evidence that the health benefits of complementary and alternative therapies are conferred independent of the placebo effect, although this fact is less well demonstrated with some forms of therapy such as homeopathy and guided imagery. Medical science could point to the fact that homeopathic agents are over 99% inert—just like the placebos used in clinical trials. However, there are clinical indications that homeopathy's benefits are *not* solely mediated by the placebo effect (see Section IV).

Guided imagery and the placebo effect can be linked by the fact that placebos are a physical representation of a therapy that is not materially present, whereas imagery draws upon a mental representation of something that is not materially present. Alternatively, placebos may have always exerted their effect by being a form of imagery—with the imagery itself serving as a bridge between the mind and the body that creates the conditions needed to promote healing (see Chapter 10). Like placebos, guided imagery can bring about a wide variety of benefits, including the reduction of pain and anxiety, improved immune responses, accelerated wound healing, and even reduction in the size of cancerous tumors (Simonton et al, 1980; Stephens, 1993). Imagery may also elicit nocebo-type effects if negative images are conjured. It seems likely that both imagery and placebos mobilize cognitive, emotional, and psychoneuroimmunological processes that activate the self-healing potential within individuals (Benson, 1996).

SUMMARY

The use of placebos widely affects clinical research as well as the integrity of professional practice in health care. Investigative methods and protocols should be modified to control for the placebo effect while minimizing false interpretations of data and undesired nocebo responses. Placebos should never be employed merely for convenience, to placate the patient, or in lieu of a consultation with or intervention by a relevant medical specialist (e.g., a pain specialist or psychologist). Health care organizations should recognize the potential harm and liability that can result from the uncontrolled use of placebos.

It should be remembered that the placebo effect is an active, physiologically real phenomenon, albeit nonspecific, and a component of the healing response common to all (allopathic and complementary alternative medicine) therapies. As we have seen, patients vary considerably in the degree to which they are susceptible to the influence of placebos. Because the effect cannot be counted upon to occur on cue, the best therapies available should be used for the patient's specific condition. Utilizing the safest and most effective treatments in which practitioners have confidence will (ironically) engage placebo effects in those patients who are most responsive.

The accumulated evidence suggests that the placebo effect is elicited by a variety of factors: (1) the physician's warmth, caring, and confidence; (2) the patient's degree of expectation; (3) operant conditioning; (4) the patient's potential for suggestibility, dissociation, and absorption; and (5) his or her "boundary thinness" and ability to make imagery physiologically "real." Health care providers should recognize the power of the placebo effect, taking the uniqueness of patients fully into account and seeking to engage with them as positively as possible in order to optimize the effect of interventions. Simple encouragement on the part of the health professional can often add 15% efficacy to the treatment—a substantial return on a modest investment.

Promoting health in a holistic manner can promote innate self-healing processes in the body and mind. To this end, the professional who spends time *talking* with patients so that they better understand both their condition and the chosen mode(s) of treatment is most likely to prompt a beneficial placebo effect. (Awareness of the patient's misperceptions or unrealistic expectations also helps the professional avoid a common cause of therapeutic failure.) And, whenever patient trust or confidence is undermined, the relationship may take on toxic rather than therapeutic characteristics, with the possibility of nocebo rather than placebo effects.

Health care is an art, science and ethical obligation that compels its practitioners to stay abreast of the latest knowledge and professional skills, while honing their interpersonal ability and remaining committed to healing. The placebo effect, which has so much to teach about the interplay of body and mind, physiology and psychology, cognition and emotion, has equivalent lessons to impart concerning the interplay of physician and patient and the uniqueness of each therapeutic relationship and encounter.

References

Agency for Health Care Policy and Research: *Management of Cancer Pain Clinical Practice Guideline number 9*, 1994, pp 69, 223. Publication No. 94-0592.

Alagaratnam WJ: Pain and the nature of the placebo effect. Oct 28, 1883-4, *Nurs Times* 1981.

Amanzio M, Pollo A, Maggi G, Benedetti F: Response variability to analgesics: a role for non-specific activation of endogenous opioids, *Pain* 90(3):205–215, 2001.

American Pain Society: *Principles of Analgesic Use in The Treatment of Acute and Cancer Pain*, ed 3, Skokie, IL, 1992, p 25.

Bandura A, O'Leary A, Taylor CB, et al: Perceived self-efficacy and pain control: opioid and non-opioid mechanisms, *J Pers Soc Psychol* 53(3):563–571, 1987.

Beecher HK: The powerful placebo, *JAMA* 159(17):1602–1606, 1955.

Benson H: *Timeless Healing: The power and biology of belief*, New York, 1996, Scribner.

Benson H, et al: Relaxation good for your genes, *PLoS ONE* 2013.

Benson H, Epstein MD: The placebo effect: A neglected asset in the care of patients, *JAMA* 232(12):1225–1227, 1975.

Blanchard J, Ramamurthy S, Walsh N, et al: Intravenous regional sympatholysis: a double-blind comparison of guanethidinne, reserpine and normal saline, *J Pain Symptom Manage* 5(6):357–361, 1990.

Bok S: The ethics of giving placebos, *Sci Am* 231(5):17–23, 1974.

Brider P: Jury says neglect of pain is worth $15 million award, *AJN* 110, 1991.

Brody H: *Placebos and the philosophy of medicine*, ed 2, Chicago, 1980, The University of Chicago Press.

Chiodo GT, Tolle SW, Bevan L: Placebo-controlled trials: good science or medical neglect? *West J Med* 172(4):271–273, 2000.

Cobb LA, Thomas GI, Dillard DH, et al: An evaluation of internal-mammary-artery-ligation by a double-blind technique, *NEJM* 260:1115–1118, 1959.

Diers D: The effect of nursing interaction on patients in pain, *Nurs Res* 21(5):419–428, 1972.

Eaker E, Pinsky L, Castelli WP: Myocardial infarction and coronary death among women: psychosocial predictors from a 20-year follow-up of women in the Framingham Study, *Am J Epidemiol* 135:854–864, 1992.

Elander G: Ethical conflicts in placebo treatment, *J Adv Nurs* 16(8):947–951, 1991.

Enserink M: Psychiatry. Are placebo-controlled drug trials ethical? *Science* 288(5465):416, 2000.

Evans FJ: The power of the sugar pill, *Psychol Today* 7:55–61, 1974.

Fine PG, Roberts WJ, Gillette RG, Child TR: Slowly developing placebo responses confound tests of intravenous phentolamine to determine mechanisms underlying idiopathic chronic low back pain, *Pain* 56(2):235–242, 1994.

Fox AE: Confronting the use of placebos for pain, *AJN* 42–45, 1994.

Freedman David H: The Triumph of New-Age Medicine, *Atlantic* 2001.

Ganiats TG: What to do until the POEMS arrive, *J Fam Pract* 49(4):362–368, 2000.

Geden EA: A perspective on the proper use of placebos in research and therapy, *AORN J* 40(6):912–916, 1984.

Gladwell Malcolm: *The Tipping Point*, New York, 2000, Little, Brown and Company.

Goodwin JS, Goodwin JM, Vogel AA: Knowledge and use of placebos by house officers and nurses, *Ann Intern Med* 91:106–110, 1979.

Gowdy CW: A guide to the pharmacology of placebos, *CMAJ* 128:921–925, 1983.

Graceley RH, Dubner R, Deeter WR, Wolskee PJ: Clinicians' expectations influence placebo analgesia, *Lancet* 331(1):43, 1985.

Hahn RA: The nocebo phenomenon: scope and foundations. In Harrington A, editor: *The placebo effect: an interdisciplinary exploration*, Cambridge, MA., 1997, Harvard University Press.

Hartmann Ernest: *Boundaries in the Mind: A New Dimension of Personality*, New York, 1991, Basic Books.

Hojat M, Gonella JS, Mangione S, et al: Physician empathy in medical education and practice, *Semin Integr Med* 1(1):25–41, 2003.

Jones JH: *Bad Blood: The Tuskegee Syphilis Experiment*, ed 2, New York, 1993, The Free Press.

Kaufman M: *Homeopathy in America: the rise and fall of medical heresy*, Baltimore, 1971, The Johns Hopkins Press.

Kleinman I, Brown P, Librach L: Placebo pain medications: Ethical and practical considerations, *Arch Fam Med* 3(5):453–457, 1994.

Kong J, Spaeth R, Cook A, et al: Are All Placebo Effects Equal? Placebo Pills, Sham Acupuncture, Cue Conditioning and Their Association, *PLoS ONE* 8(7):e67485, 2013.

Krishnan KR: Efficient trial designs to reduce placebo requirements, *Biol Psychiatry* 47(8):724–726, 2000.

Lasagna L: The placebo effect, *J Allergy Clin Immun* 78:161–165, 1986.

Lavin MR: Placebo effects on the mind and body, *JAMA* 265:1753–1754, 1991.

LeVasseur SA, Helme RD: A double-blind study to compare the efficacy of an active based cream against placebo cream for the treatment of pressure ulcers, *J Adv Nurs* 16(8):952–956, 1991.

Levine JD, Gordon NC, Fields HL: The mechanism of placebo analgesia, *Lancet* 2:654–657, 1978.

Lipmann JJ, Miller BE, Mays KS, et al: Peak β endorphin concentration in cerebrospinal fluid: reduced in chronic pain patients & increased during the placebo response, *Psychopharmacology (Berl)* 102(1):112–116, 1990.

Meehan TC: Therapeutic Touch and postoperative pain, *Nurs Sci Q* 6(2):69–78, 1993.

Micozzi M: Forensic Pathology, Toxicology & Pathophysiology in Medical-Legal Death Investigation in *Rubin's Textbook of Pathology*, ed 7, Philadelphia, 2015, Wolters Kluwer/Lippincott Williams & Wilkins.

Murray TH: Medical ethics, moral philosophy and moral tradition, *Soc Sci Med* 25(6):637–644, 1987.

Osler W: *Aequanimitas*, ed 3, New York, 1953, Blakiston.

Seeley D: Selected nonpharmacologic therapies for chronic pain: the therapeutic use of the placebo effect, *J Am Acad Nurse Pract* 2(1):10–16, 1990.

Simonton OC, Matthews-Simonton S, Sparks TF: Psychological intervention in the treatment of cancer, *Psychosomatics* 21(3): 226–233, 1980.

Spiegel H: Nocebo: The power of suggestibility, *Prev Med* 26:616–621, 1997.

Stefano GB, Fricchione GL, Slingsby BT, Benson H: The placebo effect and relaxation response: neural processes and the coupling to constitutive nitric oxide, *Brain Res Rev* 35:1–19, 2001.

Stephens RL: Imagery: A strategic intervention to empower clients part 1, *Clin Nurse Spec* 7(4):170–174, 1993.

Tejedor-Real P, Mico JA, Malsonado R, et al: Implications of endogenous opioid system in the learned helplessness model of depression, *Pharmacol Biochem Behav* 52(1):145–152, 1995.

Tellegen Auke, Atkinson Gilbert: Openness to Absorbing and Self-Altering Experiences ('Absorption'), a Trait Related to Hypnotic Susceptibility, *J Abnorm Psychol* 83(3):276, 1974.

Tesh SN: *Hidden arguments: Political ideologies and disease prevention*, New Brunswick, 1983, Rutgers University Press, pp 154–177.

Thomas KB: General practice consultations: Is there any point to being positive? *BMJ* 294:1200–1202, 1987.

Tsolka P, Morris RW, Preiskel HW: Occlusion therapy for craniomandibular disorders: a clinical assessment by a double blind method, *J Prosthet Dent* 68(6):957–964, 1992.

Turner JA, Deyo RA, Loeser JD, et al: The importance of placebo effects in pain treatment and research, *JAMA* 271(20):1609–1614, 1994.

Verdugo RJ, Campero M, Ochoa JL: Phentolamine sympathetic block in painful polyneuropathies: Questioning the concept of Sympathetically Maintained Pain, *Neurology* 44(6):1010–1014, 1994.

Wall PD: The placebo effect: an unpopular topic, *Pain* 51:1–3, 1992.

Wolf S, Pinsky RH: Effect of placebo administration and occurrence of toxic reactions, *JAMA* 155:339–341, 1954.

Further Readings

Jaffe DT, Bresler DE: Guided imagery: Healing through the mind's eye. In Shorr J, Sobel G, Pennee R, Conelly J, editors: *Imagery: Its Many Dimensions and Applications*, New York, 1980, Plenum Press, pp 253–266.

McCrae Robert R, Costa Paul T Jr: Conceptions and Correlates of Openness to Experience. In Hogan R, Johnson JA, Briggs SR, editors: *Handbook of Personality Psychology*, Orlando, Fl., 1997, Academic Press, pp 825–847.

Vines SW: The therapeutics of guided imagery, *Holist Nurs Pract* 2(3):34–44, 1988.

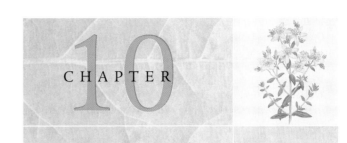

CHAPTER 10

Mind–Body Therapies, Stress, and Psychometrics

MARC S. MICOZZI

MICHAEL A. JAWER

In modern medicine, various forms of psychotherapy have been the preferred methods for addressing psychological, emotional, and mental health issues. To the extent that it is, at times, formally attempted to access a spiritual dimension, it also lies within this realm of mainstream medicine. In the approaches taken in this text, and this section, we can see that various forms of stress create changes and enlist responses in a kind of mind–body–spirit continuum. This chapter begins with a brief review of psychotherapeutic approaches in context.

PSYCHOTHERAPY

The word *psychotherapy* is derived from Greek words meaning "healing of the soul" and refers to treatment involving emotional and mental health, which is interwoven with physical health. Psychotherapy encompasses a wide range of specific treatments, from talk therapy and combination of medication with discussion of the patient's concerns, to more active behavioral and emotional approaches. Psychotherapy has evolved through a succession of concepts that also relate to complementary and alternative medical approaches. (Some of the major figures and the relevant concepts for which they are most known are listed in Box 10-1.)

An average of one in every five people in the United States experiences a major psychological disorder every six months—most commonly anxiety, depression, substance abuse, or acute confusion (Strain, 1993). This rate is believed to be even higher among patients with a chronic illness and among elderly patients. Approximately three-fifths of patients with psychological problems are seen only by primary care physicians, many of whom are not adequately trained in psychotherapy and most of whom do not have adequate time to spend discussing patients' psychological issues. Despite the enormous need for different forms of psychological care, most people who display the greatest need for such care receive less than adequate screening and treatment for their conditions.

It is generally considered that primary care physicians recognize cases of depression in only one-quarter to one-half of the patients who experience it, and they recognize other types of mental illness in less than one-quarter of cases. However, these same physicians write most of the prescriptions for antidepressant and antianxiety drugs and may often prescribe them inappropriately. Clearly, there is a significant need for better recognition and management of the mental and emotional issues that can often result in serious illness.

Methods of Psychotherapy

Mental health professionals are paying more attention to features shared by all effective forms of psychotherapy, especially collaboration between the therapist and patient in developing an account of the patient's emotional life that promotes confidence, heightens well-being, and suggests ways to overcome cognitive or emotional difficulties. A primary aim of psychotherapy is to transform the meaning of the patient's experience by improving emotional state through an intimate relationship with a helpful professional. Conventional psychotherapy is conducted primarily through psychological methods such as suggestion, persuasion, psychoanalysis, and reframing. Although research suggests that the methods do not differ greatly in effectiveness, several hundred types of psychotherapy are available, used individually or in groups. In general, most forms of psychotherapy fall into categories listed below.

Carl Jung

Unconscious
Collective unconscious
Archetypes

Abraham Maslow

Humanistic psychology
Self-actualization
Hierarchy of needs

Carl Rogers

Person-centered psychotherapy
Humanistic psychology

Milton Erikson

Unconscious
Hypnosis
Family system therapy

- **Psychodynamic therapy.** Psychodynamic therapy is derived from psychoanalysis and seeks to understand and resolve emotional conflicts that originate in childhood relationships with patterns that repeat themselves in adult life. Sessions usually are devoted to exploring current emotional reactions from past situations. This approach works best if the patient's goal is to make fundamental changes in personality patterns rather than to change one specific behavior. Psychodynamic therapy is often called *interpretive therapy* or *expressive therapy*.
- **Behavior therapy.** Behavior therapy emphasizes changing specific behavior, such as a phobia, by stopping what has been reinforcing it or by replacing it with a more desirable response. Sessions are usually devoted to analyzing the behavior and devising ways to change it, with specific instructions carried out between sessions. Behavior therapy is more effective with focused problems, such as a fear of public speaking.
- **Cognitive therapy.** Cognitive therapy is similar to behavior therapy in changing specific habits; however, it emphasizes the habitual thoughts that underlie those habits. The general strategy is similar to that of behavior therapy, and the two approaches are often used together. Cognitive therapy is generally effective for treating depression and low self-esteem.
- **Systems therapy.** Systems therapy focuses on relationship patterns, either in couples, between parents and children, or within the whole family. This approach requires that everyone involved attend therapy sessions and often entails experiential practice aimed at changing problem-causing patterns. Systems therapies work well for a troubled marriage or intense conflicts between parents and children, where the problem is in the relationship between them.
- **Supportive therapy.** Supportive therapy concentrates on helping people who are in an intense emotional

crisis, such as a deep depression, and may be used in combination with pharmacological support. It focuses on building tools to handle overwhelming day-to-day situations.

- **Body-oriented therapy.** Body-oriented therapy hypothesizes that emotions are encoded in and may be expressed as tension and restriction in various parts of the body. Various methods, including breath work, movement, and manual pressure, are used to help release emotions that are believed to be held in the muscles and tissues (see also Section III).

Underlining the relationship between mind and body, psychotherapeutic treatment can hasten recovery from a medical crisis and, in some cases, is the best treatment for it. Brief psychotherapy sessions reduce time spent in hospitals for elderly patients with broken hips by an average of 2 days; these patients returned to the hospital fewer times and spent fewer days in rehabilitation (Strain, 1993). Other studies show that psychotherapy is most effective when started soon after a patient is admitted to a hospital. At present, however, most psychological problems associated with physical illnesses remain undiagnosed or are not identified until near the end of a hospital stay.

One of the most common emotional problems of medical patients is "reactive" anxiety and depression—the distress stemming from a patient's normative reaction to a medical diagnosis. Those with serious or terminal illnesses are particularly vulnerable. In other cases, psychological symptoms are a direct result of the patient's physical disease. Still other patients experience a shift in their mental or emotional state as a direct result of a specific medication. For example, some patients taking high levels of steroids may react psychotically, whereas others may experience severe depression, or even periods of euphoria.

COST EFFECTIVENESS

Psychotherapy has been shown to speed patients' recovery from illness. Faster recovery leads to reduced costs and fewer return visits to medical practitioners. In one study, patients who frequently visited medical clinics and accepted short-term psychotherapy had significant declines in visits to their doctors, days spent in the hospital, emergency department visits, diagnostic procedures, and drug prescriptions. Their overall health care costs decreased by 10% to 20% in the years after brief psychotherapy (Cummings & Bragman, 1988).

A more specific example of cost effectiveness was provided by a 1991 study where participation in 10 group sessions of 90 minutes of psychotherapy and relaxation techniques significantly reduced the severity of pain. In patients with chronic pain, those who participated in the outpatient behavioral medicine program had 36% fewer clinic visits than those who did not (Caudill et al, 1991).

In a 1987 study conducted jointly by Mount Sinai Hospital and Northwestern Memorial Hospital, psychiatrist George Fulop of Mount Sinai and his colleagues observed that patients hospitalized for medical or surgical reasons had significantly longer hospital stays if they also had concurrent psychiatric problems, especially if they were elderly. In other words, a patient who had a heart attack and who was also depressed tended to remain in the hospital for more days than a similar heart attack patient whose mood was normal. Fulop's study suggested that treating a medical patient's emotional state with psychotherapy in conjunction with medication could improve psychological well-being in tandem with the patient's physical condition (Fulop et al, 1987).

Another well-known study, published in 1983 by psychologists Herbert J. Schlesinger and Emily Mumford and their colleagues at the University of Colorado School of Medicine, investigated patients with four common chronic diseases: asthma, diabetes, coronary heart disease, and high blood pressure. The researchers examined a group that underwent some form of psychotherapy after having been identified as having one of these four physical conditions, compared with a control group who did not receive psychological treatment after similar diagnoses were made (Schlesinger et al, 1983). Three years after they received their medical diagnoses, patients who had undergone 7 to 20 mental health treatment visits had incurred lower medical costs than those who did not have psychological treatment. The total charges for the psychotherapy group, including those incurred for psychotherapy and counseling, were more than $300 less than for the control group. The savings on medical bills offered by psychotherapy, therefore, more than compensated for its costs. After 21 sessions the savings began to diminish as the cumulative cost of mental health care increased.

Although this study is often cited as proof of psychotherapy's financial advantages for medically ill patients, it was a retrospective study rather than prospective study. Additional research is needed in which subjects are selected at random from the beginning of treatment and closely followed after treatment. Another limitation of this particular study was that the investigators could not delineate the type of mental health problems the patients experienced nor the specific treatment they received (a wide variety of psychological interventions was covered).

More rigorous research on specific forms of psychotherapy, including precise diagnoses, will be needed to reach firm conclusions about the economic benefits of psychological treatment for medically ill patients. However, there is already sufficient evidence to suggest that this cost–benefit research is important to pursue. It was generally observed during the period from 1965 to 1980 that patients who underwent psychotherapy used other medical services significantly less than patients who did not receive psychotherapy.

The concept of what constitutes appropriate areas for psychological intervention could also be expanded, because many health care professionals and academics now consider psychotherapeutic intervention in physical illness a peripheral concern. The studies we have touched on here, as well as others, however, suggest that psychological

intervention is often beneficial. Such treatment is most effective when used early in the disease process; it can even affect mortality (Micozzi, 2015). Further research is needed to disclose the myriad ways the mind and body are connected and how methods that make use of these connections can potentially improve health and limit costs simultaneously.

SOCIAL SUPPORT AND PSYCHOLOGICAL COUNSELING

Psychologists have known since World War II that social support and group consciousness greatly aid people in their attitudes and emotional resiliency. Over the past 10 years, especially, clinical studies have shown that social support has a significant influence on symptoms of stress for patients with chronic illnesses (Chapter 4).

In a study of patients with coronary artery disease, group support and psychological counseling were combined with diet and exercise. Symptoms such as angina pectoris rapidly diminished or disappeared, and after 1 year the coronary arteries were less obstructed. This evidence strongly suggests that heart disease, the most deadly and costly U.S. health care problem, is reversible through a complementary, noninvasive, diet and behavioral modification approach that emphasizes group psychotherapy and social support (Ornish, 1990).

A landmark case study was conducted in 1989 by David Spiegel, a professor of psychiatry and behavioral sciences at Stanford School of Medicine, in which he investigated the benefits of social support on women with metastatic breast cancer. The women who participated in the group psychotherapy lived an average of 18 months longer than those who did not participate, doubling their survival time. The added survival time was longer than that of any medication or other known medical treatment for women with advanced breast cancer. The intense social support the women experienced in these sessions appeared to influence the way their bodies coped with the illness, which showed that quality of life affects longevity (Spiegel et al, 1989).

In 1999, Spiegel conducted a multicenter feasibility study to examine the benefits of a supportive-expressive group psychotherapy intervention for patients with recently diagnosed breast cancer. The study recruited 111 patients with breast cancer within 1 year of diagnosis from 10 geographically diverse sites of the Community Clinical Oncology Program of the National Cancer Institute and two academic medical centers. Each patient who participated in the expressive psychotherapy group met for 12 weekly sessions of 90 minutes each. Results indicated a significant decrease in mood disturbance scores, anxiety, and depression in group session participants (Spiegel et al, 1999).

A similar study was conducted involving 102 women with metastatic breast cancer who were randomly selected to receive 1 year of weekly supportive-expressive group therapy and educational materials. Control participants received education materials only. Those who received group therapy showed a significantly greater decline in traumatic stress symptoms and total mood disturbance (Classen et al, 2001).

Maintenance of emotional well-being is critical to cardiovascular health. People who feel lonely, depressed, and isolated are more likely to suffer illnesses and die prematurely of cardiovascular diseases than those who have adequate social support (Williams et al, 1999). Consequently, the development of appropriate interventions to improve the emotional health of people with certain psychosocial risk factors is essential. It is anticipated that such interventions will increase life expectancy of people at risk and may also save millions of dollars in medical care costs.

A cross-sectional study conducted at Stanford University examined whether coping styles of emotional suppression and "fighting spirit" were associated with mood disturbance in 121 cancer patients participating in professionally led, community-based support groups. The investigators concluded that expression of negative affect and an attitude of realistic optimism may enhance adjustment and reduce stress for patients with cancer in support groups (Cordova et al, 2003).

Psychological support studies lead to a convergence of significant emotional, health behavior, and biological benefits for cancer patients. An Ohio State University study tested the hypothesis that a psychological intervention could reduce emotional distress, improve health behavior, and enhance immune responses; 227 women who had undergone breast cancer surgery were randomly assigned to receive an intervention that included strategies to reduce stress, improve mood, alter health behaviors, and maintain adherence to cancer treatment. The control group received no intervention. The treatment group met in weekly sessions for 4 months. Patients who attended the weekly support group sessions showed significant lowering of anxiety, improvements in perceived social support, improved dietary habits, and reduction in smoking. Immune responses for the intervention group paralleled their psychological and behavioral improvements. T-lymphocyte proliferation remained stable or increased in the treatment group, whereas this response declined in the control group (Andersen et al, 2004).

SOCIAL SUPPORT AND MORTALITY

A growing number of large-scale studies evidence a link between social support and physical well-being. This research shows that having many close social relationships is associated with a lower risk of dying at any age. Research focused specifically on sick people shows that, once serious illness strikes, social support continues to affect the chances of staying alive.

Over 40 years ago, medical researchers were drawn to the tight-knit Italian-American community of Roseto in northeastern Pennsylvania. Its late-middle-aged citizens seemed nearly immune to heart disease, seemingly in defiance of medical logic. The men of the town smoked and drank wine freely. (This same effect observed in Europe would later become known as the *French Paradox.*) They worked in slate quarries 200 feet down in the earth. At home their tables were laden with Italian food modified in a way that would horrify a dietitian. To save money, they had replaced olive oil with . . . lard! Yet their hefty bodies contained healthy hearts. Why?

Every aspect of their health was examined in a comprehensive series of tests, observations, and interviews; however, traditional medical science did not offer any answer.

The answer lay in social science, not medicine. Stated simply, it was found that people nourish other people. The households in Roseto contained three generations; furthermore, everyone had a well-established place in their society. The community had stability and predictability. Similar "Roseto effects" have been documented from Israel to Borneo, as well as in France (as noted above).

Even the success of the Ornish diet in preventing and reversing heart disease has been thought by some observers to be due primarily to the social support of the dieters' cooking, eating, and interacting together (especially because the diet itself is simply too high in carbohydrates for optimal health; see Chapter 26) (Egolf et al, 1992).

The researchers who came to study this community also predicted that the Roseto effect would disappear. Indeed, as suburbs arose, with their fenced-in yards and satellite dishes, the rate of heart attacks in Roseto came to reflect the national averages (Chicago Tribune, 1996, "A new 'Roseto Effect'").

Elsewhere, internist James Goodwin at the Medical College of Wisconsin studied cancer survival in several thousand patients. The married cancer patients did better medically and had lower mortality rates than the unmarried patients (Goodwin et al, 1987). Similarly, in a study of 1368 patients with coronary artery disease, Redford Williams at Duke University found that having a spouse or other close confidant tripled the chances that a patient would be alive 5 years later (Williams et al, 1999).

In 1990, epidemiologists Peggy Reynolds and George Kaplan at the California Department of Health Services studied the number of social contacts that cancer patients had each day. Women with the least amount of social contact were 2.2 times more likely to die of cancer over a 17-year period than were the most socially connected women (Reynolds & Kaplan, 1990).

In a review of research concerning mortality and social relationships, James House observed that the relationship between social isolation and early death is stronger statistically than the relationship between dying and smoking or dying and having a high serum cholesterol level. International observations from the World Health Organization, among individual countries, and in the United States have consistently shown that low serum cholesterol is a poor measure or predictor of better health or longevity (Hite et al, 2010). It is more important to one's health to be socially integrated than it is to stop smoking or to reduce one's cholesterol level (House et al, 1988).

People who feel lonely, depressed, and isolated have been found to be significantly more likely to experience illnesses and to die prematurely (i.e., before their 70s) than those who have adequate social support (Williams et al, 1999). Of course, other social factors may account for why one patient survives longer than another. Most such studies have been careful to eliminate the "usual" confounding variables, such as smoking and alcohol use, differences in socioeconomic status, and access to health care.

Understanding Stress Reduction

However, a lack of understanding of the individual nature of stress, and apparent stress-reducing benefits of moderate alcohol consumption and even light tobacco use, limit the precision of such approaches. After all, natural tobacco originated as a common Native American herbal remedy that was also used in *social settings* and widely observed to reduce stress, granting the peaceful effects of the proverbial "peace pipe." While modern interpretations seem to associate the widely used term "peace pipe" to express an association with communally sharing a tobacco pipe to commemorate a "peace" treaty (most of which treaties had no more lasting effects than the evanescent puffs of smoke on the wind), the cultural transliteration of the term "peace" relates to the clear physiologic effects of sharing "a smoke." Tobacco still is seen as a medicinal as well as mystical plant by indigenous peoples. Among hunting-gathering Neolithic tribes on the banks of the Upper Amazon, as soon as agriculture in introduced fields are cleared for planting, tobacco was the first plant grown (see Section VI).

In general, studies consistently show that increased and better social support from family, friends, and community is associated with lower odds of dying at any given age. Although the relation between social support and health outcome has been largely underestimated by medical science, two studies examining social support and its relationship to mortality are noteworthy. The Department of Community and Preventative Medicine at the University of Rochester School of Medicine found that certain aspects of informal caregiving are important factors in enhancing the survival of frail nursing home residents. Several social support variables were statistically significant predictors of mortality. Participants whose primary caregiver was their spouse had a significantly lower risk of mortality than those whose caregiver was not their spouse (Temkin-Greener et al, 2004). Researchers at the Mayo Clinic confirmed many of these findings in a systematic review of evidence related to social support, specifically the role of social support in cardiovascular disease-related outcomes (Mookadam & Arthur, 2004).

A number of studies have demonstrated a relationship among low perceived social support and depression, as well as low perceived social support and mortality in patients with heart disease. Evidence also suggests that depression increases the risk of acute myocardial infarction along with the level of resulting morbidity and mortality (Malach & Imperato, 2004).

STRESS REDUCTION AND RELAXATION THERAPIES

Stress Management

The term *stress* was brought into popular use by Professor Hans Selye, director of the Institute of Experimental Medicine and Surgery at the University of Montreal. He defined stress as "the rate of wear and tear on the body." Confusion and debate continue as to whether stress is the factor that causes the wear and tear and/or is the resulting damage. Selye described a "general adaptation syndrome," which has three phases: an alarm reaction, a stage of resistance, and a stage of exhaustion. A stress cause, or stressor, activates the sympathetic branch of the autonomic nervous system. Hormones bring about physiological changes in the body, often referred to as the "fight-or-flight response" (Selye, 1978).

The problem of stress receives wide publicity in the media today. A constant cliché held that "stress" was the epidemic of the 1980s, and then the 1990s, and we can only imagine the dimensions of this pandemic in the twenty-first century. As early as 1970, Alvin Toffler (the first self-proclaimed futurist) proclaimed that "future shock" would leave us all in a state of discombobulation. Consequently, the term *stress* has also become a buzzword and acquired a highly negative connotation. Much advice has also been dispensed, from all manner of sources, gurus, and even "management consultants," about the many approaches to controlling stress. (One approach is to quit doing real work and *become* a management consultant or self-help guru). A key missing element, however, is an understanding that different stress-reduction techniques have different degrees of effectiveness for each individual. Apart from the psychometric evaluation of personality type, there is simply no good way to predict (see the final portion of this chapter).

All the alarmist and negative publicity has stimulated further anxiety and concern in many people's minds—a fear of stress, which in itself can lead to further stress. Having become aware of it, everyone now wants to manage his or her stress, and many cater to this growing demand. This rapidly expanding market is served by various self-proclaimed experts, consultants, and therapists, as well as assorted management "gurus" who place showmanship over science. Vitamin regimens, herbal supplements, fitness programs, relaxation techniques, and personal development courses are all on offer in the name of *stress management*. Numerous experts, both qualified and self-appointed, are convinced that their particular product or service will banish stress for good. But none yet has a clue as to how to match the right approach to each individual versus one-size-fits-all approaches (see Psychometrics section of this chapter).

The fact remains that there are no magic cures and no magic bullets. Harmful stress is essentially the result of an interaction between a negative environment, unhealthful lifestyle, and self-defeating attitudes and beliefs. Therefore, in contrast to what we would be led to believe by stress management consultants, no one particular technique, method, program, or regimen can reduce long-term stress for everyone or any "group" of individuals.

THE SUBJECTIVE NATURE OF STRESS

Stress can also be viewed as the outside pressures and problems that encroach on our busy lives: deadlines, excessive workload, noise, traffic, problems with spouse or children, as well as any excessive demands made by others or even placed upon ourselves. Seen in this light, stress is the unconscious response to a demand. However, stress is not solely "those things out there," but rather what happens inside the mind and body as we react unconsciously to circumstances, events, or people. Normally, we experience some degree of stress in everything we do and everything that happens to us. Our bodies continuously react to even the most minute changes. This process occurs all the time, whether we are consciously aware of it or not.

There are also indisputably positive aspects to stress, however. In *Magical Child*, Joseph Chilton Pearce writes, "Stress is the way intelligence grows." He explains that, under stress, the brain immediately grows massive numbers of new connections among the neurons that enable learning. Although the stressed mind/brain grows in ability and the unstressed mind lags behind, the *over*stressed brain can collapse into refractory physiological shock. Balance is therefore essential to maintain an optimal level of stress—an ideal method for gaining balance being what we call relaxation (Pearce, 1992).

When the stress response is minor, we do not notice any symptoms. But the greater the stimulation, the more symptoms we notice. Holmes and Rahe's scale of life changes provides a guide to the amount of stress attached to major events, such as marriage, relocation, emigration, loss of a job, death of a spouse, or birth of a child. These significant life events, whether objectively positive or negative, can quickly overload our ability to cope and maintain balance (Holmes & Rahe, 1967).

In *The Human Zoo*, Desmond Morris posits that modern humans are engaged in the "stimulus struggle": "If we abandon it, or tackle it badly, we are in serious trouble." Each of us is trying to maintain the *optimal* level of stimulation—not the maximum, but a balance that is most beneficial, somewhere between understimulation and overstimulation (Morris, 1995).

We all continuously adjust to changing conditions, beginning with homeostatic mechanisms, rather like an air conditioner controlled by a thermostat. As the temperature outside increases, the thermostat turns on the air conditioner, which begins to bring the interior temperature back to a specified normal level of comfort. The greater the changes outside, the harder the machine has to work to keep up with them. If the external temperature moves into extreme ranges, the machine will be pushed to the limit. If it exceeds its specified limit, it will eventually break down, and the motor will burn out.

Stress becomes a problem when it reaches excessive levels, when the demands exceed our ability to respond or to cope effectively. When we are under excessive, prolonged stress and no longer able to cope or adjust, the "stress" becomes "distress." Symptoms then develop that lead to stress-induced illnesses. The physical body (our "engine") begins to rev at high speed. Over extended periods, constant wear and tear will take its toll, and disease can creep into the body.

We learn to manage our responses to stress by developing the ability to exert control over our attitudes and behaviors. When we become more aware of this innate ability, we naturally begin to assert control over the life situations that seem to be stressful. It is not this stress itself that is harmful but our reactions to it that create havoc in the body and mind.

The greatest stressor that most people experience daily is change. Indeed, the only constant today *is* change. To update the words of Franklin Delano Roosevelt, however, we need not fear "change itself." Shifting life events are inevitable and require us to adapt. If we do not adapt by modifying our attitudes and expectations, our minds and bodies will suffer. When changes take place in our immediate environment, career, or personal relationships, it becomes essential to learn new styles of thinking, feeling, and behaving in order to cope with the new situation effectively.

Taking a longer view, adaptation to environmental stress can be accomplished during the growth period (ontogenetic), by learning and sharing new behaviors in a community or society (cultural) and, eventually, by shifts in gene frequency (evolutionary) (see Chapter 2).

Different people respond differently to stress and to different mind-body techniques for stress and disease management. We know people who can appear cool, calm, and collected under the most trying circumstances, and we know others who seem unable to cope when faced with even minor contingencies. The difference is the aggregate result of variations in genetics, upbringing, personal understandings, attitudes, beliefs, values, perceptions, and coping skills—all of which develop over years and even generations. Furthermore, when individuals experience distress, the symptoms they develop also vary; different people seem to channel their excessive stress into different parts of the body. The long-term effects of such differing responses include physical illnesses such as ulcers, headaches, chronic backaches, and high blood pressure. These responses can ultimately result in heart disease, cancer, or other chronic disorders.

Using a psychometric method for evaluating different personality types, we can come a long way toward better gauging who will be more or less susceptible to various stress-related illnesses, and who will respond best to which mind–body therapies (see the final portion of this chapter).

It stands to reason—and studies have found—that people who learn to manage stress are more resilient, experience fewer symptoms, and experience an improved quality of life (Kabat-Zinn, 1990). Still, in evaluating 26 randomized controlled trials testing the effect of cognitive-behavioral techniques (including meditation) on hypertension, Eisenberg et al (1993) found that no single technique appears to be more effective than any other in treating the condition. He had no method, however, for evaluating personality type that would have allowed matching each person with the mind–body treatment most likely to be effective. Without discriminating between personality types, such research results in "noise." The benefit for patients, indeed, is unlikely to be as evident or effective as it is for standard antihypertensive pharmacotherapy, unless integrative medical approaches do a better job of matching the right mind–body therapies to the right patients.

Relaxation Response

Harvard School of Medicine cardiologist Herbert Benson began investigating the benefits of relaxation in the late 1960s and continues to research the effects of stress on various disease-specific populations. For example, Benson's group has examined the effects of stress on cardiovascular diseases and neurodegenerative diseases (Esch et al, 2002a, 2000b). They found that stress has a major impact on the circulatory and nervous systems, playing a significant role in susceptibility, progress, and outcome of both cardiovascular and neurodegenerative diseases. However, they also found that some amounts of stress ("positive" stress, or *eustress*) can actually improve performance and thus can be beneficial in certain cases. Recently, Benson's group used the latest molecular genetic techniques to demonstrate that relaxation regulates the expression of different genes, turning some on and others off. Although many observers hold out hope that new biotechnology research will yet lead to new gene therapies, instead it is serving to demonstrate the mechanisms of action for age-old approaches like mind–body medicine, as well as nutritional factors (Chapters 9 and 26).

Once he was able to demonstrate that meditation could lower high blood pressure, Benson continued research into a variety of psychological and physiological effects that appear to be common among many mind–body practices. He eventually identified the "relaxation response," which is essentially the same response common to meditation, prayer, autogenic training, and some forms of hypnosis (Benson, 1975).

Benson's research indicates that excessive stress causes or aggravates hypertension and thus related diseases of atherosclerosis, coronary heart disease, and stroke. He then examined the nature of the relaxation response, showing that physiological changes, opposite to but as prominent as those seen in the fight-or-flight response, also occur during true relaxation, including a decrease in oxygen con-sumption, metabolic rate, heart rate, and blood pressure, as well as increased production of alpha brain waves. A marked decrease in blood lactate level was also found. Blood lactate has often been linked with muscle tension and anxiety.

According to Benson, following these guidelines can help achieve the relaxation response:
1. Try to find 10 to 20 minutes in your daily routine.
2. Sit comfortably.
3. For the period you will practice, try to arrange your life so that you will have no distractions. For example, let the answering machine handle the phone, or ask someone to watch the children.
4. Time yourself by glancing periodically at a clock or watch (but do not set an alarm). Commit yourself to a specific length of practice.

Expanding on these guidelines, the following is one approach to elicit the relaxation response:

Step 1: Pick a focus word or short phrase firmly rooted in your personal belief system. For example, a nonreligious individual might choose a neutral word such as *one, peace,* or *love.* A Buddhist could repeat *om.* A Christian could recite the opening words of Psalm 23, "The Lord is my shepherd"; a Jew could choose *shalom,* a Muslim, *salaam.*

Step 2: Sit quietly in a comfortable position.

Step 3: Close your eyes.

Step 4: Relax your muscles.

Step 5: Breathe slowly and naturally, repeating your focus word or phrase silently as you exhale.

Step 6: Throughout, assume a passive attitude. Do not worry about how well you are doing. When other thoughts come to mind, simply say to yourself, "Oh, well," and gently return to the repetition.

Step 7: Continue for 10 to 20 minutes. You may open your eyes to check the time, but do not use an alarm. When you finish, sit quietly for a minute or so, at first with your eyes closed and later with your eyes open. Then do not stand for 1 or 2 minutes.

Step 8: Practice the technique once or twice a day.

Benson's subsequent research into the relaxation response investigated several efficient techniques of relaxation training, including Transcendental Meditation, Zen and yoga, autogenic training, progression relaxation, hypnosis, and sentic cycles (Table 10-1). He found that these methods had four common elements: a quiet environment, an object on which to focus the mind, a passive attitude, and a comfortable position. Some practices are more effective than others, and some are easier to learn and practice than others (Benson, 1993).

Benson's group also found that patients with chronic pain who meditated regularly had a net reduction in general health care costs, which suggests that the use of relaxation techniques is cost effective (Caudill et al, 1991).

Deepak et al (1994) found that 11 patients with drug-resistant epilepsy who practiced Benson's relaxation response for 20 minutes each day experienced a decrease in

TABLE 10-1 *Relaxation Response*

Technique	Oxygen consumption	Respiratory rate	Heart rate	Alpha waves	Blood pressure	Muscle tension
Transcendental meditation	Decreases	Decreases	Decreases	Increase	Decreases[a]	(Not measured)
Zen and yoga	Decreases	Decreases	Decreases	Increase	Decreases[a]	
Autogenic training	(Not measured)	Decreases	Decreases	Increase	Inconclusive	Decreases
Progressive relaxation	(Not measured)	(Not measured)	(Not measured)	(Not measured)	Inconclusive	Decreases
Hypnosis with suggested deep relaxation	Decreases	Decreases	Decreases	(Not measured)	Inconclusive	(Not measured)

[a]In patients with elevated blood pressure.

absolute frequency of seizures, and that the decrease became significant at between 6 and 12 months of continued practice. Duration of seizures declined over the 12 months to a more significant degree than did frequency of seizures.

The value of Benson's technique for patients with congestive heart failure was evidenced in a study of 57 veterans who received relaxation response training. Approximately half the group reported physical improvements that went beyond disease management and into lifestyle changes and improved relationships (Chang et al, 2004).

EXERCISE

Michael Sacks, MD, professor of psychiatry at Cornell University Medical College, found that various forms of exercise are powerful methods of relaxation and are effective for dealing with the stress of daily life. Researchers have found in various studies that exercise can decrease anxiety and depression, improve an individual's self-image, and buffer people from the effects of stress. Not every study has shown the precise benefits for which researchers were looking, but taken as a whole, the research strongly supports the common experience that exercise can elevate mood and reduce anxiety and stress (Sacks, 1993).

Although most research has focused on the physical benefits of exercise, any exercise can help people feel more focused and relaxed as long as the activity remains enjoyable. Regular exercise does seem to affect the ability to withstand stress. Exercise and physical fitness act as a buffer against stress, so that stressful events have a less negative impact on psychological and physical health.

MEDITATION

The Centers for Disease Control and Prevention (2003) released data showing chronic diseases afflict more than 90 million Americans accounting for one-third of the years of potential life lost before age 65 years. The financial burden of treating chronic diseases now amounts to nearly two-thirds of the total medical care costs in the United States. Evidence is accumulating that chronically ill patients derive great benefits from using meditation, including a decrease in the number of visits to physicians (Sobel, 1992).

Complementary and alternative medicine (CAM) is often defined as encompassing a broad group of interventions, such as meditation, that are not taught widely at U.S. medical schools or generally available at U.S. hospitals (see Chapter 1). This appears to be a curious definition when, as early as 1997, more than 42% of the adult U.S. population used CAM to manage cancer and other chronic diseases, and meditation is one of the most common practices among them (Eisenberg et al, 2001).

Although various practices of meditation are ancient in their roots, the science of meditation and its physiological effects is still in its infancy. Only recently has the concept of meditation been introduced into the realm of modern Western medicine. As a result of the Cartesian split between the mind and body in the early seventeenth century, science came to emphasize the body and medicine followed the direction of science. The term *mind–body connection* relates to an understanding that the two are not separate (they have always been together) and have an interactive influence on each other. Meditation is said to realign the two, balancing the consciousness within the physical body, creating more harmonious interactions.

Like the word *medicine*, the word *meditation* suggests something to do with healing. The root in Latin means "to cure" but at its deepest root means "to measure" (Bohm, 1983). But what does medicine or meditation have to do with measure? The ancient Greeks said, "Man is the measure of all things." According to Jon Kabat-Zinn, PhD, founder and director of the Stress Reduction Clinic at the University of Massachusetts Medical Center, meditation has to do with the "platonic notion that every shape, every being, and every thing has its right inward measure. In other words, a tree has its own quality of wholeness that gives it particular properties. A human being has an individual right inward measure, when everything is balanced and physiologically homeostatic. That is the totality of the individual at that point in time" (Kabat-Zinn, 1993a, 1993b, 1993c). He believes that medicine is the science and art of restoring right inward measure when it is thrown off balance. From the meditative perspective and from the perspective of the new mind–body medicine, health does not have a finite or static destination. Health is a dynamic energy flow that changes from day-to-day, and over a lifetime, with health and illness coexisting.

Although there is a strong home-grown tradition in Great Britain and America of contemplative thought and practice (see Chapter 7), many meditative practices came to the West from Asian religious practices, particularly those of India, Tibet, China, and Japan. Others can be traced to other ethnomedical traditions around the world. Although Western meditators practice a *contemplative* form of meditation, there are also many *active* forms of meditation, such as the Chinese martial art t'ai chi, the Japanese martial art aikido, and the walking meditations of Zen Buddhism.

Until recently, the primary purpose of meditation has been religious or spiritual in nature. During the past 30 years, however, meditation has been explored as a method for reducing stress on both mind and body. Many studies have found that various practices of meditation appear to produce physical and psychological changes. Meditation is a self-directed practice for the purpose of relaxing and calming the mind and body. Many methods of meditation include focusing on a single thought or word for a specific time. Some forms of meditation focus on a physical experience, such as the breath or a specific sound or mantra. All forms of meditation have the common objective of stilling the restlessness of the mind so that the focus can be directed inwardly.

Meditation is thus a technique that can be used to calm mental activity, endless thoughts, and ways of reacting to one's circumstances. As long as these accumulated impressions linger in the inner recesses of the mind, pushing for attention, it remains difficult to experience an inner state of peace, calm, and health. Fast-paced Western society, filled with external stimuli, has conditioned us to push our minds and bodies to the point of exhaustion, often to the detriment of our own well-being. To be still, to experience the peace and contentment that lies within, we must free ourselves from this external materiality. Meditation is a process for calming and releasing the distractions from the mind for the purpose of opening up and awakening to our true inner natures.

ASIAN TECHNIQUES AND TRANSCENDENTAL MEDITATION

In the mid-1960s, a popular trend in meditation called *Transcendental Meditation (TM)* began to emerge. The Vedic philosophy and practice was brought from India to the United States by its founder, Maharishi Mahesh Yogi. The Maharishi had eliminated ancient yogic elements that he considered would be unpopular in a contemporary twentieth century Western society. Omitting difficult physical postures, procedures and mental exercises, his modified version became more easily understood, accepted, and practiced by Westerners (see Chapters 3, 7).

TM is relatively simple in application. A student is given a mantra (a word or sound) to repeat silently over and over again while sitting in a comfortable position. The purpose of repeating the sound or word is to prevent distracting thoughts from entering the mind. Students are instructed to be passive and, if thoughts other than the mantra come to mind, to note them and return the attention to the mantra. TM is generally practiced in the morning and in the evening for approximately 20 minutes.

On the Maharishi's first visit to America in 1959, a San Francisco newspaper heralded TM as a "nonmedicinal tranquilizer" and praised it as a promising cure for insomnia. TM soon began to ride a crest of popularity, with almost half a million Americans learning the technique by 1975, and it was embraced by many celebrities of that day, such as the Beatles. It is estimated that more than 2 million people currently practice TM.

In 1968, Benson was asked by the Maharishi International University in Fairfield, Iowa, to test TM practitioners on their ability to lower their own blood pressure. Benson initially refused to participate but was later persuaded to do so. Benson's studies and other research showed that TM was associated with reduced health care costs, increased longevity, and better quality of life (Benson et al, 1977); reduced anxiety, lowered blood pressure, and reduced serum cholesterol levels (Cooper & Aygen, 1978); viable treatment of post-traumatic stress syndrome in Vietnam War veterans (Brooks & Scarano, 1985); and reduction in chronic pain (Kabat-Zinn et al, 1986).

In a study aimed at linking TM practice to longevity, 73 elders were randomly assigned to either a TM program, mindfulness training, a relaxation program, or no treatment. Both the TM and mindfulness training groups showed significant reductions in systolic blood pressure compared with those receiving mental relaxation training or no training. As reported by the nursing staff, TM and mindfulness training improved patients' mental health. Longevity was defined as the subjects' survival rate over a 36-month period, which was found to be greater for those using TM than for those receiving mental relaxation training and control subjects (Alexander et al, 1989).

Additional research showed the effectiveness of TM in the reduction of substance abuse (Sharma et al, 1991), blood pressure reduction in African Americans (Schneider et al, 1992), and lowering of blood cortisol levels initially raised by stress (MacLean et al, 1992).

In a follow-up study of 127 African American elders, Schneider again found that blood pressure decreased significantly in those practicing both TM and progressive muscle relaxation compared with the control group, and that TM was significantly more effective than progressive muscle relaxation techniques (Schneider et al, 1995).

In a study to examine the effects of TM on nine women with symptoms of cardiac syndrome X, those who practiced TM for 3 months showed an improvement in quality of life, exercise tolerance, and angina episodes (Cunningham et al, 2000). An experiment to determine the effects of TM-based stress reduction on carotid atherosclerosis in 60 hypertensive African Americans used B-mode ultrasound to measure carotid intima media thickness, a surrogate measure of coronary atherosclerosis. The group practicing the TM technique group showed a significant decrease in thickness, whereas thickness increased in the control group (Castillo-Richmond et al, 2000).

Herron and Hillis (2000) broke new economic ground by conducting a quasi-experimental, longitudinal study of the impact of a TM program on government payments to physicians in Quebec. They found that payments to physicians treating practitioners of TM were lower than payments to physicians treating a randomly selected and matched control group over a 6-year period, with a 13.78% mean annual difference in payments. A true experimental design with randomization would be needed to control for social factors that may have confounded study results.

WESTERN TECHNIQUES AND MINDFULNESS MEDITATION

The term *mindfulness* was coined by Jon Kabat-Zinn, known for his work using mindfulness meditation to help medical patients with chronic pain and stress-related disorders (Kabat-Zinn, 1993a, 1993b). Like other mind–body therapies, mindfulness meditation can induce deep states of relaxation, at times can directly improve physical symptoms, and can help patients lead fuller and more satisfying lives. Although Asian forms of meditation involve focusing on a sound, phrase, or prayer to minimize distraction, the practice of mindfulness does the opposite. In mindfulness meditation, "distractions" are not ignored but are focused on. This form of meditation practice can ultimately be traced originally back to the Buddhist tradition and is about 2500 years old. The method was developed as a means of cultivating greater awareness and wisdom, with the aim of helping people live each moment of their lives as fully as possible in a state of awareness of the present moment (McCown & Micozzi, 2012).

Kabat-Zinn points out that mindfulness is about more than feeling relaxed or stress free. Its true aim is to nurture an inner balance of mind that allows an individual to face life situations with greater clarity, stability, and understanding and to respond more effectively from that sense of clarity.

An integral part of mindfulness practice is to accept and welcome stress, pain, anger, frustration, disappointment, and insecurity when those feelings are present. Kabat-Zinn believes that acknowledgment is paramount. Whether pleasant or unpleasant, admission is the first step toward transforming that reality.

Kabat-Zinn founded the Stress Reduction Clinic at the University of Massachusetts Medical Center in Worcester. The Center for Mindfulness in Medicine, Health Care, and Society, established in 1995, is an outgrowth of the clinic. Since the clinic was founded, more than 10,000 medical patients have gone through Kabat-Zinn's mindfulness meditation programs, almost all referred by their physicians.

The Center for Mindfulness has produced several peer-reviewed papers on mindfulness-based stress reduction. Research pursuits of the center have included a prostate cancer study funded by the U.S. Department of Defense; a cost-effectiveness study; development of an innovative substance abuse recovery program for young, low-income, inner city mothers; and a wide variety of other collaborative research endeavors.

Unlike standard medical and psychological approaches, the clinic does not categorize and treat patients differently depending on their illnesses. Their 8-week courses offer the same training program in mindfulness and stress reduction to everyone. They emphasize what is "right" with their patients, rather than what is "wrong" with them, focusing on mobilizing their inner strengths and changing their behaviors in new and innovative ways. Facilitators maintain that the programs are not held out as some kind of magical cure when other approaches have failed; rather, they provide a sensible and straightforward way for people to experience and understand the mind–body connection firsthand and use that knowledge to better cope with their illnesses.

In the practice of mindfulness, the patient begins by using one-pointed attention to cultivate calmness and stability. When thoughts and feelings arise, it is important not to ignore or suppress them or analyze or judge them by their content; rather, the thoughts are observed intentionally and nonjudgmentally, moment by moment, as events in the field of awareness.

This inclusive noting of thoughts, coming and going in the mind, can lead to a detachment from them, which allows a deeper perspective about the stresses of life to emerge. By observing the thoughts from this vantage point, one gains a new frame of reference. In this way, valuable insight can be allowed to surface. The key to mindfulness is not the topic focused on but the quality of awareness brought into each moment. Observing the thought processes, without intellectualizing them and without judgment, creates greater clarity. The goal of mindfulness is to become more aware, more in touch with life and what is happening at the time it is happening, in the present.

Acceptance does not mean passivity or resignation. Accepting what each moment offers provides the opportunity to experience life more completely. In this manner, the individual can respond to any situation with greater confidence and clarity.

One way to envision how mindfulness works is to think of the mind as the surface of a lake or ocean. Many people think the goal of meditation is to stop the waves so that the water will be flat, peaceful, and tranquil. The spirit of mindfulness practice is to experience the waves.

The consistent practice of mindfulness meditation has been shown to decrease the subjective experience of pain and stress in a variety of research settings. One study found a 65% improvement in pain symptoms and an approximately 60% improvement in sleep and fatigue levels in a sample of 77 patients with fibromyalgia, an illness believed to have psychosomatic components (Kaplan et al, 1993).

Dunn et al (1999) used electroencephalographic recordings to differentiate between two types of meditation, concentration and mindfulness, and a normal relaxation control condition. They found significant differences between readings at numerous cortical sites, which suggests that concentration and mindfulness meditations may be unique forms of consciousness and not merely degrees of a state of relaxation.

In a pilot study using mindfulness of movement as a coping strategy for multiple sclerosis, patients attended six individual one-on-one sessions of mindfulness training. Results showed that balance improved significantly in those who underwent the training compared with those who did not (Mills & Allen, 2000).

Eighty cancer patients were followed for 6 months after attending a mindfulness meditation group for 90 minutes each week for 7 weeks. They were also asked to practice meditation at home on a daily basis. Results showed significantly lower mood disturbances and fewer symptoms of stress at the 6-month follow-up for both male and female participants. The greatest improvement, however, occurred on subscales measuring depression, anxiety, and anger. Results for various mindfulness meditation techniques are consistent with those for other meditation-based interventions (Carlson et al, 2001).

Nurses are often known to make mindfulness practice part of their continuing education. They find that this technique often prevents compassion fatigue and burnout, enhances health, and increases awareness of holism within the self.

HYPNOSIS

Modern hypnosis is said to have begun in the late eighteenth century with Franz Anton Mesmer, who used what he called "magnetic healing" to treat a variety of psychological and psychophysiological disorders, such as hysterical blindness, paralysis, headaches, and joint pains (see Chapter 15). The famous Austrian neuropathologist and psychotherapist Sigmund Freud initially found hypnosis to be extremely effective in treating hysteria, and then, troubled (if not actually hysterical) about the sudden catharsis of powerful emotions by his patients, abandoned its use.

The word *hypnosis* is derived from the Greek word *hypnos*, meaning "sleep." It is thought that hypnotic suggestion has been a part of ancient healing traditions for centuries. The induction of trance states and the use of therapeutic suggestion were a central feature of the early Greek healing temples, and variations of these techniques were practiced throughout the ancient world.

In more recent years, hypnosis has experienced a resurgence. Initially, this form of therapy became popular within mainstream medicine among physicians and dentists. At present, hypnosis is widely used by mental health professionals for the treatment of addictions, anxiety disorders, and phobias and for pain control. During hypnosis a patient enters a state of attentive and focused concentration and becomes relatively unaware of the immediate surroundings. While in this state of deep concentration, the individual is highly responsive to suggestion. Contrary to popular folklore, however, people cannot be hypnotized against their will or involuntarily, or "regressed" to earlier ages of cognitive functioning. As Canadian-U.S. psychiatrist and hypnotist Martin Orne, MD, taught, a patient hypnotically regressed to the age of 5 years will behave the way that person *thinks* a 5-year-old child would behave, but neurologically the mind remains that of an adult. Thus, the power of suggestion. The patient must be willing to concentrate all thoughts and to follow the suggestions offered. Essentially, all forms of hypnotherapy are actually forms of self-hypnosis.

HYPNOTIC SUGGESTIBILITY AND SUSCEPTIBILITY

It has been well established through the development and use of the Speigel Hypnotic Susceptibility Scales (developed by Drs. Speigel, father and son at Stanford University; see above) that hypnotic susceptibility falls along a spectrum with 10% extremely susceptible, 10% relatively impervious, and everyone else falling somewhere in between. Thus, hypnosis can work for up to 90% of patients, but it works best among the 10% of those who are most susceptible.

This pattern is the same as what we (the authors of this chapter) found to be true for six other common mind-body techniques, falling along a spectrum of personality types as evaluated by a standard psychometric method. In the personality type analysis, patients susceptible to hypnosis are also those who fall at the "thin" end of the *personality boundary type* spectrum. Details are given at the end of this chapter. We have suggested for many years that the field of CAM and integrative medicine develop "susceptibility scales" like this one for each and all of the myriad varieties of CAM as the single simplest and most clinically useful step that could be taken to help overcome the problem that not all CAM therapies are equally effective for everyone (see also Chapter 3 for a discussion on reasons why CAM does not always work for this and other reasons).

HYPNOTIC STATES

Hypnosis has three major components: *absorption* (in the words or images presented by the hypnotherapist), *dissociation* (from one's ordinary critical faculties), and *responsiveness*. A hypnotherapist either leads patients through relaxation, mental imagery, and suggestions, or teaches patients to perform the techniques on themselves. Many hypnotherapists provide guided audiotapes for their patients so that they can practice the therapy at home. The images presented are specifically tailored to the particular patient's needs and may use one or all of the senses.

Physiologically, hypnosis resembles other forms of *deep relaxation*. It is known to decrease sympathetic nervous system activity, decrease oxygen consumption and carbon dioxide elimination, and lower blood pressure and heart rate, and it is linked to increase or decrease in certain types of brain wave activity.

Hypnotherapy's effectiveness lies in the complex connections between the mind and the body. It is now well understood that illness can affect one's emotional state and, conversely, that one's emotional state can affect one's physical state. For example, an emotional reaction to stress can make heart disease worse, and heart disease, a physical condition, can cause depression.

Hypnosis carries this connection to the next logical step by using the power of the mind to bring about change in the body. No one is quite sure how hypnosis works, but with more sophisticated brain imaging techniques, that understanding is changing. But even if we do not fully understand the mechanism of action, we can take a more scientific approach to its clinical application by using the susceptibility scales and personality boundary types that have been proven to predict its effectiveness (see details at end of this chapter).

CLINICAL APPLICATIONS

One of the most dramatic early uses of hypnosis was for treatment of skin disorders. In the mid-1950s an anesthesiologist, Arthur Mason, used hypnosis to effectively treat a 16-year-old patient who had warts. Within 10 days after the youth underwent hypnosis, the warts fell off and normal skin replaced it (Mason & Black, 1958). Since that time, hypnosis has been used to dramatically improve other skin disorders, such as ichthyosis, and the importance of the role of the skin in the development of the immune system has been long recognized (see Chapter 8).

Depending on the individual's situation, hypnotherapy can be used as a complement to medical care or as a primary treatment. Many people find that the benefits of hypnotherapy are enhanced by the use of *biofeedback* to induce physiological changes. Biofeedback helps patients see that they can control certain bodily functions simply by altering their thoughts, and the added confidence helps them improve more rapidly.

There is little doubt that the regular practice of self-hypnosis is helpful to people with chronic diseases. The benefits include reduction of anxiety and fear, decreased requirements for analgesics, increased comfort during medical procedures, and greater stability of functions controlled by the autonomic nervous system, such as blood pressure. Training in self-hypnosis also enhances the patient's sense of control, which is often affected by chronic illness. Hypnotherapy may also have direct clinical effects on certain chronic diseases, such as reducing bleeding in hemophiliac patients, stabilizing blood glucose level in diabetic patients, and reducing the severity of asthmatic attacks (Weintraub & Micozzi, 2008).

For many years, W.M. Gonsalkorale has been researching the benefits of hypnotherapy for management of irritable bowel syndrome at the University Hospital of South Manchester, United Kingdom. In only 3 months, symptoms such as pain and bloating, as well as the level of "disease interference" with life, improved profoundly for most of the 232 patients who underwent hypnotherapy (Gonsalkorale et al, 2002). Good evidence now supports the long-term benefits for up to 6 years following hypnotherapy. In 204 patients, of the 71% who responded to therapy, 81% maintained their improvements and the remaining 19% claimed that deterioration of symptoms had been slight (Gonsalkorale et al, 2003). Besides improving physical symptoms, hypnotherapy has also been shown to decrease cognitive symptoms such as anxiety and depression, and to improve quality of life (Gonsalkorale et al, 2004).

Preoperative and Postoperative Therapy

In 1997, Mehmet Oz, a cardiothoracic surgeon at Columbia Presbyterian Medical Center (who is now better known for other, less scientific, pursuits), was receiving a great deal of attention, even then, for advocating, learning (from an earlier edition of this textbook), and using complementary medical approaches in his surgical practice. Oz took 32 patients scheduled for coronary bypass surgery and randomly assigned them to two groups. One group received instruction on self-hypnosis relaxation techniques before surgery, and the other group received no instruction. Results showed that patients who practiced the self-hypnosis techniques were significantly more relaxed than the control subjects in the days after surgery (Ashton et al, 1997). We also had discussions about having the surgical nurses perform "healing touch" therapy before, after, and even during open heart surgery. However, there was no significant difference between the two groups in length of hospital stay and postoperative morbidity and mortality.

Carol Ginandes, a Harvard instructor, did investigate how hypnotherapy can help people heal more quickly after surgery. Each of 18 women undergoing breast reduction surgery was placed in one of three groups. One group received standard surgical care. The second group received the same care and also received psychological support. The third group underwent hypnosis before and after surgery in addition to receiving standard care. Those who underwent hypnosis healed more rapidly, felt less discomfort, and had fewer complications (Ginandes et al, 2003).

Pain Control

Hypnosis can also be effective in reducing the fear and anxiety that accompanies pain. It is said that anxiety increases pain, and hypnotherapy helps a patient gain control over the fear and anxiety, thereby reducing the psychic dimensions of pain. Many controlled studies have demonstrated that hypnosis is an effective way to reduce migraine attacks in children and teenagers. In one experiment, 30 schoolchildren were randomly assigned to receive a placebo or propranolol (a blood pressure–lowering agent) or were taught self-hypnosis. Only the children who used the self-hypnosis techniques experienced a significant decrease in severity and frequency of headaches (Olness & Gardner, 1988). A study of chronically ill patients reported a 113% increase in pain tolerance among highly hypnotizable individuals compared with members of a control group who did not receive hypnosis (Debenedittis et al, 1989).

Researchers at Virginia Polytechnic Institute found that during induction of a hypnotic state aimed at bringing about pain control, the prefrontal cortex of the brain directed other areas of the brain to reduce or eliminate their awareness of pain (Gordon, 2004). A technique used for pain control during surgery in people with little or no tolerance for chemical anesthesia, called "spinal anesthesia illusion," was developed by Philip Ament, a dentist and psychologist from Buffalo, New York. In this method a deep state of relaxation is induced by having the patient count mentally or focus on a specific image. The patient is given the suggestion that he or she will feel a growing numbness begin to spread from the navel to the toes as he or she counts to a higher and higher number. Once the patient feels numb, the surgery can proceed. After the surgery the therapist gives the patient suggestions that lead to the gradual return of normal sensations (Perlman, 1999).

Dentistry

Some people have learned to tolerate dental work (e.g., drilling, extraction, periodontal surgery) using the safe alternative of hypnosis as the sole anesthesia. Even when an anesthetic is used, hypnotherapy can also be used to reduce fear and anxiety, control bleeding and salivation, and lessen postoperative discomfort. Used with children, hypnosis can decrease the chances of developing a dental phobia (Perlman, 1999).

Pregnancy and Delivery

It is believed that Lamaze and other popular breathing techniques used during labor and delivery may actually work by inducing a hypnotic state. Women who have used hypnosis before delivery tend to have a shorter labor and more comfortable delivery than other pregnant women. There are even reports of cesarean sections being performed with hypnosis as the sole anesthesia. Women are taught to take advantage of their body's natural anesthetic abilities to make childbirth a less painful, more positive experience (Goldman, 1999).

Anxiety

Hypnosis can be used to establish a new kind of response to specific anxiety-causing stimuli, such as in the treatment of stage fright, fear of airplane flight, and other phobias.

Typically, the hypnotherapist helps the patient undo a conditioned physiological response, such as hyperventilation or nausea. This method can also be used to help calm athletes who are preparing to compete. Hypnotherapy can be used to quell almost any fear, whether associated with examinations, public speaking, or social interactions.

Allergies and Asthma

Ran Anbar, a pediatric pulmonologist at the State University of New York's Upstate Medical University in Syracuse, teaches children self-hypnosis to help them control their allergies and asthma (Gordon, 2004).

BIOFEEDBACK

Biofeedback therapies emerged in the 1960s and 1970s, when advances in psychological and medical research converged with developments in biomedical technology. Improved electronic instruments could convey information to patients about their autonomic nervous system functions and their neuromuscular and circulatory responsiveness in the form of audio and visual signals that patients could understand. The word *biofeedback* became the general term to define the procedures and treatments that make use of these instruments (Green et al, 1977).

Biofeedback therapy uses special instruments and methods to expand the body's natural internal feedback systems. By watching a monitoring device, patients can learn empirically, by trial and error, to adjust their thinking and other mental processes to control bodily processes previously thought to be involuntary, such as blood pressure, temperature, gastrointestinal functioning, and brain wave activity. In fact, biofeedback can be used to influence almost any bodily process that can be measured accurately.

Biofeedback does not belong to any particular field of health care and is used in many disciplines, including internal medicine, dentistry, physical therapy and rehabilitation, psychology and psychiatry, and pain management. As with other forms of therapy, biofeedback is more useful in addressing some clinical problems than others and works better for some individuals than others, also according to personality boundary type. For example, biofeedback is a useful treatment in Raynaud disease, a painful and potentially dangerous spasm of the small arteries, and certain types of fecal and urinary incontinence. It has also become an integral part of the treatment of many other disorders, including headaches, anxiety, high blood pressure, teeth clenching, asthma, and muscle disorders.

Researchers have also been experimenting with biofeedback treatments for conditions believed to stem from irregular brain wave patterns, such as epilepsy, attention-deficit disorder, and attention-deficit/hyperactivity disorder in children, with promising results.

Biofeedback is successful in helping people learn to regulate many physical conditions, partly because it puts them in better contact with specific parts of their bodies. For example, biofeedback can help teach people to tighten the muscles at the neck of the bladder to better control impaired bladder function. It can help postoperative patients learn to reuse the muscles of the legs and arms. It can help teach stroke patients to use alternative muscles to move a limb if the primary ones can no longer do the job. Biofeedback is also helpful in training patients to use artificial limbs after amputation, and to deal with the problem of "phantom limb" syndrome and phantom pain.

In a normal biofeedback session, electrodes are attached to the area being monitored. These electrodes feed the information to a small monitoring box that registers the results aurally by a tone that varies in pitch or visually by a light that varies in brightness as the function being monitored decreases or increases. A biofeedback therapist leads the patient in mental exercises to help the patient reach the desired result. Through trial and error, patients gradually train themselves to control the inner mechanism involved. For some disorders, training requires 8 to 10 sessions; however, a single session can often provide symptomatic relief. Patients with long-term or severe disorders may require longer therapy. The aim of the treatment is to teach patients to regulate their own inner mental and bodily processes without the help of a machine.

FIVE COMMON FORMS OF BIOFEEDBACK THERAPY

1. **Electromyographic biofeedback** measures muscular tension. Sensors are attached to the skin to detect electrical activity related to muscle tension in a given area. The biofeedback instrument amplifies and converts this activity into useful information, displaying the various degrees of muscle tension. This form of biofeedback therapy is most often used for reduction of tension headaches, physical rehabilitation, treatment of chronic muscle pain, management of incontinence, and promotion of general relaxation.

2. **Thermal biofeedback therapy** measures skin temperature as an index of changes in blood flow from the constriction and dilation of blood vessels. Low skin temperature usually means decreased blood flow in that area. A temperature-sensitive probe is taped to the skin, often on a finger. The instrument converts information into feedback that can be seen and heard and can be used to reduce or increase blood flow to the hands and feet. Thermal biofeedback is often used for management of Raynaud disease, migraine headaches, hypertension, and anxiety disorders, and to promote general relaxation.

3. **Electrodermal activity therapy** measures changes in sweat activity that are too minimal to feel. Two sensors are attached to the palm side of the fingers or hand to measure sweat activity. They produce a tiny electrical current that measures skin conductance on the basis of the amount of moisture present. Increased sweat can mean arousal of part of the autonomic nervous system. Electrodermal activity devices can be used to measure the sweat output stemming from stressful thoughts or rapid deep breathing. Electrodermal activity therapy is most often used in the treatment of anxiety and hyperhidrosis.

4. **Finger pulse therapy** measures pulse rate and force. A sensor is attached to a finger and helps measure heart activity as a sign of arousal of part of the autonomic nervous system. Finger pulse therapy is most often used for management of hypertension, anxiety, and some cardiac arrhythmias.

5. **Breathing biofeedback therapy** measures the rate, volume, rhythm, and location of breathing. Sensors are placed around the chest and abdomen to measure air flow from the mouth and nose. The feedback is usually visual, and patients learn to take deeper, slower, lower, and more regular breaths using abdominal muscles. This simple form of biofeedback is most often used for management of asthma and other respiratory conditions, hyperventilation, and anxiety.

A more recent acoustic technique for measuring the microwaves of sound generating in joints could potentially be used to guide patients to less stressful use of the musculoskeletal system in carrying out physical movements and exercise in those with arthritis, and to measure the effectiveness of various joint therapies.

APPLICATIONS

The general goal of biofeedback therapy is to lower body tension and to modify faulty biological patterns to reduce symptoms. Many people can and do reach goals of relaxation without the use of biofeedback. Although biofeedback may not be necessary, it can potentially add something useful to any treatment.

A major reason that many patients find biofeedback training appealing is that, as with behavioral approaches in general, it puts the patient in charge, giving the patient a sense of mastery and self-reliance with regard to the illness. It is believed that such an attitude can play a critical role in shortening recovery time, reducing incidence, and lowering health care costs. This kind of approach works better with patients who appreciate the concrete feedback provided and like to be in control of their condition, which can be effectively assessed through the personality type evaluation.

RESEARCH AND COST-EFFECTIVENESS CONSIDERATIONS

Biofeedback-assisted relaxation training has been associated with a decrease in medical care costs, a decrease in the number of claims and costs to insurers in claims payments, reduction in medication and physician use, reduction in hospital stays and re-hospitalization, reduction of mortality and morbidity, and enhanced quality of life.

An unpublished study involving 241 employees of a Siberian metal company showed promising results for the integration of biofeedback training into occupational medicine as a method to increase workers' ability to work with fewer errors while increasing labor productivity levels. The employees had psychosomatic disorders presenting with symptoms of headache, sleepiness, and periodic blood pressure fluctuations. Workers attended 10- to 40-minute biofeedback sessions over 2 weeks. The results clearly indicated that the workers were able to control the brain's blood flow. Furthermore, a follow-up biofeedback session was repeated 1 month later and showed that all workers in the initial group could recall their strategies for producing positive change.

In another study, 30 patients with fibromyalgia syndrome received biofeedback and experienced statistically significant improvements in mental clarity, mood, and sleep (Mueller et al, 2001). However, additional research using controlled trials would be useful to better understand disease mechanisms.

Biofeedback, both sensory and augmented, has been used with some degree of success to treat patients with fecal incontinence. Forty women with fecal incontinence were randomly assigned to receive either augmented biofeedback or sensory biofeedback. After 12 weeks of treatment, the augmented form of biofeedback was found to be superior, although fecal incontinence improved in both treatment groups (Fynes et al, 1999). Another study compared biofeedback to standard care for treatment of fecal incontinence. Results showed that biofeedback was not superior to standard care in improving incontinence, but those who received biofeedback had significantly better scores on tests of hospital anxiety and depression (Norton et al, 2003).

More recently, 92 patients with systemic lupus erythematosus were assigned randomly to receive biofeedback-assisted cognitive-behavioral treatment, a symptom-monitoring support intervention, or usual medical care. Those who received biofeedback experienced significantly greater reductions in pain and psychological dysfunction than those who did not receive the biofeedback-assisted therapy. At 9-month follow-up, the biofeedback group continued to exhibit relative benefit compared with the control group (Greco et al, 2004).

In a randomized United Kingdom study, 38 patients with fecal incontinence were assigned to undergo sphincter repair or sphincter repair plus biofeedback. Although the results were not statistically significant, continence and satisfaction scores improved in the biofeedback group, and these improvements were sustained over time. Quality of life measures also improved in the biofeedback group (Davis et al, 2004).

The Department of Psychiatry at Robert Wood Johnson Medical School in New Jersey evaluated the effectiveness of heart rate variability (HRV) biofeedback as a complementary treatment in 94 patients with asthma (Lehrer et al, 2004; see also Mayor & Micozzi, 2011). Patients in the two groups receiving biofeedback were prescribed less medication than those in the two control groups (placebo and wait list), which indicates that HRV biofeedback may be a useful adjunct to asthma treatment and may help to reduce dependence on steroid medications (Lehrer et al, 2004). Biofeedback techniques have also been used with some success to treat epilepsy and attention problems, such as sleeplessness, fatigue, and body pain.

Research on exactly *how* biofeedback works is somewhat inconclusive. Some studies link its benefits directly to physiological changes that the patient learns to make voluntarily. Other experiments find benefits even for patients who do not make the desired changes in the physiological measures. Biofeedback appears to help some patients increase their sense of control, heighten their optimism, and lessen feelings of hopelessness triggered by chronic health problems (Hatch et al, 1987). It appears that biofeedback used as adjunct therapy could add something beneficial to an existing therapy.

GUIDED IMAGERY

Since human societies began analyzing human experiences, philosophers have tried to define and explain the interior processes, including visualizations of the mind in "the mind's eye"—all those experiences that are invisible to another person because they do not have physical referents. Philosophers have speculated at length on the nature of mental imagery, and scientists have found the phenomenon difficult to verify or measure. Behavioral psychologists of the 1920s went so far as to say that mental images simply do not exist.

Since 1960, psychologists have done a great amount of work exploring and categorizing mental imagery and inner processes. Contemporary psychologists distinguish several types of imagery. Probably the most common form of imagery that people experience is memory. If a person tries to remember a friend, the bed in his or her room, or the feel of the seats of his or her car, that person immediately perceives an image in his or her mind, the "mind's eye." People refer to this experience as "forming a mental picture." Some people believe that they do not "see" the scene but simply have a strong sense of such a scene and simply "know" what it would actually "look like."

Imagery can be used to refer to both a mental process and to a wide variety of procedures used in therapy to encourage changes in attitudes, behaviors, or physiological reactions. As a mental process, it is often defined as "any thought representing a sensory quality" (Horowitz, 1983). In addition to the visual sense, it includes all the senses: aural, tactile, olfactory, proprioceptive, and kinesthetic. *Imagery* is often used synonymously with *visualization*. However, visualization refers only to "seeing" something in the mind's eye, whereas imagery can use one sense or combination of senses to produce a mental visual image.

Creating images with the mind is also a way of communicating with the deeper-than-conscious aspects of the mind. This phenomenon is apparent when considering the dream state, which communicates mainly in images that are then interpreted to create a coherent narrative, or story.

This communicative quality of imagery is important, because feelings and behaviors are primarily motivated by subconscious and unconscious factors.

Imagery can be taught either individually or in groups, and the therapist often uses it to accomplish a particular result, such as cessation of addictive behavior or bolstering of the immune system to attack cancer cells. Because it often involves directed concentration, imagery can also be regarded as a form of guided meditation.

Many practices discussed in this book use a component of imagery. Psychotherapy, hypnosis, and biofeedback all use various elements of this process, as well as "shamanic healing" discussed in the last section of this book. Any therapy that relies on the imagination to stimulate, communicate, solve problems, or evoke a heightened awareness or sensitivity could be described as a form of imagery.

Numerous early studies indicated that mental imagery brings about significant physiological and biochemical changes. These findings have encouraged the development of imagery as a health care tool. Imagery was found to have the capacity to affect dramatically the oxygen supply in tissues (Olness & Gardner, 1988), cardiovascular parameters (Barber, 1969), vascular or thermal parameters (Green et al, 1977), the pupil and cochlear reflexes, heart rate and galvanic skin response (Jordan & Lenington, 1979), and salivation (Barber, 1984; White, 1978).

CLINICAL APPLICATIONS

Communication with the unconscious had previously been the domain only of hypnosis, which basically consists of two components: (1) the use of a technique to induce a state of consciousness in which there is freer access to the deeper part of the mind; and (2) a method of communicating with that deeper part of the mind. Often this communication involves making suggestions to the inner depths and recesses of the mind, suggesting items or behaviors that the individual desires for his or her betterment. In guided imagery, different techniques are used to induce the necessary state of consciousness, some quite similar to more common relaxation techniques and to meditation techniques (Jordan & Lenington, 1979).

SELF-DIRECTED IMAGERY

Increased attention is being focused on the ability of individuals to use the principles of guided imagery. Through the practice of effective *deep relaxation* techniques, individuals can bring themselves into a state of consciousness in which they have increased access to deeper parts of the mind. Then, using imagery, they can "reprogram" into new healthier images (Achterberg, 1985).

Self-directed imagery is a powerful way in which individuals can have more control over their healing processes. Imagery can be used to contribute to the healing of physical problems and has been used extensively in the area of pain control. In one method the individual allows an image for his or her pain to emerge. For example, an individual may create an image that characterizes the area of pain,

then create a second image to *counteract* the pain image. Once the images are formed, the individual uses a relaxation or meditation technique to open access to the levels where his or her self-healing potential resides and to imagine the healing image. This process can be repeated as often as necessary, allowing changes in the healing image that either might appear spontaneously or might be appropriate if the image associated with the pain were to change.

Self-directed imagery can also be used to stimulate personal growth and change by repeatedly entering a relaxed or meditative state, and strongly imaging a new desired behavior. Similarly, when one repeatedly images oneself as having already achieved a desired goal, the deeper mind gradually accepts this new image and works to bring it into reality.

Carl O. Simonton, MD, often regarded as founder of guided imagery, and his wife, Stephanie, brought to popular attention the use of meditation and imagery for cancer self-help. They emphasized several aspects characteristic of a powerful healing image: (1) the image is created by the "healee" himself or herself; (2) it involves as many sensory modalities as possible; and (3) it has as much dynamism and energy behind it as possible. The image must be vital, because that vitality is what stimulates the image to take root (Simonton et al, 1978).

RESEARCH CONSIDERATIONS

Early studies suggest a direct relationship between imagery and its corresponding effects on the body. Findings include the following:

1. Correlations were found between levels of various types of immune system white blood cells and components of cancer patients' images of their disease, treatment, and immune system (Achterberg & Lawlis, 1984).
2. "Natural killer" cell function, first identified by Dr Jerry Thornthwaite, was enhanced in geriatric patients (Kiecolt-Glaser et al, 1985) and in adult cancer patients with metastatic disease (Gruber et al, 1988) after engaging in a relaxation and imagery procedure.
3. Specificity of imagery training was suggested by a study in which patients were trained in cell-specific imagery of either T lymphocyte or neutrophil white blood cells. The effects of training, assessed after 6 weeks, were statistically associated with the type of imagery procedure used (Achterberg et al, 1989).

Of all the many mind-body modalities, guided imagery appears to be the most widely used and accepted in many nursing departments. The University of Akron College of Nursing conducted a study demonstrating that guided imagery was an effective intervention for enhancing comfort in women undergoing radiation therapy for early stage breast cancer. In this study, 53 women were randomly assigned to either a control group or a treatment group. The experimental group listened to a guided imagery tape once a day for the duration of the study. The guided imagery group demonstrated significantly improved comfort compared with the control group, with the treatment group experiencing greater comfort over time (Kolcaba & Fox, 1999).

A community-based nursing study was recently conducted in Sydney, Australia, where 56 people with advanced cancer experiencing anxiety and depression were randomly assigned to one of four treatment conditions: (1) progressive muscle relaxation training; (2) guided imagery training; (3) both types of training; and (4) no training (control). Patients were tested for anxiety, depression, and quality of life. The guided imagery training led to no significant improvement in anxiety but was associated with significant positive changes in depression and quality of life (Sloman, 2002).

Nurses at Ephrata Community Hospital in Pennsylvania found that offering their patients guided imagery compact discs (CDs) was effective in a variety of ways. They reported that guided imagery (1) helped patients relieve pain and anxiety before and after surgery; (2) helped patients relax and sleep better during evening hours; (3) helped to lower blood pressure; and (4) reduced the need for breathing and respiratory devices. Nurses also reported that the CDs were often more effective than sedation for easing confusion in older patients. Each bedside had a packet of CDs and a CD player with earphones. Each CD focused on a major component of a successful hospital stay (e.g., health and healing, comfort, peaceful rest, courage, serenity). In addition, all the staff nurses, therapists, social workers, and managers were trained in the use of the CDs and employed them for their personal benefit (Miller, 2003).

Differences in pain perception with guided imagery were examined at Kent State's College of Nursing, where 42 patients were randomly assigned to treatment (guided imagery) and control (no imagery) groups. Those who participated in guided imagery experienced decreased pain during the last 2 days of the 4-day trial (Lewandowski, 2004).

A 1993 study conducted by Bennett compared the effectiveness of various types of guided imagery in preoperative patients. Three outcomes were examined: intraoperative blood loss, length of hospital stay, and use of postoperative pain medication. A population of 335 surgical patients were randomly assigned to five groups. Each of the four experimental groups was provided with a guided imagery audiotape created by four different therapists. The control group received an audiotape with a "whooshing" noise that produced no meaningful physiological effect. Results showed that use of three of the four guided imagery audiotapes yielded no significant beneficial effects on any of the medical outcomes examined. By contrast, use of the guided imagery audiotape produced by Belleruth Naparstek, a highly regarded therapist and imagery practitioner, led to highly significant results for two outcomes, reduced postoperative blood loss and length of stay. Bennett found that Naparstek's tape was much more sophisticated than the others. Her imagery had been scored with specially composed music designed to highlight and accompany each image, with an emphasis on spiritual connectedness. Naparstek included visualizations of positive outcomes, faster wound healing, less pain, and no nausea (Bennett, 1996).

In two unpublished studies, guided imagery was used to reduce menopausal symptoms. The University Hospital in Linkoping, Sweden, found that menopausal women using guided imagery averaged 73% fewer hot flashes over 6 months and had a significant reduction in other symptoms. A study at New England Deaconess Hospital involving 33 menopausal women who were not using hormone replacement therapy found that guided imagery strategies produced a significant reduction in hot-flash intensity, tension and anxiety, and depression.

Cleveland Clinic researchers assessed 130 colorectal surgery patients for anxiety levels, pain perceptions, and narcotic medication requirements (Tusek et al, 1997). The treatment group listened to guided imagery tapes for 3 days before their surgery, during anesthesia induction, intraoperatively, after anesthesia, and for 6 days after surgery; the control group received routine perioperative care. Patients in the guided imagery group experienced considerably less preoperative and postoperative anxiety and pain, and they required 50% less narcotic medication after surgery than patients in the control group.

Not only has the use of guided imagery been shown to be effective for reducing pain and anxiety preoperatively and postoperatively, it is now proving to be cost effective. In 1999, a cardiac surgery team implemented a guided imagery program and compared cardiac surgical outcomes in those who participated in guided imagery and those who did not. Patients who completed the guided imagery program had a shorter average length of hospital stay, a decrease in average direct pharmacy costs, and a decrease in average direct pain medication costs, while overall patient satisfaction with the care and treatment provided remained high (Halpin et al, 2002).

MENTAL HEALING

The idea that consciousness can affect the physical body is a time-honored concept with a respected historical base (see Chapter 6). The observation that "there is a measure of consciousness throughout the body" is scattered about in the 2000-year-old Hippocratic writings. Before the ancient Greeks, Persians had also expounded on this concept, insisting that a person's mind can intervene not just in his or her own body but also in that of another individual located far away. The great Muslim physician Abu Ali ibn Sina (Avicenna in Latinized form, AD 980-1037) later postulated that it was the faculty of imagination that humans use to make themselves ill or to restore health (Amri, Abu-Asab, & Micozzi, 2013).

The attitudes of the ancient Greeks, Persians, and Islamic physicians toward the interaction between mind and body eventually gave rise to two very different types of healing: local and nonlocal. The Greeks believed that the action of the mind on the body was a "local" event in the here and now. The Persians, however, viewed the mind–body relationship as "nonlocal." They held that the mind was not localized or confined to the body but extended beyond the body. This implied that the mind was capable of affecting any physical body, local or nonlocal. A modern example is when someone prays for the benefit of another (see below, and Chapter 11).

IMPLICATIONS OF NONLOCALITY

Modern physicists have long recognized the concept of nonlocality. These developments rest largely on an idea in physics called "Bell's theorem," introduced in 1964 by the Irish physicist John Stewart Bell and supported by subsequent experiments (see also Chapter 14, and Mayor & Micozzi, 2011). Bell showed that if distant objects have once been in contact, a change thereafter in one causes an immediate change in the other, even were they to be separated to the opposite ends of the universe. Thus it is important to realize that nonlocality is not just a theoretical idea in fundamental physics, but that its proof rests on the results of actual experiments.

The idea prevalent in contemporary science is that the mind and consciousness are entirely local phenomenon, and specifically localized to the mind and confined to the present moment in time. From this perspective nonlocal healing cannot occur in principle because the mind is bound by the "here and now." Research studies examining distant mental influence challenge these modern-day assumptions. Dozens of experiments conducted over the past 30 years suggest that the mind can bring about changes in nonlocal physical bodies, even when shielded from all sensory and electromagnetic influences. This suggests that what we have called "mind" and "consciousness" may not be located at fixed points in space (Braud, 1992; Braud & Schlitz, 1991; Jahn & Dunn, 1987).

Some physicists believe that nonlocality applies not just to the domain of electrons and other subatomic particles, but also to our familiar world consisting of dense matter. A growing number of physicists think that nonlocality may apply to the mind. Physicist Nick Herbert, in his book *Quantum Reality,* states, "Bell's theorem requires our quantum knowledge to be nonlocal, instantly linked to everything it has previously touched" (Herbert, 1987; Chapter 14).

For the Western model of medicine, the implications of a nonlocal concept are profound and include the following:

1. Nonlocal models of the mind could be helpful in understanding the actual dynamics of the healing process. They may help to explain why in some patients a cure suddenly appears unexpectedly, "spontaneously," or a healing appears to be influenced by events occurring nonlocally.
2. Nonlocal manifestations of consciousness complicate traditional experimental designs, which cannot account for them (see Chapter 14) and require innovative

research methods, because the mental state of the healer may influence the experiment's outcome, even under "blind," "controlled" conditions (Solfvin, 1984).

Nonlocality assumptions give rise to the idea that consciousness could prevail after the death of the body/brain, which suggests that some aspect of the psyche is not bound only to specific points in space or time. This idea in turn leads toward a nonlocal model of consciousness, which allows for the possibility of distant healing exchange.

This nonlocal model of consciousness implies that at some level of the psyche, no fundamental separations exist between individual minds. Nobel physicist Erwin Schroedinger suggested that at some level and in some sense there may be unity and oneness of all minds (Schroedinger, 1969). In the nonlocal model, distance is not fundamental but is completely overcome. In other words, because of the unification of consciousness, the healer and the patient are not separated by physical distance.

For 40 years, psychologist Lawrence LeShan investigated the local and nonlocal effects of prayer and mental healing. He taught these techniques to more than 400 people and ultimately became a healer himself. He maintained that healing changes were observed to have occurred 15% to 20% of the time but never could be predicted in advance of any specific healing (LeShan, 1966). LeShan found that mental-spiritual healing methods can be categorized into the following two main types:

- *Type I (nonlocal).* The healer enters a prayerful, altered state of consciousness in which he or she views himself or herself and the patient as a single entity. There is no physical contact or any attempt to offer anything of a physical nature to the person in need, only the desire to connect and unite. These healers emphasize the importance of empathy, love, and caring in this process. When the healing takes place, it does so in the context of unity, compassion, and love. This type of healing is considered a natural process and merely speeds up the normal healing processes.
- *Type II (local).* The healer does touch the patient and may imagine some "flow of energy" through his or her hands to the area of the patient receiving the healing. Feelings of heat are common in both the healer and patient. In this mode, unlike type I, the healer holds the intention for healing.

Research into the origins of consciousness and how it relates to the physical brain has been practically nonexistent. Although hypotheses purporting to explain consciousness do exist, there is no agreement among researchers as to its nature, local or nonlocal (see Chapter 14).

SPIRITUALITY AND HEALING

Throughout the ages, ancient mystical traditions have valued the spiritual qualities of humans over the physical, emphasizing the transcendence of one over the other. In the background of most mystical traditions is the idea that the body is somehow at odds with the spirit. A war wages, and one must battle the war to achieve an enlightened status. Still other theologians postulate that the greatest spiritual achievement of all may lie in the realization that the spiritual and the physical are but one, and that perhaps the ultimate spiritual goal is not to *transcend* anything but to realize the integration and oneness of being. Such a truth would seem to obviate the need for Western Transcendentalism, or for Eastern Transcendental Meditation, once realized.

A new quality of spiritual awakening has been emerging worldwide over the past 40 years. This innovative approach encourages people to develop faith in their own capacity to create their own reality in partnership with a "G-d-force within." In many cultures, both Eastern and Western, prayer-based spiritual healing is an integral part of modern religious practices.

The premise of creating our own reality is, in essence, a spiritual one. This concept is sometimes contrary to many fundamental religious positions that embrace God as an external being, because spirituality also emphasizes a "G-d-within" reality, or duality. Transcending the boundaries and limitations of specific religions, a spiritual practice honors a relation between the individual and the G-d-force as a kind of partnership.

When people consider the possibility that they create their own realities, the question that invariably arises is, "Through what source? What is the source of this power of creation that runs through my being?" The answer to this question is found not externally but internally. This internal source seeking to understand our own nature is considered divinity in action, incarnated in each person.

The blending of spirituality with the tenets of alternative and complementary therapies provides individuals with a means of understanding how they contribute to the creation of their illness and to their healing. This understanding does not come from a place of self-blame and does not view illness as a result of the will of G-d but rather is an attempt to understand a spiritual purpose for suffering in a physical body. The relationship that is cultivated ultimately transcends the human value system of punishment versus reward and grows into a relationship based on principles of co-creation and co-responsibility. Therefore the journey of healing for patients, as well as the journey of life, is freed of the burden of feeling victimized by fate, circumstances, or God, and patients are free to have faith and hope not only in G-d but in themselves as well.

Research in the last 20 years has made an indelible mark on the way health care professionals think about the role of spirituality and religion in physical, mental, and social health. Hundreds of studies have explored the relations between body and spirit. Most studies have been cross-sectional, but some have also been longitudinal. Many studies now document an association between religious involvement and lower anxiety, fewer psychotic symptoms, less substance abuse, and better coping mechanisms. A comprehensive review found that 478 of 742 quantitative studies (66%) reported a statistically significant relationship between religious involvement and better mental health and greater social support. The review also found that almost 80% of those who are religious have significantly greater well-being, hope, and optimism compared with those who are less religious (Koenig et al, 2001).

At Duke University, studies were conducted examining the effects of religiousness on the course of depression in 850 hospitalized patients over age 60. Results showed that religious coping predicted lower levels of depressive symptoms at baseline and at 6 months after discharge (Koenig et al, 1992).

Koenig's studies and others have shown that spirituality and religiosity are clearly associated with longer survival, healthier behaviors, and less distress and are believed to have an effect on coping (Pargament et al, 1998; Tix & Frazier, 1997), anxiety (Koenig et al, 1993), success in aging (Crowther et al, 2002), end-of-life issues (Daaleman & VandeCreek, 2000), and cortisol levels in patients with human immunodeficiency virus infection and acquired immunodeficiency syndrome (Ironson et al, 2002).

POWER OF PRAYER

The use of prayer in healing may have begun in human prehistory and continues to this day as an underlying tenet in almost all religions. The records of many of the great religious traditions, including the mystical traditions of Christianity, Daoism, Hinduism, Buddhism, and Islam, give the strong impression that enlightenment comes when one begins to explore the dynamic qualities of interrelation and interconnection between the self and the source of all being.

The word *prayer* comes from the Latin *precarious,* "obtained by begging," and *precari,* "to entreat"—to ask earnestly, beseech, implore. This suggests two of the most common forms of prayer: *petition,* asking something for one's self, and *intercession,* asking something for others.

Prayer is a genuinely nonlocal event, not confined to a specific place in space or to a specific moment in time. Prayer reaches outside the here and now; it operates at a distance and outside the present moment. Prayer is initiated by mental action and intention which implies that some aspect of our psyche also is genuinely nonlocal. Nonlocality implies infinitude in space and time, because a limited nonlocality is a contradiction in terms. In the West, this infinite aspect of the psyche has been referred to as the *soul* (see also Chapter 6). Empirical evidence for the power of prayer therefore may be seen as indirect evidence for the soul.

Scientific attempts to assess the effects of prayer and spiritual practices on health began in the nineteenth century with Sir Francis Galton's treatise *Statistical Inquiries into the Efficacy of Prayer* (Galton, 1872). Galton, a nephew of Charles Darwin, is considered the founder of modern statistics. He initially used these new methods to study human growth, but believed that statistical analysis could be brought to any topic even when the "mechanism of action" was unknown, such as in the example of prayer. This also helps make the point that useful statistical, psychometric profiles can be brought to the study and application of any mind–body therapy such as hypnosis where there is no known "mechanism" for how and why it works for whom.

Galton assessed the longevity of people who were frequently prayed for, such as clergy, monarchs, and heads of state. He concluded that there was no demonstrable effect of prayer on longevity. By current scientific standards, Galton's study was flawed. He was successful, however, in promoting the idea that prayer is subject to empirical scrutiny. Galton did acknowledge that praying could make a person feel better. In the end he maintained that although his attempts to prove the efficacy of prayer had failed, he could see no good reason to abandon prayer (reminiscent of Pascal's wager).

Those who practice healing with prayer claim uniformly that the effects are not diminished with distance; therefore it falls within the nonlocal perspective discussed earlier. Claims about the effectiveness of prayer do not rely on anecdote or single case studies; numerous controlled studies have validated the nonlocal nature of prayer. Moreover, much of this evidence suggests that praying individuals, or people involved in compassionate imagery or mental intent, whether or not it is called "prayer," can purposefully affect the physiology of distant people without the awareness of the receiver.

The medical community has begun to acknowledge the importance of exploring the association between spirituality and medicine. Many medical schools now offer courses in religion, spirituality, and health. According to a 1994 survey, 98% of hospitalized patients ascribe to a belief in God or some higher power, and 96% acknowledge a personal use of prayer to aid in the healing process. In addition, 77% of 203 hospitalized family practice patients believed that their physicians should consider their spiritual needs. In contrast, only 32% of the patients' family physicians actually discussed spirituality with their patients (King & Bushwick, 1994).

Anecdotal accounts of the power of prayer are legendary, and countless books on the subject are available; however, literature of scientific value is still limited.

The now-famous prayer study involving humans was published in 1988 by Randolph Byrd, a staff cardiologist at San Francisco School of Medicine, University of California. Byrd randomly assigned 393 patients in the coronary care unit either to a group receiving intercessory prayer or to a control group receiving no prayer. Intercessory prayer was offered through interventions outside the hospital. They were not instructed how often to pray but were told to pray as they saw fit. In this double-blind study, the prayed-for patients did better on several counts. Although the results were not statistically significant, there were fewer deaths in the prayer group; these patients were less likely to require intubation and ventilator support; they required fewer potent drugs; they experienced a lower incidence of pulmo-

nary edema; and they required cardiopulmonary resuscitation less often (Byrd, 1988).

In 1999, W.E. Harris attempted to replicate Byrd's findings at the Mid America Heart Institute in Kansas City. Although the study did not produce statistically significant results, the researchers reported that patients received significant benefit from intercessory prayer, as reflected by a coronary care unit outcome measure (Harris et al, 1999). Critics have charged that performing controlled studies on prayer is impossible, because extraneous prayer for the control group cannot be eliminated. So, according to such critics, if available methods cannot be used to study something, it should not be studied. This anti-science attitude was famously documented in Thomas Kuhn's classic treatise, *The Structure of Scientific Revolutions*, which points out that the prevailing scientific paradigm is always limited by the questions that can asked based upon the only scientific tools and methods that are available, or considered acceptable.

Other studies have been conducted to assess the effect of intercessory prayer on the treatment of alcohol abuse and dependence (Walker et al, 1997), the well-being of kidney dialysis patients (Matthews et al, 2001), and feelings of self-esteem (O'Laoire, 1997). A prospective study of 40 patients with class II or III rheumatoid arthritis compared the effects of direct-contact intercessory prayer with distance intercessory prayer. Persons receiving direct-contact prayer showed significant overall improvement at the 1-year follow-up. The group receiving distant prayer showed no additional benefits (Matthews et al, 2000).

The benefits of spiritual healing were examined in 120 patients with chronic pain at the Department of Complementary Medicine at the University of Exeter, United Kingdom. Patients were randomly assigned to face-to-face healing or simulated face-to-face healing for 30 minutes per week for 8 weeks or to distant healing or no healing for the same time. Although subjects in both healing groups reported significantly more "unusual experiences" during the sessions, the clinical relevance of this is unclear. It was concluded that a specific effect of face-to-face or distant healing on chronic pain could not be demonstrated over eight treatment sessions in these patients (Abbot et al, 2002).

Although research problems are difficult to overcome in evaluating the power of prayer, Byrd's initial prayer study broke significant ground in medical research. Many questions still remain unanswered, and further study is warranted to define the effects of intercessory prayer on quantitative and qualitative outcomes and to identify end points that best measure efficacy.

Although validated evidence continues to build concerning the efficacy of prayer, Dossey (1993) has maintained that serious questions arise in the wake of these experiments. Evidence shows that mental activity can be used to influence people nonlocally, at a distance, without their knowledge. Scores of experiments on prayer also show that it can be used to great effect without the subject's awareness. There is a question as to whether it is ethical to use these techniques if recipients are unaware that they are being used. This question becomes even more compelling as one considers the possibility that prayer, or any other form of mind-to-mind communication, may also be used at a distance to harm people without their knowledge. Institutional review committees that oversee the design of experiments involving humans to ensure their safety have rarely had to consider these types of ethical questions.

COMBINED APPROACHES

Although evidence continues to mount regarding the efficacy of mind–body approaches used individually, more researchers and clinicians are beginning to combine various approaches to create a synergistic healing process.

Combining hypnosis with guided imagery yielded impressive results in improving the postoperative course of pediatric surgical patients. Fifty-two children were randomly assigned to an experimental group or control group. Children in the experimental group were taught imagery, which included hypnotic suggestions for a favorable postoperative course; children in the control group received no such training. The children in the imagery group had significantly lower postoperative pain ratings and shorter hospital stays than those in the control group. State anxiety was decreased in the guided imagery group but increased in the control group (Lambert, 1996).

A study at the University of Texas (Houston) School of Public Health was conducted to differentiate the effects of imagery and support on coping, life attitudes, immune function, quality of life, and emotional well-being after breast cancer. Forty-seven breast cancer survivors were randomly assigned to: (1) standard care only; (2) standard care with six weekly social support sessions: or (3) standard care with guided imagery sessions. For women in both active treatment groups, interferon-γ levels increased, neopterin levels decreased, quality of life improved, and natural killer cell activity remained unchanged. Compared with standard care only, both social support and guided imagery interventions improved coping skills, increased perceived social support, and generally enhanced feelings of meaning in life. Imagery participants had less stress, increased vigor, and improved functional and social quality of life compared with the support group (Richardson et al, 1997).

In another study, Harvard University Mind/Body Institute randomly assigned 128 otherwise healthy college students to an experimental group or a wait-list control group. The experimental group received six 90-minute group training sessions in the relaxation response and cognitive-behavioral skills; the control group received no training. Significantly greater reductions in psychological distress, state anxiety, and perceived stress were found in the treatment group compared with the control group (Deckro et al, 2002).

California Pacific Medical Center conducted a study funded by the U.S. Department of Defense that examined the outcomes for 181 women with breast cancer. Women were randomly assigned to participate in a 12-week "mind, body, and spirit" support group or a standard support group. The women in the mind, body, and spirit group were taught meditation, affirmations, imagery, and ritual. In the standard group, cognitive-behavioral approaches were combined with group sharing and support. Both interventions were found to be associated with improved quality of life, decreased depression and anxiety, and spiritual well-being. Only women in the mind, body, and spirit group, however, showed significant increases in measures of spiritual integration. At the end of the intervention, those in the mind, body, and spirit group showed higher satisfaction and the group had fewer dropouts than the standard group (Targ & Levine, 2002).

Kinney et al (2003) conducted a similar intervention for breast cancer survivors using a mind, body, and spirit self-empowerment program. Fifty-one women participated in a 12-week psychospiritual supportive program that included multiple strategies for creating a balance among spiritual, mental, emotional, and physical health. Components included meditation, visualization, guided imagery, affirmations, and dream work. Statistically significant improvements were seen in depression, perceived wellness, quality of life, and spiritual well-being.

Guided imagery and progressive relaxation techniques were the focus of a recent study at New Jersey Goryeb Children's Hospital. Eighteen children between the ages of 5 and 12 years with chronic abdominal pain were taught guided imagery and progressive relaxation techniques over 9 months. Abdominal pain improved in 89% of the patients, weekly pain episodes decreased, pain intensity decreased, days missed from school decreased, and physician office contacts decreased. In addition, social activities increased and quality of life improved (Youssef et al, 2004).

A recent Korean study examined the effectiveness of a combination of guided imagery and progressive relaxation techniques in reducing the chemotherapy side effects of anticipatory nausea and vomiting and postchemotherapy nausea and vomiting in 30 patients with breast cancer; the effects on patients' quality of life was also measured. Both therapies combined produced improvements on all measures (Yoo et al, 2005). Mind–body pathways and therapeutic modalities have been difficult to understand and interpret in Western biomedicine.

PSYCHOMETRIC APPROACH TO SELECTING CAM THERAPIES

The science of psychometric analysis, widely used in the business and management world, has yet to be widely applied to CAM despite decades of research showing individual variation in susceptibility to various illnesses and responses to different therapies (as highlighted throughout this chapter and textbook).

One important exception is hypnosis—for which susceptibility scales have long been developed and which accurately predict therapeutic response. The same principles promise to apply to other mind–body therapies.

As discussed below, validated psychometric profiles can and should be developed to both aid in clinical therapy and guide relevant research.

PERSONALITY TYPE, SUSCEPTIBILITY TO CHRONIC ILLNESS, AND APPROPRIATE COMPLEMENTARY AND ALTERNATIVE MEDICINE TREATMENTS

Sir William Osler offered a great insight when he stated, "Variability is the law of life and, as no two faces are the same, so no two bodies are alike, and no two individuals react alike and behave alike under the abnormal conditions we know as disease" (Osler, 1953). This observation applies to susceptibility to both disease and treatment approaches.

Utilizing a well-researched psychometric method—Hartmann's Boundary Questionnaire—to categorize personality type, Jawer and Micozzi (2009, 2011) found that personality type explains why certain people get specific chronic illnesses and what forms of CAM can best treat these conditions. We reviewed thousands of research studies and dozens of textbooks on various aspects of CAM, published over the last 20 years, and ranked the relative effectiveness of each of seven common mind–body modalities in treating each of 12 common illnesses that have a strong mind–body component.

The evidence led us to focus on 12 chronic illnesses that in most cases are not life-threatening but can profoundly diminish quality of life. Included in the list are asthma and allergies, chronic fatigue syndrome, depression, fibromyalgia, hypertension, irritable bowel syndrome, migraine headache, phantom pain, post-traumatic stress disorder, rheumatoid arthritis, skin conditions such as eczema and psoriasis, and ulcers. Multiple studies also convincingly demonstrated that each of these 12 disorders involves deep-seated body-mind interactions; each also poses major challenges for conventional medicine, which struggles to understand these illnesses and devise and apply effective treatments. In many cases, CAM approaches appear to be the best fit for people with these conditions—it is then up to the practitioner or therapist to apply the given treatment to the right person.

Central to this approach is the boundary spectrum developed by psychiatrist Ernest Hartmann, of Tufts University, in which personalities are characterized along a continuum from "thick" to "thin" (Hartman, 1991). The boundaries construct also provides a practical frame of reference for a variety of health conditions. Based on where someone falls on this thick/thin spectrum, the types of illnesses to which they will be susceptible, as well as the therapies most likely to be helpful, can be discerned. This offers an authentic form of personalized medicine that differs from genetically based "personalized medicine," which many in conventional medicine and the pharmaceutical industry still hold out as promising future therapeutic breakthroughs.

Unlike the genomic version, our psychometric method is available now through an inexpensive, noninvasive survey instrument that takes 10 to 15 minutes to complete (short version) or up to one hour for the long version. Using factorial analysis, the short version captures over 90% of the variability implicit in the longer version. Psychometric analysis has been used for decades with tens of millions of people for vocational, management, and sociological applications. It does not require the time, expense, dangers, or privacy violations necessitated by creating and ingesting drugs or "fingerprinting" someone's DNA; indeed, only a paper and pencil are involved.

According to Hartmann's model, thin boundary people are highly sensitive in a variety of ways from an early age. They react more strongly than other individuals to sensory stimuli and can become agitated when exposed to bright lights, to loud sounds, or to particular aromas, tastes and textures. They respond more strongly to physical and emotional pain in themselves as well as in others. They can become stressed or fatigued due to an overload of sensory or emotional input. They are more allergic, and their immune systems are seemingly more reactive.

In contrast, thick boundary people are described as stolid, rigid, implacable, or thick-skinned. They tend to brush aside emotional upset in favor of simply 'handling' the situation and maintain a calm demeanor. In practice, they suppress or deny strong feelings. They may experience an ongoing sense of ennui, of emptiness and detachment. Experiments show, however, that thick boundary people *do not actually feel their feelings any less*. Bodily indicators (heart rate, blood pressure, blood flow, hand temperature, muscle tension) betray their considerable agitation despite surface claims of being "unruffled."

Examples of the relation between chronic illness and thick/thin boundaries include chronic fatigue syndrome and rheumatoid arthritis as "thick" conditions and irritable bowel syndrome, seasonal allergies, and allergic eczema as "thin" conditions (Table 10-2 and Figure 10-1).

The seemingly intractable mystery of fibromyalgia syndrome/chronic fatigue syndrome (FMS/CFS) was elucidated for the first time through the thick-thin model. Like the boundary types themselves, FMS/CFS exists along a spectrum. Our analysis revealed that given the same risk factors and exposures, thin boundary types express the illness as fibromyalgia, whereas thick boundary types express it as chronic fatigue. The psychometric analysis is more than an academic exercise as it points both patient and therapist in the direction of the most helpful CAM therapies.

As introduced in Chapter 3, with the exception of hypnosis (and the associated Spiegel Hypnotic Susceptibility Scales), there are no objective, standardized methods for assessing which individuals are most likely to benefit from

| Thick boundary conditions | | | | | | |
Disorder	Hypnosis	Acupuncture	Biofeedback	Meditation/Yoga	Guided imagery	Stress reduction
Rheumatoid Arthritis		3	3	4		3
CFS		3	3	3	3	
Hypertension	2	1	4	5	2	4
Phantom Pain	1	4	2	2		
Psoriasis	2		3			
Ulcer						3

| Thin boundary conditions | | | | | | |
Disorder	Hypnosis	Acupuncture	Biofeedback	Meditation/Yoga	Guided imagery	Stress reduction
Asthma/Allergies	4	5	4	2		
Eczema	4					
Fibromyalgia		3				3
IBS	4	4	3			
Migraine	3	4	5	3	3	2
PTSD	2	3	2	3		3

| Boundary-independent conditions | | | | | | |
Disorder	Hypnosis	Acupuncture	Biofeedback	Meditation/Yoga	Guided imagery	Stress reduction
Depression	4	3	5	5	3	3
Pain	5	4	5	4	2	3

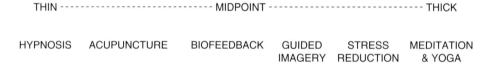

THIN ------------------------------ MIDPOINT ------------------------------ THICK

HYPNOSIS · ACUPUNCTURE · BIOFEEDBACK · GUIDED IMAGERY · STRESS REDUCTION · MEDITATION & YOGA

Figure 10-1 Spectrum of mind–body boundary types and therapies.

the bewildering variety of CAM therapies available today. Practitioners seem content to take a 'shot in the dark' when it comes to choosing therapies, or perhaps simply prescribe what happens to be available within the scope of their own practices.

As discussed in Chapter 3, although the CAM therapies included in this text have all been demonstrated to be effective through historical usage as well as contemporary clinical trials, it is also common knowledge that not all CAM therapies work equally well for everyone (and may not work at all for some).

One of the major barriers to widespread acceptance and utilization of CAM therapies is the need to effectively match individual to treatment. Otherwise, CAM, especially when practiced as "integrative medicine," is subject to the same "one-size-fits-all" conundrum that is characteristic of today's mainstream health care system. A sound matching of personality type, chronic condition, and form of treatment—through the psychometric analysis described—will finally help address this serious limitation of integrative medicine as currently practiced.

Acknowledgments

Denise Rodgers for earlier versions of this chapter in prior editions

References

Abbot NC, Harkness EF, Stevinson C, et al: Spiritual healing as a therapy for chronic pain: a randomized clinical trial, *Pain* 91(1/2):79, 2002.

Achterberg J: *Imagery in healing: shamanism and modern medicine*, Boston, 1985, Shambhala.

Achterberg J, Lawlis GF: *Imagery and disease: diagnostic tools*, Champaign, Ill, 1984, Institute for Personality and Ability Testing.

Achterberg J, Lawlis GF, Rider MS: The effects of music-mediated imagery on neutrophils and lymphocytes, *Biofeedback Self Regul* 114:247, 1989.

Alexander CN, Langer EJ, Newman RI, et al: Transcendental meditation, mindfulness, and longevity: an experimental study with the elderly, *J Pers Soc Psychol* 57(6):950, 1989.

Amri H, Abu-Asab M, Micozzi MS: *Avicenna's Canon of Medicine New Translation*, Rochester VT, 2013, Healing Arts Press.

Andersen BL, Farrar WB, Golden-Kreutz DM, et al: Psychological, behavioral, and immune changes after a psychological intervention: a clinical trial, *J Clin Oncol* 22(17):3570, 2004.

Ashton C, Whitworth GC, Seldomridge JA, et al: Self-hypnosis reduces anxiety following coronary artery bypass surgery: a prospective, randomized trial, *J Cardiovasc Surg* 38:69, 1997.

Barber TX: *A scientific approach*, New York, 1969, Van Nostrand.

Barber TX: Changing "unchangeable" bodily processes by hypnotic suggestions: a new look at hypnosis, imaging and the mind/body problem, *Advances* 1(2):7, 1984.

Bennett HL: *A comparison of audiotaped preparations for surgery: evaluation and outcomes*. Paper presented at the Annual Meeting of the Society of Clinical and Experimental Hypnosis, Tampa, Fla, 1996.

Benson H: *The relaxation response*, New York, 1975, Morrow.

Benson HR: The relaxation response. In Goleman D, Gurin J, editors: *Mind–body medicine*, New York, 1993, Consumer Reports Books.

Benson H, Kotch JB, Crassweller KD: Relaxation response: bridge between psychiatry and medicine, *Med Clin North Am* 61:929, 1977.

Bohm D: *Wholeness and implicate order*, London, 1983, Routledge & Kegan Paul.

Braud WG: Human interconnectedness: research indications, *ReVision* 14:140, 1992.

Braud WG, Schlitz M: Consciousness interactions with remote biological systems: anomalous intentionality effects, *Subtle Energies* 2(1):1, 1991.

Brooks JS, Scarano T: Transcendental meditation in the treatment of post-Vietnam adjustment, *J Couns Dev* 65:212, 1985.

Byrd RC: Positive therapeutic effects of intercessory prayer in a coronary care unit population, *South Med J* 81(7):826, 1988.

Carlson LE, Ursuliak Z, Goodey E, et al: The effects of a mindfulness meditation–based stress reduction program on mood and symptoms of stress in cancer outpatients: 6-month follow-up, *Support Care Cancer* 9:112, 2001.

Castillo-Richmond A, Schneider RH, Alexander CN, et al: Effects of stress reduction on carotid atherosclerosis in hypertensive African Americans, *Stroke* 31(3):568, 2000.

Caudill M, Schnable R, Zuttermeister P, et al: Decreased clinic use by chronic pain patients: response to behavioral medicine intervention, *J Chronic Pain* 7:305, 1991.

Centers for Disease Control and Prevention: *About chronic disease: definition, overall burden, and cost effectiveness of prevention*, 2003. Available at: http://www.cdc.gov/nccdphp/about.htm.

Chang KC, Jones D, Hendricks A, et al: Relaxation response for veterans affairs with congestive heart failure: results from a qualitative study within a clinical trial, *Prev Cardiol* 7(2):64, 2004.

Chicago Tribune: *Editorial: A new "Roseto Effect"*, 1996.

Classen C, Butler LD, Koopman C, et al: Supportive-expressive group therapy and distress in patients with metastatic breast cancer, *Arch Gen Psychiatry* 58:494, 2001.

Cooper M, Aygen M: Effects of meditation on blood cholesterol and blood pressure, *J Israel Med Assoc* 95:1, 1978.

Cordova MJ, Giese-Davis J, Golant M, et al: Mood disturbance in community cancer support groups: the role of emotional suppression and fighting spirit, *J Psychosom Res* 55(5):461, 2003.

Crowther MR, Parker MW, Achenbaum WA, et al: Rowe and Kahn's model of successful aging revisited: positive spirituality—the forgotten factor, *Gerontologist* 42(5):613, 2002.

Cummings NA, Bragman JI: Triaging the "somatizer" out of the medical system into psychological system. In Stern EM, Stern F, editors: *Psychotherapy and the somatizing patient*, New York, 1988, Hayward Press.

Cunningham C, Brown S, Kaski JC: Effects of transcendental meditation on symptoms and electrocardiographic changes in patients with cardiac syndrome X, *Am J Cardiol* 85(5):653, 2000.

Daaleman TP, VandeCreek P: Placing religion and spirituality in end-of-life care, *JAMA* 284:2514, 2000.

Davis KJ, Kumar D, Poloniecki J: Adjuvant biofeedback following anal sphincter repair: a randomized study, *Aliment Pharmacol Ther* 20(5):539, 2004.

Debenedittis C, Panerai AA, Villamira MA: Effect of hypnotic analgesia and hypnotizability on experimental ischemic pain, *Int J Clin Exp Hypn* 37:55, 1989.

Deckro GR, Ballinger KM, Hoyt M, et al: The evaluation of a mind/body intervention to reduce psychological distress and perceived stress in college students, *J Am Coll Health* 50(6):281, 2002.

Deepak KK, Manchanda SK, Maheshwari MC: Effects of meditation on the clinicoencephalographic activity of drug-resistant epileptics, *Biofeedback Self Regul* 19(1):25, 1994.

Dossey L: *Healing words: the power of prayer and the practice of medicine*, San Francisco, 1993, Harper.

Dunn BR, Hartigan JA, Mikulas WL: Concentration and mindfulness meditations: unique forms of consciousness? *Appl Psychophysiol Biofeedback* 24(3):147, 1999.

Egolf B, Lasker J, Wolf S, et al: The Roseto effect: a 50-year comparison of mortality rates, *Am J Public Health* 82(8):1089, 1992. Available at: http://www.pubmedcentral.nih.gov/articlerender.fcgi?artid=1695733.

Eisenberg DM, Kessler RC, Foster C, et al: Unconventional medicine in the United States, *N Engl J Med* 238(4):246, 1993.

Eisenberg DM, Kessler RC, Van Rompay MI, et al: Perceptions about complementary therapies relative to conventional therapies among adults who use both: results from a national survey, *Ann Intern Med* 135(5):344, 2001.

Esch T, Stefano GB, Fricchione GL, et al: Stress in cardiovascular diseases, *Med Sci Monit* 8(5):RA93, 2000a.

Esch T, Stefano GB, Fricchione GL, et al: The role of stress in neurodegenerative diseases and mental disorders, *Neuro Endocrinol Lett* 23(2):199, 2000b.

Fulop G, Strain JJ, Vita J, et al: Impact of psychiatric comorbidity on length of stay for medical/surgical patients: a preliminary report, *Am J Psychiatry* 144:878, 1987.

Fynes MM, Marshall K, Cassidy M, et al: A prospective, randomized study comparing the effects of augmented biofeedback with sensory biofeedback alone on fecal incontinence after obstetric trauma, *Dis Colon Rectum* 42(6):753, 1999.

Galton F: Statistical inquiries into the efficacy of prayer, *Fortn Rev* 12:11225, 1872.

Ginandes C, Brooks P, Sando W, et al: Can medical hypnosis accelerate post-surgical wound healing? Results of a clinical trial, *Am J Clin Hypn* 45(4):333, 2003.

Goldman L: Hypnosis in obstetrics and gynecology. In Temes R, editor: *Medical hypnosis: an introduction and clinical guide*, New York and Edinburgh, 1999, Churchill Livingstone, p 65.

Gonsalkorale WM, Houghton LA, Whorwell PJ: Hypnotherapy in irritable bowel syndrome: a large-scale audit of a clinical service with examination of factors influencing responsiveness, *Am J Gastroenterol* 97:954, 2002.

Gonsalkorale WM, Miller V, Afzal A, et al: Long term benefits of hypnotherapy for irritable bowel syndrome, *Gut* 52(11):1623, 2003.

Gonsalkorale WM, Toner BB, Whorwell PJ: Cognitive change in patients undergoing hypnotherapy for irritable bowel syndrome, *J Psychosom Res* 56(3):271, 2004.

Goodwin JS, Hunt WC, Key CR, Samet JM: The effect of marital status on stage, treatment and survival of cancer patients, *JAMA* 258:3125, 1987.

Gordon D: *The fresh face of hypnosis: an old practice finds new uses*, 2004, Better Homes & Gardens.

Greco CM, Rudy TE, Manzi S: Effects of a stress-reduction program on psychological function, pain, and physical function of systemic lupus erythematosus patients: a randomized controlled trial, *Arthritis Rheum* 51(4):625, 2004.

Green E, Green A: *Beyond biofeedback*, New York, 1977, Delta.

Gruber BL, Hall NR, Hersh SP, et al: Immune system and psychological changes in metastatic cancer patients using relaxation and guided imagery: a pilot study, *Scand J Behav Ther* 17:25, 1988.

Halpin LS, Speir AM, CapoBianco P, Barnett SD: Guided imagery in cardiac surgery, *Outcomes Manag* 6(3):132, 2002.

Harris WS, Gowda M, Kolb JW, et al: A randomized, controlled trial of the effects of remote, intercessory prayer on outcomes in patients admitted to the coronary care unit, *Arch Intern Med* 159(19):2272, 1999.

Hartmann E: *Boundaries in the Mind: A New Dimension of Personality*, New York, 1991, Basic Books.

Hatch JP, Fisher JG, Rugh JD: *Biofeedback: studies in clinical efficacy*, New York, 1987, Plenum.

Herbert N: *Quantum reality*, Garden City, NY, 1987, Anchor/Doubleday.

Herron RE, Hillis SL: The impact of the transcendental meditation program on government payments to physicians in Quebec: an update, *Am J Health Promot* 14(5):284, 2000.

Hite AH, Feinman RD, Guzman GE, et al: In the face of contradictory evidence: Report of the Dietary Guidelines for Americans Committee, *Nutrition* 26(10):915–924, 2010.

Holmes TH, Rahe RH: The social readjustment rating scale, *J Psychosom Res* 11:213, 1967.

Horowitz M: *Image formation*, New York, 1983, Jason Aronson.

House J, Landis KR, Umberson D: Social relationships and health, *Science* 241:540, 1988.

Ironson G, Solomon GF, Balbin EG, et al: The Ironson Woods Spirituality/Religious Index is associated with long survival, health behaviors less stress, and low cortisol in people with HIV/AIDS, *Ann Behav Med* 24(1):34, 2002.

Jahn RG, Dunn BJ: *Precognitive remote perception. In Margins of reality: the role of consciousness in the physical world*, New York, 1987, Harcourt Brace, p 149.

Jawer M, Micozzi MS: *The Spiritual Anatomy of Emotion*, Rochester VT, 2009, Park Street Press.

Jawer M, Micozzi MS: *Your Emotional Type*, Rochester VT, 2011, Healing Arts Press.

Jordan CS, Lenington KT: Psychological correlates of eidetic imagery and induced anxiety, *J Ment Imagery* 3:31, 1979.

Kabat-Zinn J: *Full catastrophe living*, New York, 1990, Delacorte Press.

Kabat-Zinn J: Meditation. In Flowers BS, Grubin D, Meryman-Bruner E, editors: *Healing and the mind*, New York, 1993a, Bantam/Doubleday.

Kabat-Zinn J: Mindfulness meditation. In Goleman D, Gurin J, editors: *Mind–body medicine*, New York, 1993b, Consumer Reports Books.

Kabat-Zinn J: *Wherever you go, there you are: mindfulness meditation in everyday life*, New York, 1993c, Hyperion.

Kabat-Zinn J, Lipworth L, Burney R, et al: Four-year follow-up of a meditation-based program for the self-regulation of chronic pain, *J Behav Med* 8:163, 1986.

Kaplan KH, Goldenberg DL, Galvin-Nadeau M: The impact of a meditation-based stress reduction program on fibromyalgia, *Gen Hosp Psychiatry* 15(5):284, 1993.

Kiecolt-Glaser JK, Glaser R, Williger D, et al: Psychosocial enhancement of immunocompetence in a geriatric population, *Health Psychol* 4:25, 1985.

King DE, Bushwick B: Beliefs and attitudes of hospital inpatients about faith healing and prayer, *J Fam Pract* 39:349, 1994.

Kinney CK, Rodgers DM, Nash KA, et al: Holistic healing for women with breast cancer through a mind, body, and spirit self-empowerment program, *J Holist Nurs* 21(3):260, 2003.

Koenig HG, Cohen HJ, Blazer DG, et al: Religious coping and depression in elderly hospitalized medically ill men, *Am J Psychiatry* 149:1693, 1992.

Koenig HG, Ford S, George LK, et al: Religion and anxiety disorder: an examination and comparison of associations in young, middle-aged, and elderly adults, *J Anxiety Disord* 7:321, 1993.

Koenig HG, McCullough M, Larson DB: *Handbook of religion and health: a century of research reviewed*, New York, 2001, Oxford University Press.

Kolcaba K, Fox C: The effects of guided imagery on comfort of women with early stage breast cancer undergoing radiation therapy, *Oncol Nurs Forum* 26(1):67, 1999.

Lambert SA: The effects of hypnosis/guided imagery on the postoperative course of children, *J Dev Behav Pediatr* 17(5):307, 1996.

Lehrer PM, Vaschillo E, Vashchillo B, et al: Biofeedback treatment in asthma, *Chest* 126(2):352, 2004.

LeShan L: *The medium, the mystic, and the physicist*, New York, 1966, Viking.

Lewandowski WA: Patterning of pain and power with guided imagery, *Nurs Sci Q* 17(3):233, 2004.

MacLean CRK, Walton KG, Wenneberg SR, et al: *Altered cortisol response to stress after four months' practice of the transcendental meditation program.* Paper presented at the 18th Annual Meeting of the Society for Neuroscience, Anaheim, Calif, 1992.

Malach M, Imperato PJ: Depression and acute myocardial infarction, *Prev Cardiol* 7(2):83, 2004.

Mason AA, Black S: Allergic skin responses abolished under treatment of asthma and hay fever by hypnosis, *Lancet* 1:877, 1958.

Matthews DA, Conti JM, Sireci SG: The effects of intercessory prayer, positive visualization, and expectancy on the well-being of kidney dialysis patients, *Altern Ther Health Med* 7(5):42, 2001.

Matthews DA, Marlowe SM, MacNutt FS: Effects of intercessory prayer on patients with rheumatoid arthritis, *South Med J* 93(12):1177, 2000.

Mayor D, Micozzi MS: *Energy Medicine*, London, 2011, Elsevier Health Sciences.

McCown D, Micozzi MS: *New World Mindfulness: From the Founding Fathers, Emerson, and Thoreau to Your Personal Practice*, Rochester VT, 2012, Healing Arts Press/Inner Traditions, p 288.

Micozzi MS: Forensic Pathology, Toxicology and Pathophysiology in Medical-Legal Death Investigation. In Rubin E, Strayer D, editors: *Rubin's Textbook of Pathology*, Philadelphia, 2015, Wolters Kluwer/Raven Lippincott, Williams & Wilkins.

Miller R: Nurses at community hospital welcome guided imagery, *Dimens Crit Care Nurs* 22(5):225, 2003.

Mills H, Allen J: Mindfulness of movement as a coping strategy in multiple sclerosis: a pilot study, *Gen Hosp Psychiatry* 22(6):425, 2000.

Mookadam F, Arthur HM: Social support and its relationship to morbidity and mortality after acute myocardial infarction: systematic overview, *Arch Intern Med* 164(14):1514, 2004.

Morris D: *The human zoo*, New York, 1995, Oxford University Press.

Mueller HH, Donaldson CC, Nelson DV, et al: Treatment of fibromyalgia incorporating EEG-driven stimulation: a clinical outcomes study, *J Clin Psychol* 57(7):933, 2001.

Norton C, Chelvanayagam S, Wilson-Barnett J, et al: Randomized controlled trial of biofeedback for fecal incontinence, *Gastroenterology* 125(5):1320, 2003.

O'Laoire S: An experimental study of the effects of distant, intercessory prayer on self-esteem, anxiety, and depression, *Altern Ther Health Med* 3(6):38, 1997.

Olness K, Gardner GG: *Hypnosis and hypnotherapy with children*, ed 2, Philadelphia, 1988, Saunders.

Ornish D: Can lifestyle changes reverse coronary artery disease? *Lancet* 336:129, 1990.

Osler W: *Aequanimitas*, ed 3, New York, 1953, Blakiston.

Pargament KI, Smith BW, Koenig HG, et al: Patterns of positive and negative religious coping with major life stressors, *J Sci Study Relig* 37:710, 1998.

Pearce JC: *The magical child*, New York, 1992, Penguin Books.

Perlman S: Dentistry. In Temes & Micozzi, editor: *Medical Hypnosis*, London, 1999, Churchill Livingston, pp 131–140.

Reynolds P, Kaplan GA: Social connections and risk for cancer: prospective evidence from the Alameda County Study, *Behav Med* 16(3):101, 1990.

Richardson MA, Post-White J, Grimm EA, et al: Coping, life attitudes, immune responses to imagery and group support after breast cancer treatment, *J Altern Ther Health Med* 3(5):62, 1997.

Sacks M: Exercise for stress control. In Goleman D, Gurin J, editors: *Mind–body medicine*, New York, 1993, Consumer Reports Books.

Schlesinger HJ, Mumford E, Glass GV: Mental health treatment and medical care utilization in a fee-for-service system: outpatient mental health treatment following onset of a chronic disease, *Am J Public Health* 73:422, 1983.

Schneider RH, Alexander CN, Wallace RK, et al: In search of an optimal behavioral treatment for hypertension: a review and focus on transcendental meditation. In Johnson EH, editor: *Hypertension*, Washington, DC, 1992, Hemisphere.

Schneider RH, Staggers F, Alexander CN, et al: A randomized controlled trial of stress reduction for hypertension in older African Americans, *Hypertension* 26(5):820, 1995.

Schroedinger E: *What is life? And mind and matter*, London, 1969, Cambridge University Press.

Selye H: *The stress of life*, New York, 1978, McGraw-Hill.

Sharma HM, Triguna BD, Chopra D: Maharishi Ayur-Veda: modern insights into ancient meditation, *JAMA* 265:2633, 1991.

Simonton OC, Simonton S, Creighton J: *Getting well again*, Los Angeles, 1978, Tarcher.

Sloman R: Relaxation and imagery for anxiety and depression control in community patients with advanced cancer, *Cancer Nurs* 25(6):432, 2002.

Sobel DS: *Mind matters and money matters: is clinical behavioral medicine cost effective?* Paper presented at the Fourth International Conference on the Psychology of Health, Immunity and Disease, Hilton Head, SC, 1992.

Solfvin J: Mental healing. In Krippner S, editor: *Advances in parapsychological research* (vol 4), Jefferson, NC, 1984, McFarland.

Spiegel D, Bloom JR, Kraemer HC, Gottheil E: Effect of psychosocial treatment on survival of patients with metastatic breast cancer, *Lancet* 2(8668):888, 1989.

Spiegel D, Morrow GR, Classen C, et al: Group psychotherapy for recently diagnosed breast cancer patients: a multicenter feasibility study, *Psychooncology* 8:482, 1999.

Strain JJ: Psychotherapy and medical conditions. In Goleman D, Gurin J, editors: *Mind–body medicine*, New York, 1993, Consumer Reports Books.

Targ EF, Levine EG: The efficacy of a mind–body–spirit group for women with breast cancer: a randomized controlled trial, *Gen Hosp Psychiatry* 24:238, 2002.

Temkin-Greener H, Bajorska A, Peterson DR, et al: Social support and risk-adjusted mortality in a frail older population, *Med Care* 42(8):779, 2004.

Tix AP, Frazier PA: The use of religious coping during stressful life events: main effects, moderation, and meditation, *J Consult Clin Psychol* 66:411, 1997.

Tusek D, Church JM, Fazio VW: Guided imagery as a coping strategy for perioperative patients, *AORN J* 66(4):644, 1997.

Walker SR, Tonigan JS, Miller WR, et al: Intercessory prayer in the treatment of alcohol abuse and dependence: a pilot investigation, *Altern Ther Health Med* 3(6):79, 1997.

Weintraub MI, Micozzi MS: *Complementary and Integrative Medicine in Pain Management*, New York, 2008, Springer, p 440.

White KD: Salivation: the significance of imagery in its voluntary control, *Psychophysiology* 15(3):196, 1978.

Williams R, Kiecolt-Glasser J, Legato MJ, et al: The impact of emotions on cardiovascular health, *J Gend Specif Med* 2(5):52, 1999.

Yoo HJ, Ahn SH, Kim SB, et al: Efficacy of progressive muscle relaxation training and guided imagery in reducing chemotherapy side effects in patients with breast cancer and in improving their quality of life, *Support Care Cancer* 13(10):826, 2005. [Epub April 23, 2005].

Youssef NN, Rosh JR, Loughran M, et al: Treatment of functional abdominal pain in childhood with cognitive behavioral strategies, *J Pediatr Gastroenterol Nutr* 39(2):192, 2004.

Suggested Readings

Ader R: Conditioned immunomodulation: research needs and directions, *Brain Behav Immun* 17(Suppl 1):S51, 2003.

Ader R, Cohen N: *Psychoneuroimmunology*, ed 2, San Diego, 1991, Academic Press.

Baskins TW, Tierney SC, Minami T, Wampold BE: Establishing specificity in psychotherapy: a meta-analysis of structural equivalence of placebo controls, *J Consult Clin Psychol* 71(6):973, 2003.

Benson H: *Timeless healing: the power and biology of belief*, New York, 1996, Scribner.

Chopra D: *Quantum healing: exploring the frontiers of mind/body medicine*, New York, 1990, Bantam Books.

Dossey L: *Recovering the soul: a scientific and spiritual approach*, New York, 1989, Bantam Books.

Flowers BS, Grubin D, Meryman-Brunner E, editors: *Healing and the mind*, New York, 1993, Bantam/Doubleday.

Holbrook A, Goldsmith D: Placebos: our most effective therapy? *Can J Clin Pharmacol* 11(1):e39, 2004. [Epub April 1, 2004].

Hyman SE: *Briefing on the brain-body connection*, Bethesda, MD, 1998, National Institute of Mental Health. Available at: http://lecerveau.mcgill.ca/flash/capsules/articles_pdf/circuit_fear.pdf.

Locke S, Hornig-Rohan M: *Mind and immunity: behavioral immunology*, New York, 1983, Institute for the Advancement of Health.

McCown D, Micozzi MS: *Teaching Mindfulness: A Practical Guide for Clinicians and Educators*, ed 1, New York, 2010, Springer, p 250.

Naperstek B: *Staying well with guided imagery*, New York, 1994, Warner Books.

Pert CB: *Molecules of emotion*, New York, 1997, Simon & Schuster.

Schlitz M, Amorok T, Micozzi MS: *Consciousness and healing: integral approaches to mind–body medicine*, St Louis, 2005, Elsevier.

Schwartz J: American Institute of Stress, New York Times, p A15, 2004.

Simonton OC, Henson R: *The healing journey*, New York, 1994, Bantam Books.

CHAPTER 11

Prayer, Religion, and Spirituality

MARC S. MICOZZI

DAVID LARSON

INTRODUCTION

Although spirituality and religion are frequently used interchangeably, the two could also be viewed as unique but complementary entities. Spirituality could be seen as a search for something beyond oneself. Martin Buber, a Jewish philosopher, defined it as "[relating] beyond the reliable world of density and duration and to enter into a dialogical encounter with something beyond yourself" (Buber, 1970). For Buber, it is the transcendence of ordinary life experience into a journey for meaning, value, and purpose. Spiritual issues may include but are not limited to the following questions: Does life have any meaning? Does death have meaning? Why is there evil in this world? What is my purpose in being here? Why is there suffering? Is there a God?

In contrast, religion can be viewed as one type of infrastructure through which many may choose to address spiritual issues. For many, it is the practical outworking of their spirituality. Harold Koenig defined religion as an organized system of beliefs, practices, rituals, and symbols designed (1) to facilitate closeness to the sacred and (2) to foster an understanding of one's relationship and responsibility to others in living together in a community (Koenig et al, 2001). Thus for Western religious traditions, religion involves God, who is the supreme being, and religious practices involve rituals, creeds, ceremonies, or participative communities that help mediate one's relationship or harmony with God.

Although this chapter deals with both religion and spirituality in the life of the patient, much of the research in this field, especially the initial work that is highlighted here, regards religion and the patient. Therefore, as the field is re-emerging in the West, we highlight these studies

on religion. Future research is needed to look at the extent spirituality may be separate from religion at least from the standpoint of health and healing and how these two dimensions may or not differ.

SPIRITUALITY AND RELIGION IN AMERICA

The popular Gallup polls (e.g., Gallup, 2001) reveal that 95% of Americans believe in God, a number that has remained relatively static since these polls were begun in 1944. During that period of time, a belief in the afterlife as well as acceptance in the divinity of Jesus have both remained virtually unchanged, at about 75%. Nearly 60% of respondents report that religion plays a very important role in their lives and about 50% attend a worship service on a weekly basis. Americans are largely Protestant (56%) or Catholic (26%), with a smaller proportion of Jewish (2%), Muslim (2%), persons affiliating with other religious beliefs (5%), or no religious preference (9%). Since the mid-1950s, the number and proportion of Protestants has declined and has now fallen below half for the first time in our nation's history. Southern Baptists and Assemblies of God, two more conservative denominational groups, have continued to grow within this group. Over this same period of time, Catholic traditions, in contrast, have shown gradual growth, largely because of the immigration of Mexicans and Central and South Americans, among whom Catholicism is robust. Overall, however, since the mid-1960s, church attendance has surprisingly not changed measurably. Of all medical studies on religion and chronic diseases, there has been particular focus on cancer, perhaps because it is generally a chronic condition that profoundly impacts the patient over some period of time (without "sudden deaths" as healthy people may experience with cardiovascular diseases such as heart attack, pulmonary embolism, or stroke, or sudden traumatic accidents). It is also seen as a "fatal" disease, although not at all the case with many cancers, and there is a strong "fear" factor associated with the disease. It is seen as a condition whereby the body "turns against us," with strong psychological components. Accordingly, there is also strong evidence that various mind–body techniques, such as guided imagery, meditation, and others, may be associated with prolonged survival and improved quality of life, as well as the occasional "spontaneous remission" (Chapters 9, 10).

CHRONIC DISEASES AND CANCER IN AMERICA

Chronic diseases and cancer are of much concern to many Americans. It is not only the second leading cause of death in America, but also the leading cause of death among Americans between the ages of 25 and 64 years. According to the Cancer Registry, the incidence of cancer has been on a steady rise since 1973, although cancer mortality has remained relatively stable (Howe et al, 2001). Really winning the "war on cancer" would mean reducing mortality rates, and over 550,000 people die each year, with 1.1 million cases diagnosed annually. In addition, over 8 million Americans are living with cancer or have previously received a diagnosis of cancer. According to the National Center for Health Statistics and the Centers for Disease Control and Prevention, approximately 80% of patients with a cancer diagnosis also resort to the use of one or more complementary/alternative therapies. Cases of cancer of the lung, breast, prostate, melanoma, and lymphoma have been increasing, whereas those of colorectal, endometrial, cervical, and stomach cancer have been stable or decreasing. The age-adjusted mortality ratio for males to females for all cancers has been 1.1 and for incidence (i.e., initial diagnosis) also 1.1. The mortality ratio of black people to white people in the same years for all cancers has been 1.25 and the incidence of newly diagnosed cancers 1.1. The risk for developing cancer for a newborn over a lifetime is estimated at 45%, somewhat surprisingly similar to the lifetime risk for persons aged 45 (i.e., 44%). By the age of 65, the risk decreases to 35%, probably reflecting competing risks from heart disease, diabetes, and strokes.

Lung cancer remains the greatest threat for cancer mortality risk, accounting for about 30% of deaths related to cancer, with an estimated 165,000 deaths per year. In contrast, lung cancers are proportionally 13%, or about one-seventh, of all cancer diagnoses. Thus, the mortality rate remains very high for lung cancer. Although the 1-year survival rate was up from 32% to 41% over 20 years, the 5-year survival rate remained the same over both years at 14% (Howe et al, 2001). The strongest single risk factor for lung cancer is excessive cigarette smoking (more than one-half pack per day). Although other important risk factors are involved, for over 30 years the government's focus has been exclusively on smoking cessation and prevention.

Colon cancer is the second leading cause of death from cancer, with over 55,000 deaths a year, accounting for 10% of all deaths from cancer and a similar 11% of diagnoses (Howe et al, 2001). Survival rates for colon cancer vary based on spread of disease, age, symptoms at presentation, and history of perforation of the bowel. Ironically, the younger patient with colorectal cancer appears to have a lower rate of survival, as these patients tend to have more aggressive tumors. This observation is similar to other conditions, such as breast cancer and heart attacks, whereby the fatality is higher at younger ages due to the aggressiveness of the disease. At the same time, at older ages it takes on average 15 years for a precancerous polyp found on colonoscopy to become cancerous. Aside from the pros and cons of colonoscopy screenings, patients who present with actual symptoms (rectal bleeding, abdominal pain, change of stool habits, etc.) and/or perforation of the bowel have a poorer prognosis, because of the advancement of the disease. Risk factors for colon cancer include genetic mutations leading to polyposis syndromes, inflammatory bowel disease, history of pelvic irradiation and other environmental mutagens such as fecal mutagens (substances either ingested or produced by bacteria that promote cancer) that interfere with normal intestinal flora (probiotics) and the microbiome.

Breast cancer is the third leading cause of death, numbering over 40,000 per year and constituting 8% of deaths from cancer and a somewhat higher 16% of diagnoses (Howe et al, 2001). However, breast cancer is the leading cause of death among women ages 40 to 55 years. Over 210,000 new cases are diagnosed each year. Risk factors for breast cancer include age, genetics (presence of the *BRCA1* or *BRCA2* gene), past history of breast cancer, nulliparity (or late or low parity), not breastfeeding. Dietary factors and oral contraceptives have also been long discussed and debated as risk factors (Harris et al, 1996). However, to date, there is little evidence that adult diet has an influence on the risk of breast cancer.

CHRONIC DISEASES AND CANCER AMONG RELIGIOUS GROUPS

Initial research on religion classified disease risk by religious denominational groups such as Jewish, Catholic, Protestant, and other smaller denominational groups (e.g., Seventh-Day Adventist, Latter-Day Saints, and Hutterite Christian groups). Findings on these earlier religious denominational studies are shown below.

JUDAISM

Early studies show a mixed prevalence rate of specific cancer in the Jewish population. Wolbarst (1932) looked at an ethnically diverse group of 40,709 patients across 205 hospitals in the United States, 1628 (4.4%) of whom were of Jewish origin. A total of 830 patients of the 40,709 were diagnosed with penile cancer. Importantly, none of those with penile cancer were Jewish. The author also examined the total number of cases of penile cancer reported in the United States, India, and Java, and found that of the 2517 cases of penile cancer, 2484 (98%) were found among uncircumcised men. The authors concluded that the ceremonial practice of circumcision probably afforded Jewish men a lower risk for penile cancer.

That same year Hoffman (1932) reported a lower rate of uterine, stomach, laryngeal, and esophageal cancer among the Jewish population, but they also found a higher rate of liver, gallbladder, rectal, ovarian, and breast cancer. Similarly, Wolff (1939) found that overall cancer rates in Berlin were nearly the same for Jewish as for non-Jewish subjects, but the distribution of cancer did vary. Again, esophageal, uterine, and stomach cancer rates were lower but those of colorectal, lung, ovarian and breast cancer were higher. It was later postulated that differences in smoking, sexual practices, and intake of alcohol may have accounted for the different rates of cancer for Jewish versus non-Jewish U.S. samples. In addition, it was postulated that genetic factors may contribute to higher ovarian and breast cancer rates in Jewish versus non-Jewish women.

Specifically, Egan et al (1996) examined 6611 women with breast cancer and compared them to 9026 controls without breast cancer, and found that Jewish women were at a slightly increased overall risk for breast cancer but had a significantly higher risk if a first-degree relative had breast cancer (RR 3.78, 95% CI, $p < 0.001$). Similarly, Toniolo and Kato (1996) found that Jewish women age 50 or younger with a family history of breast cancer had a higher risk (RR 2.33, 95% CI) than similarly aged women of other religious groups.

Steinberg et al (1998) compared 471 women with ovarian cancer to 4025 without ovarian cancer in a case-control study and found that Jewish women with a first-degree relative were more likely than non-Jewish women to have familial ovarian cancer (OR 8.8). We now believe that many of these Jewish women probably carry specific genetic mutations (*BRCA1* and *BRCA2*) that increase their risk for breast and ovarian cancer. A brief review of the potential impact of these mutations is discussed in a later section (see p. 179).

To summarize, it appears that Jewish persons are at a lower risk of uterine, cervical, and penile cancer (possibly related to behavioral factors such as sexual practice and circumcision status) as well as some gastrointestinal tumors (unknown reasons) but are at an increased risk for breast and ovarian cancers (possibly related to genetic factors). Religious tradition may be highly correlated to genetic background, particularly among certain religions such as Judaism, and must be considered in these observations.

SEVENTH-DAY ADVENTISTS

Seventh-Day Adventists (SDAs) are a Christian denominational group founded in the mid-19th century whose basic belief system is Christian but also includes a distinctive apocalyptic belief emphasis (i.e., *advent* referring to the conviction in the nearness of the return of Jesus Christ, or the "Second Coming"). Unlike most Christian groups that worship on Sunday (the day of Christ's resurrection), SDAs worship on the seventh day or Saturday (i.e., Sabbath day). SDAs promote a close community of believers who foster some healthy and protective lifestyle practices, including diet and sexual practices. Smoking and alcohol are expressly prohibited, as is pork and fish without fins and scales. In contrast, fruits, vegetables and plenty of fluids are encouraged. Although not mandatory, some practice lacto-ovo-vegetarianism, or strict vegetarianism (vegan), excluding animal products such as meat, eggs, and milk. Such diets are by definition not balanced in terms of human nutrition and risk serious nutritional deficiencies of B vitamins and the fat-soluble vitamins A, D, and E (see Chapter 26).

Wynder et al (1959) were the first to report that cancer and coronary artery disease rates were lower in California SDAs than in the general population. Phillips et al later published a 17-year follow-up study concerning a cohort of 23,000 SDAs from California, 59 of whom had developed colorectal cancer, 24 of whom developed lung cancer, and 120 of whom developed breast cancer. The age- and sex-adjusted mortality ratios were significantly lower for SDA men and women with colorectal and lung cancer than the rest of the Californian sample. However, mortality ratios were also lower for SDAs of both sexes when compared to non-SDA nonsmokers with colorectal and lung cancer. The authors concluded that abstinence from smoking was only a partial explanation for lower rates of colorectal and lung cancer, and suggested that other aspects of the SDA lifestyle also play an important role (Phillips et al, 1980).

Similarly, Berkel and deWaard (1983) found a 50% reduction in the likelihood of death from cancer in Dutch SDAs compared to the general Dutch population. Thus it appears that, as in the Jewish population, safer health practices promoted by religious practices such as smoking abstinence, healthier diets, and other yet unidentified practices or other roles of religion seem to promote a lower incidence and mortality from cancer.

CHURCH OF JESUS CHRIST OF LATTER-DAY SAINTS

Mormons, also known as members of The Church of Jesus Christ of Latter-Day Saints, are a Christian group founded by Joseph Smith and his brother, Hyrum, in the early nineteenth century. In addition to the standard Christian canon of Scripture, Mormons believe in a subsequent revelation encompassed in the Book of Mormon. They are also a religious group whose religion forbids tobacco, alcohol, coffee, tea, and other "addictive" drugs; furthermore, they stress a well-balanced diet, a strong family life, and education (Word of Wisdom 5–18).

Enstrom (1975) was the first investigator to examine the relative cancer rates for Mormons as he examined 360,000 California Mormons from all across the state and compared them to the general California population. He found a lower mortality from lung, many gastrointestinal and genitourinary tumors for men, and for women lower mortality from breast and uterine cancers. Lyon et al (1976) sampled 10,641 cancer deaths in Utah from 1966 to 1970 and found an overall lower incidence of cancer, especially breast, cervical, and ovarian cancer among Mormon women. Much higher fertility in Mormon women is strongly protective against breast cancer.

Enstrom (1989) published the most recent mortality study concerning Mormons and found that the 3119 Mormons sampled had a lower death rate from cancer, especially from lung cancer. Interestingly, among the controls who attended weekly worship services (i.e., mainly people of Protestant and Catholic faith but some people of Jewish and Muslim faith as well) and engaged in three or more health-related practices (i.e., smoking abstinence, exercise, and at least 8 hours of sleep at night), the rates of cancer were comparable to those who were Mormon, implying that religiously active persons regardless of denomination appear to have the same low cancer risk as Mormons.

Hutterites

Hutterites also are Christian in their beliefs but are quite small in number compared to SDAs and Latter-Day Saints. They originated in Europe (Switzerland, Germany, Italy, and Austria) and are now largely represented in Canada and the mid-western United States. Although their beliefs are close to those of the Baptist tradition, they stress communal living and are seen in essence to be an inbred social isolate (Steinberg et al, 1967). Inbreeding increases the probability of expression of otherwise rare genes and allows scientists opportunities to understand the role of genes in the development of disease, as represented within a specific religious group.

Martin et al (1980) studied over 12,000 Hutterites to investigate the frequency of recessive genes for various cancers. He found that Hutterites had significantly fewer deaths from cancer and that most of the difference could be explained by fewer lung cancers (only 1 patient died from lung cancer while 13 were expected). The latter was attributed to the prohibition of smoking. Also, Martin noted that the low frequency of cervical cancer (only 1 woman developed cervical cancer) is consistent with evidence of an inverse association between cervical cancer and promiscuity. He did note that there was an increased incidence of childhood leukemia and that the coefficient of inbreeding was twice as high in these patients than in the general Hutterite population, implying a possible genetic mutation that is passed down in these patients, which could be true for other cancers as well.

RELIGIOUS COMMITMENT

Rates of cancer in several religious groups show consistent relations between religiously encouraged, or even proscribed, healthy lifestyles and a generally lower incidence of at least several diseases. In this section, we examine the relations between the religiousness of U.S. samples and the development of cancer, as well as the subsequent diagnosis of cancer and how patients utilize religious beliefs or practices to cope with their cancers.

DEVELOPMENT

When examining the relationship between religiousness or religious commitment and prevalence and mortality of cancer, researchers have most frequently assessed religiousness using single-item measures of worship attendance. Although a rather simplistic approach for measuring religious commitment, there is a generally a relationship between religiousness and cancer outcomes.

Monk et al (1962) examined patients with colorectal cancer in an age-, gender-, and race-matched population and found that those with rectal cancer were less likely to associate with a worship congregation, but the authors did not find a similar relationship in the analogous colon cancer population.

Naguib et al (1966) examined close to 4200 women 30 to 45 years of age from Washington County, Maryland, and reported an inverse relationship between frequency of their worship attendance and rates of abnormal Pap smears. Among the women who identified themselves as Christian (the authors did not delineate from which denominations), those who attended worship services less than twice a year were more than twice as likely to have a positive Pap smear than those who attended weekly. The authors note that there were "too few Jewish women in the study to justify conclusions." However, Comstock and Partridge (1972), in their prospective study of over 50,000 women also from Washington County, did not find a survival advantage for frequent church-goers when compared to infrequent attendees.

To further complicate the picture, two mortality studies that found somewhat conflicting results (Enstrom 1989) analyzed 5231 Mormon high priests and 4613 wives of the high priests and compared them to a representative sample of 3119 adults in Alameda County, California. The standardized mortality ratios (SMR) for all cancers for the high priests was 47% and for the wives was 72%. The authors then defined a subgroup (whom they called "active Mormon-like persons") from among the 3119 control subjects who were religious (those who attended worship services weekly) and did not smoke. The SMR for men in this group was 51% and for women was 54%, comparable to the Mormon high priests and wives. Furthermore, for those "active Mormon-like persons" who incorporated general health practices such as regular exercise and 7 to 8 hours of sleep, the SMR was 0% for males and 21% for females, considerably lower than the SMR for nonreligious nonsmokers, which was 58% for males and 59% for females. The authors report that in their sample, lifestyles that incorporate weekly worship attendance, no smoking, and routine general health practices, such as exercise and regular sleep, "could result in a major reduction in cancer mortality."

In contrast, Reynolds and Kaplan (1990) reported, in a 17-year follow-up study of close to 7000 patients from the same population pool as Enstrom used, that women who were socially isolated were at greater risk of cancer mortality (relative hazard, 2.2, and smoking-related cancers relative hazard, 5.7), and no association was found between worship service attendance and rates of cancer or cancer mortality.

Hummer et al (1999) evaluated a nationally representative sample of 22,080 U.S. adults from the National Health Interview Survey and found that worship service attendance was associated with lower all-cause mortality in a graded fashion (i.e., people who never attended worship services exhibited a higher risk of death in the follow-up period than those who attended less than once a week, who in turn exhibited a higher risk of death in the follow-up period than those who attended church weekly). When subjected to multivariate analysis for cause-specific models for mortality, the authors reported that when controlled for age, gender, race, region, social ties, and health behaviors, the risk for mortality from cancer (hazards ratio 1.25, $p < 0.10$) and circulatory diseases (hazards ratio 1.32, $p < 0.10$) was not significantly different in subjects who never attended a worship service than for those who attended weekly. The greatest differences were observed in mortality from respiratory disease (hazards ratio 2.1, $p < 0.05$), diabetes (hazards ratio 2.1, $p < 0.05$), and infectious disease (hazards ratio 2.9, $p < 0.05$). The authors conclude that "religious involvement is strongly associated with adult mortality in a graded fashion. Those who never attend services exhibit the highest risk of death, and those who attend more than once a week exhibit the lowest risk" but fail to show this strong association in the case of all-cause cancer mortality. However, as the authors did not examine mortality rates for individual cancers, it is possible that a significant difference might exist, as shown in the above studies for various specific cancers.

Another method used to examine the relationship between religiousness or religious commitment and risk of cancer mortality is by assessing clergy or religious orders—the assumption being that these groups are at least, if not more, religious than the general population. In an early study, Taylor et al (1959) examined cancer rates from three orders of nuns. He reported that the nuns experienced a lower rate of gynecological malignancies as well as lowered total cancer mortality for nuns aged between 20 and 59 years, but the researchers also found that the nuns over 60 years of age had a higher rate of gastrointestinal and ovarian cancer when compared to age-matched controls. When combining all age groups 20 years and older, the total overall mortality among all ages was unchanged. The

conclusions observed are consistent with the observation that gynecological malignancies for younger women in part tend to occur associated with risky sexual habits (e.g., promiscuity and early intercourse). Furthermore, the authors' conclusion is also consistent with reports that married women are at a lower risk of developing ovarian cancer than single women and that multiparity affords a decreased risk compared to nulliparity (Chiaffarino et al, 2001).

King and Locke (1980) examined a sample of 28,000 clergy from Protestant churches over a 10-year period and examined cancer death rates from among the 5200 deaths that occurred during that same 10-year period of time. They reported that the clergy were 46% less likely than the general population to die of cancer and 60% less likely to die from lung cancer.

Similarly, Ogata et al (1984) studied 4300 Japanese male Zen-Buddhist priests and found that lung and other respiratory tract cancer rates were significantly reduced when compared to those of the general Japanese population, as were other medical conditions such as cardiovascular disease, peptic ulcers, and cirrhosis. The study also found that the priests smoked less, ate less, and lived in less polluted areas while still drinking similar levels of alcohol as similarly aged Japanese males.

In summary, in assessing the relations between religiousness or religious commitment with cancer incidence, researchers have examined both worship attendance and clergy and religious orders. Conclusions from studies utilizing single item assessments of religion have tended to be mixed. However, studies examining clergy or religious orders and cancer mortality appear to show a relationship between clergy and religious commitment and mortality from cancer.

RELIGION AND COPING

Upon receiving a diagnosis, the patient is faced with not only the physical manifestations of the disease but also stress, fears, and anxiety concerning the future as well as coping with pain, discomfort, and fatigue—and finally nagging anxieties about death. To examine the question of how frequently patients use religion to cope with cancer, Johnson and Spilka (1991) surveyed 103 women from Colorado with breast cancer. Eighty percent of these women reported that religion was very helpful in their coping with cancer, whereas only 12% considered religion unimportant. The authors examined the relationship between intrinsic (IR) and extrinsic (ER) religiousness. IR is regarded as the search for God or a Higher Power or personal meaning through one's faith or religion, whereas ER is more utilitarian and instrumental, a faith or religion more motivated by external factors (e.g., tradition, family, friends, and job). The authors concluded that although ER was found to be unrelated to religious coping, IR was. Factors predicting these outcomes included: (1) greater involvement with clergy; (2) belief that God was concerned with their illness; and (3) greater satisfaction from the use of religion as a coping behavior.

Similarly, Carver et al (1993) also looked at a cohort of 59 women with breast cancer and concluded that religious coping, along with acceptance and positive reframing of the cancer diagnosis, were employed most readily as preoperative strategies to cope with psychological distress. The authors noted that use of religious coping became less frequent postoperatively through a 12-month follow-up.

Roberts et al (1997) at the University of Michigan surveyed 108 women with gynecological malignancies and found that 93% believed that religious commitment helped them sustain their hopes and 76% found their religious commitment important to them. Nearly half had become more religious since diagnosed with cancer. The authors concluded that women with gynecological cancer are dealing with fear as a primary problem and that they depend on their religious convictions and experiences as an important means to cope with their disease. It appears evident from these few studies that women who have cancer do seem to employ religion as a coping strategy.

Torbjornsen et al (2000) sampled a population of 107 roughly equal numbers of male and female Norwegians with Hodgkin's lymphoma. At baseline, the patients' attitudes to religion differed little from those of the Norwegian population at large. In this study, 15% of the Norwegian patients defined themselves as atheists, 14% as agnostics, 23% as deists (defined by the authors as those who believe in "an impersonal supreme power"), and only 48% as theists (defined by the authors as those who believe in "a personal God"). However, the authors found that 40 of their patients (38%) changed their religious beliefs in part because of their illness, 33 becoming more religious, resulting in 58% of the respondents praying to God for a cure of their illness. The authors concluded that in their sample, cancer activated religiousness and seemed to help many patients cope with their illness.

A question that logically follows would be how helpful is religion to patients who employ religion to cope with their cancer. Acklin et al (1983) examined 26 patients with a recent diagnosis of cancer (20 females and 6 males) and measured IR and church attendance, as well as their coping strategies and their psychological well-being using the Grief Experience Inventory. The authors reported that IR and church attendance were related to greater transcendent meaning, less anger and hostility, and reduced social isolation.

Similarly, Jenkins and Pargament (1988) found that 62 patients they studied with cancer perceived that God had some control over their disease. Their disease course was generally found to be linked with higher self-esteem and less maladjustment scores as rated by a group of nurses. Also, Pargament et al (1988) found that positive mental health status related to a problem-solving process involving active give-and-take between the individual and God.

Regarding anxiety, Kaczorowski (1989) reported that among the 114 cancer hospice patients they surveyed,

religious well-being and anxiety were inversely related. Similarly regarding hope, Raleigh (1992) examined 90 chronically ill patients, half of whom had cancer. The authors concluded that the most common sources to support hopefulness were family, friends, and religious beliefs.

We can conclude, then, that many, but not all, patients with cancer may use their personal religiousness to cope with their illnesses and that as a result many of them may seem to enjoy higher levels of psychological well-being, self-esteem, and general mental health as a result.

RELIGIOUS PATTERNS OF COPING

A diagnosis of cancer presents a multitude of challenges to the patient. The cancer patient may use religion to cope with these threatening or difficult situations in a number of ways. According to Musick et al (1998), at least four have been identified and include the following: (1) changing one's perceived locus of control from self to God; (2) relying on one's religious worldview; (3) employing religious practices; and (4) using religious social support.

Those faced with cancer have been found to struggle with loss of control, which in turn can lead to increased psychological distress (Folkman, 1988). Similarly, higher levels of perceived control can be associated with improved adjustment to a stressful context. In an effort to regain control, patients have, for example, options that include employing primary control ("things are under my control") or secondary control ("things are under the control of God, chance, nature, other people, etc."). Jenkins and Pargament (1988) showed that patients who use secondary God perceptions as a method of coping had higher levels of self-esteem and lower levels of psychological distress than whose who employed primary control or other nonreligious means of secondary control. The authors observe that subjects tended to describe an active process of exchange with God rather than a passive submission to an external force. They conclude that those who coped most effectively tended to institute a "problem-solving" process involving an active give-and-take between the individual and God.

In 1999, Cole and Pargament (1999) reported a pilot psychotherapy program in which an intervention designed to redirect primary control to secondary control was instituted in 10 patients. Nine of the 10 patients reported preference for this support program over traditional nonspiritual approaches such as psychotherapy programs.

In addition to changing one's locus of control, patients may utilize a philosophical or theological interpretive framework, a worldview or a system of beliefs, through which to interpret their disease. For example, using a sample of 1610 subjects, Brady et al (1999) assessed the relationship of transcendent meaning to quality of life in patients with cancer and HIV, using questionnaires that evaluated functional status (level of fatigue and pain) and spiritual well-being. From these questionnaires, the authors were able to derive a "meaning/peace" score that correlated with the sense of meaning, harmony, and peacefulness in one's life. Similarly, the authors were able to derive a "faith" score that was related with one's strength and comfort in drawing from one's faith. Finally, the respondents were then asked a simple question: "Do you enjoy life right now?"

Of the group of patients that reported high levels of pain, 48% with higher meaning/peace scores answered that they enjoyed life compared to a much smaller 9% with low meaning/peace scores. Of those who reported no pain, 77% with high meaning/peace scores reported that they enjoyed life compared to only 25% with low meaning/peace scores. Similar results were observed for fatigue levels. Also, similar findings were found when looking at faith scores instead of meaning/peace scores. The authors conclude that patients need a metaphysical framework through which to interpret their disease and that despite symptoms, "spirituality might operate so as to help people continue to value themselves and their lives . . . as well as maintain strength to endure the symptom[s]."

Furthermore, Baider et al (1999) surveyed a group of 100 malignant melanoma patients in Israel over a 6-month period and measured coping, psychological distress, and social support. They found that their patient sample used their system of beliefs to engage in an active-cognitive coping strategy and that strategy also was associated with lower levels of anxiety and depression. The authors concluded that "a system of beliefs actually helps reduce the degree of psychological stress brought on by a life-threatening illness . . . they increase psychological health and serve as a source of effective coping." Their study supported previous research that had shown that religious beliefs were associated with lower levels of anxiety and greater activity and flexibility in dealing with illness (Baider et al, 1997).

A third method of religion as a coping mechanism used by cancer patients could be viewed as utilizing personal religious practices. These religious practices have been referred to as "ways to encounter the God of transcendence, order and freedom—ways that are explicitly set aside, designated, and tried-and-true" (Underwood, 1985). Sodestrom and Martinson (1987) found that the most frequently cited coping strategies by hospitalized cancer patients were personal prayer and prayer of others. The second most common activity was reading religious literature such as the Bible and other religious books and listening to religious broadcasts. Furthermore, Halstead and Fernsler (1994) found that prayer was the most frequently cited coping strategy in their sample of patients diagnosed with cancer.

Similarly, Johnson and Spilka (1991), in the study noted earlier, evaluated the value of religion in 103 women with breast cancer by administering questionnaires before and after clergy visits. The authors found that on open-ended questions, "the words 'care' or 'caring' were repeatedly employed . . . and was repeatedly associated with prayer."

The fourth and final means that cancer patients might use in coping with their diagnosis is the use of social

support groups through the local or religious communities. Musick et al (1998) note that community/social support may help the cancer patient by: (1) allowing more contact with others of a similar fate bolster their own faith; (2) meeting with people and obtaining their promises to pray; (3) being part of a social group that may provide instrumental help or assistance; and (4) reminding the patient that she or he is part of a caring community (Chapter 4).

Dunkel-Schetter et al (1992) examined 603 cancer patients to evaluate coping strategies and found that social support and focusing on the positive was associated with less emotional distress. The use of social support as a coping mechanism was more prevalent in patients with a greater perceived stress from cancer and those who more frequently worried about their disease. As the investigators followed the patients longitudinally through their disease course, coping through social support was associated with decreased emotional distress. Distancing (e.g., "making light of the disease" and "trying not to think about it"), although the most utilized coping strategy, was also found to be linked with more emotional distress.

In the first of two important interventional studies on social support, Spiegel et al (1989) examined 86 women with metastatic breast cancer and randomized them to weekly supportive group therapy meetings to discuss side effects of therapy and self-hypnosis for pain management versus a no intervention comparison group. The study time period was 1 year with multiyear follow-up. According to the authors, developing strong relations among members lessened the potential for social isolation. After 10 years, the average survival for the intervention group was 33.6 months compared with 18.9 months for women in the control group ($p < 0.0001$). In addition, the authors reported that the time from first metastasis to death was also prolonged for the intervention group (58.4 months) compared to the control group (43.2 months, $p < 0.02$). The authors conclude that social support appears to be an important factor in survival of breast cancer patients. They suggest that the cancer support group "may have allowed patients to mobilize their resources better, perhaps by complying more vigorously with medical treatment or by improving appetite and diet through reduced depression. Treated patients learned about hypnosis for pain control and therefore may have been more able to maintain exercise and other routine activities." The authors furthermore conclude that neuroendocrine and immune systems may be a mediating link between emotional processes and cancer course. Critics of this study have cited sampling error as a problem (Fox, 1998) and have called for other studies to replicate Spiegel's work (see Chapter 10).

Subsequently, Fawzy et al (1990, 1993) conducted a similar study in patients with melanoma and randomly assigned patients to weekly support groups to help patients better cope with illness or else to a comparison group of routine care. The intervention group showed significant increases in large granular lymphocytes, natural killer (NK) cells, and NK cell activity compared with the control group. (These are cells that function in identifying and killing cancer cells.) In addition, in a clinical follow-up study in 1993, the intervention group had a lower rate of cancer recurrence (21% to 38%) and a lower rate of likelihood of death (9% to 29%).

BIOLOGICAL MEDIATING FACTORS

This chapter has examined research revealing potential links between spirituality, particularly religion, and cancer. We now look at potential biological explanations, although much work remains to be done to elucidate the potential biological pathways and connections. For example, it appears that psychological state as well as the progression of cancer and survival are mediated at a biological level by neuroendocrine and inflammatory cytokine status. The neuroendocrine system is where the nervous system interacts with and helps regulate the release of hormones into the circulatory system. Inflammatory cytokines are proteins secreted by white blood cells that help signal for and mediate an immune response (see Chapter 8). Here is a brief discussion of these relations as well as the potential roles religion might play.

STRESS, NEUROENDOCRINE, AND IMMUNE STATUS

Psychological stress in the form of anxiety and depression has been shown to increase the production of cortisol by the adrenal glands (Felten et al, 1987). This increase is accomplished by stimulating the production of corticotropic releasing factor (CRF) in the hypothalamus, which then stimulates the pituitary gland to produce adrenocorticotropic hormone (ACTH), which in turn signals the adrenal gland to produce cortisol.

Cortisol helps activate the sympathetic central nervous system and is important in an acute "fight-or-flight" response. It raises blood pressure, heart rate, mental awareness, regulates glucose level, and recirculates white blood cells, all of which are important in an acutely stressful event. However, chronic stress and activation of this CNS-mediated pathway has been shown to impair immunity. Repeated "hits" on this sympathetic nervous system may affect a compensatory hyperactivity of other mediators, including cytokines, which then downregulate the immune system (McEwen et al, 1997).

Cacioppo et al (1995) showed that brief psychological stressors elicit autonomic and neuroendocrine responses. This same study revealed that subjects who were characterized by high cardiac sympathetic reactivity to brief stressors also showed high stress-induced changes in plasma cortisol and ACTH levels, suggesting a relative activation of the hypothalamic–pituitary–adrenocortical system in these subjects. Kiecolt-Glaser et al (1993) observed that conflict and marital discord was strongly associated with fluctuation in cortisol, ACTH, and norepinephrine levels among female spouses.

In addition, Rassnick et al (1994) showed in the locus coeruleus of the brain in awake rats that the stimulation of the autonomic nervous system with CRF caused not only cortisol levels but also interleuken-6 (IL-6) levels to rise. The role of IL-6 is briefly discussed below. The authors also observed that T-lymphocyte responses were decreased. They conclude that the central nervous system/adrenal axis is involved in stressor-induced immune suppression.

Both "humoral" and "cell-mediated" immunity are part of an overall "adaptive" immune system that responds to cancer. The humoral system immune response is mediated by antibodies, whereas the cell-mediated immune response does not involve humoral antibodies. Specifically, the humoral system helps signal and trigger tumor-specific cytotoxic T lymphocytes (CTL), T-helper cells (Th), as well as "natural killer" (NK) cells. Often, when a cell mutates into cancer, this adaptive system can keep the cancer from growing and spreading and may eliminate the cancer altogether. The "innate" immune system also responds to cancer and is made up of NK cells that have cell-specific receptors that generate recognition of tumor cells and initiate cell signals that mediate cytotoxicity of tumor cells. Both the adaptive and innate immune systems appear to be depressed in the presence of psychological stressors, as stated previously, possibly through a CNS-mediated pathway.

Early studies performed in animals focused on how stress affects the humoral immune system. Gisler (1974) reported that mice that were stressed by either restraint or crowding had blunted antibody responses over the first 3 days of exposure to the stressor. However, with repeated stimulus, the antibody responses eventually returned back to prestressor baseline levels. Similarly, Monjan and Collector (1977) exposed mice to auditory stress and measured antibody responses of lymphocytes to bacterial lipopolysaccharide, a protein on the surface of various bacteria and reported that in their mice the antibody responses were suppressed for up to 20 days.

Subsequent studies began to evaluate the role of stress on cell-mediated immunity. Reite et al (1981) subjected pigtailed monkeys to maternal and peer separation for 2-week intervals and measured T-lymphocyte mitogen responses and reported, similarly to previous work, that these acute stressors elicited a degree of suppression of T-cell function that normalized only after reunion with peer monkeys. Maternal and peer separation represents an animal model for grief and loss-related depression (Reite et al, 1978). Similar studies have been performed demonstrating a relationship between the intensity of the stressor and the degree of suppression of T-lymphocyte function in rats. Keller et al (1981) reported that both the number and function of T lymphocytes appear to be suppressed progressively more in rats as the level of electrical shock delivered to the rats increased.

In humans, Schleifer et al (1983) showed the suppression of mitogen-induced lymphocyte proliferation (a process by which lymphocytes are stimulated to reproduce) after the loss of a spouse. The investigators measured lymphocyte function in 15 men before and after the deaths of their spouses from breast cancer and discovered markedly lowered immune responses during the first 2 months postbereavement. In a similar work on bereavement, Zisook et al (1994) reported on a sample of 21 female widows who were evaluated for 13 months postbereavement. The subset of widows who met DSM-III-R criteria for major depressive disorders also demonstrated lower NK cell activity and lower mitogen stimulation compared to those who did not meet these criteria.

Furthermore, depression has been shown to correlate with increased oxidative damage to DNA, a process critical in tumor development and progression (Jackson & Loeb, 2001). Adachi et al (1993) reported increased levels of a biomarker for cancer-related DNA damage in rats that had been subjected to multiple electrical shocks over control, unshocked rats, which provided the first evidence of such damage induced by psychological stress. This finding was replicated in human studies; Irie et al (2001) reported that in their sample population of 362 healthy adults (276 males and 86 females), after adjusting for body mass index, cigarette smoking, and alcohol use, there were positive relationships of the biomarker for DNA damage to average working hours, a self-blame coping strategy, and recent loss of a close family member in male subjects.

Taken together, psychological stressors have been observed to result in: (1) DNA damage thereby contributing to carcinogenesis; (2) suppressed humoral and cell-mediated immune responses; and (3) decreased NK cell number and function. All three may promote cancer growth and metastasis.

Increased incidence and mortality of cancer has been theorized to occur in populations with higher levels of psychological stressors. In fact, Shekelle et al (1981) examined 2000 men for 17 years and after controlling for sociodemographic and preexisting medical morbidities found that the likelihood of death from cancer was twice as high in men who were depressed compared to men who were not depressed.

In similar fashion, Levy et al (1991) reported that in their sample of 90 women with early-stage (stage I or II) breast cancer followed for 5 years, fatigue/depression and lack of social support predicted levels of NK cell activity and disease-free survival and rate of disease progression for those who relapsed. Mood as measured by the Profile of Mood States and perceived familial social support predicted rate of disease progression for the women who did eventually relapse.

RELIGION, STRESS, AND THE IMMUNE SYSTEM

A few studies have examined the relationship between religion, stress, and immune function. Two studies assessed the potential for religious factors to be linked with reduced stress and lower cortisol levels in cancer patients. For example, Katz et al (1970) evaluated 30 women with known breast masses awaiting breast biopsies for possible cancer and assessed them for their approaches to coping and cortisol levels. The authors noted that the women employed one or more of five coping strategies (i.e., displacement, projection, denial, fatalism, and/or prayer/faith). They concluded that those women who employed prayer and faith as coping mechanisms tended to have lower cortisol levels compared to those using other coping strategies ($p < 0.02$). Similarly, Schaal et al (1998) evaluated 112 women with metastatic breast cancer and measured attendance at worship services, religious or spiritual expression, and diurnal salivary cortisol levels. The authors found that although overall salivary cortisol levels did not associate with worship service attendance, evening cortisol levels were significantly lower among women who scored higher on religious expression.

In an effort to examine the relationship between stress, religion, and immune function, cytokine markers such as IL-6 have been studied. IL-6 is a small protein involved in the acute inflammatory response which stimulates the growth and differentiation of B lymphocytes. Furthermore, it is elevated in cancer cachexia (i.e., cancer wasting syndromes). High levels of IL-6 have been found in various cancers, such as plasmacytomas, Hodgkin's lymphoma, and kidney and head and neck cancers (Blay et al, 1994; Ershler et al, 1994; Ur et al, 1992). Some research groups have suggested that IL-6 might serve as a marker for a "stable immune system" (Koenig et al, 2001).

Koenig et al (1997) measured IL-6 levels in 1718 elderly persons in North Carolina. The authors found that IL-6 levels correlated with frequency of religious attendance. Subjects who attended religious services were 49% less likely than nonattenders to have high IL-6 levels (>5 pg/ mL). It is possible, however, that those who were healthier to begin with (lower IL-6 levels) were the individuals who were able to go to church, whereas those who were sicker (higher IL-6 levels) were not.

Lutgendorf (2001) examined the relationship between religious beliefs and behavior and IL-6 in 55 adults in Iowa (age range 65 to 89 years). Half of the subjects were moving from their homes to senior housing (considered in the study as a stressful event) and IL-6 levels as well as religious and spiritual coping were measured before, during, and after the key stressful event. The authors found that levels of IL-6 were inversely related to greater use of spiritual coping, independent of whether seniors were stressed.

Sephton et al (2001) examined the effect of spirituality on the immune system of 112 patients with breast cancer and found that spirituality was associated with greater numbers of circulating white blood cells, total lymphocytes, helper T cells, and cytotoxic T cells.

There is also evidence to suggest that there are neurologic changes that occur during spiritual and religious activity. Newberg et al (2001) studied nuns and monks during meditation and prayer using single-photon emission computed tomography, which images blood flow to various parts of the brain. They reported that both the Franciscan nuns and Buddhist monks experienced decreased brain activity in the left orientation association areas (posterior superior parietal lobes) during the height of meditation. Scientists tell us that the parietal lobe is important to establish our physical relationship to the outside world.

It could be that spirituality or, in particular, religiousness may, in essence, lead to lowered levels of stress and psychological distress and thereby may lower neurologic and/or neuroendocrine stimulation and normalize immune functioning (at least as represented by IL-6 levels). Although much further work remains to be done, preliminary data suggest a potential positive correlation between healthy immune systems to fight cancer (i.e., increased level and function of cytotoxic T lymphocytes and NK cells and lower IL-6, cortisol, and ACTH levels) and religious practice.

GENETIC FACTORS AND RELIGION

Genetic associations of cancer risk may be related to ethnicity and religion. At present, much is known about the role of genetic factors in cancer. Below we highlight some of the studies done in this area as it relates to religion. When a small religious group maintains over time similar family participants, there is increased chance for intermarriage or, in essence, inbreeding to occur, and genetic factors may come to play an increased role. Similar groups from nearby locations with similar cultures and beliefs marry and may, over time, "intermarry." In this manner, genes are passed down, including unwanted mutations. Under this premise, the Hutterites, as previously highlighted, have been studied as a familial aggregate and deemed to be a human isolate. In Martin et al's study, the authors suggested that there was an association between inbreeding in these Hutterite populations and incidence of childhood leukemia, suggesting the existence of a gene or multiple genes responsible for the development of certain childhood leukemias (Martin et al, 1980).

Simpson et al (1981) studied this same population of Hutterites and examined 177 cases of cancer, specifically addressing the relationship of inbreeding to incidence of breast cancer. The coefficient of inbreeding (F) can be seen as the proportion of alleles (genes) that are homozygous (paired together) by descent from a common ancestor, that is, the probability that a person with two identical genes received each individual gene from the same ancestor. The higher the F, the more likely that recessive gene(s) will be expressed. The authors conclude that a higher F was present in women with early breast cancer (before the age of 45) when compared to age-matched controls and suggest the presence of recessive gene(s) that may cause a select subpopulation of breast cancer. Until recently, however, no specific gene(s) have been characterized.

BREAST CANCER

The cause of early familial breast cancer has now been in part elucidated. Hall et al (1990) reported that the genes responsible for this form of breast cancer, up to 10% of all cases, is located on chromosome 17q21 and was later named BRCA1 and BRCA2 (BReast CAncer). The presence of these mutations are a risk for early breast cancer and are thought to be histologically more aggressive in that they are highly proliferative, tend not to express hormone receptors (estrogen receptor/progesterone receptor), and are aneuploid—meaning they are chromosomally complicated and disrupted (Bertwistle & Ashworth, 1999).

Jewish women appear to have slightly higher risks for breast and ovarian cancer compared to the general population, and significantly higher risk if a young, first-degree relative has breast cancer. Individuals of Ashkenazi Jewish descent who bear the BRCA mutant gene usually carry one of three common mutations in either BRCA1 or BRCA2 (Beller et al, 1997). In Ashkenazi Jews, the carrier rate is 1.2% and 1.5%, respectively, for these BRCA1 and BRCA2 mutations. Two of these BRCA1 mutations can be found in 6.9% of Ashkenazi women with breast cancer (Robson et al, 1999). Thirteen percent of Ashkenazi women diagnosed by age 65 (Gershoni-Baruch et al, 1997) and up to 24% of these same women diagnosed before age 42 years have one of these mutations (Gershoni-Baruch et al, 1997; Offit et al, 1996).

It appears that these mutations can negatively affect survival in Ashkenazi women. Foulkes et al (1998), in a group of 117 Ashkenazi women, found that disease-free survival at 5 years was significantly higher in non-BRCA associated tumors than in BRCA mutated ones (88.7% versus 68.2%). The overall survival was also significantly lower (95.7% versus 64.3%). The mutation appears to affect the cell's ability to repair itself (Bhattacharyya et al, 2000). Specifically, the BRCA1 protein binds with another protein, Rad51, which is involved in DNA repair. The cell harboring this complex (labeled BRCA1:Rad51) has a decreased ability to repair DNA damage and ultimately leads to cell death.

This process of programmed cell death, or apoptosis, is mediated by a gene called p53 and is very important so as to disallow dysfunctional cells (cells with the BRCA mutation) to continue to proliferate. However, it has also been discovered that an inordinately high number of p53 mutations are found in the very same Ashkenazi Jewish population that go on to develop breast cancer, thus explaining why not all Ashkenazi Jews with a BRCA1 or BRCA2 mutation develop cancer and supporting the concept of a multistep process of carcinogenesis (Hilakivi-Clarke, 2000). In other words, it appears that a series of mutations are necessary to originate and promulgate cancer and that BRCA1 or BRCA2 mutations provide but a single step along the way.

RELIGION AND NEGATIVE HEALTH OUTCOMES

Thus far, we have discussed what in essence are generally health-enhancing or the health benefits of religious affiliation or commitment. However, the fact remains that the derivation of favorable health from religion is neither simple nor straightforward and not always the case. Religious beliefs, practices, and coping strategies have also been found to negatively affect physical and mental health status.

The first means by which a negative association may occur is inculcating *unhealthy practices*. One example is replacing religious healing practices for indicated medical treatment and care. For example, Lannin et al (1998) reported over 500 women with newly diagnosed breast cancer who were compared with 400 demographically matched controls and found that cultural beliefs (including religious beliefs) and socioeconomic factors were both significant predictors of late-stage diagnosis. The authors viewed that faith played a problematic role. They concluded that for a number of reasons many in their study failed to seek early medical attention despite recognizing a breast lump and, although well-intended in their hopes and beliefs, felt "perhaps most importantly [that] prayer and a reliance on God [would] heal the disorder."

Other examples in which religion might reduce use of appropriate medical care include the refusing of blood transfusions (Jehovah's Witnesses), childhood immunizations (although many parents are convinced that risk outweighs benefits for newer vaccines, such as HPV and influenza), prenatal care, medically assisted birthing (Faith Assembly), and traditional mental health care (more orthodox Protestant groups). Although the intent of these religious practices is benevolent, overlooking some appropriate and indicated medical treatments can lead to unfavorable clinical outcomes. When the practice of regular medicine conflicts with the theology and doctrines of the religious order, these institutions and individuals may choose to reject medical care which may otherwise be appropriate.

Another means by which religion can negatively influence health status is by using negative religious coping strategies. Koenig et al (1998) reported that coping strategies in which God is viewed as benevolent or as a collaborative partner in coping with life's stresses tended to be associated with better mental health outcomes; in contrast, coping in which God is viewed as a punishing or a rejecting deity were associated with poorer mental health outcomes. The authors note that this study was cross-sectional study and that preexistent psychological distress may have been responsible for such beliefs.

Pargament et al (2001) published a 2-year longitudinal study of 600 medical inpatients and concluded that some forms of religious coping leading to religious struggle or conflict may actually increase the risk of earlier death. The patients who employed negative religious coping (e.g., "God has abandoned me because of a lack of devotion" and "God does not love me") had higher risk ratios for mortality than did patients who employed positive religious coping strategies. Even after controlling for demographics, illness severity, church attendance, depressed mood, and quality of life, these negative types of religious struggle continued to predict increased risk of mortality.

A third example of the negative effects of religion on health can be illustrated in "all-or-nothing" extremist cult groups. Dein and Littlewood (2000) report that violence and suicide among cult members became somewhat more frequent, especially in light of a "divine millennium"–the end of the world or the return of God—not yet materializing. Upon this disappointment and because they may consider themselves immune to death, they often choose to attempt to exit their physical bodies and go to a better "spiritual" world. An example of these religious cults was the Heaven's Gate cult, whose members believed that aliens resided on the Hale–Bopp comet and committed mass suicide in an effort to be initiated into a higher existence. Likewise, the members of the Solar Temple, realizing that the New Age as promised by their leader did not come to pass, and believing that a spaceship would collect their souls and deliver them to another planet, committed mass suicide. Also, during the mid-1990s, the Branch Davidians—a breakaway group from the Seventh-Day Adventists—believed that their leader, David Koresh, would usher in the end of the world and that the American government represented an evil enemy state. In the end, they were only half-right and it was an aggressive and overreaching federal government that brought about their demise.

Furthermore, the above authors report in their review of these extremist apocalyptic groups that commonalities exist among these various extremist cults: (1) they teach a strong dualistic philosophy (i.e., an evil physical world and a good spiritual world); (2) they have charismatic leaders with total control; and (3) they promote an isolationism among the members that makes it exceedingly difficult to object to the teachings or to leave the group. The authors argue that health professionals need to understand the belief system and pattern of leadership before working with members of these groups. Not all groups are so extremist. Anyone leaving such a movement might also undergo stress, if not conflict, sometimes severe, in attempting to reconcile their past and present worldviews.

CLINICAL IMPLICATIONS

Day-to-day care of cancer patients by helping to deal with the spiritual aspects of their condition makes clinical sense. If not just for supporting a patient's spirituality when it gives them hope or support, it also makes sense when a patient has spiritual distress with the potential for such distress to worsen physical or psychological problems that may intercalate with depression, hopelessness, worthlessness, and/or meaninglessness. Furthermore, pain, fatigue and the rigors and side effects of treatment may compound the anguish. Therefore it is important for the clinician to be aware of the potential for the spiritual distress or existential angst of their patient and to recognize the importance of questions such as: Where is God when I need him? Why has he abandoned me? Where am I going when/if I die? Is God punishing me? When there is such distress, it is very important to consult with a chaplain or an indicated health care consultant who can better address such spiritual issues.

Toward this end, clinicians need to develop some skills in addressing spiritual needs. Below are propose two necessary skills: (1) establishing rapport and a dialogue with patients about their needs; and (2) recognizing the appropriate time for referrals to professional religious workers, particularly chaplains.

SPIRITUAL DIALOGUE

Addressing the importance of the role of dialogue in spiritual matters, Roberts et al (1997) surveyed over 100 women with gynecological malignancies and found that a majority of these women placed greater emphasis on receiving "straight talk" (96%) from their physician, which was more important than compassion (64%). Over three-quarters of the women (76%) viewed religion as very important to them and of these, nearly half (49%) reported an increase in their religiousness after the diagnosis of cancer. Over 90% felt that religious commitment helped them sustain their hopes and 41% felt that it helped them sustain their worth. The authors concluded that women with gynecological cancer "depend on their religious convictions and experiences as they cope with disease" and that physicians should "aim to educate their patients sufficiently for them to exercise control over their experience, to allay fears and make personal decisions that further their aspirations."

Furthermore, King and Bushwick (1994) interviewed 203 medical inpatients about their religious and health behavior and found that 77% of the patients wanted their physicians to consider their spiritual needs. Somewhat surprisingly, 48% wanted their physicians to pray with them; however, 68% of their physicians had never discussed religious beliefs with patients.

Ehman et al (1999) interviewed 177 pulmonary medicine patients and found that 51% described themselves as religious and 90% believed that prayer may sometimes influence recovery from an illness. Of those, 94% felt that physicians ought to ask them of their religious beliefs should they become gravely ill. Interestingly, of the 49% who did not describe themselves as religious, still about half felt that that physicians ought to ask them of their religious beliefs should they become gravely ill.

Moadel et al (1999) addressed what cancer patients desire from their physicians regarding spiritual care. They interviewed 268 ethnically diverse patients in an urban oncology center and found that 51% of patients wanted assistance in overcoming their fears in life (referring to existential fears about life), 42% wanted assistance in seeking hope, 40% wanted help in finding meaning in life, and 39% looked to their physicians for spiritual resources.

Because patients are willing to discuss spiritual issues with their clinicians, the latter must be able to formulate relevant open-ended questions while communicating a nonjudgmental respect for that patient's beliefs and struggles (Post et al, 2000). Puchalski (1999) offers one approach using the mnemonic FICA in obtaining a spiritual history from the patient. This tool incorporates questions dealing with the patients' *Faith*, the *Importance* or influence of this faith, the religious *Community* they are in, and how it is the clinician can *Address* any needs.

Furthermore, the American College of Physicians–American Society of Internal Medicine Concensus Panel Statement on End-of-life Issues (Lo et al, 1999) outlines an unassuming method to begin to open discussion, explore, and discuss spiritual and existential issues and answers objections to this approach. Open-ended questions such as "What are your hopes, your expectations, your fears for the future?" or "As you think about the future, what is most important for you?" Physicians and caretakers are encouraged to pursue an honest dialogue if patients appear available and willing.

Further questions such as "Is faith (religion, spirituality) important to you?" or "Do you have someone to talk to about religious matters?" More direct questions such as "What thoughts have you had about why you got this illness at this time?" or "What do you still want to accomplish during your life?" are also included. The consensus report authors note four important points for the caretakers to keep in mind: (1) uncovering painful emotions may increase short-term suffering but may lessen fear and anxiety in the long term; (2) open and honest dialogue by both the physician and patient may lead to a connectedness between the two individuals; (3) caretakers can clarify their own roles, noting they are "fellow travelers" who may not have all the answers but who can listen and try to understand; and (4) caretakers do not have sole responsibilities for the patients suffering but can call on nurses, social workers, chaplains, psychologists, and psychiatrists for help.

REFERRALS TO CHAPLAINS

The clinician should be thinking of referral for spiritual issues when: (1) they are uncomfortable; (2) when there is spiritual distress; (3) the spiritual issues are complex; or (4) addressing these particular issues will take more time than allotted. The emergence of spiritual distress in particular in the life of a patient may be the culmination of a lifetime of struggle, disappointment, or pain and will not be adequately addressed with a few platitudes or prosaic phrases. Opening a dialogue with the patient is important for the clinician as much to diagnose the spiritual problem as to begin addressing it. Under these conditions it is best for the physician to refer to a chaplain or a spiritual care provider.

The clinician may want to invest some time in creating their network of support staff by establishing relationships through a local ministerial association, contract, volunteer arrangement, or pastoral care department of a local hospital or by working with students from local religious educational facilities (Harris & Satterly, 1998). Because patients may have a diversity of cultural and religious backgrounds, clinicians need to keep in mind that one size may not fit all. That is, it is important for the clinician to be aware of a number of different spiritual or religious professionals with different backgrounds and different strengths so as to be able to refer patients with unique needs to the appropriate resource(s), like making any referral. More importantly, chaplains can often work with patients of different faith traditions and when needed make linkages among these traditions.

EFFICACY OF CLINICIANS AS HEALERS

Although it is becoming increasingly clear that patients desire their caretakers to address religious and spiritual issues, whether supportive or stressful, it appears that physicians and nurses may not integrate this level of care into their practice as frequently as they would like. Kristeller et al (1999) surveyed 94 oncologists and 267 oncology nurses regarding attitudes and practices regarding patient care, specifically spiritual distress. Of the oncologists and nurses surveyed, 37.5% and 47.5%, respectively, reported identifying themselves as the primary clinician responsible for addressing spiritual distress. However, only 11.8% and 8.5%, respectively, ranked spiritual distress as one of the top three psychosocial issues that they would actually address. Furthermore, although over 85% of these caretakers believed a chaplain to be the ideal person to address these issues, very few of them actually made a formal referral for spiritual distress (25% and 37% for MDs and nurses, respectively).

The Joint Commission has now begun to address spiritual issues in health care settings. They require physicians to respond to spiritual issues in end of life care (RI.I.2), refer to pastoral counseling or chaplains when appropriate (RI.I.2.7), make an initial spiritual assessment to dying patients (PE.I.I), and address spiritual orientation when treating drug and alcohol dependency (PE.7). Toward this end, physicians are presently being better trained in taking a spiritual history as over 60 of the 126 medical schools presently have courses that specifically address this issue.

SUMMARY AND CONCLUSION

Dealing with illness can be an important aspect in the lives of Americans. Cancer remains a leading cause of morbidity and mortality today as lung, colorectal, and breast cancer continue to rank as the top three cancer-related causes of mortality each year. Overall, cancer is the second leading killer of Americans. Since the early 1970s, when the "war on cancer" was declared, overall cancer incidence has been on a steady rise while cancer mortality has generally not declined. The rates of other chronic diseases such as diabetes and dementia have increased, while there has been some stabilization in cardiovascular diseases.

Probably because of the nature and meaning of cancer as a disease and diagnosis, studies on religion and spirituality have been weight to addressing this condition. Religion remains important in the lives of Americans with levels of religious practices and beliefs remaining high and some-

what constant since the early 1950s. A majority of Americans believe in God and attend houses of worship on a regular basis.

Certain religious groups have been of particular research interest given their differential prevalence and mortality rates from cancer. For example, the Jewish population appears to have a lower incidence of penile cancer (circumcision) and uterine and cervical cancer (safer sexual habits) but slightly higher rates of breast and ovarian cancer (genetic mutations and higher SES). Seventh-Day Adventists have a lower rate of colorectal and lung cancer (dietary and smoking-related practices) and Mormons similarly have lower rates of colorectal, lung, and genitourinary cancers (dietary, smoking, and possibly other health-related practices). Finally, Hutterites have been found to have lower lung cancer and cervical cancer rates (smoking-related and safer sexual habits). Thus, it appears that various religious groups tend to promote safer and healthier lifestyles and these maybe translate into lower prevalence and mortality from cancer, aside from the purely spiritual aspects.

In addition to lifestyle modifications for certain religious groups, religious commitment also appears to provide health benefits on a more spiritual basis. Regular worship attendance has been found to protect against all-cause mortality in general, as well as cancer mortality specifically. Furthermore, in the studies discussed in this chapter, it appears that clergy and religious professionals tend to have a lower cancer prevalence and mortality. Following the diagnosis of cancer, religion may provide additional health-related roles as it may be frequently employed successfully as a positive coping strategy to potentially reduce psychological distress and increase adjustment to serious illness. For example, cancer patients may employ secondary control, utilizing their system of beliefs, supported by their personal religious practices, as well as accessing social support through their congregational settings.

The potential clinical benefits may be mediated by a psychoneuroimmunological model involving the stress response as well as inflammatory cytokine cascades (Chapter 8). Psychological stressors may induce DNA damage thereby contributing to carcinogenesis, suppressed humoral and cell-mediated immune responses, as well as decreased NK cell number and function, all of which may promote cancer growth and metastasis.

Religion may reduce psychological distress, which may in turn mediate its beneficial effects by way of the immune system.

Religion may also, however, have a negative impact on health as it may promote unhealthy beliefs about oneself and God and, in turn, increase potential for psychological distress and negatively impact survival. Furthermore, religion may promulgate potentially unhealthy practices such as avoiding or substituting religious ritual for regular medical care, including the appropriate resort to surgery, antibiotics, chemotherapy, blood transfusion, and certain immunizations. On a case-by-case basis, resistance to using any or all of these approaches, based upon informed awareness of risks, costs and benefits, may also be a matter of simple logic and reason regardless of religious beliefs.

Considering the complicating issues surrounding religion and health, patients appear to desire that their physicians address spiritual issues and their spiritual distress. Skills necessary in this process can be as simple as asking a few questions, and opening a dialogue with patients to ascertain the role of spiritual issues in their lives. When the physician has limited time, the issues are complex, or there is spiritual distress, subsequent appropriate referrals can be made to spiritual care providers such as chaplains. There is increasing need in areas such as oncology for specialists to address these areas of concern, and to educate and equip the clinician to be a genuine, capable provider of care to the whole person—body, mind, and spirit.

Acknowledgment

Prior contributions for this chapter were received from David Larsen, PhD, deceased, 1948–2002.

References

Acklin MW, Brown EC, Mauger PA: The role of religious values and coping with cancer, *J Relig Health* 22:322–333, 1983.

Adachi S, Kawamura K, Takemoto K: Oxidative damage of nuclear DNA in liver of rats exposed to psychological stress, *Cancer Res* 53(18):4153–4155, 1993.

Baider L, Perry S, Sison A, et al: The role of psychological variables in a group of melanoma patients. An Israeli sample, *Psychosomatics* 38(1):45–53, 1997.

Baider L, Russak SM, Perry S, et al: The role of religious and spiritual beliefs in coping with malignant melanoma: an Israeli sample, *Psychooncology* 8(1):27–35, 1999.

Beller U, Halle D, Catane R, et al: High frequency of BRCA1 and BRCA2 germline mutations in Ashkenazi Jewish ovarian cancer patients, regardless of family history, *Gynecol Oncol* 67(2):123–126, 1997.

Berkel J: deWaard F: Mortality patterns and life expectancy of Seventh-Day Adventists in the Netherlands, *Int J Epidemiol* 12:455–459, 1983.

Bertwistle D, Ashworth A: The pathology of familial breast cancer: How do the functions of BRCA1 and BRCA2 relate to breast tumour pathology, *Breast Cancer Res* 1(1):41–47, 1999.

Bhattacharyya A, Ear US, Koller BH, et al: The breast cancer susceptibility gene BRCA1 is required for subnuclear assembly of Rad51 and survival following treatment with the DNA cross-linking agent cisplatin, *J Biol Chem* 275(31):23899–23903, 2000.

Blay JY, Schemann S, Favrot MC: Local production of interleukin 6 by renal adenocarcinoma in vivo, *J Natl Cancer Inst* 86(3):238, 1994.

Brady MJ, Peterman AH, Fitchett G, et al: A case for including spirituality in quality of life measurement in oncology, *Psychooncology* 8(5):417–428, 1999.

Buber M: *I and thou*, New York, 1970, Charles Scribner's Sons.

Cacioppo JT, Malarkey WB, Kiecolt-Glaser JK, et al: Heterogeneity in neuroendocrine and immune responses to brief psychological stressors as a function of autonomic cardiac activation, *Psychosom Med* 57(2):154–164, 1995.

Carver CS, Pozo C, Harris SD, et al: How coping mediates the effect of optimism on distress: A study of women with early stage breast cancer, *J Pers Soc Psychol* 65(2):375–390, 1993.

Chiaffarino F, Pelucchi C, Parazzini F, et al: Reproductive and hormonal factors and ovarian cancer, *Ann Oncol* 12(3):337–341, 2001.

Cole B, Pargament K: Re-creating your life: A spiritual/psychotherapeutic intervention for people diagnosed with cancer, *Psychooncology* 8(5):395–407, 1999.

Comstock GW, Partridge KB: Church attendance and health, *J Chronic Dis* 25(12):665–672, 1972.

Dein S, Littlewood R: Apocalyptic suicide, *Ment Health Relig Cult* 3(2):109–114, 2000.

Dunkel-Schetter C, Fernstein LG, Taylor SE, Falke RL: Patterns of coping with cancer, *Health Psychol* 11:79–87, 1992.

Egan KM, Newcomb PA, Longnecker MP, et al: Jewish religion and risk of breast cancer, *Lancet* 347(9016):1645–1646, 1996.

Ehman JW, Ott BB, Short TH, et al: Do patients want physicians to inquire about their spiritual or religious beliefs if they become gravely ill, *Arch Intl Med* 159(15):1803–1806, 1999.

Enstrom JE: Cancer mortality among Mormons, *Cancer* 36(3):825–841, 1975.

Enstrom JE: Health practices and cancer mortality among active California Mormons, *J Natl Cancer Inst* 81(23):1807–1814, 1989.

Ershler WB, Sun WH, Binkley N: The role of interleukin-6 in certain age-related diseases, *Drugs Aging* 5(5):358–365, 1994.

Fawzy FI, Fawzy NW, Hyun CS, et al: Malignant melanoma: Effects of an early structured psychiatric intervention, coping, and affective state on recurrence and survival 6 years later, *Arch Gen Psychiatry* 50(9):681–689, 1993.

Fawzy FI, Kemeny ME, Fawzy NW, et al: A structured psychiatric intervention for cancer patients. II. Changes over time in immunological measures, *Arch Gen Psychiatry* 47(8):729–835, 1990.

Felten DL, Felten SY, Bellinger DL, et al: Noradrenergic sympathetic neural interactions with the immune system: Structure and function, *Immunol Rev* 100:225–260, 1987.

Folkman S: Personal control and stress and coping processes: A theoretical analysis, *Kango Kenkyu* 21(3):243–260, 1988.

Foulkes WD, Wong N, Rozen F, et al: Survival of patients with breast cancer and BRCA1 mutations, *Lancet* 351(9112):1359–1360, 1998.

Fox BH: A hypothesis about Spiegel et al.'s 1989 paper on psychosocial intervention and breast cancer survival, *Psychooncology* 7(5):361–370, 1998.

Gershoni-Baruch R, Dagan E, Kepten I, Freid G: Co-segregation of BRCA1 185delAG mutation and BRCA2 6174delT in one single family, *Eur J Cancer* 33(13):2283–2284, 1997.

Gisler RH: Stress and the hormonal regulation of the immune response in mice, *Psychother Psychosom* 23(1–6):197–208, 1974.

Hall JM, Lee MK, Newman B, et al: Linkage of early-onset familial breast cancer to chromosome 17q21, *Science* 250(4988):1684–1689, 1990.

Halstead MT, Fernsler JI: Coping strategies of long-term cancer survivors, *Cancer Nurs* 17(2):94–100, 1994.

Harris JR, Lippman ME, Morrow M, Hellman S: *Diseases of the breast*, Philadelphia, PA, 1996, Lippencott-Raven.

Harris MD, Satterly LR: The chaplain as a member of the hospice team, *Home Health Nurse* 16(9):591–593, 1998.

Hilakivi-Clarke L: Estrogens, BRCA1, and breast cancer, *Cancer Res* 60(18):4993–5001, 2000.

Hoffman FL: The cancer mortality of Amsterdam, Holland, by religious sects, *Am J Cancer* 17:142–153, 1932.

Howe HL, Wingo PA, Thun MJ, et al: The annual report to the nation on the status of cancer (1973 through 1998), featuring cancers with recent increasing trends, *J Natl Cancer Inst* 93(11):824–842, 2001.

Hummer RA, Rogers RG, Nam CB, Ellison CG: Religious involvement and U.S. adult mortality, *Demography* 36(2):273–285, 1999.

Irie M, Asami S, Nagata S, et al: Psychosocial factors as a potential trigger of oxidative DNA damage in human leukocytes, *Jpn J Cancer Res* 92(3):367–376, 2001.

Jackson AL, Loeb LA: The contribution of endogenous sources of DNA damage to the multiple mutations in cancer, *Mutat Res* 477(1–2):7–21, 2001.

Jenkins RA, Pargament KI: Cognitive appraisals in cancer patients, *Soc Sci Med* 26(6):625–633, 1998.

Johnson SC, Spilka B: Coping with breast cancer: The roles of clergy and faith, *J Relig Health* 30:21–33, 1991.

Kaczorowski JM: Spiritual well-being and anxiety in adults diagnosed with cancer, *Hosp J* 5(3–4):105–116, 1989.

Katz JL, Weiner H, Gallagher TF, Hellman L: Stress, distress, and ego defenses: Psychoendocrine response to impending breast tumor biopsy, *Arch Gen Psychiatry* 23(2):131–142, 1970.

Keller SE, Weiss JM, Schleifer SJ, et al: Suppression of immunity by stress: Effect of a graded series of stressors on lymphocyte stimulation in the rat, *Science* 213(4514):1397–1400, 1981.

Kiecolt-Glaser JK, Malarkey WB, Chee M, et al: Negative behavior during marital conflict is associated with immunological down-regulation, *Psychosom Med* 55(5):395–409, 1993.

King DE, Bushwick B: Beliefs and attitudes of hospital inpatients about faith healing and prayer, *J Fam Pract* 39(4):349–352, 1994.

King H, Locke FB: American white Protestant clergy as a low-risk population for mortality research, *J Natl Cancer Inst* 65(5):1115–1124, 1980.

Koenig HG, Cohen HJ, George LK, et al: Attendance at religious services, interleukin-6, and other biological parameters of immune function in older adults, *Int J Psychiatry Med* 27(3):233–250, 1997.

Koenig HG, McCullough ME, Larson DB: *Handbook of Religion and Health*, New York, 2001, Oxford University Press.

Koenig HG, Pargament KI, Nielsen J: Religious coping and health status in medically ill hospitalized older adults, *J Nerv Ment Dis* 186(9):513–521, 1998.

Kristeller JL, Zumbrun CS, Schilling RF: 'I would if I could': How oncologists and oncology nurses address spiritual distress in cancer patients, *Psychooncology* 8(5):451–458, 1999.

Lannin DR, Mathews HF, Mitchell J, et al: Influence of socioeconomic and cultural factors on racial differences in late-stage presentation of breast cancer, *JAMA* 279(22):1801–1807, 1998.

Levy SM, Herberman RB, Lippman M, et al: Immunological and psychosocial predictors of disease recurrence in patients with early-stage breast cancer, *Behav Med* 17(2):67–75, 1991.

Lo B, Quill T, Tulsky J: Discussing palliative care with patients. ACP-ASIM End-of-Life Care Consensus Panel. American College of Physicians-American Society of Internal Medicine, *Ann Intern Med* 130(9):744–749, 1999.

Lyon JL, Klauber MR, Gardner JW, Smart CR: Cancer incidence in Mormons and non-Mormons in Utah, 1966–1970, *N Eng J Med* 294(3):129–133, 1976.

Lutgendorf S: IL-6 level, stress and spiritual support in older adults: Personal communication. In Koenig HG, McCullough ME, Larson DB, editors: *Handbook of religion and health*, New York, 2001, Oxford University Press.

Martin AO, Dunn JK, Simpson JL, et al: Cancer mortality in a human isolate, *J Natl Cancer Inst* 65(5):1109–1113, 1980.

McEwen BS, Biron CA, Brunson KW, et al: The role of adrenocorticoids as modulators of immune function in health and disease: neural, endocrine and immune interactions, *Brain Res Rev* 23(1–2):79–133, 1997.

Moadel A, Morgan C, Fatone A, et al: Seeking meaning and hope: Self-reported spiritual and existential needs among an ethnically-diverse cancer patient population, *Psychooncology* 8(5):378–385, 1999.

Monjan AA, Collector MI: Stress-induced modulation of the immune response, *Science* 196(4287):307–308, 1977.

Monk M, Lilienfield A, Mendeloff A: *Preliminary report of an epidemiologic study of cancers of the colon and rectum*, 1962. Paper presented at the meeting of the epidemiologic section of the American Public Health Association.

Musick MA, Koenig HG, Larson DB, Matthews D: Holland J, editor: *Textbook of psycho-oncology*, New York, 1998, Oxford University Press.

Naguib SM, Lundin FE Jr, Davis HJ: Relation of various epidemiologic factors to cervical cancer as determined by a screening program, *Obstet Gynecol* 28(4):451–459, 1966.

Newberg A, D'Aquili E, Rause V: *Why God won't go away: Brain science and the biology of belief*, New York, 2001, Ballantine.

Offit K, Gilewski T, McGuire P, et al: Germline BRCA1 185delAG mutations in Jewish women with breast cancer, *Lancet* 347(9016):1643–1645, 1996.

Ogata A, Ideda M, Kuratsune MB: Mortality among Japanese Zen priests, *J Epidemiol Community Health* 38:161–166, 1984.

Pargament KI, Kennell J, Hathaway W, et al: Religion and the problem solving process: three styles of coping, *J Sci Study Relig* 27:90–104, 1988.

Pargament KI, Koenig HG, Tarakeshwar N, Hahn J: Religious struggle as a predictor of mortality among medically ill elderly patients: A 2-year longitudinal study, *Arch Intern Med* 161(15):1881–1885, 2001.

Phillips RL, Kuzma JW, Beeson WL, Lotz T: Influence of selection versus lifestyle on risk of fatal cancer and cardiovascular disease among Seventh-day Adventists, *Am J Epidemiol* 112(2):296–314, 1980.

Post SG, Puchalski CM, Larson DB: Physicians and patient spirituality: Professional boundaries, competency, and ethics, *Ann Intern Med* 132(7):578–583, 2000.

Puchalski CM: Taking a spiritual history: FICA, *Spiritual Med Connect* 3(1):1999.

Raleigh ED: Sources of hope in chronic illness, *Oncol Nurs Forum* 19(3):443–448, 1992.

Rassnick S, Sved AF, Rabin BS: Locus coeruleus stimulation by corticotropin-releasing hormone suppresses in vitro cellular immune responses, *J Neurosci* 10:6033–6040, 1994.

Reite M, Harbeck R, Hoffman A: Altered cellular immune response following peer separation, *Life Sci* 29(11):1133–1136, 1981.

Reite M, Short R, Kaufman IC, et al: Heart rate and body temperature in separated monkey infants, *Biol Psychiatry* 13(1):91–105, 1978.

Reynolds P, Kaplan GA: Social connections and risk for cancer: Prospective evidence from the Alameda County Study, *Behav Med* 16(3):101–110, 1990.

Roberts JA, Brown D, Elkins T, Larson DB: Factors influencing views of patients with gynecologic cancer about end-of-life decisions, *Am J Obstet Gynecol* 176(1 Pt 1):166–172, 1997.

Robson M, Levin D, Federici M, et al: Breast conservation therapy for invasive breast cancer in Ashkenazi women with BRCA gene founder mutations, *J Natl Cancer Inst* 91(24):2112–2117, 1999.

Schaal MD, Sephton SE, Thoreson C, et al: *Religious expression and immune competence in women with advanced cancer*, San Francisco, 1998. Presented at the meeting of the American Psychological Association.

Schleifer SJ, Keller SE, Camerino M, et al: Suppression of lymphocyte stimulation following bereavement, *JAMA* 250(3):374–377, 1983.

Sephton SE, Koopman C, Schaal M: Spiritual expression and immune status in women with metastatic breast cancer: An exploratory study, *Breast J* 7:345–353, 2001.

Shekelle RB, Raynor WJ Jr, Ostfeld AM, et al: Psychological depression and 17-year risk of death from cancer, *Psychosom Med* 43(2):117–125, 1981.

Simpson JL, Martin AO, Elias S, et al: Cancers of the breast and female genital system: Search for recessive genetic factors through analysis of human isolate, *Am J Obstet Gynecol* 141(6):629–636, 1981.

Sodestrom KE, Martinson IM: Patients' spiritual coping strategies: a study of nurse and patient perspectives, *Oncol Nurs Forum* 14(2):41–46, 1987.

Spiegel D, Bloom JR, Kraemer HC, Gottheil E: Effect of psychosocial treatment on survival of patients with metastatic breast cancer, *Lancet* 2(8668):888–891, 1989.

Steinberg AG, Bleibtreu HK, Kurczynski TW, Kurczynski EM: Genetic studies on an inbred human isolate. In Crow JF, Neel JV, editors: *Proceedings of the third national congress of human genetics*, Baltimore, 1967, Johns Hopkins University Press.

Steinberg KK, Pernarelli JM, Marcus M, et al: Increased risk for familial ovarian cancer among Jewish women: A population-based case-control study, *Genet Epidemiol* 15(1):51–59, 1998.

Taylor RS, Carroll BE, Lloyd JW: Mortality among women in 3 Catholic religious orders with special reference to cancer, *Cancer* 12:1207–1225, 1959.

Toniolo PG, Kato I: Jewish religion and risk of breast cancer, *Lancet* 348(9029):760, 1996.

Torbjornsen T, Stifoss-Hanssen H, Abrahamsen AF, Hannisdal E: Cancer and religiosity—A follow up of patients with Hodgkin's disease, *Tidsskr Nor Laegeforen* 120(3):346–348, 2000.

Underwood R: The presence of God in pastoral care ministry, *Austin Pres Theol Sem Bulletin* 61(4):7, 1985.

Ur E, White PD, Grossman A: Hypothesis: Cytokines may be activated to cause depressive illness and chronic fatigue syndrome, *Eur Arch Psychiatry Clin Neurosci* 241(5):317–322, 1992.

Wolbarst AL: Circumcision and penile cancer in men, *Lancet* 1:150–153, 1932.

Wolff G: Cancer and race with special reference to the Jews, *Am J Hyg* 29:121–137, 1939.

Wynder EL, Lemon FR, Bross IJ: Cancer and coronary artery disease among Seventh-Day Adventists, *Cancer* 12:1016–1028, 1959.

Zisook S, Shuchter SR, Irwin M, et al: Bereavement, depression, and immune function, *Psychiatry Res* 52(1):1–10, 1994.

Suggested Readings

Fahey JL: A structured psychiatric intervention for cancer patients. II. Changes over time in immunological measures, *Arch Gen Psychiatry* 47(8):729–735, 1990.

Gallup G: Americans more religious now than ten years ago, but less so than in 1950s and 1960s. March, *Gallup News Serv* 2001.

Hojat M, Gonnella JS, Mangione K, et al: Physician empathy in medical education and practice, *Semin Integr Med* 1(1):25–41, 2003.

Jawer M, Micozzi MS: *The Spiritual Anatomy of Emotion*, Rochester VT, 2009, Park Street Press/Inner Traditions.

Jawer M, Micozzi MS: *Your Emotional Type*, Rochester, 2011, Healing Arts Press/Inner Traditions.

Marchbanks PA: Increased risk for familial ovarian cancer among Jewish women: A population-based case-control study, *Genet Epidemiol* 15(1):51–59, 1998.

Mayor D: Elemental souls and vernacular: Some attributes of what moves us. In Mayor D, Micozzi MS, editors: *Energy Medicine East and West*, Edinburgh & London, 2011, Churchill Livingstone/Elsevier, pp 23–48.

McCown DM, Reibel D, Micozzi MS: *Teaching Mindfulness*, New York NY, 2009, Springer.

McCown DM, Micozzi MS: *New World Mindfulness*, 2011, Healing Arts Press/Inner Traditions.

Micozzi MS: *Celestial Healing*, London, 2011, Singing Dragon Press.

Micozzi MS, McCown DM: *Vital Healing*, London, 2011, Singing Dragon Press.

Schlitz M, Amorok T, Micozzi MS: *Consciousness & Healing*, St Louis, 2005, Elsevier.

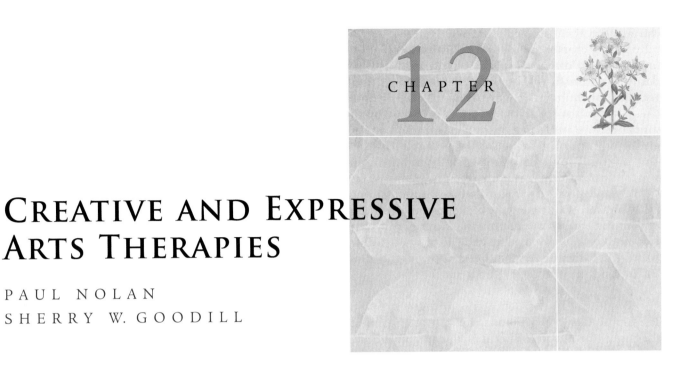

CHAPTER 12

CREATIVE AND EXPRESSIVE ARTS THERAPIES

PAUL NOLAN
SHERRY W. GOODILL

This chapter describes arts-based approaches to health care. The creative arts therapies—specifically art, dance/ movement, drama/psychodrama, music, and poetry therapies—are each separate arts-based integrative medicine health care disciplines. The chapter also discusses expressive arts therapy and the *arts in health care* movement as additional approaches involving the arts within a health care system or environment. The term *creative arts therapy* refers to an arts-based therapy performed by a credentialed creative arts therapist under the auspices of the national organization representing that treatment modality.

A creative arts therapist demonstrates aesthetic competencies in his or her respective arts modality (i.e., art, dance, music) and has received extensive education and training in that art form prior to entering into study and clinical training in one of the creative arts therapies. Expressive arts therapists use "the expressive art—movement, art, music, writing, sound and improvisation—in a supportive setting to facilitate growth and healing" (Rogers, 1993). Expressive arts therapists use any of these arts in varying sequences in order to express the emotional and intuitive aspects of the self. Expressive arts therapists can become registered practitioners but are not required to demonstrate artistic ability in any of the arts. *Arts in health care* is a multidisciplinary global movement with aim to promote the integration of arts into several aspects of patient care and health care systems.

The chapter covers professional, theoretical, clinical, and research areas, providing brief descriptions and discussing similarities and differences between the creative arts therapies, expressive arts therapy, and the arts in health care.

ARTS IN HEALTH CARE, EXPRESSIVE ART THERAPY, AND CREATIVE ARTS THERAPIES

The creative arts therapies, expressive arts therapy, and arts in health care are all established approaches that invoke the therapeutic uses of the arts. Various professionals and authors use these three terms interchangeably, if not precisely. It is important to understand the differences in their purposes and the ways in which they are used. Many titles and terms are used in relation to the arts within the health care arena. These include *arts therapies, expressive arts therapies, therapeutic arts, creative arts therapy* (or *creative arts in therapy*), *expressive therapies, arts psychotherapy,* and *arts in health care* to name a few. Until the mid-1990s many of these terms had been used interchangeably by many in the health care communities. Over time the differences were reflected in the education and training programs, professional qualifications, and literature. The separateness between the creative arts therapies and the expressive arts therapies approaches became most apparent. This difference was manifested by a more consistent distinction in the use of the two titles "creative arts therapist" and "expressive therapist/expressive arts therapist." However, the term *expressive therapy* occasionally appears in the psychotherapy literature without a connection to any of the arts. Unfortunately, Internet sites such as Wikipedia undo any attempts at clarity by jumbling up these terms into an interchangeable and incorrect muddle.

The creative arts therapies are distinguished from expressive arts therapy and arts in health care, two other established approaches that invoke the therapeutic uses of the arts. For example, Levine and Levine (1999), in their introductory chapter to the book *The Foundations of Expressive Arts Therapy*, describe expressive arts therapy as growing out of the expressive therapy movement in the 1970s to establish a multimodal use of the arts in healing as an alternative to the single arts modality employed by the various creative arts therapy disciplines. Malchiodi (2005), on the other hand, 6 years later in her book, *Expressive Therapies*, refers to the creative arts therapies with expressive arts therapy (formerly called expressive therapies) collectively as *expressive therapies*. This merging of distinct disciplines into the single *expressive therapies* identifier continues to be a reality for educators, health care administrators, and consumers, but differences in their education/ training, accreditation/registration, and scope of practice and methods are important to understand.

ARTS IN HEALTH CARE

The Global Alliance for Arts and Health (GAAH; formerly the Society for Arts in Healthcare) promotes the growing multidisciplinary field of arts in health care as an umbrella for the many disciplines that are concerned with the intersection of arts and health care systems. According to the GAAH, there are five loci: patient care; caregiver support; community well-being; the education of health care professionals about the arts; and creation of healing environments (Global Alliance for Arts and Health, 2011). The first three of these have potential overlap with the expressive arts therapy and the creative arts therapies. Specifically, *arts in health care* includes the work of artists in any form who provide performances, classes, and supportive experiences to patients and their caregivers in health care or community settings (see Chapter 4). Training for work as an artist in health care is currently unregulated and within the offerings there is a wide range in-depth and length of study. Programs are currently usually offered in certificate programs, although university degree programs exist and are growing in number. The GAAH has published the international peer-reviewed journal *Arts & Health* since 2009. There is a broad range of research occurring in the arts in health care spectrum, examples of which will be discussed in this chapter.

It is important to be clear about scope of practices. Including the arts in medical settings has proven attractive to various health care professionals, including physicians, nurses, and occupational therapists, among others, who refer to their own use of music, art, poetry, or dance/ movement as "therapy." For example, the nursing literature, in particular, contains published reports of many studies in which recorded music was played to achieve a temporary therapeutic effect. This practice is frequently incorrectly labeled as *music therapy* in that it falls outside of the established definition and ethical practice of music therapy and is used by a non-credentialed artist.

These types of uses of an art form may have positive effects, and the research reports are helpful. However, the good intentions of the practitioner may result in a negative effect as well. Every person has a highly personal, subjective response to the arts and develops mental associations that can trigger powerful emotional responses. A health care worker untrained in the psychological effects of the arts may rely on his or her own preferences or personal beliefs in presenting arts experiences to health care consumers. It is not unusual for a well-intentioned health care worker to present an arts experience to an unattended seriously ill patient only to have the result be a more anxious or, worse yet, confused and disoriented patient. Patients in medical settings who have anxiety-producing medical problems are sometimes unable to defend against the unexpected emotionally overwhelming experience induced by arts stimuli, especially if the patient is left alone during the arts experience (Nolan, 2006). The use of the arts stimulus by a credentialed creative arts therapist allows for modulation and modification of the arts depending on treatment goals and patient response.

EXPRESSIVE ARTS THERAPY

Expressive therapy is a term that is continuing to evolve and broaden from its original usage in the 1960s, developed by Natalie Rogers. Initially the term implied the multiple use of various arts by an expressive therapist, for human growth. In 1994, the term changed to *expressive arts therapy*, retaining its emphasis on a practitioner's use of multiple art forms. The International Expressive Arts Therapy Association (IEATA; www.ieata.org) website defines the expressive arts therapy as: "The expressive arts combine the visual arts, movement, drama, music, writing and other creative processes to foster deep personal growth and community development. IEATA encourages an evolving multimodal approach within psychology, organizational development, community arts and education. By integrating the arts processes and allowing one to flow into another, we gain access to our inner resources for healing, clarity, illumination and creativity."

THE CREATIVE ARTS THERAPIES

Theoretical Foundations

Creative arts therapists incorporate art products into the therapeutic relationship and rely on the client's inner process of creativity and art making in relation to the client's developmental level and clinical needs. Nolan, in a 1989 unpublished manuscript, identified the following as some of the commonalities within the different creative arts therapies. They all:

- Have ancient roots and have been used as part of health care since antiquity.
- Use esthetically guided arts experiences within a clinically structured therapeutic relationship, informed by systematic assessment, to invoke a wide range of physical, psychological, and spiritual responses in the client.
- Rely on nonverbal and verbal processes.
- Use imagery, associations, metaphor, symbolization, and affective and body processes.

- Use the arts to stimulate unconscious processes.
- Use, promote, and nurture creative processes.
- Follow clinical guidelines, codes of ethics, and educational requirements of a governing body.
- Work as either primary or adjunctive therapies.

It is important to note that clinical work in the creative arts therapies is far from strictly nonverbal. Poetry, drama therapy, and psychodrama focus very much on spoken or written language. Music therapy's techniques of song writing engage the "poet within" for creation of lyrics. Dance/movement therapists and art therapists engage their clients in the exchange of words and observations during the movement or art making, and also afterward. Initially, the nondiscursive use of spoken or written language is actually key to the integration of felt, sensory, *unlanguaged* arts experiences. Consequent discussion with the therapy group or with the therapist helps a patient generalize discoveries made in the creative process to everyday life and the treatment concerns that brought him or her to therapy in the first place.

Creativity is the common basis of all of the creative arts therapies. One distinction in current discussions of creativity is the differences between eminent and everyday creativity. Eminent creativity in the arts and sciences leaves a lasting mark and influence on a culture (Simonton, 2010). Everyday creativity (Runco & Richards, 1998), defined as original and meaningful, is related to improved psychological and physical health. Everyday creativity is applied in problem solving, from creating a meal to solving an interpersonal problem. It is generally assumed that this "distinct and independent capacity" (Runco, 2007) can be found, to a greater or lesser degree, in all humans. A general assumption of these therapies is that the activation of a client's potential for everyday creativity enhances adaptation, provides motivation, encourages the tendency toward self-actualization, and improves quality of life. Creativity is both a means for conducting therapy and a client goal. Creative arts therapists may model creativity within their own arts therapy modality, recognize and support spontaneous patient/client creative processes and behaviors, or employ arts therapy-based techniques to activate creative thinking in their patients/clients.

These therapies focus on the intrapersonal and interpersonal processes of arts expression and reception within a therapeutic relationship with a creative arts therapist. The actual art product, such as a drawing, song, or dance, although representing a client creation and a statement about the person at a given point in time, is not typically the goal in the creative arts therapies. Searle and Streng (2001) describe the use of the arts product, or artifact, in therapy to "illustrate particular feelings or dynamics, to aid verbal integration, and as tools of assessment" (p. 5). The use of an art product, such as a drawing, a musical theme or song, or a personally symbolized movement, adds a new and unique dimension to psychotherapeutic applications as a "third party" or as a bridge that connects the client's inner and outer worlds. Searle and Streng (2001) refer to a triangular relationship, in that the art product adds a third point in a client–therapist–art product triangle. This third element in therapy provides for variations in the dynamics of the therapeutic relationship, in which both participants may be active within what Winnicott (1971) conceptualized as the "potential space," or that psychic area in which subjectivity and objectivity interact.

The creative arts therapies continually deal with the relationship between "healing" and "treatment" in that they attempt to "retain the healing properties of the Creative Arts while developing a science of Arts Therapies" (Zwerling, 1984, p. 16). Zwerling disagreed that the healing function of the arts defines the creative arts therapies; he also addressed the dangers in obliterating the potential healing impact of the arts modality. In addressing their healing and treatment roles, he believed that the arts therapies needed to address the issue "How will we use the arts modalities in an organized, systematic, deliberate way to bring about change in somebody who needs change?" (p. 32).

Thus, the healing properties of the creative art therapies, in that their use "attracts that which is well within a patient" (Nolan, as cited in Pratt, 1992), may represent their short-term, or therapeutic, effect. This effect can be described as a change, usually for a short period of time, of a mental, affective, and/or physical state in the client. These changes seem to be related to the effect of the arts experience itself on the client, in the sense of the *arts as therapy* approach used by many expressive therapists, whereas the use of the arts within a therapeutic relationship to address persistent problems in living in the social, occupational, and self-esteem domains describes the arts psychotherapy model used by most creative arts therapists.

Although the arts have been described as having "healing power," the way that the arts are used within a therapeutic relationship "is a crucial factor that determines whether or not therapeutic transformation can occur" (Karkou & Sanderson, 2006, p. 53). Although one may experience a short-term, healing effect from exposure to the arts on a regular basis, within the creative arts therapies, the role of the therapeutic relationship is integral to the longer-term healing transformation, as in a psychotherapeutic effect.

In the last decade all of the creative arts therapy disciplines have been focusing theoretical, clinical, and research attention to multicultural aspects of the work, including a special issue of the *Arts in Psychotherapy* journal devoted to social justice (Sajnani & Kaplan, 2012). One transition is that arts expressions, once romanticized as "the universal" languages, are now understood as highly inflected with cultural identity, norms, and values. Accordingly, most creative arts therapy education and training now includes coursework and experiences that encourage awareness of self and others from a multicultural standpoint, as well as knowledge and skills for using the arts media in culturally sensitive ways.

To place the creative arts therapies in the context of complementary and alternative medicine (CAM), one may look back to the early 1990s, when Congress mandated that the National Institutes of Health establish the Office of Alternative Medicine (OAM; now the National Center for Complementary and Alternative Medicine, or NCCAM). The creative arts therapies were listed under the mind–body intervention category (just as they appear in the mind–body section of this text, although this text does not generally follow the bureaucratic taxonomy of the National Institutes of Health), and the inaugural round of field investigations funded by the OAM included two creative arts therapy studies (see Goodill, 2005a). Today, there is a resurgence of interest in the creative arts therapies, especially in the complementary and integrative medicine arena, evidenced by scholarly contributions and research funding announcements from the NCCAM that include the creative arts therapies.

Each creative arts therapy specialty has organized itself professionally with its own educational standards, credentials, codes of ethics, and standards of practice, research, and scholarship. All provide continuing education to members and interested others through national and regional conferences and, increasingly, through online formats. Currently, creative arts therapists are licensed in many states under various mental health titles, including Licensed Professional Counselor, Licensed Mental Health Counselor and Licensed Creative Arts Therapist, and occasionally with discipline-specific licensure titles.

The following sections summarize the state of the various fields from an organizational standpoint. Specific information about training and credentials is provided to assist the reader who seeks clinical services, consultation, education, training, or collaboration with a creative arts therapist. The information provided here covers the predominant groups in the United States. All six of the identified creative arts therapies are international in scope as well, with lively collegial and interdisciplinary networking.

American Dance Therapy Association

The American Dance Therapy Association (ADTA; www.adta.org) is the primary national organization for dance/movement therapy. The entry-level degree for dance/movement therapy, also known as dance therapy, is the master's degree. Established in 1966, the ADTA confers professional credentials in a two-tiered system: the R-DMT (Registered Dance/Movement Therapist) for clinicians with new master's degrees, and the BC-DMT (Board Certified Dance/Movement Therapist) for advanced clinicians, supervisors, and instructors of dance/movement therapy. The Dance/Movement Therapy Certification Board upholds the standards for these clinical credentials. The ADTA upholds educational standards in masters programs through its regulatory Committee on Approval. The *American Journal of Dance Therapy,* a peer-reviewed journal, has been in regular publication since 1977.

American Art Therapy Association

The American Art Therapy Association (AATA; www.arttherapy.org) was established in 1969. As with dance/movement therapy, a master's degree is required for entry into the field of art therapy. At career entry, art therapists are credentialed with the designation ATR (Art Therapist Registered), and the Art Therapy Certification Board conducts examination-based certification to confer the designation ATR-BC (Art Therapist Registered–Board Certified) on advanced practitioners. Educational programs are regulated by AATA's Education Program Approval Board, and *Art Therapy: Journal of the American Art Therapy Association* publishes peer-reviewed articles.

American Music Therapy Association

The American Music Therapy Association (AMTA; www.musictherapy.org) is now the predominant professional organization for music therapy. The field of music therapy was organized in the United States with the founding of the National Association of Music Therapy in 1950 and the American Association of Music Therapy in 1971. The merger of these in 1998 formed AMTA, which publishes two peer-reviewed journals, the research-oriented *Journal of Music Therapy* and the practice-oriented *Music Therapy Perspectives.*

Music therapists can obtain practice credentials with a bachelor's degree and can sit for the certification examination given by the Certification Board for Music Therapists. Board-certified music therapists are so designated with the MT-BC (Music Therapist-Board Certified) credential. A graduate degree in music therapy provides for more advanced levels of practice. Doctorate degrees that are field specific are just beginning to develop.

National Association for Poetry Therapy

The National Association for Poetry Therapy (NAPT; www.poetrytherapy.org), incorporated in 1981, defines poetry therapy as "the interactive use of literature and/or writing to promote growth and healing" and uses the umbrella term *poetry therapy* to encompass related modalities, including applied poetry facilitation, journal therapy, bibliotherapy, biblio/poetry therapy, and poetry/journal therapy. Preparation of poetry therapists is regulated by the National Federation for Biblio/Poetry Therapy and is not degree based, but emphasizes specific didactic and supervisory plans of study with practical training. There are separate requirements and credentials for those with a bachelor's degree (the Certified Applied Poetry Facilitator, or CAPF) and those with a mental health master's degree (the Certified Poetry Therapist, or CPT). Requirements include knowledge of psychology, group dynamics, and literature, among other topics. The NAPT also publishes the *Journal of Poetry Therapy: The Interdisciplinary Journal of Practice, Theory, Research and Education.*

North American Drama Therapy Association

Although drama therapy and psychodrama are often combined in the literature and sometimes in practice, they are distinct disciplines. Each has unique training standards and credentialing bodies, and each is organized by a different professional association. Drama therapy has been defined as the "intentional and systematic use of drama/theater processes to achieve psychological growth and change" (Emunah, 1994, p. 3).

The North American Drama Therapy Association (NADTA; http://www.nadta.org) incorporated in 1979 and has since maintained standards of professional competence in this discipline. Drama therapy training requires a master's or doctoral degree, either in drama therapy or in another related area. A handful of drama therapy graduate degree programs exist, but drama therapists also train through institute and individual plans of study regulated by the NADTA. The NADTA maintains a professional registry and, at the time of writing this chapter, the NADTA is in the process of developing a certification examination. Drama therapy literature is found in various publications, including the journals *Dramatherapy* and *The Arts in Psychotherapy*. A peer-reviewed journal is currently in development.

American Society of Group Psychotherapy and Psychodrama

The American Society of Group Psychotherapy and Psychodrama (ASGPP) is the main professional organization for those who practice psychodrama in the United States. Psychodrama has its roots in the seminal work of J.L. Moreno and encompasses the use of the therapeutic structures of psychodrama (in which the scene is developed around the needs of an individual) and sociodrama (in which the focus is on the needs and understanding of the group). Training (chiefly institute based) is regulated by the American Board of Examiners in Psychodrama, Sociometry and Group Psychotherapy, with a master's degree required along with specific didactic and practical education in psychodrama. Certification in psychodrama is two tiered with the designations Certified Practitioner (CP) for beginning clinicians and Trainer, Educator, Practitioner (TEP) for advanced practitioners. The peer-reviewed *Journal of Group Psychotherapy, Psychodrama and Sociometry* is one venue for literature in this specialty.

National Coalition of Creative Arts Therapies Associations

The National Coalition of Creative Arts Therapies Associations (NCCATA; www.nccata.org), as an alliance of associations, has joined the aforementioned six creative arts therapy specialties together for the primary purpose of educating the public and governmental entities about the creative arts therapies (lobbying for more government funding and public relations). In terms of scholarship, the journal *Arts in Psychotherapy* publishes research, theory, and clinical practice pieces in all of these disciplines.

Although many creative arts therapists have doctoral-level preparation, doctoral education is not regulated in these professions. A handful of doctoral programs do exist, and because these programs generate scholarship and

research, they are critical to the viability of these professions. NCCATA was founded in 1979 as an alliance of the creative arts therapy professional associations and represents over 15,000 individual members of six creative arts therapies associations nationwide. The creative arts therapy members include music therapy, art therapy, dance/movement therapy, drama therapy, poetry therapy, and psychodrama.

CLINICAL AND RESEARCH LITERATURE

This section provides a survey of the clinical and research literature in the creative arts therapies, arts in health care, and expressive arts therapy to illustrate the range of work. The four categories used here are something of a contrivance. Patterns of comorbidity among physical and psychological disorders are many, and distinctions among domains of functioning, treatment settings, and diagnoses are influenced by culture, public policy, institutional structures, and local and regional systems. We have selected four areas of recent concern in the society: trauma, behavioral and psychosocial problems in children and teens, mental illness, and applications in medical settings. Patients' names, when used in vignettes, are pseudonyms.

TRAUMA AND POST-TRAUMATIC STRESS DISORDER

Johnson (2009) reports that creative arts therapies have been applied to the treatment of acute trauma, specifically in accessing memories of the trauma or the abuse, treating chronic post-traumatic stress disorder (PTSD), and performing cross-cultural interventions with survivors of war, torture, and disasters. From a theoretical standpoint, in relation to alexithymia (a frequent problem for traumatized individuals), Miller and Johnson (2011) found that in participants with PTSD, the capacity for symbolic representation was higher and the capacity for lexical (verbal) representation lower, when compared to participants without PTSD. Extrapolating from this evidence, clinical methods of assessment and treatment that employ symbolic mental imagery and nonverbal forms of representation (e.g., the creative arts therapists) would reach for the strengths of those with trauma and enable the necessary expression of feelings, thoughts, and experiences.

Significant reduction of PTSD symptoms and reduced frequency of nightmares were reported by Morgan and Johnson (1995).

Art therapy was found to be the most effective treatment for veterans with PTSD symptoms in a single-session design in which art therapy was 1 of 15 treatment components in an inpatient PTSD program. Art therapy produced significant short-term symptom reduction and lowered distress, possibly related to the focus of attention onto interpersonal or external stimuli, which allowed traumatic material to be processed differently than through verbal means (Johnson et al, 1997). Art therapy has also been used to treat individuals who have experienced mass trauma. One example is the work of Gonzalez-Dolginko (2002), which had a community focus, after the attack on the World Trade Center in New York City.

Music therapy approaches to trauma include music therapist Austin's vocal holding (Austin, 2001, 2002) and vocal psychotherapy (Austin, 2007b) for adult survivors of sexual and physical assault and abuse, and trauma by neglect. Austin (2007a) also describes an approach used with adolescents who were victims of childhood trauma such as physical, sexual, or emotional abuse, which for many continued in the foster homes. As a result, these adolescents have great difficulty trusting others and forming attachments. They often suffer from intense feelings of anxiety, rage, and depression. Unconsciously they may blame themselves for the situation in which they find themselves. Listening to music, singing, writing songs, and playing improvised music proved effective in facilitating self-expression and nonviolent communication and in creating a safe and playful environment in which relationships could grow and community could flourish.

Amir (2004) used music therapy improvisational methods with adult survivors of childhood sexual abuse. She described a case involving 2 years of therapy with a 32-year-old woman who had difficulty in making and keeping relationships as an adult. Music therapy improvisation was used to develop a supportive therapeutic relationship in which the client was able to re-create memories and gain mastery over the abuse within the musical improvisations.

Loewy and Frisch Hara (2002) edited a book describing a 9-week program that combined music psychotherapy and trauma training used in New York City after the terrorist attacks of September 11, 2001. The book presented several music therapy approaches by various authors that were used to help individuals coping with the events and aftermath of a traumatic experience. Reports of working with a self-selected group of adult caregivers seeking support in dealing with their experiences of the traumatic events of 9/11 stressed the roles of music and music therapy in encouraging self-care.

Lang and McInerney (2002) described a different experience in trauma therapy, working in a postwar environment at the Pavarotti Music Center in Bosnia–Herzegovina. They found that many of their clients "did not have the words to say what was clearly expressed through the nonverbal medium of music" (p. 172). The clients were able to re-experience the feelings associated with the traumatic events of war that they had witnessed. The music making served as a support for their feelings, which led to an acknowledgment and acceptance. The therapists observed that, over time, their clients were able gradually to retake control over some aspects of their lives.

Mills and Daniluk (2002) conducted a phenomenological investigation of the experience of five women, all of whom were sexually abused as girls and had been treated using dance/movement therapy for issues related to that early abuse. The researchers were interested in the women's own perceptions of how dance/movement therapy may have played a role in their psychological healing. The six themes that emerged from analysis of in-depth interviews about the therapy were that women felt a sense of *struggle* in the therapy (vulnerability, challenge, discomfort, and efforts to keep from being overwhelmed) yet also reported a sense of *spontaneity, freedom,* and *permission to play;* a sense of *intimate connection* with others; and a *reconnection to their own bodies* as a result of the dance/movement therapy experience. A direct quote captures one participant's appreciation of the mind–body integrative aspect of this modality: "Dance therapy was one of the first experiences of discovering how much was stored in my body . . . I discovered that there were whole aspects of my body and my experiences that I hadn't gone into . . . it was a powerful way of getting connected to myself" (p. 80).

Gray (2001) presented a case study of dance/movement therapy with an adult survivor of political torture. The story of the therapy, 19 individual sessions given over 6 months, is an impressive narrative of healing and courage. The patient, Rita, began with symptoms of PTSD and in the context of the psychotherapeutic relationship explored her emotional pain, sense of helplessness and disconnection, body-level trauma, depression, and shame. Using images arising from the bodily felt experience, symbolization in posture and gesture, integration of verbal and nonverbal expression, and "titration" of the intensity and pace of the work (p. 35), the therapist guided Rita's recall of the traumatic events, the rebuilding of a capacity to trust, and the rekindling of a will to live. With this, many of the crippling symptoms of PTSD subsided.

Harris (2007) reported two group case studies of dance/movement therapy with children traumatized by war. In the first, he developed culturally sensitive dance groups for teens who had been among the Lost Boys of Sudan and had resettled in the United States. In the second, dance/movement therapy was the primary method used in psychosocial rehabilitation of adolescent boys who had been conscripted as child soldiers in the civil war in Sierra Leone. In both groups, Harris demonstrated through detailed and vivid descriptions of therapeutic methods and patient responses how the integrated focus of dance/movement therapy on embodiment, creativity, and group process brought about healing and recovery for these young people.

Johnson's seminal work in drama therapy for survivors of trauma has focused largely on the needs and treatment of combat veterans. The increasing incidence of PTSD among men and women returning from combat zones has become a growing challenge to the public health care system in the United States. The clinical discoveries made by Johnson and his colleagues constitute an effective way to address the complex ways that trauma interferes with functioning (James & Johnson, 1997). The intensity of the war experience is brought home in the intensity of residual memories—feelings that are difficult to access, much less express verbally. The drama therapy creates a theater in which the stark reality can be visited from a psychologically safer distance in role playing, character, and symbols.

It is key, the authors emphasize, that drama therapists working with this population "preserve the play space, that is, the sense that the group exists within an imaginary, pretend environment in which feelings can be played out" (James & Johnson, 1997, p. 385). In this space, in which reality is suspended briefly, the feelings emerge and are examined as patients move through what the authors term "developmental transformations." There are three necessary and sequential phases to this treatment: the acknowledgment and expression of anger; the working through of shame; and, finally, the cultivation of an empathic stance toward others. Working through the anger and shame phases may involve actions and interactions that recall unspeakable events, and the therapist must be prepared to work with the passion and the imagery that the veterans carry in to the treatment sessions.

As one group entered into the empathic phase, the image of a cauldron formed, and into it the men threw "hate, anger, fear, shame, guilt, sadness and regret" (p. 392). They chanted and stirred the pot until the imaginary substance from the pot splatted out like clay, and the concomitant emotion was labeled "shame." Under the improvisatory guidance of the therapist, the clay was formed into a person, dubbed "Being," who spoke through the voices of the men in the group, confessing to the atrocities of war. As Being was joined in exclaiming "We have killed! We have all killed! You are not alone!" (p. 393), the men joined each other in weeping and holding. At that point, without the veil of the role or the imaginal, the therapist could support the group members in open interaction focused on sharing one another's pain and burdens. Following this they discussed the process verbally, wrote in their journals, and made the first steps toward translating the gains made through symbols and imagery into their behavioral repertoires and everyday relationships. This example, given here in condensed form, shows vividly how the drama-related methods bring the internal experience out and into a social context where is it accessible to group therapeutic and healing processes.

After the horrific massacre at Columbine High School in Colorado, poetry therapist Catherine O'Neill Thorn and several colleagues worked with surviving students at Columbine. The outpouring of emotion, shaped by the teens' resilient and inherent aesthetic sense in the context of a psychologically safe group writing environment, yielded a collection of heart-wrenching yet beautiful poetry, *Screams Aren't Enough* (O'Neill Thorn, 1999). More importantly, the teens involved show through their poetry how their process of healing evolved from pure shock to anger and confusion to a search for faith in the face of pain in the world. This collection of poetry by four of the young women in their project attests to the healing power of expressive writing and the poetry form. One excerpt, from a poem by Jocelyn Heckler, age 16, brings this to life (p. 24):

As I lay my head down
I feel the brisk coolness of crisp sheets
Surround my body
And, as I feel the heat from my body
Flowing to make my bed of equal warmth
I remember that I am alive. . . . And in the deepest void
    of darkness
I take refuge in the melodious song
Of my pen scratching paper
As it creates a masterpiece of words
And I remember
that I am alive.

Lai (2011) published an expressive arts therapy approach that combined artistic creation, psychodrama techniques, and a concluding ceremony for mothers and children who were traumatized survivors of domestic violence. The approach was adapted for the Chinese culture. This approach allows for a preparation of the clients to participate in a four-step model through creating art productions of personal strengths. Then participants used sociodrama and drawings that explored the traumatic aspects of domestic violence. Further stems help to transform their perceptions toward a new family outlook.

CHILDREN AND ADOLESCENTS

This section includes creative art therapy work with children and adolescents conducted in both clinical mental health and educational settings.

A study by Harvey (1989) with a repeated measures design investigated the use of art therapy, music therapy, and dance/movement therapy in a classroom-based program intended to provide affective education. Specific goals were to enhance self-concept, creative thinking, intrinsic motivation, and reading comprehension in a sample of second- and fourth-graders ($n = 58$). Creative arts therapists trained in each of the three disciplines worked together in 30-minute sessions held twice weekly for 12 weeks. Standardized measures were used to assess each target area of child functioning, and statistically significant increases in reading comprehension ($p = 0.000$), verbal originality ($p = 0.014$), and figural creative originality ($p = 0.023$) were seen after intervention. Additional analysis led the researcher to conclude that "interventions designed specifically to address persona/social affective conflict produce positive gains in creative thinking and school achievement" (p. 98) and that "young students can become aware of their creative abilities and can begin to relate their perceptions of mastery, challenge, and cognitive competency to these creative abilities following the use of creative arts therapies" (p. 98).

Hervey and Kornblum (2006) published a mixed-method program evaluation of Kornblum's (2002) dance/movement therapy curriculum "Disarming the Playground: Violence Prevention Through Movement and Prosocial Skills." The program served 56 children in three second-grade classrooms, 33% to 50% of whom had special needs or were identified as at risk. Children received weekly group sessions of 45 minutes for one-half, three-quarters, or a full school year, depending on the classroom. Mean scores on the Behavior Rating Index for Children, an assessment scale completed by the classroom teachers, showed significant decreases in problematic behaviors over the year that the program was given ($p = 0.002$). The children themselves described their gains from the program in terms of the pro-social skills that they continued to use independently, at home and in school. These included the skills of ignoring, making "I" statements, slowing and calming oneself, moving away or leaving a tense or provocative situation, and using the "Four Bs," a simple sequence for interrupting escalating energy and reorienting (Hervey & Kornblum, 2006, p. 125). It is notable that these outcomes are the result of a body-centered intervention using creative movement and dance therapy methods.

In their evaluation of a mixed-method violence prevention program, Koshland & Wittaker (2004) reported on a 12-week dance/movement therapy intervention used with a sample of 54 children. At the end of the dance/movement therapy program, statistically significant decreases were seen in the incidence of several problem behaviors among children participating in the program: instigating fights ($p = 0.041$), failing to calm down ($p = 0.029$), being short tempered and quick to anger ($p = 0.017$), throwing articles ($p = 0.041$), becoming upset when something desired could not be done immediately ($p = 0.029$), and acting aggravated or abusive when frustrated ($p = 0.048$). The number of aggressive incidents that were reported to the principal's office decreased significantly more in the group undergoing the dance/movement therapy program than among children in the same school who did not participate in the program ($p < 0.001$).

The role theory that informs drama therapy has been articulated by Landy et al (2003) as follows:

> Role is a set of archetypal qualities representing one aspect of a person, an aspect that relates to others and when taken together, provides a meaningful and coherent view of self . . . A human personality, in turn, is essentially an amalgamation of the roles a person takes on and plays out. According to role theory human beings are motivated to seek balance among their often discrepant roles. Implicit here is the notion that humans have access to an internal system of roles and that they may call upon those roles as they are needed. (p. 152)

As in any mainstream, alternative, or complementary therapy, good practice begins with assessment. Landy's use of his Role Profile Assessment with a 13-year-old girl called Dakota shows how this unique drama therapy assessment can bring out important and previously unacknowledged concerns. In this method the client sorts a stack of 70 cards, each labeled with a role, into four stacks: "I am this," "I am not this," "I am not sure if I am this," and "I want to be this." Dakota's work in completing the assessment caused family issues to surface. A child of divorce, Dakota struggled with the role cards for Orphan and Daughter, exploring how she was indeed a biological daughter, but

felt like an orphan in relation to a mother with whom she could neither identify nor share. Working with the Sister card, she revealed a wish for someone who could experience what she did and who could understand her (Landy et al, 2003). It is well known among therapists that it is sometimes difficult to engage adolescents in the therapy process. As illustrated here, this brief drama therapy assessment can indicate clear directions for therapy in a nonthreatening manner and engage teens in exchanges about real issues in their lives.

Music therapy approaches with children with autism and a wide variety of developmental disorders were pioneered in the United States by Nordoff and Robbins (1971). Their approach and results led to the establishment of training centers on four continents. Their music-based approach was founded on the premise that all children, regardless of handicap, are musically sensitive and possess musical capabilities, which in turn can be used to promote communication and a wide range of other developmental improvements. Their work is focused largely on enhancing humanness and improving communication, and relies on clinical case studies.

Another poetry therapy program involving adolescent girls in residential mental health treatment focused on the goals of "uncovering and processing interpersonal conflict, exploring resistance to therapy, and deepening positive support among group members" (Gillespie, 2005, p. 222). Group sessions began with an affirmation of confidentiality by the group and a report by each girl on her current feeling state and any immediate concerns. "Warm-ups" focused on collaboration, with creation of a group story in which each member moved the story line forward by adding a line or two to what had come before. The story built improvisationally, and afterward the therapist helped the group discuss the story and the group or personal issues that might have arisen from the story. From collaborative story creation the group moved to collaborative poem writing, beginning with first lines provided by the therapist and elaborated by the group members as they passed the poems around and contributed line by line. In this way, the group created several poems together, then read them aloud and explored personal meanings. The therapist facilitated the linking of these responses to individual treatment objectives, helping the patients draw analogies to their lives outside the poetry sessions.

An expressive arts therapy approach referred to as group sand tray play therapy for children with mental health problems is described by Hunter (2009) for use within schools, shelters, camps, and other child-oriented locations. The approach is a group model that combines creating a "free and protected space," having the therapist witness the play, and facilitating the group toward an emphasis upon a Jungian perspective of imaginative symbolic meanings.

MENTAL HEALTH

In a contemporary biopsychosocial paradigm, mental health is an essential component of health, as in the World

Health Organization definition of health: "Health is a state of complete physical, mental and social well-being and not merely the absence of disease or infirmity." Mental health populations are the group most served by all creative arts therapy disciplines in the United States linked with their inception as health care disciplines beginning in the post–World War II era.

Art therapy has developed a wide range of clinical approaches in the treatment of mental disorders over the last four decades. In most applications art therapy is informed by psychodynamic orientations. Other orientations being developed more fully are cognitive–behavioral and humanistic perspectives. The art psychotherapy approach has been in use since the publication in 1966 of Naumburg's book on the topic, which further developed the concept that artwork contains both manifest and latent content (Naumburg, 1966). Judith Rubin (1987), Cathy Malchiodi (1990), and Helen Landgarten (1981) are some of the developers of current art therapy practice in mental health.

Dally (2008) reported on innovative uses of art therapy in a multidisciplinary team approach to work with adolescents with eating disorders and their families, using clay sculptures to depict the family. This process leads to easier and better awareness and articulation of family struggles. Also, art therapy has been used in prisons to reduce depression among inmates. In Gussak's 2007 study, a significant decrease in depression was seen among inmates participating in art therapy as measured by the Beck Depression Inventory (Gussak, 2007). This author again published (Gussak, 2009) a pre-test, post-test control group design with prisoners, this time including male ($n = 37$) and female subjects ($n = 76$) with 25 men and 20 women in the control group. In addition to significant decreases in depression scores, there were significant decreases in external locus of control for all experimental groups.

Erhardt et al (1989) conducted an interesting study involving outpatients who had been in dance/movement therapy as part of multidisciplinary treatment for chronic and persistent mental illness. Through interviews, video review, and the use of a modified Q-sort method, the interviewers were able to determine what aspects of group dance/movement therapy the patients found most beneficial. To test a theoretical model proposed by Schmais (1985) on curative factors in group dance/movement therapy, the researchers followed the well-established wisdom on the effectiveness of psychotherapy: namely, that the patient's perception of change and benefit is a strong predictor of such positive effects. Of the eight factors included—expression, rhythm, synchrony, vitalization, relaxation, exercise, music, and cohesion—patients gave the highest ranking to vitalization, defined here as "an increase of energy that mobilizes the entire body" (Erhardt et al, 1989, p. 49).

Koch et al (2007) investigated the important question of the differential benefits of a circle dance intervention, a music listening session, and exercise. This study, with a three-group repeated measures design, examined mood-related variables (depression, vitality, and affect) in a group of psychiatric patients ($n = 31$), all of whom carried some diagnosis of depression and who were assigned to one of the three treatment groups. A single session of each intervention was given under well-controlled conditions. As revealed by a comparison of scores on a self-report measure before and after the intervention, the patients in the dance group showed a significant decrease in depression compared with both the music group ($p < 0.001$) and the exercise group ($p < 0.05$), and a significant increase in vitality compared with the music group ($p < 0.05$).

A recent study by Bräuninger (2012) demonstrated the effectiveness of dance/movement therapy for stress reduction in a randomized controlled trial of 162 adults who self-assessed as suffering from stress. The multisite project administered group dance/movement therapy in ten 90-minute sessions over 3 months, and measured outcome variables with standardized instruments at pre-test, post-test and 6 months following the therapy. When compared to the control group, the intervention group showed statistically significant improvements in stress management at both post-test ($p < 0.005$) and follow-up ($p < 0.05$), with statistically significant reductions in depression, anxiety, phobic anxiety, positive symptom distress, and obsessive-compulsive behaviors at post-test (Bräuninger, 2012, pp. 447–48).

An early meta-analysis of studies of dance/movement therapy (Cruz & Sabers, 1998) showed overall effect sizes for dance/movement therapy in the moderate range, a magnitude of change similar to that reported for other approaches such as verbal psychotherapy, meditation methods, cognitive–behavioral therapy, and exercise. The Cruz and Sabers (1998) meta-analysis focused on studies with treatment outcomes addressing the variables of anxiety, depression, vitality, and self-concept in psychiatric populations. Since the publication of this meta-analysis, other studies have been completed showing benefits of this modality on various aspects of mood (see, for example, Dibbel-Hope, 2000; Erwin-Grabner et al, 1999).

One meta-analysis of the effectiveness of psychodrama techniques has been conducted (Kipper & Ritchie, 2003), and it is quite instructive. The researchers gathered data from 25 controlled trials of psychodrama sessions (including some studies of several-session courses of therapy and some of single-session exposure) representing a total combined sample size of 281 study participants. They analyzed for differential effects of four main psychodrama techniques: role reversal, doubling, role playing, and the combination of multiple techniques. The total overall adjusted median effect size for all techniques combined was 0.85, which indicates a large intervention effect, according to Cohen's benchmarks (Kipper & Ritchie, 2003, p. 19). Calculating separately the effect sizes for each of the four techniques, the researcher found that the techniques of role reversal and doubling each had large mean effect sizes, whereas the techniques of role playing and combination of multiple techniques had effect sizes in the small to moderate range (again, as defined by Cohen). Importantly, post hoc analyses revealed that these effects were as strong for mental health patients, prisoners, and special needs populations as they were for healthy participants, and that there were no differences in effect for male and female participants. This meta-analysis advanced research in the area by studying the critical question of which creative arts therapy methods are most effective with which populations.

Music therapy uses a wide range of receptive methods, including music-assisted relaxation, song lyric analysis, elicitation of mental imagery for self-management or psychotherapy, and recreational listening. Expressive methods can include singing, song writing, ensemble instrumental playing with or without singing, movement to music, action games using music, instrumental and vocal improvisation, and music composition. Individuals with mental disorders represent the largest clinical population served by music therapists around the world. Much of the literature describes clinical methods or uses case studies to illustrate how outcomes are reached. As more doctoral programs in music therapy are established, additional research designs are being developed, including designs for qualitative and quantitative outcome studies.

Gold et al (2005) compiled a Cochrane Review on the effects of music therapy in individuals with schizophrenia. For the four studies that met the inclusion criteria, they found that music therapy improved overall mental functioning and reduced negative symptoms, which are usually medication resistant. In their Cochrane abstract, they state, "Music therapy as an addition to standard care helps people with schizophrenia to improve their global state and may also improve mental state and functioning if a sufficient number of music therapy sessions are provided. Further research should address the dose effect relationship and the long-term effects of music therapy."

Music therapy approaches using live (expressive or active) and recorded (receptive) music to help individuals with eating disorders have been developed incorporating a wide range of psychotherapeutic perspectives, including ego psychology (Nolan, 1989a, 1989b), psychodrama (Parente, 1989a, 1989b), object relations (Robarts & Sloboda, 1994), behavior therapy (Justice, 1994), Jungian psychology (Sloboda, 1995), and modified cognitive-behavioral approaches (Hilliard, 2001).

In a randomized study, Perez et al (2010) compared the effects of music therapy and psychotherapy in a group of subjects with low and medium levels of depression from a city in Mexico. The authors based their research "on the fact that music can stimulate and activate signal pathways, which can, in turn, modulate chemical mediators; thus facilitating recovery from depression or diminishing its symptoms" (p 388). The music therapy sessions consisted of a receptive approach during which 50 minutes of music from the baroque and classical periods were used in

self-administrations at the subjects' ($n = 41$) homes, with one of the sessions taking place in a group setting at the clinic. Between the seventh and eighth weekly sessions, improvement in the scores on the Hamilton Depression Scale were observed in 29 participants, with a lack of improvement in 4 of the remaining music therapy subjects. Results from the psychotherapy group showed improvement of 12 subjects, 16 without improvement, and 10 abandoned the study. The music therapy results were understood to have resulted from selected areas of brain activation and changes in brain chemistry producing positive emotions. However, durational differences in the conditions as well as other control biases may have had some effect on the results as well.

Approaches to music psychotherapy that were developed in the 1970s, such as the Bonny Method of Guided Imagery and Music, have since been the subject of increasingly more sophisticated study, from outcomes assessment to the development of specific measuring tools (Bruscia, 2000).

All of the creative arts therapies rely on images, metaphors, and symbols as representations of the inner life and carriers of the therapeutic process, and accept that images can be manifested in words, graphic elements, the kinesthetic sense (Serlin et al, 2000), and sounds. The poetry therapy described by Springer (2006) for those in recovery from substance addictions and for trauma survivors offers examples of metaphor as an agent of insight and change. Springer cautions that in using poetry therapeutically it is important to explicitly relax the rules of poetry writing and recommends the use of "sense poems" when clients are invited to imagine an abstract phenomenon in terms of concrete sensory qualities: "What is the color of addiction? What does it sound like? What does it smell like? What does it look like? What does it feel like?" (p. 74). In setting the stage for behavioral change, the poetry therapist helps the patient enter the imaginal realm where a different life can be envisioned. The imagined then becomes a plan, and the authenticity of plans that spring from the creative process can buoy the recovering person over the sometimes rough seas of therapeutic work.

Poetry therapist Amanda Meunier's case study of George, a 45-year-old man with schizophrenia in short-term treatment, illustrates beautifully the weaving together of patient-created poems, attention to specific treatment goals, dialogue about both the poetry and the individual's life, and study of published works that is poetry therapy. In this case, George articulated his own treatment foci: "gain better identification and acceptance of his negative feelings, particularly anger . . . [find] constructive outlets for dealing with his anger . . . [accept] his own morality and discuss parental loss" (Meunier, 2003, p. 231). Meunier described the course of therapy in four phases: (1) the *supportive* phase, in which goals were set and she used the structured of published poems and directed journaling with George; (2) the *apperceptive* phase, in which George's poetry and their discussions probed his anger, family relationships and feelings about death; (3) the *action* phase, marked by poetry that evidenced an understanding of life's cyclic nature and by intentions to make healthy changes in his life; and (4) the *integrative* phase, in which George openly worked toward autonomously applying the gains and insights made during this brief therapy.

Another report of poetry therapy (Reiter, 2010) describes the Poets-Behind-Bars project, a collaboration between a state maximum security prison and a poetry therapy training program. This innovative program, directed by a poetry therapist/mentor-supervisor (PTR/MS), paired 12 inmate poets with 12 poetry therapy trainees who worked as mentors through e-mail with the incarcerated poets. To preserve interpersonal and professional boundaries for the trainee mentors, the distance model for interaction was mediated through the educational director of state prison, and poets and mentors knew each other only by first names. The work had the quality of an extended tutorial, taught to a curriculum but tailored to the particular interests and responses of the poets in prison. Program evaluation was conducted through qualitative reflections by the prison education director, the poetry therapy trainees, and the poetry therapy education director. Questionnaires designed for this project were administered to the inmates at the beginning and conclusion of the project. Despite many challenges resulting from the realities of prison life, there were apparent benefits for the poets as evidenced in some of the statements from the final questionnaires, excerpted below:

- "This program helped me to be more open and expressive."
- "It gave me better creativity."
- "I reached my goal of writing in a poetically structured manner."
- "Poetry helps me to bless a whole lot of people."
- "It helped me to write poems that did not rhyme."
- "I felt there was someone who wanted to hear what I had to say."

Senroy (2009) used expressive arts therapy including dance, drama, music, and visual arts with young male offenders recovering from substance abuse in India. Vignettes of group sessions focused on accessing the authentic self and providing strength to bridge from the literal self to the imagination where life stories could be written in mythic and symbolic form in order to create a therapeutic environment for recovery.

From the arts in health care arena, the study by Daykin et al (2010) on the impact of a large environmental arts project in the UK entitled "Moving On," is an excellent example of work in the area of healing environments. The project improved 16 mental health units with commissioned art (including landscaping) using a participatory process with unit staff, the mental health service users (consumers), and other stakeholders. Researchers used multiple qualitative methods in a robust, triangulated data collection plan that included discourse analysis of 400 documents and photos generated by various aspects of

"Moving On," followed by the conduct and analysis of 55 qualitative interviews with artists, staff, mental health service users, carers, and other stakeholders, including three focus groups. The following impacts were discovered through this inductive investigation: modernization, stimulation, relaxation, an increased sense of privacy, and an increased contact with nature that was valued by mental health service users. In addition, the theme of participation emerged, along with decreases in institutionalization and stigmatization. Opportunities for engagement, the sense of empowerment and with that, a perceived impact on identity for the mental health service users: "Participation in arts processes as well as the strategic development of the project seemed to give service users access to a range of identities other than the stigmatized and relatively powerless one of 'patient'" (p. 43).

The arts in health care literature also reports a study conducted in a community setting. This project, conducted in Texas, focused on the health benefits of a community-based art education program for older adults (Greer et al, 2012), who constitute a growing and diverse sector of the population and who are the focus of much holistic and arts in health care programming. The program offered painting classes at beginning and intermediate levels, taught by a professional art educator in a museum's studio setting. Classes met once per week for 2 hours and were instructed with a flexible structure that permitted both individual artistic guidance for each participant and a social atmosphere in which people could focus on their own creative process.

The program evaluation focused on 11 individuals (10 women and 1 man, age range 66-79 years) who attended the classes for at least 3 months. Five participants self-identified as African American and three as Hispanic; 10 identified as Christian. Qualitative data were generated through semistructured interviews conducted at 1, 6, and 12 months after starting the classes, field notes on observations of social interaction during the classes, and the artwork itself. The impacts and outcomes of the class were many, and focused on psychosocial benefits for the participants. Specifically, data analysis identified increased relaxation with a sense of calm and peace, increased social engagement and a sense of belonging in a community, increased self-awareness and self-understanding, empowerment through the creative process, and altered perspectives of others and their surroundings. Finally and perhaps most meaningfully, new dimensions of family relationships developed, reinforcing and reshaping the connections between the older parents and their adult children. It appeared that the mastery, the productivity, and the art itself opened up new and positive areas for discussion, heartfelt sharing, and inspiration in the parent-child relationships. Researchers offered a theory of change based on motivation, that "a positive feedback loop ensued, whereby the outcomes produced positive motivations to ongoing class attendance" and autonomous engagement with the art process as well (p. 271).

MEDICAL SETTINGS

When arts services are provided as part of holistic, integrated health care, generally the goals have to do with increasing quality of life variables, improving the ability to cope, providing psychosocial support, and sometimes reducing pain or anxiety.

Art therapy has developed many approaches for working in medical settings. The randomized study by Monti et al (2006) used a mindfulness approach to art therapy in groups of women with breast cancer. Their results showed significant improvement in quality of life and reduction in indicators of distress. Creative arts therapy clinical work for people with neurological disorders is directed at physical problems and symptoms associated with the disorders. An example of the latter is an art therapy study in which people with Parkinson disease ($n = 19$) and a control group without Parkinson disease (caregivers and volunteers) were asked to mold clay into recognizable shapes. Post-treatment scores on the Brief Symptom Inventory indicated a decrease in symptoms in all areas in both groups. The Parkinson group showed improvements that were significant and, overall, higher than those of the control group in somatic and emotional areas including depression, anxiety, average level of distress, and obsessive-compulsive symptoms. Choice of clay color seemed to be related to creation of human figures and affective response.

In a randomized trial of art therapy for children with asthma, Bebee et al (2010) reported their work with 22 children randomized for art therapy or wait-control groups for 7 weeks of one 60-minute art therapy session per week. Sessions included art therapy tasks focused on encouraging expression, discussion, and problem solving in response the stress of having a chronic illness. Results showed a "reduction of parent-reported and child-reported worry scores from the PedsQL questionnaires; a reduction in the anxiety score and an increase in the self-concept score from the child-reported Beck Inventories; and improvements in the color, logic, and details scores from the FEATS in the intervention group compared with the control group." Six-month follow up showed fewer asthma exacerbations in the art therapy group.

Berrol et al (1997) conducted a multisite, mixed-methodology demonstration project showing the impact of group dance/movement therapy in older adults who had experienced stroke, cerebral aneurysm, or traumatic brain injury. The study used a randomized controlled trial design ($n = 107$) with qualitative analysis of data from videotapes of treatment sessions and content analysis of both patient responses to satisfaction questionnaires and therapists' reports. Compared with patients in the control group, those in the treatment group showed significantly greater positive changes in two dimensions of perceptual–motor functioning, dynamic balance (walking backward and walking sideways to the left), and in one range-of-motion item (reaching down from a seated position to cross the midline right to left). The treatment group also showed

significant improvement in cognitive performance (decision making, ability to make oneself understood, and short-term memory) ($p = 0.006$) and in components of social interaction (ease with others, involvement in social/group activities, planned/structured activities, acceptance of invitations, self-initiated activities, and interaction with others) ($p = 0.0027$).

Studies on the benefits of dance/movement therapy for adults with cancer have shown that breast cancer patients in particular seem to profit from this modality. Sandel et al (2005) found significant improvement in breast cancer-specific quality of life (as measured with the Functional Assessment of Cancer Therapy–Breast [FACT-B] questionnaire) in women in the group dance treatment condition compared with a wait-list group. Serlin et al (2000) used patient ratings on the Profile of Mood States inventory as one indicator of treatment effectiveness of a group dance/movement therapy program and reported that "significant improvement was found on the fatigue, vigor and tension subscales, while depression and anxiety decreased" (p. 130). In addition, compelling qualitative findings were noted in the way the women participants described the bodily changes they felt in themselves after existentially oriented supportive dance/movement therapy.

Creative arts therapy programs for medically ill children are sometimes integrated with child life and pediatric psychology services. An example is the Hackensack University Medical Center, New Jersey, where dance/movement therapy is part of the holistically oriented treatment for children with hematologic and oncologic diseases. Cohen and Walco (1999) described this work as a developmentally sensitive approach to helping children through the challenges of serious illness by providing creative explorations of feelings, relationships, the body image, and ways of coping. Their goal was to use both structured and improvisational movement expression not only to bring out children's fears and concerns, but also to encourage the maintenance or resumption of normal development. This work can be done at the bedside, even when little movement is possible, or in outpatient programs. An example of the latter was the dance/movement therapy-based support group for teens (boys and girls) with cancer. The group called themselves "The Braves," and with the guidance of Cohen, their therapist, they tackled the difficult issues of emerging sexuality, peer dynamics, body image, trust, and mortality in playful yet serious psychophysical expression.

Music therapy studies in medical settings with adults and children have increased greatly in the last decade. This section presents brief examples in the areas of cancer, palliative care, neurological rehabilitation, pain reduction, and neonatal intensive care. Clinical use of music therapy in patients with cancer is well described in empirical and clinical case studies. The literature related to music therapy in hospice and palliative care is fairly large and growing. The primary use of supportive music psychotherapy is to improve the individual's quality of life, decrease pain, reduce anxiety and depression, encourage expression, improve communication (especially between family members), and enhance spiritual well-being. Music therapists often continue to work with families after the patient's death for bereavement support (Dileo & Loewy, 2005; Hilliard, 2003; Magill & Luzzato, 2002; O'Callaghan, 1996, 1997).

In Hilliard's 2003 study, 80 individuals living in their homes and receiving hospice care were randomly assigned to receive standard care plus music therapy (live music) or standard care alone. Quality of life was shown to be higher in the music therapy group (Hilliard, 2003).

Music therapy has a wide range of applications in pediatric medical environments. Music therapy researchers and educators Jayne Standley and Jennifer Whipple conducted a meta-analysis of the use of music therapy in pediatric settings. A range of music therapy populations and applications was studied, including all major specializations from the neonatal intensive care unit (NICU) through pediatric hospice care (Standley & Whipple, 2003).

Although music has historically been linked with pain reduction, it is only recently that empirical studies by music therapists have been published. Standley, in her 1986 meta-analysis of all empirical studies using music in dental and medical treatments, found that "music conditions enhanced medical objectives whether measured by physiological (ES [effect size] = 0.97), psychological/self-report (ES = 0.85), or behavioral (ES = 1.10) parameters" (p. 79). Standley (1986) added that most of the studies included participant's pain as a variable. Loewy et al (2005) compared the sedating effects of live music to the effects of chloral hydrate in children undergoing electroencephalographic (EEG) testing. Sixty children between the ages of 1 and 5 years were assigned to either the music group or the chloral hydrate group. Of the children in the music group, 97% needed no other intervention to complete the EEG recording, whereas 50% of the children in the chloral hydrate group required additional interventions to finish the EEG testing. Those in the music group achieved sedation more quickly and were able to leave the hospital much sooner than those in the chloral hydrate group.

NICUs employ music therapy to increase nonnutritive sucking (Standley, 2000), to improve physiological measures, including reducing heart and respiration rates and increasing blood oxygen saturation using infant-directed singing and simulated womb sounds, and to alter the overall NICU sound environment (Stewart & Schneider, 2000).

Loewy et al (2013) used live infant-directed music therapy in the NICU. In a multisite, randomized clinical trial, 272 infants, 32 weeks or older, each with sepsis, respiratory distress syndrome, and/or small for gestational age received three music therapy interventions per week for 2 weeks. From the conclusions section of the article: "The informed, intentional therapeutic use of live sound and parent-preferred lullabies applied by a certified music therapist can influence cardiac and respiratory function. Entrained with a premature infant's observed vital signs,

sound and lullaby may improve feeding behaviors and sucking patterns and may increase prolonged periods of quiet-alert states. Parent-preferred lullabies, sung live, can enhance bonding, thus decreasing the stress parent's associate with premature infant care."

In music therapy and cancer research, Bradt et al (2011) compiled an analysis for the Cochrane Review for music interventions for improving psychological and physical outcomes in cancer patients. The authors included a review that included 30 trials of 1891 participants. From the review: "the findings suggest that music therapy and music medicine interventions may have a beneficial effect on anxiety, pain, mood, quality of life, heart rate, respiratory rate, and blood pressure in cancer patients. Most trials were at high risk of bias and, therefore, these results need to be interpreted with caution" (Bradt et al, 2011, p. 2).

Music therapy clinical work and studies have increased in all the rehabilitative sciences in parallel with the rapid growth of neurosciences in the last 25 years. Neuroscientists are very interested in the human response to music, because music is processed in many different areas of the brain. By studying the response to music scientists are learning much more about the way the brain works. Clinicians, educators, and developmental specialists are learning how music affects the individual's physical, cognitive, interpersonal, emotional, and spiritual life in ways that were unimaginable three decades ago. Perhaps the best current examples of the effects of music on the whole person from a neurological perspective come from Oliver Sacks (2007), a strong advocate for the creative arts therapies, who, in working with music therapist and researcher Concetta Tomaino at the Institute for Music and Neurologic Function in New York City, has sparked worldwide interest in the areas of music and memory, neural plasticity, and the reactivation of nerve pathways in people with a wide range of chronic neurological disorders.

Research on the uses of music, specifically rhythmic auditory stimulation (RAS) for gait training in stroke patients, is demonstrated in the prolific research of Michael Thaut. In a recent study (Thaut et al, 2007), RAS and neurodevelopmental therapy (NDT)/Bobath-based training were used in two groups of hemiparetic stroke patients. The study included 78 patients who had experienced a stroke 3 weeks earlier (43 in the group receiving RAS, and 35 in the group receiving NDT/Bobath training). Over a 3-week period of daily gait training, the RAS group outperformed the NDT group in velocity, stride length, and steps per minute.

Living with a chronic medical condition impacts all aspects of life—vocational, spiritual, relational, sexual, emotional, and psychological—and when cure is elusive, comprehensive care must equip people to live as full and satisfying a life as possible (Goodill, 2005b, 2006). Baker and Mazza (2004) show how this can be accomplished with poetry therapy and therapeutic writing in their case study of a woman with systemic lupus erythematosis who was also a breast cancer survivor. Anna struggled with chronic pain and fatigue, but also with a sense of hopelessness and a belief that her own need for therapy was a weakness in herself. The disease had damaged both her marriage and her career. As described in the case study, therapeutic writing, performed in the context of an empathic ongoing therapeutic relationship, enabled her to first accept her limitations and then build into her life the supports she needed to function optimally. Baker and Mazza (2004) quote from the patient's journal: "I have decided to replace my stubbornness with determination. I am determined not to be defined by my disease. It is a part of my life but not all of it" (p. 150).

Consistent with the definition of poetry therapy as including therapeutic writing, some of the work in poetry therapy, as in the case study described earlier, draws on the curative properties of creating a narrative by writing out one's troubling thoughts and feelings. This effect has been extensively researched by psychologist James Pennebaker and his many collaborators. Among the related studies is that by Krantz and Pennebaker (2007) in which dance/movement was shown to confer similar health benefits.

In a pilot feasibility study of poetry therapy for women with cancer, Tegnera et al (2009) conducted a small randomized trial with a crossover (waiting-list control) design. Twelve women age 50 years and over participated in a group poetry therapy intervention that met 1.5 hours weekly for 6 weeks in a cancer support center. All women continued their usual medical treatment throughout the study period. The intervention was delivered by a CPT and focused on creating "a safe space for the participants to share their thoughts and feelings" (p. 125) through verbal and written responses to poems chosen for this particular group. The hypothesis "that an intervention of poetry therapy will increase the emotional resilience of cancer patients by encouraging expression of emotion, and in particular negative emotions, thus improving psychological well-being as measured by lower mood disturbance" (p. 123) was informed by extant research (Berry & Pennebaker, 1993) on the health and psychosocial benefits of expressive writing, particularly the expression of troubling emotions through expressive writing tasks.

Pre-test and post-tests self-report assessments measured depression, adjustment to cancer, post-traumatic growth, and the degree to which participants constrained expression of emotions. Changes from pre-test to post-test were examined separately for the experimental and the control groups using non-parametric tests. Nine participants received the intervention and their data were included in experimental group analyses, and the delayed intervention group included control data from six participants. The control group evidenced significant reduction in anxious preoccupation ($p = 0.039$), a component of adjustment to cancer and a subscale on the Mini-Mental Adjustment to Cancer Scale. The experimental group showed significant reductions in restraint of emotions as measured by the Courtauld Emotional Control Scale (CECS) in the anger subscale ($p = 0.034$) and for total CECS scores ($p = 0.050$).

In addition, after experiencing poetry therapy, participants reported significant reductions in depression on the Hospital Assessment of Depression Scale ($p = 0.035$). No significant changes in post-traumatic growth were found after this brief intervention. Researchers recommended replicating the study with larger samples, the measurement of potential moderating variables such as disease status, and the use of mixed methods to integrate qualitative data.

Application of poetry therapy as a crisis intervention tool in a day treatment program for people living with human immunodeficiency virus infection was described by Schweitert (2004). In a descriptive case study, she tells of Wilberto, who, despite making good progress in the program, nearly relapsed into drug use when frustrated by the challenges of a new employment situation. When Wilberto stormed into the clinic, anxious and angry, the poetry therapist quickly recognized the crisis and the danger this situation presented to Wilberto. Within a few minutes the therapist structured the collaborative writing of a "calm-down" poem using sentence stems. As Schweitert reports, "the finished product was stunning" (p. 191):

Stem (by the therapist)	Line completion (by the patient)
When I get angry	I need to get away!
If I can just	take myself outside
Then I will	watch the squirrels having fun
And maybe	find a cool, quiet lake
Where I can	calm my mind and feel peace
That would be	perfect.

The patient, visibly calmer, kept the poem with him and, as the case study documents, began a new initiative in both therapy and work. Four months later he had avoided relapse and was actively addressing issues related to living with human immunodeficiency virus.

Ferris and Stein (2002) employed expressive arts therapy within a 10-week workshop for cancer survivors called Cancer, Courage and Creativity, developed at Living Arts, a non-profit organization in Montana. The project uses art, drama, poetry, movement, ritual, myth, and mask making to promote inner personal change. The expressive arts therapy was used to invoke metaphors, symbols, and myth in order to build bridges from the past through a heroic journey toward an expanded life journey toward a future, new life beyond cancer.

Expressive arts therapies were used as a complementary treatment for 20 women with breast cancer in an integrative support group (Klagsbrun et al, 2005). The format included a centering tool (*Focusing*), or turning the attention inward, and expressive arts therapy (dance/movement, visual art, and creative writing). *Clearing a Space* followed to allow for the women to symbolize their inner felt experience toward a goal of improved quality of life.

Scales that developed from humanistic psychology studies, including the Experiencing Scale and the Clearing a Space checklist, were used with quality-of-life scales and qualitative research (e.g., informed interviews). Positive results were demonstrated via most measures. The 6-week follow-up interviews indicated that many of the women used the methods taught in the support group and felt that they contributed to an increase in quality of life.

SCOPE OF STUDIES AND PRACTICE

The array of study topics and methodologies demonstrate that scholars in arts in health care, expressive arts therapy, and the creative arts therapies engage in all forms of systematic inquiry, including quantitative, qualitative, mixed-method, and arts-based studies. The research agendas for these disciplines may differ but have identified the following as priorities: the evaluation of clinical outcomes, comparison and refinement of treatment methods, theory testing, derivation of theories, psychosocial assessment using art forms and media, definition of best practices in therapist preparation and education, and investigation of basic research questions linking creative arts therapy practice with findings from other disciplines.

An example of the development of a systematic research agenda is provided by the recent Delphi study conducted by Kaiser and Deaver (2013) for the field of art therapy. A Delphi study is basically a group communication process that is established so that many individuals (in this case, art therapy researchers) may deal with a complex problem (the future of art therapy research). Art therapy research panelists ($n = 26$) were asked to "identify the most important areas of investigation, research questions, methods, and populations or conditions that should be studied" (p. 114). A first round of open-ended questions was sent to participants that contained the questions: "What areas are important to research in art therapy and why?"; "What research questions are important to address?"; and "What methods should be used to study the areas and questions you have identified?" A second round of questions asked for a rank ordering of the prior responses. Following the rank-orderings, a third solicitation was sent to weigh the items. The researchers concluded:

> Of the areas panelists thought were most important to study, outcome research received the most endorsements, followed by art therapy and neuroscience, the processes and mechanisms in art therapy, research that establishes the validity and reliability of art therapy assessments, cross-cultural and multicultural approaches to art therapy assessment and practice, and the establishment of a database of normative artwork across the lifespan (Kaiser & Deaver, 2013, p. 115).

As these disciplines develop and grow, the arts remain at the core of practice while creativity remains the underlying drive. Healing, or becoming whole, occurs through a process of activation of the person's creative potential through the arts. The similarities appear in the innate responses to the arts as well as in the individual's use of creativity and the arts to form human relationships. As psychologist Ernest Rossi (1999) posits, creative activity is one way to stimulate endogenous mind–body healing processes.

However, as noted in the opening sections of this chapter, there are distinctions. For example, in contrast to the multimodal use of the arts in expressive arts therapy practice (Klagsbrun et al, 2005), the creative arts therapies advocate for specialists' use of each art form, grounded in the uniqueness of the media themselves. We can recognize these distinctive processes in the following examples: the music therapist's song in the NICU that activates the neonate's inherent creative tendency to "find" the transformational effect in the therapist's voice; the art therapist's facilitation of a client's natural desire to create and show others a visual representation of his or her inner world; the dance/movement therapist's use of an expressive gesture to convey empathy in response to the client's movement depiction of uncovered individuality; the drama therapist's moving a patient out of a role play at precisely the moment when the patient is ready to express authentic feelings; or the poetry therapist's selection of a starter poem that can reflect the as-yet-unspoken language of the heart.

The clinical and research discoveries of these arts-based service professions point to future investigations in little explored but increasingly important areas such as the neuroscience (see Chapter 8) and psychological interfaces with the effects of the experience of beauty on health, physiological responses to arts experiences, spiritual dimensions of the arts, and the impact of the instillation of hope through the arts. Concerted effort and interdisciplinary collaboration, scholarship, and advocacy for these practices will make arts-based services accessible to more patients and clients in the future.

References

Amir D: Giving trauma a voice: The role of improvisational music therapy in exposing, dealing with, and healing a traumatic experience of sexual abuse, *Music Ther Perspect* 22:96, 2004.

Austin D: In search of self: the use of vocal holding techniques with adults traumatized as children, *Music Ther Perspect* 19(1): 22, 2001.

Austin D: The voice of trauma: a wounded healer's perspective. In Sutton J, editor: *Music, music therapy and trauma*, Philadelphia, 2002, Jessica Kingsley, p 231.

Austin D: Lifesongs: music therapy with adolescents in foster care. In Camilleri VA, editor: *Healing the inner city child: creative arts therapies with at-risk youth*, London, 2007a, Jessica Kingsley, p 92.

Austin D: Vocal psychotherapy. In Crowe B, Colwell C, editors: *Music therapy for children, adolescents, and adults with mental disorders: using music to maximize mental health, AMTA monograph series, Effective Clinical Practice in Music Therapy*, Silver Spring, Md, 2007b, American Music Therapy Association.

Baker KC, Mazza N: The healing power of writing: applying the expressive/creative component of poetry therapy, *J Poetry Ther* 17:141–154, 2004.

Bebee A, Gelfand EW, Bender B: A randomized trial to test the effectiveness of art therapy for children with trauma, *J Allergy Clin Immun* 126:263, 2010.

Berrol CF, Ooi WL, Katz SS: Dance/movement therapy with older adults who have sustained neurological insult: a demonstration project, *Am J Dance Ther* 19(2):135–160, 1997.

Berry DS, Pennebaker JW: Nonverbal and verbal emotional expression and health, *Psychother Psychosom* 59:11–19, 1993.

Bradt J, Dileo C, Grocke D, Magill L: Music interventions for improving psychological and physical outcomes for cancer patients, *The Cochrane Library* 2011. doi: 10.1002/14651858.CD006911:11.

Bräuninger I: Dance/movement therapy group intervention in stress treatment: A randomized controlled trial (RCT), *Art Psychothep* 39:443–450, 2012.

Bruscia KE: A scale for assessing responsiveness to guided imagery and music, *J Assoc Music Imagery* 7:1, 2000.

Cohen SO, Walco GA: Dance/movement therapy for children and adolescents with cancer, *Cancer Pract* 7(1):34–42, 1999.

Cruz R, Sabers D: Dance/movement therapy is more effective than previously reported, *Arts Psychother* 25:101, 1998.

Dibbel-Hope S: The use of dance/movement therapy in psychological adaptation to breast cancer, *Arts Psychother* 27(1):51, 2000.

Dally T: "I wonder if I exist?": a multi-family approach to the treatment of anorexia in adolescence. In Case C, editor: *Art therapy with children: from infancy to adolescence*, New York, 2008, Routledge/Taylor & Francis Group, p 215.

Daykin N, Byrne E, Soteriou T, O'Connor S: Using arts to enhance mental healthcare environments: Findings from qualitative research, *Arts & Health* 2(1):33–46, 2010.

Dileo C, Loewy JV: *Music therapy at the end of life*, Cherry Hill, NJ, 2005, Jeffrey Books.

Emunah R: *Acting for real: drama therapy process, technique and performance*, New York, 1994, Brunner/Mazel.

Erhardt BT, Hearne MB, Novak C: Outpatient clients' attitudes towards healing processes in dance therapy, *Am J Dance Ther* 11(1):39, 1989.

Erwin-Grabner T, Goodill S, Schelly Hill E, et al: Effectiveness of dance/movement therapy on reducing test anxiety, *Am J Dance Ther* 21(1):19–34, 1999.

Ferris B, Stein Y: Care beyond cancer: the culture of creativity, *Illn Crisis Loss* 10:42, 2002.

Gillespie C: The use of collaborative poetry as a method of deepening interpersonal communication among adolescent girls, *J Poetry Ther* 18(4):221, 2005.

Global Alliance for Arts and Health: *What is Arts and Health?* 2011. http://thesah.org/doc/Definition_FINALNovember2011.pdf. Accessed on: 9/21/2012.

Gold C, Heldal TO, Dahle T, et al: Music therapy for schizophrenia or schizophrenia-like illnesses, *Cochrane Database Syst Rev* (2):CD004025, 2005. doi: 10.1002/14651858.CD004025.pub2.

Gonzalez-Dolginko B: In the shadows of terror: a community neighboring the World Trade Center disaster uses art therapy to process trauma, *Art Ther* 19(3):120, 2002.

Goodill S: Research letter: dance/movement therapy for adults with cystic fibrosis: pilot data on mood and adherence, *Altern Ther Health Med* 11(1):76, 2005a.

Goodill S: *An introduction to medical dance/movement therapy: Health care in motion*, London, 2005b, Jessica Kingsley Publishers, Inc.

Goodill S: Dance/Movement Therapy for Adults with Chronic Medical Illness. In Koch S, Brauninger I, editors: *Advances in Dance/Movement Therapy: Theoretical perspectives and empirical findings*, Berlin, 2006, Logos Verlag Berlin.

Gray AE: The body remembers: dance/movement therapy with an adult survivor of torture, *Am J Dance Ther* 23(1):29, 2001.

Greer N, Fleuriet KJ, Cantu AG: Acrylic Rx: A program evaluation of a professional taught painting class among older Americans, *Arts & Health* 4(3):262–273, 2012.

Gussak D: The effectiveness of art therapy in reducing depression in prison populations, *Int J Offender Ther Comp Criminol* 51(4):444, 2007.

Gussak D: The effects of art therapy on male and female inmates: Advancing the research base, *Arts Psychother* 36:5, 2009.

Harris DA: Dance/movement therapy approaches to fostering resilience and recovery among African adolescent torture survivors, *Torture* 17(2):134, 2007.

Harvey S: Creative arts therapies in the classroom: a study of cognitive, emotional, and motivational changes, *AJDT* 11(2):85, 1989.

Hervey L, Kornblum R: An evaluation of Kornblum's body-based violence prevention curriculum for children, *Arts Psychother* 33:113, 2006.

Hilliard RB: The use of cognitive-behavioral music therapy in the treatment of women with eating disorders, *Music Ther Perspect* 19(2):109, 2001.

Hilliard RB: The effects of music therapy on the quality and length of life of people diagnosed with terminal cancer, *J Music Ther* 40(2):113, 2003.

Hunter L: Group sandtray play therapy. In Kaduson HG, Schaefer CE, editors: *Short-term play therapy for children*, New York, 2009, The Guilford Press.

James M, Johnson DR: Drama therapy in the treatment of combat-related post-traumatic stress disorder, *Arts Psychother* 23(5):383, 1997.

Johnson D, Lubin H, Hale K, et al: Single session effects of treatment components within a specialized inpatient posttraumatic stress disorder program, *J Trauma Stress* 10:377, 1997.

Johnson DR: Creative therapies for adults. In Foa E, Keane TM, Friedman MJ, et al, editors: *Effective treatments for PTSD*, New York, 2009, Guilford Press, p 479.

Justice RW: Music therapy interventions for people with eating disorders in an inpatient setting, *Music Ther Perspect* 12(2):104, 1994.

Kaiser D, Deaver S: Establishing a Research Agenda for Art Therapy: A Delphi Study, *Art Ther J Am Art Assoc* 30(3):114–121, 2013. http://eric.ed.gov/?q=%22Kaiser+Donna%22&id=EJ1021917.

Karkou V, Sanderson P: *Arts therapies: a research based map of the field*, Edinburgh, 2006, Elsevier Churchill Livingstone.

Kipper DA, Ritchie TD: The effectiveness of psychodramatic techniques: a meta-analysis, *Group Dyn* 7(1):13, 2003.

Klagsbrun J, Rappaport L, Speiser V, et al: Focusing and expressive arts therapy as a complimentary treatment for women with breast cancer, *JCMH* 1:107, 2005.

Koch S, Morlinghaus K, Fuchs T: The joy dance: specific effects of single dance intervention on psychiatric patients with depression, *Arts in Psychother* 34(4):340–349, 2007.

Kornblum R: *Disarming the playground: violence prevention through movement and pro-social skills*, Oklahoma City, Okla, 2002, Wood & Barnes.

Koshland L, Wittaker JWB: PEACE through dance/movement: evaluating a violence prevention program, *Am J Dance Ther* 26(2):69, 2004.

Krantz AM, Pennebaker JW: Expressive dance, writing, trauma, and health: when words have a body. In Sonke-Henderson J, Brandman R, Serlin I, et al, editors: *The arts and health*, vol 3, Westport, Conn, 2007, Praeger Perspectives, p 201.

Lai NG: Expressive arts therapy for mother-child relationship (EAT-MCR): A novel model for domestic violence survivors in Chinese culture, *Arts Psychother* 38:305, 2011.

Landgarten H: *Clinical art therapy: a comprehensive guide*, New York, 1981, Brunner/Mazel.

Landy RJ, Luck B, Conner E, et al: Role profiles: a drama therapy assessment instrument, *Arts Pyschother* 30:151, 2003.

Lang L, McInerney U: A music therapy service in a post-war environment. In Sutton J, editor: *Music, music therapy and trauma*, Philadelphia, 2002, Jessica Kingsley, p 153.

Levine SK, Levine EG, editors: *Foundations of expressive arts therapy: theoretical and clinical perspectives*, London and Philadelphia, 1999, Jessica Kingsley Press, p 9.

Loewy J, Frisch Hara A, editors: *Caring for the caregiver: the use of music therapy on grief and trauma*, Silver Spring, Md, 2002, American Music Therapy Association.

Loewy JV, Hallan C, Friedman E, et al: Sleep/sedation in children undergoing EEG testing: a comparison of chloral hydrate and music therapy, *J Perianesth Nurs* 3(5):323, 2005.

Loewy J, Stewart K, Dassler AM, et al: The effect of music therapy on vital signs, feeding, and sleep in pre-mature infants, *Pediatrics* 131:902, 2013.

Magill L, Luzzato P: Music therapy and art therapy. In Berger A, Portenoy R, Weissman D, editors: *Principles and practice of palliative care and supportive oncology*, ed 2, Philadelphia, 2002, Lippincott Williams & Wilkins, p 993.

Malchiodi CA: *Breaking the silence: art therapy with children from violent homes*, New York, 1990, Brunner/Mazel.

Malchiodi CA: *Expressive therapies*, New York, 2005, Guilford Press, p 2.

Meunier A: The expressive/creative mode of poetry therapy in short-term treatment: a case study, *J Poetry Ther* 16(4):229, 2003.

Miller JM, Johnson DR: The capacity for symbolization in Post-traumatic Stress Disorder, *Psychol Trauma* 2011. doi: 10.1037/a0021580. Advance online publication.

Mills LJ, Daniluk JC: Her body speaks: the experience of dance therapy for women survivors of child sexual abuse, *J Couns Devel* 80:77, 2002.

Monti DA, Peterson C, Kunkel E, et al: A randomized controlled trial of mindfulness-based art therapy (MBAT) for women with cancer, *Psychooncology* 15(5):363, 2006.

Morgan C, Johnson D: Use of a drawing task in the treatment of nightmares in combat—related PTSD, *Art Ther* 12:253, 1995.

Naumburg M: *Dynamically oriented art therapy: its principles and practice*, Oxford, 1966, Grune & Stratton.

Nolan P: Music as a transitional object in the treatment of bulimia, *Music Ther Perspect* 6:48, 1989a.

Nolan P: Music therapy improvisation techniques with bulimic patients. In Hornyak LM, Baker EK, editors: *Experiential therapies for eating disorders*, London, 1989b, Guilford Press, p 167.

Nolan P: What to do until the music therapist arrives, *Holist Nurs Pract* 20(1):37, 2006.

Nordoff P, Robbins C: *Therapy in music for handicapped children*, New York, 1971, St Martins Press.

O'Callaghan C: Complementary therapies in terminal care: pain, music, creativity, and music therapy in palliative care, *Am J Hosp Palliat Care* 13:43–49, 1996.

O'Callaghan C: Therapeutic opportunities associated with music when using song writing in palliative care, *Music Ther Perspect* 15:32, 1997.

O'Neill Thorn C: *Screams aren't enough: poems by Devon Adams, Jocelyn Heckler, Alex Marsh, Allison Carter*, Indian Hills, Colo, 1999, O'Neill.

Parente A: Feeding the hungry soul: music as a therapeutic modality in the treatment of anorexia nervosa, *Music Thera Perspect* 6:44, 1989a.

Parente A: Music as a therapeutic tool in treating anorexia nervosa. In Hornyak LM, Baker EK, editors: *Experiential therapies for eating disorders*, London, 1989b, Guilford Press, p 305.

Perez SC, Perez VG, Velasco MC, et al: Effects of music therapy on depression compared to psychotherapy, *Arts Psychother* 37:387, 2010.

Pratt RR: Healing and art, *Int J Arts Med* 1(2):3, 1992.

Reiter S: Poets-behind-bars: A creative "righting" project for prisoners and poetry therapists-in-training, *J Poetry Ther* 23(4):215–238, 2010. doi: 10.1080/08893675.2010.528221.

Robarts J, Sloboda A: Perspectives on music therapy with people suffering from anorexia nervosa, *J Br Music Ther* 8(1):7, 1994.

Rogers N: Person-centered expressive arts therapy, *Creation Spirituality* 28, 1993.

Rossi E: *An introduction to clinical hypnosis and mind/body healing: a psychobiological approach to the hypnotherapeutic arts (3-day course with institute certificate)*, 1999. Paper presented at Psychology of Consciousness, Energy Medicine and Dynamic Change, Third International Conference of the National Institute for the Clinical Application of Behavioral Medicine, Hilton Head, SC, March 8–10.

Rubin JA, editor: *Approaches to art therapy: theory and technique*, New York, 1987, Brunner/Mazel.

Runco MA: *Creativity theories and themes: research, development, and practice*, Burlington, MA, 2007, Elsevier Academic Press.

Runco MA, Richards R, editors: *Eminent creativity and everyday creativity, and health*, Greenwich, CT, 1998, Ablex.

Sacks OW: *Musicophilia: tales of music and the brain*, New York, 2007, Alfred A Knopf.

Schmais C: Healing processes in group dance therapy, *Am J Dance Ther* 8:17, 1985.

Sajnani N, Kaplan FF: The creative arts therapies and social justice: A conversation between the editors of this special issue, *Art Psychother* 39(3):165–167, 2012.

Sandel S, Judge J, Landry N, et al: Dance and movement program improves quality-of-life measures in breast cancer survivors, *Cancer Nurs* 28(4):301, 2005.

Schweitert JA: The use of poetry therapy in crisis intervention and short-term treatment: two case studies, *J Poetry Ther* 17(4):189, 2004.

Searle Y, Streng I: *Where analysis meets the arts: the integration of the arts therapies with psychoanalytic theory*, London, 2001, Karnac Books.

Senroy P: Using expressive arts therapy with young male offenders recovering from substance abuse in a de-addiction setup in India. In Brooke SL, editor: *The use of creative therapies in chemical dependency issues*, Springfield, IL, 2009, Charles C Thomas, p 175.

Serlin IA, Classen C, Frances B, et al: Symposium: Support groups for women with breast cancer: traditional and alternative expressive approaches, *Arts Psychother* 27(2):123, 2000.

Simonton DK: Creativity in highly eminent individuals. In Kaufman JC, Sternberg RJ, editors: *The cambridge handbook of creativity*, New York, 2010, Cambridge University Press.

Sloboda A: Individual music therapy with anorexia and bulimia patients. In Dokter D, editor: *Arts therapies and clients with eating disorders*, London, 1995, Jessica Kingsley, p 247.

Springer W: Poetry in therapy: a way to heal for trauma survivors and clients in recovery from addiction, *J Poetry Ther* 19(2):69, 2006.

Standley JM: Music research in medical/dental treatment: meta analysis and clinical applications, *J Music Ther* 25(2):56, 1986.

Standley JM: The effect of contingent music to increase non-nutritive sucking of pre-mature infants, *Pediatr Nurs* 26(5):493, 2000.

Standley JM, Whipple J: Music therapy with pediatric patients: a meta-analysis. In Robb SL, editor: *Music therapy in pediatric health care: research and evidence-based practice*, Silver Spring, Md, 2003, American Music Therapy Association, p 1.

Stewart K, Schneider S: The effects of music therapy on the sound environment in the NICU: a pilot study. In Loewy JV, editor: *Music therapy in the neonatal intensive care unit*, New York, 2000, Satchnote Press, p 85.

Tegnera I, Fox J, Philipp R, Thorne P: Evaluating the use of poetry to improve well-being and emotional resilience in cancer patients, *J Poetry Ther* 22(3):121–131, 2009. doi: 10.1080/08893670903198383.

Thaut MH, Leins AK, Rice RR, et al: Rhythmic auditory stimulation improves gait more than NDT/Bobath training in near-ambulatory patients early poststroke: a single-blind, randomized trial, *Neurorehabil Neural Repair* 21(5):455, 2007.

Winnicott DW: *Playing and Reality*, London, 1971, Tavistock.

Zwerling I: *Looking ahead, planning together: the creative arts in therapy as an integral part of treatment for the 90's: proceedings from a symposium sponsored by the Creative Arts in Therapy Program, Hahnemann University*, Philadelphia, Pennsylvania, 1984, The University, p 17.

Suggested Readings

Elkis-Abuhoff DL, Goldblatt RB, Gaydos M, et al: Effects of clay manipulation on somatic dysfunction and emotional distress in patients with Parkinson's disease, *Art Ther* 25(3):122, 2008.

Farr M: The role of dance/movement therapy in treating at-risk African American adolescents, *Arts Psychother* 24(2):183, 1997.

World Health Organization: *Constitution of the World Health Organization*, 1946. http://apps.who.int/gb/bd/PDF/bd47/EN/constitution-en.pdf. Accessed on: 9/30/13.

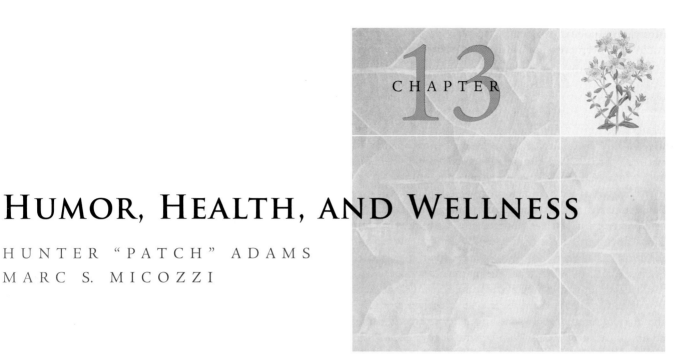

CHAPTER 13

HUMOR, HEALTH, AND WELLNESS

HUNTER "PATCH" ADAMS
MARC S. MICOZZI

The arrival of a good clown exercises a more beneficial influence upon the health of a town than of twenty asses laden with drugs.

—Thomas Sydenham, MD
(seventeenth-century English physician)

The first two sections of the book have provided an introduction and what can be considered the basic sciences for complementary/alternative medicine. In this final chapter, before proceeding to each specific alternative/complementary therapy and what may be considered their clinical sciences and applications, we provide some review, further introduction of the next sections, and synthesis.

Before tackling what humor therapy might be, we would like to introduce where it fits into complementary and alternative medicine in the context of wellness and preventive medicine. Allopathic medicine has generally ignored this field. What could be more complementary to any system of disease care than a sound emphasis on being well? And a traditional sense of well-being is conveyed by the concept of good humor. As the ancient sages originally proposed in terms of the role of "humors" in the body (see Chapters 1 and 2), the word has come down to indicate something more profound than just comedy. As the economic crisis in medicine worsens, it seems both prudent and inevitable that we focus much greater attention on living healthful lives. Regarding Dr. Sydenham's comment above, we are now seeing government and industry getting more involved in health care than ever before, so we have a surfeit of all three of the components of his original equation (clowns, asses, and drugs) in our health care system, but we will get them in the right proportion?

The complementary therapies all have a greater emphasis on health and wellness because they fit into a more holistic approach (see Chapter 1). Often, when more time is spent with patients, the intimacy that happens leads to a compassionate desire to help the patient feel better. Primary care health providers clearly see the differences between their responses to illness between healthy people in a wellness program and people who do not engage in wellness. They also see less frequent illness in people on wellness programs.

WELLNESS—RECOGNIZING WHOLE POTENTIAL

Exercise and recreation are as necessary as reading. I will say rather more necessary because health is worth more than learning.

—THOMAS JEFFERSON

The practice of medicine can sometimes be an exercise in frustration. Current medical education, research, and practice largely focus on disease care: a patient comes to the doctor sick, does the prescribed treatment, and returns to the world. Why he or she really got sick in the first place is glossed over with a few quick questions, partly because during the short dialogue now sanctioned between physician and patient (see Foreword by the late former U.S. Surgeon General C. Everett Koop), there is no time to address the patient's lifestyle. One of the authors (Patch Adams) has chosen to spend long hours with patients for these past 40 years to try to understand the processes that lead to illness. In medical school, "health" was defined as the absence of disease, so those not complaining of symptoms were considered healthy. Yet, so few adults to whom I have spoken actually speak of life as a wondrous zestful journey. Most illnesses seen by a family doctor have a huge lifestyle component, frustrating the physician because they could have been prevented with some greater self-care and self-consciousness.

HEALTH

Health is obviously so much more than a disease-free interlude in life. To be healthy is to have a body toned to its optimal performance potential, a clear mind exploding with wonder and curiosity, and a spirit happy and at peace with the world. Most adults, however, exist in a gray area between health and sickness, a zone where people say, "I'm fine," when ritually asked how they are, and how they feel. This "fine" can be chock full of diseases as diverse and inhibiting as: (1) the chronic fatigue or "blah" experienced because of those labile fluctuations in blood sugar as a result of a high-sugar diet; (2) the foot problems that come from wearing shoes geared for fashion, not fitness; and (3) the distraction and anger that linger in the air after poor communication with a spouse or friend. In fact, our lifestyle is assaulting us now and anticipating future expression in disease in hundreds of silent ways.

Because wellness can be seen as the summation of all factors leading us to being healthier, this chapter can only touch, ever so briefly, on some of those of paramount importance, ideally stimulating a thirst in each person to discover individual parameters. In the wellness model, patients become responsible for their own health, because health results from an active participation that only the self can give (see Chapter 1). The health professional's role then shifts from that of a mechanic fixing the breakdowns to that of a gardener nurturing growth, as in one Chinese metaphor and model of the body (see Chapter 2).

Much of illness, from minor to profound, has a powerful stress component (see Chapters 9 and 10). An intention of wellness is to offer many insights and paths to eliminate unhealthy stress and make good use of positive stress to "lighten up" and live life in deepest appreciation of all its gifts.

Wellness is a great investment with many positive repercussions. A long-term investment in good health opens the door to a lifetime of quality living for the investor. The physical body becomes the vehicle for indulging in every activity one desires, never limited because of being out of shape. However, the benefits of wellness extend far beyond the self. Family life can become a rich, creative, and happy experience on the train of communication and cooperation. The workplace can become a fun place, as a "well-dressed" attitude and personality help make all employees a team and every task a delight.

Separating self, family, and work is arbitrary and possibly even dangerous, because the health of one so obviously has an impact on all the others. People who are at maximum health will be happier and more loving in all their relationships and thus also prepared to give their best work performance. An individual striving to be healthy, full of caring and curiosity, brings loving management and creativity to the workplace. A body in tone and at proper weight is ready for the tasks at hand. If any of these areas is ignored in one's pursuit of health, the others will suffer. Studies have shown that emphasizing a human-centered, healthy workplace and providing space and time to exercise cuts absenteeism and turnover and increases honesty and productivity.

Unfortunately, one of life's ironies is that wisdom mostly comes with age. By the time we realize that a habit has profoundly hurt us, we feel helpless to change the habit, even justifying it as intrinsic to our nature. Luckily the design of a great organism is such that it can recover remarkably well; in fact, it begins to repair itself as soon as we alter the unhealthy habit through self-healing (see Chapter 1). Wellness is not some kind of "end product"; it is a process, a journey in which each day presents its unique face, and we must choose among many options which paths to follow. We cannot rest on the health of our past, because it must be renewed each day.

Life is a cascade of choices, and we are an expression of both the short-term and the long-term choices we make. To manage the number of choices we have to make daily, we fall into habits, and following a routine substitutes for making a choice. These habits can be a double-edged sword: although it is true we do not have to concern ourselves any longer with making an immediate choice, once entrenched, a habit is incredibly hard to break. When the habit is an unhealthy one and we want to break it, the task is arduous. Wellness seems like an emerging system to help people restructure or balance habits, so how we live becomes healthy, not as a task of effort but simply as a collection of positive, intentional habits. As medical practitioners focus on the causes and prevention of illness, they are finding that many major diseases could have been prevented or dramatically postponed through lifestyle changes. Most of this information has been reiterated throughout the medical literature from Hippocrates to the present.

NUTRITION

Take nutrition, for example. Simplified, we are a sack of water with chemicals in solution. How these chemicals interact determines what our health is to be, but in many of the interactions, chemicals are used up or altered and must be replenished. Nutrition consists of the proper consumption and assimilation of foods containing those necessary chemicals. Because few foods contain all or most of the needed nutrients, we have to obtain them in a variety of foods. As people have moved farther from food sources, and as food companies have changed the foods grown to have longer shelf life, our diets have changed dramatically. For about the last 100 years, synthetic chemicals, refined foods, sugar, and salt have replaced many of the natural foods our ancestors ate (see Chapter 26).

Refined simple sugars so dominate our lives that they are ubiquitous, present even in some table salt. In the United States 100 years ago, we consumed 3 lb of sugar per person per year; we now consume 180 lb. After being considered "safe" (aside from the excess calories), research is now showing that sugar in any form has a profound effect on our health. Certainly it plays a major role in one of the most devastating diseases—obesity. The federal government has stepped in to encourage some nutritional changes: (1) dramatic cutbacks in sugar and salt consumption; (2) increased consumption of foods containing fiber; and (3) a decrease in consumption of whole milk products and other animal fat products. We should expand on this to say: eat mostly whole grains, fresh fruit and vegetables, and lean meat, fish, and poultry.

EXERCISE

If nutrition is the fuel, exercise is the "toner" for the body. Modern civilization has changed few things in our lives as severely as the type and amount of exercise we get. We have never been as sedentary as we are today, and this circumstance, combined with dietary changes, has made much of our adult population overweight and flabby. There is a popular quip that says, "If you do not use it, you lose it." The interplay of muscles, bones, tendons, ligaments, and joints demands consistent stimulation to stay in tone. Being in shape does not mean simply being slender but having all the muscles toned.

There are four types of exercise to consider. The body's internal toner in *heart-lung (aerobic) exercise* strengthens the heart, exercises the bellows to supply oxygen to the body and rid it of carbon dioxide, and tones the muscles used in exercise, all giving the body endurance. Joint *flexibility exercises,* such as stretching or yoga-style exercises, keep the body limber and relaxed. *Strength exercises* are important to tone those muscles not covered in the heart-lung exercises. *Balancing exercises,* such as dance, gymnastics, or circus skills, add another dimension to maximum performance.

Being in shape has obvious rewards in being physically able to do whatever you want to do, and regular exercise has other benefits. It has been shown to lower blood pressure, to have a positive effect on mental health, to diminish stress, and to aid digestion. We believe that regular exercise does such good for the body that it appears to slow the aging process. Most of these benefits come from just moderate exercise, and only a small percentage of benefit is added by extreme or over-strenuous exercise (which, in turn, ultimately contributes to wear-and-tear and stress on the joints especially).

EMOTIONAL LIFE

Just as we must exercise our bodies to be fit, so must we exercise our minds to keep awake and alert. Among the greatest instruments for the mind's stimulation are wonder and curiosity. Boredom is a major cognitive "disease," eroding the health of many adults who over time narrow their spheres of interest and activities. Wonder and curiosity are the tools that all children carry with them in their interactions with the world. In fact, that wonder and curiosity are what make kids seem so alive. For adults, somewhere along the line, sunsets and moonrises become routine and life's pace too hectic.

But wonder and curiosity can be recaptured. There are no stimulants that begin to awaken a person like a new interest captivating one's life or consuming ongoing exploration. The next time a person is excited about something, instead of turning it off, jump right into it and share in their interest. Carry your wonder and curiosity into your older years and you take your youth with you. Often, having such a vibrant interest is a major impetus and motivation for staying healthy, so the exploration goes unimpeded.

It goes without saying that love is one of the most important wellness factors in sustaining a healthy, happy life. Love, that passionate abstract, has captured the imagination of all the creative, expressive, and fine arts from the beginning of history, as they attempted in turn to capture love, to define and elucidate it. Love has profound beneficial effects, yet no scientist has ever measured it or reproduced it in a test tube; nonetheless, it has healing power and some health practitioners have learned to apply it. As a healing force, *love* can be defined as that unconditional surrender to the overwhelming wonderful feeling experienced in giving to or receiving from an object or subject. We most often express love toward family, friends, God, self, lovers, pets, nature, or hobbies. By "surrender" is meant to lose oneself in awe, trust, respect, fun, and tenderness for the object of surrender. In striving for maximum wellness, one could pursue love in all the parameters just mentioned. It appears that the more one submits to unconditional love toward one object, the easier it is to do so for others. The unconditional aspect is so important, because without it, love is often lost to expectations, doubts, and fears.

If love is the foundation for happiness, then fun, play, and laughter are among the vehicles for its expression. The great physician Sir William Osler said that laughter is the "music of life." The physicians of the ancient world and the doctors of the Middle Ages still regarded music as medicine as well (see Chapters 1 and 2), while their medical works remained guided by faith.

FAITH

Faith is the cornerstone of our inner strength. Faith is a personal, passionate, immutable belief in something of inexhaustible power and mystery. Whenever we have to face any kind of devastating change without some kind of solid belief, we become prey to confusion, fear, and panic. Often these crises present questions that have no answers; the discomfort arising from this uncertainty is healed in the domain of our beliefs. Faith has no physical characteristics, no external requirements; it is not a commodity. To acquire a belief, one simply needs to have an interest and a willingness to submit to its mystery. While there are many great religious traditions that promote a common interpretation of belief, and in turn hold many beliefs in common, each person also has to find an individual, meaningful faith and their own sense of spirituality. Faith and spirituality are not summarized by a label but expressed by an inner experience of strength that lives in each of us, day by day.

NATURE

Whereas faith and love are intangible, requiring sweet surrender, nature is a physical, sensual tangible surrounding. Our relationship with nature has had great historical significance as part of our healthy life. It is of little surprise that most symbols in early religions were from nature. Our moods are often described in terms of nature: a synonym for "happy" is "sunny." The first warm, bright day after winter universally and consistently heightens spirits as few days of the year can do. Love has a metaphorical connection to the moon. Most early spiritual observations and celebrations grew out of ties with and reliance on the seasons. We have such strong needs to connect with nature that billions of dollars are spent to bring nature into our homes in the form of pets and house plants. Medical literature is currently peppered with the therapeutic significance of putting pets in the lives of elderly and mentally ill patients, and for benefits in reducing blood pressure and heart disease.

Flowers are a major communication of love at sickbeds, deaths, marriages, and special occasions. The few days we take during a year to relax on vacation are mostly spent with a natural setting in mind: the beach or the mountains, for instance. Let's face it—nature is the mother of wonder. If we are to be fully well, we need a daily communion with nature, from the daily spectacular sunsets and moonrise, to the tenacious blade of grass as it pushes up through the urban or suburban sidewalk.

CREATIVITY

Our imaginations, hands, and senses are the tools for the next major wellness factor—creativity. Life is experienced as a rich journey if we believe we have a creative hand in its passage. Creativity is not just expressed through hobbies and arts but can touch every aspect of life: our work, family, and even how we wait in line—"the art of living." The importance seems to be in the enjoyment of the process rather than in the quality of the final product. Creativity works like our muscles: the more it is exercised, the greater its tone. Explore the next idea, activity, or interest in your life that catches your eye. Whenever exploring, do not settle for one point of view; set it aside and insist on other perspectives. Explore the spontaneous. The key here is to be open and susceptible. Do not catalog your hobbies and interests as indulgences; respect them as major medicines. Our interests often decline with age, which can be deadly. Try to see each day as a building block to the next. Be sure to take advantage of all the human creativity in existence, because the arts give such a sense of well-being (see Chapter 12).

SERVICE

As soon as people recognize how fortunate they are to be well, there arises the urge to give thanks. The healthy expression of that thanks is in service. Unless individuals believe they live a life of service, in whatever form suits them, they will have a difficult time feeling that life is ultimately fulfilling. For example, with respect to yoga, although in the United States we favor the physical form of Hatha Yoga (see Chapter 21), the other forms of yoga practice all emphasize service and devotion (such as Bahkti and Karma Yoga).

The seventeenth-century metaphysician–physician John Donne (see the Front Matter) also wrote, "No man is an island, Entire to himself. . . . Send not to seek for whom the bell tolls, it tolls for thee," in turn drawing on Chaucer's great work of the fifteenth century. As great twentieth-century authors like Hemingway also acknowledged, we are all connected in some way. It is through helping others that we find this deepest interdependence. It is important that this service be done out of thanks in the joy of giving, and living, because service can easily slide into a debit-and-credit accounting mentality. Service can take many forms, from simply being a loving friend or parent to stopping to help someone in need, to teaching others to help themselves. These are very personal forms of service. There is also an important wellness connection to our community and to our planet. When increasingly large, intrusive governments create new programs to provide services that were formerly provided by church, civic, and volunteers, we certainly lose the personal dimension and replace it with impersonal (and often disinterested and incompetent) bureaucracy; the same is happening with our "official" health care system in general.

SYNERGY

To these components of wellness could be added passion, hope, relaxation, wisdom, and peace. In the wellness lifestyle, each of these components suggests a context in which men and women can live their lives so that they can feel healthy, as well as a context that dramatically softens the experience when they do become sick. It is safe to say that these components of wellness, regularly practiced, are healthy for individuals and families. When these two are healthier, it helps make the community and society healthier.

All these wellness components act uniquely in each person with his or her own personalities, and within specific cultures, and they all act together in a person at the same time without a measurement of "relative value" (see Chapter 10).

Each of these wellness components is dramatically affected by the others; for example, humor is different in a jolly, friendly person than in an angry, lonely one. If one were to use these components in a therapeutic way, it would make sense to have the medical environment exude these qualities to create a context of love, wonder, curiosity, and humor. This atmosphere would have a positive health effect on patients, staff, and visitors, whether in an office or in a hospital.

The examination of these wellness qualities, until modern times, has not been addressed by science, but rather by art, philosophy, and religions. However, some exciting research in medicine today is finding the connections in biochemistry and physiology between the mind and its thoughts, and the health of the body. This new field is evolving and the practice is now popularly called *mind-body medicine* (see Chapters 9 and 10) and the basic science behind it, *psychoneuroimmunology* (see Chapter 8).

HUMOR AND LAUGHTER

This chapter looks at one component of wellness in detail—humor. Many of the wellness components (e.g., love, passion, faith) are difficult to measure with some scientific precision or standard. Humor is thought to be somewhat different because it has one handle to measure it—laughter. Laughter has wide variation within genders, ages, personalities, and cultures, which means actual studies point to a direction rather than establish a fact. This research is one area of study in which anecdotal experience may have to count as science. One who uses humor in therapy does not do so because he or she found that laboratory studies showed its value.

Humor therapy is not a static regimen of memorized (unlike much of medical education) jokes and numbers of chuckles per hour. Humor therapy comes out when therapists decide to let their humorous parts enjoin their interactions with a patient. This approach can be expressed in many forms, such as laughter, theater, and verbal and physical play. With humor, the one who practices (whether laugher, funny person, clown, or comic) the craft in the "laboratory of laughter" is the patient, audience, or friend. All of one's past experience in that laboratory is brought to the spontaneous act with the patient, and if it is effective, smiling and laughter occur. This positive feedback is the determining feature in reproducing the gesture, statement, or behavior that elicited the laughter. When a patient says, "My doctor has a good bedside manner," he or she is speaking not about scientific and technical expertise, but about qualities of interaction. A friendly, playful sense of humor is at the core of a good bedside manner. The patient's appreciation perpetuates the behavior. Friendship is the safest context for humor in which to work, so when humor has missed its mark, instead of giving offense, forgiveness is felt. It is noteworthy that this dimension of "friendship" is also felt to be important by experts in sorting our relations among teacher, student and patient, among practitioners of "mindfulness-based" interventions (McCown et al, 2010).

> A merry heart doeth good like a medicine.
> —Proverbs 17:22

BOX 13-1 *Herbert's Spencer's Laughter as "Survival of the Fittest"*

The *first to* make the suggestion that laughter is a discharge mechanism for "nervous energy" seems to have been Herbert Spencer, a nineteenth-century British social scientist and philosopher who is paradoxically credited with coining the term "survival of the fittest." He based this term on his interpretation of Charles Darwin's work on evolutionary biology. (Darwin himself never used the term.) Nonetheless, Spencer's concept certainly provided ample reasons for humans in society to be "nervous" and thus have the need to discharge "nervous energy."

Spencer's essay the "Physiology of Laughter" (1860) starts with the proposition: "Nervous energy always tends to beget muscular motion; and when it rises to a certain intensity always does beget it. . . . Emotions and sensations tend to generate bodily movements, and . . . the movements are violent in proportion as the emotions or sensations are intense." Hence, he concludes, "when consciousness is unawares transferred from great things to small" the "liberated nerve force" will expand itself along the channels of least resistance, which are the muscular movements of laughter.

One searches in such descriptions for something to appear that may be useful in helping patients or caregivers in the delivery of care. For this we turn to research done in the twentieth century.

HISTORY

There is little recorded history of the use of laughter therapy; much of it is being made now (Box 13-1). However, there is a large body of comments on humor and laughter from literature, philosophy, religion, and the arts.

Arthur Koestler (1964) summarizes a fraction of these comments in his book *The Act of Creation:*

> Among the theories of laughter that have been proposed since the days of Aristotle, the "theory of degradation" appears as the most persistent. For Aristotle himself laughter was closely related to ugliness and debasement; for Cicero "the province of the ridiculous . . . lies in certain baseness and deformity"; for Descartes laughter is a manifestation of joy "mixed with surprise or hate or sometimes with both"; in Francis Bacon's list of laughable objects, the first place is taken by "deformity."

The essence of the "theory of degradation" is defined in Thomas Hobbes's seventeenth-century classic on man and society, *Leviathan:*

> The passion of laughter is nothing else but sudden glory arising from a sudden conception of some eminency in ourselves by comparison with the infirmity of others, or with our own formerly.

Regarding this view, Hobbes's own description of his birth in 1588, the year the Spanish Armada was threatening to invade England: "Born in 1588, Armada Year; Twin came forth, myself and fear."

Bainey (1993), one of the founders of modern psychology, largely followed the same theory:

> Not in physical effects alone, but in everything where a man can achieve a stroke of superiority, in surpassing or discomforting a rival, is the disposition of laughter apparent.

For Bergson (1911), laughter is the corrective punishment inflicted by society upon the unsocial individual: "In laughter we always find an unavowed intention to humiliate and consequently to correct our neighbor." The early-twentieth-century humorist Max Beerbohm found "two elements in the public's humour: delight in suffering, contempt for the unfamiliar." McDougall believed that "laughter has been evolved in the human race as an antidote to sympathy, a protective reaction shielding us from the depressive influence of the shortcomings of our fellow men."

RESEARCH

According to Ruxton (1988), humor can help establish rapport and verbalize emotionally charged interpersonal events. Using humor, patients may find it easier to express embarrassing or frightening parts of their history, and when nurses use funny anecdotes and are more vulnerable with a patient, it appears to strengthen the staff–patient bond.

Coser (1959) looked closely at a hospital's social structure and found that humor helped relieve tension, reassure, transfer information, and draw people together. Publisher Norman Cousins (1979) put humor back on the therapeutic map when he laughed himself well from a profound painful chronic illness, dramatically reducing the pain of his ankylosing spondylitis. He spent the rest of his life working with the University of California School of Medicine investigating the positive emotions and their relations to health. Dr. William Fry studied humor for 50 years and believed it is an exercise for the body. Mirthful laughter exercises the diaphragm and cardiovascular systems. Initially it causes an increase in heart rate and blood pressure, but after a short while it produces a much longer lasting decrease in heart rate and blood pressure, a relaxation response. Paskind (1932) first showed that skeletal muscle tone was diminished during mirthful laughter in muscles not actually participating in the laughter. Lloyd (1938) showed an expiratory predominance with mirthful laughter manifesting in a decrease in residual air in the lungs and increased oxygenation of the blood. Based on work done by Schachter and Wheeler (1962) and Levi (1965), catecholamine levels appear to be elevated with mirthful laughter. Researchers later found the body's immune response to laughter (see Chapter 8).

Sigmund Freud had originally suggested that the psychotherapeutic use of humor causes a release of stress,

BOX 13-2 *Medical Humor*

- The Doctor gave a man 6 months to live. The man could not pay his bill, so the doctor gave him another 6 months.
- The Doctor called the patient, saying, "Madame, your check came back." The patient answered, "So did my arthritis!"
- *Doctor:* "You'll live to be 60!" *Patient:* "I am 60!" *Doctor:* "See! What did I tell you?"
- A doctor held a stethoscope up to a man's chest. The man asks, "Doc, how do I stand?" The doctor says, "That's what puzzles me!"
- *Patient:* "I have a ringing in my ears." *Doctor:* "Don't answer!"
- *Patient:* "It hurts when I do this." *Doctor:* "Don't do that."

tension, and anxiety. Psychotherapists use humor to facilitate insight (through metaphor, joke, or story) and offer a sense of detachment or perspective. Humor can build a closer relationship between therapist and patient. Humor can be offered as a tool for coping with life's troubles (Box 13-2).

Mahrer and Gervaize (1974) looked at their review of the research literature on laughter in psychotherapy and found that strong laughter is a valuable indication of the presence of strong feelings and is seen by most therapeutic approaches as a desirable event. Strong laughter seems to correlate with increased self-esteem and heightened experiencing.

Although research has not conclusively shown a release of endorphins with mirthful laughter, the anecdotal literature about laughter's pain-killing properties is massive. Cousins (1979) opened this door. The Clemson University nurses' program did a study with elderly residents in a long-term care facility. The residents were divided into two groups. One group watched a comedy video nightly for 6 weeks; the other watched a serious drama. The nurses checked the need for analgesics. There were fewer requests for painkillers from the comedy group. Texas Tech University School of Medicine did another study in which research participants were shown comedy or serious material for just 20 minutes; relaxation therapy was given to a third group. The researchers then determined the participants' pain thresholds using inflated blood pressure cuffs. The comedy group had the greatest pain tolerance of the three groups.

One of us (Patch Adams) would here like to relate a powerful story of a time when humor quite clearly was a painkiller.

CONTEXT

I have been doing street clowning almost daily for 40 years, increasingly all over the world. In my 45 years of being a physician, I have always practiced in a humorous context.

With a group called Gesundheit Institute, we are building the first hospital to fully incorporate humor. Although the idea is disconcerting at first, in the many lectures to lay and medical audiences I have given for the last 25 years about our work, when asked which ward they would choose—a serious, solemn one or a fun, silly one—more than 85% have chosen the fun one. Few people need more than their personal experience to be completely convinced that humor is necessary for their personal health and the health of their relationships.

The primary practice of medicine is a delicate balance between science and art. Ideally, this relationship is one of friendship in which, although the parties have radically different approaches, there is a mutual appreciation of the value of all parties involved and a thankfulness and a necessity that they can work together in harmony. Science and art play different roles in the healing interaction. Medical science works at tackling the disease (the organ or systems afflicted) using a well-mapped-out series of thought processes, tests, and treatments. The "art of medicine" is concerned with how the disease affects the patient, the family, and their society—the larger repercussions of the disease. These concepts are beautifully discussed in *The Illness Narratives* (Kleinman, 1988) and *The Nature of Suffering* (Cassell, 1991). The art of medicine comes from the intuition and inherent magic found in compassion, love, humor, wonder, and curiosity. For these reasons, one is hard put to break down the components or mechanics of what is working in the art of medicine. Simply put, science serves reductionism, and art serves holism. For this reason, when I do clowning, I am free to explore all these healing abstractions. I use all of these approaches in a multitude of combinations, not because they are well mapped out but because they can more freely arise within the clown persona.

I am both a professional clown and a physician. Each discipline took about the same number of years to master. The difficulties in becoming each were also similar. In one, I had to master information and the ability to synthesize information to make responsible decisions; and in the other, I had to master the art of spontaneity and freedom of behavior. I could never say which parts of my clown persona did the trick in a healing interaction, and I bet the patient could not either. I can only say that my character brings a blatant expression of love, innocence, fun, joy, and friendliness to which people readily respond.

I believe humor and love are at the core of good bedside manner, burnout prevention, and malpractice prevention, and for these reasons alone, humor deserves a central place in a medical practice. But let us not deny its value in just raw fun. Despite my long, deep experiences with humor, I still can be brought to tears of joy over its power.

This power was all brought home to me in November 1991 in a children's burn unit in a hospital in Tallinn, the capital of Estonia, which at that time, was just becoming independent from the collapsing former USSR.

 Case Study

For many years I have taken a group of clowns to the former Soviet Union, now Russia, to promote good relations between our countries, to spread good cheer, and to provide a 2-week seminar in clowning for both beginners and professionals. We clown in hospitals, orphanages, prisons, and schools, and we perform a tremendous amount in the street. Everywhere we go, patients, staff, and clowns are tremendously uplifted; at times it even seems to help their medical problems.

Estonia was the footnote to a trip that normally just visits Moscow and St. Petersburg. I added it in 1991 so that we could explore a new country. We arrived 25-clowns strong at the burn hospital, where right off I noticed a woman crying outside a closed door. My medical training told me that this was a mother agonizing over a severely ill child. I knew that to touch her pain I should not clown with her—but with her child. Against strong protestations from the smiling staff, I went inside the room.

I walked in on three women (one physician and two assistants) who had just begun to change dressings and perform debridement on a 5-year-old boy, Raido, who had at least 60% third-degree burns solid from ears to knees on both sides of his body. He was in his third week of recovery. I was first struck by the medical supply and pharmaceutical shortages so devastating in the former Soviet Union, where the Communist government had run the health care system, in the winter of 1991. There were no masks or gloves and no strong painkillers, but the work had to be done. With the utmost in loving tenderness on the staff's part and commanding bravery on the boy's part, I watched the bandages come off his wound, revealing a bloody exudative, meaty field, slowly healing from the edges with no evidence of grafts. The silence was punctuated by Raido's screams with each tug of the bandages. At first I felt the horror of a parent for his suffering. From this feeling came a gushing empathy moving the clown to act instinctively; to love, comfort, care for, and bring forth laughter. Without fear.

I watched only for the first third of removal because I was not sure how to proceed. Raido's neck involvement prevented him from looking up at me. When they took a short break, I went over, dressed in full clown regalia, bent over him, and smiled. Spontaneously he looked surprised and delighted and said in Estonian, "You look beautiful." My heart was captured. I immediately went around to the head of his stretcher and spent the next hour stroking his face and hair, smiling and laughing and talking with him. We played. He stopped screaming entirely. I was only 1 foot from his small, unburned face, and I fell in love with him (having a 4-year-old son at that time, myself). I had never seen humor's power so raw. I kept telling him he was beautiful and strong and that he was going to live.

Continued

Case Study—cont'd

It is clear that the child is the one who changed himself from being sad to being cheerful. I was my clown self. His response "you're beautiful" came as a surprise. My character is not "beautiful" in terms of the Western standards of pulchritude. It was his willingness to let me inside that made me be of beauty and value to him. Another child could have been spooked and cried. Unlike a surgical operation, the impact of humor on the patient wholly has to do with the individual patient.

I cannot say what specifically I did that was, in this case, the catalyst for a pain-free experience. Was it the sparkle in my eye, the duck hat on my head, the soothing stroking of his head, the words of love and encouragement—or was it simply skilled diversion—like a magician?

Raido asked me to come back to his room, so I wheeled his mummy-wrapped body (bandages already bloody) back to his bed. There for 1 hour I entertained him with clown silliness, still peering into his sky-blue eyes and stroking his face. I do not know who benefited more, because my whole body shook, thrilled for being there. I left most of my toys with Raido, even dressing up his dad like a clown while Raido laughed heartily. It was hard to leave him; I felt like he had given me so much.

HUMOR AS THERAPY

So what is humor therapy? In its broadest sense it is whatever one does to put mirth into a patient encounter or hospital setting. This field is still new, and many are exploring how to add humor to the medical setting.

Ruth Hamilton has been using humor carts at Duke University Medical Center since 1989. Peggy Bushey is a nurse who has used the same carts in the intensive care unit (ICU) at Medical Hospital of Vermont for several years. These carts have comic videos and cassettes, funny and cartoon books, props, makeup, and costumes, and a host of volunteers are called in on consultation for patients or staff who request it. Patients have given wonderful feedback on the pain-killing and relaxing results of cart use. There is a suggestion that they improve communication, help visitors to hospitals to relax, and even increase motivation in rehabilitation programs. Greater staff relaxation may also be a factor.

Other hospitals, such as Dekalb Medical Center near Atlanta, have created lively rooms, similar to an expanded cart, with all the same items and a place to use them. Carts and rooms do not make humor, however, so the volunteer becomes the key.

In 1990, Michael Christensen of the Big Apple Circus started taking clowns into children's hospitals to make regular, three-times-a-week rounds to the children. What started out as a whim for him has become a full-time passion. He now has 45 clowns in six hospitals in New York City. Clowns who have worked for him have since set up similar programs in France, Germany, and Holland. The wonderful, positive feedback by staff, patients, and family keeps this program alive.

Others, like Annette Goodheart, insist that they do "laughing therapy," not humor therapy. There are laughter meditations and workshops on laughter and play. For many the decision has simply been how to bring more laughter, play, and levity to the medical setting. It suggests a broader view for humor therapy. In our society, which harbors alienation, depression, anxiety, and boredom, one could decide to be indiscriminately humorous and joyous to try to add these elements to every human encounter. It would help our general societal health.

Humor therapy could include wearing a loud bow tie, singing on the ward, engaging in word play, posting cartoons around the hospital, and even inviting comedians to come into the hospital. One note of caution: some believe humor can be harmful in some situations, especially in psychotherapy. I would certainly suggest humor that is not racist or sexist. I suggest first becoming quite close to your patients and having them be sure of your tenderness and sincerity, so that if a funny situation or joke hurts, someone can simply apologize. It behooves the medical history taker to make an exploration into the patient's sense of humor and act on it. Because humor in therapy is new to medicine, at least "officially," we have asked a half-dozen of the leading voices in humor today to make a few statements about their place in the use of humor. I also encourage people considering putting more humor in their practice to consult the resources at the end of this chapter for greater depth.

HUMOR THERAPY IN PRACTICE

BIG APPLE CIRCUS CLOWN CARE UNIT

The Big Apple Circus Clown Care Unit (CCU) is a community outreach program of the Big Apple Circus, a not-for-profit performing arts organization presenting the finest classic circus in America. The CCU transforms the performance of classic circus arts to aid in the care and healing of hospitalized children and teens, and their parents and caregivers.

Just as classic circus defines a specific body of knowledge, so too does classic clowning. Three classic clown types of the *Comedia dell'Arte*, White, Auguste, and Eccentric, appeared as horsemen, acrobats, jugglers, dancers, musicians and, of course, actors and actresses. Using all these skills, they had a singular focus: to make people laugh. To this end, they used parody. They parodied all circus acts, rules, structures, and authority as symbolized in one circus figure: the black-booted, top-hatted, red-coated, riding-cropped ringmaster.

For the Big Apple Circus CCU, the hospital room replaces the circus ring; the physician replaces the ringmaster; and all the rules, charts, formulas, procedures, machines, and straight-laced, white-washed corridors of the hospital become the source of endless parody. The focus is still to bring laughter to patients' hearts.

Using juggling, mime, music, and magic, 35 specially trained "doctors of delight" bring the joy and excitement of classic circus to the bedsides of hospitalized children 2 and 3 days each week, 50 weeks a year. The Big Apple CCU makes "clown rounds," a parody of medical rounds in which the healing power of laughter is the chief medical treatment. Using sophisticated medical-clown techniques (including red-nose "transplants," "rubber chicken" soup, and "kitty" cat scans), professional CCU performers work one-on-one with hospitalized children, their parents, and caregivers to ease the stress of serious illness by reintroducing laughter and fun as natural parts of life.

In the Beginning

The CCU was created in 1986 by Michael Christensen, director of clowning at the Big Apple Circus, in cooperation with the medical staff at Babies and Children's Hospital of New York at New York–Presbyterian/Columbia University Medical Center. The first CCU clowns, "Dr. Stubs" and "Disorderly Gordoon," learned that they could reduce children's fears about their hospital experiences by using medical instruments as props (e.g., blowing bubbles through a stethoscope) or performing silly medical procedures that echo real medical procedures (e.g., chocolate milk transfusions). The red-nose "transplant," for example, was created specifically to ease the fears of heart transplant patients at Babies and Children's Hospital.

At every CCU host hospital, the medical staff has recognized the healing effect of the CCU—how joy and delight relieve the stress of pediatric patients and their worried parents; how music, magic, and mayhem in the halls make patients easier to treat and enhance the effectiveness of the medical staff; and how a happy child appears to get better faster. Dr. Driscoll, chairman of pediatrics at Babies and Children's Hospital of New York, states, "When a child begins to laugh, it means he's probably beginning to feel better. I see the clowns as healers. When someone gets around to studying it, I would not be at all surprised to see a connection between programs like the CCU and shorter hospital stays."

In addition to being the subject of numerous news articles and television features, Michael Christensen and the CCU have received wide public recognition for their innovative work in the field of health and humor, including the prestigious Raoul Wallenberg Humanitarian Award, the Red Skelton Award, and the Northeast Clown Convention's annual Gold Nose Award.

Resident Hospital Programs

The Big Apple Circus currently operates CCU programs in seven prominent metropolitan hospitals: Babies and Children's Hospital of New York at Columbia–Presbyterian Medical Center, Harlem Hospital Center, the Hospital for Special Surgery, Memorial Sloan-Kettering Cancer Center, Mount Sinai Medical Center, New York University Medical Center, and Schneider Children's Hospital of Long Island Jewish Medical Center. Each CCU clown team works under the direct supervision of the hospital's chief of pediatrics.

In addition, the CCU is resident each summer at Queens Hospital Center and Paul Newman's Hole in the Wall Gang Camp for children with cancer and chronic blood diseases.

Working in close partnership with the medical staff at each hospital, the CCU tailors its activities to meet the special needs of each facility. The supervising clown consults daily with nurses, child life staff, and chief residents on the status of individual children. The clown team visits children in all areas of the hospital, including at their bedsides in wards, in ICUs, and in clinic and acute care waiting rooms. The CCU clowns also visit specialty clinics such as the bone marrow transplant unit at Memorial Sloan-Kettering Cancer Center and the human immunodeficiency virus/acquired immunodeficiency syndrome (HIV/AIDS) clinic at Harlem Hospital.

All CCU clowns are professional performers who have auditioned and have been selected for their professionalism, artistry, and sensitivity. They undergo a rigorous CCU training program to prepare them to work safely and appropriately in the hospital environment. The CCU continually improves its level of quality through rehearsals, continuing education, and procedural and artistic reviews.

The CCU has plans to expand to preeminent children's hospitals in major cities throughout the country. Affiliate programs begun by Big Apple Circus CCU–trained performers currently operate in France (Paris), Brazil (São Paulo), and Germany (Wiesbaden).

If you would like further information about the CCU, see www.bigapplecircus.org/clown-care or contact Big Apple Circus Clown Care Unit, 35 West 35th Street, 9th Floor, New York, NY 10001; (212) 268-2500.

LAUGHING SPIRIT LISTENING CIRCLES

The potential for healing laughter bubbles deep within us like natural hot springs. It just is. For *laughing spirit listening circles*, humor therapy is about providing the safe space that allows us to erupt in our uniquely unpredictable, often socially unacceptable way, fluidly carrying warm chuckles, hot guffaws, and tender tears to the places within and without that serve our body, our soul, and our community.

The laughter that is the best medicine is that which lies beneath seriousness and respects gravity, sadness, fear, frustration, and anger. It is not the surface, over-the-counter, diluted gigglery we call "lightening up."

Robust tears are no less potent than lusty laughter, and when "lightening up" is even slightly more valued over "getting heavy," therapy is dead and community is crippled.

Humor therapy in the form called *laughing spirit listening circles* involves participants in a group of 6 to 10, each of whom gets equal time to receive absolute positive, silent attention, first for 3 minutes, then for 5 minutes. The guidelines are "dare to be boring." You do not even have to speak. When you do, just tell the truth without trying to be funny. Stay in connection with individuals when you speak. Receive your support, rather than trying to give. The first time around is often serious, even grave, as people feel the safety and respect and build the integrity of the community. By the second time around, laughter and tears often flow, sometimes interchangeably.

Laugh Mobile Program

The Carolina Health and Humor Association (Carolina Ha Ha) is an educational service organization dedicated to promoting humor in health care and for personal growth. The Duke Humor Project started with the Duke Oncology Recreation Therapy department in 1986. At Duke University Medical Center in Durham, North Carolina, oncology patients may come for as long as 6 weeks for various cancer treatments. One difficulty with recreational programming is that patients must feel well enough to attend a group craft or entertainment program. Often the patient is too ill to leave the room during the intensive treatments. The Laugh Mobile was created to bring humorous media bedside to these patients. Volunteers from Carolina Health and Humor Association use the Laugh Mobile to deliver bedside laughs and to initiate a *humor intervention*. A humor intervention may be described as a plan to promote joy and laughter in the treatment program for patient care.

The Duke Humor Project continues to bring joy bedside to cancer patients at Duke University Medical Center. The Laugh Mobile delivers humorous media bedside to patients and family twice weekly. Humor volunteers engage in yo-yo demonstrations, guitar playing, and practical jokes. For example, the patient may want to set up a "whoopee cushion" under the covers of his or her bed and then invite the doctor "to have a seat and take a load off." Water guns are also dispensed to allow the patient a way to fight back. It is all in the interest of building fun-loving relationships, and the staff is highly receptive to any humor statements from the patient, especially practical jokes.

One of the evolving aspects of the Duke Humor Project and the Laugh Mobile Program is the referral procedure used for targeting the patients. The professional oncology recreation staff attends grand rounds and gathers information about the patients who may be most receptive to humor. Background information is provided in a notebook that goes with the Laugh Mobile. This report contains pertinent information on the patient and suggestions for the best approach. For example, the staff may relate that the patient is hard of hearing or that the patient may enjoy learning to juggle scarves. The humor volunteer comes in and sees each patient on referral. The volunteer reports back to the staff about how the humor intervention worked. This gives the hospital staff an opportunity to follow up between Laugh Mobile visits.

Humor and intentional laughter programs are expanding to reach patients in all stages of recovery with volunteers who work with the cancer patients weekly. New avenues for spreading the humor programming include the design of programs for bone marrow transplant and cardiac care patients. Each illness seems to have its own set of humorous episodes and strategies requiring exploration with patients as to the areas that need more humor and to suggest funny coping strategies. A challenge is continually to seek new ways for the "humor impaired" to laugh and to invite the medical staff to enjoy more playfulness. Community-based groups such as Carolina Ha Ha, which offers both trained volunteers and professional program implementation, continue to plant the seeds of comic caring and loving laughter.

THE GROWING WORLD OF HUMOR

When Dr. William Fry first started humor studies in 1953, there was a dearth of scientific investigation of the subject. Literary analyses of humor and comedy abounded, and there was ample hypothesizing and theorizing, particularly about the identity of the crucial element of humor that precipitates the mirthful reaction. Also, a few psychological and anthropological studies had carried out examinations of humor preferences, humor values, interactive uses of humor, communication, and humor; this was as close as we got to science. Mind you, it was not a complete wasteland, but it looked like an Edward Hopper canvas; it certainly was not Times Square at midnight on New Year's Eve.

Fry entered the field through the gate of humor and communications, as a member of ethnologist Gregory Bateson's research team (Bateson was married to American anthropologist Margaret Mead, who did fieldwork in the South Pacific, following the great European anthropologist Bronislow Malinoswski, and became better known for it). The research team had been originally assembled by Bateson to explore the roles of the "paradoxes of logical type" in communication (Fry, 1971). As a psychiatrist, Fry was the team member with training most closely related to the so-called hard sciences, with university classes in a large variety of chemistries, physics, embryology, bacteriology, laboratory technology, physiology, and biochemistry. The scientific method had been portrayed as the criterion for research purity and rigor. Psychiatric residency exercised understanding of scientific discipline by designing, conducting, and reporting in the literature a postdoctoral psychophysiological study of schizophrenia.

In the 1950s a certain excitement had been stirred in the humor studies field by psychologist D.E. Berlyne, a very talented and innovative scholar. Up to the time of his contributions, humor theory was strongly dominated by the views Freud had adopted from nineteenth-century social philosopher Herbert Spencer's "discharge of energy" postulate (see Box 13-1), who was the first to originate the concept expressed as "survival of the fittest" (a term never actually used by Darwin).

This dominance theory directed most views of humor to observing it primarily as a cathartic phenomenon, a sudden diminution of repressed psychic energy involving a release from inhibition. Berlyne's contribution shifted emphasis to the state of arousal, which he proposed to be the dominant element of the humor response: "laughter . . . is restricted to situations in which a spell or moment of aversely high arousal is followed by sudden and pronounced arousal reduction" (Berlyne, 1972). Needless to say, this attempt to supplant Freud's doctrine aroused much controversy and energy. Some of the energy was channeled into research procedures aimed at proving or disproving one or another of the main themes and their various corollaries. As these experiments proceeded and were reported in the scientific literature, it became increasingly perceived they were using defective protocols, in that much of the test ratings were based on subjective, vaguely defined, and arbitrary criteria; in many instances, test results were measured by degrees of humor identified as "much," "moderate," or "slight," or by some similar system. Conclusions based on these studies were flawed by deficiencies of objectivity.

A readily available source of objectivity in humor experimentation would be the physiological phenomena that both the Freudians and the Berlynians agreed accompany the perception of humor and the experiencing of reactive mirth. A National Institute of Mental Health small grant in 1963–1964 made it possible to develop an answer to the question of whether it is possible to observe experimentally the somewhat ephemeral physiology of mirth in such artificial and rigid environments as those that often develop in scientific pursuits (when the fun of science is lost sight of, or is ignored).

During the 1960s, the unhumorous Vietnam War buildup made it futile to try to obtain financial support from government scientific agencies (when armaments had so much greater priority than laughter). Fry instead worked on designing and carrying out a series of basic science studies of the physiology of mirth and laughter during the following approximately 15 years.

Fry and colleagues in those studies were able to perform contributive research in most of the human body's major physiology system areas (Fry, 1994) to demonstrate significant impacts of mirth and mirthful laughter in the cardiovascular, respiratory, muscular, immune, endocrine, and central nervous systems. With that basic science information established and disseminated, many other professionals subsequently have found it possible and desirable to extend their speculations and practice outside spheres of scholarly study in a number of directions, many of them relating to health issues, both in prevention of disease and in uses of humor as adjunctive therapy to traditional treatment procedures.

During the 1960s, 1970s, and 1980s, several other themes and ventures were forming, developing, building, expanding, and arousing the interest and participation of more and more persons throughout North America, in the United Kingdom, and to a certain extent in Europe, especially in France, the Netherlands, and Belgium. This process was a vital component of a truly revolutionary movement throughout the world. The worldwide movement has been designated by several different titles, depending on the specific location or years being considered.

Broader titles identify this movement as a modern renaissance, a new style of life, and the deconstruction era; more specific titles designated the hippy revolution, the free speech movement, and an overturning of old values. The period for a while was called the age of Aquarius. Other, less enthusiastic designations characterized the new era as being a time of Satan's dominance over humankind or an ascendancy of evil and libertine practices. Whatever the values ascribed, there is little argument over the presence of new beliefs, values, and social practices, over the revolutions of social customs, garb, artistic expression, communication, lifestyles, music, interpersonal interactions of many varieties, and religious practices. This revolution undoubtedly was built on the shoulders of earlier times, as is the way of the world. However, this era was a watershed, providing a parametric cultural shift (see Chapter 7).

Tons of paper and miles of words have been exchanged during the past 50 years regarding this parametric revolution. Discussion of the underlying implications, and dealing with issues of the past and future of humanity, is beyond the scope of this chapter. Suffice it to say that a vast proportion of the revolutionary changes has been associated with what can be called the "pragmatics" of human life and human behavior. Changes brought during these turbulent years have involved more the everyday ways of humans, less so a consideration of the many and deep implications of the turbulence and its innovative consequences. To be sure, these implications have received some attention, but to a large extent in the more traditional manner of analysis and consideration. The changes in lifestyle and performance have been huge and have been little inhibited by the paucity of reflective attention turned toward them. There has been much change in daily ways of life, and not only in so-called developed cultures; the revolution has been universal over the globe, with varied intensities and varied specifics of behavior—called by some, "a new world order" (anticipated by the U.S. Founding Fathers as *novum ordus seculorum*; see Chapter 1).

Returning to the issues of humor in health care, it is apparent that part of this revolution has been a process of reshaping the pragmatics of health care, making it possible to consider many new features of health care, including interrelationships between health care and humor, in which humor takes adjunctive roles such as cited previously. Underlying the pragmatics that predominate with this development is new emphasis on the principle of one's personal responsibility for one's own health care (Cousins, 1979).

More so than many other products of this social revolutionary era, the issue of health care responsibility received more and more attention since the 1970s and 1980s. With this expanding orientation, and under the title of "holistic medicine," implementation of adjunctive roles in healing and health care for humor, as well as many other alternative, complementary, and integrative nontraditional medical practices, became not only possible, but also realized. Many opportunities for using humor and mirthful laughter have been created and taken advantage of successfully. Dr. Fry identified one of us (Patch Adams) as one of the luminous pioneers in this humor movement. The movement has spread throughout areas of the world where humans attempt to improve the quality of their lives, both in health and at times of illness.

The nature of many humor–health care innovations is such that adjunctive use of humor, mirth, and laughter is having increasingly interesting application. Facilities have been established in hospitals, convalescent homes, day care centers, long-term care units, and rehabilitation centers in which sources of humor are made available. These humor sources are usually intended primarily for the patient or resident, but this practice has also brought forth recognition that benefits of humor can be experienced by others in the broader health care environment. As studies have demonstrated, staff members, patients' family members, volunteers, and community contacts all have benefited by having humor "tonics" available at times when they are beset by the various "negative emotions" so common in such circumstances. Patient benefits are demonstrated to come doubly, both from direct impact and from the energizing and positive effects on those who are participating with the patient in his or her struggle for return to or maintenance of health. It is indicative of this "double value" that much of the encouragement for humor facility establishment in health care institutions has come from nursing staffs who routinely experience a greater degree of patient–provider interaction, both in terms of quantity and intensity.

This use of humor in health care facilities as adjunctive therapy to other, more traditional medical procedures and practices does not stand alone in the new orientation concerning humor in health care. A rising enthusiasm for humor in wider use, beyond institutional use and beyond the age-old popularity of humor as an important source of entertainment and amusement, is fueling spread of humor forms among populations throughout the world (Berger, 1993). This enthusiasm has broken down many of the customary prejudices against humor, which have previously characterized humor as frivolous, unimportant, or vulgar and reprehensible. People have shaken the sense of guilt or shame or flippancy that earlier restricted their access to their natural, genetically inculcated sense of humor (Morreall, 1983).

Individuals in their inner lives, in their relationships with family members, in the workplace, and in their public activities increasingly avail themselves of this element of their biological inheritance to enrich their existence and to make unexpected discoveries about the complexities of life (Blumenfeld and Alpern, 1994; Klein, 1989). Work-shops, seminars, lectures, and discussion groups throughout the world explore new and beneficial values of humor and laughter for enabling people to lead healthful lives, for helping patients recover from illness, and for helping patients maintain higher quality of life during illness. Humor was even admitted into the quiet privacy of psychotherapy and counseling (Fry et al, 1993).

Humor continues to be a major source of entertainment, a major component of the array of pleasures to be enjoyed in this world. All evidence indicates sturdy continuation of that status. Humor and laughter, with new knowledge and new attitudes about their values and benefits, now increasingly spread their magic into areas of human experience not previously visualized as appropriate places for their presence.

THREE MYTHS ABOUT LAUGHTER THAT KEEP US FROM LAUGHING

The *first major myth* about laughter that prevents us from laughing as much as we need to is that "we must have a reason to laugh." The people who respond to laughter with great seriousness may feel that there is no reason to be laughing, or if there is, they missed it. Not only must we have a reason to laugh, according to this myth, but the reason must be so good that when someone challenges us with "Why are you laughing? What is so funny?" when we explain it, they will "get it" and they too will laugh. (There is an old joke: "Did you hear about the duck that got social security?" Response: "You will when you're 65"—maybe.) If they do not get it, and do not laugh, very often we are presented with a puzzled face and a remark, such as, "That was it? Wow, you have a weird sense of humor!"

Many of us unconsciously censor our laughter because at some level we think our reason for laughing is not good enough. It is important to note here that the reality is that laughter is unreasonable, illogical, and irrational. We do not need a reason to laugh. When we see a 6-month-old baby laughing, we do not demand, "What's so funny?" but rather delight in the response and often join in. We can do so with adults as well. Insisting on a reason to laugh is an excellent way of stopping someone, or ourselves, from laughing. This is important to remember when we are in situations in which laughter is inappropriate. We may want to ask ourselves, "Why am I laughing right now?" so that we can stop, for example, if we get the giggles when pulled over by a policeman for speeding or some other minor infraction of the law.

The *second major myth* about laughter is that "we laugh because we are happy," when the reality is that we are also happy because we laugh. When asking how many feel better after they have laughed, there is always a unanimous show of hands. If laughter came out of happiness, we would not feel better after laughing—we would have already felt better *before* laughing.

Laughter has been assigned the job of indicating happiness because we have been so desperate for some outward sign of this vague, undefined, but treasured state. Actually, most people do not know what happiness is. We know that the U.S. Declaration of Independence (1776), with its "new world order," mandates us to pursue it (and, in fact, the right to do so is held to be "self-evident" except to our current government), but judging by our national behavior, we are somewhat confused about where happiness lies. If we feel better *after* we laugh, laughter must come from a source other than happiness.

Those many of us who have laughed until we have cried know that in the middle of the process, we can no longer tell which is which. We do not laugh because we are happy and cry because we are sad; we laugh or cry because we have tension, stress, or pain. Laughter and tears rebalance the biochemicals and physiology our bodies create when these distressed states are present, so we feel better after we have laughed *and/or* cried.

The *third major myth* is that "a sense of humor is the same thing as laughter." Although the two terms are used interchangeably, they are very different processes. The reality is that you do not need a sense of humor to laugh. There is much joyless, cynical, and sarcastic laughter in the world. And again, when we see a 6-month-old baby laughing, we do not remark, "Doesn't that baby have a wonderful sense of humor!" A sense of humor is learned; laughter is innate. A sense of humor is an intellectual process, whereas laughter spontaneously engages every major system in the body.

There is absolutely no agreement on what a sense of humor is or what makes something funny. Senses of humor vary according to personality, culture, age, ethnic or economic background, race, gender, and so on. One is informed on good authority that women in the ladies' room laugh at different things than do men in the men's room, including *at* the men in the men's room (and in many "progressive" jurisdictions today, at the men in the ladies' room, and vice versa). A man once raised his hand and said, "Men don't laugh in the men's room."

Many women (and some men) do not realize this fact, having spent very little time in the men's room (and certainly not as much time as the ladies spend in the ladies' room). A man once said he knew why men did not laugh in the men's room: it is hard to laugh and aim at the same time. The first week on the hospital floor, a professor in medical school advised the new students to make sure they learn the locations of all the men's rooms in the building. He said it will be the only place where you still feel like you know what you are doing.

Having a sense of humor does not guarantee laughter in the person in whom we identify that trait. Many people with great senses of humor, even comedic genius, do not laugh. Groucho Marx was known to have laughed only once, publicly or privately. He kept a straight face at all times when performing, including the occasion on the live 1950s TV show *You Bet Your Life,* when he expressed surprise (with his eyebrows) at a woman who told him she had

seven children. When she protested, "But I love my husband," Groucho responded, "I love my cigar, but I take it out of my mouth once in a while."

Often, people who make other people laugh do so because they can control when the laughter will occur. The emphasis on humor diverts us from the broad scope of laughter that is available, making laughter a specialty that is then possible only occasionally.

A DEFINITION OF HUMOR

A clear understanding of what constitutes humor and what does not, as listed next, is necessary to prevent the inevitable misunderstandings that arise when the subject is considered.

1. Humor is *not* the equivalent of laughter. Humor may or may not stimulate laughter; sometimes it is merely a quiet smile or even an inner glow of delight. Laughter may accompany humor, but it can also accompany aggression, surprise, and even grief (like Leoncavallo's *I Pagliacci,* or, if you prefer, Smokey Robinson and "The Tears of a Clown").
2. Joking makes up a minor percentage of humor experience. Only about 4% of the adult population admit to remembering and telling jokes well, whereas more than 90% consider that they have a "pretty good" sense of humor. Humor is often conveyed between persons nonverbally, such as in the eye twinkle and the smile, or Groucho's raised eyebrows.
3. Humor is *not* a form of therapy. It is a perspective and an appropriate behavior integrated in the overall conduct of our lives that can extend to health care and wellness.
4. Humor does *not* cure cancer, baldness, or major depression. Humor is a marvelous adjunct to the overall conduct of one's psychological life, especially when one is confronting illness, tragedy, or death.
5. Although the observational evidence is intriguing, humor as yet has *not* been demonstrated conclusively to release endorphins. ("Endorphins": small children without parents who live in the house all the time.)

Humor is a mature psychological response to stress in which the stressful issue is maintained in consciousness, without distortion, and is responded to with amusement when double meanings, ironies, or some other inconsistency is noted. Humor does not increase the discomfort of the individual nor those in his company.

Until the 1970s, humor was frowned upon in the conduct of medicine as being unprofessional or uncaring or even beneath the standard of care. Such an attitude could be in response to immature psychological defenses masquerading as humor (e.g., passive aggression, schizoid fantasy, projection).

Applying humor with kindness, compassion, and empathy is key. For the most part, humor in medical practice should take the form of gentle amusement, twinkling eye contact, and, only in rare situations, jokes.

The following is a short listing of specific guides to the conduct of humor (Hageseth, 1988) in a five, four, three formulation:

- **Five** mature ego mechanisms of defense:
  - Altruism
  - Humor
  - Anticipation
  - Suppression
  - Sublimation
- **Four** elements of successful communication of humor:
  - Relationship
  - Rapport
  - Setting
  - Timing
- **Three** pathways to a humor experience
  - Nonverbal interaction (e.g., smiling, eye twinkle)
  - Raising of forbidden, "taboo" subjects
  - Jokes and other forms of verbal humor

IT MAY BE SERIOUS, BUT IT NEEDN'T BE SOLEMN

These healing hot springs of holistic "laugh-tears" are what I'm after in humor therapy.
I try to be playful but others won't respond.
If I ever needed humor it is now.
I want to smile and laugh, but that upsets my family.

—Hospice patients' comments
(*American Journal of Hospice Care,* 1990)

Salt water is the cure for everything; sweat, tears and the sea

—Isak Dinesen

A couple of years ago a father-in-law was very ill. When he came home from the hospital, it was his wedding anniversary. The son-in-law suggested that they invite a few friends over for dinner and he would cook a turkey.

He managed to get out of bed to join in. He enjoyed the meal, but the strain of feeding himself and the presence of guests were obviously tiring him. Noticing this situation and knowing that he could not hear very well, his wife wrote a note and passed it to the son-in-law to give to him. She realized what she just wrote and laughed out loud:

The note said, "Happy Anniversary dear. Do you want to go to bed?"

He read what his wife had written, looked up across the table, and with a twinkle in his eye and a smile on his face slowly said to her, "I would love to dear, but we have company."

It was only a brief moment of levity in his difficult last days, but it was a moment that was long remembered after he was gone.

Looking for humor in the not-so-funny world of serious illness may seem disrespectful to those who are suffering. However, situational humor, which inevitably arises during stressful times, is very appropriate. Because of humor's ability to give a new perspective to any situation, it is an important coping tool for everyone involved in the dying process, including the physician.

Laughter is a powerful tool in otherwise powerless situations. It can give hope and an upper hand to patients who are experiencing both physical and mental loss, as well as to physicians who cannot change that loss or stop the demise of the patient.

The safest way for a physician to find that laughter is first to establish a rapport with the patient, then look for humor by listening to what the patient jokes about. Above all, do not go into a patient's room with a battery of jokes. First, jokes can be offensive, and second, when you enter a patient's room, you have no knowledge of whether they will be receptive to your kidding around. Keep in mind that humor is a wonderful bonding tool, but it can also backfire and create alienation.

Patty Wooten ("Nancy Nurse") once told a story about the time she was bathing a patient who had a rather large surgical scar down her front. The patient said, "Nurse, look at my scar. It looks just like Market Street in San Francisco." Puzzled by this remark, Patty questioned, "What do you mean, 'Market Street in San Francisco'?" "Well," replied the patient, "it goes from Twin Peaks to the waterfront." (Indeed, Market Street in San Francisco does run from Twin Peaks to the waterfront.)

Patty and the patient laughed uproariously together. Then, months later, Patty was bathing another woman who had a similar scar and told her this joke. The patient got highly insulted.

In the first case, humor came from a woman who was comfortable enough to laugh at what she had experienced; the second patient was not.

The best way to find humor when working with seriously ill patients is to listen to what they are saying. The patient is the one who will often give you the laugh lines.

One example comes from a man who had AIDS for 8 years. One day he had put up a Star of David, a crucifix, and a picture of Buddha on the wall. A friend walked into the house and said, "You're a Quaker, why do you have these opposing religious items around?" The ill man, who never missed a moment for some levity, replied, reminiscent of Pascal's Wager, "Well, you never know who's right. I'm covering all bases!"

He was someone who could joke about his illness, because he would be the first one to poke fun at his difficulties. Your patients are the ones who will let you know if it is okay to kid around with them, supply you with laughs, and help you see death as less of a grave matter.

HUMOR IN HEALTH CARE

We think of humor as just fun and play—not serious. Yet it is one of the most healthy, healing phenomena humans have. It is a cognitive, emotional, and physical response to stress. Humor gives us balance and a perspective and provides a comic relief and survival with all the seriousness of living.

Within the health care arena, which is probably one of the most stressful and craziest areas in which we can live and work, humor is a major coping mechanism for patients and staff and a powerful tool for healing. It makes a perfect mind–body connection! The humor, verbal or nonverbal, stimulates feelings of mirth and laughter, which researchers have found produces a healthy biochemical and physiological response in the body.

As an indirect form of communication, humor facilitates all the relationships and manages all the delicate situations that occur. It conveys messages and helps us get in touch with our feelings. And, when we laugh, we release those associated feelings.

Humor reduces all the social conflicts inherent in health care, and it facilitates change and survival in the system. As a major relief mechanism, humor reduces anxiety, provides a healthy outlet for anger and frustration, and is a healthy denial of all the heaviness of crises, tragedy, and death.

Humor is also a major source of coping for the caregiver and for the prevention of burnout. The health professional who can accept and value his or her need for laughter and comedy can then be comfortable using and encouraging humor with clients.

As a communication tool, humor should be an integral part of the total healing and caring process. Humor conveys our concern, understanding, warmth, and caring. As one patient said, when staff laughed and joked with him, he knew they cared.

For the health professional, key to the therapeutic use of humor is being sensitive to whose needs are being met and being sensitive to the right time, the right place, and the right amount, like a judicious dose of good medicine. Oftentimes the least medicine that works is the best medicine. And always, humor must be used in the context of caring, a laughing with and not a laughing at.

HUMOR—ANTIDOTE FOR STRESS

Humor is a perceptual quality that enables us to experience joy even when faced with adversity. Health professionals work in stress-filled environments that place demands on their physical, emotional, and spiritual well-being (Maslach, 1982). Most caregivers are compassionate and sensitive individuals working with people who are suffering. This combination too can be a source of stress. Caregivers can experience what is known as *compassion fatigue*—feeling that they have very little left to give (Ritz, 1995). Finding humor in our work and personal life can be one way to replenish ourselves from compassion fatigue (Ritz, 1995; Robinson, 1991; Wooten, 1995). This can be an effective self-care tool for the health care professional.

In his book *Stress Without Distress,* Selye (1974) clarified that a person's interpretation of stress does not depend solely on an objective external event, but also on the individual's subjective perception of the event and the meaning he or she gives it; how one looks at a situation determines whether one will respond to it as threatening or challeng-

ing (Kobassa, 1983). In this context, humor can be an empowerment tool because it gives us a different perspective on our problems, and with an attitude of detachment, we feel a sense of self-protection and control in our environment (Klein, 1989; McGhee, 1994). As comedian Bill Cosby is fond of saying, "If you can laugh at it, you can survive it."

There is a type of humor called "gallows humor" (McGhee, 1994; Robinson, 1991) that is unique to people who deal with tragedy and suffering. Those outside the caregiving professions often do not understand our sometimes desperate need to laugh and may not appreciate this type of humor. The term *gallows humor* supposedly came into being when two brothers were being executed by judicial hanging. Both were standing on the gallows, and one brother was already hanged when the other brother said, "Look at my brother there, making a spectacle of himself. Pretty soon we'll be a pair of spectacles."

This laughing bravado in the face of death is what caregivers can also use to maintain their sanity amidst the horror. It is well documented that there is more laughter in the ICU, emergency room, and operating room than in other places in the hospital setting. Much of the humor is sexual or obscene, or jokes directly about the tragedy and suffering (Ritz, 1995; Rosenburg, 1991; Wooten, 1995). This appears to be a psychological game one plays with oneself and others, in hope of communicating, "See, I'm doing okay amidst all this horror. Really. See? I'm laughing!"

An ICU nurse shared a sign that the staff had placed in the visitor waiting area to explain what might be overheard and misunderstood (Box 13-3).

We attempt to maintain balance by offsetting tragedy in our lives with comedy. Another true story of this cathartic activity was shared by an emergency room nurse:

> You saw me laugh after your father died. . . . To you I must have appeared calloused and uncaring. . . . Please understand, much of the stress health care workers suffer comes about because we do care. Sooner or later we will all

BOX 13-3 *Laughter in the Intensive Care Unit*

If you are waiting ...
You may possibly see us laughing; or even take note of some jest;
Know that we are giving your loved one our care at its very best!
There are times when tension is highest;
There are times when our systems are stressed;
We've discovered humor, a factor in keeping our sanity blessed.
So, if you're a patient in waiting, or a relative or friend of one seeing,
Don't hold our smiling against us, it's a way that we keep from screaming.
Sincerely,
The ICU Staff

laugh at the wrong time. I hope your father would understand, my laugh meant no disrespect, it was a grab at balance. I knew there was another patient who needed my full care and attention . . . my laugh was no less cleansing for me than your tears were for you. (Johnston, 1985)

Laughter can provide a cathartic release, a purifying of emotions, and a release of emotional tension. Laughter, crying, raging, and trembling are all cathartic activities that can unblock energy flow (Goodheart, 1996).

An ability to laugh at our situation or problem gives us a feeling of superiority and power. We are less likely to succumb to feelings of depression and helplessness if we are able to laugh at what is troubling us. Humor gives us a sense of perspective on our problems. Laughter provides an opportunity for the release of uncomfortable emotions, which, if held inside, may create biochemical changes that are harmful to the body.

As the famous American humorist Mark Twain once said:

> Humor is the great thing, the saving thing. After all, the moment it arises, all our hardnesses yield, our irritations and resentments slip away, and a sunny spirit takes their place. (Klein, 1989)

HEALTH CARE HUMOR IN TODAY'S WORLD—UPDATE FROM THE FIELD

So much has happened in the connection between humor and health since this chapter was first composed. [Actually, here's a funny story: the first version of this chapter was prepared for the first edition of this textbook in 1995; but somebody at the publisher's office got "cold feet"—which can be a major issue for a clown—about publishing a chapter about clowning in a new textbook on the serious subject of medicine, and the chapter did not actually appear until the second edition in 2000, for the new millenium.]

Clowns are now going strong in hospitals and nursing homes in 120 countries. There are even graduate degrees in hospital clowning. Many clowns have formed non-profit foundations so that they can help support themselves in formerly all-volunteer service. I (Patch Adams) have not. All the clowning I have done is free and I mostly work with untrained clowns between the ages 3 and 88 years from 50 countries on the six to nine clown trips we lead all over the world each year.

We have taken clowns into war zones, refugee camps, disasters (Haiti post-earthquake and Sri Lanka post-tsunami) and poverty. We have seen humor change the mood in the worst of circumstances. In Trinidad, I was asked to clown for five men who were hung the next day for capital crimes, and four loved it. (The other did not want to hang around for my act.)

For 50 years now, I have clowned every day in public to put joy in the public space, and for the last 30 years I have only worn clown clothes. I constantly see it soothe an environment, making it less alienating. I have used clowning often to stop public violence. For the last 30 years, I have been lecturing and performing 250 or more days a year in 70 countries and have seen humor alter every environment with a touching universality. I have also gone into hospitals and other institutions in 70 counties on 6 continents and been bathed in hilarity. Humor can alter the worst of suffering and it diminishes hierarchy.

I have been trying to promote the ability of clowns and of all citizens to reclaim the commons with joy and laughter. I would like to see what is being done in some U.S. hospitals spread to all human cultures. I know it would diminish depression and anxiety. In hospitals and other institutions, I encourage the staffs to use humor, joy, and love as a way of being, to help themselves not burn out, and to help hospitals be more radiant. In all my travels I have not found one happy hospital. I hear from medical students from 120 countries and all are crying out for more compassion and care. It is a deep hurt, and humor and love diffuse it (Gesundheit Institute, 2013).

After 42 years we have begun building our free hospital in West Virginia for which we have long planned (Adams, 1998). It will be the first (intentionally) silly hospital staff in history. All the permanent staff, from cleaning person to surgeon, will make the same salary, 300 dollars/month, and live together as a communal eco-village. By creating a free, humorous, joyous, loving hospital vested in cooperation, creativity, and thoughtfulness, we can attract unlimited staff to work at such low fees. This reality represents the economic value of humor and the whole design will eliminate over 90% of the cost of care. This reward is only part of value of a life in compassionate service.

Acknowledgments

The following contributed to this chapter in previous editions: William F. Fry, Lee Glickstein, Annette Goodheart, Christian Hageseth III, Ruth Hamilton, Allen Klein, Vera M. Robinson, and Patty Wooten.

References

Adams P: *House Calls,* San Francisco, 1998, Robert Reed Press, p 159.

Bainey M: *Why do we laugh and cry?* West Ryde, Australia, 1993, Sunlight Publications.

Berger AA: *An anatomy of humor,* New Brunswick, NJ, 1993, Transaction.

Bergson H: *Laughter: an essay on the meaning of the comic,* New York, 1911, Macmillan.

Berlyne DE: Humor and its kin. In Goldstein JH, McGhee PE, editors: *The psychology of humor,* New York, 1972, Academic Press.

Blumenfeld E, Alpern L: *Humor at work,* Atlanta, 1994, Peachtree.

Cassell E: *The nature of suffering,* New York, 1991, Oxford University Press.

Coser RL: Some social functions of laughter: a study of humor in a hospital setting, *Hum Relat* 12:171, 1959.

Cousins N: *Anatomy of an illness as perceived by the patient,* New York, 1979, Norton.

Fry WF: Laughter: is it the best medicine? *Stanford MD* 10(1):16, 1971.

Fry WF: The biology of humor, *Humor Int J Humor Res* 7(2):111, 1994.

Fry WF, Salameh W: *Advances in humor and psychotherapy*, Sarasota, Fla, 1993, Professional Resources Press.

Gesundheit Institute: *Clown in Kabul*, Urbana IL, 2013, Gesundheit Press.

Goodheart A: *Laughter therapy*, Santa Barbara, Calif, 1996, Stress Less Press.

Hageseth CM: *A laughing place*, Ft Collins, Colo, 1988, Berwick.

Johnston W: To the ones left behind, *Am J Nurs* 85(8):936, 1985.

Klein A: *The Healing power of humor*, Los Angeles, 1989, Tarcher.

Kleinman A: *The illness narratives*, New York, 1988, Basic Books.

Kobassa SC: Personality and social resources in stress resistance, *J Pers Soc Psychol* 45:839, 1983.

Koestler A: *The act of creation*, New York, 1964, Macmillan.

Levi L: The urinary output of adrenaline and noradrenaline during pleasant and unpleasant states, *Psychosom Med* 27:80, 1965.

Lloyd EL: The respiratory rate in laughter, *J Gen Psychol* 10:179, 1938.

Mahrer A, Gervaize P: An integrative review of strong laughter in psychotherapy: what it is and how it works, *Psychotherapy* 21:510, 1974.

Maslach C: *Burnout—the cost of caring*, Upper Saddle River, NJ, 1982, Prentice-Hall.

McCown DM, Reibel D, Micozzi MS: *Teaching Mindfulness*, New York, 2010, Springer.

McGhee P: *How to develop your sense of humor*, Dubuque, Iowa, 1994, Kendall-Hunt.

Morreall J: *Taking laughter seriously*, Albany, NY, 1983, State University of New York Press.

Paskind HA: Effect of laughter on muscle tone, *Arch Neurol Psychiatry* 23:623, 1932.

Ritz S: Survivor humor and disaster nursing. In Buxman K, editor: *Humor and nursing*, New York, 1995, Von Publishers.

Robinson V: *Humor and the health professions*, ed 2, Thorofare, NJ, 1991, Slack.

Rosenburg L: Clinical articles: a qualitative investigation of the use of humor by emergency personnel as a strategy for coping with stress, *J Emerg Nurs* 17(4):197–202; discussion 202–3. 1991.

Ruxton SP: Humor deserves our attention, *Holist Nurs Pract* 2(3):54, 1988.

Schachter S, Wheeler L: Epinephrine, chlorpromazine, and amusement, *J Abnorm Soc Psychol* 1962.

Selye H: *Stress without distress*, New York, 1974, Lippincott & Crowell.

Wooten P: Interview with Sandy Ritz, *J Nurs Jocularity* 5(1):46, 1995.

Suggested Readings

Ader R, Felten DL, Cohen N, editors: *Psychoneuroimmunology*, ed 2, San Diego, 1991, Academic Press.

Arieti S: New views on the psychology of wit and the comic, *Psychiatry* 13:43, 1950.

Averill JR: Autonomic response patterns during sadness and mirth, *Psychophysiology* 5(4):399, 1969.

Baron RA, Ball RL: The aggression-inhibition influence of non-hostile humor, *J Exp Soc Psychol* 10:23, 1974.

Barra JM: High kicks in the ICU, *RN* 49:45, 1986.

Baudelaire C: *The essence of laughter*, In Essays, New York, 1956, Meridian.

Berk LS, Felten D, Tan S, et al: Modulation of human natural killer cells by catecholamines, *Clin Res* 32(1):62–72, 1984.

Berk LS, Tan S, Napier B, et al: Eustress of mirthful laughter modifies natural killer cell activity, *Clin Res* 37(1):p. C064. 1989.

Berk LS, Tan S, Fry W, et al: Neuroendocrine and stress hormone changes during mirthful laughter, *Am J Med Sci* 296(7):390, 1989.

Berkowitz L: Aggressive humor as a stimulus to aggressive responses, *J Pers Soc Psychol* 16:710, 1970.

Beyondananda S: *When you see a sacred cow milk it for all it's worth*, Lower Lake, Calif, 1993, Aslan.

Bhargava KP: An overview of endorphins' probable role in health and disease. In Dhawan BN, editor: *Current status of centrally acting peptides*, Oxford, 1982, Pergamon Press.

Blair W: What's funny about doctors, *Perspect Biol Med* 21(1):89, 1977.

Bloch S, McGrath G: Humor in group psychotherapy, *Br J Med Psychol* 56:88, 1983.

Blumenfeld E, Alpern L: *The smile connection*, Englewood Cliffs, NJ, 1986, Prentice-Hall.

Bokun B: *Humour therapy*, London, 1986, Vita Books.

Boston R: *An anatomy of laughter*, London, 1974, Collins.

Brill AA: The mechanism of wit and humor in normal and psychopathic states, *Psychiatr Q* 14:731, 1940.

Brody MW: The meaning of laughter, *Psychoanal Q* 19:192, 1950.

Burton R: *The anatomy of melancholy*, New York, 1927, Tudor.

Buxman K: Humor in therapy for the mentally ill, *J Psychol Nurs* 29(12):15, 1991.

Byrne DE: The relationship between humor and the expression of hostility, *J Abnorm Soc Psychol* 53:84, 1956.

Byrne DE, Terril S, McReynolds P: Incongruence as a predictor of response to humor, *J Abnorm Soc Psychol* 62:435, 1961.

Cassell E: *The healer's art*, Boston, 1986, MIT Press.

Cassell J: The function of humor in the counseling process, *Rehabil Counsel* 17:240, 1974.

Chapman AJ: An experimental study of socially facilitated humorous laughter, *Psychol Rep* 35:727, 1974.

Chapman AJ, Foot HC, editors: *It's a funny thing, humour*. Reports of papers presented at the International Conference on Humor and Laughter, Oxford, 1976, Pergamon Press.

Dana B, Laurence P: *The laughter prescription*, New York, 1982, Ballantine Books.

Dearborn GVN: The nature of the smile and the laugh, *Science* 851, 1900.

Dillon KM, Minchoff B, Baker KH: Positive emotional states and enhancement of the immune system, *Int J Psychiatry Med* 15(1):13, 1985–1986.

Domis J, Fierman E: Humor and anxiety, *J Abnorm Soc Psychol* 53:59, 1956.

Elliot-Binns CP: Laughter and medicine, *J R Coll Gen Pract* 37(277):364, 1985.

Erdman L: Laughter therapy for patients with cancer, *Oncol Nurs Forum* 18(8):1359, 1991.

Euck JJ, Forter E, Whitley A, editors: *The comic in theory and practice*, New York, 1960, Appleton-Century-Crofts.

Fairbanks D: *Laugh and live*, New York, 1917, Britton.

Feibleman J: *In praise of comedy*, New York, 1970, Horizon Press.

Flugel JC: Humor and laughter. In Lindsay G, editor: *Handbook of social psychology*, Cambridge, Mass, 1954, Addison-Wesley.

Freud S: *Jokes and their relationship to the unconscious*, New York, 1964, Norton.

Fry WF Jr: *Sweet madness: a study of humor*, Palo Alto, Calif, 1963, Pacific Books.

Fry WF Jr: *Make 'em laugh*, Palo Alto, Calif, 1975, Science & Behavior Books.

Fry WF Jr: *Humor and the cardiovascular system*. Paper presented at the Second International Conference on Humor and Laughter, Los Angeles, August 1979.

Fry WF Jr, Rader C: The respiratory components of mirthful laughter, *J Biol Psychol* 19:39, 1977.

Fry WF Jr, Stoft PE: Mirth and oxygen saturation levels of peripheral blood, *Psychother Psychosom* 19:76, 1971.

Gaberson KB: The effect of humorous distraction on preoperative anxiety, *AORN J* 54(6):1258, 1991.

Greenwald H: Humor in psychotherapy, *J Contemp Psychother* 7:113, 1975.

Grotjahn M: *Beyond laughter*, New York, 1956, McGraw-Hill.

Haller B, Zarai R: *Rire c'est la sante*, Geneva, 1986, Editions Soleil.

Harlow HF: The anatomy of humor, *Impact Sci Soc* 19:225, 1969.

Hassett J, Schwartz GE: *Why can't people take humor seriously?* February 1977, New York Times Magazine.

Herth KA: Laughter: a nursing Rx, *Am J Nurs* 84(8):991, 1984.

Heuscher J: The role of humor and folklore themes of psychotherapy, *Am J Psychiatry* 137:1546, 1980.

Holden R: *Laughter is the best medicine*, London, 1993, Thorsons.

Holland N: *Laughing: the psychology of humor*, New York, 1982, Cornell University Press.

Joubert L: *Treatise on laughter*, Birmingham, 1970, University of Alabama Press.

Kaplan H, Boyd I: The social functions of humor on an open psychiatric ward, *Psychiatr Q* 39:502, 1965.

Keller D: *Humor as therapy*, Wauwatosa, Wisc, 1984, Med-Psych Publications.

Kubie LS: The destructive potential of humor in psychotherapy, *Am J Psychiatry* 127:861, 1971.

Lefcourt H, Martin R: *Humor and life stress*, New York, 1986, Springer-Verlag.

Leiber DB: Laughter and humor in critical care, *Dimens Crit Care* 5(3):162, 1986.

Levine J: Humor as a form of therapy. In Chapman AJ, Foot HC, editors: *It's a funny thing, humor*, Oxford, 1976, Pergamon Press.

McConnell J: Confessions of a scientific humorist, *Impact Sci Soc* 19:241, 1969.

McGhee P, Goldstein JH, editors: *Handbook of humor research. vol 1, Basic issues; vol 2, Applied studies*, New York, 1983, Springer-Verlag.

McHale M: Getting the joke: interpreting humor in group therapy, *J Psychol Nurs* 27(9):24, 1989.

Metcalf CW, Felible R: *Lighten up*, Reading, Mass, 1992, Addison-Wesley.

Mind H: The use and abuse of humor in psychotherapy. In Chapman AJ, Foot HC, editors: *Humor and laughter: theory, research and application*, New York, 1976, John Wiley & Sons.

Mindess H: *Laughter and liberation*, Los Angeles, 1971, Nash.

Mindess H: Laughter and humor in medical practice, *Behav Med* 1979.

Mindess H, Miller C, Turek J, et al, editors: *The Antioch humor test: Making sense of humor*, New York, 1985, Avon.

Moody RA Jr: *Laugh after laugh: the healing power of humor*, Jacksonville, Fla, 1978, Headwaters Press.

Nussbaum K, Michaux WW: Response to humor in depression: a predictor and evaluator of patient change, *Psychiatr Q* 37:527, 1963.

O'Connell WE: The adaptive functions of wit and humor, *J Abnorm Soc Psychol* 61:263, 1960.

O'Connell WE: Humor and death, *Psychol Rep* 22:391, 1968.

Pasquali EA: Learning to laugh: humor as therapy, *J Psychol Nurs* 28(3):31–5, 1990.

Pirandello L: *On humor*, Chapel Hill, 1974, University of North Carolina Press.

Poland WS: The place of humor in psychotherapy, *Am J Psychiatry* 28:635, 1971.

Potter S: *The sense of humor*, Middlesex, England, 1954, Penguin Books.

Powell BS: Laughter and healing: the use of humor in hospitals treating children, *Assoc Care Child Hosp J* 4:10, 1974.

Robinson V: Humor and health. In Goldstein JH, McGhee P, editors: *Handbook of humor research*, New York, 1983, Springer-Verlag.

Robinson VM: Humor is a serious business, *Dimens Crit Care* 5(3):132, 1986.

Rosenheim E: Humor in psychotherapy: an interactive experience, *Am J Psychother* 28:584, 1974.

Samra C: *The joyful chant: the healing power of humor*, San Francisco, 1986, Harper & Row.

Schaller CT: *Rire pour gai-rire*, Geneva, 1994, Editions Vivez Soleil.

Spenser H: *The physiology of laughter*, 1860, Macmillan's Magazine.

The healing power of laughter and play: uses of humor in the healing arts, Portola Valley, Calif, 1983, Institute for the Advancement of Human Behavior (12 tapes).

Vaillant G: *Empirical studies in ego mechanisms of defense*, Washington, DC, 1986, American Psychiatric Press.

Vaillant G: *The wisdom of the ego*, Cambridge, Mass, 1993, Harvard University Press.

Vergeer G, MacRae A: Therapeutic use of humor in occupational therapy, *Am J Occup Ther* 47(8):678–83, 1993.

Williams H: Humor and healing: therapeutic effects in geriatrics, *Gerontion* 1(3):14, 1986.

Wooten P, editor: *Heart, humor, and healing*, Mt Shasta, Calif, 1994, Commune-A-Key.

Zillman D, Rockwell S, Schweitzer K, et al: Does humor facilitate coping with physical discomfort? *Motiv Emot* 17(1):1–21, 1993.

Health and Humor Resources: Individuals, Organizations, and Publications

Alan Agins, PhD, Assistant Professor of Nursing, University of Virginia, School of Nursing, McLeod Hall, Charlottesville, VA 22903-3395, (804) 924-1647.

Steve Allen, Jr, MD, 8 LeGrand Ct, Ithaca, NY 19850; physician lecturer on humor.

Al's Magic Shop, 1012 Vermont Ave, Washington, DC 20005.

Dale Anderson, MD, 2982 West Owasso Blvd, Roseville, MN 55113; physician doing humor programs.

Lee Berk, 11645 Wiley St, Loma Linda, CA 92354; researcher into biochemistry and physiology of laughter, especially neuroimmunology.

Steve Bhaerman, "Swami Beyondananda," PO Box 110, Burnet, TX 78611, (512) 756-2791; lectures, workshops, books, tapes.

Michael Christensen, Clown Care Unit, Big Apple Circus, 35 W 35th St, New York, NY 10001; clowns who visit pediatric wards.

Clown Hall of Fame, Museum & Gifts, 212 E Walworth, Delavan, WI 53115.

Eric de Bont, Bont's Adventures in Clown Arts, Pardoestheater, postbus 419, 6800 AK Arnheim, The Netherlands; center for learning clown arts.

Mouton DeGruyter, W DeGruyter Inc, 200 Saw Mill River Road, Hawthorne, NY 10532; publishes humor.

Glenn C Ellenbogen, Wry-Bred Press, Inc, 10 Waterside Plaza, New York, NY 10010, 1985; publishes directory of humor magazines and organizations in America and Canada.

Fellowship of Merry Christians, Cal Samra, PO Box 895, Portage, MI 49081; network of Christian humorists, publishes *The Joyful Noiseletter*.

Laura Fernandez, Die Clown Doktoren, Klaren Thaler Str 3, 65197 Wiesbaden, Germany, 0611-9490981; clown who created hospital clown units in Germany.

William Fry, 156 Grove St, Nevada City, CA 95959; physician researcher on humor.

Cathy Gibbons, Fun Technicians, PO Box 160, Syracuse, NY 13215; published *Laughmaker's Magazine*.

Leslie Gibson, RN, The Comedy Connection, 323 Jeffords St, Clearwater, FL 34617, (813) 462-7842; lectures and hospital humor carts.

Lee Glickstein, Center for the Laughing Spirit, 288 Juanita Way, San Francisco, CA 94127.

Art Gliner, Humor Communications, 8902 Maine Ave, Silver Spring, MD 20910; lectures and workshops.

Annette Goodheart, PO Box 40297, Santa Barbara, CA 93103; laughter therapist, lectures and workshops.

Joel Goodman, The Humor Project, 179 Spring St, Box L, Saratoga Springs, NY 12866; publishes quarterly newsletter *Laughing Matters*, lectures, workshops, and annual humor conference.

Christian Hageseth, MD, 1113 Stoneyhill Dr, Ft Collins, CO 80525; psychotherapist doing humor programs.

Ruth Hamilton, Carolina Health and Humor Association, 5223 Revere Rd, Durham, NC 27713; newsletter and workshops.

International Humor Institute, 32362 Saddle Mt Road, Westlake Village, CA 91361, (818) 879-9085.

International Laughter Society, 16000 Glen Una Dr, Los Gatos, CA 95030.

Steve Kissel, 1227 Manchester Ave, Norfolk, VA 23508-1122.

Alan Klein, The Whole Mirth Catalog, 1034 Page St, San Francisco, CA 94117; catalogue of books and toys.

Karen Lee, The Laughter Prescription, 7720 El Camino Real B-225, Carlsbad, CA 92009, (800) RxHUMOR.

Paul McGhee, The Laughter Remedy, 380 Claremont Ave, Montclair, NJ 07042; researcher and lecturer.

CW Metcalf, The Humor Option, 2801 S Remington, Suite 2, Ft Collins, CO 80525; workshops and presentations on humor.

Jeff Moore, Orthopedic Coordinator, Physical Medicine, Saint Paul Medical Center, 5909 Harry Hines Blvd, Dallas, TX 75235; entertains patients.

Jim Pelley, Laughter Works, PO Box 1076, Fair Oaks, CA 95628; workshops and newsletter.

Dr. Karen Peterson, 1320 S Dixie Hwy, Coral Gables, FL 33146.

Caroline Simonds, Le Rire Médecin, 75 Ave Parmentier, 7509 Paris, France; French version of clown care units.

Dhyan Sutorius, MD, Secretariat of the Center in Favor of Laughter, Jupiter, 1008, NL-1115 TX, Duivendrecht, Holland.

Christian tal Schaller, 15 François Jacquier CH1235 Chene-Bourg, Geneva.

Tumor Humor, Uniquest, PO Box 97391, Raleigh, NC 27624.

Lex Van Someren, Batstangveien 81, 3200 Sandefjord Norway, 034-59644; "The Mystic Clown," teacher of workshops.

Joan White, Joygerms, PO Box 219, Syracuse, NY 13206; spreader of good cheer, resources.

Patty Wooten, RN, "Nancy Nurse," PO Box 4040, Davis, CA 95617; editor of *Heart, Humor and Healing*.

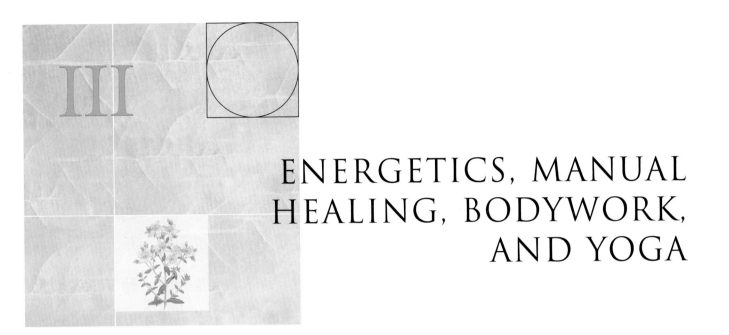

ENERGETICS, MANUAL HEALING, BODYWORK, AND YOGA

This section covers energetics, manual healing, bodywork, and yoga in continuity. In practice, many healing techniques that invoke the energy of the body in fact involve physically touching, massaging, or manipulating the body as a means of therapy. Sometimes it is just seen as the energy in the healer's hands, or the healer's intentions. Measuring this quality of energy is discussed as "Energy Medicine," followed by a review of the properties and therapeutic applications of electromagnetism, including the spectrum of electricity, light, sound, and biophysical devices that make use of these properties. Healing touch, massage, and bodywork are then addressed in continuity, followed by the American traditions of manipulative therapies founded by those who originally thought of themselves as "magnetic" or "mesmeric" healers. Yoga is addressed following the presentations of the mind–body–spirit dimensions of contemplation and meditation, as well as the effects of energy and physical posturing and inspiration, whereby the contemporary research presented is confirming all these connections.

ENERGY MEDICINE

JOHN A. IVES
WAYNE B. JONAS

We live forwards, but we understand backwards.
—William James

Nothing is so firmly believed as that which is least known.
—Michel de Montaigne

ENERGY AND ENERGY MEDICINE

In the United States, modern definitions for energy are introduced at grade school level and high school students are taught formal (mathematical) definitions for energy as part of introductory physics courses. Energy is defined as the ability to do work and has two basic forms, potential and kinetic. Potential energy is stored energy and has the latent ability to do work. Kinetic energy is, simply put, the movement of things—from air molecules to sound to the splitting of neutrons into atomic nuclei. Underlying these deceptively simple descriptions are several subtleties that have been investigated and understood to such an extent that we can harness the awesome power of atomic energy.

Thus, we can see how putting a venipuncture needle in someone's arm is an example of kinetic energy: the movement of the needle through the skin, the movement of the fluid into the lumen of the vein, and the movement of the pharmaceutical agent to the receptor of the target cell. Then, in a microburst of activity, the receptor binds the agent, often releasing potential energy that was stored in the characteristic configuration of the receptor itself. The change in receptor topology releases stored energy and helps to propel or allow the movement of molecules and atoms across the cellular membrane, in the process con-

suming potential energy stored in the molecule adenosine triphosphate (ATP), the universal coin of energy in the biology of cellular reactions and actions. ATP is the vehicle for storing energy in chemical bonds that is captured during cellular respiration, which combines oxygen with carbohydrate, yielding carbon dioxide as a byproduct, water for cellular hydration, and energy (see Chapter 26).

It is at this energetic interface that the pharmaceutical industry and much of allopathic medicine have focused their efforts. This space is where endogenous molecules as well as pharmaceutical agents ultimately interact with our physical selves. These agents cause and modulate cellular responses through interactions with a class of biomolecules called "receptors." Sometimes the agent is harvested and acquired from natural sources (materia medica), sometimes it is synthesized in a laboratory, and nearly always it interacts with a naturally occurring receptor type associated with some tissue or organ, or groups of tissues or organs. The point is that all of these steps and the downstream and sidestream consequences involve the use of energy and its transformation from potential to kinetic and back again with some loss to heat and randomness at every step. All health and healing involve these biochemical, energy-driven reactions, and thus all healing can be considered as forms of energy medicine.

Given our understanding of the nature of these biochemical reactions, we believe that all life is dependent on these reactions and that all life ceases when they fail. Certainly, life is dependent on these chemical energies, and in allopathic medicine we use the kinetic energy of objects (i.e., pharmaceuticals) to affect biological processes and, hopefully, maintain or improve health and healing.

197

SUBTLE AND VITAL ENERGY

It is also well known that different types and sources, or packets, of energy may interact, which results in a modulation or change in the energies involved. It is at this interface that energy medicine takes place, and we will describe possible models for understanding this interface.

So far we have described a conventional view of energy in healing. However, the "energy" in so-called energy medicine is not of this same nature. First and foremost, it is not directly measurable. Second, it does not appear to fall off in power with distance by the inverse square law. Finally, it is not blocked by the barriers that block conventional energy. This distinction in "energies" is important, because often these two very different concepts are used interchangeably and confusion results. Yet both types of "energy medicine" are placed in this single category by the putative experts at the National Center for Complementary and Alternative Medicine (NCCAM).

This blindsight may not be a surprise, because not long after leading members of Congress first legislated the funding to create what is now the NCCAM at the National Institutes of Health (NIH), bureaucratic managers at the NIH told Congress that the NIH "does not believe in bioenergy" (Sen. Arlen Specter R/D-PA, personal communication). It has been suggested in testimony to Congress (by the editor of this book) that the U.S. Department of Energy may be a better place to study bioenergy. We will summarize research involving both types of energy, but will make a clear distinction between the two uses of the term. We will also discuss the limits of current standards for evaluating this area and possible models to help improve our understanding of these concepts.

The intriguing and disputed (at least by Western allopathic healers) energy medicines such as qigong, reiki, and therapeutic touch are thought to involve putative forms of energy. (In this new edition of this textbook, all these topics are grouped together in this same section of the text.) There have been questions about the efficacy of these energy medicine modalities, and there have not been any unequivocal demonstrations of the involvement of either known or heretofore unknown forms of energy from the healer or between the healer and the patient. These modalities are based on philosophy, historical use, and/or tradition but without definitive modern scientific empirical evidence. These energy medicine modalities are thought to involve the interactions between the "energy field" of the patient and the *energy field* or the *intention* of the healer. We will return to this idea of intention and interaction with forms of energy when we discuss the *quantum enigma*. For now, we will consider what is meant by the use of the terms *intention* and *human energy fields* to be related and interdependent.

As hinted earlier, often missing is a rational *mechanism of action* in the practice of energy medicine. The confounding of *mechanism* with *empiricism* in the study of healing has been an ongoing challenge in medicine (see Chapter 6).

This mechanism provides a distinction between veritable forms of energy medicine such as magnetic therapy and the putative forms such as reiki (NCCAM, 2007). In spite of this gap in our understanding and knowledge, and the stress placed on understanding mechanism by the biomedical complex, it remains very difficult to find funding for basic mechanistic studies. For several years, the NCCAM dedicated over 60% of its budget to clinical research and 20% to applied research at centers, with only the remaining funds allocated to basic research (nccam.nih.gov). Further, the NCCAM continues to move more toward clinical trials (although the methodology for such trials is frequently inappropriate; see Chapters 3, 5 and 25), to the further exclusion of basic research and applied research. Thus, basic research on energy (both veritable and putative) medicine is scarce.

Although recent literature on forms of bioenergy—qi, ki, *prana*—and their biomedical application has significantly increased (see Chapter 6), the form(s) of energy involved in energy medicine remain(s) largely mysterious. There are some examples in the English-language literature of attempts to characterize this energy (Ohnishi & Ohnishi, 2008), but these studies have not been replicated by other groups. To date, the most complete, criteria-based, systematic review of this field is the book by Jonas and Crawford (2003b). An additional comprehensive survey has been compiled by Benor (2004), and a current edited volume by Mayor and Micozzi (2011).

In addition, over the past 30 years considerable work has been done on the measurement of external qi as physical energy. The majority of publications in this field is in Chinese and therefore is not easily accessible to the Western scientific community. The few English-language references dealing with bioenergy include a book by Lu (1997). A more complete review by Zha is found in the proceedings of the Samueli Institute for Information Biology meetings in Hawaii (Zha, 2001). A thorough review of previous work on physical measurements of external qi is outside the scope of this chapter, and the previous references are included as the most accessible material. It appears from these documents that the previous experiments neither had been done in a rigorously controlled way nor had utilized instruments that are currently state of the art. The documented experiments reveal, at best, very low levels of physical energy associated with external qi emission by qigong practitioners and healers (Hintz et al, 2003).

The lack of solid evidence and an accepted mechanistic explanation for the "energy" in energy medicine presents a fairly large hurdle to acceptance by Western medicine. Although there is no universal agreement as to what is meant by the "energy" in energy medicine—or even what kind it might be—terms such as "subtle energy," "qi energy," and "*prana*" are often used. There does seem to be some consensus on both sides of this discussion that, whatever it is, it is not the energy currently identified and described by traditional Western physics (see Chapter 1).

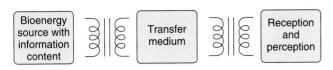

Figure 14-1 Block diagram of bioenergy transport mechanism components.

Finally, for a concept of such "energy" to be of value and to be adopted within the scientific community, there must be consilience among and with accepted physics, chemistry, and biology. Therefore, any putative bioenergy involved in energy medicine must be internally consistent and allow for consilience with the other known energies.

A cybernetic or systems analytic approach consistent with conventional descriptions of electromagnetic energies describing this system is shown in Figure 14-1. This depiction provides a level of abstraction based on the concepts of (1) information sources; (2) a medium for carrying the signal; and (3) receivers. In this view, the underlying physical layer of transfer of information is intentionally hidden to allow discussion of the transfer of bioinformation without an a priori decision about what is the physical mechanism for that transfer (Hintz et al, 2003).

In this model, we can define a bioenergy system as one that is composed of the following:
- A source that generates energy and modulates it in some manner so that it conveys information.
- A coupling mechanism connecting the bioenergy source to a transfer medium.
- A transfer medium through which the bioenergy flows.
- A coupling mechanism connecting the transfer medium to the bioenergy sink.
- A terminal sink that includes a mechanism for the perception of information.

The input and output coupling depends on properties of the source and the transfer medium, and likewise for the sink. The term *perception* (rather than *reception*) is used to imply some active process that uses some form of perceptual reasoning in processing the information based on its content.

The means by which information is transmitted and interacts with the system, in the sense that physicists understand it, is not clear. Feedback loops in biosystems are examples of information transfer. In most, if not all, cases the physical means by which the feedback is provided to the system is either understood or is assumed to involve interactions among actual physical objects. In the case of the placebo pill (see Chapter 9) and the branding study reported later, it is not self-evident how the information is transmitted but, de facto, it appears to be.

Thus, in these studies, information is able to significantly influence a biological system and its response to pain. Although we have some understanding of the biological consequences of energy medicine (Yan et al, 2008), the means by which this is done, the "energy," remains unknown. For example, qigong has been demonstrated to have antidepressive effects in patients, but although the psychological mechanisms underlying this effect have been described, the neurobiological mechanism remains unclear (Tsang & Fung, 2008). The same may be said of hypnosis, for which the clinical effects are now widely accepted (thanks in part to statistical and psychometric profiling of "susceptibility" to hypnotic "suggestion") but the neurobiological mechanism has remained unclear since the time of Mesmer (see Chapters 9 and 10). The authors conclude that further research is needed to elucidate the biology and consolidate its scientific base.

There are examples within the field of veritable energy medicine, however, in which there is a good understanding of the energies and energy fields involved. For example, the magnetic fields employed in transcranial magnetic stimulation are well characterized (see Chapter 15). Even so, the biology and biological mechanisms at work and affected by the magnetic fields are only beginning to be understood (Lopez-Ibor et al, 2008). Thus, although transcranial magnetic stimulation has been shown to be an effective alternative for the treatment of refractory neuropathic pain by epidural motor cortex stimulation, the mechanisms at work remain poorly understood (Lazorthes et al, 2007).

STANDARDS AND QUALITY

Although it is facile to recommend that complementary and alternative medicine (CAM) be held to the same standards as conventional medical science, the complexity and intricacies of CAM have been widely discussed and documented by the White House Commission on Complementary and Alternative Medicine Policy (2002). This reality is particularly true for energy medicine.

Studies are conducted in nearly all the CAM disciplines that lend themselves to the hypothesis-driven paradigm, and a search of the literature attests to that fact. Essentially, CAM scientific research is following the same standards used for conventional research, that is, the use of statistically significant numbers of subjects, specimens, or replicates; the introduction of internal and experimental controls; the definition of response specificity; and the requirement for reproducibility. The last is perhaps the most challenging criterion. In several cases, experiments have shown positive results but when repeated, sometimes in the same laboratory, do not work despite following the precautions of maintaining identical experimental conditions.

This challenge is illustrated in the work published by Yount et al (2004). They investigated the effect of 30 minutes of qigong on the healthy growth of cultured human cells. A rigorous experimental design of randomization, blinding, and controls was followed. Although both a pilot study that included 8 independent experiments and a formal study that included 28 independent experiments showed positive effects, the replication study of over 60 independent experiments showed no difference between the sham (untreated) and treated cells. This study represents an excellent example of holding basic science research on energy medicine to the highest standard of experimental methodology.

This level of rigor is rarely achieved in energy laboratory research, however (nor is it achieved in much mainstream research; see Chapter 3). The basic and clinical research in the area of distant mental influence on living systems (DMILS) and energy medicine has been reviewed. The quality of the research was quite varied. Although a few simple research models met all quality criteria, such as in mental influence on random number generators or electrodermal activity, much basic research into DMILS, qigong, prayer, and other techniques was poor (Jonas & Crawford, 2003b). In setting up these evaluations, the reviewers established basic criteria that should be met for all such laboratory research (Jonas & Crawford, 2003a; Sparber et al, 2003).

In basic scientific research, formulating the testable hypothesis is sometimes not the major issue; it is setting up and testing the practice itself. In the example of Yount et al (2004), in which they followed the most rigorous methodological and experimental designs, the practice under investigation was not a simple treatment with defined doses of a pharmaceutical compound or an antagonist of a specific receptor. Instead it was an unknown amount of energy of unknown characteristics emanating from the hands of a number of qigong practitioners, with variable levels of skills.

Acupuncture is a CAM application that lends itself to use in animal models for in vivo and ex vivo evaluation of its effects. By applying electroacupuncture, researchers are able to control the amount of energy delivered. However, the challenge here is the placement of the needles. Whereas in humans needles would be placed based on meridian (or channel) maps, in rats they must be placed so that they will not be disturbed during normal grooming while still being located along a meridian location of relevance. In addition, 20-minute electroacupuncture is often used because this method is what would be done in humans (Li et al, 2008); however, should not the time and dose parameters be adjusted to the animal's body size?

Mind-body–based therapies are often not considered energy medicine, especially when applied to oneself, although they are also considered in this light for the purposes of this book (see Section II). When the goal is to produce a change in an outside entity through meditation, for example, then we can claim this result as a form of energy medicine and, as such, very challenging to explore in a laboratory setting. There are several studies showing the effects of meditation on cell growth (Yu et al, 2003), differentiation (Ventura, 2005), water pH, and temperature change, as well as on the development time of fruit fly larvae (Tiller, 1997). We think that for these studies the necessary level of methodological rigor has not been met. Independent replication has been especially problematic.

On the other hand, some CAM applications, such as homeopathy, phytotherapy, and dietary supplements (Ayurveda and traditional Chinese medicine), are relatively easy to translate to the laboratory setting due to the fact that these practices and their products of use can be thought of as conventional interventions using pharmaceutical compounds, for which dose and time-course experiments can be designed. Later in this chapter, we will return to homeopathy considered as a form of energy medicine.

HOW GOOD IS GOOD ENOUGH?

It is appropriate to talk about levels of evidence, how we should catalogue the evidence, and at what point we should consider policy and educational changes to health care training to incorporate new information, knowledge, and understanding.

When evaluating scientific evidence, one must carefully consider the nature of the evidence itself. Figure 14-2 shows a way to categorize the types of data associated with biomedical research. This evidence pyramid illustrates how the "causal" characteristics of the data can be evaluated. Thus, randomized controlled trials are second from the peak, or best evidence, which is systematic reviews of randomized controlled trials. At the base are anecdotes, qualitative research, and case studies. Evidence of this type should not be ignored, but it should not be overinterpreted. In cases in which the information is sufficiently compelling, the therapeutic interventions are novel, or the condition has no other remedies available for patients, then further studies are often warranted. The "evidence" may be good enough to indicate the need for further research and the generation of more valid data but may not be good enough to form a basis for medical decisions.

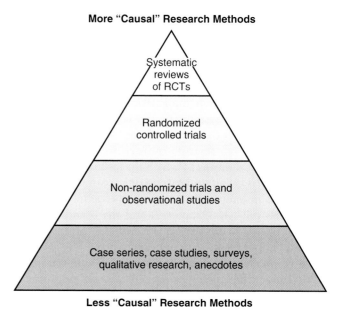

Figure 14-2 "Best" evidence hierarchy.

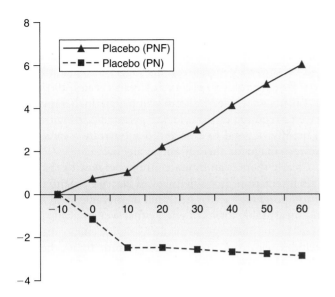

Figure 14-3 Physician knowledge affects outcome. (From Gracely RH et al: The effect of naloxone on multidimensional scales of postsurgical pain in nonsedated patients, *Soc Neurosci Abstr* 5:609, 1979.)

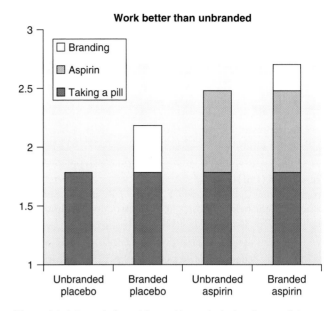

Figure 14-4 Branded aspirin and branded placebo work better than unbranded. (From Margo CE: The placebo effect, *Surv Ophthalmol* 44:31, 1999.)

ORTHODOXIES AND PLACEBO

Virtually all the doctor's healing power flows from the doctor's self-mastery.

Healing power consists only in and no more than ... bringing to bear those forces ... that already exist in the patient.

—Eric J. Cassell, MD, *The Nature of Suffering and the Goals of Medicine*, 2004

By the same token, we should always examine our orthodoxies and assumptions. For example, it would be reasonable to assume that subjects given a placebo for pain would get little to no relief. In a study reported at the 1979 Society for Neuroscience conference, R.H. Gracely showed evidence that the expectations (*intentions?*) of the physician significantly affected the outcomes (Gracely et al, 1979) (Figure 14-3). All subjects were given the same placebo, but half were given it by physicians who thought they were giving active medication. The patients of physicians who thought they were giving an active agent experienced a significant reduction in pain, whereas subjects in the other study group received no relief and in fact their pain got worse.

In 1999, the impact of expectation was further explored in a four-arm study carried out by C.E. Margo (1999). One group was given an "unbranded" placebo, another group was given a "branded" placebo, a third group was given unbranded aspirin, and the fourth group was given branded aspirin. As can be seen from Figure 14-4, there appears to be an analgesic effect just from the act of taking a pill, and this effect is significantly improved if the pill is branded. In this study, actual aspirin produced greater analgesia than branded placebo, and branded aspirin was

better than unbranded aspirin for analgesia. The author interpreted these data to indicate that taking a pill has significant analgesic effect for patients with pain, whether the pill has any conventionally defined "bioactive" agent or not. Further, branding of the pill enhances the effect whether it is a placebo or active. One can interpret this as a demonstration of the power and efficacy of therapeutic expectation (a form of *intention*) (Kirsch, 1999).

Even the color of the pill apparently makes a difference on people's expectations. Hot colors such as red, yellow, and pink have a stimulatory effect, whereas pills that are cool in color, such as blue or green, have a calming effect (Blackwell et al, 1972). It is perhaps less surprising that the number of pills taken affects healing rates. This is true, however, even when the pills are inert placebos. Placebo healing rates rise with the number of pills taken per day. In patients with stomach ulcers, subjects who took four placebo pills per day recovered faster than those who took two a day (De Craen et al, 1999). In a similar vein, switching a placebo treatment from oral to subcutaneous injection had a greater likelihood of decreasing headache severity over the course of two hours (De Craen et al, 2000). De Craen also showed that giving a treatment at the hospital compared to at home increases the placebo effect—people's expectation of an effect.

MAGNETIC THERAPY

Before we get into the more exotic forms of energy medicine, and to drive home our point about the need to evaluate the quality and type of information we have on a subject, we discuss the relatively well studied use of magnetic therapy for the treatment of pain (see Chapter 15).

TABLE 14-1 *Proportion of Subjects Reporting Improvement of Pain After 45 Minutes of Magnetic Therapy (see Chapter 15)*

	Active magnetic device ($n = 29$)	Inactive device ($n = 21$)
Pain improved	22 (76%)	4 (19%)
Pain not improved	7 (24%)	17 (81%)

Chi-squared (1 df) = 20.6, $p < 0.0001$.
From Vallbona C, Hazlewood CF, Jurida G: Response of pain to static magnetic fields in postpolio patients: a double-blind pilot study, *Arch Phys Med Rehabil* 78:1200, 1997.

Magnetic therapy is reportedly a safe, noninvasive method of applying magnetic fields to the body for therapeutic purposes. The use of magnets for relief of pain has become extremely popular, with consumer spending on such therapy exceeding $500 million in the United States and Canada and $5 billion worldwide (Weintraub et al, 2003, 2008). There have been many clinical studies of magnetic therapy. For example, Therion's Advanced Biomagnetics Database claims to contain over 300 clinical studies. However, few of these are randomized controlled trials, and the quality of the research is unknown.

It has been known for some time that magnets can reduce pain in subjects. Table 14-1 shows the data from a 1997 study by Vallbona et al (1997). A highly significant analgesic effect is demonstrated by these data. Overall, the evidence shows that patients with severe pain appear to respond better to magnetic therapy than patients with mild symptoms. There appear to be no adverse effects from application of static or dynamic pulsed magnetic therapy (Harlow et al, 2004; Segal et al, 2001; Weintraub & Cole, 2008; Weintraub et al, 2003). In a randomized, double-blind, placebo-controlled trial involving 36 symptomatic patients with refractory carpal tunnel syndrome, application of dynamic magnetic fields produced significantly greater pain relief than use of a placebo device as measured by short- and long-term pain scores, and better objective nerve conduction without changing motor strength or sensitivity to electrical current (Weintraub & Cole, 2008; Weintraub et al, 2008).

The study by Weintraub (co-author of the next chapter in this text) on magnetic therapy (Weintraub et al, 2003) was the first multicenter, double-blind, placebo-controlled study to examine the role of static magnetic fields in treatment of diabetic peripheral neuropathy and neuropathic pain. The results confirmed those of two previous pilot studies showing that the antinociceptive (pain relief) effect was significantly enhanced with long-term exposure to magnetic therapy. Since then the evidence has continued to support magnetic therapy as an effective tool for dealing with neuropathic pain (Segal et al, 2001).

Overall, 14 of 22 studies reported a significant analgesic effect of static magnets. Of the 19 better-quality studies, 12 found positive results and 6 found negative results, and in 1 there was a nonsignificant trend toward a positive analgesic effect. The weight of evidence from published, well-conducted, controlled trials suggests that static magnetic fields are able to induce analgesia (Eccles, 2005).

Taken as a whole, the studies of magnetic therapy are of the type required by the evidence pyramid (see Figure 14-2) to qualify as good to best and demonstrate a causal link between magnetic therapy and analgesia.

Clearly there is an interaction of energy with the body. This interaction probably involves electric potentials and action potentials across neuronal membranes with known and measurable forms of energy that we have called "veritable" forms of energy medicine. Veritable energy medicine includes electromagnetic, sound, and light therapies (NCCAM, 2007).

DISTANT HEALING

Let us now look at a set of studies performed to examine the effects of a healer's employing distance healing on cells in culture. This healer explained that he uses intention to focus his mind and channel "Divine love through his heart" to perform healing. This claim and similar energy medicine practices are often called "distant healing" because the practitioners do not place their hands on the patient or subject. Practitioners of this form of healing believe that the distance does not matter, although most, in fact, do their work within a foot or so of their patients. This healer usually placed his hands within inches of the person on whom he was working. As an aside, he also performs diagnosis by placing his hands near the person but without touching the person. We will return to the issue of distance later in the description of the studies' findings. The approach of this healer is typical of the so-called laying on of hands practiced in many cultures and accepted and associated traditionally with healing in Western medicine as well as Judeo-Christian tradition.

The explanation often given for any benefit seen from energy medicine of this kind is that it is a strong placebo effect that results from belief and expectation generated during the encounter (Moerman & Jonas, 2002). The investigators intended to minimize this effect by using cells grown in laboratory culture. The healer came to the laboratories one morning per week throughout much of two sequential winters. The researchers wanted to understand how he "communicated" with cells in the laboratory and influenced them with his "intention" in a positive and healthful way. The study would not involve diagnosis or even a human subject. By working with cultured cells in a laboratory setting, the investigators increased their power over the experimental and control parameters by comparing the effects of the healer to no treatment or sham treatment, comparing treatments at different doses and time periods, and examining the effects of various other environmentally controlled conditions, including the effects of expectation with blinding.

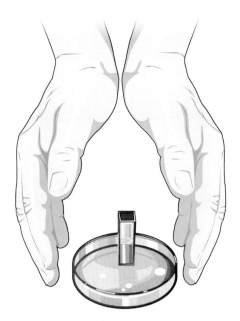

Figure 14-5 Performance of external bioenergy.

The healer was asked to alter the calcium flux in such a way as to increase the concentration of calcium ions inside the cells. Any change in cellular calcium was measured by putting the cells in a scintillation counter before and after the healer's "treatments." A demonstration of significant effect would be powerful evidence that something, some form of energy presumably, flowed from the healer to the cells and changed their biochemistry in a targeted, intentional, and specific way.

The studies used Jurkat cells, an immortalized line of T lymphocytes derived from human immune system T cells. They were established as an immortalized line in the late 1970s and are available for purchase and easy to grow and maintain in the laboratory. They have been used extensively to study mechanisms of action for human immunodeficiency virus and anticancer agents. There is, in fact, a vast literature on Jurkat cells, because they are a favorite choice for cellular immunobiologists interested in understanding cellular mechanisms of the immune system.

The setup was quite simple. Jurkat cells were grown in tissue culture dishes to near confluence, then on the day of the experiment the cells were suspended in a balanced salt solution, loaded with calcium-sensitive dye (fura-2), and placed inside a square cuvette. Because of the activity of the dye, the amount of light emitted by the cells is proportional to the amount of free calcium ions inside the cell. When the light is measured spectrofluorometrically, this technique provides an accurate and objective measure of the amount of free calcium inside the cells.

As noted earlier, the healer was asked to increase the internal concentration of calcium ions inside the cell. He told the investigators that he would need 15 minutes of relative quiet while he placed his hands near the cuvette of cells and concentrated on his intention (Figure 14-5). The experiments were repeated in six independent trials occurring on different days. Internal cellular calcium concentra-

BOX 14-1 *Summary of Results of Distant Healing Experiment*

30% increase in cellular calcium absorption in 15 minutes
Effect *not* blocked by a Faraday cage
Lingering effect for 24 hours
No effect at a distance of 10 miles

tions were significantly increased by 30% to 35% (p <0.05, Student *t*-test) compared with controls run in parallel. Varying the distance between 3 and 30 inches did not seem to have an effect on the outcome (Kiang et al, 2005).

Three independent attempts were made by the healer to affect calcium concentration in this system from approximately 10 miles away. He tried first with internal visualization, then with a photograph of the cells to focus his attention, and finally with a video camera display of a "live" version of the cells. None of these tests produced any noticeable change in the calcium concentration. Anecdotally, a few uncontrolled tests were run in which the healer's hands were kept behind his back rather than toward the cuvette of cells. This position seemed to interfere with his ability to affect calcium concentration. This occurred in spite of the fact that the researchers documented a "linger effect" in which cells put on the table where the healer had focused his intention but after he had left showed an increase in calcium concentration similar to that of the cells that had been directly subject to his intention. This linger effect disappeared over time, and within 24 hours cells placed in this way had a calcium concentration no different from that of controls.

Finally, the investigators attempted to block the healer's "energy" or intention by placing a grounded copper Faraday cage around the cuvette containing cells. Thus the healer, although still within 30 inches of the cells, had to keep his hands outside of the wire enclosure surrounding the cells. There was no significant difference in effect on the internal calcium concentration. It was still raised by the healer's 15-minute "treatment." This observation suggests that, whatever the energy is, it is not blocked by a Faraday cage the way an electric field would be (Box 14-1).

THERAPEUTIC TOUCH, HEALING TOUCH, AND ENERGY THERAPIES

Reiki, healing touch (HT), qigong, and therapeutic touch (TT) are all "energy therapies" that use gentle hand techniques thought to help repattern the patient's energy field and accelerate healing of the body, mind, and spirit. They are all based on the belief that human beings are fields of energy that are in constant interaction with other fields of energy from others and the environment. The goal of energy therapies is to purposefully use the energetic interaction between the practitioner and the patient to restore harmony to the patient's energy system. Western allopathic approaches focus on diseases and their underlying mechanisms. Cure is the end-all and be-all. Most energy therapies are based on a holistic philosophy that places the patient within the context of that patient's life and an understanding of the dynamic interconnectedness with themselves and their environment (Cassidy, 1995; see also Chapter 5). They are about healing rather than cure (Engebretson & Wardell, 2007).

The most common contemporary touch therapies used in nursing practice are TT, HT, and reiki. The first two were developed by nurses, whereas reiki comes out of pre–World War II Japan and, although not targeted for nursing, is being used today by many in hospital settings (Engebretson & Wardell, 2007; Krieger, 1993; Mentgen, 2001). Controversy has accompanied the use of these therapies, even after the inclusion of these therapies by the North American Nursing Diagnosis Association (NANDA). The controversy has not prevented their increasing popularity within the profession to promote health by reducing symptoms and ameliorating treatment side effects. Practitioners use TT and HT to improve health and healing by addressing, in the words of the official NANDA diagnosis, a patient's "Disturbed Energy Field: disruption in the flow of energy surrounding a person's being that results in a disharmony of the body, mind, and/or spirit" (NANDA, 2008).

Like many other energy therapies, TT is not designed to treat specific diseases but instead to balance the energy field of the patient or, through a boosting of energy, improve the patient's energy. TT was developed by Dolores Krieger, PhD, RN, in the 1970s. She borrowed from and mixed together ancient shamanic traditions and techniques she learned from well-known healers of her time. Like acupuncture, qigong, and yoga, HT is based on the idea that illness and poor health represent an imbalance of personal bioenergetic forces and fields that exist around and through a person's body. Rebalancing and boosting of these energies is done through a clear intention to support and harmonize the person with his or her innate energy balance. These practices, therefore, typically begin with the practitioner performing some form of ritual that clears and focuses the intention to bring harmony and balance to the person who is in need.

In a typical TT session, the practitioner begins with a centering process to calm the mind, access a sense of compassion, and become fully present with the patient. The practitioner then focuses intention on the patient's highest good and places his or her hands lightly on the patient's body or slightly away from it, often making sweeping hand motions above the body. Enough research on TT has been published in peer-reviewed journals to perform a meta-analysis of the combined results from separate studies. Two meta-analyses have determined that TT produces a moderately positive effect on psychological and physiological variables hypothesized to be influenced by TT, primarily anxiety and pain (Peters, 1999; Winstead-Fry & Kijek, 1999). A systematic review of the HT research published in 2000 included 19 randomized controlled trials involving 1122 patients (Astin et al, 2000). The reviewers found 11

studies (58%) that reported statistically significant treatment effects. Another systematic review of the literature on wound healing and TT found only four studies that met the author's criteria for quality. Of these, two showed statistically significant effects, whereas the other two found no effect from TT. The evidence is therefore insufficient to conclude that TT works for wound healing (O'Mathuna & Ashford, 2003, 2012).

Applications for which TT and HT seem to work well include reducing anxiety, improving muscle relaxation, aiding in stress reduction, promoting relaxation, enhancing a sense of well-being, promoting wound healing, and reducing pain. In addition, no serious side effects have been associated with these healing modalities (Engebretson & Wardell, 2007). One review of touch therapies looked at studies with outcomes such as pain reduction, improvement of mood, reduction of anxiety, promotion of relaxation, improvement of functional status, improvement of health status, increase in well-being, wound healing, reduction of blood pressure, and increase in immune function. The authors found that the studies were mixed in their quality and the degree of evidence supporting the effectiveness of touch therapies in influencing these outcomes (Warber et al, 2003).

Reiki was originally intended as a self-practice. Today it is often performed by practitioners to help their clients strengthen their wellness, assist them in coping with symptoms such as pain or fatigue, or support their medical care, sometimes in the case of chronic illness or at the end of life. Reiki was developed by Mikao Usui in Japan in the 1920s as a spiritual practice. One of his master students, Chujiro Hayashi, with Usui's help, extracted the healing practices from the larger body of practices. Hayashi began to teach these practices and opened a clinic to treat patients. Reiki practice itself is extremely passive. Practitioners lay their hands gently on the patient or hold them just above the body without moving their hands except to place them over another area. The reiki practitioner does not attempt to adjust the patient's energy field or actively project energy into the patient's body. Also, unlike other forms of energy medicine and more like meditation, reiki does not involve an assessment of the patient's energy field or an active attempt to reorganize or adjust the patient's energy field. Instead, reiki practitioners believe that healing energy arises from the practitioner's hand as a response to the patient's needs. It is in this way customized to the patient's needs and condition.

In one study, 23 reiki-naive healthy volunteers participated in standardized 30-minute reiki sessions. They often reported experiencing a "liminal state of awareness." This state is characterized by novel and paradoxical sensations, often symbolic in nature. The experiences run the gamut from disorientation in space and time to altered experience of self and the environment as well as relationships with people, especially the reiki master. In another study, quantitative measures of anxiety and objective measures of systolic blood pressure and salivary immunoglobulin A were altered significantly by the reiki experience; anxiety and systolic blood pressure were lowered, whereas immunoglobulin A level was increased. Skin temperature, electromyographic readings, and salivary cortisol level were all lowered but not significantly. When these results are taken together, it is apparent that in this study reiki induced states of lowered stress and anxiety and should be considered salutogenic in nature. The authors concluded that the liminal state and paradoxical experiences are related to the ritual and holistic nature of this healing practice (Engebretson & Wardell, 2002).

A 2008 systematic Cochrane Review of the literature on touch therapy for pain relief included studies of HT, TT, and reiki (So et al, 2008). The authors evaluated the literature to determine the effectiveness of these therapies for relieving both acute and chronic pain. They also looked for any adverse effects from these therapies. Randomized controlled trials and controlled clinical trials investigating the use of these therapies for treatment of pain that included a sham placebo or "no treatment" control group met the criteria for inclusion. A total of 24 studies, including 16 involving TT, 5 involving HT, and involving 3 reiki, were found that met these criteria. A small but significant average effect on pain relief (0.83 units on a scale of 0 to 10) was found. The greatest effect was seen in the reiki studies and appeared to involve the more experienced practitioners, but the authors concluded that the data were inconclusive with regard to which was more important, the level of experience or the modality of therapy. In spite of the paucity of studies, the authors concluded that the evidence supports the use of touch therapies for pain relief. Application of these therapies also decreased the use of analgesics in two studies. No statistically significant placebo effect was seen, and no adverse effects from these therapies were reported. The authors pointed out the need for higher-quality studies, especially of HT and reiki (So et al, 2008).

In one study involving a combination of HT and guided imagery (GI), 123 returning combat-exposed active duty military with significant post-traumatic stress disorder (PTSD) symptoms were randomized into a 1-month study receiving either HT+GI or treatment as usual (TAU) (Jain et al, 2012). The primary outcome measure was impact on PTSD symptoms and secondary outcome measures were depression, quality of life, and hostility. Analysis of outcomes indicated a statistically and clinically significant reduction in PTSD symptoms (effect size of 0.85 [Cohen's d]) and depression (effect size 0.70) for HT+GI compared to TAU. In addition, compared to TAU, HT+GI produced significant improvement in mental qualify of life and cynicism, equating to greater optimism. The authors conclude: "Participation in a complementary medicine intervention resulted in a clinically significant reduction in PTSD and related symptoms in a returning, combat-exposed active duty military population."

Qigong is a bioenergy modality originating in Asia, more specifically, ancient China, and has been utilized for many years to aid healing. The term *qigong* itself can be parsed to help explain its use. In China, qi is considered the universal life force described sometimes as energy. *Gong* refers to the training and cultivating of qi (Guo et al, 2008). Therefore, qigong is the practice of cultivating the universal life force. Qigong is thought to be made up of two different types of qi: internal and external. Internal qigong refers to a self-practice (typically involving stereotypical movements) to restore qi. External qi is practitioner-based, in which qigong masters exude their "qi" onto their patients to foster healing (Jahnke et al, 2010). There is no agreed upon physical evidence to show the qi is ever emitted or even that it exists at all.

The gentle movements, meditation, and controlled breathing of internal qigong exercises have evidence to support their use in physiological and psychological ailments. In a comprehensive review of tai chi (an ancient Chinese practice to improve internal qi) and qigong, evidence was evaluated for cardiopulmonary conditions as well as its effects on bones, physical function, quality of life, self-efficacy, psychological functioning, and immune function (Jahnke et al, 2010). The studies varied with regard to population under investigation, intervention length, and intervention goal. One study showed positive effect on bone density. As other reviews have reported, there were consistent findings for reducing blood pressure. When used in conjunction with antihypertensive medication, the effect is greater than just the use of medication alone (Lee et al, 2007). The evidence for qigong on lipid profiles and ejection fraction were inconclusive. Cardiopulmonary fitness outcomes varied based on the study population and the outcome measures used. Physical function outcomes were inconclusive, and improvements in two quality of life studies were not statistically significant. Psychological evidence was positive and promising.

Three studies showed significant decreases in anxiety when compared to active exercise. One study included in the review showed a significant decrease in depression symptoms compared to reading a newspaper. Biomarker studies were also examined, and qigong significantly decreased blood catecholamines and cortisol. Three studies examined immune function and inflammation, and these studies showed positive effects on these systems. One study showed an increase in antibody levels after influenza vaccinations in an aging study group compared to usual care. Another study showed positive modulation of interleukin-6. The review concluded by noting that, overall, there appear to be positive benefits of qigong in health outcomes.

There are a number of systematic reviews supporting this conclusion. Lee et al (2007) reviewed the literature on qigong for hypertension and, although they conclude that many of the studies are of poor methodological quality, they performed a meta-analysis on a subset of the better-quality studies. This analysis indicates that qigong plus antihypertensive drugs results in significantly lower blood pressure than antihypertensives alone. Another, more recent review (Guo et al, 2008) examined the effectiveness of internal qigong and its clinical effectiveness in essential hypertension. Nine studies were extracted from their search for randomized controlled trials evaluating clinical effectiveness of qigong on hypertension (stage I and II). The studies reported varied in their comparators and had other differences in methodologies. Nonetheless, the authors declare qigong to be better than nontreatment, equal or less effective compared to active controls, and has the greatest effect when used in conjunction with medication.

Recently, qigong has been shown to be of benefit for anxiety and depression in a systematic review and meta-analysis of randomized controlled trials (Wang et al, 2013). Twelve randomized controlled trials were evaluated and, although qigong showed no difference when compared to cognitive-behavioral therapy, when qigong and usual care was compared to wait lists or usual care, the high-quality studies included had results supporting the benefit of qigong for depressive symptoms. As is the case for much of the research in these areas, the authors conclude that most of the studies have a number of methodological errors. The benefits are often associated with specific populations such as cancer patients and patients suffering with Parkinson's disease.

Of note is the author's report of "Qigong-precipitated psychoses." They did not include the study reporting this observation in their analysis because of methodological weakness in the study. Even so, the authors report that these "psychoses" are thought to stem from unrealistic expectations. More typically, other reviews explicitly state that no adverse events resulted from qigong in any of the included studies in their review (Oh et al, 2013). Although these reviews, like many other CAM studies, report methodological weaknesses in the underlying studies, the overall conclusion is that qigong has benefit for some people and some conditions.

LIGHT, HEALING, AND BIOPHOTONS

Light therapy is, of course, a veritable form of energy generally not thought of as a "subtle energy" of the types we have just discussed (NCCAM, 2007; see also Chapter 15). There is good evidence that applied near-infrared (NIR) light (670 and 810 nm) can significantly improve wound healing and even promote neural regeneration in animal models (Byrnes et al, 2005; Whelan et al, 2008). The mechanisms underlying this "photobiomodulation" are not understood. Nonetheless, the therapeutic use of low-level NIR laser light is a promising area. Physiological effects that have been documented include increased rate of tissue regeneration as well as reduction in inflammation and pain. Production of reactive oxygen species by cells put under stress is lowered with NIR treatment. The application of 810-nm NIR light has been tested in an animal spinal cord injury model and has been shown to significantly increase axonal number and distance of regrowth. This light treatment also returned aspects of function to baseline levels and significantly suppressed immune cell activation and cytokine-chemokine expression. The

authors concluded that externally delivered NIR light improves recovery after injury and suggested that light will be a useful treatment for human spinal cord injury (Whelan et al, 2008).

To understand more about the role of light in biology and human health, investigators examined the spontaneous emission of ultraweak photons, often called "biophotons," in humans (Van Wijk et al, 2008). Although these photons are in the visible range (470 to 570 nm), they are at too low a level to be seen in normal background light. Thus, a very efficient photomultiplier was developed, and the experiments were run in a completely light-tight environment. Reactive oxygen species are theorized to be the principal source of the photons, because these are very reactive molecules and are involved in interactions with high enough energy to result in spontaneous photon emissions. The study found that biophotons were emitted in a generally symmetrical pattern from the human body. This pattern was not true for individuals with chronic diseases such as diabetes and arthritis, however. Further, reproducible emission patterns were demonstrated in meditating subjects, and another pattern was identified in sleeping individuals. The investigators believe this approach holds promise as a real-time, continuous, and noninvasive method for monitoring health, wellness, healing, and chronic disease, and perhaps even states of consciousness.

In a recent paper these same researchers observed ultraweak spontaneous photon emission (UPE) altering when an injury is induced in plant models. Changes in photon intensity were also seen over the course of injury and healing in animal models. In humans, differences in UPE pattern and intensity were observed to change with time of day. The authors speculate a possible correlation with acupuncture and traditional Chinese medicine (Van Wijk et al, 2013).

An important focus for future research is whether energy medicine modalities exploit these biophotonic emissions. It is not hard to imagine that some, or perhaps all, of us are able to detect these emissions. If this is possible, it is a small step to imagine that healers "learn" to detect these biophotons and their correlations with health or the lack of it. Finally, is it possible that healers interact with their clients' biophotons and use this system not only to gain information and knowledge but, in fact, to transmit biological information and instructions to their clients through these interactions? Is it possible that healers emit biophotons in patterns to which a patient's biosystems and biophotons respond and with which they interact? At this point, these are all untested hypotheses. Only by further researching these questions will we learn the answers.

THE QUANTUM ENIGMA

I cannot seriously believe in [quantum physics] because . . . physics should represent a reality in time and space, free from spooky actions at a distance.

—Albert Einstein

The universe begins to look more like a great thought than a great machine.

—Sir James Jeans

Since its inception, quantum mechanics has had a problem with consciousness—despite the fact that it is the most rigorously tested theory in all of science. Furthermore, no test ever performed has ever failed to agree completely with the theory (Rosenblum & Kuttner, 2008). So, where is the problem?

Although quantum mechanics is applied in much of our daily lives, from computers to magnetic resonance imaging, there is an aspect of it that remains counterintuitive and paradoxical. This enigma is best illustrated with light in what is called the "double-slit experiment." As the reader will recall, light has a dual (and paradoxical) nature. It can be either a wave or a particle (photon), and Nobel Prizes have been awarded both for demonstrating that light is a wave and for demonstrating that light is a particle (see Chapter 1). Which of these properties light is, at any given moment, is dependent on our conscious observation. How can this be? At this moment in time no one knows, but the evidence has never been refuted; in fact, the more sophisticated we become in our experiments and tests the more entrenched and mysterious this phenomenon becomes (Walborn et al, 2003).

The double-slit interference experiment is performed in the following way. (Because this is not a text or chapter on quantum mechanics, we will gloss over some of the details.) Light is shone into the back of two open boxes with slits on the front sides. On the wall opposite the slits, on the other side from the light source, is a projection screen. No light can reach this screen except the light that comes through the slits. If the slits are narrow enough and spaced properly, the waves of light come out the slits and, because they are made of waves with high points (peaks) and low points (valleys), the waves can interact and interfere with each other in a fashion analogous to waves on water. The light spreads out from the two slits and the waves interact where they strike the screen. Where two peaks reach the screen at the same point there is a light band. Where two valleys reach the screen at the same point there is a shadow, because no light has reached this point. What one sees, as demonstrated all the time in physics courses around the world, is a series of light and dark stripes, or "interference pattern." This pattern is considered definitive evidence for the wave nature of light.

Now here is the next part. The experiment can be run so that only a single "packet" of light exists in *both* boxes. (This part we are glossing over, but this experiment can be and has been done many times.) When this procedure is followed, the interference pattern is still generated, which demonstrates that light is a wave and that the wave of energy was distributed in both boxes. However, if there are photon detectors in both boxes, and we *observe* them while the experiment is running, only *one* of the detectors will react, and a photon (a quantum of light energy) will be found in only one box. Furthermore, the interference pattern will not appear because there is no longer a wave of light. The wave function is said to collapse and form the photon. If you find this confusing, you are in good company. No one has been able to adequately explain this undisputed phenomenon, called *complementarity*. It is important to note that no physicist disputes this phenomenon, but there is considerable controversy as to how to interpret it. The majority simply ignore it and its implications. (Editor's note: To the extent that the *mechanisms* of much of complementary medicine become understood to be based on this *quantum enigma*, it may someday be labeled "*complementarity medicine*.")

If this experiment is repeated many times, it always comes out one of two ways. If there is no photon detector, then we see the wave nature of light. If there are photon counters in both boxes that we *observe,* then we only see photons and no wave. Furthermore, the probability of finding the photon in one box or the other is exactly $50:50$. It was this phenomenon that drove Einstein to try to wish it away by saying that "God does not play dice." The reader will have noted that we used ***bold italics*** when describing the act of **observation.** This is where consciousness comes in. As strange as this sounds, the collapsing of the wave function is dependent not only on the presence of the instruments but on our conscious awareness of their output. This phenomenon is demonstrated elegantly in the established work by Walborn et al (2002, 2003) on a phenomenon called *quantum erasure*.

These same papers address another aspect of quantum physics called *entanglement*. It appears that the universe, Noah-like, makes most, if not all, things in pairs. Thus, it is possible to entangle two photons such that they have paired aspects of their quantum natures. (This entanglement is another case in which we are glossing over the technical details, but entanglement at the photon level has been demonstrated repeatedly.) Two photons thus entangled have a very strange property: without any detectable form of energy transfer or communication and in a distance-independent manner, whatever is done to one photon *immediately,* without time delay and no matter the distance separating them, affects the other entangled photon. This effect is not causal. Observation and the observer do not cause the effect. Rather, the effect is said to be a *nonlocal connectivity* or nonlocal correlation (Hyland, 2003).

Where does that leave us? Light has a dual nature, and which of its two natures it demonstrates depends on **how we look at it.** When photons, and apparently other very small quanta, are entangled, they remain entangled regardless of the distance between them. Furthermore, whatever happens to one is immediately reflected in the other without any time delay and with no detectable or explainable form of energy or information transfer. We conclude, as do some physicists (Rosenblum & Kuttner, 2008), that these phenomena demonstrate **interaction among consciousness and energy and matter** that appears to go beyond currently understood principles of physics, and that there are ways to transfer information that are independent of distance and through means that physics has not yet determined.

We think that the incorporation of quantum physics into the discussion on energy medicine provides a possible explanation for some of the empirical observations, anomalies, and hallmarks of this therapy. In addition to helping to explain the role of consciousness and intention in healing, and in energy medicine in particular, quantum mechanics and physics may explain some of the anomalous observations that have been made in aspects of energy medicine such as *distant healing*.

INVERSE SQUARE LAW

Most forms of energy obey an *inverse square law*. That is, the effect or force drops as an inverse square of the distance. Quantum effects do not show this drop-off with distance. Furthermore, all other energies exert their influence either at or below the speed of light. Quantum effects, however, like many phenomena in energy medicine, seem to happen immediately without an appreciable time delay. Thus, two of the anomalous aspects of energy medicine, *independence of time* and *independence of distance,* are also observed in quantum effects (Julsgaard et al, 2001). In this way we may explain the exchange of healing information, or "subtle energy," between healer and patient from a distance (Bennett & DiVincenzo, 2000).

We are not alone in making this connection. Smith (1998) has postulated that the body functions as a macroscopic quantum system. This idea may also be applicable to related fields of energy medicine (Mayor & Micozzi, 2011). The data reported by Smith in his 2003 paper suggest that the acupuncture meridian system is made up of quantum domains and networks (Smith, 2003). Even the proposition that consciousness and intention are connected through quantum mechanical means to our body's healing potentials has been proposed by others (Jahn & Dunne, 1986).

There are serious problems with this hypothesis, however. Specifically, quantum effects have only been demonstrated at an extremely small scale and are thought by most physicists not to be applicable in domains larger than Planck's constant (i.e., photons and electrons) and that only traditional Newtonian mechanics applies to domains we experience in everyday life. Smith proposes that there is a hierarchical series of networks and domains in which quantum effects are transmitted to molecules through their quantum particles, and that molecules transfer this information to cells, and so on, until the intact organism is involved and influenced by quantum effects.

HOMEOPATHY AS ENERGY MEDICINE

Homeopathy is defined as yet another form of energy medicine by the NIH (NCCAM, 2007). This may make

sense, because standard pharmacology is surely *not* at work in what are called "high-potency" remedies. These are remedies in which the original active substance is diluted to such an extent that there is no possibility than any of the original constituents are present. Dilutions of 30,000-fold, 100,000-fold, or even a millionfold are quite common in this type of homeopathy. Quantum theory is currently in vogue, and perhaps partly because of its mysterious nature, it is sometimes invoked to explain all aspects of energy medicine, or medicines that have an energetic aspect, including homeopathy. This application is usually not done in a formal mathematical way and is often done by novices to the world of quantum mechanics.

Harald Walach and his colleagues have addressed this gap using a formal mathematical approach, however, and published a paper in *Foundations of Physics* in 2002 in which they describe how quantum mechanics and quantum theory could be applied to macro environments and to nonphysical properties such as intention and thoughts. Their theory, called "weak quantum theory and generalized entanglement," demonstrates that, mathematically at least, transfer of information between consciousnesses in a nonphysical way is possible (Atmanspacher et al, 2002).

Walach has also produced experimental data to support this hypothesis that need independent replication, by presenting a case for the application of weak quantum theory and generalized entanglement to homeopathy (Walach, 2003). He contends that the remedies are entangled with both the system and the condition (symptoms) and that even when the original substance has been diluted out of the solution, the entanglement remains. Further, he proposes that this "entanglement" explains both the efficacy of homeopathy when it works and the difficulty conventional researchers have in demonstrating this efficacy in clinical trials. Milgrom has also developed formal models for mapping how quantum mechanics could be used to explain the effects of homeopathy and has made suggestions for testing these models in clinical settings (Milgrom, 2006, 2008a, 2008b).

Entanglement is not fully understood, may not operate inside the normal boundaries of time and space, and is certainly complex and counterintuitive. Thus, conventional, linear, cause-and-effect experiments may not properly test the system as it actually exists: *entangled*. Certainly physicists have demonstrated how counterintuitive and mysterious this property can be, and how difficult it is to show, even when one knows what one is looking for and specifically set up sophisticated experiments to demonstrate the existence of entanglement. Standard biomedical research methods and study designs, including randomized controlled trials, would not be able to demonstrate entanglement.

> From the quantum mechanical perspective, to measure the position of an electron is not to find out where it is but to cause it to be somewhere.
>
> —Louisa Gilder
> *The Age of Entanglement*

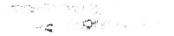

Walach believes that weak *quantum effects and entanglement underlie much of CAM practices and especially energy medicine* (Walach, 2005). If this supposition is true, it would explain the difficulty in demonstrating the efficacy of energy medicine using conventional experimental approaches and would simultaneously provide an explanation for the effects that are clinically observed empirically but without apparent causal connections. For example, two salient characteristics of energy medicine are the apparent lack of dissipation of the effect of "subtle energy" with distance and our inability to block the effects with conventional energy barriers (Astin et al, 2000). This same pair of phenomena is observed in entangled quantum effects. Thinking in this way and designing tests to support or refute the weak quantum theory and entanglement hypothesis represent important directions for future research.

Recently, Bell and Koithan (2012) speculated that homeopathic remedies work by "mobilizing hormesis and time-dependent sensitizations via nonpharmalogical effects on specific biological adaptive and amplification mechanism." Hormesis is defined as a nonlinear dose response relationship in which low doses of a given agent or stressor can exert effects in opposite directions (Calabrese et al, 2007).

Along a similar line of reasoning, we have proposed that nanoparticles are playing an important if not critical role in homeopathic remedies (Bell et al, 2014). Nanoparticles are extremely small particles in the nanometer range that are biologically super-potent. The impact of nanoparticles on biological systems could be electromagnetic, thermal, optical, biochemical, or even quantum. Perhaps this field is the connection between the macrophysical and the quantum nanoparticles. In fact, nanoparticles have, unexpectedly, been found in commercial homeopathic preparations, even at dilutions (10^{-400} molar) thought to have no chance of the starting material still being present (Chikramane et al, 2012).

PLACEBO AND BIOFIELD

We are not so bold as to suggest that we know *the* mechanism for energy medicine. On the contrary, we contend that there is legitimate debate as to whether there even is such a thing as "subtle energy." Our goal in this chapter has been to present some of the discussion that is occurring in the field and the literature around energy medicine. There are at least three theories as to the underlying mechanisms giving rise to the observed effects of energy medicine: (1) a *conventional energy* explanation; (2) an explanation based on *placebo* effects; and (3) a *quantum entanglement* explanation. Just what the mechanism of the well-established placebo effect may be is not addressed in this distinction. We have devoted attention in this chapter on the quantum mechanics approach, not because we feel that it is the most correct one, but because it is the most novel and perhaps least understood of the theories, and it

also best fits all the best data collected so far regarding all forms of energy medicine.

A mechanism that also might explain the effects of energy medicine is the *placebo* effect. That is, whatever is going on is the result of patients' convincing themselves that they are healing or being healed—they feel less pain, they have fewer complaints, and so on—but "nothing really happened" between healer and patient. However, this explanation is not really more satisfactory and also does not fit some of the best data. The placebo effect itself, while unquestionably real and clinically meaningful, is not well understood or well defined and thus still begs the question of mechanism. Second, if patients actually experience healing and/or feeling better, then something "really" is happening *consciously,* and we are back to our first point of still not knowing the underlying mechanism while in fact having authentic healing. Thus, we find invoking the placebo effect to be equivalent to confessing that something really is happening with the patient but that we do not know how, or whether it is coming from within or from without. In addition, the known mechanisms of placebo, such as belief, expectancy, and conditioning, do not account for some of the best-replicated data on the direct effects of intention in living and nonliving systems and blinded distant effects (Jonas & Crawford, 2003b).

The idea of a "vital force" has been a core aspect of traditional healing practices for millennia and has often been used to explain therapeutic practices in the West such as mesmerism, magnetic healing, and faith healing (see Chapters 2 and 6). It has also been part of discussions in modern Western science at least since 1907, when Henri Bergson proposed it as an explanation for why organic molecules could not be synthesized at the time (Bergson, 1911). Part of this thinking held that electricity—the physics and engineering wonder of the time—was somehow connected with this vital force. Thousands of years earlier, Chinese and Indian healers had another idea, which has lately been seen as equivalent, called "qi" or "*prana*." Clearly such an idea has been around a long time.

A modern expression of this idea is often called the "biofield hypothesis" (Rubik, 2002). For our discussion here the important aspect of the biofield hypothesis is its dependence on classical electromagnetic fields and forces. (See Rubik's paper for a more thorough description of this concept and discussion.) As Rubik points out, "The biofield is a useful construct consistent with bioelectromagnetics and the physics of nonlinear, dynamical, nonequilibrium living systems." Although some aspects of energy medicine may be explained by the biofield and it is completely consistent with and even sufficient to explain magnetic therapy, there are at least two aspects of some forms of energy medicine that it does not adequately explain. One is the apparent distance independence. The other is the apparent instantaneous state change (like quantum entanglement) that forms part of some forms of energy medicine. This factor is the second anomaly of subtle energy medicine: it often happens faster than classical mechanisms could explain.

It is possible that these anomalies, as well as the very fundamental aspects of energy medicine, have their explanation and source in quantum physics. We acknowledge that others disagree with this idea (May, 2003). Still others think that, although it is not the whole explanation, some aspects of quantum physics may be relevant and may play a role in energy medicine (Dossey, 2003). If it is true that energy medicine is often working through nonclassical and quantum forms of energy, it is now possible to visualize a future in which energy medicine uses a combination of classical and quantum energy fields and forces to target and regulate endogenous processes and fields within the body to affect healing and salutogenesis.

If energy medicine and distant healing are fundamentally forms of information transfer, then quantum mechanics may provide the explanation and means for this process. In addition to explaining the transfer of healing energy between people, it may underlie the natural self-healing process itself. Rein (2004) has proposed that this information flow within the body is necessary for health and that when it is impeded, ill health and disease result. In this thinking, energy medicine is also the flow of information through quantum effects between healer and patient. In an analogous fashion, salutogenesis and health is the free flow and transfer of information within the body and the interchange of information with the environment to augment this flow. Thus, we believe that the fields of information and quantum models will be important areas of focus for future research and practice. Indeed, if testable theoretical models can be developed that explain data from both veritable and putative forms of energy medicine, a new paradigm of understanding in science and health care may emerge that is as important and revolutionary as molecular biological and biochemical models were in the twentieth century.

References

Astin JA, Harkness E, Ernst E: The efficacy of "distant healing": a systematic review of randomized trials, *Ann Intern Med* 132(11):903, 2000.

Atmanspacher H, Romer H, Walach H: Weak quantum theory: complementarity and entanglement in physics and beyond, *Found Phys* 32(3):379, 2002.

Bell I, Koithan M: A model for homeopathic remedy effects: low dose nanoparticles, allostatic cross-adaptation, and time-dependent sensitization in a complex adaptive system, *BMC Complement Altern Med* 12:191, 2012.

Bell IR, Ives JA, Jonas WB: *Nonlinear effects of nanoparticles: Biological variability from hermetic doses, small particle sizes, and dynamic adaptive interactions, Dose Response* 12(2):202–32, 2013 Nov 7.

Bennett CH, DiVincenzo DP: Quantum information and computation, *Nature* 404(6775):247, 2000.

Benor DJ: *Consciousness bioenergy and healing: self-healing and energy medicine for the 21st century,* vol 2, Medford, NJ, 2004, Wholistic Healing.

Bergson H: *Creative evolution,* New York, 1911, Henry Holt (translated by Arthur Mitchell).

Blackwell B, Bloomfield SS, Buncher CR: Demonstration to medical students of placebo responses and non-drug factors, *Lancet* 1:1279–1282, 1972.

Byrnes K, Waynant RW, Ilev IK, et al: Light promotes regeneration and functional recovery and alters the immune response after spinal cord injury, *Lasers Surg Med* 36(3):171, 2005.

Calabrese EJ, Bachmann KA, Bailer AJ, et al: Biological stress response terminology: Integrating the concepts of adaptive response and preconditioning stress within a hormetic dose-response framework, *Toxicol Appl Pharmacol* 222:122–128, 2007.

Cassidy CM: Social science theory and methods in the study of alternative and complementary medicine, *J Altern Complement Med* 1(1):19, 1995.

Chikramane PS, Kalita D, Suresh AK, et al: Why extreme dilutions reach non-zero asymptotes: a nanoparticulate hypothesis based on froth flotation, *Langmuir* 28:15864–15875, 2012.

de Craen AJM, Moerman DE, Heisterkamp SH, et al: Placebo effect in the treatment of duodenal ulcer, *Br J Clin Pharmacol* 48:853–860, 1999.

de Craen AJ, Tijssen JG, de Gans J, Kleijnen J: Placebo effect in the acute treatment of migraine: subcutaneous placebos are better than oral placebos, *J Neurol* 247:183–188, 2000.

Dossey L: Signal versus information in DMILS research protocols (response to Kevin Chen), *J Non-Locality Remote Ment Interact* 2(1):2003. Available at: http://www.emergentmind.org/letters1.htm#7.%20The%20problem%20of%20intelligent%20signals:%20expanding%20the%20quantum%20envelope%20(response%20to%20Larry%20Dossey.

Eccles NK: A critical review of randomized controlled trials of static magnets for pain relief, *J Altern Complement Med* 11(3):495, 2005.

Engebretson J, Wardell DW: Experience of a reiki session, *Altern Ther Health Med* 8(2):48, 2002.

Engebretson J, Wardell DW: Energy-based modalities, *Nurs Clin North Am* 42(2):243, 2007.

Gracely RH, Deeter WR, Wolskee PJ, et al: The effect of naloxone on multidimensional scales of postsurgical pain in nonsedated patients, *Soc Neurosci Abstr* 5:609, 1979.

Guo X, Zhou B, Nishimura T, et al: Clinical effect of Qigong practice on essential hypertension: a meta-analysis of randomized controlled trials, *J Altern Complement Med* 14:27–37, 2008.

Harlow T, Greaves C, White A, et al: Randomised controlled trial of magnetic bracelets for relieving pain in osteoarthritis of the hip and knee, *BMJ* 329(7480):1450, 2004.

Hintz KJ, Yount GL, Kadar I, et al: Bioenergy definitions and research guidelines, *Altern Ther Health Med* 9(3 Suppl):A13, 2003.

Hyland ME: The meaning(s) of entanglement in entanglement theory. In Walach H, Schneider R, Chez RA, editors: *Proceedings: generalized entanglement from a multidisciplinary perspective, Freiburg, Germany, October 9-11, 2003,* Alexandria, Va, 2003, Samueli Institute, p 117.

Jahn RG, Dunne BJ: On the quantum mechanics of consciousness, with applications to anomalous phenomena, *Found Phys* 16:721, 1986.

Jahnke R, Larkey L, Rogers C, et al: A comprehensive review of health benefits of qigong and tai chi, *Am J Health Promot* 24:e1–e25, 2010.

Jain S, McMahon GF, Hasen P, et al: Healing Touch with Guided Imagery for PTSD in returning active duty military: a randomized controlled trial, *Mil Med* 177:1015–1021, 2012.

Jonas WB, Crawford CC: Science and spiritual healing: a critical review of spiritual healing, "energy" medicine, and intentionality, *Altern Ther Health Med* 9(2):56, 2003a.

Jonas WB, Crawford CC, editors: *Healing, intention and energy medicine: science, research methods and clinical implications*, London, 2003b, Churchill Livingstone.

Julsgaard B, Kozhekin A, Polzik ES: Experimental long-lived entanglement of two macroscopic objects, *Nature* 413(6854): 400, 2001.

Kiang JG, Ives JA, Jonas WB: External bioenergy-induced increases in intracellular free calcium concentrations are mediated by Na$^+$/Ca^{2+} exchanger and L-type calcium channel, *Mol Cell Biochem* 271(1–2):51, 2005.

Kirsch I, editor: *How expectancies shape experience*, Washington, DC, 1999, American Psychological Association.

Kreiger D: *Accepting your power to heal*, Santa Fe, NM, 1993, Bear.

Lazorthes Y, Sol JC, Fowo S, et al: Motor cortex stimulation for neuropathic pain, *Acta Neurochir Suppl* 97(Pt 2):37, 2007.

Lee MS, Pittler MH, Guo R, Ernst E: Qigong for hypertension: a systematic review of randomized clinical trials, *J Hypertens* 25:1525–1532, 2007.

Li A, Lao L, Wang Y, et al: Electroacupuncture activates corticotrophin-releasing hormone-containing neurons in the paraventricular nucleus of the hypothalmmus to alleviate edema in a rat model of inflammation, *BMC Complement Altern Med* 8:20, 2008.

Lopez-Ibor JJ, Lopez-Ibor MI, Pastrana JI: Transcranial magnetic stimulation, *Curr Opin Psychiatry* 21(6):640, 2008.

Lu Z: *Scientific qigong exploration: the wonders and mysteries of qi*, Malvern, Pa, 1997, Amber Leaf Press.

Margo CE: The placebo effect, *Surv Ophthalmol* 44(1):31, 1999.

May E: Challenges for healing and intentionality research: causation and information. In Jonas WB, Crawford CC, editors: *Healing, intention and energy medicine: science, research methods and clinical implications*, London, 2003, Churchill Livingstone, p 283.

Mayor DF, Micozzi MS, editors: *Energy Medicine East and West: A Natural History of Qi*, Edinburgh, 2011, Churchill Livingstone.

Mentgen JL: Healing touch, *Nurs Clin North Am* 36(1):143, 2001.

Milgrom LR: Towards a new model of the homeopathic process based on quantum field theory, *Forsch Komplementmed* 13(3): 174, 2006.

Milgrom LR: A new geometrical description of entanglement and the curative homeopathic process, *J Altern Complement Med* 14(3):329, 2008a.

Milgrom LR: Treating Leick with like: response to criticisms of the use of entanglement to illustrate homeopathy, *Homeopathy* 97(2):96, 2008b.

Moerman DE, Jonas WB: Deconstructing the placebo effect and finding the meaning response, *Ann Intern Med* 136:471, 2002.

National Center for Complementary and Alternative Medicine (NCCAM): Energy medicine: an overview, 2007. Available at: http://nccam.nih.gov/health/whatiscam/energy/energymed .htm.

North American Nursing Diagnosis Association (NANDA): *Nursing diagnoses: definitions and classifications, 2007–2008*, Philadelphia, 2008, The Association.

Oh B, Choi SM, Inamori A, et al: Effects of qigong on depression: a systemic review, *Evid Based Complement Altern Med Epub* 2013.

Ohnishi ST, Ohnishi T: Philosophy, psychology, physics and practice of ki, *Evid Based Complement Alternat Med* 6(2):175, 2008.

O'Mathuna DP, Ashford RL: Therapeutic touch for healing acute wounds, *Cochrane Database Syst Rev* (4):CD002766, 2003.

O'Mathuna DP, Ashford RL: Therapeutic touch for healing acute wounds, *Cochrane Database Syst Rev* CD002766, 2012.

Peters RM: The effectiveness of therapeutic touch: a meta-analytic review, *Nurs Sci Q* 12(1):52, 1999.

Rein G: Bioinformation within the biofield: beyond bioelectromagnetics, *J Altern Complement Med* 10(1):59, 2004.

Rosenblum B, Kuttner F: *Quantum enigma: physics encounters consciousness*, New York, 2008, Oxford University Press.

Rubik B: The biofield hypothesis: its biophysical basis and role in medicine, *J Altern Complement Med* 8(6):703, 2002.

Segal NA, Toda Y, Huston J, et al: Two configurations of static magnetic fields for treating rheumatoid arthritis of the knee: a double-blind clinical trial, *Arch Phys Med Rehabil* 82(10):1453, 2001.

Smith CW: Is a living system a macroscopic quantum system?, *Frontier Perspect* 7:9, 1998.

Smith CW: Straws in the wind, *J Altern Complement Med* 9(1):1, 2003.

So PS, Jiang Y, Qin Y: Touch therapies for pain relief in adults, *Cochrane Database Syst Rev* (4):CD006535, 2008.

Sparber AG, Crawford CC, Jonas WB: Laboratory research on bioenergy healing. In Jonas WB, Crawford CC, editors: *Healing, intention and energy medicine: science, research methods and clinical implications*, London, 2003, Churchill Livingstone, p 139.

Tiller WA: *Science and human transformation: subtle energies, intentionality and consciousness*, Walnut Creek, Calif, 1997, Pavior.

Tsang HW, Fung KM: A review on neurobiological and psychological mechanisms underlying the anti-depressive effect of qigong exercise, *J Health Psychol* 13(7):857, 2008.

Vallbona C, Hazlewood CF, Jurida G: Response of pain to static magnetic fields in postpolio patients: a double-blind pilot study, *Arch Phys Med Rehabil* 78(11):1200, 1997.

Van Wijk R, Van Wijk EP, Wiegant FA, Ives J: Free radicals and low-level photon emission in human pathogenesis: state of the art, *Indian J Exp Biol* 46(5):273, 2008.

Van Wijk E: Imaging human spontaneous photo emission: Historical development, recent data, and perspectives, *Trends in Photochemistry & Photobiology* 15:27–40, 2013.

Ventura C: CAM and cell fate targeting: molecular and energetic insights into cell growth and differentiation, *Evid Based Complement Alternat Med* 2(3):277, 2005.

Walach H: Entanglement model of homeopathy as an example of generalized entanglement predicted by weak quantum theory, *Forsch Komplementarmed Klass Naturheilkd* 10(4):192, 2003.

Walach H: Generalized entanglement: a new theoretical model for understanding the effects of complementary and alternative medicine, *J Altern Complement Med* 11(3):549, 2005.

Walborn SP, Cunha MO, Padua S, et al: Double-slit quantum erasure, *Phys Rev A* 65(033818):1, 2002.

Walborn SP, Cunha MO, Padua S, et al: Quantum erasure, *Am Sci* 91:336, 2003.

Wang F, Man JK, Lee EK, et al: The effects of qigong on anxiety, depression, and psychological well-being: a systematic review and meta-analysis, *Evid Based Complement Alternat Med* [*Epub* Jan 14, 2013].

Warber SL, Gordon A, Gillespie BW, et al: Standards for conducting clinical biofield energy healing research, *Altern Ther Health Med* 9(3 Suppl):A54, 2003.

Weintraub MI, Cole SP: A randomized controlled trial of the effects of a combination of static and dynamic magnetic fields on carpal tunnel syndrome, *Pain Med* 9(5):493, 2008.

Weintraub MI, Mamtani R, Micozzi MS: *Complementary and integrative medicine in pain management*, New York, 2008, Springer, p 69.

Weintraub MI, Wolfe GI, Barohn RA, et al: Static magnetic field therapy for symptomatic diabetic neuropathy: a randomized, double-blind, placebo-controlled trial, *Arch Phys Med Rehabil* 84(5):736, 2003.

Whelan H, Desmet K, Buchmann E, et al: Harnessing the cell's own ability to repair and prevent neurodegenerative disease, *SPIE Newsroom* 2008. doi: 10.1117/2.1200802.1014.

White House Commission on Complementary and Alternative Medicine Policy: *Final report*, 2002. Available at: http://www.whccamp.hhs.gov.

Winstead-Fry P, Kijek J: An integrative review and meta-analysis of therapeutic touch research, *Altern Ther Health Med* 5(6):58, 1999.

Yan X, Shen H, Jiang H, et al: External qi of yan xin qigong induces G2/M arrest and apoptosis of androgen-independent prostate cancer cells by inhibiting Akt and Nf-Kappa B pathways, *Mol Cell Biochem* 310(1-2):227, 2008.

Yount G, Solfin J, Moore D, et al: In vitro test of external qigong, *BMC Complement Altern Med* 4:5, 2004.

Yu T, Tsai HL, Hwang ML: Suppressing tumor progression of in vitro prostate cancer cells by emitted psychosomatic power through Zen meditation, *Am J Chin Med* 31(3):499, 2003.

Zha L: Review of history, findings and implications of research on exceptional functions of the human body in China. In *Proceedings: bridging worlds and filling gaps in the science of spiritual healing, Keauhou Beach Resort, Kona, Hawaii, November 29–December 4, 2001*, Alexandria, Va, 2001, Samueli Institute.

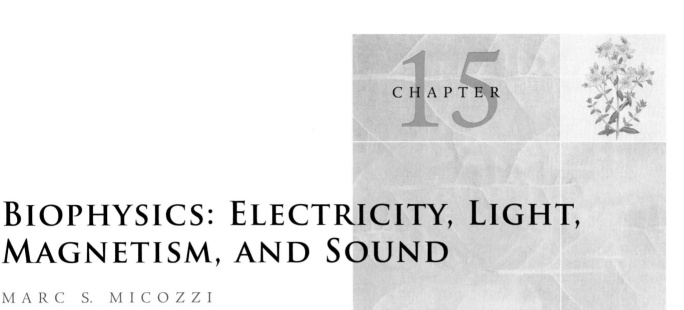

Biophysics: Electricity, Light, Magnetism, and Sound

MARC S. MICOZZI

MICHAEL I. WEINTRAUB

JENNIFER GEHL

There is a biophysical aspect to many healing modalities that has long been observed clinically. Contemporary fundamental physics is now in the process of providing explanatory models, mechanisms, and paradigms for the biophysical basis for many healing phenomena. These biophysical characteristics extend beyond the currently established basis of biomedical science in reductionist biochemical, molecular biological, and anatomical terms. Further, biophysics is consistent with many biomedical observations in whole-organism biology, physiology, and homeostasis.

Contemporary biophysics is important for understanding the basis of many contemporary diagnostic and therapeutic approaches. Biophysics, rather than using only biochemistry or molecular biology, may better provide explanatory mechanisms for the observed effectiveness of such clinical practices as acupuncture, herbalism (e.g., Bach Flower Remedies), homeopathy, touch, and meditation.

For example, nonthermal, nonionizing electromagnetic fields in low frequencies have been observed to have the following effects on the physical body: stimulation of bone repair, nerve stimulation, promotion of soft tissue wound healing, treatment of osteoarthritis, tissue regeneration, immune system stimulation, and neuroendocrine modulation.

Contemporary biophysically based diagnostic/therapeutic modalities include electrodermal screening, applied kinesiology, bioresonance, and radionics. Utilization of these approaches requires the availability of devices and practitioners.

Many well-established historical healing traditions have drawn on diagnostic and therapeutic approaches that may now be interpreted in the light of contemporary biophysics. The ancient and complex healing traditions of China and India make reference to and use practices based on biophysical modalities. Acupuncture, acupressure, *jin shin do*, t'ai chi, reiki, qigong, tui na, and yoga may be seen today to operate on a biophysical basis, but these methods have developed over three millennia in widespread clinical practice and observation. Contemporary outcomes-based clinical trials are demonstrating the efficacy of these modalities in management of many medical conditions. In addition, Asian medical systems have used sound, light, and color for their healing properties, which may be viewed in biophysical perspective (see Chapter 2).

WESTERN SCHOOLS OF THOUGHT AND PRACTICE

Biophysical medical modalities have also been prominent in the history of American medicine. Several schools of thought were created in the United States, or brought from Europe, that center around healing approaches which we may now associate in whole or in part with emerging biophysical explanations. Such schools and their founders have often influenced each other through time (Box 15-1).

In addition, interpretations of herbal, nutritional, and even pharmacological therapies have been extended to include "vibrational energy" as a potential mechanism of action.

There have been many adherents, practitioners, and clinical observations of these schools of thought and practice over time. They have been outside the realm of regular medical practice partially because the mechanisms of

213

BOX 15-1 *Schools and Their Founders with Influence on the Development of Biophysics (in Chronological Order)*

· Homeopathy (Samuel Hahnemann, Germany, 1830–1860)
· Faith healing (Phineas Quimby, 1830–1860)
· Christian Science (Mary Baker Eddy, 1861–1880)
· Theosophy (Helena Blavatsky and Henry Steel Olcott, 1861–1880)
· Movement therapy (Matthias Alexander, 1861–1880)
· Iridology (Nils Liljequist and Ignaz von Peczely, 1861–1900)
· Zone therapy/reflexology (William Fitzgerald, 1901–1920)
· Anthroposophical medicine (Madame Blavatsky and Rudolf Steiner, 1901–1920)
· Polarity therapy (Randolph Stone, 1921–1940)
· Bach flower remedies (Edward Bach, 1921–1940)
· Electromagnetism (Semyon and Valentine Kirlian, 1921–1940)
· Movement therapy (Moshé Feldenkrais, 1941–1960)
· Shiatsu (Tokujiro Namikoshi, 1941–1960)
· *Jin shin jyutsu* (Jiro Murai, 1941–1960)
· Orgone therapy (Wilhelm Reich, 1941–1960)
· Structural integration (Ida Rolf, 1960–1980)

action of these approaches have not been explained within the prevailing biomedical paradigm. Hypnosis is an example of an effective therapeutic modality with widespread effectiveness and acceptance within medicine. However, there remains no explanation for its mechanism of action. An alternative approach to explaining hypnosis has been developed on a statistical basis, describing the profile of clients and conditions likely to benefit, and developing "hypnotic susceptibility scales." This same approach is available for the clinical study of any therapeutic modality with observable outcomes in the absence of an identified "mechanism of action." Application of the science of psychometrics provides an approach similar to that of hypnosis, which has been successfully applied to a spectrum of "mind–body" approaches, as well as acupuncture (Jawer & Micozzi, 2011; see Chapter 10).

Concepts of mechanism of action are always bounded by the prevailing scientific paradigm and may not be the most clinically useful question (see Chapter 5). With the development of new scientific observations, a new paradigm emerges that is more inclusive in its explanation of observed phenomena.

INDIVIDUAL PRACTITIONERS

In addition to the fairly widespread, organized schools of thought and practice, there are many intuitive healers whose practices are highly individualized and highly eclectic. These practitioners represent important approaches used by many clients. The knowledge and practices of such gifted healers must be passed on or they will be lost. This represents a situation in the contemporary United States that is analogous to that of herbal remedies in the rain forest. Environmentalists are rightly concerned about the loss of biodiversity when unique plants disappear; ethnobotanists are concerned about the loss of the peoples whose cultural knowledge alone can convert the rain forest plants to cures.

EMPIRICAL ASSUMPTIONS OF BIOPHYSICALLY BASED MODALITIES

1. The human body has a biophysical component.
2. What has been scientifically defined as the "mind" is biophysically linked to the human body.
3. Every part of the human body is biophysically linked to every other part of the body.
4. Mental states (thoughts, emotions) generate physiological responses in the human body through neurological, hormonal, and immunological mechanisms (psychoneuroimmunology).
5. Biophysically based modalities are noninvasive by currently measurable and clinically observable criteria.

LIGHT

The application of light for medicinal purposes (healing) has been understood for thousands of years. The ancient Greeks observed that exposure to sunlight induced strength and health. During the Middle Ages, the disinfectant properties of sunlight were used to combat plague and other illnesses, and in the nineteenth century, cutaneous tuberculosis (scrofula) was treated with ultraviolet light exposure, as well as more general exposure to light and sunshine as part of the popular nature cure for a wide range of ailments (see Chapters 3 and 23). Currently, light therapy is used to treat psoriasis, hyperbilirubinemia, seasonal affective disorder, and vitamin D deficiency.

 The Light Cure and Vitamin D

Although the biochemistry of vitamin D has been understood only relatively recently, it has been a part of biology for a very long time. A microorganism that is estimated to have lived in the oceans for 750 million years is able to synthesize vitamin D, which possibly makes vitamin D the oldest hormone on the planet (see Chapter 26).

It was recognized over 150 years ago that people, especially children, who lived and worked in dark urban areas where there was little light were susceptible to bone diseases such as rickets. In Boston in 1889, it was estimated that 80% of infants had rickets. This pattern marked a shift away from a U.S. population that was primarily engaged in agriculture (Thomas Jefferson's idea of an agrarian democracy) during the 1800s and exposed to

The Light Cure and Vitamin D—cont'd

plenty of light on the farms and in the fields. The lack of light in dank, dark urban environments was compounded by the unavailability of fresh foods and lack of food distribution.

At that time it was noted that an extended visit to the country with clean air, clean water, abundant sunlight, and the benefits of nature would often cure medical disorders. Thus the idea of the nature cure was born (see Chapter 2). One of the many famous beneficiaries of the nature cure in the late 1800s was future president Theodore Roosevelt, who was well known for saying that he was literally "Dee-lighted" with any number of things, including the results of his cure for his lung disease. One of the most common lung diseases in the late 1800s was tuberculosis (TB). Sanitoriums and solariums were created in wilderness areas away from the cities so that TB patients could benefit from the nature cure. Although no antibiotic treatments were available at that time, many patients with TB benefitted from exposure to nature, including sunlight.

As early as 1849, cod liver oil was also used in the treatment of TB, according to the *Brompton Hospital Records*, Volume 38 (Table 15-1). We now know cod liver oil to be one of the few dietary sources of vitamin D. We also now know that vitamin D activates the immune system cells that can fight TB. So the nature cure of sun and fish oil (also known to sailors as the "sun-fish" cure), which delivered increased vitamin D, was the right treatment for the times.

The direct connection between sunlight and bone metabolism was also established in 1919 when Huldschinsky treated rickets with exposure to a mercury arc lamp. In 1921, Hess and Unger observed that sun exposure cured rickets.

In the 1930s, medicine began to directly appreciate the connection between sunlight and the metabolic activities we now associate with vitamin D. This was also the decade that saw the actual identification and labeling of the many metabolically active constituents we now call vitamins. Vitamin D was discovered in the early 1920s by Windaus, who was later awarded the Nobel Prize for synthesizing vitamin D in the laboratory by replicating the photoactivation process that occurs in the skin.

In the 1930s, the federal government set up an agency to recommend to parents, especially those living in the Northeast, that they send their children outside to play and get some sun exposure.

Fortification of milk with vitamin D also began at that time. Unfortunately, the last 40 years have actually seen a reversal of some of the sensible public health recommendations regarding adequate vitamin D and sun exposure.

Vitamin D and Dermatology: There Goes the Sun

Many physicians and public health organizations, including the biomedically oriented World Health Organization, have been trying to go one better on *Moby Dick*'s Captain Ahab, who said he "would strike the sun if it insulted me." For 40 years there has been a concerted campaign to make people avoid sun exposure. Because ultraviolet B (UVB) light from the sun is responsible for the photoactivation of vitamin D in the skin, sun blockers that "protect" the skin also virtually eliminate photoactivation of vitamin D. A sunscreen with a sun protection factor (SPF) of 8 is supposed to absorb 92.5% of UVB light, whereas doubling the SPF to 16 absorbs 99%. This essentially shuts down vitamin D production. (It also demonstrates that SPF formulations above 16 have little marginal utility and calls into question the appropriateness of the ever-increasing SPF numbers found on the pharmacy shelves.) People have become photophobic, and dermatologists have been on a campaign to "strike the sun."

A study in Australia, which has high levels of sunlight and high rates of skin cancer, found 100% of dermatologists to be deficient in vitamin D. In fact, most people should go outside in the sun for reasonable periods of time to get the many benefits of sunlight (Box 15-2). It is always wise to protect the face and head with a hat and

TABLE 15-1 *Historic Milestones in Recognition of the Relations among Sunlight, Vitamin D Activity, and Health*

Year	Observation/milestone	Vitamin D pioneers
1849	Cod liver oil (vitamin D) treats tuberculosis	Brompton Hospital
1889	Nature cure treats rickets	S. Weir Mitchell et al
1919	Mercury arc lamp (ultraviolet B light) treats rickets	Huldschinsky
1921	Sun exposure cures rickets	Hess and Unger
1920s	Vitamin D discovered	Adolf Windaus
1920s	Vitamin D photosynthesized in laboratory	Adolf Windaus (Nobel Prize, 1928)
1940s	Sunlight protects *against* cancer	Apperly
1970	25-Hydroxyvitamin D_3 isolated	Holick
1971	1,25-Dihydroxyvitamin D_3 isolated	Holick
1979	Vitamin D receptors found	De Luca et al
1980	Vitamin D treats psoriasis	Holick et al
2002	Vitamin D regulates blood pressure	Li et al

Continued

BOX 15-2 *Get Some Sun: Benefits of Sunlight*

- Improves bone health
- Improves mental health
- Improves heart health
- Prevents many common cancers
- Alleviates skin disorders
- Decreases risk of autoimmune disorders
- Decreases risk of multiple sclerosis
- Decreases risk of diabetes

 The Light Cure and Vitamin D—cont'd

sunglasses, because less than 10% of UVB light absorption happens above the neck and the face is the most cosmetically sensitive. It is best to expose the entire body in a bathing suit for 10 to 15 minutes at least three times per week. African Americans require more sun exposure because their natural skin pigmentation provides an SPF equivalent of 8 to 15.

Global Dimensions of D-ficiency

Essentially little or no active vitamin D is available from regular dietary sources. It is principally found in fish oils, sun-dried mushrooms, and fortified foods like milk and orange juice. However, many countries worldwide forbid the fortification of foods. There is potentially plenty of vitamin D in the food chain, because both phytoplankton and zooplankton exposed to sunlight make vitamin D. Wild-caught salmon, which feed on natural food sources, for example, has available vitamin D. However, farmed salmon fed food pellets with little nutritional value have only 10% of the vitamin D of wild fish. The "perfect storm" of photophobia, lack of exposure to sunlight, and insufficiency of available dietary vitamin D has led to a national and worldwide epidemic of vitamin D deficiency.

Estimates are that at least 30% and as much as 80% of the U.S. population is vitamin D deficient. In the United States, at latitudes north of Atlanta, the skin does not make (photoconvert) any vitamin D from November through March (i.e., essentially outside of daylight savings time; so although we shift the clock around, it does not salvage vitamin D synthesis). During this season the angle of the sun in the sky is too low to allow UVB light to penetrate the atmosphere, and it is absorbed by the ozone layer. Even in the late spring, summer, and early fall, most vitamin D is made between 10 AM and 3 PM when UVB from the sun penetrates the atmosphere and reaches the earth's surface.

It might be expected that vitamin D deficiency would be a problem limited to northern latitudes.

In Bangor, Maine, among young girls 9 to 11 years old, nearly 50% were deficient at the end of winter and nearly 20% remained deficient at the end of summer. At Boston Children's Hospital, over 50% of adolescent girls and African American and Hispanic boys were found to be vitamin D deficient year round. In another study in Boston, 34% of whites, 40% of Hispanics, and 84% of African American adults over age 50 were found to be deficient.

Vitamin D deficiency is also a national problem, however. The U.S. Centers for Disease Control and Prevention completed a national survey at the end of winter and found that nearly 50% of African American women aged 15 to 49 years were deficient. These are women in the critical childbearing years. A growing fetus must receive adequate vitamin D from the mother, especially because breast milk does not provide adequate vitamin D. A study of pregnant women in Boston found that in 40 mother–infant pairs at the time of labor and delivery, over 75% of mothers and 80% of newborns were deficient. This observation was made despite the fact that pregnant women were instructed to take a prenatal vitamin that included 400 IU of vitamin D and to drink two glasses of milk per day.

Further, vitamin D deficiency is a global problem. Even in India, home to 1 billion of the earth's people, where there is plenty of sun, 30% to 50% of children, 50% to 80% of adults, and 90% of physicians are deficient. In South Africa, vitamin D deficiency is also a problem even though Cape Town is situated at 34 degrees latitude.

Although there are many new bilateral and multilateral governmental and private efforts to export Western medical technology and pharmaceuticals to the Third World to combat infectious diseases such as acquired immunodeficiency syndrome (AIDS), there is no comparable effort to acknowledge and address the global dimensions of the vitamin D deficiency epidemic. The U.S. Congress and president deemed it as a great achievement to give $40 billion to U.S. pharmaceutical companies to send expensive drug treatments for AIDS (a preventable disease) overseas. By contrast, addressing the vitamin D deficiency epidemic could be accomplished with much safer and less expensive nutritional supplements together with sunlight, the only source of energy that is still free. ∞

THE IDENTITY OF LIGHT

Light has one identity as electromagnetic waves characterized by wavelength but also exists as tiny energy bundles, or photons. As discussed in Chapter 1, and the previous chapter, light is paradoxically both a particle and a wave. Visible light, called the "visual spectrum," is electromagnetic radiation at wavelengths of 400 to 700 nanometers (nm) appreciated by the human eye. The human eye is sensitive to approximately 90% of the spectrum of electromagnetic radiation that propagates through the atmosphere and reaches the earth's surface. As a sensory organ, the eye evolved to detect that portion of the electromagnetic spectrum that is there to be seen in the terrestrial environment. Due to the elevation of the path of the sun through the sky at different times of year (seasons) at different latitudes, beneficial and/or harmful wavelengths may or may not penetrate the atmosphere. In the temperate zones of the planet (between the Arctic and Tropic circles), the months and weeks around the time of the equinoxes generally provide a good balance of healthful wavelengths without harmful wavelengths of light passing through the atmosphere.

One nanometer equals one billionth of a meter. The shorter the wavelength, the higher the energy (from Planck's law, the energy level is the inverse of the wavelength multiplied by the Planck constant) and the greater the ability of light to penetrate tissues. For example, a blue-violet light has a shorter wavelength, and a red light has a longer wavelength. Infrared light is even longer in wavelength (lower energy) and ultraviolet light is even shorter in wavelength (higher energy) than the visible spectrum. This is the reason for the concern of dermatologists that DNA-damaging ultraviolet light with a shorter wavelength and higher "ionizing" energy is dangerous, and for the notion that using infrared light with a longer wavelength and lower energy for tanning is a "safer" form of exposure. (See the sidebar "The Light Cure and Vitamin D.")

X-rays, gamma rays, ultraviolet rays, cosmic rays, and others all fall below visible light on the electromagnetic spectrum. Longer wavelengths such as infrared rays, microwaves, television signals, and FM/AM radio waves have different characteristics. Laser beams are a particular kind of amplified light. The atomic models that led to the discovery of lasers were conceptualized and developed in 1917 by Albert Einstein. His discovery became known as "LASER" for *l*ight *a*mplification by *s*timulated *e*mission of *r*adiation. When an atom is in an excited state and an incoming light particle reaches it, it may eject an additional photon instead of absorbing the particle. This theory was a revolutionary concept that proved to be true, and Einstein received the Nobel Prize for explaining the photoelectric effect. By 1960, the first practical ruby red laser was developed by T.H. Maiman, who used crystals and mirrors to produce a monochromatic, nondivergent light beam in which all waves were parallel and in phase (Maiman, 1960). These characteristics were subsequently referred to as "monochromaticity," "collimation," and "coherence," respectively. The original ruby red beam was a visible red light with a wavelength of 694 nm. Since then, various crystals and gases have been used to develop lasers in other regions of the electromagnetic spectrum, including infrared and visible-light lasers (Box 15-3).

THE EFFECTS OF LIGHT

Every object has optical properties that determine the reflectiveness of light and the interaction of light with that object. For example, the light from mid-infrared and

BOX 15-3 *LASER (Light Amplification by Stimulated Emission of Radiation)*

When light is directed onto an object, one (or more) of the following occurs:
1. The light is reflected
2. The light is transmitted
3. The light is scattered
4. The light is absorbed

far-infrared lasers, such as carbon dioxide, holmium, and yttrium-aluminum-garnet lasers, is primarily absorbed by water in the tissues. This absorption of the infrared light energy produces heat, which leads to local vaporization that does not spread. The light from near-infrared and visible-light lasers such as neodymium and argon lasers is poorly absorbed by water but is rapidly absorbed by pigments such as hemoglobin and melanin. This optical property makes these lasers effective in the destruction of tissues that are rich in pigment, such as retina, gastric mucosa, and pigmented cutaneous lesions. It is easy to see how these so-called high-powered surgical lasers, using heat and energy, lead to specific tissue changes. Over the past 30 years, numerous animal and laboratory experiments were carried out using these high-energy lasers. These experiments produced results that ultimately led to human testing and approval by the FDA of the use of lasers in humans.

Despite more than 30 years of similar experiments using weak or low-level nonthermal lasers, there is still controversy concerning the effectiveness of low-level laser therapy (LLLT) as a treatment modality because of a lack of randomized, double-blind, placebo-controlled trials and publication of findings in peer-reviewed journals. Various articles have made claims, but the studies reported by many have flawed methodology, use different time and dosage schedules, and do not have a strict placebo-controlled design. Despite all these shortcomings, several investigations were brought to the attention of the FDA, and in 2002 the FDA approved an application for the use of laser light as a therapeutic device for pain relief.

Cold laser therapy, or LLLT, is based on the idea that monochromatic light energy, which depends on wavelength for its penetration, can alter cellular functions. Because the original European studies on wound healing in animals yielded positive results, the technique was described as "biostimulation." Mester et al (1982) and Lyons et al (1987) found that light could be stimulatory at low power and could elicit an opposite inhibitory effect at higher power. In addition, the cumulative dosages of the radiation could sometimes be inhibitory. Today a variety of lasers are available, but the two most popular are helium-neon (HeNe) (632 nm) and gallium-aluminum-arsenide (GaAlAs) (830 nm). In practice, these visible and infrared lasers have powers of 30 to 90 mW and deliver from 1 to

9 J/cm^2 to treatment sites. To date, they have been shown to be safe within this range, but they have also been used at higher doses.

TISSUE OPTICAL PROPERTIES

Musculoskeletal tissues appear to have optical properties that respond to light between 500 and 1000 nm. Sufficient specific laser dose and the number of treatments needed are still the subject of controversy. It is hypothesized that light-sensitive organelles, or chromatophores, absorb light (Walsh, 1997) and that ultimately the energy produces a biological reaction. It has been suggested that chromatophores are present on the myelin sheath and in mitochondria, and that it is the monochromatic wavelength properties, rather than the coherency and collimation of laser light, that induce biological changes. It is presumed that the collimation and coherency lead to rapid degradation by scatter. Others have theorized that the primary photoreceptors are the flavins and porphyrins and that the therapeutic benefit of pain reduction produced by a combination of red and near-infrared light is caused by an increase in β-endorphins, blocking depolarization of C-fiber afferents, a reduction in bradykinin levels, and ionic channel stabilization.

Tissue penetration depends on the wavelength. The shorter HeNe laser beam (632 nm) penetrates several millimeters into tissue, whereas the GaAlAs (830 nm) at 30 mW allows photons to penetrate more than an inch (3 cm). Several authors have stated that an infrared laser beam travels about 2 mm into tissue and that this represents one penetration depth with a loss of $1/e$ (37%) of beam intensity (Basford, 1998). However, the shorter visible HeNe red beam is attenuated the same amount in 0.5 to 1 mm (Anderson & Parish, 1981; Basford, 1995; Kolari, 1985). How does one measure the decay in the amount of energy with distance? At the surface of the skin, the laser delivers from 1 to 9 J/cm^2. Karu (1987) has demonstrated that light of 0.01 J/cm^2 can alter cellular processes. As a result, approximately six penetration depths (3 to 6 mm for HeNe red light and about 24 mm for GaAlAs infrared light) are possible before the strength of the beam stream drops from 9 J/cm^2 to 0.01 J/cm^2. Thus, the threshold and specific therapeutic amount needed for stimulation differs for the superficial nerves and tissues and for the deeper structures. There is also a scattering of energy that influences nonneural adjacent tissues (i.e., flexor tendons in the forearm and wrist with stimulation at the level of the carpal tunnel).

PENETRATION, PAIN, AND THRESHOLDS

It has been stated that tissue penetration and saturation with pulsed frequency settings of 1 to 100 Hz influenced pain and neuralgia, whereas setting of 1000 Hz influenced edema and swelling and 5000 Hz influenced inflammation. Light from a superpulsed laser using a gallium arsenide (GaAs) infrared diode provides the deepest penetration

in body tissues. It operates at a wavelength of 904 nm. Superpulsing is defined as the generation of continuous bursts of very-high-power pulses of light energy (10 to 100 Watts) that are of extremely short duration (100 to 200 nanoseconds). This allows GaAs penetration to tissue depths of 3 to 5 cm and deeper. Some versions of GaAs therapeutic lasers actually penetrate to tissue depths of 10 to 14 cm (Kneebone, 2007). There have been many claims and studies regarding LLLT, but the varied quality of trials has led to controversy. Basford (1986, 1995, 1998), a major critic of the deficiencies of many studies, notes that LLLT research has developed along the following three separate lines:
1. Cellular function
2. Animal studies
3. Human trials.

Effects on Cellular Functions

Perhaps the strongest and most well-established research has been on changes in cellular functions. There is a strong body of direct evidence indicating that LLLT can significantly alter cellular processes. The following are specific areas of treatment in which benefits have been claimed:
- Stimulation of collagen formation leading to stronger scars (Mester et al, 1985), increased recruitment of fibroblasts and formation of granulation tissue (Mester & Jaszsagi-Nagy, 1973), increased neovascularization (Mester et al, 1982), and faster wound healing (Lam et al, 1986; Lyons et al, 1987; Rochkind et al, 1987)
- Pain relief and reduced firing frequency of nociceptors (Mezawa et al, 1988)
- Enhanced remodeling and repair of bone (Rochkind et al, 1987; Walsh, 1997)
- Stimulation of endorphin release (Yamada, 1991)
- Modulation of the immune system via prostaglandin synthesis (Kubasova et al, 1984; Mester et al, 1982).

Basic animal and cellular research with red-beam low-level lasers has produced both positive and negative results. Passarella (1989) believes that the optical properties of mitochondria are influenced by HeNe laser irradiation, with new mitochondrial conformations produced that ultimately lead to increased oxygen consumption. Walker (1983) has suggested that HeNe laser light affects serotonin metabolism, and Yu et al (1997) has demonstrated an increased phosphate potential and energy charge with light exposure. Further research continues at the cellular level. Fibroblast, lymphocyte, monocyte, and macrophage cells have been studied, and bacterial cell lines of *Escherichia coli* have served as models for investigation (Karu, 1988). The most popular laser in such cellular research has been the HeNe laser with a wavelength of 632.8 nm. However, some major discrepancies are found in the results reported in the existing literature because of the wide variation in the laser parameters employed, particularly dose and treatment time. Because imprecise dosimetry has clouded the issues, the optimal dose for achieving a biological benefit has yet to be determined.

Animal Studies

Despite the problems posed by a lack of standardization, lack of controls, and imprecise dose and treatment schedules for in vivo experimental work, results from cellular research were extrapolated to research on animals. Subsequently, a wide variety of animal models were employed to assess the putative biostimulatory effects of laser irradiation on wound healing. Small, loose-skinned rodents such as mice, rats, and guinea pigs have been used most often, but studies using pig models have led to different results. It has been argued that pigskin represents a more suitable model for extrapolation to humans, because it is similar in character to human skin, which has led to its use in human skin grafts, for example (Basford, 1986; Hunter et al, 1984).

Baxter (1997) provides an excellent review of the animal models used in the wound-healing literature. The details of experimental and irradiation procedures are so numerous and variable, however, that reproduction of results and intertrial comparisons are usually not practical. Research groups reported either acceleration in healing or no effect on the healing process. Two criteria frequently used to assess wound healing were collagen content and tensile strength. Rochkind et al (1989) conducted one of the largest series of controlled animal trials, comparing the recovery of LLLT-treated crushed sciatic nerves with that of nonirradiated nerves in rats. Constant low-intensity laser irradiation (7.6 to 10 J/cm^2 daily for up to 20 days) demonstrated highly beneficial effects as judged from recordings of compound action potentials. Wound-healing rates in both irradiated and nonirradiated wounds were accelerated, but the amplitude of action potentials in crushed sciatic nerves was raised substantially only in the irradiated groups. The laser treatment also greatly reduced the degeneration of motor neurons, which suggested that these results might be extrapolated for application in human research trials.

The information gained from trials of in vivo animal exposure to laser photobiostimulation indicated that, in certain animal models, wound healing could be achieved. The reader is cautioned to remain both critical and skeptical, however, because variations existed in methodology, techniques, dosimetry, exposure time, and frequency of treatments.

Human Trials

Despite the aforementioned controversy and limitations, many clinicians were persuaded by the cellular and animal data to attempt human trials. A number of disorders, including neurological, rheumatological, and musculoskeletal conditions, have been treated with LLLT with various claims regarding results. The FDA had previously been a major obstacle because of the absence of randomized, placebo-controlled trials and the varying methodology, varying dosages and techniques, and absence of objective parameters. However, as described earlier, in February 2002 the FDA approved the application for the use of LLLT for pain relief.

Carpal tunnel syndrome Carpal tunnel syndrome is a common clinical disorder, seen in 5% to 10% of the population, and is caused by compression of the median nerve at the wrist. Acroparesthesia (numbness, tingling, and burning) in the first three fingers often arises and may interfere with sleep. When resistant to conservative treatment, the disorder often progresses, with weakness and atrophy. There are nine flexor tendons adjacent to the median nerve, and they often intersect the nerve fascicles in the carpal tunnel. Thus, nerve compression or tendinitis may serve as a cause.

Basford et al (1993), using laser light of only 1 J of energy, found that both sensory and motor distal latencies could be significantly decreased in normal volunteers. Basford et al's study was a double-blind controlled trial using a GaAlAs percutaneous laser. Weintraub (1997), who used a similar laser but at higher energy levels of 9 J and measured compound motor nerve action potential/sensory nerve action potential electrophysiological parameters, reported a nearly 80% success rate in resolving the symptoms of carpal tunnel syndrome with laser therapy. There were no control subjects in the study, but almost 1000 sensory and motor nerve latencies were analyzed before and after each treatment. Particularly interesting was the fact that the distal latency was prolonged in 40% of subjects, yet they remained asymptomatic. This prolonged latency suggests that nonneural tissues were stimulated and could be responsible for symptoms of tendonitis. At the dose used, a significant number of individuals showed immediate prolongation of distal latency (nerve conduction). They remained asymptomatic, however, and by the next visit, the distal latency was back to baseline or improved. A similar observation has also been made by others (Snyder-Mackler & Bork, 1988). Padua et al (1998) validated Weintraub's study, and currently three placebo-controlled trials are being conducted with preliminary reports of 70% success (Lasermedics, 1999). In addition, several reports of studies using higher doses of 10 to 12 J of infrared laser light (40 to 50 mW) revealed alterations in conduction in both the median and superficial radial nerves (Baxter et al, 1994; Bork & Snyder-Mackler, 1988; Walsh et al, 1991).

Naeser et al (1996) and Branco and Naeser (1999) used a combination of two noninvasive, painless treatment modalities—red-beam laser and microampere-level transcutaneous electrical nerve stimulation (TENS)—to stimulate acupuncture points on the hand of patients with carpal tunnel syndrome or wrist pain. Sham treatments were used as a control. A significant reduction in median nerve sensory latencies in the treated hand and a 92% reduction in pain were observed. Postoperative failures also decreased with this protocol. Weintraub (n.d.) used his original laser treatment protocol (9 J/cm^2) and also stimulated various acupressure points as did Naeser et al (1996) and Branco and Naeser (1999) as well as the flexor tendons in the upper wrist. Up to 85% improvement in wrist pain was achieved in patients with carpal tunnel syndrome.

Other nerve pain Other superficial nerves also respond to laser biostimulation. Disorders such as meralgia paresthetica, cubital tunnel syndrome, tarsal tunnel syndrome, radial nerve palsy, and traumatic digital neuralgias have responded to this treatment (Weintraub, 1998). Because of the small number of individuals treated, these observations are to be considered anecdotal. However, Weintraub believes that his observations that nonneural structures play an important yet unappreciated role in symptomatic carpal tunnel syndrome, and probably other nerve entrapments, are indeed significant. For example, the distal latency of the median nerve could be longer than 5 milliseconds in patients who have become asymptomatic with laser treatment. Either a threshold exists for the median nerve, or the tendons and blood vessels surrounding the median nerve exert some influence. Franzblau and Werner (1999) raised similar issues in a provocative editorial titled "What Is Carpal Tunnel Syndrome?"

The efficacy of laser therapy in treating various pain syndromes has been investigated by several groups. Preliminary double-blind studies by Walker (1983) demonstrated improvement in seven out of nine patients with trigeminal neuralgia. Two out of five patients with postherpetic neuralgia showed improvement, and five out of six patients with radiculopathy improved. Baxter et al (1991) also believed that laser therapy was effective for postherpetic neuralgia. Moore et al (1988) investigated the efficacy of GaAlAs laser therapy in the treatment of postherpetic neuralgia in a double-blind crossover trial involving 20 patients. The result was an apparently significant reduction in pain. Hong et al (1990) validated these results in their study, in which 60% of patients with postherpetic neuralgia felt improvement within 10 minutes. Friedman et al (1994) used an intraoral HeNe laser directed at a specific maxillary alveolar tender point to significantly abort atypical facial pain.

Trigeminal neuralgia was successfully treated with a HeNe laser by Walker et al (1986). In the 35 patients studied in this double-blind, placebo-controlled trial, a significant difference was found in visual analogue scale pain ratings between patients receiving active laser treatment and placebo-treated patients.

Using an intraoral HeNe laser directed at a specific maxillary alveolar tender point, Weintraub (1996) was able to abort acute migraine headaches in 85% of cases in a study that included a sham-treatment control condition. These findings support the trigeminovascular theory of migraine with a maxillary (V2) provocative site. The results achieved rival those of pharmacotherapy. Interestingly, Friedman (1998) used cryotherapy (cold water) applied to the same maxillary alveolar tender point to treat atypical facial pain and migraine headache. The treatment produced a striking reduction in discomfort.

Several groups have investigated the efficacy of laser therapy in the treatment of radicular and pseudoradicular pain syndromes. Bieglio and Bisschop (1986) and Mizokami et al (1990) reported positive effects in treating these conditions. Low-power laser therapy has also been used successfully to induce preoperative anesthesia in both veterinary practice and dental surgery (Christensen, 1989). In contrast to the numerous clinical human studies of laser-mediated analgesia, there have been relatively few laboratory studies. Most of the experiments have been completed in China in a variety of animals, including rats, goats, rabbits, sheep, and horses. There are no English abstracts or translations of most of these works. Other studies in animals that were published in English and used tail-flick methodology to assess pain have reported variable findings.

Arthritis Laser acupuncture using an HeNe diode was reported to be successful in the treatment of experimentally induced arthritis in rats. Vocalization and limb withdrawal in response to noxious stimulation were the parameters measured (Zhu et al, 1990). Although it is clear that problems exist in extrapolating the findings of laboratory work to humans, as noted earlier Naeser et al (1996) and Branco and Naeser (1999) were successful in applying this procedure to treatment of carpal tunnel syndrome. Similarly, Weintraub (1997) saw additional improvement when he combined Naeser's acupressure points with his protocol in treating this syndrome.

One of the major economic burdens in the United States has been caused by the high incidence of soft tissue injuries and low back pain and subsequent work disability. Numerous studies using HeNe and infrared laser diodes (830 nm) have reported varying results (Basford, 1986, 1995; Gam et al, 1993; Klein & Eek, 1990), but randomized controlled and blinded studies have been difficult to carry out.

Rheumatologists in the United States have found encouraging results in laser treatment of rheumatoid arthritis (Goldman et al, 1980), and similar results have been reported in the Soviet Union/Russia, Eastern Europe, and Japan. Walker et al (1986) reported success after a 10-week course of treatment with HeNe lasers. Using a GaAlAs 830-nm laser, Asada et al (1989) found 90% improvement in an uncontrolled trial in 170 patients with rheumatoid arthritis. Despite these generally positive results, Bliddal et al (1987) did not see any significant change in symptoms of morning stiffness or joint function in such patients. However, slight improvement was noted in pain scale ratings. Similar positive results for laser therapy have been reported for osteoarthritis and other conditions. Critics have argued, however, that because rheumatoid arthritis is a disease of exacerbation and remission, it is difficult to assess the efficacy of the therapy.

Sports medicine A number of reports document the apparent efficacy of laser therapy in reducing pain associated with sports injuries. These reports initially came from Russia and Eastern Europe, but the results were subsequently confirmed by Morselli et al (1985) and Emmanoulidis et al (1986). It is notable that in the latter study, improvement was accompanied by a decrease in thermographic readings.

The use of laser therapy to treat tendinopathies, especially lateral humeral epicondylitis (tennis elbow), has been studied by numerous groups. There has usually been a relatively rapid response to therapy; however, Haker and Lundberg (1990) failed to show any effect of laser acupuncture treatment on tennis elbow.

Chronic neck pain is common and is often associated specifically with a herniated disk, degenerative disk disease, degenerative spine disease, spinal stenosis, or facet joint dysfunction. The small C-nociceptive afferents and the larger myelinated A delta fibers usually innervate these areas. Local chemical dysfunction with release of substance P, phospholipase A, cytokines, nitric oxide, and so on is probably also involved. It is theorized that direct photoreception by cytochromes produces elevated production of adenosine triphosphate and changes in cell membrane permeability. Antiedema effects and antiinflammatory responses have been alleged to occur in response to laser therapy through reduction in bradykinin levels and increase in β-endorphin levels. Both the depth of penetration and the total dose influence the success of the laser treatment at the target tissue level. Thus, combinations of high-output (centiwatt) GaAlAs and GaAs (superpulsing) lasers can achieve penetration of 3 to 5 cm and even deeper (10 to 14 cm). In addition, acupressure point stimulation (2 to 4 J of energy) to the ear, hand, or body should be used.

Low back pain Low back pain syndrome is the most common cause of disability in the United States, affecting 75% to 85% of Americans at some point in their lifetimes. Low back pain provides an example in which a host of noninvasive, nonsurgical therapies have been shown to be more effective and cost-effective, such as spinal manual therapy, acupuncture, bodywork and massage, physical therapy, active herbal ingredients for joints (such as *Bosewellia*), and biophysical modalities. Common causes include herniated disks, spinal stenosis, spondylosis, facet joint dysfunction, and failed back syndrome secondary to surgery. As with chronic neck pain, the small C-nociceptive afferents and A delta fibers are involved, with localized chemical dysfunction producing altered signal transduction. Use of a high-output GaAlAs infrared laser at 9 J/cm and/or a GaAs superpulsed infrared laser may be effective in treating the deeper tissues. Usually the nerve irritation occurs deep, around 60 mm, secondary to a herniated disk. Acupressure point stimulation should also be used.

Cerebral circulation, migraine, and auditory and vestibular function Naeser et al (1995) improved blood flow in stroke patients using laser acupuncture treatment and noted improvement in symptoms.

One of us (Weintraub, personal observation) has achieved benefit by stimulating naguien acupressure points with an 830-nm laser. Naeser (1999), in a review of the highlights of the Second Congress of the World Association for Laser Therapy, reported that Wilden treated inner ear disorders, including vertigo, tinnitus, and hearing loss, with a combination of 630- to 700-nm and 830-nm lasers.

The total dose was at least 4000 J. Daily, 1-hour laser treatments to both ears were performed for at least 3 weeks. The lasers were applied to the auditory canal and the mastoid and petrosal bones. Wilden said that he used this approach for more than 9 years in 800 patients, and except in very severe cases, most patients reported improvement in hearing.

Application of laser light to the *hegu* point on the side contralateral to the pain may be effective for treating migraine headaches. Treatment with an intraoral HeNe laser directed along the zone of maxillary alveolar tenderness also achieves success in the range of 78%. Stimulation is repeated three times at intervals of 1 minute to 90 seconds.

Lower limbs Meralgia paresthetica is an often disabling symptom that is caused by compression of the lateral anterior femoral cutaneous nerve at the level of the inguinal ligament. The author (Weintraub) has treated 10 patients with this condition by applying laser stimulation from the level of the inguinal ligament to the level of the knee anterolaterally. Significant pain reduction was noted in 8 of the 10 patients by the fourth treatment, but there have been recurrences.

The soles of the feet and various acupressure points were stimulated by laser without providing relief in 10 cases of nondiabetic peripheral neuropathy. However, the use of monochromatic infrared and visible light phototherapy to treat diabetic peripheral neuropathy has been reported to be successful in inducing temporary or permanent relief from pain and inflammation (Leonard et al, 2004).

PRECAUTIONS

No detrimental effects are produced by low-output nonthermal lasers, although it is obvious that direct retinal exposure is to be avoided. Pregnancy does not appear to be a contraindication with LLLT, but investigators have been advised to avoid treating pregnant women and individuals with local tumors in the area of treatment. Individuals who are taking photosensitizing drugs such as tetracycline or who have photosensitive skin should probably avoid this treatment. It has also been suggested that the use of phototherapy after steroid injections is contraindicated, because antiinflammatory medicine is well documented to reduce the effectiveness of photobiostimulation (Lopes-Martins et al, 2006).

APPEAL OF PHOTOTHERAPY

Medicine is faced with many conditions that respond poorly or marginally to pharmacological therapy in addition to the side effects inherent. Thus, the appeal of noninvasive therapeutic laser and other phototherapy devices, that are both effective and safe, is evident. They are a most welcome addition to the physician's armamentarium. Therapeutic laser treatment has been used successfully in a number of fields and is a popular modality worldwide.

Critical analysis of the literature indicates that the majority of studies suffer from methodological flaws such as the absence of controls, variable duration and intensity of laser treatment, and poor quality. Consequently, the majority of observations are to be considered anecdotal until appropriate randomized control trials have been undertaken. In the interim, laser therapy appears to be safe and worthy of further investigation for the management of pain and other medical conditions.

SOUND

Jennifer Gehl

From ancient Greek traditions, to Chinese and Ayurvedic medicine, to sound therapy, music therapy and creative arts therapies today (see Chapter 12), there has always been an abiding belief that sound and music have the power to heal. Simultaneously, there has been a profound feeling that all life is connected and intertwined among seemingly invisible lines of energy that lie, not only within the physical body (channels, or meridians), but also within and beyond the earth into the realms of space.

Carey et al (2010) describe the vast body of knowledge comprised of archetypes, myths, mysticism, and science that informs the cosmology of an organized form of sound healing, practices as "acutonics." Drawing from Taoism and the acupuncture system, sound healing recognizes a connection between the microcosm (physical body) and the macrocosm (universe). They are not only connected to each other, but reflect many similarities and parallels between the electromagnetic fabric of the universe and the invisible lines that conduct energy in the body, known here as the 12 meridians. The meridians may act like electrical current grids that when activated via the "plug" or acupuncture point, mediate the flow of qi, blood and body fluids. In acupuncture, these currents of energy are stimulated through the process of inserting needles in a particular point or points (Mayor & Micozzi, 2011), as well as deeper reservoirs of energy known as the Eight Extraordinary Vessels (EV). As mentioned in Chapters 2 and 32, observations have been made when merely holding needles *over* the points results in effects.

The eight vessels are considered "extraordinary" because they regulate the flow of qi among the internal organs and 12 meridians when ordinary methods fail. Whereas the 12 meridians behave like electrical currents, the EV behave more like water, the conductor of electricity, thereby responding to sound much more readily (Carey & de Muynck, 2007).

Depending on overall health, the body itself is 70% water. Therefore it is an excellent resonator for sound. An interpretation of the word "person" goes back to Greek roots *per*, meaning "through," and *son*, meaning "sound," implying that to be a person means to have sound passing through us (Shipley, 1945). Many of the ancient systems that now fall under the umbrella of complementary and alternative medicine (CAM) acknowledged the healing power of sound. As early as sixth century BC, Pythagoras, who in the West is known more for his mathematics than for his "music of the spheres," recognized that vibration is subject to universal laws and mathematical proportions that represent the foundation and fabric of the universe itself (Carey et al, 2010). (The music of the spheres later held interest for leading figures, scientists, and musicians of the Enlightenment Era, who also searched for a "vital energy" [see Chapters 1 and 2]. Leading lights, from musician Wolfgang Amadeus Mozart, to scientist Alexander von Humboldt, as well as many of the Founding Fathers of the United States, spoke in terms of a divine design or plan and natural order for the conduct of human affairs, science, and the universe. These connections are explored, for example, in *The Music of the Spheres: Music, Science and the Natural Order of the Universe,* by Jamie James [New York: Copernicus/Springer Verlag, 1993].)

The concepts that all life and matter are composed of the same substances, and that energy waves, such as sound, represent a universal and unifying principle of all life, is now gaining recognition in fundamental physics with respect to string theory and the unified field of consciousness. Recent studies that have analyzed material from an interstellar comet compared it to the chemistry of DNA are finding some intriguing similarities (Carey et al, 2010).

Referring to Hippocrates (see Chapter 2 on holism), Hofman (2009) discussed the four humors as they relate to the building blocks of the cosmos: fire (fire), solids (earth), gases (air) and liquids (water). Each individual carries a signature of these humors, much like a bottle of wine retains the notes of the grapes within its content.

In Chinese medicine, each one of the internal organs is seen to fall under the properties of one of these elements, with the fifth element (wood) representing creativity and growth (as in the tree that grows). Fire feeds earth as wood burns to the ground, earth feeds metal by creating minerals, minerals nourish the water, and water nourishes wood. This can be related to the 5-element or 5-phase system seen in Chinese medicine.

Notice that this element is not present in the individual's humoral signature, and many speculate it is because the creative principle is what allows the other elements to change from one into the other, and what connects humans to divinity, which is infinitely creating. Whether an entire galaxy, planet, or a microscopic cell, everything in the universe has a vibrational energy (Kairos Institute of Sound Healing, 2011). Carey was able to apply a system of sound healing that uses precision-calibrated tuning forks to be applied in pairs on the EV points and/or on the meridian points to restore health. She brought together influences from Johannes Kepler's historic work on the laws of planetary motion, and Hans Cousto's work on transposing the *music of the spheres* from frequencies outside the range of human hearing into an octave and range the human ear can discern (Carey & De Muynck, 2007). However, it is also important to note that the body perceives and interprets vibration with more than just the ears. It is constantly receiving, interpreting, and transmitting vibration at every metabolic level such as cells, organ systems, the five sensory organs, and at the level of emotion and spirit (Carey et al, 2010).

Maciocia (1989) lists the correspondences of elements, organs and planets in Five Element Theory: Mars/fire (heart and small intestine), Saturn/Earth (stomach and spleen), Venus/metal or air (lung and large intestine), Mercury/water (kidney and urinary bladder) and Jupiter (liver and gallbladder). Fire activates energy as the heart pumps blood through the body and also enables the transformation of energy that nourishes earth. Earth breaks down the food we consume, transforming it into "food qi" for the body and nutrients that create minerals, feeding metal/air. Metal/air helps to carry away toxins in the body, either through the lung's exhalation of CO_2 or through the large intestine's elimination of waste. Metal also represents the minerals that feed and nourish our water system, hence the kidneys and urinary bladder in the body. Water (kidney and bladder) are responsible for pH balance in the body and for carrying waste away through the urinary system. Water is also the element that feeds wood (liver and gallbladder), the trees on earth and our creative natures. Wood, in turn, feeds fire, thereby starting the cycle all over again.

The planetary system is seen to fit into this concept of the flow of energy. Mars activates energy, aiding in the process of fire and transformation of qi; Saturn's boundaries represent the earthly, material world. Venus represents the magnetic qualities of metal, with an archetypal nature that wants to connect and attract. Mercury is the messenger that behaves much like a chameleon ("mercurial"), taking on the shape of its environment, which is how water and fluid behave (liquid metal). Jupiter is the planet of expansion and abundance, creating more of whatever it touches. Its schematic relationship with wood and the liver and gallbladder can be related to the liver's role in moving qi up and out everywhere, ensuring the smooth flow of energy among all the organs (Clogstoun-Willmott, 1985).

Carey et al (2010) have taken the acutonics sound healing system beyond the bounds of the ancient Chinese, with the five planetary correspondences of the ancient world, to schematically include all the currently known planetary bodies (together with their healing archetypes), namely, Neptune, Uranus, Pluto, Sedna (discovered in 2003), and more. The acutonics sound healing practitioner aims to combine the frequencies of the precision-calibrated tuning forks (seen to vibrate in harmony with the planetary frequencies) with those of the EV points. In an Acutonics session, there is simultaneously a calming, centering and grounded feeling of being utterly present in the body and the moment (like "mindfulness"), and a feeling of being safe, and aware of the body, as well as realization and expansion into subtle realms of spirit and cosmos. The individual literally becomes an instrument that resonates with his/her environment a little more each cycle: body, mind, and spirit; earth and universe. The beauty and eloquence of this system can be genuinely experienced as a reflection of the elegant order of all life as it should be: in harmony.

MAGNETISM

Human awareness of magnetism also extends back in time, with extravagant claims of "magnetic" healing traced back more than 4000 years. In more recent times, attempts to explain the efficacy of this invisible force by invoking unique and unfounded scientific principles and claims, as well as the commercial efforts to sell these products, produced an interesting history of pseudoscience, sensationalism, and controversy. Today, in the twenty-first century, despite the fact that permanent magnets and electromagnetic therapies are currently riding the crest of public enthusiasm, it is not surprising that the scientific community remains somewhat skeptical of the current widespread claims. A major obstacle has been an inability to determine a mechanism of action. In addition, fundamental questions regarding efficacy can only be resolved by rigorous, randomized, double-blind, placebo-controlled trials, which have only recently come about in the scientific community. The scientific community can now look at this subject objectively and perhaps reverse the entrenched skepticism.

Historical perspectives on magnetism and healing are provided by a number of sources (Armstrong & Armstrong, 1991; Geddes, 1991; Macklis, 1993; Markov, 2007; Mourino, 1991; Rosch, 2004; Weintraub, 2001, 2004a, 2004b), which include several excellent reviews of this rich history. According to the *Yellow Emperor's Classic* (or *Canon of Internal Medicine* (or the *Yellow Emperor's "Inner Classic"*), magnetic stones (lodestones) were applied to acupressure points as a means of pain reduction. Similarly, the ancient Hindu Vedas ascribed therapeutic powers of ashmana and siktavati (instruments of stone).

THE WORD MAGNET

The term *magnet* was probably derived from Magnes, a shepherd who, according to legend, was walking on Mount Ida when suddenly the metallic tacks in his sandals were drawn to specific rocks. These rocks were mineral lodestones that contained magnetite, a magnetic oxide of iron (Fe_3O_4). These natural magnetic stones were noted to influence other similar adjacent stones that were brought into close proximity, producing movement.

HERCULEAN STONES

The ancients called them *alive stones* or *Herculean stones* because they were meant to lead the way. Various powers were attributed to these stones as noted in the writings and artifacts of the ancient Greek and Roman civilizations. For example, Plato, Euripides, and others indicated that these invisible powers of movement could be put to practical use, such as by building ships with iron nails and destroying opposing military ships and navies by maneuvering them close to magnetic mountains or magnetic rock.

Medicinal and healing properties were also attributed to these lodestones. Various magnetic rings and necklaces were sold in the marketplace in Samothrace around AD 200 to treat arthritis and pain. Similarly, lodestones were ground up to make powders and salves to treat various conditions. Numerous claims and anecdotal stories led to the public embrace of these magical devices. In 1289, the first major treatise on magnetism was written by Peter Peregrinus. He ascribed to lodestone curative properties for treating gout, baldness, and arthritis and spoke about its strong aphrodisiac powers. He also described drawing poison from wounds with close application. His work contains the first drawing and description of a compass in the Western world.

Medieval Myths

The Middle Ages in Europe witnessed the emergence of numerous myths that persist in certain segments of society. For example, it was believed that magnets could extract gold from wells and that application or ingestion of garlic could neutralize magnetic properties. The idea that magnets could be used therapeutically resurfaced in the early sixteenth century when Paracelsus (Philippus Aureolus Theophrastus Bombastus von Hohenheim), considered to be one of the most influential physicians and alchemists of his time, used lodestones (magnets) to treat conditions such as epilepsy, diarrhea, and hemorrhage. He believed that every person is a living magnet, that they can attract good and evil, and that magnets are an important elixir of life.

Enlightenment about Magnetism

Scientific enlightenment in the seventeenth century on this topic began with the work of Dr. William Gilbert, physician to Queen Elizabeth I of England. He wrote his classic text *De Magnete* in 1600 describing hundreds of detailed experiments concerning electricity and also terrestrial magnetism. He debunked many medicinal applications and was responsible for laying the groundwork for future research and study. Despite the fact that Luigi Galvani and Alessandro Volta made significant contributions, for the next 100 years there were no major advancements in the study of magnetism.

In the early eighteenth century, there was significant interest in both magnetism and electricity. Francis Hauksbee, in 1705, invented an electrostatic engine that, by rotating and spinning an attached globe, could transfer an electronic charge to various metallic objects brought close to it, such as chain, wire, and metal. This procedure induced electrical shocks. Refinements in this machine led to more general usage, and in 1743, traveling circuses throughout Europe and the American colonies provided individuals with shocks for a small fee.

Benjamin Franklin Again

Legend suggests that Benjamin Franklin witnessed an "electrified boy" exhibition in a traveling circus in the mid-1700s, and thus first became interested in his life-long experiments on both electricity and magnetic phenomena. Franklin is also famed for his later experiments on electricity, by capturing lightning, in which he attached a key to an airborne kite during a thunderstorm (as depicted in the heroic portrait by Benjamin West known as *Benjamin Franklin Drawing Electricity from the Sky*) (see Figure 2-1, p. 14). In fact, it was actually Franklin's young son who he sent out into the lightning storm with the kite, risking the exhibition of Franklin's own version of his own "electrified boy." (It appears Franklin did not like his son. Later, when the son was serving as British Colonial Governor of New Jersey during the Revolutionary War, the father had him arrested and jailed.)

Much of the current magnetic terminology regarding electricity originated with Franklin, such as charge, discharge, condenser, electric shock, electrician, positive, negative, plus and minus, and so on. Franklin distinguished himself in studies primarily of electric "fluid" and charges, and concluded that all matter contained magnetic fields that are uniformly distributed throughout the body. He believed that when an object is magnetized, the fluid condenses in one of its extremities. That extremity becomes positively magnetized, whereas the donor region of the object becomes negatively magnetized. He thought that the degree to which an object can be magnetized depends on the force necessary to start the fluid moving within it.

Back to Europe

The scientific revolution brought to Europe the development of carbon-steel magnets (1743 to 1751). Father Maximilian Hell and, later, his student, Franz Anton Mesmer, applied these magnetic devices to patients, many of whom were experiencing hysterical or psychosomatic symptoms (see Chapters 6 and 9). In his major treatise, "On the Medicinal Uses of the Magnet," Mesmer described how he fed a patient iron filings and then applied specially designed magnets over the vital organs to generally stop uncontrolled seizures. His cures were not only astounding but also good theater, because they were performed in front of large groups (see Chapter 10).

It was the "power of suggestion" that was clearly being displayed as it was ultimately transferred to nonferric objects such as paper, wood, silk, and stone. Mesmer reasoned that he was not dealing with ordinary mineral magnetism but rather with a special *animal magnetism*. The term *mesmerization* is often applied to his displays of people overcoming illness and disease by *mesmerizing* their bodies' innate magnetic poles to induce a crisis, often in the form of convulsions. After this crisis, health would be restored. Mesmer hailed this animal magnetism as a specific natural force of healing. Later, during the nineteenth century, such approaches would be referred to as "magnetic healing," or "mesmeric healing (see Section IV).

REVOLUTIONARY DEVELOPMENTS

Mesmer's claims of success infuriated his conservative colleagues and motivated the French Academy of Sciences under King Louis XVI to convene a special study in 1784. The panel for this study included such distinguished figures Antoine-Laurent Lavoisier, Joseph-Ignace Guillotin, and Benjamin Franklin (again), ambassador to France from the newly independent United States of America. In a controlled set of experiments, blindfolded patients were to be exposed to a series of magnets or sham magnetic objects and asked to describe the induced sensation. Although there remains controversy as to whether and what experimental observations were actually made, the committee "lost their heads" (a process that was soon to be facilitated in reality by the invention of one of their members, Dr. Guillotin, in the coming French Revolution) in bickering about mechanisms of action.

The royal panel concluded that the efficacy of the magnetic healing resided entirely within the mind of the individual and that any healing was due to suggestion. Based on these conclusions, the medical establishment declared Mesmer's theories fraudulent, and mesmerism was equated with medical quackery. Mesmer left France in disgrace. Some members of the panel who remained in France, such as Lavoisier, literally lost their heads.

In Europe, Hans Christian Ørsted (1777–1851), a physicist, continued studies and noted that a compass needle was deflected when a current flowed through a nearby wire. He also discovered that a current-carrying wire coil exerts a force on a magnet, and a magnet exerts a force on the coil of wire, inducing an electrical current. The coil behaves like a magnet, as if it possessed magnetic north and south poles. Magnetism and electricity were somehow connected.

AMPING UP RESEARCH

Ørsted was instrumental in creating a proper scientific environment that led to further study, with André-Marie Ampère, deducing the quantitative relation between magnetic force and electric current. In the 1820s, Michael Faraday and Joseph Henry (later founding secretary of the Smithsonian Institution in the 1850s) demonstrated more connections between magnetism and electricity, showing that a changing magnetic field could induce an electrical field perpendicularly.

In 1896, Arsène D'Arsonval reported to the Société de Biologie in Paris that when a subject's head was placed in a strong time-varying magnetic field, phosphenes (sensations of light caused by retinal stimulation) were perceived. Some 15 years later, Silvanus P. Thompson (1910) confirmed that not only could phosphenes be induced, but that exposure to a strong alternating magnetic field also produced taste sensation. Various coils were constructed by Dunlap and later Magnusson and Stevens. They noted that magnetophosphenes were brightest at a low frequency of about 25 Hz and became fainter at higher frequencies.

MAGNETIC HEALING IN THE UNITED STATES

Meanwhile, in the United States magnetic therapy flourished, with significant sales of magnets, magnetic salves, and liniments by traveling magnetic healers. Later in the nineteenth century Daniel David Palmer, the founder of chiropractic and self-described "magnetic healer," stated that putting down his hands for physical manipulation of the patient produced better results than the simple "laying on of hands" (see Chapter 19).

By 1886, the Sears catalogue advertised numerous magnetic products such as magnetic rings, belts, caps, soles for boots, and girdles. In the 1920s, Thacher created a mail-order catalogue advertising over 700 specific magnetic garments and devices and products that he described as a "plain road to health without the use of medicine and was dependent on the magnetic energy of the sun." He believed that the iron content of the blood made it the primary magnetic conductor of the body, and thus the most efficient way to *recharge* the body's magnetic field was by wearing his magnetic garments. The complete set was said to "furnish full and complete protection of all the vital organs of the body." *Collier's Weekly* dubbed Thacher the "king of the magnetic quacks." There was no government regulation of these devices or claims, and thus these types of promotion fueled skepticism. The U.S. Food and Drug Administration (FDA) had no jurisdiction over medical devices at that time, and there were no good scientific trials, although problems with the purity of drugs had led to the passage of the Pure Food and Drug Act of 1906 and the subsequent formation of the FDA.

POST-WW II RESEARCH WORLDWIDE

After World War II, there was heightened interest and research in magnetotherapy in Japan and the former Soviet Union. Specifically, in Japan magnetotherapeutic devices were accepted under the Drug Regulation Act of 1961, and by 1976, various devices were commonly and commercially employed to treat various illnesses and promote health. Similar interest in Bulgaria, Romania, and Russia led to development of various therapeutic approaches, so that the physician had available the use of magnetic fields to assist in treating disease. Today, Germany, Japan, Russia, Israel, and at least 45 other countries consider magnetic therapy to be an accepted medical procedure for the treatment of various neurological and inflammatory conditions (Whitaker & Adderly, 1998). By contrast, magnetotherapy had limited acceptance in Western medicine. Unwarranted claims and its promotion by charlatans only led to further public and scientific skepticism.

MODERN MEDICAL MAGNETISM

The modern era of magnetic stimulation began with the work of R.G. Bickford and colleagues (Bickford &

Fremming, 1965) who considered the possibility of stimulation of the nervous system (frog nerve and human peripheral nerves). He also discussed the generation of eddy currents in the brain that could reach a certain magnitude to stimulate cortical structures through an intact cranium (Bickford & Fremming, 1965). Barker and colleagues at the University of Sheffield developed the first commercial cranial magnetic stimulator in 1985 (Barker, 1991; Barker et al, 1987). They gave a practical demonstration at Queen's Square by stimulating "Dr. Merton's brain," which caused muscle twitches. As might be expected, the physiological and clinical possibilities became obvious (Merton, 1980). Although there were technical challenges, they were met with the development of devices capable of stimulating the brain focally at frequencies of up to 100 Hz using specific coil configurations (i.e., circular). Adaptations for focal therapy were created. Thus, a new discipline developed using high and low repetitive stimulation frequencies directed to previously inaccessible areas of the brain and body (George et al, 2003; Kobayashi & Pascual-Leone, 2003; Pascual-Leone et al, 1994). By the end of the twentieth century, over 6000 publications existed that dealt with basic neurophysiology, clinical syndromes, and therapeutic implications. Although most of the initial papers were the results of open-label (nonplacebo) observations, many current publications report on randomized, double-blind, placebo-controlled trials. Thus, when all of this information is pooled, both experimental and clinical, the data strongly suggest that the application of exogenous magnetic fields at low levels does indeed induce a biological effect on a variety of systems, especially pain sensation and the musculoskeletal system.

TERMINOLOGY AND PRINCIPLES

Essential terms must be defined to understand the role of magnetism. *Biomagnetics* refers to the field of science dealing with the application of magnetic fields to living organisms. Basic research on cells in culture as well as clinical trials have provided a better understanding of mechanisms of action (Adey, 1992, 2004; Lednev, 1991; Markov, 2004; Markov & Colbert, 2001; Pilla, 2003; Pilla et al, 1997; Timmel et al, 1998). Human tissues are dielectric and conductive and therefore can respond to electrical and magnetic fields that are oscillating or static. Cell membranes consist of paramagnetic and diamagnetic lipoprotein materials that respond to magnetic fields and serve as signaling (transduction) pathways by which external stimuli are sent and conveyed to the cell interior. Calcium ions are very important in transduction coupling at the cell membrane level. Electromagnetic fields can also alter the configuration of atoms and molecules in dielectric and paramagnetic-diamagnetic substances. Thus atoms in these substances polarize, to some degree, when placed in an electromagnetic field and act as a dipole and align accordingly (Adey, 1988, 1992; Blumenthal et al, 1997; DeLoecker et al, 1990; Engstrom & Fitzsimmons, 1999; Farndale et al, 1987; Lednev, 1991; Maccabee et al, 1991;

Pilla et al, 1997; Repacholi & Greenebaum, 1999; Rosen, 1992; Rossini et al, 1994; Timmel et al, 1998). Adey thinks that free radicals are important for signal transduction.

THE CHEMISTRY OF MAGNETISM

Chemical bonds are essentially electromagnetic bonds formed between adjacent atoms. The breaking of the chemical bonds of a singlet pair allows electrons to influence adjacent electrons with similar or opposite spins, which thereby become triplet pairs, and so on. Thus, by imposing magnetic fields in this medium, one may influence the rate and amount of communication between cells. At the cell membrane level, free radicals of nitric oxide may play an essential role in this regulation of receptors specifically (Adey, 1988, 1992, 2004). It is known that free radicals are involved in the normal regulatory mechanisms in many tissues and that certain disorders are associated with disordered free radical regulation producing oxidative stress. These include Alzheimer disease, Parkinson disease, cancer, and coronary artery disease. This entire area is still incompletely understood yet under intense research scrutiny.

MAGNETIC FIELDS

Magnetic field strength is indicated by magnetic flux density, which is the number of field lines (flux) that cross a unit of surface area. It is usually described in terms of the unit gauss (G) or tesla (T). There are 10,000 G in 1 T. Because there is an exponential decay of field strength with distance from a magnetic source according the inverse square law, the objective is to apply a static magnetic device as close to the skin as possible and to ensure that a magnet of sufficient size and surface field is used when the target is in deep tissue areas. *Magnetotherapy* is defined as the use of time-varying magnetic fields of low-frequency values (3 Hz to 3 KHz) to induce a sufficiently strong current to stimulate living tissue.

Faraday's law (1831) defines the fundamental relationship between a changing magnetic field and a conductor (any medium that carries electrically charged particles). When a wire is used as an example of a conductor, Faraday's law basically states that any change in the magnetic environment of the coil of wire with time will cause a voltage to be induced in the wire. No matter how the change is produced, a voltage will be generated. Thus, magnetic field amplitude may be varied by powering the electromagnet with sinusoidal or pulsing current or by moving a permanent magnet toward or away from the wire, moving the wire toward or away from the magnetic field, rotating the wire relative to the magnet, and so on (DeLoecker et al, 1990; Goodman & Blank, 2002; Serway, 1998; Smith, 1996; Wittig & Engstrom, 2002).

Lenz's law states that the polarity of the voltage induced according to Faraday's law is such that it produces a current whose magnetic field opposes the applied magnetic field (back EMF, or electromagnetic field). Therefore, if a current is passed through a coil that creates an expanding magnetic field around the coil, the induced voltage and associated current flow produce a magnetic field in opposition to the directly induced magnetic field.

Eddy currents are induced by the voltage generated according to Faraday's law in any conducting medium. When the conducting medium does not contain defined current pathways, there is no induced current, only induced voltage. There is movement in a spiral, swirling fashion, and this in turn potentially penetrates the membranes of the neurons. If the induced current is of sufficient amplitude, an action potential or an excitatory or inhibitory postsynaptic potential may be produced.

The Hall effect and the Lorentz force are related to the same physical phenomenon of electromagnetism. In the Hall effect, when charged particles in a conductor move along a path that is transverse to a magnetic field, the particles experience a force that pushes them toward the outer walls of the conductor. The positively charged particles move to one side and the negatively charged particles move to the other side. This produces a voltage across the conductor known as the "Hall voltage." Because the human body is replete with charged ions, the Hall effect would certainly occur to varying degrees when a magnetic field is passed through the body. The strength of the Hall voltage produced depends on three factors: (1) the strength of the magnetic field; (2) the number of charged particles moving transverse to the magnetic field; and (3) the velocity of movement of the charged particles (ions). The pulsing and static magnetic fields in current therapeutic applications are much too weak and the endogenous currents much too small for the Hall effect to be of any significance in magnetic field bioeffects (Pilla et al, 1992, 1993). However, this is somewhat controversial and not universally accepted. Clearly, cellular and neural components in the body provide conductive pathways for ions, so it is reasonable to assume that these components would be prime objects of attention in attempting to observe the Hall effect. It is presumed that this voltage might add to the nerve's resting potential of −70 mV and make it harder to depolarize. Once the resting potential rises from its normal undisturbed voltage of about −70 mV to a voltage of approximately −55 mV (threshold potential), an action potential spike is initiated. When ions move under the influence of a voltage, they become an electric current the magnitude of which is determined by Ohm's law, which states that electric current equals voltage divided by resistance.

This phenomenon predicts the effects of ions exposed to a combination of exogenous AC/DC magnetic fields at approximately 0.1 G and the dynamics of ions in a binding site. A bound ion in a static magnetic field will precess at the Larmour frequency and will accelerate faster to preferred orientations in the binding site with increased magnetic field strength. Thus, an increased binding rate can occur with a resultant acceleration in the downstream biochemical cascade.

Magnetic fields can penetrate all tissues, including epidermis, dermis, and subcutaneous tissue as well as tendons, muscles, and even bone. The specific amount of magnetic energy and its effect at the target organ depends on the size, strength, and duration of contact of the device. Magnetic fields fall into two broad categories: (1) *static* (DC) and (2) *time varying* (AC).

The strength of *static magnetic* devices varies from 1 to 4000 G. Static fields have zero frequency, because the polarity and field strength do not change with time but rather remain constant. Permanent magnets produce only static fields unless they are rotated or otherwise moved, which causes the magnetic field amplitude to change with time at the tissue target. Static magnetic fields that are either permanent or electromagnetic are in the range of 1 to 4000 G and have been reported to have significant biological effects (Colbert, 2004; Markov & Colbert, 2001; Pilla, 2003; Pilla & Muehsam, 2003). The most common static magnets sold to the public are known as refrigerator or flat-button magnets. They are made of various materials and also have different designs. Configuration can be unidirectional so that only one magnetic pole is represented on one side of the surface (whereas the opposite pole is on the opposite side away from the applied surface) or the surface can have a bipolar north–south design that appears repetitively as concentric ring, multitriangular, or quadripolar configurations.

The term *bipolar magnets* refers to a repetitive north–south polarity created on the same side of a ceramic or plastic alloy or neodymium material, whereas the term *unipolar* refers to only one magnetic pole at a given surface, that is, north or south. Multipolar alterations of north and south have also been employed. Each specific manufacturer makes claims as to the superiority of its product. However, the most important characteristic of the magnetic field is the field strength at the target site and also the duration of exposure that leads to biological effects. It is thought that tissues, cells, and other structures have a "biological window" within which they can interact with these invisible fields. Static magnetic fields of 5 to 20 G have been felt to be pertinent. Thus, the gauss rating and field strength at the surface are irrelevant in predicting biological response. Bipolar magnets, using a small arc, are capable of inducing biologically significant fields at a relatively short distance from the surface (1 to 1.5 cm), whereas the penetration of unipolar magnets is much deeper (4 to 8 cm) (Markov, 2007).

BIOLOGIC EFFECTS AND PAIN

As indicated earlier, review of the literature reveals that static magnetic fields in the 1 to 4000 G range have been reported to have significant biological effect. Basic science has demonstrated that static magnetic fields ranging from 23 to 3000 G can alter the electrical properties of solutions. In addition, weak static magnetic fields can modulate myosin phosphorylation at the molecular level in a cell-free preparation (Markov & Pilla, 1997). At a cellular level, exposure to 300 G doubled alkaline phosphatase activity in osteoblast-like cells (McDonald, 1993). Neurite outgrowth from embryonic chick ganglia was significantly increased by exposure to 225 to 900 G (Macias et al, 2000; Sisken et al, 1993). McLean et al (1995), in several experiments using unidirectional and multipolar magnets, demonstrated a blockade of sensory nociceptive neuron action potentials by exposure to a static magnetic field in the 10 mT range. A minimum magnetic field gradient of 15 G/mm was required to cause approximately 80% action potential blockade in isolated nerve preparations (McLean et al, 1995). This blockade reversed when the magnetic exposure was removed. Protection against kainic acid–induced neuronal swelling was also demonstrated with magnetic exposure (McLean et al, 2003). Others have demonstrated a biphasic response of the acute microcirculation in rabbits exposed to static magnetic fields (10 G) (Ohkubo & Xu, 1997; Okano et al, 1999). Despite all this provocative and promising data in both in vitro and in vivo studies, skepticism prevails because of design flaws (Holcomb et al, 2002; Ramey, 1998). Specifically, a rigorous randomized, placebo-controlled, double-blind design has been lacking; basic mechanisms of action have not been identified; and optimum target dosage and optimum polarity have yet to be determined. The absence of nonmagnetic placebos as controls has also been described as a problem.

Colbert (2004) reviewed 22 therapeutic trials reported in the U.S. literature from 1982 to 2002. Clinical improvement in subjects who wore permanent magnets on various parts of their bodies was demonstrated in 15 studies, whereas 7 reported limited or no benefit. Magnetic field strength varied from 68 to 2000 G and time exposure varied from 45 minutes to constant wearing for 4 months. Thus the optimum treatment duration, as well as the optimal polarity (unidirectional, multipolar, etc.), has yet to be established. Complicating the issue even further is the observation by Blechman et al (2001) that a significant number of the static magnets sold to the public had lower field flux density measurements than the manufacturers claimed. It is known that a large amount of cancellation occurs in multipolar arrays. Similarly, Eccles (2005) conducted a critical review of the randomized controlled trials that used static magnets for pain relief. He found a 73% statistical reduction in pain. He also commented on the difficulty in performing double-blind studies using static magnets because of the obvious interaction with metallic objects.

Specific clinical trials using a double-blind, placebo-controlled design include that of Vallbona et al (1997), who applied 300- to 500-G concentric-circle bipolar magnets over painful joints in patients with postpolio syndrome for 45 minutes and reduced pain by 76%. Carter et al (2002) applied unipolar 1000-G static magnets and placebos over the carpal tunnel for 45 minutes and both groups experienced significant pain reduction. This was felt to represent a placebo effect. Unidirectional magnetic pads (150 to 400 G) were placed over liposuction sites immediately after the procedure and kept in place for 14 days; this treatment produced a 40% to 70% reduction of pain, edema, and discoloration (Man et al, 1999). Brown et al (2002) demonstrated statistical reduction of pelvic pain with magnetic therapy. Patients with fibromyalgia who slept on a unidirectional magnetic mattress pad (800-G ceramic magnets) for 4 months experienced a 40% improvement (Colbert et al, 1999). Weintraub (1999) noted a 90% reduction in neuropathic pain in patients with diabetic peripheral neuropathy with constant wearing of multipolar 475-G insole devices. There was also a 30% reduction in neuropathic pain associated with nondiabetic peripheral neuropathy (Man et al, 1999; Weintraub, 1999). A nationwide study using placebo controls also confirmed these results in 275 patients with diabetic peripheral neuropathy (Weintraub et al, 2003).

Hinman et al (2002) found a 30% response to short-term application of unipolar static magnets positioned over painful knees. Greater movement was also noted. Holcomb et al (2002), using a quadripolar array of static magnets with alternating polarity, demonstrated analgesic benefit in patients with low back pain and knee pain.

Saygili et al (1992), in an investigation of the effect of magnetic retention systems in dental prostheses on buccal mucosal blood flow, failed to detect changes in capillary blood flow after continuous exposure to a magnetic field for 45 days. Hong et al (1982) had 101 patients with chronic neck and shoulder pain wear magnetic necklaces or placebos for 3 consecutive weeks after baseline electrodiagnostic studies, but no significant improvement was seen in the magnetic therapy group. In a study using a randomized placebo crossover design, Martel et al (2002) could not identify any change in forearm blood flow after 30 minutes of exposure to bipolar magnets. Other randomized placebo-controlled trials producing negative results should be mentioned, including the use of bipolar devices in patients with chronic low back pain (Collacott et al, 2000) and the use of magnetic insoles by patients with plantar fasciitis (Winemiller et al, 2003). Weintraub and others commented on design flaws in both of these studies (Weintraub, 2000, 2004a, 2004b). Simultaneous application of static magnets to the back and feet in patient with failed back syndrome was also ineffective (Weintraub et al, 2005). Pilla (2003) independently assessed the strength of the magnetic devices and found them to be less than the manufacturer's claims, thereby confirming the observations of Blechman et al (2001) regarding the discrepancy between claimed and measured field flux densities.

It is assumed that the biological benefits from static magnetic fields are similar to those from pulsed electromagnetic fields, but the correlation has been imperfect. The specific mechanism of biological benefit remains to be determined. At present, the most generally accepted theory is that static magnetic fields on the order of 1 to 10 G can affect ion-ligand binding, producing modulation (Pilla, 2003; Pilla & Muehsam, 2003; Pilla et al, 1997). There may also be physical realignment and translational movement of diamagnetically anisotropic molecules. Despite these theoretical and scientific rationales for benefit, the criticisms and skepticism prevail. Critics allege that it is all placebo effects, yet a more enlightened and open-minded appraisal would accept the positive in vitro and in vivo observations. Ramey (1998), a veterinarian, has been a noted critic of static magnetic therapy, yet these devices are used extensively in veterinary medicine (e.g., magnetic blankets for race horses).

The World Health Organization has stated that there are no adverse effects on human health from exposure to static magnetic fields, even up to 2 T, which equals 20,000 G (United Nations Environment Programme MF, 1987). Similarly, in 2003 the FDA extended nonsignificant risk status to magnetic resonance imaging (MRI) using flux densities of up to 8 T (U.S. Food and Drug Administration, 2003).

PULSED ELECTROMAGNETIC FIELDS

The generation of pulsed electromagnetic fields (PEMFs) require an electric current to produce a pulsating (time-varying) magnetic field. This is because the coil that produces the magnetic field is stationary. Regardless of how the waveforms are transmitted through the coil, the ensuing magnetic flux lines appear in space in exactly the same manner as the flux lines from a permanent magnet. The magnetic field penetrates biological tissues without modification, and the induced electrical fields are produced at right angles to the flux lines. The ensuing current flow is determined by the tissue's electrical properties (impedance) and determines the final spacial dosimetry. Peak magnetic fields from PEMF devices are typically 5 to 30 G at the target tissue with varying specific shapes and amplitudes of fields.

Cellular studies (in vitro, in vivo) have been most provocative. In reviewing this work, Markov has summarized various cellular and structural changes in response to this PEMF exposure (Markov, 2004; Markov & Colbert, 2001). Specifically, changes in fibrinogen, fibroblasts, leukocytes, platelets, fibrin, cytokines, collagen, elastin, keratinocytes, osteoblasts, and free radicals are noted. In addition, magnetic fields influence vasoconstriction, vasodilatation, phagocytosis, cell proliferation, epithelialization, and scar formation.

Bone Repair

Similarly, in a series of reviews, Pilla has summarized the effects of these weak PEMFs on both signal transduction and growth factor synthesis as it relates to fractures (Pilla, 2003; Pilla & Muehsam, 2003; Pilla et al, 1992, 1993). He noted that there is upregulation of growth factor production, calcium ion transport, self-proliferation, insulin-like growth factor II release, and insulin-like growth factor II receptor expression in osteoblasts as a mechanism for bone repair. He also cited an increase in both transforming growth factor-β1 messenger RNA and protein in osteoblast cultures, producing an effect on a calcium/calmodulin-dependent pathway. Other studies with chondrocytes confirm similar increases in transforming growth factor-β1 messenger RNA and protein synthesis with PEMF exposure, which suggests a therapeutic application for joint

repair (Ciombor et al, 2002; Pilla et al, 1996). PEMFs have also been successfully applied to stimulate nerve regeneration. Neurite outgrowth has been demonstrated in cell cultures exposed to electromagnetic fields. Eddy currents are generated that can depolarize, hyperpolarize, and repolarize nerve cells, which suggests that neuromodulation potentially can arise.

In 1979, the FDA approved the use of PEMF as a means of stimulating and recruiting osteoblast cells at a fracture site. Application of coils around the cast induces current flows through the fracture site, producing 80% success. It became apparent after early testing that intermittent exposure, rather continuous exposure, was the optimal technique. Currently, there are four FDA-approved devices for treatment of non-union fractures, and each has specific signal parameters, treatment time, and so on. It is not yet clear how long PEMF exposure must last to trigger a bioelectrical effect. Effective waveforms tend to be asymmetric, biphasic, and quasi-rectangular or quasi-triangular in shape. This indicates that tissues have various windows of vulnerability and susceptibility to PEMF. Based on the high success rate of PEMF therapy, it is currently considered part of the standard armamentarium of orthopedic spine surgeons and is recommended as an adjunct to standard fracture management. In addition, the results are equivalent to those of surgical repair with minimal risk, and the treatment is more cost effective.

PEMF therapy has also been used to treat other orthopedic conditions as well as painful musculoskeletal disorders. These include aseptic necrosis of the hips, osteoporosis, osteoarthritis, osteogenesis imperfecta, rotator cuff dysfunction, and low back pain (Aaron et al, 1989; Binder et al, 1984; Fukada & Yasuda, 1957; Jacobson et al, 2001; Linovitz et al, 2000; Mooney, 1990; Pipitone & Scott, 2001; Pujol et al, 1998; Wilson & Jagadeesh, 1974; Zdeblic, 1993). In his reviews, Markov (2004, 2007; Markov & Colbert, 2001), stated that with the exception of periarthritis, for which no difference was reported between treatment and control groups, reduced pain scores were noted in carpal tunnel pain (93%) (Battisti et al, 1998) and rotator cuff tendinitis (83%) (Binder et al, 1984), and 70% of multiple sclerosis patients had reduced spasticity (Lappin et al, 2003). Pilla reports double-blind studies claiming benefit for chronic wound repair (Battisti et al, 1998; Kloth et al, 1999; Mayrovitz & Larsen, 1995; Todd et al, 1991), acute ankle sprain (Ciombor et al, 2002; Pilla et al, 1996), and acute whiplash injuries (Foley-Nolan et al, 1990, 1992).

Pain Relief

Pujol et al (1998) targeted musculoskeletal pain using magnetic coils, which produced a benefit compared with placebo. Weintraub and Cole (2004) applied nine consecutive 1-hour treatments to patients with peripheral neuropathy, which induced a greater than 50% reduction in neuropathic pain. This was an open-label, nonplacebo trial.

Pickering et al (2003) demonstrated that gentamicin's effect against *Staphylococcus epidermidis* could be augmented by exposure to a PEMF. In other research with a double-blind, placebo-controlled design, use of pulsed high-frequency (27-MHz) electromagnetic therapy to treat persistent neck pain produced significant improvement by the second week of therapy (Foley-Nolan et al, 1990, 1992).

In 1983, Raji and Bowden applied 27-MHz pulsed electromagnetic therapy to the transected common peroneal nerve of rats; 15 minutes of treatment daily produced accelerated healing with reduced scar tissue, increased growth of blood vessels, and maturation of myelin (Fukada & Yasuda, 1957).

Mechanism of action

Despite all the convincing data, the use of PEMF therapy does not enjoy universal acceptance. In addition, the large number of different commercially available PEMF devices, which generate low-frequency fields of different shapes and amplitudes, are a major variable in attempting to understand and analyze the putative biological clinical effects. It has been speculated that the target area receives 5 to 30 G and that each tissue has its own biophysical window and specific encoding susceptibility (Pilla & Muehsam, 2003).

Despite all these provocative data, there is considerable uncertainty about the specific mechanisms involved as well as the optimal approach in terms of frequency, amplitude, and duration of exposure. Of course, this issue may be moot based on available data, because several different devices generating different frequencies and amplitudes and used for different durations have been successful in producing similar nonunion fracture healing. In addition, there is an abundance of experimental and clinical data demonstrating that extremely low frequency and static magnetic fields can have a profound effect on a large variety of biological systems, organisms, and tissues as well as cellular and subcellular structures. It is assumed that the target is the cell membrane with ion and ligand binding and that even small changes in transmembrane voltage can induce a significant modulation of cellular function. In a recent review, Pilla (2003) attempted to provide a unifying approach for static and pulsating magnetic fields, as well as weak ultrasound, which also induces electrical fields comparable to those associated with PEMFs. Pilla has also employed pulsed (nonthermal) radiofrequency fields at 27.12 Hz and has achieved soft tissue healing, reduction of edema, and postoperative pain relief. Pulsed radiofrequency therapy has recently been approved by the FDA (Mayrovitz & Larsen, 1995).

A novel device has now been developed with time-varying, biaxial rotation that generates simultaneous static (DC) and oscillating (AC) fields. The fields are constantly changing and thus produce variable exposure to tissues and varying amplitudes at the target tissue. Weintraub and coworkers have recently found this type of therapy to be effective in reducing neuropathic pain from diabetic peripheral neuropathy and carpal tunnel syndrome (Weintraub & Cole, 2007a, 2007b).

TRANSCRANIAL MAGNETIC STIMULATION

Transcranial magnetic stimulation (TMS) is a specific adaptation of PEMF that creates a time-varying magnetic field over the surface of the head and depolarizes underlying superficial neurons, which induce electrical currents in the brain. High-intensity current is rapidly turned on and off in the electromagnetic coil through the discharge of capacitors. Thus, brief (microseconds) and powerful magnetic fields are produced, which in turn induce current in the brain. Two magnetic stimuli delivered in close sequence to the same cortical region through a single stimulating coil are used. The first is a conditioning stimulus at submotor threshold intensity that influences the intracortical neurons and exerts a significant modulating effect on the amplitude of the motor evoked potential induced by the second, supramotor threshold stimulus. This modulating effect depends on the interval between the stimuli. Cortical inhibition consistently occurs at intervals between 1 and 5 ms, and facilitation is seen at intervals between 10 and 20 ms. TMS is simple to perform, inexpensive, generally safe, and provides useful measures of neuronal excitability. It has also been used along the neuraxis and continues to provide important insights into basic neurological functions, neurophysiology, and neurobiology. Although TMS is generally used as a research tool, it has been proposed that the therapeutic use of TMS be considered. The abnormalities that are revealed by TMS are not disease specific and need clinical correlation. Initially, stimulation directed to the primary motor cortex in individuals with a number of movement disorders helped investigators appreciate the role of the basal ganglia.

Neurological Disorders and Procedures

Specific TMS studies looked at Parkinson disease, dystonia, Huntington chorea, essential tremor, Tourette syndrome, myoclonus, restless legs syndrome, progressive supranuclear palsy, Wilson disease, stiff-person syndrome, and Rett syndrome, among others. The results were promising, which suggests that future large multicenter trials are warranted.

TMS has also proved useful in investigating the mechanisms of epilepsy, and repetitive TMS may prove to have a therapeutic role in the future (Osenbach, 2006).

TMS also is used in preoperative assessment of specific brain areas to optimize the surgical procedure. Both inhibitory and facilitatory interactions in the cortex can be studied by combining a subthreshold conditioning stimulus with a suprathreshold test stimulus at different short (1 to 20 ms) intervals through the same coil. In addition, this paired-pulse TMS approach is used to investigate potential central nervous system–activating drugs, various neurological and psychological diseases, and so on. Left and right hemispheres often react differently (Cahn & Herzog, 2003). The clinical utility of this aspect has not yet been demonstrated. If TMS pulses are delivered repetitively and rhythmically, the process is called "repetitive TMS" (rTMS) and can be modified further to induce excitatory or inhibitory effects. In rare cases seizures may be provoked in epileptic patients as well as in normal volunteers (Abbruzzese & Trompetto, 2002; Amassian et al, 1989; Cantello, 2002; Chae et al, in press; George et al, 1999; Kobayashi & Pascual-Leone, 2003; Lisamby et al, 2001; Pascual-Leone et al, 2002; Rollnik et al, 2002; Terao & Ugawa, 2002; Theodore, 2003; Wasserman, 1998; Walsh & Rushworth, 1999).

Repetitive TMS (rTMS) leads to modulation of cortical excitability. For example, high-frequency rTMS of the dominant hemisphere, but not the nondominant hemisphere, can induce speech arrest (Orpin, 1982). This effect also correlates with results of the Wada test. The higher the stimulation frequency, the greater the disruption of cortical function. Lower frequencies of rTMS in a 1-Hz range can suppress excitability of the motor cortex, whereas 20-Hz stimulation trains lead to a temporary increase in cortical excitability. Pascual-Leone and coworkers have been studying these effects in patients with neurological disorders such as Parkinson disease, dystonia, epilepsy, and stroke. Osenbach (2006) provides a comprehensive review of the use of motor cortex stimulation (MCS) to manage intractable pain, concluding "there is little doubt that MCS provides excellent relief in carefully selected patients with a variety of neuropathic pain but leaves many unanswered questions." Tinnitus has been recalcitrant to many therapies, but there has been increasing use of magnetic and electrical stimulation of the auditory cortex with benefit (DeRidder et al, 2004; Whitaker & Adderly, 1998). Psychiatric conditions, including anxiety, mania, depression, and schizophrenia, are also being treated with TMS (George et al, 1999, 2003, 2004). These early observations and data suggest a rich potential therapeutic utility heretofore not known. Elucidation of the underlying neurobiology is still a work in progress in various neuropsychiatric syndromes. Creating sham TMS is difficult, and there is some evidence to suggest that tilting of the coils produces some biological effect on the brain with (George et al, 2004).

Side Effects

A controversial and legitimate concern relates to the possibility that exposure of living tissue to an electromagnetic field may play a causative role in malignancy and birth defects. Specifically, this concern has been raised because of the foci of childhood leukemia cases reported adjacent to high-power lines. During a 5-year period (1991 to 1996), Congress appropriated $60 million for dedicated research to look for such a causal association. The result was that no significant risk from power line frequencies could be confirmed and the fears did not appear justified. *No funding* was made available to explore and expand the beneficial effects of magnetics and electromagnetic fields! The facts are that there is now a 30-year experience with and history of the approved use of PEMF in promoting repair of recalcitrant fractures with not one adverse effect reported. Similarly, static magnetic fields have been employed for

therapeutic uses for centuries, and no adverse effects have been reported.

The FDA has received a number of reports and complaints through its Medical Device Reporting system concerning electromagnetic field interference with a variety of medical devices, such as pacemakers and defibrillators. In addition, the development of advanced magnetic resonance technology using ultra-high magnetic field systems of more than 3 T, although they were considered safe, led to a reassessment of biomedical implant devices, which were previously judged to be safe to use at 1.5 T. Of the 109 implants and devices tested, 4% were considered to have a magnetic field interaction at 3 T and were potentially unsafe to use with fields of this magnitude (Shellock, 2002). Because of potential concerns regarding radiofrequency-induced magnetic fields with thermal effects at the cellular and molecular levels, the FDA has limited switching rates for generation of these gradient fields to a factor of three below the mean threshold of peripheral nerve stimulation (Shellock & Crues, 2004). Recently, Weintraub et al (2007) looked at the biological effects of 3-T MRI machines compared with 1.5-T and 0.6-T machines and found that 14% of subjects experienced sensory symptoms (new or altered) with both the 3-T and 1.5-T systems.

PROFESSIONALIZATION

The study of magnetic fields (static and pulsed) has evolved from a medical curiosity into investigation of significant and specific medical applications.

There are at least five major professional and scientific societies involved in the study of the biological and clinical effects of electromagnetic fields (Markov & Colbert, 2001): (1) the Bioelectromagnetics Society (BEMS); (2) the European Bioelectromagnetics Association (EBEA); (3) the Bioelectrochemical Society (BES); (4) the Society for Physical Regulation in Biology and Medicine (SPRBM); and (5) Engineering in Medicine and Biology (IEMB).

That PEMF and TMS can influence biological functions and serve as a therapeutic intervention is not in dispute. However, judging the efficacy of static magnets for treatment of various clinical conditions remains challenging, particularly because the important dosimetry component has not been documented. The ultimate question is what it will take to convince the scientific community of the merits of static magnetotherapy. Although the debate continues, more attention must be focused on creating strong randomized, placebo-controlled designs and looking for biological markers. This step should help reduce the skepticism of the medical community.

A major obstacle to future progress has been the lack of research funding, especially National Institutes of Health (NIH) funding. When the late senator Arlen Specter (R/D-PA), a senior member of the Senate Appropriations Subcommittee on Health and Education, which had just doubled the NIH budget, asked the leadership of the NIH about funding research on bioenergy, he was told that the NIH "does not believe in bioenergy." Perhaps the U.S.

Department of Energy should sponsor research in this field. Its leaders cannot respond that they do not believe in energy. The medical device industry has been willing to support many innovative studies, but if major advancement of knowledge is to occur in the field of magnetotherapy, recent history shows that it will require a combination.

NONINVASIVE DEVICES FOR DIAGNOSIS AND TREATMENT

Practitioners using biophysical modalities employ a number of noninvasive devices (i.e., devices that do not penetrate the skin) to measure electrical charges and magnetic fields of particular low frequencies. Such devices are also believed to promote healing by interacting with the body.

Biophysical properties of the body have long been observed and utilized in healing. For example, these properties have been known as *qi* (*chi*) in traditional Chinese medicine, *prana* in Ayurvedic medicine, and *vital force* in homeopathy. Acupuncturists, homeopathic doctors, chiropractors, and practitioners of biophysical medicine and magnetic field therapy (including medical doctors) are among the practitioners who use noninvasive devices to detect and influence biophysical properties of the body.

Although conventional medicine recognizes the presence of electrical charges and magnetic forces in the body, certain biophysical properties, also referenced as "subtle energy," have not generally been studied or utilized by Western science and medicine.

Unlike other medical devices regulated by the FDA, many of the noninvasive devices used to detect and influence these biophysical properties fall into a gray area from a regulatory standpoint. In 1976 the FDA set standards for the regulation of acupuncture needles as an experimental device, and the needle was reclassified as a therapeutic device in 1996, based partly on clinical evidence published in a series of articles that one of us (Micozzi) as editor published in the new *Journal of Alternative and Complementary Medicine: Research on Paradigm, Practice and Policy* during 1995. The FDA team working on reclassification specifically requested the founding editor of the journal at that time (the editor of this textbook) to provide lists of references to accelerate the review process. That FDA action occurred before the NIH Consensus Conference on Acupuncture in 1997. However, the FDA did not adopt standards for electroacupuncture devices, a major category of biophysical devices. One of the challenges continues to be the inability of Western science to measure these biophysical properties. As a result, such devices, when cleared by the FDA, are generally approved for use for "investigational" or experimental, purposes, as in research studies, but not in the diagnosis or treatment of illness.

The following sections discuss four categories of devices: (1) electrical and magnetic devices used in conventional medicine for conventional purposes; (2) conventional devices used in innovative applications; (3) conventional devices used for both innovative and conventional applications; and (4) unconventional devices.

ELECTRICAL AND MAGNETIC DEVICES USED CONVENTIONALLY IN BIOMEDICINE

Devices that measure the electrical and magnetic properties of the physical body have been used conventionally in biomedicine for many years. These electrical devices include the electrocardiograph (ECG, EKG), electroencephalograph (EEG), and electromyograph (EMG), used to measure heart, brain, and muscle activity, respectively, and skin galvanic response, for diagnostic purposes. The ECG reads the electrical rhythms of the heart, the EEG records electrical brain waves, and the EMG measures electrical properties of the muscles, which may be correlated to muscle performance. The EMG is often used in physical (rehabilitative) medicine to diagnose conditions that cause pain, weakness, and numbness.

In addition to devices that measure electrical charges, conventionally, biomedicine has made increasing use of magnetic resonance imaging (MRI) for diagnostic purposes. MRI measures the magnetic fields of the body to create images for the diagnosis of physical abnormalities. Another magnetic device, the superconducting quantum interference device (SQUID), combines magnetic flux quantization and Josephson tunneling to measure magnetic heart signals complementary to ECG signals.

CONVENTIONAL BIOMEDICAL DEVICES IN INNOVATIVE APPLICATIONS

Some of the devices just described have also been used in innovative ways (not as originally intended) for treatment purposes, such as the use of the ECG and EEG in biofeedback to monitor subconscious processes and "feedback" this information to support behavioral change. The ECG is also the basis of the Flexyx Neurotherapy System, an innovative approach to the modulation of central perception and the processing of afferent signals from the physical receptors in the body (pressure, pain, heat, cold).

MRI, used to diagnose a variety of medical abnormalities, is also being used in a number of innovative ways, as in neuroscience to show brain activity during performance of different tasks, such as reading or other language tasks, and during acupuncture. At the NIH, basic science researchers are currently investigating innovative uses of MRI to measure physiological changes, such as those involved in eye movement or brain activity.

CONVENTIONAL DEVICES USED FOR TREATMENT IN BOTH BIOMEDICINE AND BIOPHYSICAL MEDICINE

Some devices that utilize electrical charges and magnetic fields are being used by both conventional and biophysical medical practitioners.

Superconducting quantum interference device In addition to its use in conventional medicine, the SQUID has also been used to measure weak magnetic fields of the brain. In other studies, it has been used to measure large, frequency-pulsing biomagnetic fields that emanate from certain practitioners, such as polarity therapists. This biomagnetic field is thought to trigger biological processes at the cellular and molecular levels, helping the body repair itself.

Transcutaneous electrical nerve stimulation unit Developed by Dr. C. Norman Shealy, the TENS unit is used by both conventional medical and biophysical practitioners for pain relief. The FDA approved the TENS unit as a device for pain management in the 1970s. The electronic unit sends pulsed currents to electrodes attached to the skin, displacing pain signals from the affected nerves and preventing the pain message from reaching the brain.

TENS has been suggested to stimulate the production of endorphins as one proposed mechanism of action. In 1990, TENS was the subject of a study published in the *New England Journal of Medicine*. Although it was found ineffective in this study, other studies have found TENS helpful for mild to moderate pain. TENS may have better results in relieving skin and connective tissue pain than muscle or bone pain.

Electro-Acuscope Using a lower amplitude electrical current than the TENS unit, the Electro-Acuscope device reduces pain by stimulating tissue rather than by stimulating the nerves or causing muscle contractions. It is thought to relieve pain by running currents through damaged tissues. Medical doctors, chiropractors, and physical therapists use the Electro-Acuscope for treatment of muscle spasms, migraines, jaw pain, bursitis, arthritis, surgical incisions, sprains and strains, neuralgia, shingles, and bruises. As with the TENS unit, the Electro-Acuscope has been approved by the FDA as a device for pain management.

Diapulse The Diapulse device emits radio waves that produce short, intense electromagnetic pulses which penetrate the tissue. It is said to improve blood flow, reduce pain, and promote healing. The Diapulse is used in a variety of health care settings, especially in the treatment of postoperative swelling and pain.

UNCONVENTIONAL DEVICES USED IN BIOPHYSICAL MEDICINE

The following devices are some of the more popular devices used in biophysical medicine. The FDA has not set standards for these devices, but some may be registered with the FDA as "biofeedback" devices.

Electroacupuncture Devices

Dermatron Voll, a German physician, introduced the Dermatron in the 1940s. Voll believed that acupuncture points have electrical conductivity, and he used this device to measure electrical changes in the body. This technique became known as "electroacupuncture according to Voll" (EAV) and is currently termed *electroacupuncture biofeedback*. Used for diagnosis, the Dermatron became the basis for a number of devices manufactured in Germany, France, Russia, Japan, Korea, the United Kingdom, and the United States.

Vega Another modified electroacupuncture device similar to the Voll device, the Vega works much faster and is also used for diagnosis. Based on the belief that the first sign of abnormality in the body is a change in electrical charge, this device records the change in skin conductivity after the application of a small voltage. Computers have been added to recent models using different names, such as the Computron.

Mora Franz Morel, MD, a colleague of Voll, developed the Mora, another variation of the Voll device. Morel believed that electromagnetic signals could be described by a complex waveform. The Mora reads "wave" information from the body. Proponents believe that the Mora can relieve headaches, migraines, muscular aches and pains, circulation disorders, and skin disease.

Other devices Modern variations of Voll's electroacupuncture devices include the Accupath 1000, Biotron, Computron, DiagnoMetre, Eclosion, Elast, Interro, LISTEN System, Omega AcuBase, Omega Vision, Prophyle, and Punctos III.

Devices Using Light and Sound Energy

Cymatic instruments In addition to the electroacupuncture, biofeedback, and other devices that measure electrical charges described earlier, there are also therapeutic *cymatic* devices, in which a sound transducer replaces the electrodes of the EAV devices. Each organ and tissue in the body emits sound at a particular harmonic frequency. The cymatic device recognizes and records the emitted sound patterns associated with each body part and bathes the affected area with sound to balance the disturbance. These devices are used for diagnosis and treatment.

Sound probe The sound probe emits a pulsed tone of three alternating frequencies. This device is thought to destroy bacteria, viruses, and fungi that are not in resonance with the body.

Light beam generator The light beam generator is thought to work by emitting photons of light that help to restore a normal energy state at the cellular level, allowing the body to heal. The light beam generator is believed to promote healing throughout the body and to help correct such problems as depression, insomnia, headaches, and menstrual disorders.

Infratronic QGM The Infratronic QGM uses electroacoustical technology to direct massage-like waves into the body. This device is employed as an effective pain management tool in China, Japan, Taiwan, Singapore, France, Spain, Mexico, and Argentina. The FDA has approved this device for therapeutic massage in the United States.

Teslar watch Named after the researcher Nikola Tesla, the Teslar watch was developed to modulate the harmful effects of "electronic" pollution from modern sources, such as computers, cell phones, televisions, hair dryers, and electric blankets. It is thought that these products create magnetic energy that may destabilize the body's electromagnetic field. Although this energy is at extremely low frequencies, which range from 1 to 100 Hz, it is thought to affect humans adversely over time.

Kirlian camera The Kirlian camera records and measures high-frequency, high-voltage electrons using the *gas visualization discharge* technique, also called the "corona discharge technique." The most experienced researchers in this technique are Russian; Seymon and Valentina Kirlian pioneered this research in the 1970s. Other contributors include Nikola Tesla in the United States, J.J. Narkiewich-Jodko in Russia, and Pratt and Schlemmer in the Czech Republic. In 1995, Konstantin Korotkov and his team in St. Petersburg developed a new Kirlian camera using a Crown TV.

References

Aaron RK, Lennox D, Bunce GE, et al: The conservative treatment of osteonecrosis of the femoral head. a comparison of core decompression and pulsing electromagnetic fields, *Clin Orthop Relat Res* 249:209, 1989.

Abbruzzese G, Trompetto C: Clinical and research methods for evaluating cortical excitability, *J Clin Neurophysiol* 19:307, 2002.

Adey WR: Physiological signaling across cell membranes and cooperative influences of extremely low frequency electromagnetic fields. In Frohlich H, editor: *Biological coherence and response to external stimuli*, 1988, Springer-Verlag, p 148.

Adey WR: *Resonance and other interactions of electromagnetic fields with living organisms*, 1992, Oxford University Press. Edited by C. Ramel, B Norden.

Adey WR: Potential therapeutic applications of non-thermal electromagnetic fields: ensemble organization of cells in tissue as a factor in biological field sensing. In Rosch PJ, Markov MS, editors: *Bioelectromagnetic medicine*, New York, 2004, Marcel Dekker, p 1.

Amassian VE, Cracco RQ, Maccabee PJ: Focal stimulation of human cerebral cortex with the magnetic coil: a comparison with electrical stimulation, *Electroencephalogr Clin Neurophysiol* 74:401, 1989.

Anderson RR, Parrish JA: The optics of human skin, *J Invest Dermatol* 77:13, 1981.

Armstrong D, Armstrong EM: *The great American medicine show*, New York, 1991, Prentice-Hall.

Asada K, Yutani Y, Shimazu A: Diode laser therapy for rheumatoid arthritis: a clinical evaluation of 102 joints treated with low reactive laser therapy (LLLT), *Laser Ther* 1:147, 1989.

Barker AT: Introduction to the basic principles of magnetic nerve stimulation, *J Clin Neurophysiol* 8:26, 1991.

Barker AT, Freeston IL, Jalinous R, Jarratt JA: Magnetic stimulation of the human brain and peripheral nervous system: an introduction and the results of an initial clinical evaluation, *Neurosurgery* 20:100, 1987.

Basford J: Low-energy laser treatment of pain and wounds: hype, hokum? *Mayo Clin Proc* 61:671, 1986.

Basford JR: Low intensity laser therapy: still not an established tool, *Lasers Surg Med* 16:331, 1995.

Basford J: *Laser therapy*, Paper presented at the Fiftieth Annual Meeting of the American Academy of Neurology, Minneapolis. April 27, 1998.

Basford J, Hallman HO, Matsumoto JY, et al: Effects of 830 nm continuous wave laser diode irradiation on median nerve function in normal subjects, *Lasers Surg Med* 13:597, 1993.

Battisti E, Fortunato M, Giananneshi F, et al: Efficacy of the magnetotherapy in idiopathic carpal tunnel syndrome. In Suminic D, editor: *Proceedings of the Fourth European BioElectromagnetics Association Congress*, Zagreb, Croatia, November 19-21, 1998, p 34.

Baxter GD: *Therapeutic lasers: theory and practice*, New York, 1997, Churchill Livingstone.

Baxter GD, Bell AJ, Allen JM, Ravey J: Low level laser therapy: current clinical practice in Northern Ireland, *Physiotherapy* 77:171, 1991.

Baxter GD, Walsh DM, Allen JM, et al: Effects of low intensity infrared laser irradiation upon conduction in the human median nerve in vivo, *Exp Physiol* 79(227):1994.

Bickford RG, Fremming BD: *Neuronal stimulation by pulsed magnetic fields in animals and man*, In Digest of Sixth International Conference on Medical Electronics and Biological Engineering, 1965, p 112.

Bieglio C, Bisschop C: Physical treatment for radicular pain with low-power laser stimulation, *Lasers Surg Med* 6:173, 1986.

Binder A, Parr G, Hazelman B, et al: Pulsed electromagnetic field therapy of persistent rotator cuff tendinitis: a double-blind, controlled assessment, *Lancet* 8179:695, 1984.

Blechman AM, Oz MC, Nair V, et al: Discrepancy between claimed field flux density of some commercially available magnets and actual gaussmeter measurements, *Altern Ther Health Med* 7:92, 2001.

Bliddal H, Hellesen C, Ditlevsen P, et al: Soft laser therapy of rheumatoid arthritis, *Scand J Rheumatol* 16:225, 1987.

Blumenthal NC, Ricci J, Breger L, et al: Effects of low intensity AC and/or DC electromagnetic fields on cell attachment and induction of apoptosis, *Bioelectromagnetics* 18:264, 1997.

Bork CE, Snyder-Mackler L: Effect of helium-neon laser irradiation on peripheral sensory nerve latency, *J Am Phys Ther Assoc* 68:223, 1988.

Branco K, Naeser MA: Carpal tunnel syndrome: clinical outcome after low-level laser acupuncture, microamps transcutaneous electrical nerve stimulation and other alternative therapies: an open protocol study, *J Altern Comp Med* 5:5, 1999.

Brown CS, Ling FW, Wan JY, et al: Efficacy of static magnetic field therapy in chronic pelvic pain: a double-blind, pilot study, *Am J Obstet Gynecol* 187:1581, 2002.

Cahn SD, Herzog AG, Pascual-Leone A: Paired-pulsed transcranial magnetic stimulation: effects of hemispheric laterality, gender and handedness in normal controls, *J Clin Neurophysiol* 20:371, 2003.

Cantello R: Applications of transcranial magnetic stimulation in movement disorders, *J Clin Neurophysiol* 19:272, 2002.

Carey D, De Muynck M: *Acutonics®: There's no place like ohm, sound healing, Oriental Medicine, and the cosmic mysteries*, ed 2, Llano, NM, 2007, Devachan Press.

Carey D, Franklin E, Michelangelo F, et al: *Acutonics from galaxies to cells, planetary science, harmony, and medicine*, Llano, NM, 2010, Devachan Press.

Carter R, Aspy CB, Mold J: The effectiveness of magnet therapy for treatment of wrist pain attributed to carpal tunnel syndrome, *J Fam Pract* 51:38, 2002.

Chae JH, Nahas Z, Wasserman EM, et al: A pilot study using rTMS to probe the functional neuroanatomy of tics in Tourette's syndrome, *Neuropsychiatry Neuropsychol Behav Neurol* in press.

Christensen P: Clinical laser treatment of odontological conditions. In Kert J, Rose L, editors: *Clinical laser therapy: low level laser therapy*, Copenhagen, 1989, Scandinavian Medical Laser Technology.

Ciombor D, Lester G, Aaron R, et al: Low-frequency EMF regulates chondrocyte differentiation and expression of matrix proteins, *J Orthop Res* 20:40, 2002.

Clogstoun-Willmott J: *Western astrology & Chinese medicine*, Rochester, MA, 1985, Destiny Books.

Colbert AP: Clinical trials involving static magnetic field applications. In Rosch PJ, Markov MS, editors: *Bioelectromagnetic medicine*, New York, 2004, Marcel Dekker, p 781.

Colbert AP, Markov MS, Banerij M, et al: Magnetic mattress pad use in patients with fibromyalgia: a randomized, double-blind pilot study, *J Back Musculoskeletal Rehabil* 13:19, 1999.

Collacott EA, Zimmerman JT, White DW, et al: Bipolar permanent magnets for the treatment of low back pain: a pilot study, *JAMA* 283:1322, 2000.

DeLoecker W, Cheng N, Delport PH: Effects of pulsed electromagnetic fields on membrane transport, *Emerging Electromagn Med* 45, 1990.

DeRidder D, DeMulder G, Walsh W, et al: Magnetic and electrical stimulation of the auditory cortex for intractable tinnitus, *J Neurosurg* 100:560, 2004.

Eccles NJ: A critical review of randomized controlled trials of static magnets for pain relief, *J Altern Complement Med* 11:495, 2005.

Emmanoulidis O, Diamantopoulos C: CW IR Low-power laser applications significantly accelerates chronic pain relief rehabilitation of professional athletes: a double-blind study, *Lasers Surg Med* 6:173, 1986.

Engstrom S, Fitzsimmons R: Five hypotheses to examine the nature of magnetic field transduction in biological systems, *Bioelectromagnetics* 20:423, 1999.

Farndale RW, Maroudas A, Marsland TP: Effects of low-amplitude pulsed magnetic fields on cellular ion transport, *Bioelectromagnetics* 8:119, 1987.

Foley-Nolan D, Barry C, Coughlan RJ, et al: Pulsed high-frequency (27 MHz) electromagnetic therapy for persistent neck pain: a double-blind, placebo-controlled study of 20 patients, *Orthopaedics* 13:445, 1990.

Foley-Nolan D, Moore K, Codd M, et al: Low-energy, high-frequency, pulsed electromagnetic therapy for acute whiplash injuries: a double-blind, randomized, controlled study, *Scand J Rehabil Med* 24:51, 1992.

Franzblau A, Werner RA: What is carpal tunnel syndrome? *JAMA* 282:186, 1999.

Friedman MH: Intra-oral maxillary chilling: a non-invasive treatment in acute migraine and tension-type headache treatment, *Headache Q Curr Treat Res* 9:274, 1998.

Friedman MH, Weintraub MI, Forman S: Atypical facial pain: a localized maxillary nerve disorder? *Am J Pain Manag* 4:149, 1994.

Fukada E, Yasuda I: On the piezoelectric effect of bone, *J Phys Soc Japan* 12:121, 1957.

Gam AN, Thorsen H, Lonnberg F: The effect of low-level laser therapy on musculoskeletal pain: a meta-analysis, *Pain* 52:63, 1993.

Geddes L: History of magnetic stimulation of the nervous system, *J Clin Neurophysiol* 8:3, 1991.

George MS, Lisanby SH, Sackeim HA: Transcranial magnetic stimulation: applications in neuropsychiatry, *Arch Gen Psychiatry* 56:300, 1999.

George MS, Nahas Z, Kozel FA, et al: Mechanisms and the current state of transcranial magnetic stimulation, *CNS Spectr* 8:496, 2003.

George MS, Nahas Z, Kozel FA, et al: Repetitive transcranial magnetic stimulation (rTMS) for depression and other indications. In Rosch PJ, Markov MS, editors: *Bioelectromagnetic medicine*, New York, 2004, Marcel Dekker, p 293.

Goldman JA, Chiapella J, Casey H, et al: Laser therapy of rheumatoid arthritis, *Lasers Surg Med* 1:93, 1980.

Goodman R, Blank M: Insights into electromagnetic interaction mechanisms, *J Cell Physiol* 192:16, 2002.

Haker E, Lundberg T: Laser treatment applied to acupuncture point in lateral humeral epicondylalgia: a double-blind study, *Pain* 43:243, 1990.

Hinman MR, Ford J, Heyl H: Effects of static magnets on chronic knee pain and physical function: a double-blind study, *Altern Ther Health Med* 8:50, 2002.

Hofman O: *Classical medical astrology: Healing with the elements*, Bournemouth, UK, 2009, The Wessex Astrologer.

Holcomb RR, McLean MJ, Engstrom S, et al: Treatment of mechanical low back pain with static magnetic fields: result of a clinical trial and implications for study design, *Magnetotherapy* 171, 2002.

Hong JN, Kim TH, Lim SD: Clinical trial of low reactive level laser therapy in 20 patients with post-herpetic neuralgia, *Laser Ther* 2:167, 1990.

Hong CZ, Lin JC, Bender LF, et al: Magnetic necklace: its therapeutic effectiveness on neck and shoulder pain, *Arch Phys Med Rehabil* 63:462, 1982.

Hunter J, Leonard L, Wilson R, et al: Effects of low energy laser on wound healing in a porcine model, *Lasers Surg Med* 3:285, 1984.

Jacobson JI, Gorman R, Yamanashi WS, et al: Low-amplitude, extremely low frequency magnetic fields for the treatment of osteoarthritic knees: a double-blind clinical study, *Altern Ther Health Med* 7:54, 2001.

Jawer M, Micozzi MS: *Your Emotional Type*, Rochester VT, 2011, Healing Arts Press.

Kairos Institute of Sound Healing: *Acutonics from galaxies to cells*, http://www.youtube.com/watch?v=BFXvjTr2_1U. accessed on: August 3, 2013.

Karu TI: Photobiological fundamentals of low power laser therapy, *IEEE J Quantum Electron* QE-23:1703, 1987.

Karu TI: Molecular mechanisms of the therapeutic effect of low intensity laser irradiation, *Lasers Life Sci* 2:53, 1988.

Klein RG, Eek BC: Low-energy laser treatment and exercise for chronic low back pain: double-blind control trial, *Arch Phys Med Rehabil* 71:34, 1990.

Kloth LC, Berman JE, Sutton CH, et al: Effect of pulsed radiofrequency stimulation on wound healing: a double-blind, pilot clinical study. In Bersani F, editor: *Electricity and magnetism in biology and medicine*, New York, 1999, Plenum, p 875.

Kneebone WJ: Treatment of chronic neck pain utilizing low-level laser therapy, *Pract Pain Manag* 64, 2007.

Kobayashi M, Pascual-Leone A: Transcranial magnetic stimulation in neurology, *Lancet Neurol* 2:145, 2003.

Kolari PJ: Penetration of unfocused laser light into the skin, *Arch Dermatol Res* 277:342, 1985.

Kubasova T, Kovacs L, Somosy Z: Biological effect of He-Ne laser investigations on functional and micromorphological alterations of cell membranes, in vitro, *Lasers Surg Med* 4:381, 1984.

Lam TS, Abergel RP, Meeker CA, et al: Laser stimulation of collagen synthesis in human skin fibroblast cultures, *Lasers Life Sci* 1:61, 1986.

Lappin MS, Lawrie FW, Richards TL, et al: Effects of a pulsed electromagnetic therapy on multiple sclerosis, fatigue and quality of life: a double-blind, placebo-controlled trial, *Altern Ther* 9:38, 2003.

Lasermedics [now Henley Healthcare]: Personal communication, 1999.

Lednev LL: Possible mechanism of weak magnetic fields on biological systems, *Bioelectromagnetics* 12:71, 1991.

Leonard DR, Farooqi MH, Myers S: Restoration of sensation, reduced pain and improved balance in subjects with diabetic peripheral neuropathy: a double-blind, randomized, placebo-controlled study with monochromatic near-infra-red treatment, *Diabetes Care* 27:168, 2004.

Linovitz RJ, Ryaby JT, Magee FP, et al: Combined magnetic fields accelerate primary spine fusion: a double-blind, randomized, placebo-controlled study, *Proc Am Acad Orthop Surg* 67:376, 2000.

Lisamby SH, Gutman D, Lubes B, et al: Sham TMS: intracerebral measurement of the induced electrical field and the induction of motor-evoked potentials, *Biol Psychiatry* 49:460, 2001.

Lopes-Martins RA, Albertini R, Lopes-Martins PS, et al: Steroid receptor antagonist mifepristone inhibits the anti-inflammatory effect of photoradiation, *Photomed Laser Surg* 24:197, 2006.

Lyons RF, Abergel RP, White RA, et al: Biostimulation of wound healing in vivo by a helium-neon laser, *Ann Plast Surg* 18:47, 1987.

Maccabee PJ, Amassian VE, Cracco RQ, et al: Stimulation of the human nervous system using the magnetic coil, *J Clin Neurophysiol* 8:38, 1991.

Macias MY, Buttocletti JH, Sutton CH, et al: Directed and enhanced neurite growth with pulsed magnetic field stimulation, *Bioelectromagnetics* 21:272, 2000.

Maciocia G: *The Foundations of Chinese Medicine: A comprehensive text for acupuncturists and herbalists*, New York, 1989, Churchill Livingstone.

Macklis RM: Magnetic healing, quackery and the debate about the health effects of electromagnetic fields, *Ann Intern Med* 118:376, 1993.

Maiman TH: Stimulated optical radiation in ruby, *Nature* 187:493, 1960. (letter).

Man D, Man B, Plosker H: The influence of permanent magnetic field therapy on wound healing in suction lipectomy patients: a double-blind study, *Plast Reconstr Surg* 104:2261, 1999.

Markov MS: Magnetic and electromagnetic field therapy: basic principles of application for pain relief. In Rosch PJ, Markov MS, editors: *Bioelectromagnetic medicine*, New York, 2004, Marcel Dekker, p 251.

Markov MS: Magnetic field therapy: a review, *Electromagn Biol Med* 26:1, 2007.

Markov MS, Colbert AP: Magnetic and electromagnetic field therapy, *J Back Musculoskeletal Rehabil* 15:17, 2001.

Markov MS, Pilla AA: Weak static magnetic field modulation of myosin phosphorylation in a cell-free preparation: calcium dependence, *Bioelectrochem Bioenerg* 43:233, 1997.

Martel GF, Andrews SC, Roseboom CG: Comparison of static and placebo magnets on resting forearm blood flow in young, healthy men, *J Orthop Sports Phys Ther* 32:518, 2002.

Mayor DM, Micozzi MS: *Energy Medicine East and West*, London, 2011, Elsevier Health Sciences.

Mayrovitz HN, Larsen PB: A preliminary study to evaluate the effect of pulsed radiofrequency field treatment on lower extremity peri-ulcer skin microvasculature of diabetic patients, *Wounds* 7:90, 1995.

McDonald F: Effect of static magnetic fields on osteoblasts and fibroblasts in-vitro, *Bioelectromagnetics* 14:187, 1993.

McLean M, Holcomb RR, Engstrom S, et al: A static magnetic field blocks action potential firing and kainic acid-induced neuronal injury in vitro. In McLean MJ, Engstrom S, Holcomb RR, editors: *Magnetotherapy: potential therapeutic benefits and adverse effects*, New York, 2003, TFG Press, p 29.

McLean MJ, Holcomb RR, Wamil AW, et al: Blockade of sensory neuron action potentials by a static magnetic field in the mT range, *Bioelectromagnetics* 16:20, 1995.

Merton PA, Morton HB: Stimulation of the cerebral cortex in the intact human subject, *Nature* 285:227, 1980.

Mester E, Jaszsagi-Nagy E: The effect of laser radiation on wound healing and collagen synthesis, *Stud Biophys* 35:227, 1973.

Mester E, Mester AF, Mester A: The biomedical effects of laser applications, *Lasers Surg Med* 5:31, 1985.

Mester E, Toth N, Mester A: The biostimulative effect of laser beam, *Laser Basic Biomed Res* 22:4, 1982.

Mezawa S, Iwata K, Naito K, Kamogawa H: The possible analgesic effect of soft-laser irradiation on heat nociceptors in the cat tongue, *Arch Oral Biol* 33:693, 1988.

Mizokami T, Yoshii N, Uhikubo Y, et al: Effect of diode laser for pain: a clinical study on different pain types, *Laser Ther* 2:171, 1990.

Mooney V: A randomized, double-blind, prospective study of the efficacy of pulsed electromagnetic fields for interbody lumbar fusions, *Spine* 15:708, 1990.

Moore KC, Hira N, Kumar PS, et al: A double-blind crossover trial of low level laser therapy in the treatment of post-herpetic neuralgia, *Lasers Med Sci* 301, 1988. (abstract).

Morselli LS, Sorgani O, Anselmi C, Farinelli FF, et al: Very low energy-density treatment by CO_2 laser in sports medicine, *Lasers Surg Med* 5:150, 1985.

Mourino MR: From Thales to Lauterbur, or from the lodestone to MR imaging: magnetism and medicine, *Radiology* 180:593, 1991.

Naeser MA: Review of second congress: World Association for Laser Therapy (WALT) meeting, *J Altern Complement Med* 5:177, 1999.

Naeser MA, Alexander MP, Stiassny-Eder D, et al: Laser Acupuncture in the Treatment of Paralysis in Stroke Patients: A CT Scan Lesion Site Study, *Am J Acupunct* 23(1):13–28, 1995.

Naeser MA, Hahn KK, Lieberman B: Real vs. sham laser acupuncture and microamps TENS to treat carpal tunnel syndrome and worksite wrist pain: pilot study, *Lasers Surg Med Suppl* 8:7, 1996.

Ohkubo C, Xu S: Acute effects of static magnetic fields on cutaneous microcirculation in rabbits, *In Vivo* 11:221, 1997.

Okano H, Gmitrov J, Ohkubo C: Biphasic effects of static magnetic fields on cutaneous microcirculation in rabbits, *Bioelectromagnetics* 20:161, 1999.

Orpin JA: False claims for magnetotherapy, *Can Med Assoc J* 15:1375, 1982.

Osenbach RK: Motor cortex stimulation for intractable pain, *Neurosurg Focus* 21:1, 2006.

Padua L, Padua R: Laser bio-stimulation: a reply, *Muscle Nerve* 21:1232, 1998.

Pascual-Leone A, Valls-Sole J, Wasserman EM, et al: Responses to rapid-rate transcranial magnetic stimulation of the human motor cortex, *Brain* 117:847, 1994.

Pascual-Leone A, Wasserman EM, Davey NJ, editors: *Handbook of transcranial magnetic stimulation*, London, 2002, Oxford University Press.

Passarella S: HeNe laser irradiation of isolated mitochondria, *J Photochem Photobiol* 31:642, 1989.

Pickering SAW, Bayston R, Scammell BE: Electromagnetic augmentation of antibiotic efficacy in infection of orthopaedic implants, *J Bone Joint Surg* 85:588, 2003.

Pilla AA: Weak time-varying and static magnetic fields: from mechanisms to therapeutic applications. In Stavroulakis P, editor: *Biological effects of electromagnetic fields*, New York, 2003, Springer-Verlag, p 34.

Pilla AA, Nasser PR, Kaufman JJ: The sensitivity of cells and tissues to weak electromagnetic fields. In Allen MJ, Cleary SF, Sowers AE et al, editors: *Charge and field effects in biosystems—3*, Boston, 1992, Birkhäuser, p 231.

Pilla AA, Nasser PR, Kaufman JJ: The sensitivity of cells and tissues to therapeutic and environmental EMF, *Bioelectrochem Bioenerg* 30:161, 1993.

Pilla AA, Martin DE, Schuett AM, et al: Effect of pulsed radiofrequency therapy on edema from grades I and II ankle sprains: a placebo-controlled, randomized, multi-site, double-blind, clinical study, *J Athl Train* S31:53, 1996.

Pilla AA, Muehsam DJ: Pulsing and static magnetic field therapeutics: from mechanisms to clinical application, *Magnetotherapy* 119, 2003.

Pilla AA, Muehsam DJ, Markov MS: A dynamical systems/Larmor precession model for weak magnetic field bioeffects: ion binding and orientation of bound water molecules, *Bioelectrochemistry* 43:241, 1997.

Pipitone N, Scott DL: Magnetic pulsed treatment for knee osteoarthritis: a randomized, double-blind, placebo-controlled study, *Curr Med Res Opin* 17:190, 2001.

Pujol J, Pascual-Leone A, Dolz C, et al: The effect of repetitive magnetic stimulation on localized musculoskeletal pain, *Neurol Rep* 9:1745, 1998.

Raji ARM, Bowden REM: Effects of high pulsed power electromagnetic field on the degeneration and regeneration of the common peroneal nerve in rats, *J Bone Joint Surg* 65:478, 1983.

Ramey DW: Magnetic and electromagnetic therapy, *Sci Rev Altern Med* 2:13, 1998.

Repacholi MH, Greenebaum B: Interaction of static and extremely low frequency electric and magnetic fields with living systems: health effects and research needs, *Bioelectromagnetics* 20:133, 1999.

Rochkind S, Barr-Nea L, Razon N, et al: Stimulating effect of HeNe low dose laser on injured sciatic nerves of rats, *Neurosurgery* 20:843, 1987.

Rochkind S, Rousso M, Nissan M, et al: Systemic effects of low-power laser irradiation on the peripheral and central nervous system, cutaneous wounds and burns, *Lasers Surg Med* 9:174, 1989.

Rollnik JD, Wusterfeld S, Dauper J, et al: Repetitive transcranial magnetic stimulation for the treatment of chronic pain: a pilot study, *Eur Neurol* 48:6, 2002.

Rosch P: Preface. In Rosch PJ, editor: *A brief historical perspective in bioelectromagnetic medicine*, New York, 2004, Marcel Dekker, p III.

Rosen AD: Magnetic field influence on acetylcholine release at the neuromuscular junction, *Am J Physiol* 262:1418, 1992.

Rossini PM, Barker AT, Berardelli A, et al: Non-invasive electrical and magnetic stimulation of the brain, spinal cord and roots: basic principles and procedure for routine clinical application: report of an IFCN committee, *Electroencephalogr Clin Neurophysiol* 91:79, 1994.

Saygili G, Aydinlik E, Ercan MI, et al: Investigation of the effect of magnetic retention systems used in prostheses on buccal mucosal blood flow, *Int J Prosthodont* 5:326, 1992.

Serway RA: *Principles of physics*, ed 2, Fort Worth, Tex, 1998, Saunders College Publishing, p 636.

Shellock FG: Biomedical implants and devices: assessment of magnetic field interactions with a 3.0T MR system, *J Magn Reson Imaging* 16:721, 2002.

Shellock FG, Crues JV: MR procedures: biological effects, safety and patient care, *Radiology* 232:635, 2004.

Shipley JT: *Dictionary of word origins*, New York, 1945, Dorset Press.

Sisken BF, Walker J, Orgel M: Prospects on clinical applications of electrical stimulation for nerve regeneration, *J Cell Biochem* 52:404, 1993.

Smith WF: *Principles of materials science and engineering*, ed 3, New York, 1996, McGraw-Hill, p 659.

Snyder-Mackler L, Bork CE: Effect of helium-neon laser irradiation on peripheral sensory nerve latency, *Phys Ther* 68:223, 1988.

Terao Y, Ugawa Y: Basic mechanisms of TMS, *J Clin Neurophysiol* 19:322, 2002.

Theodore WH: Transcranial magnetic stimulation in epilepsy, *Epilepsy Curr* 3:191, 2003.

Timmel CR, Till U, Brocklehurst B, et al: Effects of weak magnetic fields on free radical recombination reactions, *Mol Phys* 95:71, 1998.

Todd DJ, Heylings DJ, Allen GE, et al: Treatment of chronic varicose ulcers with pulsed electromagnetic fields: a controlled pilot study, *Ir Med J* 84:54, 1991.

U.S. Food and Drug Administration, Center for Devices and Radiological Health: *MDR Data Files*, April 1, 2003. Available at: http://www.FDA.gov/CDRH/MDRFILE/html.

United Nations Environment Programme MF: *The International Labour Organization*, Geneva, 1987, World Health Organization.

Vallbona C, Hazelwood CF, Jurida G: Response of pain to static magnetic fields in post-polio patients: a double-blind pilot study, *Arch Phys Med Rehabil* 78:1200, 1997.

Walker JB: Relief from chronic pain by low-power laser irradiation, *Neurosci Lett* 43:339, 1983.

Walker JB, Akhanjee LK, Cooney MM: Laser therapy for pain of rheumatoid arthritis, *Lasers Surg Med* 6:171, 1986.

Walsh J: The current status of low level laser therapy in dentistry: part I—soft tissue applications, *Aust Dent J* 42:247, 1997.

Walsh DM, Baxter GK, Allen JM: *The effect of 820 nm laser upon nerve conduction in the superficial radial nerve*, Abstract presented at the Fifth International Biotherapy Laser Association Meeting, London, 1991.

Walsh V, Rushworth M: A primer of magnetic stimulation as a tool for neuropsychology, *Neuropsychologia* 37:125, 1999.

Wasserman EM: Risk and safety of repetitive transcranial magnetic stimulation: report and suggested guidelines from the International Workshop in the Safety of Repetitive Transcranial Magnetic Stimulation: June 5-7, 1996, *Electroencephalogr Clin Neurophysiol* 108:1, 1998.

Weintraub MI: Migraine: a maxillary nerve disorder? A novel therapy: preliminary results, *Am J Pain Manag* 6:77, 1996.

Weintraub MI: Non-invasive laser neurolysis in carpal tunnel syndrome, *Muscle Nerve* 20:1029, 1997.

Weintraub MI: Reply to Padua et al, *Muscle Nerve* 21:1233, 1998.

Weintraub MI: Magnetic bio-stimulation in painful diabetic peripheral neuropathy: a novel intervention. A randomized, double-blind, placebo, cross-over study, *Am J Pain Manag* 9:8, 1999.

Weintraub MI: Are magnets effective for pain control? *JAMA* 284:565, 2000.

Weintraub MI: Magnetic biostimulation in neurologic illness. In Weintraub MI, editor: *Alternative and complementary treatment in neurologic illness*, New York, 2001, Churchill Livingstone, p 278.

Weintraub MI: Magnetotherapy: historical background with a stimulating future, *Crit Rev Phys Rehabil Med* 16:95, 2004a.

Weintraub MI: Magnets for patients with heel pain, *JAMA* 291:43, 2004b.

Weintraub MI, Cole SP: Pulsed magnetic field therapy in refractory neuropathic pain secondary to peripheral neuropathy: electrodiagnostic parameters—pilot study, *Neurorehabil Neural Repair* 18:42, 2004.

Weintraub MI, Cole SP: Novel device generating static and time-varying magnetic fields in refractory diabetic peripheral neuropathy: subset analysis of cohort with long-term exposure in nationwide, double-blind, placebo-controlled trial, *Diabetes suppl* A-610, 2007a.

Weintraub MI, Cole SP: A randomized, controlled trial of the effects of a combination of static and dynamic magnetic fields on carpal tunnel syndrome, *Neurology* 68(Suppl 1):A180, 2007b.

Weintraub MI, Khoury A, Cole SP: Biologic effects of 3 Tesla (T) MR imaging comparing traditional 1.5 T and 0.6 T in 1023 consecutive outpatients, *J Neuroimaging* 17:241, 2007.

Weintraub MI, Steinberg RB, Cole SP: The role of cutaneous magnetic stimulation in failed back syndrome, *Semin Integr Med* 3:101, 2005.

Weintraub MI, Wolfe GI, Barohn RA, et al: Static magnetic field therapy for symptomatic diabetic neuropathy: a randomized, double-blind, placebo-controlled trial, *Arch Phys Med Rehabil* 84:736, 2003.

Whitaker J, Adderly B: *The pain relief breakthrough*, Boston, 1998, Little, Brown, pp 24–38.

Wilson DH, Jagadeesh O: The effect of pulsed electromagnetic energy on peripheral nerve regeneration, *Ann N Y Acad Sci* 238:575, 1974.

Winemiller MH, Billow RG, Laskowski ER, et al: Effect of magnetic vs. sham-magnetic insoles on plantar heel pain: a randomized controlled trial, *JAMA* 290:1474, 2003.

Wittig JE, Engstrom S: Magnetism and magnetic materials. In McLean MJ, Engstrom S, Holcomb RR, editors: *Magnetotherapy: potential therapeutic benefits and adverse effects*, New York, 2002, TFG Press, p 3.

Yamada K: Biological effects of low-power laser irradiation on clonal osteoblastic cells (MC3T-E1), *Nippon Seikeigeka Gakkai Zasshi* 65:787, 1991.

Yu W, Naim JO, McGowan M, et al: Photomodulation of oxidative metabolism and electron chain enzymes in rat liver mitochondria, *Photochem Photobiol* 66:866, 1997.

Zdeblic TD: A prospective randomized study of lumbar fusion: preliminary results, *Spine* 18:983, 1993.

Zhu L, Li C, Ji C, Li W: The effect of laser irradiation on arthritis in rats, *Pain* 5(Suppl):385, 1990.

Suggested Readings

Alfano AP, Taylor AG, Foresman PA, et al: Static magnetic fields for treatment of fibromyalgia: a randomized, controlled trial, *Altern Comp Med* 7:53, 2001.

Asagai Y, Ueno R, Miura Y, Ohshiro T: Application of low reactive-level laser therapy (LLLT) in the functional training of cerebral palsy patients, *Laser Ther* 6:195, 1994.

Bassett CA: The development and application of pulsed electromagnetic fields (PEMFs) for ununited fracture and arthrodeses, *Orthop Clin North America* 15:61, 1984.

Bassett CA: Fundamental and practical aspects of therapeutic uses of pulsed electromagnetic fields (PEMFs), *Crit Rev Biomed Eng* 17:451, 1989.

Becker RO: *Cross currents: the perils of electropollution, the promise of electromedicine*, Los Angeles, 1990, Tarcher/Perigee.

Becker RO, Selden G: *The body electric: electromagnetism and the foundation of life*, New York, 1985, Quill/Morrow.

Blank M, editor: *Electromagnetic fields: biological interactions and mechanisms*, Washington, DC, 1995, American Chemical Society. (Includes two chapters of particular interest on health effects of bioelectromagnetic fields.)

Caselli MA, Clark N, Lazarus S, et al: Evaluation of magnetic foil and PPT insoles in the treatment of heel pain, *J Am Podiatr Med Assoc* 87:11, 1997.

Galantino ML, Eke-Okoro ST, Findley TW, et al: Use of non-invasive electroacupuncture for the treatment of HIV-related peripheral neuropathy, *J Altern Complement Med* 5(2):135, 1999.

Gerber R: *Vibrational medicine: new choices for healing ourselves*, Santa Fe, NMex, 1988, Bear.

Keck ME, Sillaber I, Ebner K, et al: Acute transcranial magnetic stimulation of frontal brain regions selectively modulates the release of vasopressin, biogenic amines and amino acids in the rat brain, *Eur J Neurosci* 12:3713, 2000.

Kellaway P: The part played by electric fish in the early history of bioelectricity and electrotherapy, *Bull Hist Med* 20:112, 1946.

Leclaire R, Bourguin J: Electromagnetic treatment of shoulder periarthritis: a randomized, controlled trial of the efficacy and tolerance of magnetotherapy, *Arch Phys Med Rehabil* 72:284, 1991.

Lytle CD, Thomas BM, Gordon EA, et al: Electrostimulators for acupuncture: safety issues, *J Altern Complement Med* 6(1):37, 2000.

Naeser MA: Carpal tunnel syndrome: clinical outcome after low-level laser acupuncture, microamps transcutaneous electrical nerve stimulation, and other alternative therapies, *J Altern Complement Med* 5:1999.

Oschman JL: *Energy medicine: the scientific basis of bioenergy therapies*, New York, 2000, Churchill Livingstone.

Patterson MA, Patterson L, Patterson SI: Electrostimulation: addiction treatment for the coming millennium, *J Altern Complement Med* 2:485, 1996.

Richards TL, Lappin MS, Acosta-Urquidi J, et al: Double-blind study of pulsing magnetic field effects on multiple sclerosis, *J Altern Complement Med* 3:21, 1997.

Rispoli FP, Corolla FM, Mussner R: The use of low frequency pulsing electromagnetic fields in patients with painful hip prostheses, *J Bioelectric* 7:181, 1988.

Ryaby JT: Electromagnetic stimulation in orthopedics: biochemical mechanisms to clinical applications. In Rosch PJ, Markov MS, editors: *Bioelectromagnetic medicine*, New York, 2004, Marcel Dekker, p 411.

Schlitz M, Amorok T, Micozzi M: *Consciousness and healing: integral approaches to mind-body medicine*, St Louis, 2005, Churchill Livingstone.

Segal NA, Toda Y, Huston J, et al: Two configurations of static magnetic fields for testing rheumatoid arthritis of the knee: a double-blind clinical trial, *Arch Phys Med Rehabil* 82:1453, 2001.

Thuile CH, Walzl M: Evaluation of electromagnetic fields in the treatment of pain in patients with lumbar radiculopathy or the whiplash syndrome, *Neurol Rehabil* 17:63, 2002.

Walleczek J: Bioelectromagnetics: the question of subtle energies, *Noetic Sci Rev* 28, 1993.

Weintraub MI, Cole SP: Time-Varying, Biaxial Magnetic Stimulation in Refractory Carpal Tunnel Syndrome: A Novel Approach. A Pilot Study, *Semin Integr Med* 3(4):123–128, 2005.

Resources

Professional Organizations

BioElectroMagnetics Institute
John Zimmerman, PhD, President
2490 W Moana Lane
Reno, NV 89509-7801, USA

John E. Fetzer Institute
9292 West KL Avenue
Kalamazoo, MI 49009, USA

Institute of Noetic Sciences
PO Box 909
Sausalito, CA 94966, USA

International Society for the Study of Subtle Energies and Energy Medicine (ISSSEEM)
11005 Ralston Road, #100 D
Arvada, CO 80004, USA
E-mail: issseem@compuserve.com

Websites

John E. Fetzer Institute: http://www.fetzer.org
International Society for the Study of Subtle Energies and Energy Medicine (ISSSEEM): http://www.ISSSEEM.org

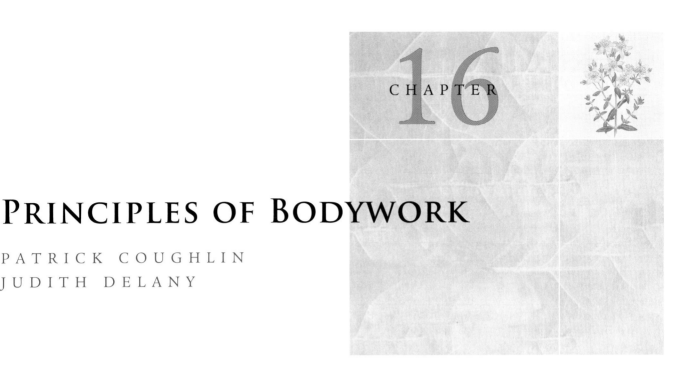

CHAPTER 16

PRINCIPLES OF BODYWORK

PATRICK COUGHLIN

JUDITH DELANY

Modalities that involve touching, massaging, and manipulating the physical body provide a pathway to healing that are also thought to draw on the connection between body and mind, as well as energetic aspects of healing. Such approaches have great antiquity. The well-known abilities of touch to heal are widely recognized in modern medicine in the tradition of "laying on of hands." The "hands-on" therapies have been well organized and widely available as contemporary systematic therapeutic practice systems. This chapter presents the basic physiologic principles that underlie the manual therapies, and the remaining chapters in this section explain each specific system that makes use of manual and manipulative modalities of healing.

As with other complementary or alternative therapies, bodywork espouses a holistic philosophy that has the following outstanding tenets:
1. The body is a unit.
2. Structure and function are interrelated.
3. The body has an inherent ability to heal itself.
4. When normal adaptability is disrupted, disease may ensue.

Based on these defining principles, bodywork seeks to reverse structural imbalances to optimize the body's ability to self-correct or repair itself, which includes the defense against invasion from foreign substances or organisms.

CONCEPTS OF BODYWORK AND MANUAL HEALING

A number of concepts based on physical laws and anatomical principles universally apply to manipulative and bodywork practices. These concepts are briefly described here so

that they can be associated with the various forms (styles) of manipulative therapy, providing the reader with a greater understanding of the reasons for applying or seeking this type of treatment.

CONCEPT 1: BILATERAL SYMMETRY

The musculoskeletal system is usually described as being bilaterally symmetrical. That is, if the body is divided in half by a slice made from top to bottom and front to back along the midline (midsagittal plane), the right-hand side should be a mirror image of the left-hand side. This image is an idealized assumption, of course, because few if any human bodies are truly symmetrical. This point is readily evident when one considers the nonsymmetrical arrangement of the visceral organs, the viscera's impact on internal weight distribution, and its potential for distortion of the skeleton, such as is often seen with the liver's expansion of the overlying right-sided ribs. Certain behaviors in which we engage, both consciously and unconsciously, are specifically designed to compensate for a lack of bilateral symmetry, particularly in regards to the skeletal frame.

CONCEPT 2: GRAVITY

The human organism is similar to all other organisms in that we are subject to the laws of physics. Thus, the way we interact with planet Earth is governed by the pull of the Earth on our bodies: the force of gravity. Because of this constant force, and because our bodies have mass, we are given the weight that we must carry as we go about our activities. Additionally, we must accommodate any weight added by items we carry, and those often are not at optimal placement in relation to our center of gravity. Theories of

240

energetic and manual healing have long considered the influences of gravity (see Chapter 6) as do contemporary analysis of yoga (Chapter 21) and meditative practices (McCown & Micozzi, 2012).

CONCEPT 3: TENSEGRITY

Tensegrity was developed as a concept in the late 1940s by the architect Buckminster Fuller and the sculptor Kenneth Snelson. The basic premise of *tensegrity* (tensional integrity) is that in many systems a balance exists between compression and tension. Tensegrity is "an architectural system in which structures stabilize themselves by balancing the counteracting forces of compression and tension which gives shape and strength to both natural and artificial forms." Architectural systems such as suspension bridges employ this concept, but it also is seen in biological systems, including the musculoskeletal system. The muscles and other soft tissues (e.g., joint capsules, tendons, and ligaments) act as tensional elements, whereas the bones act as spacers and resist the compression of weight bearing. By maximizing the ratio of tensional elements to compression elements, such a system enables the organism to maintain balance and move with a minimum amount of energy expenditure.

CONCEPT 4: POSTURAL MAINTENANCE AND COORDINATED MOVEMENT

As the human body evolved from a quadrupedal (four-legged) to a bipedal (two-legged) stance, we became able to "manipulate" our environment because our hands were freed up, but we also became more unstable (visualize the result of removing two legs of a four-legged table; even the Eiffel Tower has four legs). From an architectural point of view, we became a buttressed arch system (the feet, legs, and pelvic girdle) supporting an elongated tower (the spine and head), with two cantilevered upper appendages (the arms) that can assist with balance. However, we are designed for movement (which is necessary for survival) and are rarely stationary, even when seated. Consider the act of walking: for about 40% of the time allotted to the normal gait cycle (the period of two strides), we are moving with only one foot on the ground. Because we engage in considerable movement, we are constantly adapting to our position relative to the Earth, which exerts its gravitational pull. Accordingly, we have programmed into our neuromusculoskeletal system a device that lets us know what that position is at all times and also directs the constant physical adjustments that we make. This is commonly referred to as the "equilibrial triad," which consists of the proprioceptive system, vestibular system, and visual system.

The *proprioceptive* system gives us positional information based on the state of contraction of each muscle in the body, as well as the position of each joint. The *vestibular* system is our "gyroscope," which gives us information on the position of the head and how it and the rest of the body are rotating or accelerating in space. The *visual* system allows us to be well aware of our surroundings and position because we can "see" where we are. In fact, because the visual system is so important in our normal range of activity, the other two parts of the triad act to support it. The proprioceptive and vestibular systems sense the position of the head relative to the body and adjust the posture so that the head is situated with the eyes aligned parallel to the horizon. Together, these three systems act with the motor system to produce coordinated movement, balanced posture, and a properly aligned head.

CONCEPT 5: CONNECTIVE TISSUE (FASCIA)

Connective tissue can be highly organized, as in the case of joint capsules, ligaments, tendons, the meninges of the central nervous system (CNS), intervertebral discs, and articular cartilage, or it can be more diffuse and seemingly less organized. *Fascia* is another name for the connective tissue that surrounds and gives architectural form to the tissues and organs of the body.

Fascia can be divided into two major components: superficial fascia and deep fascia. The *superficial* fascia resides just under the skin (the hypodermis) and serves as a staging center for the immune system (large quantities of antigens from the skin are presented to immune cells in this layer) and as a fat storage depot (the cause of significant attention). The *deep* fascia is much more extensive than the superficial fascia and exists throughout the body, serving to "connect" virtually all the tissues and organs. Skeletal muscles are surrounded by capsules of deep fascia, as are nerves and blood vessels (e.g., neurovascular bundles are wrapped in deep fascia). In this sense the deep fascia forms compartments that separate these tissues, but it also forms a structural continuum, and if physical stress is applied to one area of fascia, this continuity will result in effects' being "felt" in other areas or fascial layers as well (Figure 16-1). The compartmentalization of tissues by the deep fascia also results in the formation of specific pathways for, and limits to, the spread of infection (i.e., along fascial planes), as well as for the accumulation of fluid. Both superficial fascia and deep fascia are richly supplied by blood and lymphatic vessels and by nerves (especially pain fibers).

On the molecular level, fascia is composed of a fibrous component (primarily the macromolecular proteins collagen and elastin) and a soluble, gel-like component, mostly water. The combination of fibrous and soluble components of the fascia creates, in effect, a molecular sieve through which chemical compounds diffuse to and from the cells of the body. Therefore fascia has a great impact on the function of the organs it surrounds and infiltrates. Cells also reside in the fascia, including fat and immune cells in the superficial fascia. *Fibroblasts,* a major population of connective tissue cells, are responsible for the secretion of fibrous proteins that make up the scaffold of the fascia. Immune cells constantly patrol the fascia, seeking out foreign antigens as well as ingesting and destroying extracellular debris, including used constituents of the fibrous

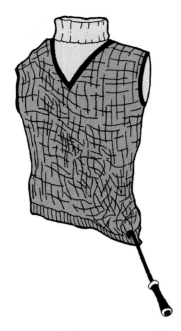

Figure 16-1 A force applied to one part of the fascial continuum affects the entire system.

matrix. This creates a significant turnover in the components of the fascia and contributes to its innate adaptability to changing body conditions. The cellular component of the fascia can be significantly altered by a state of inflammation, in which large numbers of immune cells migrate into the area in response to tissue damage or antigenic challenge. Inflammation also stimulates fibroblasts to secrete larger amounts of collagen to reseal any breaches in the continuum, which results in scar formation or fibrosis.

Not only is the fascia very adaptable to the ever-changing internal environment, but it is also significantly affected by the aging process. As the human body ages, the chemical bonds that bind collagen molecules together, known as *cross-links,* become more prevalent. As this occurs, less space is available in the fascia for water and the other soluble components. The end result is a loss of tissue water and an increase in the fibrous component, which in turn decreases the relative elasticity and physical adaptability of the tissue. In other words, the tissues dry up and become more brittle. This leaves the musculoskeletal system, in particular, significantly more susceptible to microtrauma and macrotrauma.

The physical properties of fascia have stimulated manual therapy practitioners to devise specific techniques to address these properties and the relations among the fascia and the tissue it surrounds. Just as the fascial matrix can become distorted from the forces brought to bear on it, it also can be restored to its original structural relationships by manual means. In addition, because of the continuity of the fascia throughout the body, local fascial distortions can produce distant effects. This is especially true in the case of muscle-associated deep fascia, which, if distorted, can alter the vector and function of that muscle.

The gel-like consistency of the soluble component of the fascia enables it to behave as a colloid, which resists force in direct proportion to its velocity. On the other hand, because of this property, fascia, like a colloid, will respond much more readily if force is applied slowly and gently. In addition, gentle application of force results in gradual yet sustained realignment of the fibrous component of the fascia, which can be palpated in the form of a "release." This is the rationale behind the development of myofascial, craniosacral, and other low-velocity techniques.

Recent research has led to the discovery of myofibroblasts which lends a further basis to this concept, as discussed in Chapter 17.

CONCEPT 6: SEGMENTATION (FUNCTIONAL SPINAL UNIT)

Anatomically, the human body is arranged lengthwise as a series of building blocks or segments. This can be observed most directly by the looking at the individual vertebrae that make up the spinal column, which extends from the base of the skull to the coccyx ("tailbone"). Just above the coccyx is the sacrum, a single bone resulting from the fusion of five vertebrae. This fusion is significant, because the sacrum articulates with the pelvic bones, which in turn articulate with the femurs. This relationship produces an arch that has the sacrum as its keystone.

Passing between the vertebrae and going from the spinal cord to the periphery are 31 pairs of spinal nerves (one for each side, with the exception of the coccygeal nerve, which is fused at the midline of the body). Each of these spinal nerves contains sensory and motor nerve fibers that are distributed around the body (Figure 16-2).

Most nerves are accompanied by arteries that supply blood to the same region supplied by the spinal nerve. In addition, the *neurovascular bundle* contains veins and lymphatic vessels, which serve to drain away waste products from the same territory. Thus, each segment of the body receives information (and is sending information back to the CNS) as well as nourishment, and each is being drained of waste products. It might appear that each segment functions as a separate entity, but such is not the case. Because of significant overlap both inside and outside the CNS, each segment is "aware" of what is transpiring in the segments adjacent to it.

The individual spinal nerve and all the tissues that it innervates, called the *segment* or the *spinal segment,* is also referred to as the *functional spinal unit* (FSU). The FSU thus includes two adjacent vertebrae and the spinal nerves, skeletal muscles, and fascia between them; other bones, muscles, and fascia associated with the segment (e.g., ribs, intercostal muscles); the blood and lymphatic vessels that supply these tissues; and visceral structures within the body cavities that receive innervation from the autonomic portion of the spinal nerves.

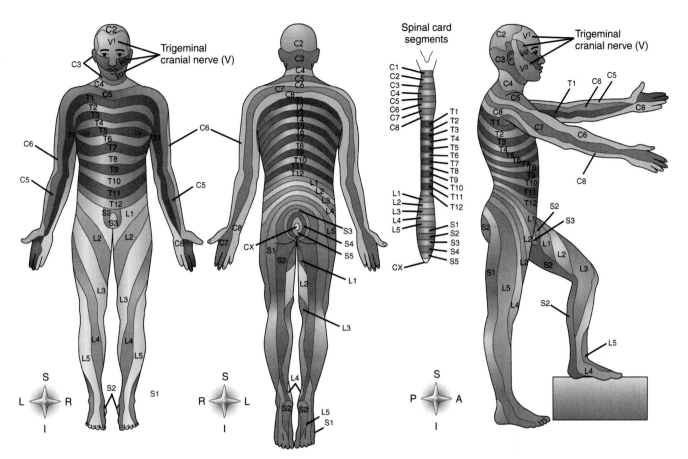

Figure 16-2 Spinal nerves and dermatomes. (Modified from Thibodeau GA, Patton KT: *Anatomy and Physiology,* ed 7, St. Louis: Mosby, 2010.)

CONCEPT 7: REFLEXES AND AUTONOMIC NERVOUS SYSTEM

The CNS, consisting of the brain and spinal cord, can be compared to a computer in that it is designed to integrate and process information. This information basically takes two forms: sensory (input) and motor (output). The most fundamental unit of information processing is the *reflex.* Information enters the CNS through a sensory neuron and is processed in the spinal cord or brain stem through an interaction between the sensory neuron and the motor neuron at a location known as a *synapse.* Motor information then leaves the CNS directly through a motor neuron to effect a response in a skeletal muscle. The most common example of this type of reflex (called *somatic* for the type of tissue involved) is the withdrawal response when a painful stimulus is encountered (e.g., when the hand touches a hot burner). The pain information is relayed through the spinal cord and out to the muscles, which causes the hand's removal before the sensation reaches the cerebral cortex and is perceived.

Although much of the sensory information coming into the CNS reaches consciousness (is perceived), much does not, and we go about our business neither knowing nor feeling what is happening. The same is true of motor activity, which can be voluntary or involuntary (see the discus-sion of the autonomic nervous system later and in Chapter 8). An example of this involuntary phenomenon is the digestive system, which, under normal circumstances, functions without our conscious awareness (with the important daily exception of elimination). With respect to postural maintenance, if we are asked to attend to our position, we are usually able to do so (a test of this system [conscious proprioception] is to ask an individual to close her or his eyes and state the location and position of differ-ent parts, such as the hands and feet). However, we usually are not particularly attentive to our position (unless we lose our balance), and there is an entire division of the pro-prioceptive system (unconscious proprioception) that is never perceived. In short, we are constantly adjusting our-selves to adapt to the gravitational pull of the Earth and our position relative to it, and most of this activity takes place at the level of the reflex.

The autonomic nervous system has as one of its respon-sibilities the unconscious control of visceral structures. These structures include smooth muscle (e.g., surrounding blood vessels and the bronchial tubes), cardiac (heart) muscle, glands, and lymphoid (immune) tissue. There are two divisions of the autonomic nervous system that have opposite actions: the *sympathetic* (thoracolumbar) division, responsible for arousal, or the "fight-or-flight" reaction; and the *parasympathetic* (craniosacral) division, responsible for (among other functions) stimulating the activity of the digestive system, or the "rest and digest" function. Although each division predominates in certain situations, the two divisions normally coexist in balance with one another to maintain a state of homeostasis, which is a form of internal equilibrium. The names "thoracolumbar" and "craniosacral" indicate the origin of the motor nerves of each division. Therefore the spinal nerves of the thoracolumbar region contain both somatic and sympathetic nerve fibers, whereas some of the cranial nerves and sacral nerves contain both somatic and parasympathetic nerve fibers.

Within the CNS, interactions between sensory and motor nerves are constantly taking place through reflexes. Although it has been long known that somatic and visceral reflexes occur, it has only recently been discovered that the two types of reflex loops overlap with one another. That is, stimulation of a visceral structure can produce a somatic response, and stimulation of a somatic structure can elicit a visceral response. This discovery is of extreme importance to the practitioners of manipulation, because it essentially validates the claim that manipulation has global effects on the body, especially with the maintenance or reestablishment of proper blood and lymphatic flow. In fact, it is quite arguable that manipulation of somatic structures (the musculoskeletal system) is entirely capable of restoring proper blood flow to visceral structures through reflexes mediated through the CNS.

CONCEPT 8: PAIN AND GUARDING, MUSCLE SPASM, AND FACILITATION

Patient: "Doc, it hurts when I do this."
Doctor: "Then don't do that!"

Pain is the result of a noxious stimulus that produces tissue damage. This stimulus can come from outside the body, such as a thermal or chemical burn, which is perceived at the skin and produces a classic withdrawal response. The stimulus can also come from inside the body, such as a sprained ankle, in which the damage is perceived at a muscle, joint or ligament.

If pain results from damage to a bone, joint, or ligament, a natural response is for the surrounding muscles to contract reflexively, producing a natural splinting of the area. This is also known as *guarding*. Another result of this type of damage is an altered gait pattern (a limp), which is merely an attempt by the body to "get off" the affected joint if weight bearing causes additional pain. This can also happen when a paravertebral muscle is overstretched from a bending or lifting maneuver. Proprioceptors in that muscle report the stretch, causing a reflex contraction of that muscle. If the amount of damage is sufficient, the reflex contraction becomes stronger, and other muscles in the area are recruited to "guard" against further stretching and damage. The involved muscles are now considered to be in *spasm*. This reaction can spread (through reflex spread within the CNS) until much of the back musculature is

involved. This is what happens when the back "goes out" and the person suffers back spasms. Because of the altered position of the body away from the norm and the prolonged spastic contraction, the involved muscles are required to do much more work than normal, which results in fatigue. When this occurs, muscle contraction results in the compression of local blood vessels, which in turn affects the nutrition of local tissue; this then exacerbates the problem by increasing localized ischemia and can lead to the development of articular dysfunction of associated joints, myofascial trigger points, and associated referred sensations, including pain.

Over time, as more and more sensory input is being fed to the CNS, the nerves that are reporting this information, as well as the nerves that are reacting (the motor neurons), become more sensitive. That is, their threshold for activity becomes significantly reduced. This situation is known as *facilitation,* which can be responsible for neural sensitization in the peripheral as well as central nervous system.

Presumably, muscle spasm lasts until the injury is healed and the surrounding muscles are allowed to release their grip on the area. Sooner or later the spasm will usually resolve on its own. However, this is not always the case, and the spasm can persist on a reduced level. This can cause the vertebrae normally moved by that muscle to become fixed in a certain position. The vertebrae may remain in that fixed position even when the muscle spasm is completely resolved. This also creates a need for a compensatory reaction or altered behavior to avoid the generation of more pain, as with a limp (see discussion in Concept 9). In many patients it is possible to interrupt this cycle by the application of manipulative therapy.

CONCEPT 9: COMPENSATION AND DECOMPENSATION

As mentioned, the proprioceptive system is constantly reporting sensory information to the CNS regarding body position so that postural adjustments can be made, primarily to maintain the eyes parallel to the horizon (horizontal gaze). However, such compensatory behavior becomes more prolonged in certain situations. For example, in a person with one leg longer than the other (asymmetry), the pelvis on the "longer" side would be elevated relative to the other side. Because the sacrum is strongly connected to the pelvic bones, the base on which the fifth lumbar vertebra (L5) rests would be tilted toward the short side. This information would be reported by the proprioceptive system, and a compensation that alters alignment would ensue. The pelvis might move into a pattern of distortion that ultimately levels the sacral plateau or the FSU above the L4–L5 level might produce a compensatory reaction (through muscular contraction) to move the spine back into vertical alignment, creating a scoliotic curve. These compensatory reactions can occur all the way up the spine, as long as the result is a level head. This creates an overall increased load on the musculoskeletal system as a whole and significantly increases the amount of work needed to maintain proper alignment.

In most cases, these responses work well, and no pain or damage is produced. This is especially true in younger people. As a person ages, however, changes in body tissues, most notably loss of water and reduced elasticity, alter the mechanical properties of the body as a whole. Eventually the system fails and begins to decompensate. This results in an increase in the amount and number of compensatory reactions as the system becomes further decompensated; this may eventually lead to tissue damage (usually on the microscopic level), which ultimately leads to pain that may become chronic. This scenario explains in part the preponderance of complaints of low back and neck pain in the general population. In fact, musculoskeletal complaints cause about one third of all the office visits to physicians in the United States. On a holistic or preventive level, intervention to correct a musculoskeletal problem or dysfunction before it becomes chronic or debilitating would be sensible and cost effective in the long run. This is where manipulative therapy is indicated and most effective.

CONCEPT 10: RANGE OF MOTION AND BARRIER CONCEPT

Each joint of the body has a normal direction and amount of motion associated with it. This is referred to as *range of motion* (ROM). When motion is outside of this normal range (a statistical norm that can vary considerably), that joint is said to be "hypermobile" or "hypomobile." In addition, joints with a greater ROM are generally less stable than those with less ROM (e.g., shoulder compared to hip). In the spine the lumbar and cervical areas have the greatest ROM, which establishes an increased probability of instability and injury, especially in the lumbar spine, where significantly greater weight is being borne. This is the principal reason for the relative frequency of lumbar and cervical problems in the general population.

Typically, if there is pain around a joint for any reason, ROM will be decreased or limited. In this case, motion is said to be "restricted." The restriction of motion in a particular direction or plane of space produces a "barrier" to normal motion. However, motion barriers may not necessarily be accompanied by or be the result of pain. In fact, barriers to motion exist under normal circumstances as "anatomical" barriers or "physiological" barriers. A good example of an anatomical barrier is seen in the elbow joint, where the olecranon process of the ulna locks into the olecranon fossa of the humerus, thus preventing overextension of the joint. Therefore the bones themselves present a motion barrier. Joint capsules and ligaments also create anatomical barriers. Physiological barriers are produced by the normal tone of the muscles around a joint, which also act in balance with one another, so that no individual muscle becomes too taut or stretched, as there are conditions that might affects its ability to perform. The proprio-

ceptive system plays an important role in maintaining physiological barriers. If a guarding reaction is present, or if a muscle is in spasm, a temporary physiological motion barrier can be established, in this case referred to as a *restrictive barrier*. In this situation, as previously noted, manipulation can be effective in reducing or eliminating musculoskeletal dysfunction and restoring normal motion.

CONCEPT 11: ACTIVE VERSUS PASSIVE AND DIRECT VERSUS INDIRECT

In treating musculoskeletal disorders with manipulation, two approaches can be used in a variety of techniques. *Active* versus *passive* refers to the activity level of the patient: is the patient actively participating in the treatment, or is the practitioner doing the mechanical work?

Direct versus *indirect* refers to the motion barrier and the practitioner's approach to it. As discussed, a motion barrier is a decrease in normal ROM caused by an increase in the normal physiological motion barrier. The practitioner seeks to remove or release this barrier and restore normal motion. The technique employed can move the affected joint either toward the motion barrier (direct) or away from the barrier (indirect). As a simple example, consider a case in which the flexors of the elbow joint are in spasm, holding the elbow in flexion (bent) and creating a barrier to extension (straightening). A direct technique would be an attempt to move the joint into extension, that is, into or toward the motion barrier. An indirect technique would be to move the elbow joint further into flexion, producing a change in the position of the joint, which would be reported by the muscle and joint proprioceptors. Over a short time, this causes a reflex release of the spastic contraction of the flexor muscles, thereby eliminating the motion barrier. These concepts are incorporated in the manual application of positional release, strain–counterstrain, and other techniques.

The various techniques and healing traditions relating to manual and physical manipulations described in this section have their effects based on these eleven principles, which describe the movement of the human body as an object in space and living on Earth. In addition, many of these "hands-on" techniques consider the human body to have an energetic component whereby physical manipulations also affect the energy of the body, as well as the "mind–body." It is useful to keep in mind this duality of human beings (both as physical bodies and as energetic bodies) when reading the chapters of this section.

SUMMARY

In summary, the practitioner of manual therapy seeks to restore proper anatomical and physiological balance in the patient. At least three types and subtypes of balance are potential targets of the various styles and techniques employed, as follows:

1. The restoration of proper joint range of motion and body symmetry

2. The restoration of balance of nervous activity
   a. Between sensory and motor systems
   b. Between somatic and autonomic nerves
   c. Between the sympathetic and parasympathetic divisions of the autonomic nervous system
3. The restoration of proper arterial flow and venous and lymphatic drainage for proper nutrition to and drainage of all tissues of the body.

References

McCown DM, Micozzi MS: *New World Mindfulness*, Rochester, VT, 2012, Healing Arts Press/Inner Traditions.

Thibodeau GA, Patton KT: *Anatomy and Physiology*, ed 7, St. Louis, 2010, Mosby.

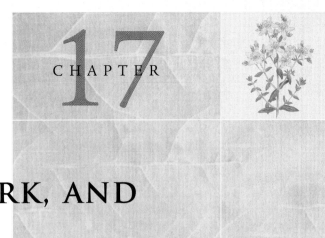

CHAPTER 17

Massage, Bodywork, and Touch Therapies

JUDITH DELANY

Massage and other interventions that use therapeutic touch include a wide variety of approaches that fall under a simplistic definition of "manual therapies." These manual modalities use the practitioner's hands, as well as elbows, forearms, and even feet, to directly apply techniques (sometimes called "manual manipulation") to the patient's body for the purpose of enhancing health and well-being. Chiropractic (Chapter 19) and osteopathic (Chapter 18) techniques as well as many aspects of physical, occupational therapy, and athletic training would, in the broadest sense, fit within this definition. These modalities are often combined with massage and other touch therapies to synergistically enhance healing.

Within the modality of massage, there is a diverse spectrum of therapeutic applications that offer a broad range of viewpoints. That is, a variety of "lenses" can be used to view the body, such as through structure, function, movement, neural communication, or energetic means. The practitioner's perspective will influence which application is chosen and that, in turn, will determine which techniques will be employed to best achieve the goals. Factors as diverse as the rate of speed of movement of the hand on the skin, the depth of pressure used, whether lubrication is employed, or whether the hand even contacts the body will combine to shape the desired outcomes for a given session.

Manual manipulation as a therapeutic practice has existed for thousands of years and is as natural to life as taking a breath. Mennell (1951) stated, "Beyond all doubt the use of the human hand, as a method of reducing human suffering, is the oldest remedy known to man; historically no date can be given for its adoption." Although the date of origin of the earliest forms of manipulative therapy is unknown, it has been recorded that Hippocrates was skilled in the use of manipulation and taught it in his school of medicine, more than 2000 years ago. A few cherished drawings tell stories of the use of manual therapies prior to written historical records. In China, the history of manual therapy (tui na) predates the development of the technology necessary to produce the needles used for acupuncture, 3000 to 5000 years ago (Figure 17-1).

All the world's cultures can demonstrate the use of manual manipulation as a form of therapy. However, much of this information has been passed on as an oral rather than a written tradition, so documentation is difficult or impossible to obtain in many cases. Consequently, the types of manipulative therapy presented here are those for which information is readily available. In modern times, manual therapies include applications from all over the world, with numerous ways to learn them. In addition to traditional live class or apprentice formats, techniques are taught on DVD, online, in webinars, and through international live broadcasts. The evolution of science-based platforms and research-based investigations reflect a deep need for ongoing inquiry and an ever-evolving understanding of the body and the way that manual therapies affect it. This chapter describes the basic principles and theories of many well-known modalities; it is not totally inclusive of all that exist, nor does it include an extensive discussion of some that are mentioned.

THE BODY'S MATRIX—FASCIA

Whether the modality targets the osseous, muscular, visceral, or even acupuncture structures, it affects, in one way or another, a common integral component—fascia, the

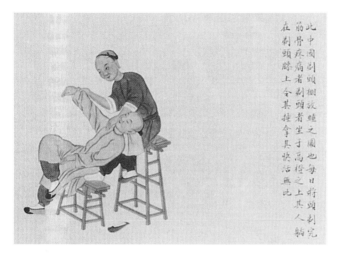

Figure 17-1 A patient receiving manipulation of the shoulder. Joint manipulation has always been an important feature of Chinese medical treatment. (Courtesy The Wellcome Trustees, London.)

colloidal matrix of the body. Fascia comprises one integrated and totally connected network, from the soles of the feet to the attachments on the inner aspects of the skull, and divides the body by diaphragms, septa, and sheaths. However, fascia is so much more than just a background element with an obvious supporting role. It is a ubiquitous, tenacious, living tissue that is deeply involved in almost all of the body's fundamental processes, including its structure, function, and metabolism.

In therapeutic terms, there can be little logic in trying to consider muscles as separate structures from fascia because they are so intimately related. Chaitow and DeLany (2008) note the following:

- Fascia attaches extensively to and invests into muscles, by providing individual muscle fibers with an envelope of endomysium that blends into the stronger perimysium surrounding the fasciculi, which, in turn, merges into an even stronger epimysium that surrounds the muscle as a whole and attaches to fascial tissues nearby. The fascial planes provide pathways for nerves, blood, and lymphatic vessels and a supporting matrix for more highly organized structures, such as the viscera.
- Fascia comprises the intermuscular septa and interosseous membranes, which provide surfaces used for muscular attachment. Restraining mechanisms, such as retention bands, fibrous pulleys, and check ligaments, are invested with fascia that assists in the production and control of movement. Where the texture is loose, it allows movement between adjacent structures and it can also mitigate the effects of pressure by forming fluid-filled sacs, called bursae, which reduce friction of tendons against underlying bones.
- Fibroblastic activity in fascia aids in the repair of injuries by the deposition of collagenous fibers (scar tissue); superficial fascia allows for the storage of fat

(panniculus adiposis), which aids in the conservation of body heat.
- Connective tissue houses nearly a quarter of all body fluids, providing an essential medium through which the cellular elements of other tissues are brought into functional relation with blood and lymph; fluids and infectious processes often travel along fascial planes. Phagocytic activity of the histiocytes in fascia provides an important defense mechanism against bacterial invasion and plays a role as scavengers in removing cell debris and foreign material.
- Remove connective tissue from the scene and any muscle left would be a jelly-like structure without form and no longer capable of performing its function.

When any part of the fascial network becomes distorted, resultant and compensating adaptive stresses can be imposed elsewhere on the structures that it divides, envelops, enmeshes, and supports, and with which it connects. The consequences of a structural cascade are not limited to the structural elements of muscle, tendon, ligament, bone, and disk. Pressure can also be imposed on the neural, blood, and lymph components, which course alongside and through them, and on the visceral organs and glands. Varying degrees of fascial entrapment of neural structures can, in turn, produce a wide range of symptoms and dysfunctions, such as by triggering the neural receptors within the fascia that report to the central nervous system (CNS) as part of any adaptation process. The sources of such signaling might include the pacinian corpuscles, which inform the CNS about the rate of acceleration of movement taking place in the area; the highly specialized, sensitive mechanoreceptors and proprioceptive reporting stations contained in the tendons and ligaments; or the hormones excreted by the glands, which serve as the chemical messengers of metabolism.

Massage and other manual techniques can be used to manipulate the connective tissues, which affect the fascia by altering its ground substance, elongates shortened tissues, and improves the biochemical environment of the cells. A diverse array of massage techniques and systems of application can offer a variety of effects on isolated tissues, overall structural integrity, and general well-being of the individual.

MASSAGE APPLICATION

As with other manipulative forms of therapy, some uses of massage may predate written history (Figure 17-2). The Greek physician Aesculapius, historically credited as the inventor of the art of gymnastics (Nissen, 1889), became perhaps the first practitioner of the "one cause, one cure" approach when he abandoned other forms of contemporary medical treatment in favor of massage to restore the free movement of body fluids and return the patient to a state of health. During the Renaissance, physician Ambroise Paré, author of a widely used surgery text, espoused the application of massage and manipulation and was

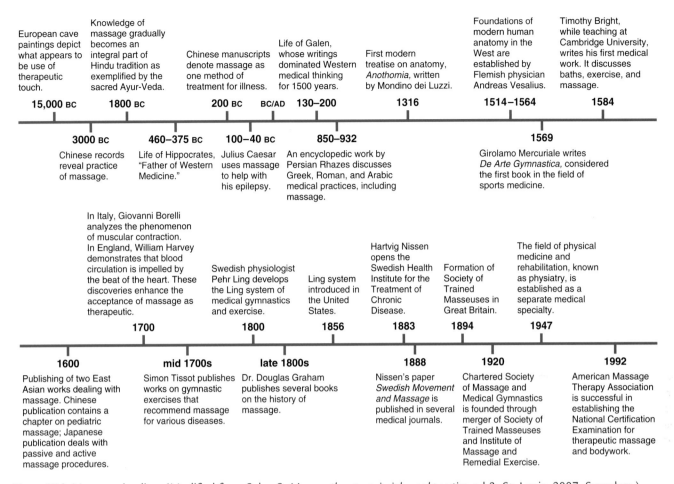

Figure 17-2 Massage timeline. (Modified from Salvo S: *Massage therapy: principles and practice,* ed 3, St. Louis, 2007, Saunders.)

reportedly the first to use the term *subluxation.* In 1813, Pehr Henrik Ling, a gymnastics instructor, founded the Royal Gymnastic Central Institute, where his systematic routine of formal movements and passive gymnastics (Swedish Movement Cure) was developed. Although his work contained minimal massage techniques, it is often erroneously given credit as the forerunner of contemporary Swedish massage, which might be better appropriated to one of his students, Johann Georg Metzger (Casanelia & Stelfox, 2010; Pettman, 2007). Even so, Ling is still considered by many to be the founder of modern massage.

Metzger, a Dutch physician, developed a basic classification of massage techniques. Although Metzger's work was never published, his students von Mosengeil and Helleday wrote and published descriptions of the techniques and the classifications, using the French terms still used today (effleurage, pétrissage, tapotement, etc.) (Orstrom, 1918). In the late nineteenth century, the prominent French physician Marie Marcellin Lucas-Championnière advocated the use of massage therapy in the treatment of fractures, arguing the case for consideration of soft tissue union in the healing process. His students, English physicians William Bennett and Robert Jones, effectively brought massage to England. Bennett incorporated the use of massage at St. George's Hospital in London around 1899,

and Jones used massage therapy at the Southern Hospital in Liverpool. Jones taught both James Mennell, author of the text *Physical Treatment by Movement, Manipulation, and Massage* (1917) and a tireless advocate of massage, and Mary McMillan, who was very influential in the introduction and promotion of massage in the United States. Around the turn of the twentieth century, Isidor Zabludowski, a professor of massage at the University of Berlin in Germany, brought science and credibility to the application of massage, while Dr. John Harvey Kellogg (see Chapter 22) completed extensive documentation as to the effects of massage at his "nature cure" institute in Battle Creek, Michigan, USA.

There are many others who contributed both to the development of massage techniques and to documentation of massage through research and writing. Early in the twentieth century, several made significant and long-lasting contributions:

- Albert Hoffa's techniques, described in his text *Technik der Massage*, published in 1900, are still in use today. Hoffa advocated the limitation of massage to 15-minute treatments, with no pain experienced by the patient. Like Ling, Hoffa stated that massage should be applied from distal to proximal, with the point of reference being the heart. His adaptations included knuckling and circular effleurage, two-finger pétrissage, and other forms.

- Mary McMillan is credited with the categorization of massage into its five basic techniques. In each of those categories, she introduced innovative variations. She advocated the use of olive oil as a lubricant for its nutritional value when absorbed through the skin. Her influence in the development of massage is universally recognized, and her techniques have been widely adopted by massage therapists in the United States and elsewhere.

- Elisabeth Dicke, proponent of Bindegewebsmassage ("binding webs" massage) was a student of Hoffa who described massage based on the connective tissue system of the body. She described areas of referred pain on the back that indicate internal pathology but do not necessarily correspond to segmental distribution. Areas of tenderness do correspond to certain acupuncture points. Treatment is given with the middle finger in a series of sequenced strokes without lubricant.

- James Cyriax was a strong advocate of friction as the most effective technique in massage. He developed the "transverse friction massage" technique, which is widely used by manual therapists. Deep friction massage is used to stimulate increased circulation to the affected area. It can be applied to muscles, tendons, ligaments, and bones. Cyriax (1984) described these methods in detail in his book *Textbook of Orthopaedic Medicine*, volume 2.

- Janet Travell (one of President John F. Kennedy's physicians in the early 1960s) and David Simons, both medical doctors in the United States, researched myofascial trigger points for half a century, documenting their locations and patterns of referral. Their extensive efforts produced two significant textbooks: *Myofacial Pain and Dysfunction: The Trigger Point Manual, vol 1: The Upper Half of Body* and *Volume 2: The Lower Extremities* (Simons et al, 1999; Travell & Simons, 1992). Their work provided the foundation for a new branch of medicine and fodder for researchers worldwide who are continuing to uncover new elements of understanding of myofascia.

DEVELOPMENT OF ESSENTIAL THEORIES OF MASSAGE

As awareness of this form of treatment grew, so did the science of physiology, and the two entities became intertwined with the growth of the Western scientific basis of medicine. Some authors attribute the development of the physical therapy profession as being an outgrowth of massage. Many other forms of so-called bodywork, an assortment of which are discussed in this chapter, are also outgrowths of massage and its various techniques and styles.

One essential theory of massage therapy is based on the principle that the tissues of the body will function at optimal levels when arterial supply and venous and lymphatic drainage are unimpeded ("rule of the artery"). When this flow becomes unbalanced for any reason, muscle tightness and changes in the nearby skin and fascia will ensue, which may result in pain. The basic techniques of massage are designed to re-establish proper fluid dynamics and are directed at the skin, muscles, and fascia, although nerve pathways occasionally are included. In general, aside from passive or active range of motion, articulations are not directly addressed in this form of therapy, although they certainly may be affected by the applied techniques.

Obvious contraindications to massage or areas to avoid during the application of massage include skin infections or melanoma, bleeding (especially within 48 hours of a traumatic event causing bleeding into tissues), acute inflammation (e.g., rheumatoid arthritis, appendicitis), thrombophlebitis, atherosclerosis, varicose veins, and immunocompromised state (to avoid transmission of infection from massage practitioner to patient). Certain procedures (e.g., radiation therapy), medications (e.g., blood thinners), or conditions (e.g., osteoporosis, recent fractures) may contraindicate deeper pressure, friction, or range-of-motion work. In addition, a number of endangerment sites require that extra caution be exercised, such as the region of the carotid artery, suboccipital triangle, supraclavicular fossa, posterior knee, femoral triangle, and abdominal cavity. Specific training may also be required, such as for intraoral applications or for work with lymphedema and cancer patients.

The techniques of massage are generally applied in the direction of the heart to stimulate increased venous and lymphatic drainage from the involved tissues. Muscles are addressed in groups, with one group usually being treated before advancing to the next. Different combinations of techniques are used depending on the objectives of treatment. Treatment typically begins with more gentle, superficial techniques before progressing to deeper, or more aggressive applications. Traditional massage is often performed with a powder, oil, or other type of lubricant applied to the skin of the patient (client), who lies prone, supine, or laterally on a table, or who may be seated in a massage chair. A variety of techniques also exist that use no lubricant or only a thin film (e.g., Rolfing™, structural bodywork), and entire approaches may be performed without lubrication (e.g., lymphatic drainage, craniosacral therapy). Verbal communication between the practitioner and patient is important, because the practitioner will use the cues given by the patient as a guide during the treatment.

The visceral effects of massage include general vasoactivity in somatic tissues as regulated by the autonomic nervous system. Also, effects on blood pressure and/or heart rate (usually decreases in both) can be observed as the person relaxes during the treatment.

MASSAGE TECHNIQUES

In its simplest form, there are five basic techniques of massage, and all are of the passive variety (i.e., the practitioner does the work). These techniques are effleurage, pétrissage, friction, tapotement, and vibration. There are numerous variations of these basic techniques, which may create different outcomes within the tissue. For instance, effleurage applied at a moderate pace with lubrication increases blood flow and lymphatic drainage. However, effleurage applied with almost no lubrication at a very slow pace produces a shearing force on the tissue that focuses more on changing the ground substance of the fascia. These variations in application provide a vast array of styles, methods, and versions of massage, each with its own foundational platform, despite their common roots in the basic techniques.

- Effleurage is the most frequently applied massage technique and is typically used to begin a treatment session and introduce the patient to the process of touching (Figure 17-3). Effleurage is a gliding stroke applied with light to moderate pressure (superficial or deep), serving to modulate the arterial supply and venous and lymphatic drainage of the tissues contacted. The amount of pressure applied determines the layer of the body contacted; very light pressure affects primarily the skin, deeper pressure the superficial fascia, even deeper pressure the deep fascia, and so on. The thumbs, fingers, or entire palmar surface of the hand is used. A "knuckling" technique may be employed, or the proximal half of the ulna can provide a very broad surface of application.

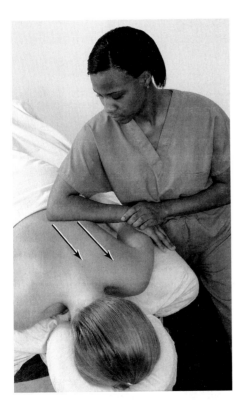

Figure 17-3 Effleurage can be applied with thumbs, fingers, palms, or forearm (as shown here). (Modified from Salvo S: *Massage therapy: principles and practice,* ed 3, St. Louis, 2007, Saunders.)

When used during the initial stages of treatment, effleurage is also used as a palpation diagnostic tool, as the practitioner searches for areas of altered texture or density, asymmetry, or tenderness. Specific long strokes are often used at the conclusion of treatment, especially if sleep induction is desired.

- Pétrissage is somewhat more aggressive than effleurage, with the thumb and fingers working together to lift and "milk" the underlying fascia and muscles in a kneading motion. Care is taken not to pinch or produce bruising. The effect of pétrissage is to increase venous and lymphatic drainage of the muscles and to break up adhesions (small areas of local fibrosis) that may be present in the fascia. Depending on the direction of application and vector of motion restriction (if any), this technique can be considered direct or indirect.

- Friction (frottage) can be the most deeply applied massage technique (Figure 17-4). The tips of the fingers or thumb are used in a circular, longitudinal, or transverse movement. If deeper pressure is desired, or if the practitioner is easily fatigued, the heel of the hand, or sometimes even the elbow, can be used. Friction can be employed when production of heat is desired, when adhesions are present, or when the target tissue is too deep for pétrissage. Cyriax developed the technique of transverse friction massage, which is widely used by physical therapists. As with pétrissage, the direction of the applied technique, relative to any motion restriction, will determine whether the application is direct or indirect.

- Tapotement, often seen in classic boxing films, involves rapid, repeated blows of varying strength delivered with the tips of the fingers, with the sides or palms of the hands, with the hands cupped, or with the fists. Occasionally, rapid pinching of the skin is done. The purpose of tapotement is to stimulate arterial circulation to the area; however, its ability to inhibit reflexive spasms or to restore tone to hypotonic muscles should not be underestimated. Again, the technique should not produce bruising and is not applied over the area of the kidneys or on the chest, or over any recent incisions or areas of inflammation or contusion.

- Vibration that is manually applied is usually considered to be one of the more difficult of the massage techniques to master or to perform without becoming fatigued. The modern application of vibration typically employs a mechanical vibrator or oscillator of some type. When the hands are used, a light, rhythmic, quivering effect is achieved. Brisk snapping or strumming across certain tissues, such as erector spinae muscles, can also be considered a form of vibration, an effect that is similar to the vibration of a guitar string when strummed.

In addition, forces may be applied to the tissue that alters its length, mobility, and density. For instance, a shear force can be applied to a superficial muscle layer to slide it laterally across the underlying muscle and disengage it from a

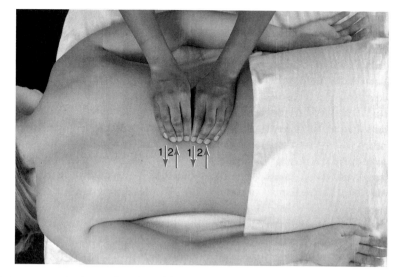

Figure 17-4 Friction applied to paraspinal muscles. (Modified from Salvo S: *Massage therapy: principles and practice,* ed 3, St. Louis, 2007, Saunders.)

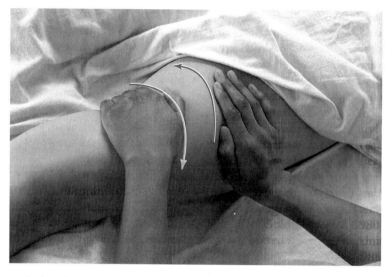

Figure 17-5 Shearing forces applied to the fascia of the anterior thigh. (Modified from Salvo S: *Massage therapy: principles and practice,* ed 3, St. Louis, 2007, Saunders.)

deeper layer, which results in more mobility between the two (Figure 17-5). Stretching a muscle's fibers can elongate the muscle and result in decompression of the associated joint(s). Elongation of a fascial plane might alter postural alignment and result in improved biomechanics of the region or of the structure body as a whole.

VARIATIONS IN APPLICATION OF TECHNIQUES

As mentioned previously, variations of these basic techniques produce different outcomes within the tissue. As a result, a multitude of methods, versions, and styles of massage have emerged, with many having broad perspectives regarding application.

In *TouchAbilities® Essential Connections,* Burman and Friedland (2006) suggest that these basic techniques form a central, unifying skill set for all massage applications that crosses global, cultural, philosophical, and theoretical foundations. Although the depth of pressure, tension applied, sequence, order, and even the inclusion of some techniques, varies among the applications, or even within an application, the techniques themselves contribute to this fundamental set of skills.

Burman and Friedland (2006) suggest that the skill set can be distilled to eight components that identify and define the main aspects of relating to and engaging with the body. They state that within those categories, 26 core skills (listed below) serve as the building blocks of all techniques that are utilized by the various massage applications. DeLany (2012) offers the following succinct list from Burman and Friedland's work.

1. BREATHING (tracking, directing, pacing) engages the mechanism of respiration, which creates waves that affect every system of the body.
2. COGNITIVE (visualizing, inquiring, intending, focusing transmitting) are tools for assessment, enhancement, modification, and change.
3. ENERGY (sensing, intuiting, balancing) is effective in detecting distortions and assisting the body to establish balance.
4. COMPRESSION (pressing/pushing, squeezing/pinching, twisting/wringing) applies a force to the body, reducing the space within and between structures and pressing fluid out.
5. EXPANSION (pulling, lifting, rolling) opens up space within and between the structures, bringing fluid into them.
6. KINETICS (holding/supporting, mobilizing, letting go/dropping, stabilizing) focuses on the movement relationship between segments of the body.
7. OSCILLATION (vibrating, shaking, striking) initiates waves by applying intermittent or continuous vibratory contact.
8. GLIDING (sliding/planing, rubbing) follows the contours of skin, muscle, tendon, ligament, bone, and fascial layers.

To achieve any intended outcome for a given application, the practitioner simply blends these basic elements to achieve the desired change within the myofascial tissues. Whether one views massage as simply five basic techniques, or prefers to categorize all tangible and intangible components as suggested above, the aim is the same. That is, with practice, the practitioner can move seamlessly from one technique or skill to another as needed, with decisions being driven in the moment by what is discovered within the tissues.

Although some of the concepts discussed later in the synopsis of various types of massage may seem foreign to the reader, it is worth remembering that many of these applications are centuries, if not millennia, old, far exceeding the experience in the practice of modern medicine. In particular, the Eastern theoretical platforms may contain concepts that do not appear to relate to Western understanding, especially those involving energy, meridians, and mysterious acupuncture points. However, with open and curious minds, even those most academically rooted in the Western paradigm can find evidence to support the Eastern principles. The following discussion (after Chaitow & DeLany, 2008) provides one example of how Eastern ideas can fit easily into a Western model when research provides physiological support.

Many experts believe that trigger points (see neuromuscular therapy discussion, p. 264) and acupuncture points are the same phenomenon (Kawakita et al, 2002; Melzack et al, 1977; Plummer, 1980). When traditional and ah shi acupuncture points are both included, approximately 80% of common trigger point sites have been claimed to lie precisely where traditional acupuncture points are situated on meridian maps (Wall & Melzack, 1990). Some (Birch, 2003; Hong, 2000) find this percentage to be flawed, particularly when the trigger points are correlated with acupuncture points that are seen to be "fixed" anatomically, as on myofascial meridian maps. When examining the validity of the findings reported by Birch (2003), Dorsher (2008) reviewed references and literature to conclude that the overlap is significant, perhaps as high as 95%. Although this debate of percentage of overlap may never be settled, most of these authors agree that so-called acupuncture points may well represent the same phenomenon as trigger points.

Ah shi points do not appear on the classical acupuncture meridian maps, but refer to "spontaneously tender" points that, when pressed, create a response in the patient of, "Oh yes!" (*ah shi*). In Chinese medicine, ah shi points are treated as "honorary acupuncture points" and, when tender or painful, are addressed in the same way as regular acupuncture points (see Chapter 29). Could they be, in all but name, identical to trigger points?

It is clearly important, therefore, in attempting to understand trigger points more fully, to pay attention to current research into acupuncture points and connective tissue in general. Ongoing research at the University of Vermont, led by Dr. Helene Langevin, has produced remarkable new information regarding the function of fascia/connective tissue as well as its relation to the location of acupuncture points and energy meridians (Ahn et al, 2010; Langevin & Yandow, 2002; Langevin et al, 2001, 2002, 2004, 2005).

Langevin and colleagues present evidence that links the network of acupuncture points and meridians to a network formed by interstitial connective tissue. Using a unique dissection and charting method for location of connective tissue (fascial) planes, acupuncture points and acupuncture meridians of the arm, they note that, overall, more than 80% of acupuncture points and 50% of meridian intersections of the arm appeared to coincide with intermuscular or intramuscular connective tissue planes (Langevin & Yandow, 2002).

Langevin's research further shows microscopic evidence that when an acupuncture needle is inserted and rotated (as is classically performed in acupuncture treatment), a "whorl" of connective tissue forms around the needle, thereby creating a tight mechanical coupling between the tissue and the needle. The tension placed on the connective tissue as a result of further movements of the needle delivers a mechanical stimulus at the cellular level. They note that changes in the extracellular matrix may, in turn, influence the various cell populations sharing this connective tissue matrix (e.g., fibroblasts, sensory afferents, immune and vascular cells).

Chaitow and DeLany (2008) summarize the key elements of Langevin's research as follows:

- Acupuncture points, and many of the effects of acupuncture, seem to relate to the fact that most of these localized "points" lie directly over areas where there is fascial cleavage, where sheets of fascia diverge to separate, surround, and support different muscle bundles (Langevin et al, 2001).

- Connective tissue is a communication system of as yet unknown potential. Ingber and Folkman (1989), Ingber (1993), and Chen and Ingber (1999) demonstrated integrins (tiny projections emerging from each cell) to comprise a cellular signaling system that modify their function depending on the relative normality of the shape of cells. The structural integrity (shape) of cells depends on the overall state of normality (e.g., deformed, stretched) of the fascia as a whole.

- Langevin et al (2004) report: "'Loose' connective tissue forms a network extending throughout the body including subcutaneous and interstitial connective tissues. The existence of a cellular network of fibroblasts within loose connective tissue may have considerable significance as it may support yet unknown body-wide cellular signaling systems. . . . Our findings indicate that soft tissue fibroblasts form an extensively interconnected cellular network, suggesting they may have important, and so far unsuspected integrative functions at the level of the whole body."

- Perhaps the most fascinating research in this remarkable series of discoveries is that cells change their shape and behavior following stretching (and crowding or deformation). The observation of these researchers is that "the dynamic, cytoskeleton-dependent responses of fibroblasts to changes in tissue length demonstrated in this study have important implications for our understanding of normal movement and posture, as well as therapies using mechanical stimulation of connective tissue, including physical therapy, massage and acupuncture" (Langevin et al, 2005).

As more clinicians seek to understand the role that fascia plays in chronic pain, structural deterioration, and illness, researchers will respond with evidence of cellular, structural, and systemic components of this complex matrix. The International Fascia Research Congress, composed of scientists, researchers, and clinicians worldwide who share an interest in human fascial tissues, meets every two or three years to share the latest global scientific research on fascia. More information can be found at www.fasciacongress.org.

Additionally, as one can readily observe everywhere, there are many "less than ideal" outcomes in modern patient care. It is important to consider that the following methods often offer significant relief to the suffering patient, with virtually no risk for potential injury or death. In an environment in which the costs of health care are out of control, the promised government-mandated "affordable" care is proving to more expensive still, and the potential for medical error is seriously increasing, use of these therapeutic interventions is proving to be practical, prudent, and economical.

The various massage styles and methods included in the following discussion are arranged alphabetically, with no indication as to which is most useful or more popular. The method's inclusion in the list and the length of any particular discussion only indicates the authors' familiarity with and/or interest in the method and does not imply its success, value, or appropriate use. Similarly, exclusion from this list simply indicates the vast diversity of this modality and the obvious restrictions applied in writing a chapter for this book, one that can only touch, so to speak, on the value, range, and scope of manual techniques. All appropriate touch therapies have intrinsic value, the degree of which is likely to be dependent on the practitioner's degree of mastery and the patient's receptivity.

ACUPRESSURE AND JIN SHIN DO

Acupressure is the application of the fingers to acupuncture points on the body, or "acupuncture without needles." It is based on the meridian or channel system, which permeates Asian medical arts and philosophy. According to this system, there are 12 major channels through which the body's energy, or qi (chi), flows. Although most of the channels are named for specific organs, they do not necessarily correspond to the anatomical body part, but rather are more functional in nature. Interruptions in the flow of qi (*prana*, ki, vital energy, as described in other cultures) cause functional aberrations associated with that particular channel. These interruptions can be released by specific application of needles or fingers.

Jin shin do, or the "way of the compassionate spirit," was developed by psychotherapist Iona Teeguarden (1978). It is a form of acupressure in which the fingers are used to apply deep pressure to hypersensitive acupuncture points. *Jin shin do* represents a synthesis of Taoist philosophy, psychology, breathing, and acupressure techniques. In accordance with this philosophy, the body is linked to the mind and spirit, and tender points found in the body can represent expressions of emotional trauma or locked memories (i.e., the somatoemotional component) (Figure 17-6).

The theory of *jin shin do* states that various stimuli cause energy to accumulate in acupuncture points. Repeated stress in turn causes a layering of tension at the point, known as *armoring*. The most painful point is termed the *local point* as a frame of reference. Other related tender points are referred to as *distal points*. Deep pressure applied to the point ultimately causes a release, and the tension dissipates. The overall effect is to reestablish flow in the channel and balance body energy. The context of the *jin shin do* treatment is as much psychological as physical and reiterates the importance of the body–mind–spirit philosophy of this treatment form.

During the treatment session the practitioner identifies a local point and "asks permission" nonverbally to treat it. A finger is placed on the local point while another finger is applied to a distal point. Gradually increasing pressure is applied to the local point. After 1 or 2 minutes, the practitioner feels the muscle relaxing, followed by a pulsation (practitioners of craniosacral therapy refer to this

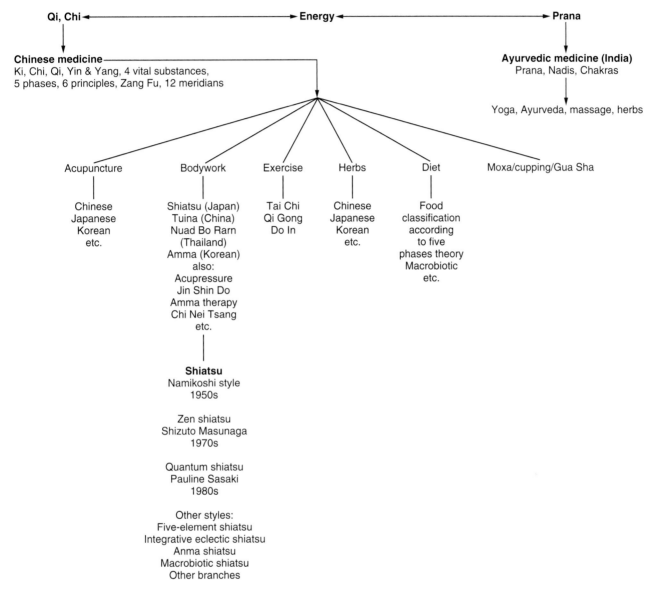

Traditional Asian Medicine
2500 to 4000 years old

Figure 17-6 Traditional Asian medicine focuses on the assessment and balancing of energetic systems. (Modified from Salvo S: *Massage therapy: principles and practice,* ed 3, St. Louis, 2007, Saunders.)

phenomenon as the "therapeutic pulse"). When the pulsing stops, the patient usually reports a decreased sensitivity at the point, indicating a successful treatment. Myofascial releases are sometimes accompanied by emotional releases as painful or emotional memories are brought to consciousness.

AYURVEDIC MANIPULATION

In Sanskrit, *Ayurveda* means "the study or science of life." As a healing art, Ayurveda is one of the world's oldest and, like the Indian culture, probably predates traditional Chinese medicine (TCM). As with TCM, Ayurveda has

many concepts and components, as discussed elsewhere in this book (Chapter 31). However, several principles pervade Ayurveda (as they do in TCM) and apply to the manual component of Ayurvedic treatment.

Both Ayurvedic and Chinese theory present five basic elements. In contrast to those of Chinese theory (fire, water, earth, wood, metal), however, Ayurveda defines space (ether), air, fire, water, and earth as the five basic elements. These elements flow through the body with one or more predominating in certain areas, corresponding to specific organs, emotions, and other categories. *Prana,* or the life force (cf. qi, ki), also flows through the body, permeating the organs and tissues, and is especially concentrated at various points along the midline of the body, known as *chakras*.

The unity and balance of body, mind, and spirit have deep cultural roots in Ayurveda. Body structure and a person's actions, feelings, and beliefs all reflect, and are reflected in, his or her constitution. The human constitution is based on the relative proportions and strengths of these three constituents (mind, body, spirit) and the five elements. Three basic types of constitutions (*doshas*) are recognized, which are based on different combinations of the five elements. The first, *vata*, is a combination of air and space and is reflected in kinetic energy. The second, *pitta*, combines fire and water and reflects a balance between kinetic and potential (stored) energy, which is expressed in the third constitution, *kapha*, a combination of earth and water.

The manipulative treatment developed within the Ayurvedic tradition offers three types of touch. *Tamasic* is strong and solid, firmly rooted in the earth (and might be well suited for a kapha constitution). The application is fast, and time is needed for the mind and spirit to "catch up." Tamasic might correspond to a high-velocity low-amplitude technique (osteopathy, chiropractic), tapotement (massage), or rubbing and thumb rocking (TCM). The second type of touch, *rajasic*, is slower and is used to expand and integrate initial manual explorations and findings. It is more in resonance with the mind and spirit. As mentioned earlier, greater depth can be achieved with less tissue resistance due to the makeup of the body fascia. Effleurage (massage) and myofascial release (osteopathy, massage) might correspond to this type of touch, which in turn might be more suited to a pitta constitution. The vata constitution might benefit from the third type of touch, *satvic*, in which the application is very slow and gentle and can follow the intention of the mind and spirit. This might correspond to cranial osteopathy, sacro-occipital technique (chiropractic), counterstrain (osteopathy), Trager work, the Feldenkrais method, or healing or therapeutic touch (massage).

In a massage-oriented treatment, different essential oils are used as lubricants according to the constitution of the individual and the problem to be treated. The patient is prone or supine, lying on either side, or sitting up, with the positions arranged in a specific sequence. Strokes are applied either toward or away from the heart, also in a specific sequence. Another technique, which is rarely encountered, uses the feet to perform the manipulation. The practitioner stands above the patient, who is lying prone on a reed mat, and applies the technique with the feet. Oils again are used as lubricants and, to maintain balance, the practitioner holds onto a cord strung lengthwise above the patient. The strokes go from the sacrum up the spine and out to the fingers, then back down to the feet. One side is done, then the other. The patient then lies supine, and the process is repeated.

Techniques can be direct or indirect relative to motion barriers. They can also be active or passive. Both the patient and the practitioner act as partners during treatment, exploring tissue and motion in an attempt to unlock the body and restore the unimpeded flow of prana and constitutional balance. Visualization, nonverbal communication, and mind intent are elements of treatment, regardless of the technique employed.

CRANIOSACRAL THERAPY

Craniosacral therapy originated from cranial osteopathy (osteopathic techniques applied to the cranium), as developed by W.G. Sutherland in the mid-1900s. (See also osseous techniques later in this chapter, and Chapter 18.) Sutherland's work was based on the observation that the joints between the skull bones are meant to permit motion just as do joints in other areas of the body. While palpating these bones and joints, he discovered the existence of a very subtle rhythm in the body unrelated to cardiovascular or breathing rhythms. Sutherland named this rhythm the cranial rhythmic impulse (CRI). This impulse, he learned, was capable of moving the cranial bones through a range of motion (ROM) that, although very small, was palpable to well-trained hands (Figure 17-7). Cranial theory posits that there is inherent motility of the CNS, resulting in fluctuations of the cerebrospinal fluid, which bathes the brain and spinal cord. This fluctuation, in turn, moves the cranial bones through their small yet palpable ROM.

These concepts were expanded further in the 1970s by the findings of a research team at Michigan State University, supervised by Dr. John Upledger. They confirmed that the motion associated with this rhythm is not restricted to the cranial bones and that, because the cranium is linked to the sacrum by the dural membranes, which cover the CNS, the motion is palpable in the sacrum as well. In addition, through the fascial–fluid system, this motion has effects all over the body. Motion restrictions in this system can be palpated and corrected (either directly or indirectly) through very gentle manipulation, also with global effects. Based on these concepts, craniosacral therapy has emerged as a separate and distinct modality.

As releases are produced in this fascial system and throughout the body, memories (sometimes emotionally painful) can be reawakened and produce "somatoemotional release," a form of mind–body connection. Clinical experience suggests that these experiences occur frequently, although it is not understood at this time whether this is due to the proximity of the membranes to the brain, stimulation of associated neural circuitry in peripheral tissues, or some other mechanism.

Craniosacral therapy has been controversial from its inception because of the lack of definitive, objective experimental evidence. Because research studies that could conclusively evaluate the effectiveness of cranial therapies have not been performed to date, evidence of effectiveness comes almost exclusively in the form of clinical case reports and testimonials. Successes have been reported in improving a variety of conditions, including chronic headache, cerebral

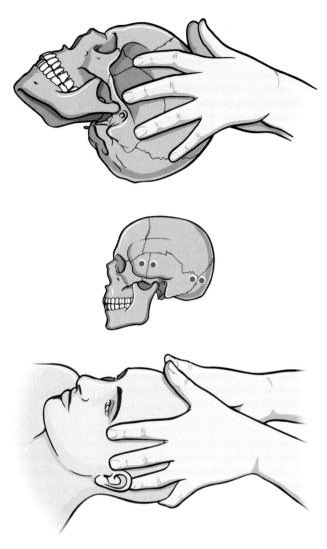

Figure 17-7 Vault hold for cranial palpation. (Borrowed with permission from Chaitow L, DeLany J: *Clinical application of neuromuscular techniques,* vol 1, ed 2, Edinburgh, 2008, Churchill Livingstone.)

palsy, autism, and behavioral disturbances. Data are now being gathered through feasibility studies (Mann et al, 2012) and outcome-based studies that lend credence to its effectiveness (Mehl-Madrona et al, 2007; Raviv et al, 2009).

Because of the time and effort necessary to develop this skill, relatively few osteopaths in the United States practice cranial osteopathy. The practice of craniosacral therapy, however, has expanded to other manual therapy fields, including chiropractic, physical and massage therapies, and dentistry, with training being offered by the Upledger Institute (Palm Beach Gardens, Florida) and others.

ENERGY WORK

Energy work refers to the techniques that have developed either as part of ancient traditions (e.g., qigong, Qi Gong) or as recently "discovered" methods in which the practitioner manipulates the bioenergy of the patient. The theory of bioenergy basically states that a life force, or vital energy, permeates the entire universe. This energy flows through all living things in distinct patterns. These patterns of flow are reflected in the meridian system (where qi, or chi, is the name of the life force) originally conceived by the Chinese and in the chakra system of Hindu tradition (where the word *prana* is used to indicate this force). Various forms of exercise have been developed for the cultivation of bioenergy, including yoga, internal qigong, and t'ai chi.

Three basic concepts are important in understanding energy work: intent, cooperation, and the tripartite nature of the human. *Intent* is important in that the practitioner projects his or her mind intent to heal into the patient. For this reason, that intent must go one step further than the proscriptive "do no harm" doctrine of Western therapeutics to an affirmative attitude of love and concern. Intent also assumes a high level of visualization. *Cooperation* implies the partnership between the practitioner and patient as participants in the healing process, with neither being exclusively active or passive. The *tripartite concept* refers to the acceptance of three parts of the human: body, mind, and spirit. This concept is envisioned in the much older Asian cultures as going beyond religion, whereas Western cultures have relied on belief systems driven by faith. In addition, the "scientific," reductionist approach of conventional Western medicine is rather dismissive of spiritual aspects and has only recently acknowledged the mind–body connection. Although there are many systems of energy work, four are included here, two rooted in Eastern teachings and two developed in Western application.

The Chinese term *qigong* (or qi gong, Qigong, Qi Gong) refers to the manipulation of bioenergy and loosely translated means "qi work." Qigong can be internal, in which an individual can strengthen and balance the flow of qi within the self, or external, in which a trained practitioner can project his or her qi into a patient to induce a therapeutic effect (see Chapter 28).

Although the vast majority of the vital energy of an organism is contained within the body, some of it radiates off the skin, producing the "aura," which has been visualized using Kirlian photography (Chapter 15). The qigong practitioner is able to palpate the meridian system through this aura, locate points of blockage, and free these blockages by projecting his or her qi into the patient, using intent and visualization. As in Trager work, the Feldenkrais method, and yoga, specific "external qigong" exercises have been developed that, when performed by an individual, serve to cultivate qi within the self. Qigong is also a natural result of long-term "internal" martial arts training, in which practitioners are capable of seemingly superhuman feats of strength and balance.

Reiki (literally "universal energy") is a method that may have originated from qigong as practiced by the Chinese Taoists and Buddhists. If ever practiced as such, it disappeared from practice in Japan at some point, only to be "rediscovered" (or created) by Dr. Mikao Usui in the mid-nineteenth century. Usui was interested in determining the nature of spiritually oriented healing power, as expressed through such individuals as Jesus Christ and Gautama the Buddha. After much study, including a doctorate from the University of Chicago, he began an extended period of fasting and meditation. At the end of this period, he reportedly received a vision and the ability to channel "reiki" through his body to effect healing in others. From that point, he continued healing, eventually training others in his method. Usui handed the title of Grand Master to Dr. Hiyashi Chugiro, who in turn passed it to Hawayo Takata, a Hawaiian woman of Japanese descent. In this way, reiki was exported from Japan to the West. There have also been attempts to trace some of the roots of reiki back to Shintoism, an early spiritual practice in Japan prior to acculturation to China. Shintoism itself had no formal organization until it was later formulated for political reasons to enhance the lineage of the Meiji emperors and the Meiji "Restoration" in Japan.

For practitioners, reiki must be "received" from a master or teacher. Only then is an individual able to effect healing. There are three degrees of reiki training. The first-degree practitioner is capable of giving a basic treatment with the hands on the patient, or about 1 inch away from the skin if touching is not possible. The second-degree practitioner can effect healing with the hands removed from the body, and treatments can be given at a faster rate. The third-degree practitioner is referred to as a "master" and is qualified to teach reiki.

The objective of reiki treatment is to restore internal harmony to the body and to release any blockages, which may be physical or emotional. The five principles of reiki are as follows:

1. Today I give thanks for my many blessings.
2. Just for today, I will not worry.
3. Today I will not be angry.
4. Today I will do my work honestly.
5. Today I will be kind to my neighbor and to every living thing.

During a reiki treatment the hands of the practitioner are placed with the fingers together on the patient. As energy is transferred from giver to receiver, the hands and the area treated become warm, which indicates a release of tension in the area and an increase in the blood flow. The head of the patient is treated first (four locations or positions), followed by the front (five positions) and back (five positions) of the body. Each position is held for 8 to 10 minutes (or less, if the practitioner is above first degree). Problem areas may be held longer until a result is sensed. The hand positions correspond to the energy points, or chakras, identified in Hindu tradition, as well as other points. The treatment is completed with a series of general myofascial techniques, including kneading, counterforce, and stroking (effleurage), to close the energy channels.

As with other energy-oriented manipulative techniques, reiki requires significant verbal and nonverbal communication between the giver and receiver, who act in partnership.

Permission must be granted both consciously and subconsciously for healing to be successful. Somatoemotional release is quite possible in this treatment.

Therapeutic touch is another form of energy work that was developed by Dr. Dolores Krieger (1992) and Dora Kunz in the late 1960s and early 1970s. In this style of bodywork, energy is directed through the hands of the "giver" (either on or off the body, but usually off) to activate the healing process of the "receiver." The therapist essentially acts as a support system to facilitate the process. Therapeutic touch treatments typically last 20 to 25 minutes and are accompanied by a relaxation response and a decrease in perceived pain. Although skeptics have claimed that this technique merely elicits a placebo effect (an interesting concept in itself, see Chapter 9), successes have also been reported with comatose patients, patients under anesthesia, and premature infants.

Therapeutic touch posits that humans are open energy systems, bilaterally symmetrical, and that illness is the result of an imbalance in the patient's energy field. The healer places himself or herself between the patient's illness and the patient's energy field to effect the healing process. The receiver must accept the energy of the healer and the necessity of change for the healing to occur. This should happen both consciously and subconsciously.

There are two phases of the treatment: assessment and balancing. Before balancing, the practitioner "centers" himself or herself, entering a state of relaxation and awareness. The hands are moved around the patient's body at a distance of 2 to 3 inches. The patient's energy field is encountered and assessed by feeling for changes in temperature, pressure, rhythm, or a tingling sensation. Simultaneously, the practitioner nonverbally requests the permission of the patient to enter the patient's field and effect a change. During the balancing phase, the healer (sometimes referred to as the "sender") then attempts to bring the two energy fields into a harmonic resonance through intent and visualization.

The attitude of the sender is one of empathy and compassion. The intent of the treatment is to facilitate the flow of vital energy, to stimulate it, to dissipate areas of congestion, and to dampen any areas of increased activity. In addition, the concept of rhythm and vibration is used, with color observed as a product of different frequencies within the field. At the beginning of the treatment, at the end of the treatment, or at both times, the practitioner "smoothes" out the patient's energy field by running the hands from head to toe. This sometimes has a cooling effect and is referred to as *unruffling*.

Healing touch, as developed by Barbara Brennan (1988), is similar to therapeutic touch in that the healer seeks to balance the energy field of the patient. A specific sequence of techniques is used in which the healer encounters, assesses, and treats different layers of the patient's visible "aura," correcting any imbalances and smoothing out the field. Healing touch is somewhat more spiritually oriented than therapeutic touch, using techniques such as channeling and employing colors and crystals to assist in the process.

These "energy-based" techniques (in addition to many of the other techniques mentioned) emphasize the importance of psychoemotional cooperation and participation by the patient (i.e., the mind–body connection) for successful application. In addition, the mind intent of the manipulator comes into play as the director of his or her internal energy outward and into the patient. This concept is quite controversial by standards of Western scientific analysis.

Although critics have referred to these and other manipulative techniques as "pseudoscience" because of a perceived lack of supportive evidence, the power of the technique and of the mind are not to be undervalued. Clinical outcomes studies have indicated that the intent of both the patient and the clinician have a demonstrable effect in determining treatment outcome. This evidence sheds new and interesting light on the placebo effect as a real phenomenon (especially in light of the fact that placebos are "effective" in randomized drug trials about 30% of the time). It also indicates that treatment of the somatic component of disease can be approached effectively through acknowledgment of the "three-legged stool" model of the human: body, mind, and spirit.

FELDENKRAIS METHOD® (AWARENESS THROUGH MOVEMENT, FUNCTIONAL INTEGRATION)

Moshé Feldenkrais (1904–1984) was an Israeli physicist who developed a system of movement and manipulation over several decades (Feldenkrais, 1991; Rywerant, 2011). The Feldenkrais Method® is divided into two "educational" processes. The first, *awareness through movement,* is a sensorimotor balancing technique that is taught to "students" who are active participants in this process. The students are verbally guided through a series of very slow movements designed to create a heightened awareness of motion patterns and to reeducate the CNS to new patterns, approaches, and possibilities (as in learning t'ai chi).

The second process is referred to as *functional integration.* This process employs a passive technique using a didactic approach, not at all unlike Trager table work (see discussion later in this chapter). The practitioner acts as "teacher" and the patient as "student." The teacher brings the student through a series of manipulons to reestablish proper neuromotor patterning and balance. *Manipulons* are a manipulative sequence of information, action (as initiated by the practitioner), and response. They are gentle and are treated as exploratory, with the therapist introducing new motion patterns to the patient. Manipulons are referred to as "positioning," "confining," "single," or "repetitive." They can also be "oscillating." In all cases the teacher plays a supportive and guiding role while creating a nonthreatening

environment for change. Functional integration can be considered a combination of passive, articulatory, or functional techniques.

HYDROTHERAPY AND THERMAL THERAPY

Hydrotherapy and thermal therapy are often considered to be an adjunct treatment to massage and other manual techniques, as well as part of traditional nature cure, naturopathy, and naturopathic medicine (see Chapter 22). They may be applied prior to, during, or after manual therapies, or may be stand-alone treatments in some cases. Some, such as aquatic massage, include techniques that may achieve significant results similar to that of massage.

Hydrotherapy is the use of water, in its many forms, either internally or externally, as a medical treatment. This modality is broadly defined and includes diverse options, such as application of or submersion in hot, cold, or neutral temperature water, application of vapocoolant spray or ice, or floating in a saltwater tank or on top of a pool of water. Which application to use depends upon the case presentations, type of trauma, consistency and fluid levels in the tissues, and desired outcome goals. A few general guidelines help prevent injury and may increase desired results.

In general, muscles relax and blood vessels dilate when anything *warm or hot is applied* to tissues, resulting in increased blood flow and oxygen levels, and decreased nociceptive metabolites, segmental reflexes, and sympathetic tone. Unless there is a contraindication, such as recent trauma or tissue bruising, vasodilation is beneficial in many ways, reducing muscle spasms and joint stiffness, as well as in softening muscles, connective tissues, and adhesions. After the application of heat, the tissues may become congested unless light exercise or gliding strokes of effleurage massage are applied. Alternatively, cold application of some sort can follow application of heat to decongest the area.

When a *cold* application is applied to tissues, it causes vasoconstriction of the local blood vessels, and will increase small-fiber activity, flooding afferent pathways and causing brain stem inhibition of nociception. After the removal of the cold pack, blood vessels dilate slowly and tissues are again flushed with fresh, oxygen-rich blood. Additional benefits may include a reduction of inflammation and swelling of tissue that is often associated with trauma.

A particularly effective thermotherapy application is alternately applied hot and cold, or contrast hydrotherapy, where heating and cooling the tissues is (usually rapidly) alternately applied to stimulate a profound flushing of blood and lymph in muscles, skin, or organs.

The general principles of hot and cold applications are as follows.

- Cold is defined as 55–65° F or 12.7–18.3° C; anything colder is considered to be very cold and may damage the skin if inappropriately applied.

- Short cold applications (less than 1 minute) stimulate circulation; long cold applications (greater than 1 minute) depress circulation and metabolism.
- Hot is defined as 98–104° F or 36.7–40° C; anything hotter than that is undesirable and dangerous.
- Short hot applications (less than 5 minutes) stimulate circulation; long hot applications (more than 5 minutes) vasodilate so well that they can result in congestion and require a cold application or massage to drain the area.
- Short hot followed by short cold applications cause alternation of circulation and may produce a profound flushing of the tissues.
- Cool is defined as 66–80° F or 18.5–26.5° C, and tepid is defined as 81–92° F or 26.5–33.3° C
- Neutral/warm (93–97° F or 33.8–36.1° C) applications or baths at body heat are very soothing and relaxing.

Hot/cold packs, hot tubs, steam rooms, saunas, and cold plunges are the most commonly used applications of thermal therapy. Though ancient in origin, massage applied with hot and/or cold stones is now enjoying popularity in modern times. Stones (usually smooth river rocks) of varying sizes allow for precise placement on small portions of a muscle. The stones are heated or cooled, and then placed in strategic locations to alter the temperature of the skin and influence the underlying muscles (Wuttke, 2012).

Cryotherapy agents, such as vapocoolant sprays, are used as surface anesthetics in the treatment of trigger points. Spray and stretch technique (S&S) can be seamlessly integrated with trigger point pressure release and other techniques to release stubborn trigger points, spasm, or ischemia that is not easily responding to manual techniques. The goal of S&S is to inhibit pain signals of short, painful muscles or from trigger points, which then allows the tissues to be manually lengthened. Among other effects, it is thought to provoke a continual barrage of alarming impulses perceived and transmitted by A-Delta fibers (cutaneous thermal receptors), which has an inhibitory effect on C-fibers (transmit pain) and on facilitated neural pathways. It is suggested that counterirritants, such as Biofreeze®, work under a similar principle.

Sensory deprivation tanks, or flotation tanks, have been used to suspend the body in a solution of heavily salted water, which causes the body to float (as can be found in the Great Salt Lake or the Dead Sea). Coupled with darkness and lack of sound, this weightless suspension from gravitational forces induces a deep relaxation effect.

Similarly, aquatic bodywork, such as Watsu™, is conducted in a fluid matrix that is usually a swimming pool or lake, and may include equipment, such as jets or waterfalls. The patient is usually supported by specially designed, strategically placed flotation devices, and moved in the water by one or more trained practitioners. Friedland (2012) describes this unusual therapy: "Specific movements, rhythms, patterns, and wave forms are created by the therapist's own kinetic actions and transmitted to the patient. These movements, rhythms, patterns, and wave forms rebound onto, across, through, around, and out from the patient and are countered by the practitioner, who responds by transmitting more movements, rhythms, waves, and patterns. . . . One of the greatest advantages of using the water is that it allows individuals with many types of injuries to receive treatment."

SPECIAL APPLICATIONS (INFANT, ELDERLY, ONCOLOGY, AND HOSPICE-CARE MASSAGE)

Age-related and condition-specific care has been a growing part of the manual therapies professions for decades. Although these special patients may require techniques from the many styles given in the chapter, they also have unique characteristics that require approaches based on age-related factors or medical conditions. Each of these require special training and an ongoing requirement for the practitioner to stay current regarding information, techniques, medications, and other pertinent data for these special circumstances.

Prenatal massage is therapeutic massage and bodywork that is given during pregnancy to promote both maternal and fetal well-being. Although cultures around the world show various forms of the use of prenatal and perinatal touch, pregnancy massage was considered as contraindicated until as recent as the 1970s.

Noted author and instructor Carole Osborne (2012) tells how this has changed. "In the last few decades, women and some maternity professions have increasingly demanded a more holistic and woman-centered approach to childbearing." As a result, in many circumstances, partners and other family members are now in close physical contact with the birthing mother. Labor assistants, or doulas, provide continuous physical and emotional support to laboring women, with impressive positive results for mothers, babies, hospitals, and other birth settings.

Beginning in the 1980s, several massage therapists and instructors began an in-depth exploration of massage therapy for childbearing concerns. Most notably, Carole Osborne, Kate Jordan, Suzanne Yates, Elaine Stillerman, and Claire Marie Miller each developed their own guidelines for safe prenatal applications of massage therapy."

As massage therapy resumes its place in integrated health care and at multidisciplinary clinics, prenatal massage therapy has surfaced as an optimal specialization. It is strongly suggested that those working with pregnant clients study with an experienced instructor and stay current with developing research and continuing education in regard to this field.

Infant massage is a unique style whose main purpose is to create and support the emotional bond between parent and child (McClure, 2012). Additionally, gastrointestinal, respiratory, and circulatory functions may be enhanced. Although massage therapists may offer infant massage, a long-lasting standard is for a parent to be trained to apply the techniques. This is usually accomplished while sitting on the floor with the adult's legs crossed and baby lying on the floor in front of him/her. McClure writes, "If the baby becomes fussy, they are comforted, and then the massage is continued. If the baby indicates they have 'had enough', the parent ends the massage with a positive, soothing movement that is familiar to the baby, and often the baby will drift off to sleep. If the baby is enjoying the massage, after massaging the face and arms, the baby is turned over and strokes are completed on the back and buttocks. During the massage, the parent often gently stops stroking and lays their hands on the baby's body, a movement called 'resting hands.'"

Considerable research has been conducted in the field of infant massage, particularly in the area of weight gain in premature infants and in prenatal substance abuse. A considerable amount of favorable research has been published regarding research conducted by Dr. Tiffany Field and others at the Touch Research Institute, Miami, Florida. A complete list can be found at www6.miami.edu/touch-research.

As the body ages into elderly years, conditions such as thinning skin, changes in muscle tone, joint deterioration, osteoporosis, and sensorineural deficits may warrant specific approaches and precautions. Elderly care training will help to ensure appropriate strategies are used for those who face the issues of aging, such as being frail and less mobile. In the United States, there are three main organizations that conduct training specific to elderly care: Day-Break Geriatric Massage Institute, Comfort Touch™, and Compassionate Touch™.

When discussing elderly care, author Susan Salvo (2012) shares, "The elderly may present the therapist with unique challenges. There are obvious physical changes, such as thinning skin, reduced muscle mass, and impairments of vision and hearing. Sensorineural deficits may also predispose the elderly to accidental injury, such as slips and falls. This population faces lifestyle and emotional changes, such as retirement, reduced income, and loss of loved ones. To better serve the elderly, the therapist needs to cultivate attitudes of patience, tolerance, loving kindness, and attentiveness."

Oncology massage designates a special set of skills used in the care of a person affected by cancer and its related treatments. Patients may be in active treatment, recovery, survivorship, or at the end of life. Practitioners pursuing this field need to develop a broad understanding of the pathophysiology of cancer, side effects of treatment (medications, radiation, chemotherapy, surgery), and an ability to modify protocols to adapt for each unique case, such as for the presence of lymphedema or with scar mobilization. Treatments may take place in private practice, a patient's home, oncology clinics, hospitals, and in hospice care.

Johnette du Rand (2012) addresses the myth that massage is contraindicated for cancer patients. "Earlier massage training did not take into consideration the pathophysiology of the disease, and mistakenly hypothesized that pressure could stimulate the spread of cancer.

Cancer starts and spreads because of a highly complicated accumulation of mutations on a genetic level in a cell's DNA and/or RNA. There is currently no evidence that massage will influence the development or proliferation of this mutation." While that debate continues in some arena, the effectiveness of massage therapy at reducing symptoms such as pain and anxiety has been demonstrated in ongoing research and clinical studies, with strong implications that massage will also reduce fatigue, stress, nausea, and depression associated with cancer treatments.

For those joining the field of oncology massage, qualified training with supervised instruction is a must. Although textbooks, articles, and webinars offer a strong support for comprehensive understanding, there is no substitute for a qualified, experienced oncology massage instructor and ongoing continuing education to stay abreast of the latest information in this ever-changing field.

Death is an integral part of life, and at the end stage for terminally ill people and their families, intensive palliative care that provides a loving touch, comfort, pain relief, and peaceful rest is priceless. With a history of more than 50 years in the United States, hospice care has provided physical, emotional, psychological, and spiritual support for those approaching the end of their lives. Hospice-based massage therapy is a natural and integral part of this care.

Sharon Puszko (2012) shares her insights: "The hospice patient receiving massage therapy may experience more immediately noticeable psychosocial benefits than physical benefits. The reason why touch is so powerful is based on the recognition that tactile experiences are the first sensations that greet us at the time of birth, and are the last perception to leave us at the end of life. Touch can penetrate the semi-comatose state produced by a painkiller, giving the treatment a modicum of human contact and reminding the patient that they are not alone. In fact, patients sometimes reduce their demand for drugs when massage is an integral part of the treatment protocol."

Puszko suggests that gentle massage reduces feelings of isolation and loneliness and supports self-acceptance and self-esteem when the body has been invaded by a debilitating disease. "The benefit of massage therapy for the hospice patient is to experience peace, joy, and love, and general feelings of comfort while actively dying."

Massage touches the lives at all ages, from birth to death, and offers specific and effective techniques to those who suffer from chronic illness, express themselves through athletics or the arts, or just live a normal life with the distortions, bumps, and bruises that come with modern life. Whatever the individual's lifestyle or life circumstances, massage can be an integral part of living it comfortably and to the fullest.

LYMPH DRAINAGE TECHNIQUES

Manually applied lymph drainage techniques incorporate application of light pressure to the skin and superficial fascia in a particular pattern that encourages an increase in

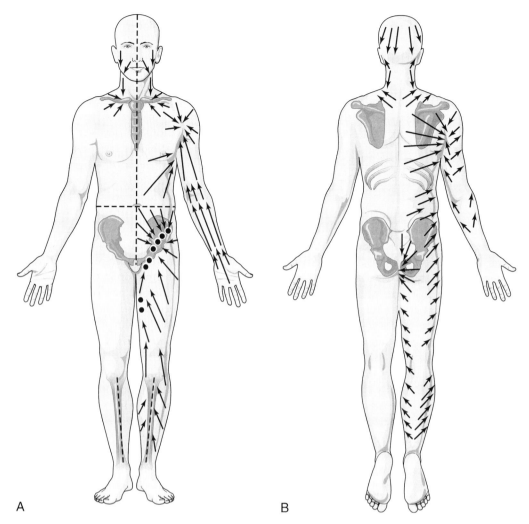

Figure 17-8 Lymphatic flow can be enhanced with manual lymph drainage techniques. (Borrowed with permission from Chaitow L, DeLany J: *Clinical application of neuromuscular techniques: practical case study exercises,* Edinburgh, 2006, Churchill Livingstone.)

the movement of lymph. In addition, lymphatic pumps are rhythmic techniques applied over organs, such as the liver and spleen, to increase drainage. The thoracic diaphragm is also sometimes used as a lymphatic pump, because movement of this structure creates increased abdominal pressure, which "pumps" the nearby cisterna chyli, a dilated portion of the thoracic lymph duct that serves as a temporary reservoir for lymph from the lower half of the body (Figure 17-8).

The hand stroke used in lymph drainage is distinctly different from effleurage. Effleurage that is applied in the direction of the heart can also increase the venous and lymphatic drainage of the involved structure(s). However, deeply applied effleurage can inhibit lymph movement and even result in damage to the lymphatic vessels, particularly if the region is already engorged with excessive lymph. Using very light pressure, lymph drainage applies a rhythmic short stroke that creates a short pulling action on the skin and superficial fascia, which is then abruptly released. A turgoring effect encourages the movement of lymph into the lymph capillary. The lymph then moves along the

vessels, which empty into progressively larger lymph vessels, until the lymph eventually rejoins the vascular system at the subclavian veins.

Lymph drainage therapy is useful in a variety of clinical settings to encourage overall health and is profoundly useful in postsurgical and post-trauma care. The edema associated with sprains, strains, and a variety of sport injuries can often be quickly reduced with these techniques. The Vodder method (manual lymph drainage, MLD®) and the Chikly method (lymph drainage therapy, LDT) are the two most popular methods in this highly effective and broadly applicable modality. Although the aims of the two methods are similar, the styles of application and of teaching are moderately different. Developers of both methods have published textbooks and journal articles to support their concepts.

MUSCLE ENERGY TECHNIQUE

Muscle energy technique (MET) can be applied directly or indirectly to individual muscles as well as to muscle groups

(Chaitow, 2013). When MET is applied *directly* (i.e., toward the motion barrier, or in an attempt to lengthen a shortened or spastic muscle), the technique is based on the principle of *reciprocal inhibition*, which states that a muscle (e.g., flexor) reflexively relaxes as its antagonist (the associated extensor) contracts. Conversely, if a muscle in spasm is contracted against resistance and then relaxed, the effect often results in increased ROM, or reduction of the motion barrier. This *indirect* application is based on the principle of *postisometric relaxation* (also known as *postcontraction relaxation*) (Lewit & Simons, 1984).

This technique is one of the few "active" techniques in manual therapy: that is, the patient does the work. A distinction of MET is the amount of effort exerted by the patient. Usually, less than 20% of the total strength of the muscle is brought to bear during the interval of contraction. Another way of showing this is through the "one-finger rule," in which the amount of force necessary is the force needed to move a single finger of the practitioner when the practitioner lightly resists the contraction. This is in contradistinction to the proprioceptive neuromuscular facilitation technique often used in physical therapy, which employs a maximal muscle contraction and may expose the patient to risk of injury. A thorough knowledge of muscle attachments and their motion vectors is necessary to apply MET effectively and efficiently.

MYOFASCIAL RELEASE

Myofascial release is a gentle technique that uses knowledge of the physical properties of the fascia as it relates to muscles (Figure 17-9). Although some skill is necessary to apply this technique effectively, it is simple to learn and easily applied. The practitioner uses light and deep pressure, depending on the target structures, to palpate motion restriction within the fascia and moves toward or away from the restriction. The position is held until a "release," or softening, is felt, the perception of which is the most difficult aspect of application. The tissues are then slowly returned to their original position. The release can be the relaxation of muscles, changes in the viscosity of the ground substance of the fascia, the slow disengagement of fascial adhesions, or the realignment of the fascia to a more appropriate orientation.

MYOFASCIAL–SOFT TISSUE TECHNIQUE

The myofascial–soft tissue technique is a combination direct-indirect massage technique for reducing muscle spasm and fascial tension. It is similar to pétrissage, except that more parts of the hand are typically employed. This technique can be used as a prelude to the high-velocity low-amplitude technique.

NEURAL MOBILIZATION/ MANIPULATION

Nerves, blood vessels, and lymphatic structures course throughout the body ensheathed in fascia. During move-

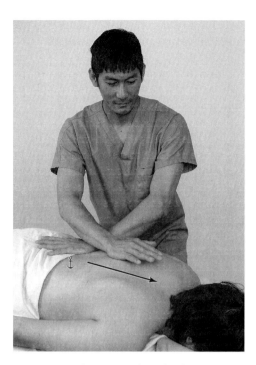

Figure 17-9 A crossed-arm myofascial release (MFR) can be applied broadly to the tissues to alter the ground substance of the fascia. (Modified from Salvo S: *Massage therapy: principles and practice,* ed 3, St. Louis, 2007, Saunders.)

ment, structures (e.g., bones, discs, muscles) and fascia, not only move, but must allow for the movement of the nerves within the sheath. The relationship of the surrounding structures to the nerves is known as the *mechanical interface.*

When tissues are strained, overused, or incur trauma, or when patterns of use require distorted movement patterns, mechanical deformation of the nerves (compression, stretching, angulation, torsion) can occur. It is also important to realize that, in addition to motor and sensory impulses that are transmitted along neural pathways, a host of important trophic substances also flow along the nerves. Any abnormality in the mechanical interface can impede axoplasmic transport, as well as interfere with normal neural firing.

A number of techniques have emerged that focus on identifying fascial and muscular restriction of the nerves. Additionally, neurodynamic testing, an assessment tool, is often coupled with the techniques. David Butler, a physical therapist from Australia, has contributed significantly through his work with neural mobilization techniques that slide, glide or "floss" the nerves through the sheaths (Butler, 1991, 2000). This is accomplished by the use of specific repetitive body movements that are performed passively or actively, which gently free the nerves from fascial restrictions.

Neural manipulation, developed by French osteopath and physical therapist Jean-Pierre Barral and fellow osteopath Alain Croibier (Barral & Croibier, 1997), focuses more directly on the neural connective tissues to create more space around the neural and vascular structures. Nerves are very important structures in the body since they are the communication between the primary control, the brain, and all other structures. If a person is feeling pain, it is because the nerves are reporting this information to the brain. Tension and injury can compress the nerves, which can result in irritation within and around the nerves. In other words, the messages of pain can be coming from problems within the nerve itself, in addition to the surrounding tissue. More importantly, the original injury or tension may have healed, but the nerve can still be compromised and still report messages of pain.

Since nerves are composed of connective tissue or fascia, the same fascial techniques that can address adhesions, restrictions, and pain in other areas can also relieve these problems in and around the nerves... Treatment of the surrounding structures could involve the tissues that the nerve supplies, such as an organ, fascia, blood vessel, or joint. Furthermore, as the nerve leaves the central nervous system through the foramina (an opening in the vertebral column), it may be compressed by the disc, vertebral fractures, or foraminal stenosis. Such elements would also need to be addressed. (Barral, 2012)

Mechanical neural lesion is often the cause of a broad range of symptoms. However, other serious conditions can mimic neuropathy, some of which are contraindicated for direct techniques. For those interested in incorporating neural assessment and treatment as discussed here, instructor-supervised training is suggested. Precise positioning as well as fundamental training will help avoid further irritation to peripheral neuropathic problems.

NEUROMUSCULAR THERAPY (NEUROMUSCULAR TECHNIQUES)

Neuromuscular therapy (NMT) is a precise and thorough examination and treatment of the soft tissues of a joint or region that is experiencing pain or dysfunction. As a medically oriented technique, it is primarily used for the treatment of chronic pain or as a treatment for recent (but not acute) trauma; however, it can also be applied to prevent injury or to enhance performance.

NMT emerged on two continents almost simultaneously, but the methods had little connection to each other until recent years. In the early twentieth century, European "neuromuscular technique" emerged, primarily through the work of Stanley Lief and Boris Chaitow. For the last several decades, it has been carried forward through the writing and teaching skills of Leon Chaitow, DO. The protocols of North American "neuromuscular therapy" also derived from a variety of sources, including chiropractic (Raymond Nimmo), myofascial trigger point therapy (Janet Travell, David Simons), and massage therapy (Judith DeLany, Paul St. John). Over the last decade, Chaitow and DeLany (2008, 2011) combined the two methods in a two-volume text that comprehensively integrates the European

and American™ versions. Neuromuscular technique (NMT) continues to evolve, with many individuals teaching the techniques worldwide.

One of the main features of NMT are step-by-step protocols that address all muscles of a region while also considering factors that may play a role in the presenting condition. Like osteopaths, neuromuscular therapists use the term *somatic dysfunction* when describing what is found during the examination. Somatic dysfunction is usually characterized by tender tissues and limited and/or painful range of motion. Causes of these lesions include, but are not limited to, connective tissue changes, ischemia, nerve compression, and postural disturbances, all of which can result from trauma, stress, and repetitive microtrauma (stress due to work and recreationally related activities). A distinct focus of treatment is the identification and treatment of *trigger points*, noxious hyperirritable nodules within the myofascia that, when provoked by applied pressure, needling, and so on, radiate sensations (usually pain) to a defined target zone (Figure 17-10). Consideration is also given to nutrition, hydration, hormonal balance, breathing patterns, and numerous other factors that affect neuromusculoskeletal health and, when indicated, professional referral for treatment of these "perpetuating factors."

Although the European and American versions have unifying philosophical threads, there are subtle, yet distinct, differences in the palpation methods. Both methods examine for taut bands that are often associated with trigger points and both use applied pressure to treat the pain-producing nodules. However, European NMT uses a slow-paced, thumb-drag method, whereas an NMT American™ version uses a medium-paced gliding stroke of the thumb or fingers. There is also a slightly different

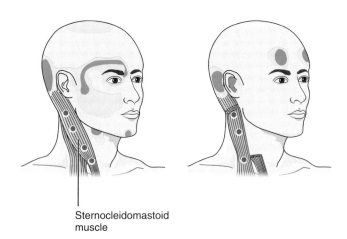

Sternocleidomastoid muscle

Figure 17-10 Neuromuscular therapy (NMT) focuses attention on locating and treating trigger points (TrPs). TrP referrals from sternocleidomastoid can produce a variety of symptoms, including facial neuralgia, headache, sore throat, voice problems, hearing loss, vertigo, ear pain, and blurred vision. (Borrowed with permission from Chaitow L, DeLany J: *Clinical application of neuromuscular techniques,* vol 1, ed 2, Edinburgh, 2008, Churchill Livingstone.)

emphasis on the manner of application of trigger point pressure release (specific compression applied to the tissues) for deactivation of trigger points. In addition, American NMT offers a more systematic method of examination and treatment, whereas European methods use less detail in palpation of deeper structures, preferring to incorporate positional release and other methods for the deeper treatment. European methods also focus significantly more on superficial tissue texture changes than their American counterparts.

Both European and American NMT support the use of hydrotherapies (hot and cold applications), movement, and self-applied (home care) therapies. Both suggest homework to encourage the patient's participation in the recovery process, which might include stretching, changes in habits of use, and alterations in lifestyle that help to eliminate perpetuating factors. Patient education may also be offered to increase awareness of static and dynamic posture in work and recreational settings, and to teach the value of healthy nutritional choices. Referral to another health care practitioner may also be considered, especially when visceral pathology is suspected.

A successful foundation includes taking a thorough case history, including the patient's account of the precipitating factors, and performing a complete examination of the soft tissues. Although many decisions will be individual to each case, the NMT protocols are performed while keeping a few basic rules in mind. Superficial tissues are treated before deeper layers, and proximal areas in an extremity are treated before distal regions. Every palpable muscle in the region is assessed, not just those whose referral patterns are consistent with the person's pain or which are thought by the practitioner to be the cause of the problem. This approach helps to reveal muscles that may be substituting for those that are dysfunctional or weak.

The first aim is to increase blood flow and soften fascia. Although gliding strokes are often the best choice, sometimes tissue manipulation (sliding the tissues between the thumb and finger to create shear) works better. Depending on the stiffness of the tissues, hot packs might be used to further encourage softening. Then the gliding strokes and manipulation can be repeated, alternating with the application of heat, or a few moments can be allowed in between for fluid exchange.

Once the tissues have become softer and more pliable, the practitioner palpates for taut bands. These bands, in which select fibers are locked in a shortened position, vary in diameter from as small as a toothpick to larger than a finger. At the center of the band there is often a thicker, denser area that is associated with central trigger point formation.

Once the fiber center is located, the region is evaluated for a trigger point, to which pressure is applied until a degree of resistance (like an "elastic barrier") is felt. Sufficient pressure is applied to match the tension, which provokes or intensifies the referral pattern to the target zone.

The applied pressure should be monitored, so that what is felt by the patient is no more than a moderate level of discomfort (7 on a scale of 1 to 10). Although the patient may feel some tenderness in the area that is being pressed, usually the focus is on the pain, tingling, numbness, burning, or other sensation in the associated target zone of the trigger point. The well-documented, common target zones are usually distant from the location of the trigger point and the zones are predictable. They have been well illustrated in numerous books and charts.

As the applied pressure is sustained, within 8 to 12 seconds the sensations being reported should begin to fade as the practitioner feels a softening of the compressed nodule or (more rarely) a profound release. The pressure can be sustained for up to approximately 20 seconds, but longer than this is not recommended because this "ischemic compression" is further reducing blood flow in tissues that are already blood-deprived.

Trigger point treatment (by pressure, needling, spray and stretch, or other method) can be repeated several times within the therapy session, with a few moments between each application to allow fluid exchange to occur. Each time treatment is re-applied, the practitioner should notice the need to increase the level of applied pressure to stimulate the same level of sensation. In some cases, the tenderness and referred sensations will be completely eliminated within one session.

As the final step, the fibers associated with the taut band should be lengthened. This might include passive or active stretching if the associated attachment sites are not too sensitive. If the attachments are moderately tender, inflammation is possible and elongation should be performed manually to avoid putting stress on the attachments. This can be achieved by using a precisely applied myofascial release or a double-thumb gliding stroke in which each thumb simultaneously slides from the central nodule to a respective attachment, applying tension to the band as the thumbs slide away from each other.

Specific training in the use of NMT protocols is necessary, because many contraindications and precautions are associated with NMT techniques. The protocols can be incorporated into any practice setting and are particularly useful when interfaced with medical procedures. Many complex conditions can benefit from the thorough protocols and treatment strategies used in NMT.

ORTHOPEDIC MASSAGE/ MEDICAL MASSAGE

Orthopedic massage is a comprehensive assessment and treatment system that, like NMT, uses a methodological approach that may incorporate several techniques. Since it has a broad application based on patient presentation, it can be incorporated into relaxation massage, sports injury care, a diverse range of medical settings, and advanced rehabilitative therapy. Although there are different styles of orthopedic massage, they all fundamentally require skills in orthopedic assessment, variability of treatment, advanced knowledge of pain and injuries and, in some cases, protocols for rehabilitation (Lowe, 2012).

Orthopedic massage drew its roots from sports massage, which emerged in the United States in the 1970s and 1980s. In particular, the standard orthopedic assessment protocols developed by James Cyriax (1984) and the orthopedic massage protocols written by Whitney Lowe (1997) provide the fundamental components that are known as orthopedic massage. Many schools have adopted Lowe's textbooks as the basis for training, resulting in a move toward standardization of orthopedic massage. Practice settings are as diverse as the application itself and include private practices, physical therapy clinics, medical settings, chiropractic offices, spas and sport facilities.

Lowe (2012) defines the core of orthopedic massage: "Assessment is at the very foundation of orthopedic massage. It is paramount to identify the tissues most likely at the root of a problem for effective management of soft tissue pain and injuries. Without an accurate assessment, there cannot be a sound or physiological rationale for the treatment and, thus, the treatment will be far less effective. . . . Skilled orthopedic massage therapists have good knowledge of what tissues are involved and which therapeutic techniques would best treat those tissues. Thus, they are not limited by their 'technique toolbag' and can employ established, as well as newly developed, techniques and methods, and hence are adaptable to the patient's condition. Their advanced education and knowledge leads to outcome-based therapeutic treatments and effective solutions."

Orthopedic massage (OM) and NMT (discussed previously) have long been established as successful medically oriented interventions that require comprehensive training and deliver highly effective results. These should not be confused with "medical massage," a term that has become popular in the last 15 years as a result of the aim of national massage organizations to standardize protocols being integrated into the medical communities. There is no one style of massage that makes up "medical massage." Clearly, OM and NMT practitioners are performing outcome-based massage targeted to specific conditions, the broad definition of medical massage. However, it is best to refer to them as orthopedic massage and neuromuscular therapy practitioners, as this better defines the degree of training they have received and the protocols that they use.

REFLEXOLOGY

In the Asian meridian system of the body, all the major meridians or channels are represented in the hands and feet. Acupuncture is usually not done on the soles of the feet in light of their sensitivity, and a system of foot massage was developed in China. William H. Fitzgerald, who called it "zone therapy," introduced this system to the United States in 1913. Now referred to by Dwight Byers

(2001) and others as *reflexology*, the technique involves the application of deep pressure to various points on the hands and feet by the thumbs and fingers of the practitioner.

The feet receive the preponderance of attention in this method, with various identified points not only noted to correspond to the energy channels of the body but also to specific organs and systems. When treatment is given, areas of tenderness or texture change are identified and pressure is applied. It is suggested that this opens the associated channel and allows body energy to flow unimpeded through its entirety. When all points are successfully treated, the energy system is flowing and balanced (see Chapter 20).

ROLFING AND OTHER STRUCTURAL INTEGRATION METHODS

Rolfing® is a form of structural integration that was developed by Ida Rolf in the middle of the twentieth century. Rolf, who had a PhD in biochemistry, sought help from an osteopath after being dissatisfied with conventional medical treatment of her pneumonia. After this experience, Dr. Rolf embarked on a lengthy period of study, including yoga study, which resulted in the manipulative system that now bears her name (Rolf, 1975, 1997; Rolf & Thompson, 1989). In 1971, she founded the Rolf Institute of Structural Integration in Boulder, Colorado, which now trains and certifies practitioners of this style.

The theory of Rolfing® is based primarily on physical consideration of the interaction of the human body with the gravitational field of the Earth. As a dynamic entity, the human body moves around and through this field in a state of equilibrium, storing potential energy and releasing kinetic energy. In this system, form (potential energy) is in direct proportion to function (kinetic energy), and the balance between the two is equivalent to the amount of energy available to the body. In simple terms, the worse the posture, the more energy we consume on a baseline level, and thus the less we have available for normal activity. Furthermore, the physical energy of the body is in direct proportion to the "vital energy" of the person. Ideally, the body is always in a position of "equipoise," but this is seldom, if ever, the case.

Rolfing® traditionally involves a 10-session treatment protocol designed to integrate the entire myofascial system of the body. Photographs are taken of the patient before and after each session or at the beginning and end of a series of treatments to evaluate progress. The body is treated as a system of integrated segments consolidated by the myofascial system. Attempts are made through "processing," as the treatment is called, to lengthen and center through the connective tissue system by a series of direct myofascial release techniques. As distortions in the system are released, the patient may experience pain. The pain experienced is not merely structural, however. It is thought that emotions are expressed through the musculoskeletal system as behavior, which is reflected in various postures and movement patterns (i.e., the widely accepted psychological concepts of Pavlovian conditioning and body language).

In other words, the musculoskeletal system is viewed as a link between the body and mind. Emotional or physical traumas are stored in the body as postures, which mirror a withdrawal response from the offending or painful agent. Over time, compensatory reactions occur, but the body ultimately decompensates (fails in adaptation to the imposed stresses), which results in somatic or visceral dysfunction. The direct technique seeks to put the energy of the practitioner into the system of the patient in an attempt to overcome the resistance to change embodied in the withdrawal response. As releases are effected through the treatment, the emotional component may also be expressed (i.e., a somatoemotional release).

The result of the treatment is a feeling of balance and "lightness" experienced by the patient. In addition, the patient should experience a heightened sense of well-being, because the treatment releases the effects of emotional trauma. Thus the feeling of lightness is more than simply an increase in the basal physical energy in the body; it is an increase in the body's vital energy as well.

From Rolf's work there were developed a number of other systems of structural integration. Among those who developed their own styles, several stand out with innovative thinking. One of these, Tom Myers, a distinguished teacher of structural integration, suggests that we consider the body to be a tensegrity structure. *Tensegrity*, a term coined by architect-engineer Buckminster Fuller, describes a system characterized by a discontinuous set of compressional elements (struts) that are held together, and/or moved, by a continuous tensional network (Chapter 16). Art student Kenneth Snelson attended Fuller's lectures and applied his concepts to build a three-dimensional tensegrity structure. His new-style sculpture was the first to exemplify the concepts of discontinuous-compression, continuous-tension structures, although Fuller usually receives the credit. The muscular system similarly supplies the tensile forces that erect the human frame by using contractile mechanisms embedded within the fascia to place tension on the compressional elements of the skeletal system, thereby providing a tensegrity structure capable of maintaining varying vertical postures, as well as carrying out significant and complex movements.

Myers (1997) has described a number of clinically useful sets of myofascial chains. He sees the fascia as continuous through the muscle and its tendinous attachments, blending with adjacent and contiguous soft tissues and with the bones, providing supportive tensional elements between the different compressional structures (bones), and thereby creating a tensegrity structure. These fascial chains are of particular importance in helping to draw attention to (for example) dysfunctional patterns in the lower limb that may affect structures in the upper body via these "long functional continuities."

Chaitow and DeLany (2008) note, "The truth, of course, is that no tissue exists in isolation but acts on, is bound to and interwoven with other structures. The body is inter- and intra-related, from top to bottom, side-to-side and front to back, by the inter-connectedness of this pervasive fascial system. When we work on a local area, we need to maintain a constant awareness of the fact that we are potentially influencing the whole body."

SHIATSU (ZEN SHIATSU)

Shiatsu means "finger pressure" in Japanese. It originally developed as a synthesis of acupuncture and Anma, a traditional Japanese massage (see Box 17-1) During the eighteenth and nineteenth centuries, Anma became more associated with carnal pleasure and subsequently lost its place as a therapeutic practice. Studies have been recently published that re-examine the therapeutic benefits of Anma (Donoyama et al, 2010, 2013). Shiatsu further diverged and became systematized in the twentieth century, with the Nippon Shiatsu School opening in the 1940s. Today, shiatsu is practiced worldwide in a multitude of practice settings. Although it has a strong root in energy-based medicine, the physical nature of its practice offers a quality more similar to massage than energy work.

As with other Asian-derived systems, shiatsu employs the meridian or channel concept of the human body. The

---

BOX 17-1 *Anma and Shiatsu*

As a healing art or treatment, Shiatsu grew from an earlier Asian form known as *Anma*. *An* denotes "pressure" and *ma* means "rubbing." This method, which was well known in China as *Tui na*, found its way to Japan and became recognized as a safe and easy way to treat the human body. In Japan, a tradition developed for it to be used and taught by blind practitioners who relied on their hands to diagnose a patient's condition.

Anma was recognized as a medical modality in Japan during the Nara period (710–784), but subsequently lost its popularity before gaining more widespread use in the Edo era (1603–1868), during which doctors were required to study Anma. During the Edo period, most practitioners were blind and provided treatments in their patients' homes. An extensive handbook on Anma was published in 1793. Anma's understanding and assessment of human structure and meridian lines were, and are still, believed to be important distinctions that separate shiatsu therapy from other healing models and massage therapies. When Western massage was introduced to Japan in the late 1880s, blind instructors dominated the many vocational schools that taught Anma. However, this very limitation stopped the further development of Anma and led to the evolution of what we recognize today as shiatsu therapy.

points along the channels are referred to as *tsubos* (Japanese for "vase"). Shiatsu theory states that when a channel becomes blocked, the tsubos along it can express a *"kyo"* state (weak energy, low vibration, cold, open) or a *"jitsu"* state (strong energy, high vibration, heat, closed). The hands are used for three purposes: for diagnosis, for treatment, and for maintenance (to strengthen the newly attained balance).

During a shiatsu treatment the practitioner (or "giver") uses acupressure to open or close jitsu or kyo tsubos, respectively. The technique is applied using the thumb, elbow, or knee, positioned perpendicular to the skin of the "receiver." The body part used by the practitioner and the duration of application depend on the state of the tsubo. Acupressure is combined systematically with passive stretching and rotation of the joints to stimulate the flow of *ki* through the channels. Treatments are described for the whole body (basic) and for each of the 12 major meridians.

Several issues have been raised in this chapter in discussing the Asian styles of manual therapy that are also relevant here to shiatsu. The intertwining of body–mind–spirit is evident as a holistic method of treatment born of an ancient philosophy. The practitioner–patient (giver-receiver) relationship is one of partnership, because each is a participant in the healing process. This is born of the yin yang principle (giver = yang, receiver = yin). The intention of the practitioner plays a major role in the effectiveness of the treatment; the giver is a nonjudgmental observer or plays an empathetic role. As opposed to the more neutral "do no harm" principle of Western caregivers, there appears to be more of a natural expression of love as a defined part of these systems (as with reiki). Intuition is also an important part of the treatment, because each session is an exploration of the process of healing and of the individuals involved (see Chapter 19).

SPORTS MASSAGE

Sports massage has emerged throughout the world as a valuable tool in prevention of and recovery from injury and for enhancing performance and increasing skills in the sport. Professional sports teams have long recognized the values of sports massage applications, employing athletic trainers, physical therapists, and massage therapists who often travel with the teams to administer care during the season and also work on team members during the off-season. The practitioners are responsible for assessing the tissues using manual techniques, but also must consider the habits of use during the associated sport, determine which dysfunctional mechanics are actually useful adaptations by the body in response to stresses imposed by the sport, and incorporate particular strategies and methods of treatment and prevention of injury, depending on what is discovered.

It is important that the practitioner understand the biomechanics of the sport and the way in which the body might adapt to the imposed stresses. What might seem like a dysfunctional mechanic to be released in a non-sporting body might be a necessary or normal occurrence for that athlete. For instance, the external and internal ROM is often displaced posteriorly in a pitcher's shoulder. This possibly occurs in the humeral shaft as a result of the torsional forces imposed on it through years of windup movements, particularly when these forces are placed on the youthful bone. If normal ROM tests are used, the external rotation would appear to be excessive and the internal ROM would appear to be reduced, although overall the degree of ROM is the same as in a nonpitching shoulder. The uninformed practitioner might attempt to increase internal ROM, believing this to be reduced, and thereby destabilize the joint and over-stretch the joint capsule, making the shoulder more vulnerable to injury.

Sports massage therapists often appear at neighborhood sport events to provide pre- and post-event massage. The techniques used warm up the tissues close to the time of event participation are significantly different from those used after the event to enhance recovery. Likewise, those used in the off-season to alter mechanics or those used in injured players differ from those used to prepare participants for play. It is important that the practitioner understand when to use which techniques, when ice and heat are appropriate, and just how much therapy is enough without overtreating the tissues. Professional sports massage training is suggested for all practitioners who work with athletes, whether in the field or in the clinic.

A number of stretching protocols can be incorporated to increase length in shortened tissues or restore balance between hypotonic and hypertonic tissues. Active isolated stretching (AIS), proprioceptive neuromuscular facilitation (PNF), and muscle energy techniques (MET) are just a few of the many stretching protocols used by manual therapists and athletic trainers to achieve greater balance within the musculoskeletal system.

In the past few decades, athletes (including Olympians) have appeared with brightly colored tape placed in unusual patterns on the skin. Kenso Kase developed the application of tape to the skin for treatment purposes, and the Kinesio Taping® Method has emerged globally as a treatment method, not only during sport and in recovery, but also in the general population.

Michael McGillicuddy (2012) explains, "Kase and others found that the Kinesio Taping applications not only reduced muscle tension, but also improved blood and lymphatic circulation and were effective in reducing neurological symptoms through skin stimulation. As Kase had studied kinesiology, he knew that muscles not only contribute to movement of the body but also help with circulation of the blood, lymphatic flow, and body temperature. By using the elastic tape, it was proposed that the muscles, fascia, and other tissues could be helped by outside assistance creating a gentle lifting of the skin, allowing for better lymphatic and vascular movement. Kase et al (2003) suggested that the application of the Kinesio Tex Tape to the skin may affect mechanical receptors, fascia, subcutaneous space, ligaments, tendons, sensory perception, and lymphatic flow."

STRAIN-COUNTERSTRAIN (POSITIONAL RELEASE TECHNIQUE)

Strain-counterstrain (SCS) technique, originally called "positional release technique (PRT)," is a very gentle, passive technique developed by Lawrence Jones, DO. The practitioner usually palpates a muscle in spasm (often associated with strain) while the patient reports on his or her sense of discomfort. The patient is next brought into a position that shortens the muscle or eases the dysfunctional joint (*counterstrain*), which exaggerates the motion restriction. The patient then reports on the level of ease. This position is held usually for 90 to 120 seconds, and the patient is then slowly returned to the original position. The technique is designed to interrupt the reflex spasm loop by altering proprioceptive input into the CNS and can be followed by gentle stretching of the involved muscle. Tender points are also treated in this manner: the patient is brought to a position of ease, held in the position until a "softening" or change in tissue texture is felt or the tenderness subsides, then slowly returned to the original position.

Similar to SCS/PRT just discussed is functional technique (functional positional release), but the latter relies a little more on the practitioner's palpation skills than on the patient's reporting. The practitioner places a hand or finger on a tender area and searches for the most distressed tissue. The patient is then positioned until a "position of ease" is produced or until the discomfort is significantly reduced, and the patient holds this position for a certain period, usually at least 90 to 120 seconds and sometimes considerably longer. The patient is then brought slowly back to the original position. It is possible that as the position of ease reduces nociceptive and aberrant proprioceptive input to the CNS, an interruption of facilitation associated with pain and spasm is achieved. Realignment of fascia is also a result of the functional technique, and it is possible that the actin and myosin filaments are able to "unlatch" due to approximation of the two ends of the fibers.

SPA-RESORT THERAPIES

"Spa" is not actually a type of massage; it is a setting in which massage and many other therapies are practiced. It is profoundly popular throughout the world, incorporates a unique atmosphere that promotes deep relaxation, and involves a number of adjunct therapies. It is appropriately included alongside many of the massage styles that are used within this setting.

Deep relaxation massage is the primary massage protocol used in most U.S.-based spas. One form, Swedish massage, was discussed earlier in this chapter, alongside the five main massage techniques that it uses: effleurage, pétrissage, friction, tapotement, and vibration. Heat, essential oils, dim lights, soft music, and other elements are often combined with the long, slow strokes and rhythmic kneading hand movements that are characteristic of relaxation massage. For many decades, this was the style of massage given at spas and was mainly reserved for the "rich and famous." In the last 30 years, massage has become openly available to a broad population, accessible in almost all communities, and marketed openly for its healing properties and as stress reduction.

Any of the styles of massage discussed in this chapter might be found in a spa. Independent as well as predominant chains may offer broad menus that include a very wide variety of massage styles, most of which are included herein. Many also offer a diverse range of classes involving exercise, healthy cooking, stress management, and self-care. Additionally, spas often incorporate skin treatments (e.g., facials, scrubs, wraps, waxing), water treatments (steam, sauna, cold plunge), and the application of an array of products that serve to exfoliate, polish, and hydrate the skin. Whether lying on a massage table, seated in a massage chair, or floating in water, the varied forms of spa-based treatment serve to relax the mind and body, and to enhance a greater sense of well-being.

THE TRAGER APPROACH® (PSYCHOPHYSICAL INTEGRATION AND MENTASTICS®)

Milton Trager, MD, was originally a boxer and gymnast and developed (almost by accident) his technique of psychophysical integration more than 50 years ago (Trager & Hammond, 1995). To obtain the credentials he believed were necessary to bring his technique to the medical community, he obtained a medical degree from the University of Guadalajara in 1955. While at medical school, he was able to demonstrate his technique and treat polio patients with a relatively high degree of success. After developing the technique over many years in his medical practice, he began to teach the method in 1975. The Trager Institute (Mill Valley, California) was founded shortly thereafter and is responsible for dissemination of information and certification programs.

The Trager® Approach is a two-tiered approach, along the lines of the Feldenkrais Method® (see previous discussion, p. 287). The psychophysical integration phase, also known as "table work," consists of a single treatment or a series of treatments. Mentastics®, as described later, is an exercise taught to patients so that they may continue the work on their own.

Psychophysical integration is essentially an indirect, functional technique. The patient lies on a table, and the practitioner applies a very gentle rocking motion to explore the body for areas of tissue tension and motion restriction. No force, stroking, or thrust is used in this technique, merely a light, rhythmic contact. The purpose is to produce a specific sensory experience for the patient, one that is positive and pleasurable. Any discomfort serves to break the continuum of "teaching" and "learning."

The focus of the treatment, however, is not on any specific anatomical structure or physiological process, but rather on the *psyche* of the patient. An attempt is made to bring the patient into a position (or motion) of ease, in which a sensation of lightness or freedom is experienced. This sensation is "learned" by the patient during the process of sensorimotor repatterning. In the words of Dr. Trager, the patient learns "how the tissue should feel when everything is right." This mind–body interaction is the core of the treatment, and plays an exceptional role to induce a change. The result is deep relaxation and increased ROM (i.e., the sense of lightness).

Patterns of behavior and posture are learned during a person's lifetime in part as reactions to trauma or withdrawal from pain, either physical or emotional (see discussion on structural integration, p. 264). Initially, the body may be able to compensate for such reactions, but it will eventually decompensate, which results in various somatic or visceral symptoms. The Trager treatment "allows" the patient to reexperience what is normal through this exploratory process.

The practitioner seeks to integrate with the patient by entering a quasi-meditative state of awareness referred to as the "hookup." This allows the practitioner to attend acutely to the work at hand and feel very subtle changes in tissue texture and movement, not unlike the level of attention necessary to practice cranial osteopathy (see p. 286). Without any specific anatomical protocol, the work is very intuitive, and "letting go" is necessary by both parties. The practitioner maintains a position of "neutrality" and makes no attempt to "make anything happen," because it is actually the patient who is sensing and learning. The practitioner's role is one of a facilitator, in which he or she seeks to provide a safe and nurturing environment for the patient to explore new and pain-free patterns of motion.

Mentastics®, the continuing phase of The Trager Approach®, is short for "mental gymnastics" and follows table work. A basic exercise set is taught, and patients are instructed to practice on their own. These exercises consist of repetitive and sequential movements of all the joints, designed to relieve tension in the body. They are to be performed in an effortless, relaxed state of awareness, in which the individual "hooks up" with the self. The basic principles of Hatha Yoga and t'ai chi are used in these exercises. Once the set is learned, individuals can then continue to explore independently, creating their own custom-designed series.

Practitioners of The Trager Approach® have reported success (not necessarily cures) in patients with multiple sclerosis, muscular dystrophy, and other debilitating diseases. Athletes have also reported significant improvements in performance as a result of applying Trager techniques.

TUI NA

Tui na is a manipulative practice within China's traditional medicine. The literal translation is "pushing and grasping." Tui na from China, is to some extent a forerunner of shiatsu in Japan. Tui na is more than 4000 years old and predates the manufacture of acupuncture needles. Tui na may be practiced by Chinese medicine physicians as part of their general practice, or they may specialize in it, as do members of the osteopathic profession.

As with other Chinese medical arts, tui na is based on the meridian or channel view of the human body, the yin-yang principle, and the five elements theory. The organs of the body exist not only as anatomical structures, but also in a functional context (e.g., the "triple burner"), as well as in relation to one another. Yin and yang, as opposite forces, coexist in equilibrium with one another. Of the 12 major meridians of the body that correspond to the organs, six are yin, the others yang.

Qi, or vital energy, is a universal force that permeates everything. It is manifest as five separate elements: fire, wood, metal, water, and earth. The organs of the body are categorized accordingly. Qi flows through all the meridians once each day in 2-hour cycles. Therefore each meridian, and thus its associated organ, has its daily strong and weak periods. When the flow of qi is impeded in any channel, that organ or function may become dysfunctional, resulting in disease.

The techniques of tui na combine soft tissue, visceral, and joint manipulation. Typically, the patient is lying on a table or is seated. Soft tissue techniques, which are applied to the limbs, trunk, and head, precede joint mobilization to prepare the joint for movement and to relax the surrounding musculature. The techniques are designed to stimulate local blood flow, venous and lymphatic drainage, and the flow of qi (see previous discussion on shiatsu). These soft tissue techniques include the following:

- *Pressing*, using the thumbs, elbows, or palms.
- *Squeezing*, using the whole hand or finger-thumb combination.
- *Kneading*, a circular pressing technique, using the thumbs, heel of the hand, elbow, or forearm.
- *Rubbing*, a high-frequency technique, using the palms, heels of the hands (chafing), or forearms.
- *Stroking* (see effleurage), moving the hand over the skin in a long stroke, in one direction only.
- *Vibration*, similar to that used in massage.
- *Thumb rocking*, for deep penetration of acupuncture points.
- *Plucking*, a transverse friction type of technique.
- *Rolling*, using the back of the hand to roll over the skin and underlying tissue.
- *Percussion* (see tapotement), which includes pummeling with the fists, hacking with the heels of the hands, and pounding with cupped hands.

Included in the joint manipulative techniques are the following:

- *Shaking,* in which traction is applied to the limb and it is shaken with high-velocity low-amplitude movements from 10 to 20 times.
- *Flexion and extension,* primarily applied to the elbow and knee joints (i.e., the hinge joints). These are both high- and low-velocity techniques designed to engage a motion barrier but not to challenge it. In addition, in some of these techniques a thumb is simultaneously applied to an acupuncture point to open a meridian.
- *Rotation,* an articulatory technique used for the ankles, wrists, hips, and shoulders. Practitioners of tui na do not apply this technique to the neck.
- *Pushing and pulling,* a low-velocity technique designed to directly engage a motion barrier, with a counterforce applied by the opposing hand in the opposite direction.
- *Stretching,* a general, low-velocity flexion-extension technique used to loosen the joints of the spine.
- *Thrust,* used on the spinal joints in a manner similar to that in osteopathic and chiropractic methods.

Tui na can be applied to virtually anyone and has few contraindications. The existing contraindications are similar to those for massage, including skin lesions or infection, skin or lymphatic cancer, and osteoporosis. In addition, it is recommended that the low back and abdomen be avoided during pregnancy.

Anatomically, tui na is applied to the musculoskeletal system and viscera, with attention being paid to the meridians and flow of qi (as specific meridians flow through specific joints, muscle groups, and visceral structures). As with other forms of manipulative treatment, tui na seeks to produce a feeling of well-being and health in the patient. In addition, as the emotional and spiritual components of the patient are addressed, emotional release can also be produced.

VISCERAL MANIPULATION

Visceral manipulation generally involves specific placement of gentle manual forces to encourage tone, mobility, and motion of the abdominopelvic viscera and their supporting connective tissue. Although not indicated in patients with tumors or inflammatory disease, visceral manipulation can be useful in stabilizing and balancing blood flow and autonomic innervation and can even dislodge certain obstructions of the gastrointestinal system.

Methods that address manual manipulation of the viscera have been a component of some therapeutic systems in Oriental medicine for centuries and are now practiced extensively by European osteopaths, physical therapists, and other manual practitioners throughout the world. Osteopath and physical therapist Jean-Pierre Barral developed a system of training and practice of this technique that is available to all manual practitioners. Contact the Barral Institute in West Palm Beach, Florida.

OSSEOUS TECHNIQUES

In addition to methods applied to the soft tissues, a variety of techniques can be used to normalize the position of the osseous structure. The prominent techniques are discussed elsewhere in this book. The techniques presented here are often used in conjunction with the aforelisted myofascial methods. Their inclusion as a supporting modality is meant to encourage the synergistic integration of manual modalities.

ARTICULATORY TECHNIQUE

In the articulatory technique, the practitioner moves the affected joint through its ROM in all planes, gently encountering motion barriers and gradually moving through them to establish normal motion. This low-velocity moderate- to high-amplitude method would be considered a passive, direct/indirect, oscillatory technique used to restore as much motion as possible to a dysfunctional joint.

CRANIAL OSTEOPATHY

Cranial osteopathy (see also Craniosacral Therapy) is the study of the anatomy and physiology of the cranium, as well as its relationship with the body as a whole. William Garner Sutherland developed and taught cranial osteopathy in the early to mid-1900s. He considered his cranial concepts to be an extension of Still's science of osteopathy and not separate from it. Where textbooks taught that cranial bones were fused and immovable, Dr. Sutherland perceived a subtle palpable movement and suggested that there was a continuity of this rhythmic fluid movement, not only throughout the cranium, but also throughout all body tissues.

The Osteopathic Cranial Academy website (www .cranialacademy.com) describes Sutherland's dilemma, "While a student at the American School of Osteopathy in 1899, Dr. Sutherland pondered the fine details of a separated or 'disarticulated' skull. He wondered about the function of this complex architecture. Dr. Still taught that every structure exists because it performs a particular function. While looking at a temporal bone, a flash of inspiration struck Dr. Sutherland: 'Beveled like the gills of a fish, indicating respiratory motion for an articular mechanism.'"

Consumed by this idea, Sutherland was inspired and motivated toward a singular, detailed, and prolonged study of the cranium, and often experimented on his own head. Over many years of intense study, he developed the concepts of "The Primary Respiratory Mechanism" with its five components: (1) the rhythmic movement of the brain and spinal cord; (2) fluctuations of cerebrospinal fluid; (3) the reciprocal tension membrane; (4) the osteoarticular mechanism; and (5) the involuntary motion of the sacrum. Dr. Sutherland described that these activities of the CNS as having a motion with "inhalation" and "exhalation" phases and that a practitioner connecting directly (through specific palpation) with the primary respiratory mechanism could bring about a therapeutic response.

Thomas Northup (1949) recognized Sutherland's work in the 1949 yearbook of the Academy of Applied Osteopathy: "Without doubt Dr. William G. Sutherland has made the greatest single contribution to the advancement of manipulative osteopathy since Dr. Andrew Taylor Still established it three quarters of a century ago and in recognition of his great contribution to the osteopathic profession we affectionately dedicate this 1949 Year Book to him." The entire issue, which contains a considerable discussion and photographs of Sutherland's techniques (Lippincott, 1949), is available online at no cost (www.lille-osteopathie.fr/upload/1949.pdf).

HIGH-VELOCITY LOW-AMPLITUDE TECHNIQUE

The high-velocity low-amplitude (HVLA) technique is probably the most publicly recognized technique of the osteopath or chiropractor. This technique is a thrust-oriented, designed to aggressively break through a motion barrier. More often than not, an audible pop is heard, the result of a brief cavitation of the involved joint. The HVLA technique can be applied directly (toward the barrier) or indirectly (away from the barrier), using short or long levers. Although often associated with manipulation of the spine, the HVLA technique can also be performed on the extremities.

Use of the HVLA technique is contraindicated in patients with osteoporosis, bone tumors, or severe atherosclerosis, and in those who are taking certain medications that make bones more brittle, such as many forms of chemotherapy. Recently, much discussion has focused on the safety of the HVLA technique when performed in the high cervical (neck) region due to potential risk to the vertebral artery. Controversy has expanded to include questions regarding the safety and accuracy of manual screening tests for vertebral artery insufficiencies (such as George's Test and the DeKlynes Test). In March 2004, all U.S. chiropractic schools agreed to abandon the teaching and use of provocation tests such as these due to the inherent risks and high level of false data. An extensive PowerPoint presentation regarding these concerns is available (Clum, 2006).

PRACTICE SETTINGS

Massage therapy is used in a variety of clinical settings, spas, private practices, and sport arenas and facilities. The expertise of the massage therapist or practitioner is essential in determining which techniques may or may not be appropriate and how the massage may be delivered. Application choices will also be based on the case presentation and may be influenced by the environment, such as a hospital vs. a spa, as well as the allocation of time, prescribed therapy, other associated modalities (e.g., stretching, exercise, biofeedback) that may be needed or desired and scope of practitioner's license. Massage is routinely applied to pediatric, adolescent, and geriatric patients. Frequently, massage therapists expand their therapeutic horizons by taking postgraduate study in other forms of bodywork or specific methods for application to certain pathologies. It is not uncommon to find a therapist who not only does Swedish massage but also employs the Trager® Approach, the Feldenkrais® method, and craniosacral therapy, moving seamlessly from one to the other, as indicated by the response of the tissues and recipient.

The application of massage therapy in medical settings has recently expanded at a dramatic rate, perhaps because of the growing use of "multidisciplinary approaches" to patient care. Massage therapists and other manual practitioners now render their skills in hospitals, physical therapy clinics, rehabilitation centers, and the offices of physicians, osteopaths, chiropractors, dentists, and multidisciplinary clinics. In professional sport arenas, Olympic competitions, and college, high school, and Little League teams, massage and manual techniques have emerged as valued tools for rehabilitation, enhancement of performance, and prevention of injury. These professions are no longer considered to be on the outskirts of medicine, but are now incorporated as an integral part of treatment options. All manual medicine modalities are areas that are ripe for research, with much being done worldwide to validate them and explore their breadth of application in patient care.

SUMMARY

In closing, it is important to note the value of the preventive aspect of manipulation as a holistic practice. Manipulative treatment can be used for proactive general maintenance as well as for reactive treatment of dysfunction. To use an automobile analogy, most consumers think nothing of periodically getting a car tuned up and paying considerable sums for the privilege. Why not do the same for their own bodies? In addition, the value of manual treatment for young persons cannot be overstated. Structural corrections can be made before fascial distortions become relatively locked in or before continuous aberrant sensory input results in facilitated sensorimotor patterning. Corrections can be made before compensatory reactions in muscles, fascia, and behavior can create unbalanced anatomy and physiology that function poorly and eventually lead to structural remodeling or a decreased resistance to disease (pathology). As Alexander Pope once proclaimed, "Just as the twig is bent, the tree's inclined."

The importance given to this information should be tied to the awareness that, as the body ages, adaptive forces cause changes in the structures of the body, with the occurrence of shortening, crowding, and distortion. With this, we can see—in real terms within our own bodies and those of our patients—the environment in which cells change shape. As they do so they change their potential for normal genetic expression, as well as their abilities to communicate and to handle nutrients efficiently.

Reversing or slowing these undesirable processes is the potential of appropriate bodywork and movement approaches. It is yet to be precisely established to what degree functional health can be modified by soft tissue techniques, such as those discussed in this chapter. However, the normalizing of structural and functional features of connective tissue by addressing myofascial trigger points, chronic muscle shortening and fibrosis, as well as perpetuating factors such as habits of use, has clear implications. Well-designed research to assess cellular, structural, and functional changes that follow the application of manual techniques is clinically relevant and sorely needed.

References

Ahn AC, Park M, Shaw JR et al: Electrical impedance of acupuncture meridians: the relevance of subcutaneous collagenous bands, *PLoS ONE* 5(7):e11907, 2010. doi: 10.1371/journal.pone.0011907.

Barral JP, Croibier A: *Approche osteopathique du traumatisme*, St. Etienne, France, 1997, Editions ATSA, CIDO & Actes Graphiques.

Barral JP: Neural manipulation. In DeLany J, editor: *3D Anatomy for massage and manual therapies*, London, 2012, Primal Pictures.

Birch S: Trigger point–acupuncture point correlations revisited, *J Altern Complement Med* 9(1):91–103, 2003.

Brennan BA: *Hands of light: a guide to healing through the human energy field*, New York, 1988, Bantam Books. (Illustrated by JA Smith.)

Burman I, Friedland S: *TouchAbilities® Essential Connections*, Clifton Park, NY, 2006, Thomson Delmar Learning.

Butler DS: *Mobilisation of the nervous system*, Melbourne, Australia, 1991, Churchill Livingstone.

Butler DS: *The sensitive nervous system*, Unley, S. Australia, 2000, Noigroup Publications.

Byers D: *Better health with foot reflexology, revised edn*, St. Petersburg FL, 2001, Ingham Publishing, Inc.

Casanelia L, Stelfox D: *Foundations of massage*, ed 3, Australia, 2010, Churchill Livingstone, Elsevier.

Chaitow L, DeLany J: *Clinical application of neuromuscular techniques* (vol 1), ed 2, *The upper body*, Edinburgh, 2008, Elsevier Health Sciences.

Chaitow L, DeLany J: *Clinical application of neuromuscular techniques* (vol 2), ed 2, *The lower body*, Edinburgh, 2011, Elsevier Health Sciences.

Chaitow L: *Muscle energy techniques*, ed 4, Edinburgh, 2013, Elsevier/Churchill Livingstone.

Chen C, Ingber D: Tensegrity and mechanoregulation: from skeleton to cytoskeleton, *Osteoarthritis Cartilage* 7(1):81–94, 1999.

Clum GW: Cervical spine adjusting and the vertebral artery, 2006, Available at: http://www.chirocolleges.org./acccva.html.

Cyriax J: *Textbook of orthopaedic medicine* (vol 2), ed 11, Treatment by manipulation, massage and injection, London, 1984, Bailliere Tindall.

Cyriax J: *Textbook of orthopaedic medicine* (vol 2), ed 2, Treatment by manipulation, massage and injection, London, 1984, WB Saunders.

DeLany J: Intro to manual therapy. In DeLany J, editor: *3D Anatomy for massage and manual therapies*, London, 2012, Primal Pictures.

Donoyama N, Manakata T, Shibasaki M: Effects of Anma therapy (traditional Japanese massage) on body and mind, *J Bodyw Mov Ther* 14(1):55–64, 2010.

Donoyama N, Satoh T, Hamano T: Effects of Anma massage therapy (Japanese massage) for gynecological cancer survivors: study protocol for a randomized controlled trial, *Trials* 14:233, 2013.

Dorsher PT: Can classical acupuncture points and trigger points be compared in the treatment of pain disorders? Birch's analysis revisited, *J Altern Complement Med* 14(4):353–359, 2008.

du Rand J: Oncology massage. In DeLany J, editor: *3D Anatomy for massage and manual therapies*, London, 2012, Primal Pictures.

Feldenkrais M: *Awareness through movement: easy-to-do health exercises to improve your posture, vision, imagination, and personal growth*, San Francisco, 1991, Harper Collins.

Friedland S: Aquatic bodywork. In DeLany J, editor: *3D Anatomy for massage and manual therapies*, London, 2012, Primal Pictures.

Hong C-Z: Myofascial trigger points: pathophysiology and correlation with acupuncture points, *Acupunct Med* 18(1):41–47, 2000.

Ingber DE: The riddle of morphogenesis: a question of solution chemistry or molecular cell engineering, *Cell* 75:1249, 1993.

Ingber DE, Folkman J: Tension and compression as basic determinants of cell form and function: utilization of a cellular tensegrity mechanism. In Stein W, Bronner F, editors: *Cell shape: determinants, regulation and regulatory role*, San Diego, 1989, Academic Press, p 1.

Kase K, Wallis J, Kase T: *Clinical therapeutic applications of the Kinesio taping method*, ed 2, Tokyo, Japan, 2003, Ken Ikai Co.

Kawakita K, Itoh K, Okada K: The polymodal receptor hypothesis of acupuncture and moxibustion, and its rational explanation of acupuncture points. In Sato A, Peng L, Campbell JL, editors: *Acupuncture—is there a physiological basis?* Exerpta Medica, International Congress Series 1238, 2002, p 63.

Krieger DK: *The therapeutic touch: how to use your hands to help or to heal*, New York, 1992, Simon & Schuster.

Langevin H, Bouffard N, Badger G et al: Dynamic fibroblast cytoskeletal response to subcutaneous tissue stretch ex vivo and in vivo, *Am J Physiol Cell Physiol* 288:C747–C756, 2005.

Langevin H, Churchill D, Cipolla M: Mechanical signaling through connective tissue: a mechanism for the therapeutic effect of acupuncture, *FASEB J* 15:2275, 2001.

Langevin H, Cornbrooks C, Taatjes D et al: Fibroblasts form a body-wide cellular network, *Histochem Cell Biol* 122(1):7, 2004.

Langevin HM, Yandow JA: Relationship of acupuncture points and meridians to connective tissue planes, *Anat Rec* 269(6):257–265, 2002.

Lewit K, Simons DG: Myofascial pain: relief by post-isometric relaxation, *Arch Phys Med Rehabil* 65(8):452, 1984.

Lippincott HA: *The osteopathic technique of Wm. G. Sutherland D.O.* Academy of Applied Osteopathy Yearbook, 1949, pp 1–24.

Lowe W: *Functional assessment in massage therapy*, ed 3, Bend, OR, USA, 1997, OMERI.

Lowe W: Orthopedic massage. In DeLany J, editor: *3D Anatomy for massage and manual therapies*, London, 2012, Primal Pictures.

Mann J, Gaylord S, Fourot K et al: Craniosacral therapy for migraine: a feasibility study, *BMC Complement Altern Med* 12(Suppl 1):111, 2012.

McClure V: Infant massage. In DeLany J, editor: *3D Anatomy for massage and manual therapies*, London, 2012, Primal Pictures.

McGillicuddy M: Kinesiotaping. In DeLany J, editor: *3D Anatomy for massage and manual therapies*, London, 2012, Primal Pictures.

Mehl-Madrona L, Kligler B, Silverman S et al: The impact of acupuncture and craniosacral therapy interventions on clinical outcomes in adults with asthma, *J Sci Healing* 3(1):28, 2007.

Melzack R, Stillwell DM, Fox EJ: Trigger points and acupuncture points for pain: correlations and implications, *Pain* 3:3, 1977.

Mennell JM: *Manual therapy*, Springfield, IL, 1951, Charles C Thomas Publisher, p 3.

Myers T: Anatomy trains, *J Body Mov Ther* 1(2):91, 1997.

Myers T: Anatomy trains, *J Body Mov Ther* 1(3):134, 1997.

Nissen H: *Swedish movement and massage treatment*, Philadelphia, 1889, FA Davis.

Northup T: Forward. Academy of Applied Osteopathy Yearbook, 1949, p ix.

Orstrom K: *Massage and the original Swedish movements*, ed 8, Philadelphia, 1918, P. Blakinston's Son & Co.

Osborne C: Prenatal massage. In DeLany J, editor: *3D Anatomy for massage and manual therapies*, London, 2012, Primal Pictures.

Pettman E: A history of manipulative therapy, *J Man Manip Ther* 15(3):165–174, 2007.

Plummer J: Anatomical findings at acupuncture loci, *Am J Chinese Med* 8:170, 1980.

Puszko S: Hospice-based massage therapy. In DeLany J, editor: *3D Anatomy for massage and manual therapies*, London, 2012, Primal Pictures.

Raviv G, Shefi S, Nizani D et al: Effect of craniosacral therapy on lower urinary tract signs and symptoms in multiple sclerosis, *Complement Ther Clin Pract* 15(2):72, 2009.

Rolf IP, Thompson R: *Rolfing: reestablishing the natural alignment and structural integration of the human body for vitality and well-being*, Rochester, VT, 1989, Inner Traditions International.

Rolf IP: *The integration of human structures*, Santa Monica, CA, 1997, Dennis-Landman.

Rolf IP: *What in the world is rolfing?* Santa Monica, CA, 1975, Dennis-Landman.

Rywerant Y, Feldenkrais M: *The Feldenkrais method*, 2011. ReadHowYouWant.com.

Salvo S: Massage of the elderly. In DeLany J, editor: *3D Anatomy for massage and manual therapies*, London, 2012, Primal Pictures.

Simons D, Travell J, Simons L: *Myofascial pain and dysfunction: the trigger point manual, vol 1: upper half of body*, Baltimore, 1999, Lippincott, Williams and Wilkins.

Teeguarden I: *Acupressure way of health: Jin Shin Do*, Tokyo, 1978, Japan Publications.

Trager M, Hammond C: *Movement as a way to agelessness: a guide to Trager mentastics*, Barrytown, NY, 1995, Station Hill Press.

Travell J, Simons D: *Myofascial pain and dysfunction: the trigger point manual, vol 2: lower half of body*, Baltimore, 1992, Williams and Wilkins.

Wall P, Melzack R: *Textbook of pain*, ed 2, Edinburgh, 1990, Churchill Livingstone.

Wuttke R: Hot/cold stone therapy. In DeLany J, editor: *3D Anatomy for massage and manual therapies*, London, 2012, Primal Pictures.

Suggested Readings

Dash VB, Dash B: *Massage therapy in Ayurveda*, New Delhi, 1992, Concept Publishing.

Dougan I, Townley A, editors: *The complete illustrated guide to reflexology: therapeutic foot massage for health and well-being*, Lanham, Md, 1999, Barnes & Noble Books. (Illustrated by P Allen, photography by G Ryecart.)

Fritz S: *Mosby's fundamentals of therapeutic massage*, ed 3, St Louis, 2005, Mosby.

Govindan SV: *Massage for health and healing: Ayurvedic and spiritual energy approach*, Columbia, Mo, 1996, South Asia Books.

Johari H: *Ayurvedic massage: traditional Indian techniques for balancing body and mind*, Rochester, VT, 1995, Inner Traditions International.

Juhan D: *Job's body: a handbook for bodywork*, Barrytown, NY, 1998, Barrytown, Ltd.

Liechti E: *The complete illustrated guide to shiatsu: the Japanese healing art of touch for health and fitness*, Rockport, Mass, 1998, Element Books.

Liskin J: *Moving medicine: the life work of Milton Trager, M.D.*, Barrytown, NY, 1995, Station Hill Press.

Liu H, Perry P: *Mastering miracles: the healing art of qi gong as taught by a master*, New York, 1997, Warner Books. (Appropriate for general reading.)

Lubeck W: *The complete reiki handbook: basic introduction and methods of natural application*, Twin Lakes, WI, 1998, Lotus Light Publications.

Lundberg P: *The book of shiatsu*, New York, 1992, Simon & Schuster. (Photography by F Dorelli.)

MacDonald G: *Medicine hands: massage therapy for people with cancer*, ed 2, Forres, UK, 2007, Findhorn Press.

Myers T: *Anatomy trains: myofascial meridians for manual and movement therapists*, ed 2, Edinburgh, UK, 2009, Churchill Livingstone, Elsevier.

Pritchard SM: *Chinese massage manual: the healing art of tui na*, Bulverde, Tex, 1999, Omni.

Rand WL, Martin SA, editors: *Reiki: the healing touch*, Southfield, Mich, 1996, Vision Publications. (Illustrated by SM Matsko.)

Rywerant Y: *The Feldenkrais method: teaching by handling*, New Canaan, CT, 1991, Keats. (Foreword by Moshé Feldenkrais; illustrated by D Mohor.)

Tappan FM, Benjamin PJ: *Tappan's handbook of healing massage techniques: classic, holistic, and emerging methods*, Norwalk, CT, 1997, Appleton & Lange.

Walton T: *Medical conditions and massage therapy: a decision tree approach*, Philadelphia, PA, 2011, Lippincott, Williams & Wilkins.

Wang S, Liu JL: *Qi gong for health and longevity: the ancient Chinese art of relaxation, meditation, physical fitness*, Tustin, CA, 1999, East Health Development Group. (Appropriate for general and professional reading.)

Wills P: *The reflexology manual: an easy-to-use illustrated guide to healing zones of the hands and feet*, Rochester, VT, 1995, Inner Traditions International. (Photography by S Atkinson.)

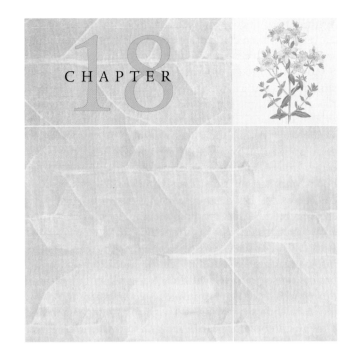

CHAPTER 18

OSTEOPATHY

J O H N   M.   J O N E S

To find health should be the object of the doctor. Anyone can find disease.

—Andrew Taylor Still, MD, DO

Osteopathic medicine began as a reform offshoot of the standard "regular" medical practices of the 1800s, when one innovative physician became disenchanted with the inadequate and harmful effects of the medicines being used by the doctors of that era.

Andrew Taylor Still, MD, DO, was born in 1828 in Jonesboro, Virginia, when this part of the country was still on the American frontier (see Chapter 1). His life experiences and observations led him to question the entire system of medicine that existed in nineteenth-century America.

Most regular medications and treatments used in that era were unresearched remedies and procedures passed on through tradition originating from the Middle Ages of Europe. Bleeding and leeching were major components of treatment when Still was trained, as were "purging" and "puking." One of the most common medications was calomel, a mercuric compound used as a purgative. It was extremely toxic, often causing patients' gums to be resorbed, teeth to fall out, and sores to break out in the mouth. Calomel contributed to many deaths and disfigured many more. Some of the most disfiguring facial injuries of the U.S. Civil War (1861-1865) were the result of giving calomel to soldiers, not just injuries form enemy bullets and artillery.

Surgery was primitive and performed without antisepsis; anesthetics were just beginning to be used in the mid-1800s. No antibiotics had been identified, and no microbial cause of infectious illness was proven until 1872. There was no knowledge of the immune system, and heart disease and cancer were not understood. Physicians were capable of diagnosing empirically, recognized patterns of illness and, in many cases, predicting outcomes. Medical treatment was often more dangerous than doing nothing. In fact, the famous seventeenth century French mathematician and philosopher Descartes (see Chapter 6) was reputed to have said, "Before, when I knew I was sick, I thought I might die; now that they are taking me to the chirurgeon, I know I shall" (Schiowitz, 1997). In England, Francis Bacon had stated simply, "The remedy is worse than the disease."

Still was seeking a philosophy of medicine and system of treatment based on scientific principles as they could be observed in nature. In one of his books, he stated that in April 1855, he began to discuss reasons "for my faith in the laws of life as given to men, worlds, and beings by the God of Nature" (Still, 1902). He was not alone in his disillusionment with the contemporary state of affairs and quest for a scientifically based philosophy of medicine. The great physician and author Oliver Wendell Holmes, for example, was often quoted from his 1860 presentation to the Massachusetts Medical Society (publisher of today's *New England Journal of Medicine*) that "if the whole of *materia medica* as now used could be sunk to the bottom of the sea, it would be all the better for mankind—and all the worse for the fishes" (Holmes, 1892). (The jurist Oliver Wendell Holmes, Jr., Supreme Court chief justice, was his son.)

By the time of the U.S. Civil War, a large number of American physicians were homeopathic or eclectic (non-standard) practitioners. In addition, many people on the frontier took care of their own medical needs (see Chapters 1 and 22). Medical education was offered in two ways, one by university degree and one by "reading medicine." At university-affiliated medical schools during the early and mid-nineteenth century, students attended a course of 4 to 6 months of morning lectures to obtain their degrees. If students voluntarily attended a second year, it was for a repeat of the same lectures.

The alternate pathway was used by many American physicians on the frontier, who learned by becoming an apprentice to an established physician. Under the physician's supervision, they read medical and scientific textbooks and accompanied him and possibly other of his colleagues on home and office visits. More specialized studies could be undertaken by arranging to work with an established expert, but most doctors did not pursue such studies. These two systems were later combined and evolved into the current system of medical education (2 years of basic science and medical didactics, followed by 2 years during which students continue to read medical books and journals while shadowing and assisting physicians in hospital and ambulatory care settings, after which the graduate physicians do an additional 3 to 7 years of supervised postgraduate hospital residencies).

Andrew Taylor Still (Figure 18-1) was the son of Abram Still, a circuit-riding Methodist minister who was also a physician, tending to his flock both spiritually and medically. Shortly after Andrew Taylor was born, the family moved from Virginia to Missouri, farther out onto the nineteenth-century frontier, so that his father could serve the needs of the Methodist Church in the West (this church had been founded by Dr. John Wesley after he returned to England from his service as chaplain in the early-eighteenth-century colony of Savannah, Georgia, and during which he wrote treatises about Native American healing and herbal remedies—see Chapter 1). Abram Still was an ardent abolitionist who sided with the small minority of Methodist ministers in Missouri who were opposed to slavery at the time of the controversial "Missouri Compromise." There were terrible insurrections in the Kansas and Missouri territories over whether they would be admitted to the Union as slave or as free states. Sen. Stephen Douglas (D-IL) worked out the historic "Missouri Compromise" to place a temporary fix on the problem. But Still's church was still split over the issue, and the elder Still moved the family to what became known as "Bleeding Kansas," over the conflict at the time, where they were able to continue to support their practice.

Like many pioneer boys, the younger Still grew up contributing to the family food supply by hunting and did much of the butchering of the animals himself. He later stated that his studies of anatomy began this way. In his autobiography, he described an intense headache that occurred when he was 10 years old. To alleviate his discomfort by taking a nap, he placed his jacket over a rope swing to construct a pillow and then lay down with the base of his skull over the other side of the rope. He fell asleep and a short time later awoke to find his headache gone. This phenomenon impressed him, and when he became a physician, the memory of it led him to think about the relationship between the body's anatomy and the disease process. He was perhaps engaging in an early form of craniosacral therapy or myofascial release (see Chapter 17).

Still obtained his medical education through the process of apprenticeship under an established physician (in Still's case, assisting his father), combined with reading the medical texts of that time. He later attended a medical school in Kansas City, Missouri, but he did not complete a degree, stating that the school had little to teach him that he did not already know.

The younger Still began his medical career by serving the local community and working with his father with the Shawnee Indian tribe. Ironically, many years earlier his maternal grandmother had been kidnapped by the Shawnee, who had also killed numerous members of that generation of her family. Still had a standard general medical practice, employing the usual medications and involving the full range of available treatment, including obstetrics and minor surgery.

Dr. Still became a battalion surgeon in the Kansas militia during the Civil War; he also served as an officer and led men into battle. He returned to his family in 1864 at the end of the western campaigns, when the Kansas militia was disbanded after the fall of Vicksburg, Mississippi, on July 4, 1863, and the Union victories of the Army of the Cumberland in the western theatre of operations.

Believing that his family was safe now that the war was over in that part of the country, he was stunned when three of his children died in an epidemic of spinal meningitis. There were no effective medications to treat such an illness.

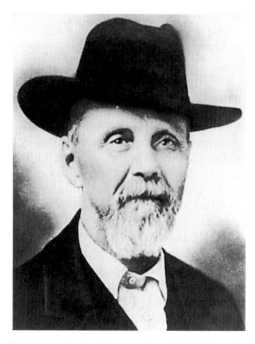

Figure 18-1 Portrait of Andrew Taylor Still, the founder of osteopathy, ca. 1900. (Courtesy Kirksville College of Osteopathy, A.T. Still Memorial Library, Archives Department, Kirksville, Mo.)

He called other physicians to attend to his family, rather than manage their cases himself, and called ministers to pray for the children as well. Nothing availed, and the children died. This event caused him to question the entire foundation of medical care in his era. He wrote, "It was when I gazed at three members of my own family—two of my own children and one adopted child—all dead from the disease, spinal meningitis, that I propounded to myself the serious questions 'In sickness has God left man in a world of guessing? Guess what is the matter? What to give, and guess the result? And when dead, guess where he goes?'" (Still, 1897, cited in Singer et al, 1962).

Seeking a more enlightened practice of medicine, Still based his reasoning on the Methodist philosophy of working to attain perfection, which seemed to him to have something in common with the new ideas of natural selection and evolution (which the English social philosopher Herbert Spencer termed "survival of the fittest," a term never actually used by Charles Darwin; see Chapter 35). The early evolutionists suggested that there existed a natural process of working toward perfection of the organism and that the human being was the highest naturally evolved life form. Still felt that the human being was perfectly constructed by the one he later referred to in his writings as the God of Nature, the Great Architect, the Great Engineer, and the Great Mechanic (comparable to the "intelligent designer" of today). If the human body was perfectly constructed as the highest form of machine, he felt it should simply need fuel and, if something went wrong, adjustment.

Like much of the general population of the nineteenth century, he had a tremendous admiration for engineering and all things mechanical. Still was also an inventor; during his life he invented an agricultural thresher and obtained patents for new types of a churn and a stove. He would eventually tell the students at the American School of Osteopathy that they were to become human engineers who knew every part and function of the body. They were to find engineering solutions to human illness and dysfunction.

Even before the Civil War, in the 1850s, Still had experimented with manual treatment of patients. But this practice was in addition to the use of standard medical practices. It was after the war, and the death of his children, that his ideas came together into a complete new philosophy regarding the etiology of illness and how to treat it. By 1897, Still wrote in his autobiography that it was on June 22, 1874, that he "flung to the breeze the banner of osteopathy" (Still, 1897, as cited in Singer et al, 1962). Apparently it was by that date that he was able to define the principles on which his philosophy and practice of medical care would be based. His new methods involved hands-on treatment, adjusting the positions of joints and levels of muscle tone; enhancing the circulation of blood, lymphatic, and cerebrospinal fluids; improving the efficiency of respiration; and therefore improving host response to disease.

Still was ostracized in Kansas for leaving the medical fold and denied the opportunity to teach his new ideas at Baker University in Baldwin, Kansas, a Methodist university where he had hoped at least to be able to discuss his ideas. He and his family had donated land to start the university, and he and his brothers had built a mill and sawed timbers for the original building. The local minister, however, indicated to the congregation that his practice was of the devil, because only Jesus was supposed to be able to "lay hands" on the sick and heal them.

After a period of time and a severe illness, he moved to back to Missouri, finally settling in Kirksville, where he said he found a few people who were willing to listen to reason. He set up a circuit practice of medicine in outlying communities. After Still had been in practice for a while, so many people began coming to Kirksville looking for him that he was able to stay in one place. He was not sure what to call his clinical practice. At first he thought his new methods, being hands on, might have something in common with magnetic healing, which was a popular nineteenth-century practice following on Mesmer's concepts of "animal magnetism" and energetic healing (see Chapters 6, 9, 10, and 15). Thus for a short time, like many others of his era (including Daniel David Palmer; see Chapter 19), Still called himself a "magnetic healer" for lack of a better, newer term. Later, he used a business card on which he called himself a "lightning bonesetter." The use of this term implies that he had heard of the folk healers who called themselves by that name. There is no evidence, however, that he ever studied with anyone who had learned this art in the usual way (i.e., it was passed from one person to the next, such as from father to son).

Still coined the term *osteopathy* (from the Greek roots *osteon* and *pathos*) sometime prior to founding the American School of Osteopathy (ASO) in 1892. This nomenclature followed the tradition of naming medical approaches after what was considered the central issue in pathology or cure (e.g., homeopathy, hydropathy, naturopathy). In the case of osteopathy, Still reasoned that malpositioning of bones and joints, especially in the spine, affected both circulation and nerve function, providing the opportunity for the development of disease in the tissues. William Smith, educated in Scotland, was another reform-minded MD who offered to teach anatomy in the new school if Still would teach him his methods. About 10 students began the first year. The school expanded rapidly, and it became impossible for Still to personally instruct all the students in his methods; thus over the next few years his first students became the new professors. Other physicians and college graduates joined the faculty as the curriculum and number of students expanded.

To further disseminate his ideas, Still wrote four books. *Autobiography of Andrew T. Still* (1897) describes his life and how he developed osteopathy. *The Philosophy of Osteopathy* (1899) and *The Philosophy and Mechanical Principles of Osteopathy* (copyrighted in 1892 but published in 1902) describe his philosophical ideas and contain a great deal of then-current simple knowledge as well as speculation about physiology, a subject poorly understood at the time. In *Osteopathy, Research and Practice* (1910), Still continued to expand on his ideas and described some of his treatment techniques.

These books reveal that he still, on occasion, used some medications—although extremely rarely. He was opposed to the use of opiates and alcohol, having seen much abuse (especially in Civil War injured and disabled), and specifically stated that it was foolish for physicians to dissolve most medications in alcohol (as tinctures), because this practice could lead to dependency. Throughout his books he recommended the use of manipulation to relieve anatomical and therefore physiological stress on the system, and return the body to a state in which it could cure itself through normal physiological processes. Still's original philosophical principles are summed up in "Our Platform," which was published in *Osteopathy, Research and Practice,* and adopted by the ASO as the foundation of its educational program.

The allopathic profession, which was becoming successful in establishing a monopoly on medical training and licensure, vigorously fought the new osteopathic profession. Still's followers, however, achieved great success in their treatment of illness in comparison with their MD counterparts, effecting cures in some "hopeless" cases and treating all types of illnesses. The new doctors also had special expertise in neuromusculoskeletal conditions at a time when no physical medicine, rehabilitation, or physical therapy was available to the public. The ASO rapidly expanded, and new schools founded by graduates helped build the osteopathic profession, which attracted supporters such as President Teddy Roosevelt, President William Howard Taft, and Mark Twain (who testified to the New York State Assembly in favor of osteopathic licensure). Osteopaths graduated with the title *Doctor of Osteopathy (DO),* which was changed at the end of the twentieth century to *Doctor of Osteopathic Medicine (DO).*

The 1910 Flexner Report, sponsored by the Carnegie Foundation, compared all American medical schools against a standard represented by the new Johns Hopkins University School of Medicine. Criticism was so devastating that about three-quarters of American medical schools closed, including many osteopathic medical schools. The surviving osteopathic medical colleges were located in Kirksville, Missouri; Kansas City, Missouri; Des Moines, Iowa; Philadelphia, Pennsylvania; Chicago, Illinois; and Los Angeles, California. None of these schools received public funding at the time. The osteopathic profession was on its own for further development.

CENTRAL CONCEPT

Still's central idea was that structural abnormality causes functional abnormality, leading to illness. To restore health, treatments were designed to use the body's own resources. He theorized that manipulation would increase

the body's efficiency, promoting appropriate delivery of blood, return of blood and lymph, delivery of neurotrophic substances, and transmission of neural impulses. Physicians had relatively few medications of value for the patient in the preantibiotic era (up to the early mid-1900s). Osteopathic manipulation, on the other hand, was a technique that a physician could employ, using his own hands, to effect physiological changes and help stimulate a host response against illness. In addition, osteopathy directly addressed a number of needs with which the medical profession had not successfully dealt: joint pain, physical rehabilitation, and soft tissue injuries.

Soon after Still's death in 1917, his new osteopathic physicians were put to the test during the Spanish influenza pandemic of 1919. The results were encouraging, while the regular medical profession had little to offer patients other than antitussives, opiates, and strychnine to stimulate the heart. Osteopathic treatment targeted autonomic changes, blood delivery, lymphatic drainage, and biomechanical improvement in respiration. Osteopathic physicians reported dramatically lower morbidity and mortality rates among their influenza patients. Following research initiated by the editor of this textbook at Walter Reed Army Medical Center in the mid-1990s, molecular biologists determined that the virulence and pathogenicity of this strain of the annual flu virus was due to the presence of genes associated with mounting a highly vigorous immune response in the host. It is therefore understandable that treatments focused on balancing the host responses would have been effective in reducing the pathogenicity of this virus.

Between the death of Still at the end of World War I in 1917 and U.S. involvement in World War II (1941–45), osteopathic colleges, like allopathic colleges, gradually improved standards. In the early 1900s, increasing practice of antiseptic procedure helped improve the safety of surgery, as did the development and use of the sulfa antibiotics beginning in the 1930s. Penicillin, although "discovered" in 1927, was not available for practical use until it was mass produced by Florey and Chain for soldiers and sailors during World War II. Even after the problems of mass production were solved, it was not readily available for the American public until after the war.

Still's students had included MDs who were less opposed to standard medications but integrated his ideas on enhancing the body's own self-healing abilities by treating the structure (anatomy) to enhance the function (physiology) and restore health. By 1928, *materia medica* (the part of medicine concerned with formulation and use of remedies or natural pharmacological preparations, taught in allopathic medical schools before the development of modern medications) was taught at all of the osteopathic medical colleges. In addition, the newly researched and efficacious antibiotics were discussed as they were developed. Osteopathic physicians, along with their MD peers, increasingly had available medications that actually worked, which they used in their general practice of medicine. From Still onward, early osteopathic physicians had included surgery in their complete practice of medicine (although, like their counterparts, not all personally performed the surgeries). DOs believed that osteopathic manipulation before and after surgery helped patients tolerate procedures better and reduced the incidence of complications, such as pneumonia, thereby resulting in a shorter recovery time.

As medical specialties and subspecialties were being developed, most osteopaths were general practitioners. American postgraduate medical specialty training programs were not generally open to DOs. A number of osteopathic specialists obtained their training in Europe from physicians who did not concern themselves with distinctions among different types of American physicians; some of these osteopathic physicians returned and set up specialty training programs within their own profession.

During World War II, osteopaths were not allowed to serve in the armed forces as physicians. Although some volunteered and served in other capacities, many stayed home and took care of patients while MDs were overseas. One result was that many families in the United States began to receive treatment from DOs. Patients were unable to see their regular physicians, and this situation helped the growth of osteopathy.

In the postwar period, as returning soldiers attended universities in record numbers on the GI Bill, osteopathic colleges enrolled record numbers of students.

By 1953, the president of the American Medical Association (AMA) had called for and received a report on the status of osteopathic medicine, which indicated that DO training was equivalent to MD training. MDs in general became less concerned with whether their osteopathic colleagues used osteopathic manipulative treatment (OMT) in the care of back pain, in sports medicine, and in rehabilitation, as long as they also prescribed new medications that were shown to be effective.

Two other events in the middle to late twentieth century helped the osteopathic profession gain acceptance. One was the merger, by government regulation, of the osteopathic profession with the allopathic medical profession in California (several members of the California state legislature had sons who were practicing osteopaths). A second was the establishment of 10 additional osteopathic medical colleges in just a little over a decade between 1969 and 1981, soon followed by others in the 1990s.

In 1961, California had more DOs than any other state. The state government, however, thought that the American Osteopathic Association (AOA) was unresponsive to its influence and decided to support a merger with the allopathic medical profession. The state osteopathic medical association worked with the California Medical Association to lobby with the public in support of this merger of professions. It was difficult at the time for DOs to obtain admission privileges in most allopathic hospitals, although osteopathic physicians had built their own hospitals. Voters were convinced to support a plan under which new osteopathic licenses would no longer be issued, with the

provision that any DO who wished to do so could trade the DO degree and $65 for an MD degree and license. More than 2000 DOs accepted MD degrees and licenses. Benefits to the new MDs included new access to hospital privileges. The largest and arguably most modern osteopathic medical school, the College of Osteopathic Physicians and Surgeons at Los Angeles, was transformed into an MD-granting institution, which shortly thereafter affiliated with the new University of California at Irvine.

The remainder of the osteopathic profession was immediately concerned that the medical establishment, unable to eliminate the osteopathic profession, was attempting to absorb it. Although there was talk of offers similar to California's in other states, there was no continuation of the process. Instead, the developments in California paved the way for further acceptance of the osteopathic medical profession. California MDs had seemingly indicated that the main differences between the two types of physicians were the letters of the degree and a $65 fee, and the osteopathic medical profession used this ammunition to approach state legislatures and other authorities in defense of osteopathic medical practice rights. Some state legislatures became convinced that it was in their interest to fund colleges of osteopathic medicine when statistics revealed that most DOs practiced general medicine and that a large proportion did so in underserved areas (small towns, rural areas, and inner cities).

The osteopathic medical profession rapidly approved the founding of numerous new osteopathic medical colleges, both public and private. Included among the state-funded colleges were schools in Michigan, Texas, Ohio, West Virginia, and Oklahoma. This rapid expansion continued the trend toward assimilation into the medical mainstream. In the latter part of the twentieth century there were insufficient numbers of osteopathic physicians to serve as role models, as well as a shortage of postgraduate training positions in osteopathic hospitals, and different interest levels in osteopathic student matriculants. The number of osteopathic graduates entering allopathic residencies increased, and young osteopathic physicians began dispersing throughout other hospitals rather than remaining concentrated in osteopathic hospitals.

In the meantime, the development of the osteopathic profession continued around the world and differed markedly from the American evolution of the profession.

OFFSHOOTS OF OSTEOPATHY

As osteopathic techniques were adapted and used by others who had become convinced of their efficacy, offshoots of the osteopathic profession developed. The first person to investigate osteopathy and found another profession was D.D. Palmer, who originated chiropractic. Palmer also initially called himself a "magnetic healer" after Mesmer and his principles of animal magnetism. In his book *The Lengthening Shadow of Dr. Andrew Taylor Still*, Arthur Hildreth, one of the first students at the ASO, mentions that Palmer was a guest of Still's, who often hosted students for dinner (Hildreth, 1942). According to Hildreth, Palmer accompanied a friend in the pioneer class who returned for his second year of instruction and appeared to be interested in becoming a student at the ASO. After learning some manipulation from Still's students, he returned to Davenport, Iowa, and later "discovered" what he called chiropractic.

Stories passed down in families in the profession suggest that Palmer may even have registered as a student for a period of time, but written evidence has not been discovered. What is clear and indisputable is that Still, a physician, practiced in northern Missouri as a magnetic healer for almost 20 years before founding his school in 1892. Davenport, Iowa, is not far from Kirksville, Missouri, and Still's reputation was attracting attention from near and far. Whether or not Palmer was a student of Still, it would not be surprising if his "serendipitous discovery" of manipulation in 1895 was based on what he had heard of Still's methods. Palmer founded his own school in 1897 (see Chapter 19).

Still's original students attempted to practice as Still himself had practiced. However, he told his students that they did not have to do exactly as he did provided they could achieve the same results. Granted this freedom to explore, they quickly developed high-velocity manipulative techniques that were passed on at the school. The original chiropractic techniques resembled the high-velocity joint-resetting techniques used and described by some of Still's original students more than the techniques Still himself used, which would support the notion that Palmer learned from the osteopathic students. By 1915, Edyth Ashmore, DO, who was in charge of teaching manipulative technique at the ASO, recommended in her published manual that the students not be taught the original methods of Still, because they were too hard for the students to learn.

Ida Rolf, the founder of *rolfing* (see Chapter 17), a method of bodywork, was clear in her writings that she learned techniques from a blind osteopath and combined them with knowledge of yoga to create a systematic protocol for whole-body structural integration.

Other adapters of osteopathic technique (and partially of osteopathic philosophy) include John Barnes, a physical therapist who studied myofascial release offered in postgraduate programs at Michigan State University (MSU) and then taught it to physical therapists, and John Upledger, a DO who mixed cranial and other manipulative techniques taught by Still's student William Garner Sutherland, DO, with light trance work and other techniques to develop what he called *craniosacral therapy*, which is now generally practiced by nonphysicians.

In addition, because of the availability of postgraduate programs such as those offered by MSU and courses offered by other osteopathic physicians, physical therapists in the United States began using osteopathic techniques such as muscle energy, myofascial release, counterstrain, and even high-velocity low-amplitude thrust. The effect of osteopathic manipulation on physical medicine, rehabilitation, sports medicine, and family practice throughout the United States has been considerable, with many health care professionals and lay personnel learning osteopathic methods of alleviating pain and enhancing physical function.

OSTEOPATHIC PHILOSOPHY

Andrew Taylor Still developed a unified philosophy of medicine in the last half of the nineteenth century, which he called *osteopathic philosophy*. The word *philosophy* often engenders an immediate visceral response in the scientific or technological mind. The scientific mind is theoretically open to processing all new ideas. The technological mind tends to reject that which has not been statistically demonstrated. Thus the connotation of "philosophy" as an organization of vague or general thoughts about the meaning of life was often antithetical to the technological mind of the twentieth century. However, some of our greatest scientists, including Einstein, spoke of the importance of ideas that are not yet statistically demonstrated (see Chapter 14).

Osteopathic philosophy is best described as a background reference system that identifies the nature of the patient, defines the physician's mission, and establishes the basic premises of the logic of diagnosis and treatment. There remains in the general medical community, which has not been exposed to this organizing system, a poor understanding of exactly what is meant by osteopathic philosophy and why doctors of osteopathic medicine consider it important.

Osteopathic medical philosophy is centered on a profound respect for the inherent ability of the human being, and particularly the body, to heal itself. This philosophy has deep roots through recorded medical history. Over time, all ideas evolve as new information is discovered. Osteopathic philosophy is no exception: time has produced a distinction between classical osteopathy, which was taught by Still, and contemporary osteopathic medical philosophy, which integrates the basic elements of Still's ideas with subsequent scientific discoveries (Box 18-1).

CLASSICAL OSTEOPATHY

Classical osteopathic philosophy identifies the human being as a unified being of body, mind, and spirit. However, Still speaks in his writings very little about how to deal with the spirit or mind, leaving that up to the individual, and confines himself in general to dealing with the body. The osteopathic perspective is that the body is a marvelous machine that will function perfectly if the structure is perfect. If a patient is sick but his body has sufficient recuperative power, the anatomy can be adjusted to the structural ideal, which assists a return to normal physiology. Surgery and obstetrics are included in this philosophy. Interestingly, Still believed that the diet of his time (completely and neccessarily "organic" in that era) was sufficient

BOX 18-1 *Traditional Versus Contemporary Osteopathy*

"Our Platform"*

It should be known where osteopathy stands and what it stands for. A political party has a platform that all may know its position in regard to matters of public importance, what it stands for and what principles it advocates. The osteopath should make his position just as clear to the public. He should let the public know, in his platform, what he advocates in his campaign against disease. Our position can be tersely stated in the following planks:

First: We believe in sanitation and hygiene.

Second: We are opposed to the use of drugs as remedial agencies.

Third: We are opposed to vaccination.

Fourth: We are opposed to the use of serums in the treatment of disease. Nature furnishes its own serums if we know how to deliver them.

Fifth: We realize that many cases require surgical treatment and therefore advocate it as a last resort. We believe many surgical operations are unnecessarily performed and that many operations can be avoided by osteopathic treatment.

Sixth: The osteopath does not depend on electricity, X-radiance, hydrotherapy or other adjuncts, but relies on osteopathic measures in the treatment of disease.

Seventh: We have a friendly feeling for other nondrug, natural methods of healing, but we do not incorporate any other methods into our system. We are all opposed to drugs; in that respect at least, all natural, unharmful methods occupy the same ground. The fundamental principles of osteopathy are different from those of any other system and the cause of disease is considered from one standpoint, viz: disease is the result of anatomical abnormalities followed by physiological discord. To cure disease the abnormal parts must be adjusted to the normal; therefore other methods that are entirely different in principle have no place in the osteopathic system.

Eighth: Osteopathy is an independent system and can be applied to all conditions of disease, including purely surgical cases, and in these cases surgery is but a branch of osteopathy.

Ninth: We believe that our therapeutic house is just large enough for osteopathy and that when other methods are brought in just that much osteopathy must move out.

Contemporary Differences with "Our Platform"

Addressing each of the planks of the platform, today's osteopathic medical physicians would have the following comments.

1. Hygienic and sanitary measures have, in fact, decreased mortality and morbidity in modern society far more than other medical measures.

2. Much of Still's criticism of the medicine of his day was provoked precisely because it was not researched and therefore, to him, without logic and not scientifically valid. However, there have been only a very few osteopathic physicians, most of them at the end of the nineteenth or beginning of the twentieth century, who were completely opposed to all medicines. Contemporary medications are often overused; there may be a higher annual number of deaths caused by medication errors and side effects than are caused by highway accidents.

3. Immunization is now achieved with standard purified doses and is better understood. Statistics have demonstrated that the morbidity and mortality rates associated with not using immunizations are considerably worse than those found when immunizations are used. Although it is impossible to predict the outcome of immunization in an individual case, assuming that the patient who succumbs to an idiosyncratic reaction to a vaccine did not have that reaction because of the sensitivity to the medium (e.g., egg protein), that patient may be the one who would have had a similar or worse reaction to the disease in an epidemic if the population were not immunized.

4. Serums or other blood parts in Still's day were much more dangerous than those found today. However, AIDS and other blood-borne diseases have demonstrated that body fluids, cells, and cell parts must be used with appropriate caution.

5. Surgery is necessary but may remain overused in the United States. Twenty-first-century medicine has improved diagnostic testing, and more conservative approaches have decreased the number of unnecessary surgeries. The use of aseptic technique, improved anesthesia, and microscopic and endoscopic and minimally invasive surgery have diminished many of surgery's historic negative consequences.

6. All therapies that are statistically demonstrated to aid patients are completely acceptable. Still was apparently never opposed to the use of x-ray studies for diagnostic purposes, because the ASO had the second diagnostic x-ray machine west of the Mississippi River. The use of radiation therapy as we know it was unknown in his time, as was the use of lasers for therapeutic purposes.

7. We are not opposed to medications, but we are opposed to inappropriate use of medications. We recognize that disease has multiple causes that were unknown in Still's day (e.g., genetic abnormality, nutritional deficiencies, radiation damage [including sunlight], psychosomatic effects) and that his unifactorial description of the cause of illness is no longer tenable.

8. The therapeutic house of the osteopathic profession, except for a few of its founding members, has always included the latest of research on medications and the expansion in medical knowledge through this past century. However, the incorporation of this expanded knowledge into medical school curricula has resulted in less available instructional time for osteopathic manipulation, leaving some physicians less skilled and neglecting its use in appropriate cases.

---

*"Our Platform" from *Osteopathy, Research and Practice* (Still, 1910).

and that the body (the machine) as an omnivore could handle any fuel as long as the machine was working correctly.

The triune nature of the human being that Still so often mentioned dates back to at least the Greeks and probably to the Egyptians. The body is anatomically apparent and needs no further definition. The mind, however, has been described both as an epiphenomenon of the brain and its biochemistry and as something that is more than the product of chemical interactions. Emotions are generally identified with the mind, but does a third factor actually exist? Although science openly questions the existence of spirit, it is perhaps obvious to say that throughout history, a third factor of human existence has been universally recognized by human societies. This factor is sometimes regarded as the most potent but the most unpredictable. Although osteopathic philosophy recognizes this factor and respects it, Still spends relatively little time on the topic of spirit in his four books. Several speculative articles indicate he gave thought to the topic, particularly after the death of his father and later his son Fred. He discussed the nature of life and death as a medical philosopher of his era, but he did not indicate that his ideas on spirit caused him to utilize any particular methods of treatment.

Still focused on what could be seen and demonstrated, particularly on the relations between structure (anatomy) and function (physiology). His methods included taking a history, observing and palpating the body, and adjusting the body's constituent parts so that they were in normal positions, with normal motion, thereby promoting normal physiology. At that point, the innate self-regulating powers of the body would accomplish what was necessary for healing to take place. Surgery and obstetrics were considered to be a normal part of osteopathic practice. Thus, Still in his writings presents osteopathic philosophy as depending on science, and not on the idea of vitalism (see Chapter 6).

EVOLUTION

All philosophies that survive must be capable of incorporating and accounting for newly discovered information. Striking differences from Still's original platform are found in contemporary osteopathic medical philosophy and practice.

Still died in 1917. But by 1911, while he was still alive, the ASO had incorporated instruction in new vaccines, serum therapy, and antitoxins into the bacteriology curriculum (Trowbridge, 1991). Also by 1911 the first modern antibiotic, the arsenic compound Salvarsan, which had been developed by Paul Erlich, had been successfully used against syphilis (infection with *Treponema pallidum*) (Singer et al, 1962). Following the success of Salvarsan, the sulfa drugs were developed by the 1930s. As new medicines were created and researched, the faculty and students at the ASO and other osteopathic medical colleges adopted and used them. By the 1930s, the osteopathic philosophy had

been expanded to include medicines that had proven their value through research, as illustrated in the following introductory quote from the 1935 edition of the "Sage Sayings of Still":

"Osteopathy is not a drugless therapy in the strict sense of the word (Chapter 19). It uses drugs that have specific scientific value, such as antiseptics, parasiticides, antidotes, anesthetics, or narcotics for the temporary relief of suffering. It is the empirical internal administration of drugs for therapeutic purposes that osteopathy opposes, substituting instead manipulation, mechanical measures and the balancing of the life essentials as more rational and more in keeping with the physiological functions of the body. The osteopathic physician is the skilled engineer of the vital human mechanism, influencing by manipulation and other osteopathic measures the activities of the nerves, cells, glands and organs, the distribution of fluids and the discharge of nerve impulses, thus normalizing tissue, fluid and function" (Webster, 1935).

Antiseptic surgical technique was developed at about the same time as osteopathy and became included in surgical procedures practiced by the new profession. One difference between the allopathic and osteopathic approaches was that patients received OMT before and after surgery. Postsurgical treatment focused on soft tissue manipulation and *rib raising*, an articulatory treatment designed to increase the efficiency of breathing while calming the sympathetic nervous system.

The development of the sulfa antibiotics (and their increased use in hospitalized patients in the 1930s) and the advent of penicillin (as noted earlier, developed in 1927 but not commercially available until after World War II in 1945) significantly changed the practice of all medicine. Except for a very few older DOs who believed manipulation was the only answer, osteopathic physicians adopted these "miracle" medicines immediately. By accepting the use of thoroughly researched, effective medicines, classical osteopathic philosophy expanded to a more comprehensive contemporary osteopathic medical philosophy.

As an indication of the evolution of osteopathic thought, George W. Northup, DO, was quoted in 1996 as saying:

It is now better understood that a given "disease" is not so easily defined as was once believed. The search for a single cause for a single disease has produced disillusionment. Even the "germ theory" is not sufficient to provide a "simple" explanation for infectious diseases. All of us live in a world of potential bacterial invasion, but relatively few become infected. There are multiple causes, even in bacterially induced diseases. Disease is a total body response. It is not merely a stomach ulcer, a broken bone, or a troublesome mother-in-law. It is a disturbance of the structure–function of the body and not an isolated or local insult. Equally important is the recognition that disease is multicausal. The understanding that multiple causes of disease can arise from remote but interconnected parts of the body will ultimately emerge into a unifying philosophy for all of medicine. When this occurs, it will embrace many of the basic principles of osteopathic medicine.

The shift in osteopathic thought embraced the progress of the scientific development of medications in the twentieth century but maintained the belief that it is not the physician who heals, but the body itself, which heals through its homeostatic mechanisms. Contemporary osteopathic medical philosophy also maintains a belief in the efficacy of manipulation to diminish or eliminate pain, improve motion, and decrease physiologic and sometimes psychological stress, thereby helping the body regain optimal homeostatic levels.

Still's original opposition to the medication of his time was due to their obvious negative effects and the lack of research to support them. One of his better-known quotes is, "Man should study and use the drugs compounded in his own body" (Still, 1897, as cited in Singer et al, 1962). This sensible approach is increasingly the method of study today: finding out how the body works and then developing medications that interact with the body's cellular receptors and that mimic or, in some cases, are identical to the compounds found in the body, such as endorphins, for example (see Chapter 8).

CONTEMPORARY OSTEOPATHY

The official definition of the term *osteopathic philosophy* at the start of the twenty-first century, published in the Educational Council on Osteopathic Principles/AACOM "Glossary of Osteopathic Terminology," is the following:

osteopathic philosophy: a concept of health care supported by expanding scientific knowledge that embraces the concept of the unity of the living organism's structure (anatomy) and function (physiology). Osteopathic philosophy emphasizes the following principles: 1. The human being is a dynamic unit of function. 2. The body possesses self-regulatory mechanisms that are self-healing in nature. 3. Structure and function are interrelated at all levels. 4. Rational treatment is based on these principles.

Contemporary osteopathic medical philosophy begins with classical osteopathy and integrates additional knowledge. Rather than application of the choice *either/or* to manipulation or medicine, *both/and* is often more appropriate. Other changes evolved including recently developed knowledge of nutrition, exercise, environmental factors, genetics and molecular biology, neuroimmunology, and psychology.

For instance, nutrition is now considered fundamentally important as with other complementary and alternative medicine (CAM) approaches. Still did not consider it significant and often recommended that patients just "eat what they want of good, plain nutritious food" (Still, 1897, as cited in Singer et al, 1962). The importance of nutrition was later added to Still's original philosophy because, although Still commented on avoiding fad diets, the food Americans ate in his age was very different from the average American diet of our times (see Chapter 26). During Still's lifetime all crops were grown organically, by definition, and most of the population of the United States was still living in a rural environment consuming locally grown foods and in most cases growing it themselves. Although he mentioned good food several times, he assumed that the average diet of that era was sufficient for nourishment.

For exercise, Still occasionally mentioned walking or horseback riding. In the preautomotive society of the majority of his life, there was little need to recommend these—all people in the United States walked or rode horseback to get where they were going. A great many labor-saving devices had not yet been invented, so normal daily living supplied most of the exercise needs of the population.

Likewise, the dangers of excessive solar radiation to health had not yet become apparent in a society in which tanning was not considered attractive, sun exposure being more commonly experienced as a "red neck" than as a Hollywood tan (see Chapter 15). Farmers often wore long-sleeved shirts and hats, and even the swim-suits of the era provided practically full covering of the body and, for women, were paired with a parasol (meaning literally, from the Spanish, "against the sun") for protection from the sun. Air pollution, water pollution, and noise pollution were not specifically identified as causes of illness, nor were workplace toxins. Radiation damage was undiscovered. However, there was a general sense that densely populated, dark, dirty urban environments were unhealthy, which led to the "nature cure" and the "west cure," meant to provide benefit from exposure to recreation in the wilderness away from civilization with fresh, clean air, water and sunlight (see Chapters 1, 2, and 22).

Genetic mutations and deficiencies also were not understood. Physicians were virtually ignorant of the science of genetics at the end of the nineteenth century. The current hopeful promotion of "biotech" research promises multiple benefits from our expanding knowledge of molecular biology. Although this knowledge has great potential for both good and harm, its application may also be seen to fit with osteopathic philosophy.

Mind–body approaches have shown considerable potential for patient applications. Biofeedback and the relaxation response have been validated by research as ways of manipulating homeostatic mechanisms to improve psychological, neurological, and immune system functions (see Section II of this book). Psychological counseling techniques have advanced the possibilities for patients to address the stresses in their psychosocial milieu.

All of these etiological factors of illness have been integrated into an expanding contemporary osteopathic philosophy while it has retained the profound respect for the body's ability to function in the face of many challenges and its inherent capacity for self-healing when injury or illness is present.

Still thought the body was basically perfect as it was and could process environmental and nutritional input without damage unless there was an injury resulting in structural damage. We now know that the human organism is continuous with the environment, and on more than one level (body: physical; mind: thought and emotion; spirit: belief).

Illness is seen by the twenty-first-century osteopathic physician as having multiple causes, any one of which can be the initiator or promoter. Nonetheless, all of these factors potentially affect the structure of the body, whether at a gross (neuromusculoskeletal) level or at a microscopic (stereochemical–bioelectrochemical) level.

Wellness therefore lies along a continuum with illness, across the time frame between the points of conception and death. Illness begins as wellness declines. Wellness indicates that the individual is capable of accepting multiple challenges without the decompensation of homeostasis to the point of interference with normal activities. As the system loses optimal homeostatic balance, less of an environmental–emotional insult is needed to precipitate a state of illness.

Problems such as nutritional deficiency, insufficient exercise or rest, and inappropriate levels of stress lie early in the continuum. If these problems are addressed while they are simple, and before the onset of "pathologic abnormality," the organism recovers and retains adaptability. On an overlapping or interactive continuum lies gross structural integrity through *tensegrity*, which involves bilateral muscle tone, balance, and function. This tensegrity system is also interactive with neural activity levels (especially in the autonomic nervous system), particularly as these factors affect the rest of the body through the respiratory, circulatory, lymphatic, endocrine, and immune systems (see Chapter 16).

Even when nothing is done, our homeostatic mechanisms may effect a recovery from illness without aid. Sometimes, however, the body does not have the ability to recover on its own. In such cases, structural dysfunction at either the gross or the microscopic levels can be compounded by the sequelae of inflammation, pain, and tissue congestion. These negative changes in the biochemical environment of the body can cause many variables in the endocrine and immune systems to swing to wider extremes and destabilize one or more of the body's systems, leading to illness. Simple problems can sometimes be solved with manipulation, lifestyle changes (e.g., exercises), or nutrition to reestablish optimal homeostatic set points.

Ideas such as these are not easily understood by a reductionistic approach to the body, in which each variable is analyzed by itself or perhaps in conjunction with one or two other variables (e.g., the balance between insulin and glucagon). Current understanding recognizes much more complexity in the interactions between many more subtle variables, such as homeostatic hormonal systems that interdependently regulate and control many body functions (see Chapter 8).

The use of a complex adaptive systems model, using *chaos theory* mathematics, has enabled greater understanding of the complexity of dynamic medical systems. Chaos theory mathematics allows us to understand how altering a single or even a few variables in one system (e.g., cardiovascular) can affect the function of other systems, and thereby the entire human being. One factor that has been noted is that a complex system has *sensitive dependence on initial conditions*. This concept has been popularized as the *butterfly effect*, which suggests that the simple motion of a butterfly's wings in the Amazon may affect the weather patterns in Moscow 3 months later (Gleick, 1987). Although this extreme example may makes us chuckle, or marvel, the mathematical models following chaos theory principles appear to be closer to predicting what actually happens in the natural world than are any previous analyses or models. Mathematicians now use similar models to explain, for example, a decompensating cycle of cardiac arrhythmia leading to fatal fibrillation (Gleick, 1987). Understanding new concepts such as point attractors, strange attractors, triviality, nontriviality, and degeneracy leads to a better understanding of the processes of homeostasis and the way in which manipulation of anatomical relations and tissue tensions may promote physiological adaptability.

Each of the body's systems is understood to be integrated with the entire body, functioning in an interactive, bidirectional manner as part of the whole person. The neuromusculoskeletal system is the largest single system in the body; it reflects the state of health of the other systems, yielding diagnostic clues for systemic or organic function or dysfunction. It can also be used as an access point for treatment, using manipulation to change the motion possible at the joints and the set points of muscle length and tone, and thereby affecting vascular and lymphatic flow and neural (particularly autonomic) tone.

OSTEOPATHIC PRINCIPLES

To an osteopathic physician, osteopathic principles are common-sense ideas that provide a milieu in which to diagnose and treat a patient. At some level, the physician should always be aware of the following considerations:

- Who is the patient? The patient is a human being like the physician, a functional unity of body (a genetically constructed grouping of cells and systems), mind (thoughts and emotions), and a third factor (identified by some as spirit), which is interactive with the environment at physical, psychosocial, and energetic levels. The human being functions by transforming thought into action through the neuromusculoskeletal system.
- Where does health arise? Health comes from within the patient.
- What is the goal of the osteopathic physician? The physician seeks health in the patient. Wellness and illness exist on a continuum, or on an interactive multidimensional group of continua. It is the physician's job to help the patient seek the highest possible level of homeostatic balance and performance within the patient's individual limitations and the current circumstances.
- How does the osteopathic physician seek health in the patient? Prevention is the best medicine; the physician encourages and teaches the patient to follow healthful practices (e.g., appropriate rest, nutrition, physical activity, breathing exercises, positive thoughts and emotions, relaxation, social interaction) and to avoid that which is

self-destructive in excess (e.g., tobacco, radiation, toxins, alcohol, drugs, eating).

- If the patient has become ill, is it possible to use treatment that will activate and/or augment the body's own self-healing processes?
- The least invasive method of treatment that can restore health in a timely fashion is preferable.

If the patient has entered the illness end of the continuum, the osteopathic physician must take a careful history, perform a physical examination, and formulate a differential diagnosis. The neuromusculoskeletal system is included as an access point for diagnostic signs that may indicate systemic problems (and later, an access for imparting information to the other systems). Tests may be needed. After arriving at a diagnosis, the physician decides on necessary treatment, bearing in mind all factors that affect the physiology and performance of the patient. The medical standard of care is included in this process, but osteopathic physicians retain a holistic rather than reductionistic focus, and include OMT when it is indicated, whether as primary or adjunct treatment.

What factors affect the physiology of the patient? Physiology (as per Hippocrates) can be affected by air, water, and food; nutritional supplements; prescription and over-the-counter medications; physical forces and impacts on the system (ranging from the effects of any movement, including exercise, to trauma); thoughts, emotions, stress, or relaxation; and energy (from gravity to sunlight to magnetic fields to subtle energies of which we may not yet be aware). All of the body's systems are integrative, but five are more easily seen as unifying systems of global body communication (cardiovascular and lymphatic, respiratory, neurologic, endocrine, and immune systems).

The host has control of vulnerability to illness through the immune system and homeostatic mechanisms (the true *vis medicatrix naturae*) (see Chapter 22). When host control decreases and the system downgrades into illness, intervention is necessary. Intervention is designed to support a system that is no longer functioning at an appropriately high level of homeostasis.

How does the osteopathic physician intervene? Just as wellness, injury, and illness exist along a continuum, so do treatment approaches. When physical or emotional force has distorted anatomical or physiological performance, the physician addresses the problems with physical approaches ranging from manipulation to surgery. When genetic limitations or illness make it impossible for the body to perform appropriate functions on its own or with the speed required, the physician uses exogenous substances such as medication, nutritional supplementation, or other proven therapies. (From the point of view of chaos mathematics and dynamical systems, the physician seeks to reverse abnormal trivial point attractors to strange attractor status.) The physician does all this in a conservative manner, bearing in mind the body's innate intelligence and the wisdom of using the least possible intervention (least invasive) for the greatest possible results.

OSTEOPATHIC TECHNIQUES

Osteopathy is not just a system of techniques, but a philosophy that is often applied through techniques of osteopathic manipulative medicine, which were developed by osteopathic physicians. Several of the more commonly recognized osteopathic diagnosis and treatment systems are described here. There are, of course, many others. Multiple techniques are generally used to achieve a single objective as part of a complete osteopathic treatment. Although some procedures relate more to joint surface apposition, others address muscle and connective tissue length and tension imbalances, promote vascular and lymphatic flow, or modulate autonomic nervous system tone. Most techniques affect more than one of those functions when applied (e.g., resetting a thoracic vertebral facet joint relaxes surrounding muscles, allows better blood and lymphatic flow through those tissues, and decreases local sympathetic tone). One technique may lead to the use of another, depending on the patient's problem, the perception and skill of the osteopathic physician, and the difficulty level in achieving the desired outcome.

Some osteopathic physicians have held that there are only two types of techniques, direct and indirect. *Direct treatment* is treatment that confronts restriction of motion, in which the body part is taken directly toward restricted motion. *Indirect treatment* is treatment in which the body part is taken in the direction of ease of motion. Once the body part is appropriately positioned, activating forces are applied to induce changes in muscle and connective tissue length and tone; central, peripheral, or autonomic nervous system tone (level of activation); joint surface apposition and motion; or vascular-lymphatic function. Treatment goals include tissue relaxation, increased physiological motion, decrease in pain, and optimization of homeostasis.

The following are examples of the more common systems of OMT. Like any form of medical treatment, manipulation in any form has both indications and contraindications, which are not discussed here and are well outlined in other specialized texts.

SOFT TISSUE AND LYMPHATIC TREATMENTS

Soft tissue treatment, generally a direct treatment, was developed by Still and his early students. It is essentially a bodywork technique and is sometimes confused with massage. The techniques focus on altering the tone (and length) of muscle and connective tissue. Soft tissue treatment relaxes muscles and connective tissue by stretching the muscle fibers in a longitudinal, perpendicular, or combined manner, decreases or removes tissue tension impediment to arterial delivery, and alters the tone of the autonomic nervous system. Whereas soft tissue treatment definitely affects the lymphatics, there are also other specific lymphatic techniques that focus on increasing lymphatic return.

HIGH-VELOCITY LOW-AMPLITUDE THRUST

In the direct method of treatment referred to as *high-velocity low-amplitude (HVLA) thrust*, the restrictive barrier is engaged by precise positioning of the body. The thrust when the body part is at the restrictive barrier is very rapid (high velocity) but operates over a very short distance (low amplitude), gapping the articulation by approximately one-eighth inch or less. This allows a reset of both joint position and muscle tension levels, which causes related neural and vascular readjustment.

ARTICULATORY TECHNIQUE

The original general articulatory technique, developed by Still and his students, takes the body part being treated to the end portion of its restricted range of motion in a gentle, repetitive fashion. The repeated motion directly increases joint range of motion while relaxing the deep intrinsic tissues and stimulating blood flow. Movements within one or more planes of motion are treated at one time. This technique can be used to treat individual joints or regions (e.g., shoulder, cervical spine).

STILL TECHNIQUE AND FACILITATED POSITIONAL RELEASE (FPR)

Still used and described (Still, 1910) specific articulation techniques that began with diagnosis, placing the body parts in the direction of ease of motion and then rotating them toward the direction of restriction. These specific articulation techniques have been called the *Still technique* (Van Buskirk, 1996). *Facilitated positional release* (Schiowitz, 1997) is also a variation of the type of work Still performed.

MUSCLE ENERGY TECHNIQUE

Muscle energy treatment was developed by Fred Mitchell, Sr., DO. It is most commonly used as a direct treatment, and the term *muscle energy* means that the patient uses his or her own energy through directed muscular cooperation with the physician. These techniques were originally designed to reposition joint surfaces. Reflexive changes in muscle tension are used in a variety of ways to allow dysfunctional, shortened muscles to lengthen; abnormally lengthened muscles to shorten; weakened muscles to strengthen; and hypertonic muscles to relax. Commonly, voluntary isometric contraction of a patient's muscles is followed by a gentle stretch of the dysfunctional, contracted tissue, which decreases abnormal restriction of motion. Other muscle energy techniques use traction on the muscle to pull an articulation back into the appropriate position, reciprocal inhibition to relax antagonists, cross-extensor reflexes to affect an opposite limb, or oculocervical reflexes (using eye motion to relax neck muscles).

COUNTERSTRAIN TECHNIQUE

Counterstrain is a passive positional technique that places the patient's dysfunctional joint (spinal or other) or tissue in a position of ease. This position arrests the inappropriate mechanoreceptor activity or nocifensive reflexes that maintain the somatic dysfunction. Marked shortening of the involved muscle or connective tissue is maintained for 90 seconds. An inappropriate strain reflex (a result of injury) is therefore inhibited by application of counterstrain. Diagnosis is primarily by palpation of areas of tenderness mapped by the originator of this system, Lawrence Jones, DO. This form of diagnosis can also be integrated with positional, movement, or tissue texture abnormalities. The tender point is indicative of inappropriate neurological balance. This system is ideal for the patient who may not respond well to articulatory techniques, such as the postsurgical patient.

MYOFASCIAL RELEASE

Myofascial release is actually a renaming of original osteopathic techniques developed by Still, which early osteopathic physicians called "fascial techniques." Anthony Chila, Robert Ward, and John Peckham developed a course in these techniques at MSU, in which they also acknowledged the importance of the muscle tissue to the treatment. This technique may be performed by either lengthening the contracted tissue (direct myofascial release) or shortening it (indirect myofascial release) and allowing the nervous and respiratory systems to facilitate changes in tension, which remain after the treatment is completed. Two physiological biomechanical tissue processes, creep and hysteresis, also play a role. Compression, traction, torsion, respiratory cooperation, or a combination may be included to facilitate treatment.

OSTEOPATHY IN THE CRANIAL FIELD

Osteopathy in the cranial field, also referred to as *OCF*, *cranial osteopathy*, and *craniosacral osteopathy*, was developed by William G. Sutherland, DO. It is usually done as a mixture of indirect and direct procedures that work with the body's inherent rhythmic motions. It is commonly used in adults as a treatment for headaches or temporomandibular joint dysfunction syndrome and in infants (whose skulls are more flexible) for treatment of symptoms related to cranial nerve compression (e.g., vomiting, poor sleep, poor feeding), for plagiocephally, or in cases in which mechanical factors can affect fluid drainage (otitis media). Although OCF techniques often focus on the skull and the sacrum, where the dura mater attaches, they can be and are commonly used throughout the body.

John Upledger, DO, taught many nonphysicians a simpler variant of the technique, which included elements not generally practiced by osteopathic physicians, and called his version *craniosacral therapy*. Because application of this technique is not medically licensed and regulated, non-osteopathic practitioners using this therapy are often doing something considerably different from and less specific than what a licensed osteopathic physician would do in practice.

VISCERAL TECHNIQUES

A variety of techniques have been developed from the beginning of the profession to address imbalance in the viscera. These approaches include stretching and balancing techniques related to ligamentous attachments, as originated by Still, and may involve use of inherent visceral motion. In the late twentieth century, Jean-Pierre Barral, a nonphysician osteopath from France, developed and taught an entire system of visceral techniques.

DIAGNOSIS AND TREATMENT

Osteopathic diagnosis and treatment are determined by the osteopathic philosophy, which makes the practice of osteopathic medicine distinctive. This philosophy and OMT should not be viewed as merely the addition of something extra to the contemporary Western medical approach, or "complementary" in this sense (see Chapter 3). Osteopathic philosophy serves as an organizer of thought that helps the physician understand what is going on in the entire organism, allows for concurrent reductionistic analysis, and then reassembles the parts into the totality of the human being, who is more than the sum of the parts.

Osteopathic structural diagnosis differs in that the osteopathic physician performs the standard orthopedic and neurological portions of the physical examination, but also includes additional tissue palpation, as well as testing of muscle and joint motion. The musculoskeletal system is examined as an access point for additional diagnostic information, not only on muscle tension but also on fluid distribution and autonomic levels of activity. Well-known neurological reflex interactions permit a physician to conclude from musculoskeletal evidence that an underlying visceral problem may exist and should be investigated. When abnormalities are noted, *somatic dysfunction* is diagnosed. It is important to note that somatic dysfunction is not tissue damage, which the body must heal. Rather, somatic dysfunction is a disorder of the body's programming for length, tension, joint surface apposition affecting mobility, tissue fluid flow efficiency, and neurological balance.

Osteopathic diagnosis expands the standard medical differential diagnosis in a number of ways. For example, consider the standard medical diagnosis of lumbalgia (lumbago) or lumbar pain. After examination, the osteopathic physician who finds the appropriate objective criteria will diagnose *lumbar somatic dysfunction*, and the physician's note will include more specific information about which of the lumbar spinal segments is (are) unable to function normally.

Four criteria are used to diagnose somatic dysfunction: tissue texture abnormalities (T), static or positional asymmetry (A), restriction of motion (R), and tenderness (T). These criteria have been referred to by the diagnostic mnemonic *TART*. When these signs are noted at particular spinal segmental levels, knowledge of reflex relationships also guides reflection on their cause. They may be evidence of viscerosomatic, somatovisceral, viscerovisceral, or somatosomatic reflexes, which are well discussed in neuroscience (see Chapter 8). Is the problem simply mechanical, or is it evidence of underlying visceral problems as well? The osteopathic physician then pays more attention to both the history and physical examination of the internal organs related to spinal cord segmental levels. These reflexes show palpatory evidence of autonomic nervous system influence at segmental levels and may produce abnormalities of tissue texture and muscle tone.

The fourth tenet of osteopathic philosophy states that treatment will be based on this knowledge of structure and function. With a primary musculoskeletal problem involving restricted motion and abnormally high muscle tone, it is common sense to decrease the tone and increase the motion to regain normal function. However, when the neuromusculoskeletal system is used as a clue in uncovering visceral dysfunction, it is recognized by the profession that lowering muscle tone related to visceral dysfunction will at the very least decrease one portion of what is now a vicious cycle from which the body is then likely to recover more rapidly. Treating musculoskeletal imbalance with OMT to improve the mechanical aspects of breathing for the patient with pneumonia is an obvious application of osteopathic principles. The same treatment will also lower inappropriate sympathetic nervous system tone and thereby enhance homeostatic balance and adaptability.

Medication or surgery may be unnecessary, depending on the severity of the problem. OMT may be used as a primary means of treatment for a problem that appears to be of nonsevere, musculoskeletal origin; as primary treatment for simple illness that requires no medication (e.g., viral upper respiratory illness); or as adjunctive therapy along with medication or surgery—again, to enhance homeostatic recovery and adaptability. Medications for symptomatic relief may or may not be used, depending on the case and the preference or needs of the patient.

Two simple case examples are presented here. These are not complete cases, but are designed to illustrate some of the osteopathic differences in approach to diagnosis and treatment. In each example, the techniques chosen did not challenge the patients with muscular effort and were selected with homeostatic effects in mind (decrease of edema, mobilization of fluids, enhancement of respiration). In many other ambulatory cases, any of the listed treatments (e.g., HVLA thrust) could be selected based on four factors: the condition of the patient, the nature of the complaint, the goals of treatment, and the skills of the physician.

 Case Example 1

A 67-year-old African American woman with a 30 pack-year history of smoking comes to the office with a productive cough that she has had for 2 weeks. She now

Continued

Case Example 1—cont'd

has a fever, and the sputum is greenish. She has pain in the ribs on the left side of the thorax and audible rhonchi when examined with the stethoscope. After a careful history taking and physical examination, the physician concludes that although the differential diagnosis includes a possible tumor, it is less likely than a community-acquired pneumonia. Radiographic studies indicate a left lingular pneumonitis, and there is an increased white blood cell count with a left shift. The physician has noted on examination that pulmonary viscerosomatic reflexes are activated in the corresponding thoracic spinal region, which is causing limitation in range of motion and tenderness, along with tissue texture changes, at several thoracic vertebral segments. Several ribs on the left have diminished mobility, and the diaphragm has decreased excursion on the left.

The physician decides to start antibiotics immediately and treats the thoracic segments and ribs with OMT, in this case choosing counterstrain because it requires no muscular effort on the part of the patient and poses minimal risk of injury to bones that may be osteoporotic. In patients who are coughing frequently, breathing mechanics are often disturbed. Treating the thoracic segments and ribs helps normalize the sympathetic nervous system activity and increases the efficiency and ease of breathing. The thoracic outlet (superior thoracic aperture) is treated to decrease soft tissue tension which can impede the flow of lymphatic fluid through the thoracic duct. The diaphragm (which often has impaired motion from the spasmodic motion of coughing) is treated with myofascial release, and the cervical region is treated with counterstrain to decrease any problems with the phrenic nerve (which innervates the diaphragm for respiration). A lymphatic pump procedure concludes the treatment. Antitussives are prescribed along with the antibiotics and an expectorant. Acetaminophen may be used for fever and pain. The patient is seen again in 3 days, at which time she is greatly improved.

The rationale behind the medical treatment is obvious: kill the bacteria, decrease the viscosity of the mucus that holds them so that they can be coughed out, and give the patient a painkiller to decrease pain. This type of treatment relies on the body to recover its optimal performance once certain negatives are canceled out. The osteopathic treatment is designed to aid normal physiological processes that augment the body's natural systems in killing the bacteria and reducing pain. OMT may enable a faster recovery for the patient—or increase the odds of survival. The osteopathic physician takes advantage of both possibilities, aiding the host's natural defenses while fighting the bacteria directly through use of antibiotics. The patient's comfort level is also increased by the use of the osteopathic manipulation. ∾

 Case Example 2

A 19-year-old white male college student comes for treatment of an apparent sprained ankle. The injury occurred during a soccer game when he reached for the ground with his foot and made a sudden turn. There is no other relevant history. The ankle is swollen, and the patient applied ice immediately after the injury. He can walk, but he keeps most of his weight off the ankle. There is pinpoint tenderness at the posteroinferior right lateral malleolus.

The physician chooses to treat with superficial indirect myofascial release and, afterward, lymphatic techniques to decrease the edema. Treatment is specifically limited to a minimal approach, which causes the patient no pain. The patient is given a set of crutches to use for a couple of days and goes to the hospital to get a radiographic study, the results of which are negative. He is to use ice at least three times a day and to keep his weight off the ankle, which is wrapped after the treatment with an elastic bandage. He is to keep the ankle elevated when possible and to use acetaminophen for pain if needed. Because the radiographic study shows no fracture, the physician continues the treatment 2 days later with counterstrain and lymphatic treatment, and the patient is allowed to discontinue use of the crutches.

Draining excess fluid and decreasing the overabundance of proinflammatory neuropeptides and other biopeptides through the use of OMT allows the hypertonic and injured tissues to return to normal more quickly. The decrease or elimination of muscle spasm allows the ankle and foot to have more normal mechanics, therefore promoting more normal lymphatic and venous drainage. Again, the osteopathic treatment is designed to enhance the body's own methods of healing, promoting a rapid return to more normal homeostatic balance by removing dysfunction. ∾

MANIPULATION

If osteopathy is a philosophy, why is the use of manipulation in the practice of medicine considered a hallmark and necessary, integral part of osteopathic medicine? The original osteopathic philosophy centers on the interaction between structure (anatomy) and function (physiology), and states that we can improve the patient's condition by manipulating his structure to change his functional level. OMT has effects at two levels, the macroscopic and the microscopic.

At the macroscopic level, it is easy to see that if there is abnormal pressure on a joint, nerve, or blood vessel, there may be resulting changes in tissue over time. For instance, if there is more pressure on the medial aspect of the right knee, over time there will be changes in the cartilage and bone to compensate. There will also be gait changes as the body attempts to rebalance itself to use the least amount of energy for posture and locomotion. Thus local dysfunction can induce global dysfunction. Manipulation, which has the local effects of adjusting the balance in the musculoskeletal system, also has global effects at a gross level.

At a microscopic level, cellular physiology depends on hydration and fluid flow. The original one-celled organisms were bathed in a solution of ancient seawater, which delivered oxygen and nutrients and also took away toxic waste products and carbon dioxide as they were produced and ejected from the cell (see Chapter 26). Multicellular organisms such as the human being contain a fluid system like an internal ocean, which has the same functions. This internal fluid system is the cardiovascular system, delivering oxygen and nutrients to each individual cell and clearing carbon dioxide and waste products (as well as excessive proteins through lymphatic drainage).

If this system is impeded in any way, cells, followed by tissues, organs, and entire systems, decrease their level of function. This form of physiological stress then makes the organism vulnerable to disease. To offer an analogy, a good fluid delivery and clearance system is like an open, clean, flowing stream or river. If the flow is blocked, there is the potential for developing a swamp. Stagnant water allows the buildup of noxious products, and the local environment is completely changed. If the blockage is cleared through manual effort, the stream reestablishes good flow and removes the toxic elements that had begun to build up. When osteopathic treatment is used to adjust tissue tensions toward the norm, the body's own elimination systems can clear toxic waste products produced by cellular damage and allowed to build up by suboptimal hydration and fluid flow.

Osteopathic manipulation is therefore a means not only of decreasing or eliminating pain, but also of adjusting the involved structures toward an optimal adaptability level of the body's *tensegrity* system. This adjustment helps prevent noxious stimulus (through compression or excessive stretching of nociceptors) at a macroscopic level, and toxic conditions (through lack of appropriate oxygen and nutrient delivery and inadequate waste clearance) in cells at a microscopic level. Manipulation is therefore a central issue for osteopathic medicine: although it cannot cure all illness, manipulation is used to help the body function at an optimal level, enhancing its ability to heal itself. The body is capable of amazing feats of self-recovery and may perform these feats more quickly and thoroughly if assisted.

Manipulation, like all forms of medical treatment, has limitations. It is possible that the body's functional levels have been so negatively, pathologically, altered that the use of manipulation alone will not be able to sufficiently enhance the body's self-adjusting systems (or perhaps not within an acceptable time) for it to regain good health without the additional assistance of medication or surgery. It may also be necessary to integrate direct psychosocial intervention to achieve recovery.

Medicines and surgery are used to effect changes in two circumstances, which occur commonly: (1) when the physi-

cian believes that preventive measures or manipulation alone will not be able to accomplish the total goal of health (e.g., when use of insulin in a patient with type 1 diabetes or narcotics in a terminally ill cancer patient is necessary); or (2) when speed is of the essence and it would be dangerous to the patient to rely solely on manipulation and/or other conservative measures and wait for solely for the body's self-healing responses (e.g., use of antibiotics to treat infection).

Those osteopathic physicians who practice holistically, but do not use manipulation (or refer patients to have that treatment if somatic dysfunction is present) are ignoring a main premise of osteopathic philosophy: eliminating functional structural impediments that decrease normal physiological function promotes the body's self-healing capabilities.

LEVELS OF IMPLEMENTATION

There have been conspicuous differences between the evolution of Still's ideas in the United States and in other parts of the world. In the United States, there is a vast spectrum of application of osteopathic principles in the practice of medicine by DOs. Internationally, the application of osteopathic philosophy through manipulative techniques has been different from that in the United States and involves multiple pathways and levels of training.

In the United States, DOs have always been considered physicians. Current practitioners implement the osteopathic medical philosophy at various levels along a continuum of medical care. Initially, all osteopathic physicians believed in the efficacy of manipulation to affect the physiology of the body in a positive way. In fact, this practice has been the hallmark of the osteopathic profession, and Still's development of osteopathic structural diagnosis and treatment was the original reason for the osteopathic profession's existence.

At one end of the continuum, the earliest osteopathic practitioners implemented a pure, classical form of osteopathy, using either manipulation or surgery but recommending *against* virtually all medications (medicines which at the time did much harm and little good). This type of practitioner is a now historical footnote in the development of osteopathic practice in America; this author knows of no such practitioners at the present time.

Some physicians accept the importance of manipulation for treatment of musculoskeletal pain but do not see it as having any value in systemic illness.

A small number of osteopathic physicians have chosen to specialize in neuromusculoskeletal medicine (osteopathic specialty: NMM). Some of their patients have primary musculoskeletal complaints, and others are given adjunctive treatment for medical conditions in conjunction with treatment by other physicians. Most of these specialists use a minimum of medications and injections, and refer patients who need additional medication or surgical care to primary care or specialty physicians.

Some primary care osteopathic physicians use osteopathic techniques in a reductionistic manner (e.g., treating only the neck if there is neck pain). This limited application is often successful and time-effective (as "formulary" approaches often can be in the use of any CAM therapy). However, such an approach will not be successful in a case in which pain is a symptom in a body region that is compensating for another problem, rather than in the region that is the primary source of the problem. The physician would be neglecting the many muscle and tissue connections between the thoracic region and the neck, as well as the sympathetic chain ganglia in the upper thoracic region that help set the tone for the cervical musculature. In addition, any other restricted region of the body may alter the body's *tensegrity* relationships, which can result in the complaint of pain in the neck. Such an approach will be successful only if the primary problem is being addressed. It is important to address the primary problem, not just compensation or annoying symptoms.

A majority of osteopathic physicians continue to work in primary care specialties, although that proportion is decreasing. There is a great range in the amount of OMT that these physicians use with their patients. Some who believe in the efficacy of OMT, but feel that they do not have time to use it in a busy day of patient care, may use it to treat a friend or relative and will refer patients who need manipulation to physicians who specialize in its use.

Remarkably, there are a number of DOs who have no belief in the clinical efficacy of OMT. Some attended an osteopathic medical college only because it was a pathway to an unrestricted medical license, and never had any interest or intention in using the osteopathic approach. These physicians are ignoring a growing body of research indicating the benefits of OMT. A subset of this group believes that the laying on of hands effect is, however, valuable for evoking either a mind–body or a placebo effect. A number of physicians are not interested in or able to perform much physical labor or are not confident in their own skill level. There are also osteopathic physicians who believe their time is better spent on prescribing medication or using surgery, and that manual therapeutics are best left to physical therapists, doctors of chiropractic and other manual or massage therapists.

Whether or not they use OMT, virtually all osteopathic physicians in the United States share a profound respect for the body's self-healing ability. They have been taught to approach their patients in a holistic manner, viewing each as a unique human being whose current circumstances are also unique to the person and interact with his or her own psychosocial and environmental milieu.

CURRENT STATUS

PRACTICE REGULATIONS

Osteopathic physicians in all 50 of the United States of America have the same practice rights as MDs. At the end

of the nineteenth and beginning of the twentieth centuries, such was not the case. Some states immediately gave full practice rights to DOs; others gave partial practice rights, which varied from the right to diagnose and treat with manual medicine without prescription of medication, to the inclusion of obstetric privileges, to full medical and surgical privileges. Most states in which osteopathic licensure was possible gave full practice rights.

Although the right to practice was guaranteed by law, it was not always easy for DOs in the early to mid-twentieth century to obtain hospital privileges. Even at the time of the 1953 Kline Report to the AMA, many MDs were unaware that osteopathic medical education was equivalent to their own and therefore blocked access to hospital privileges. Younger MDs were influenced in this regard by older physicians, whose opinions were formed at a time when DOs did not use available but highly toxic medications. There was poor understanding among MDs of the rationale behind osteopathy's early rejection of medicines: that medicines in the nineteenth and early twentieth centuries were poor in quality and generally toxic, and that their utilization was based on tradition or conjecture rather than research.

This conflict spurred DOs to build their own hospitals, thus forming a network of their own for accreditation standards. At times they used a wing of another hospital, such as the osteopathic wing of the Los Angeles County Hospital (which became the women's wing of the hospital after the osteopathic-allopathic amalgamation in 1962). Osteopathic hospitals expanded in number and size in the 1960s and 1970s. At the end of the twentieth century, many hospitals closed or merged under the purely economic pressures of managed care and health maintenance organizations. The number of osteopathic hospitals, many of which were small community hospitals, declined in the face of these changing economic conditions.

Another factor contributing to this decrease was that DOs were freely granted privileges in MD hospitals, which made independent osteopathic hospitals less necessary for patient care. The decrease in the number of independent osteopathic hospitals created a decline in osteopathic influence in graduate medical education. An increasing number of graduates of osteopathic medical schools began choosing medical specialty residencies accredited by the Accreditation Council for Graduate Medical Education (ACGME) rather than the AOA.

REQUIREMENTS FOR MATRICULATION

Prospective students who wish to apply to osteopathic medical schools should have completed a bachelor's degree with a high grade point average and successful scores on the Medical College Aptitude Test (MCAT). Interviewers at the osteopathic colleges look for students who are successful at academic tasks. Preference is given to those who also have sought relevant medical experience, such as working as a volunteer in a hospital or other medical facility, shadowing physicians, holding a job in a related field (e.g., at a hospital laboratory), or participating in medical research. Such experience suggests that an applicant has observed the work of physicians and is able to deal with the sight of blood, sick patients, and patients in pain. The colleges also look for volunteer activities that show the applicant has demonstrated a personal desire to give something back to the community through service.

The interview at an osteopathic medical school generally includes informal assessment on the part of the interviewers of the student's ability to empathize with patients. A high level value is placed on empathy with patients in osteopathic education. Because most osteopathic physicians are in general or family practice, it is a cultural value of the osteopathic profession to look for applicants who are "people persons," meaning individuals who can interact easily with others. It is believed by DOs that this

characteristic enables a physician to communicate with patients in ways that elicit information relevant to diagnosis more easily and elicit better compliance. This factor does not mean that only extraverts are accepted as students. Interviewers recognize that it is not doing a service to anyone to accept a student who has good people skills but insufficient academic strength.

Interviewers often also pay attention to whether a student has been interested enough to study the history and philosophy of medicine and osteopathic medicine.

U.S. OSTEOPATHIC MEDICAL SCHOOLS

All AOA-accredited osteopathic medical schools are listed by the World Health Organization (WHO) in its official list of United States medical schools. Table 18-1 provides additional information about these institutions.

TABLE 18-1 *U.S. Osteopathic Medical Colleges as of 2008**

College	Location	Affiliated university	First class matriculated	Public, private nonprofit, or for profit	Web address
Kirksville College of Osteopathic Medicine	Kirksville, MO	Andrew Taylor Still University (ATSU)	1892	Private	www.atsu.edu
DMU-COM	Des Moines, IA	Des Moines University	1898	Private	www.dmu.edu/com
Philadelphia College of Osteopathic Medicine (PCOM)	Philadelphia, PA	Freestanding	1899	Private	www.pcom.edu
Chicago College of Osteopathic Medicine	Downer's Grove, IL	Midwestern University	1900	Private	www.midwestern.edu/ccom
KCUMB-COM	Kansas City, MO	Kansas City University of Medicine and Biosciences	1916	Private	www.kcumb.edu
Texas College of Osteopathic Medicine	Fort Worth, TX	University of North Texas Health Science Center, Fort Worth	1970	Public	www.hsc.unt.edu/ education/tcom
MSUCOM	East Lansing, MI	Michigan State University	1970	Public	www.com.msu.edu
OSUCOM	Tulsa, OK	Oklahoma State University	1972	Public	www.healthsciences .okstate.edu/college
West Virginia School of Osteopathic Medicine	Lewisburg, WV	Freestanding	1974	Public	www.wvsom.edu
OUCOM	Athens, OH	Ohio University	1976	Public	www.oucom.ohiou.edu
New York College of Osteopathic Medicine	Old Westbury (Long Island), NY	New York Institute of Technology	1977	Private	www.nyit.edu/nycom
UMDNJSOM	Cherry Hill, NJ	University of Medicine and Dentistry New Jersey	1977	Public	www.som.umdnj.edu

Continued

TABLE 18-1 *U.S. Osteopathic Medical Colleges as of 2008*—cont'd*

College	Location	Affiliated university	First class matriculated	Public, private nonprofit, or for profit	Web address
College of Osteopathic Medicine of the Pacific	Pomona, CA	Western University of Health Sciences	1978	Private	www.westernu.edu
UNECOM	Biddeford, ME	University of New England	1978	Private	www.une.edu/com
NSU-COM	Ft. Lauderdale-Davie, FL	NOVA/Southeast University	1981	Private	www.medicine.nova.edu
Lake Erie College of Osteopathic Medicine (LECOM)	Lake Erie, PA	Freestanding	1993	Private	www.lecom.edu
Arizona College of Osteopathic Medicine	Phoenix, AZ	Midwestern University	1996	Private	www.midwestern.edu/azcom
TUCOM-CA	Vallejo, CA	Touro University	1996	Private	www.tu.edu
PCSOM	Pikeville, KY	Pikeville College	1997	Private	www.pc.edu/pcsom
Edward Via Virginia College of Osteopathic Medicine	Blacksburg, VA	Virginia Polytechnic Institute and State University	2003	Private	www.vcom.vt.edu
LECOM-B	Bradenton, FL	Branch of LECOM	2004	Private	www.lecom.edu
TUNCOM	Henderson, NV	Branch of TUCOM, Touro University Nevada	2004	Private	www.tu.edu
PCOM Georgia	Suwanee, GA.	Branch of PCOM	2005	Private	www.pcom.edu
ATSU-SOMA	Mesa, AZ	ATSU	2007	Private	www.atsu.edu/soma
LMU-DCOM	Harrogate, TN	Lincoln Memorial University	2007	Private	www.lmunet.edu/dcom
TOUROCOM	New York, NY	Touro University	2007	Private	www.touro.edu/med
PNWU-COM	Yakima, WA	Pacific North West University of Health Sciences	2008	Private	www.pnwu.org
RVU-COM	Parker, CO	Rocky Vista University	2008	For profit	www.rockyvistauniversity.org

Note: this information is now available at the AACOM website. The table lists the colleges in the order in which they began to matriculate students. *COM,* College of Osteopathic Medicine; *SOM,* School of Osteopathic Medicine.

*As of 2008, 25 U.S. osteopathic medical colleges or schools (plus three branch campuses) are currently operating. Five original private osteopathic schools form a core that dates back to the late nineteenth and early twentieth centuries (having opened from 1892 to 1916). Ten new colleges of osteopathic medicine opened their doors between 1970 and 1981. This second wave included six state-funded (public) colleges, as the states involved moved to fill a shortage of physicians, particularly primary care physicians in underserved and rural areas. A third wave of private school development began in 1992 and continues to expand. For the first time, outside entrepreneurs began to found osteopathic medical colleges for their own reasons. Touro University, a Jewish institution, founded TUCOM-CA in 1992, and followed that by opening a branch campus in Nevada (TUNCOM) in 2004 and opening a separate college of osteopathic medicine in Harlem in 2007. This was the first time a private religious university had opened an osteopathic college in the United States. In 2008, the first for-profit college of osteopathic medicine since publication of the Flexner Report in 1910 was opened, Rocky Vista University College of Osteopathic Medicine in Parker, Colorado. This was extremely controversial in the osteopathic profession, but there were no rules against it for the American Osteopathic Association to enforce.

As of 2013, 30 U.S. osteopathic medical colleges or schools were open and in operation at 40 locations, including branch campuses, in 28 states. Twenty-four of the COMs (College of Osteopathic Medicine) are private and six are public (AACOM website at www.AACOM.org). Five original private osteopathic schools form a core that dates back to the late nineteenth and early twentieth centuries (having opened from 1892 to 1916). Ten new colleges of osteopathic medicine opened their doors between 1970 and 1981. This second wave included six state-funded (public) colleges, as the states involved moved to fill a shortage of physicians, particularly primary care physicians in underserved and rural areas. A third wave of private school development began in 1992 and continues to expand.

For the first time, outside entrepreneurs began to found osteopathic medical colleges for their own reasons. Touro University, a Jewish institution, founded Touro University College of Osteopathic Medicine–California in 1992, opened a branch campus in Nevada (Touro University Nevada College of Osteopathic Medicine) in 2004, and started a separate college of osteopathic medicine in Harlem, NY, in 2007. For the first time a private religiously-affiliated university had opened an osteopathic college in the United States. In 2008, the first and only for-profit college of osteopathic medicine since publication of the Flexner Report in 1910 was opened, Rocky Vista University College of Osteopathic Medicine in Parker, Colorado. This development has been controversial in the osteopathic profession, but there are no rules against it for the AOA to enforce.

The physician shortage, particularly in rural or small-population states, has spurred additional groups to open new osteopathic medical colleges and schools. Faith-based universities have found their community's medical needs to inspire the creation of additional schools. William Carey University (WCU) is a Southern Baptist university in Mississippi, the state with the lowest physician/patient ratio in the country. When the WCUCOM matriculated the pioneer class in 2010, WCU became the second faith-based university in the country to found and operate a college of osteopathic medicine. Many of the initial applicants indicated an interest in both domestic and international medical service and missions.

Three new colleges of osteopathic medicine matriculated their first classes in the fall of 2013. Two were faith-based universities: Marian University in Indianapolis, Indiana (Roman Catholic) and Campbell University in Buies Creek, North Carolina (Baptist). The Alabama College of Osteopathic Medicine offered another new model for medical school development: Southeast Alabama Medical Center in Dothan, Alabama, became the first American hospital in recent history to found a college of osteopathic medicine based around the hospital.

Currently there are over 20,000 osteopathic medical students, which means that 20% of all U.S. medical students are attending osteopathic colleges or schools in 2013

(American Association of Colleges of Osteopathic Medicine website, www.AACOM.org). Two more colleges (both faith-based) were expected to open in 2014: Touro University is starting another COM in Middletown, New York, and Liberty University is projected to accept their first class in Lynchburg, Virginia. Several colleges are in the stage of initial study and development; additional inquiries have been sent to the AOA regarding establishing even more schools.

POSTGRADUATE EDUCATION

Medical and surgical postgraduate education consists of internships and residencies, which are training programs for general medicine, such as internal medicine or family practice, or for specialty medicine, such as cardiothoracic surgery. Throughout the twentieth century, generalists have increased the time they spend in postgraduate programs and demanded recognition for the practice of general medicine as a specialty itself, distinguishing their practices from those who did only a 1-year internship.

The rotating internship was a hallmark of the osteopathic medical profession in the twentieth century. The common understanding among osteopathic physicians was that the best specialist has a good foundation as a generalist. Competence in general medicine was believed to allow more integrated assessment of a patient's needs and to decrease the amount of "falling through the cracks" that is possible when the patient is seeing only a series of specialists. This concept remained in effect for osteopathic postgraduate programs through the last half of the twentieth century, a time when most MD specialists entered their specialty training directly after medical school. A number of states required candidates for licensure as an osteopathic physician to complete a rotating internship.

Increasingly in the last two decades, however, osteopathic medical graduates have favored omitting a year of general internship in favor of immediate pursuit of postgraduate education in a field of specialty. The AOA has responded to perceived needs of graduates by creating *tracking internships*, or internships that retain a level of general training while decreasing some of the previous requirements to allow more time within the internship for specialization. The internship is then credited as the first year of postgraduate training in the appropriate specialty. The end result is that there is still an extra requirement of general medicine and surgery in the AOA tracking internships compared with the ACGME postgraduate year 1 programs in most specialties.

Throughout the twentieth century, the osteopathic profession maintained that most physicians should be family doctors practicing general medicine and attracted students who implemented this philosophy in their choice of specialties. The profession's promotion of family medicine encouraged a number of state legislatures to fund an osteopathic medical college in the interest of their citizens, to supply more generalists and family physicians to underserved and rural areas.

A physician shortage was again predicted in the 1980s, and during the 1990s, medical schools were urged to increase the number of seats to fill that shortage. The number of available positions in osteopathic postgraduate training has not kept pace with the additional seats in the undergraduate programs as more colleges were founded and class sizes expanded. The osteopathic medical profession has continued to develop osteopathic graduate medical education (OGME) programs, including internships, residencies, and fellowships.

The AOA is expanding OGME programs to ensure that all DO graduates have a place to train once they graduate. In 2013, more than 1100 new OGME positions were created within 75 new programs, bringing the total number of available OGME positions to more than 12,000 (personal communication with Ray Stowers, president of AOA, July 19, 2013). In 2013, approximately 50% of DO graduates began AOA residencies, whereas about 50% began ACGME residencies.

When the ACGME initiated a plan to create a unified pathway for postgraduate training in the United States, the ACGME and AOA explored the possibility over the course of 18 months of discussion. At the July 2013 AOA Annual Business Meeting, the AOA and AACOM announced that the talks had so far been unsuccessful in reaching agreement on a Memorandum of Understanding for a unified graduate medical education accreditation system. Concerns on the side of the AOA included insufficient guarantees that a unified pathway would protect the distinctiveness and identity of the osteopathic medical profession. Five core principles were listed as essential by the AOA:

- The discussion is limited to GME and does not extend backward to undergraduate medical education or forward to licensing or certification.
- The osteopathic medicine licensing examination (COMLEX-USA) remains in place and viable.
- Osteopathic board certification remains in place and viable.
- Osteopathic physicians must be given an equal opportunity to participate in all training programs under any unified accreditation system.
- Any unified accreditation system must not adversely affect primary care programs in community-based settings (email communication from AOA president Ray Stowers to AOA membership, July 19, 2013).

The ACGME brought up the issue that, at this time, DO graduates are eligible to enter ACGME residencies and fellowships, but the same is not true for MD graduates who could apply for an AOA OGME position. A pathway has not been created for MD graduates to qualify by taking the additional training in osteopathic principles and practice, including osteopathic structural diagnosis and OMT. Such a pathway had been discussed and proposed in the 1990s, but it was not approved after AOA specialty colleges expressed concern that the relatively small number of certain specialty training programs accredited by the AOA

might be swamped by a large number of MD applicants with no actual background, interest in or commitment to applying osteopathic principles in their training or practice.

AOA president Ray Stowers announced in an email communication to AOA members in July 2013 that "The AOA and AACOM strongly believe that the health of the American public will benefit from a uniform path of preparation for the next generation of physicians designed to evaluate the effectiveness of GME programs in producing competent physicians."

The students favored during recruitment and interviews tend to be those who voice interest in patient care, particularly in small towns and underserved areas, and the interviews evaluate them for numerous factors including informal assessment for people skills. Matriculants are encouraged to choose primary care specialties. In addition, osteopathic colleges are community based and the majority do not have extensive research programs. One result has been that fewer graduating DOs have been interested in pursuing a career in medical research.

RESEARCH

Although the osteopathic medical profession has participated marginally in medical research from its inception, the bulk of its contribution to American health care has been through patient care. With the recent rapid increase in the number of osteopathic medical colleges, development of some state-funded institutions, and the rapid increase in the raw number of osteopathic physicians, attention to the profession's responsibility for contributing to medical research is growing.

Research at osteopathic medical schools falls into three categories. Most of the research is in either basic science or standard medical care. A small amount of research has been conducted on the scientific basis of and effects of osteopathic structural diagnosis and treatment. This third category has historically been poorly funded, because pharmaceutical companies did not appear to be inclined to sponsor research that might prove that the use of no or less medication is better or that use of natural practices is more likely to prevent side effects of medication. Until recently required by Congress, the government was not interested in funding aspects of medicine with which the medical establishment did not concern itself.

In the early to mid twentieth century, individuals such as Louisa Burns, Irvin Korr, Steadman Denslow, Beryl Arbuckle, and Viola Frymann represented a significant portion of the effort of the profession to validate the scientific and clinical basis of osteopathic manipulation. A group of researchers also came together at MSU's College of Osteopathic Medicine, which has been productive from the 1970s forward. The establishment of the Osteopathic Research Center at UNTHSC-Texas College of Osteopathic Medicine and the A.T. Still Research Institute at A.T. Still University have focused efforts on unique osteopathic research to add to and collaborate with researchers at numerous COMs and clinicians in the field.

Aside from the commercial and political nature of award grants, other factors have interfered with sufficient accumulation of research in the osteopathic profession. Only five osteopathic medical colleges continued in existence from 1916 to 1968, and all were private and had very limited if any endowment funds. Prior to 1969, no state institutions funded an osteopathic college. The colleges focused on producing practicing physicians, not researchers. Although small amounts of research were ongoing at the colleges, few researchers interested themselves in uniquely osteopathic issues. New research models had to be created to overcome the difficulty of performing double-blind studies on the use of manual medicine. Eventually this problem was addressed by the use of naive subjects, blinded physicians, and sham treatments. The increasing use of outcome and cost-effectiveness studies in the field of medicine has promoted additional interest in doing research on the unique contribution of the osteopathic profession, OMT.

In the 1980s, the AOA passed a special annual assessment that was included in membership dues to build up funds for research. Small pilot grants were distributed to the existing osteopathic colleges that applied. More recently, AOA funds were used to develop the Osteopathic Research Center at the University of North Texas Health Science Center/Texas College of Osteopathic Medicine in Fort Worth for the purpose of conducting osteopathically oriented basic science bench research, clinical research, and transitional research that bridges the gap between the two. The Osteopathic Heritage Foundation (Columbus, Ohio) has been a major contributor. The AOA Commission on Osteopathic College Accreditation requires institutions, as a part of the undergraduate accreditation process, to "make contributions to the advancement of knowledge and the development of osteopathic medicine through scientific research."

CLINICAL TRIALS RESEARCH

In 2010, a randomized controlled trial, the OSTEOPAThic Health outcomes In Chronic (OSTEOPATHIC) low back pain trial, evaluated OMT and ultrasound therapy to treat chronic low back pain. This 455-subject trial was conducted in Fort Worth, Texas, under the leadership of John Licciardone, DO, MS, MBA. Patients in the study who received ultrasound therapy did not see any improvement, but the patients who received OMT did see significant improvement in pain, used less prescription medication, and were more satisfied with their care over the 12 weeks of the study than those patients who did not receive OMT.

In study patients who received OMT, nearly two-thirds had at least a 30% reduction in their pain level, and half had at least a 50% reduction in their pain level. Patients received six treatments during the course of the study (Licciardone et al, 2013).

The Multicenter Osteopathic Pneumonia Study in the Elderly (MOPSE) was a registered, randomized controlled, double-blind clinical trial that sought to assess the impact of adjunctive osteopathic manual medicine techniques in the treatment of patients over the age of 50 years who were hospitalized with community-acquired pneumonia. The study was conducted between March 2004 and December 2006 at seven hospitals in five states: Michigan, Missouri, New Jersey, Ohio, and Texas. This clinical trial of 306 subjects who were hospitalized with community-acquired pneumonia, showed a one-day reduction in the length of hospital stay in those patients who received OMT in addition to standard medical care as compared to patients who received only conventional medical care.

Using a per protocol analysis for the subgroup of patients ages 50–74 years, patients in the conventional care group were hospitalized an average for 3.9 days, while those in the group receiving OMT in addition to conventional care were hospitalized for an average of 2.9 days. The group that received light touch (placebo manual treatment) and conventional medical care were discharged after an average of 3.5 days. An intent-to-treat analysis of patients younger than 75 years showed a significant decrease in mortality in both the OMT and light touch groups compared to the conventional care group (Noll et al, 2010).

Significant positive differences were found with OMT in a variety of conditions. In a retrospective review of postoperative ileus, Crow and Gorodinsky (2009) showed that postoperative OMT significantly decreased hospital length of stay. Baltazar et al (2013) reported the same results in a prospective study. Yurvati et al (2005) demonstrated hemodynamic changes in subjects treated with OMT immediately after coronary artery bypass surgery, while still sedated and paralyzed. Using patients as their own controls pre- and post-OMT, significant positive changes were noted in SVO_2 (an indicator of peripheral oxygen saturation), thoracic impedance (an indicator of central blood volume), and cardiac index (an indicator of cardiac function). One study showed OMT significantly improve balance in the elderly (Lopez et al, 2011). In other patients, it decreased dizziness at a significant level, as measured by the SMART Balance Master (Fraix et al, 2013).

INTERNATIONAL IMPACT

Osteopathy began as a unique American contribution to the science and art of health care. The international evolution of osteopathy became complex and diversified. Americans and international students trained in the United States around 1900, at the inception of the osteopathic medical profession, emigrated or returned to their own native countries. The early osteopath who had the most to do with spreading Still's original discovery internationally was John Martin Littlejohn, a Scottish MD who served for 2 years as Dean of Faculty at the American School of

Osteopathy while obtaining his American DO degree. Leaving Kirksville MO in 1900, he moved to Chicago and founded the American College of Osteopathic Medicine and Surgery, which is now Midwestern University. Littlejohn was a native of the United Kingdom, and he returned to the United Kingdom in 1913.

UNITED KINGDOM

In 1918, Littlejohn opened the British School of Osteopathy (BSO), founding an osteopathic profession in which the practitioners did not use surgery, medicine, or obstetrics, and it has not evolved into a profession with an unlimited medical license (Van Buskirk, 1996). The BSO's first diplomats graduated in 1925, but the practice of osteopathy in the United Kingdom remained unregulated until the last decade of the twentieth century. Based on this model, the nonphysician practice of osteopathic philosophy and manipulation spread through the British Commonwealth, was copied in other western European nations, and was disseminated from there to much of the rest of the world. Australia regulated the practice of osteopathy in 1978, and the United Kingdom in 1993.

The British government regulated the practice of osteopathy in 1993 with the Act of Osteopaths and later included nonphysician osteopathic practitioners in the national health care system. These practitioners are generally perceived as specialists in treatment of musculoskeletal pain and adjunctive treatment. They are also sometimes consulted if the patient has vague complaints and continuing physician efforts do not produce an organic diagnosis. Management of medical conditions is left to the physician. Incorporation of a limited amount of medical knowledge has increased in the education of osteopathic practitioners in the past two decades. Their diploma does not give them the education or the right to prescribe medicine or to perform or assist at surgery or childbirth. Generally, the public easily identifies this profession and respects the practitioners.

Practitioners outside the United States are often called DOs, a designation that stands for *Diploma (or Diplomat) in (or of) Osteopathy*, as opposed to the American degree of DO (which means *Doctor of Osteopathic Medicine*). The level of training and requirements for the diploma in osteopathy are not standardized in most other countries, and there is certainly no international standard. Schools in some countries offer a series of weekend courses over several years for physical therapists and others who wish to become osteopaths, whereas there are only a few international 4- to 5-year full-time programs.

FRANCE AND QUEBEC

A number of part-time osteopathic schools in France began to train physical therapists in osteopathic technique and philosophy some time after World War II, granting them a diploma of osteopathy. These diplomats continued to practice outside the law by tolerance. Although they orga-

nized and formed a national registry, they were not sanctioned by the government. As their numbers grew, they lobbied for and obtained the legal right to practice in 2002. The law specified that they could practice osteopathic diagnosis and techniques; however, the official decrees issued later specified limitations in their practice of osteopathic techniques. The Décret 2007-437 in 2007 established new educational standards that are required for the practice of osteopathy in France, allowing a time period for those already practicing to fill their deficiencies.

Returning after many years to the North American continent by way of France, osteopathy came full circle when one French citizen opened a part-time osteopathic school in Quebec. American nonphysician health care practitioners were allowed to enroll as students, and a number have made the journey to Canada, then used the knowledge gained to practice in the United States under their previously held license as a physical therapist or massage therapist. The graduates of this school receive a Diploma in Osteopathy Manual Practice [DO(MP)].

INTERNATIONAL DIVERSITY

The laws that govern the practice of physical therapy allow a great deal of leeway in choice of manual techniques. A few physical therapists have claimed that they are now the "true osteopaths" because of their part-time training in osteopathic techniques and philosophy. When challenged, however, it is clear that they do not have the right to the title *osteopath* in the United States, because this title is reserved by law for American DOs.

A unique international forum was held in Atlanta, Georgia, in 1995 by the American Academy of Osteopathy (AAO), the AOA's specialty college focused on the osteopathic philosophy and osteopathic manipulative medicine. For some years, the AAO had been receiving an increasing number of letters and contacts from international diplomats of osteopathy. A few international practitioners of osteopathy wanted to visit the birthplace of osteopathy, as well as to take courses or arrange for American DOs to offer instruction abroad. As the whole world increases its movement toward globalization, this trend grows stronger. Many international practitioners also request advice about obtaining practice rights in their own countries that do not have laws permitting osteopathic practice of any type.

The forum allowed presentations by individuals from numerous countries, and certain facts became clear:

- The majority of osteopathic education outside of the United States and the United Kingdom was on a part-time basis and not at the doctoral level.
- The vast majority of international osteopathic education was for profit and entrepreneurial.
- Australia and the United Kingdom were the only countries present that had created national laws allowing the practice of osteopathy (Australia, 1978, and the United Kingdom, 1993), but not osteopathic medicine as a full licensure including medicine and surgery.

- There were very few registries of osteopaths; in some countries there were competing registries with no government-approved status.
- Great rivalries existed in several countries as to who were the *real* osteopaths, and some competitors sought AAO validation.
- The United States was the only country with strict and extensive national standards set by a government-approved accrediting agency regarding osteopathic education for the award of a doctoral degree, national board examinations, and medical licensure (the latter granted by states).
- The United States was the only country with osteopathic physicians who were trained at the predoctoral level with the goal of full medical and surgical practice rights after graduation.
- The general population of U.S. doctors of osteopathic medicine was very different from the general population of the international diplomats of osteopathy; those in the United States have a much broader interest and training in medicine, surgery, and obstetrics.

Subsequently, the International Affairs Committee of the AAO undertook the process of creating an annual international forum. Any international DO was able to come; there were no elected delegates. The AAO realized that it would be difficult if not impossible to set up a representative group from each country, because many had more than one organization claiming its own legitimacy. In initial meetings, the focus was on reports regarding legal status and schools in the various countries. A group of cooperating individuals from various nations remained over the years to work on topics of common interest.

The AAO realized that it was not up to the United States to tell the other countries what to do in their own jurisdictions, but recognized that many were clamoring for guidance on establishing practice rights, educational standards, the vocabulary to use when discussing unique osteopathic concepts, and osteopathic research. As a result, later international forums came to include workshops and discussions on these topics. Competing groups from individual nations were encouraged to cooperate with each other in obtaining practice rights and education.

The parent organization of the AAO, the AOA, followed the AAO's initial work on international osteopathic communication, and began to explore communication with practitioners of osteopathy on common interests. Initially, the focus of the AOA had been on the American model of a complete osteopathic medical, surgical, and obstetrical practice, and on obtaining the right for U.S. DOs to practice with full medical and surgical rights in other countries.

In 2003, ten countries and 17 international organizations were represented in Chicago, Illinois, by 34 individuals who attended the American Osteopathic Association–sponsored 1st Invitational Conference to Organise an International Osteopathic Association. The Osteopathic International Alliance (OIA) was founded in 2004. OIA goals relate to international health care policy, fostering improved international health care by promoting osteopathic medicine and osteopathy. The members of the OIA are groups, and in 2013, has 70 member organizations in over 27 countries on 5 continents. A list of member organizations, the goals, bylaws, and a 2012 official report, *History and Current Context of the Osteopathic Profession,* can be accessed at www.oialliance.org). The report is a succinct summary of the state of both the American model and international model osteopathic systems.

A move toward higher standards and full-time schools for the nonphysician osteopaths is currently in process internationally, but there still are no worldwide international standards requiring full-time schooling to obtain a diploma of osteopathy. The European Union has developed legislation to give practice rights to, and set standards for, alternative medical practices, including osteopathy, throughout the member nations in Europe. The WHO created a committee in 2004 to develop suggestions for international osteopathic educational standards, and in 2010 published *Benchmarks for Training in Osteopathy* as part of its *Benchmarks for training in traditional/complementary and alternative medicine.* The document seems to relate more to standards for international diplomats of osteopathy rather than the American model osteopathic medical physicians, but there is overlap with the unique osteopathic portion of American DO training.

MDs and those with equivalent degrees from various countries (e.g., United Kingdom, France, Russia, Japan) have taken postgraduate training in osteopathic diagnosis and manipulation. These practitioners have an unlimited medical license, but may have less exposure to osteopathic medical philosophy and/or a focus on a limited range of techniques. However, they have many similarities with American DOs. Many of these physicians integrate osteopathic care into general practice, rehabilitation medicine, sports medicine, rheumatology, or neurology, or focus on the conservative treatment of musculoskeletal conditions as well as preoperative and postoperative care.

France is one country where postgraduate training in osteopathic technique exists for MDs, in large part due to teaching groups inspired by the work of Robert Maigne, MD. French physicians have long enjoyed the right to use osteopathy as part of their practice. In Russia, several osteopathic schools exist in St. Petersburg and Moscow as postgraduate training sites for physicians, including a school at the state university in St. Petersburg. The London School of Osteopathy has also had a postgraduate training program for physicians for many years. Several organizations have existed in Japan for decades that have trained both physicians and nonphysicians in osteopathic techniques and philosophy.

Opinions on the evolution of osteopathy as a nonmedical practice vary. American DOs are aware of the dangers in having an expert in manipulation who is not well trained in differential medical diagnosis. Pain might not be recognized as symptomatic of a serious underlying treatable medical or surgical condition, and appropriate treatment may be delayed until it is too late to obtain a favorable outcome. When the only tool one has is a hammer, too often every problem begins to look like a nail.

International nonmedical osteopathic practitioners, however, would be quick to point out that a significant number of American DOs who have an excellent knowledge of medical diagnosis and treatment nonetheless lack sufficient manipulative skills to effectively diagnose or treat a patient with a problem for which manipulation is clearly indicated.

American osteopathic medical physicians and international osteopaths have joined forces in the OIA to cooperate on common vocabulary, communication, educational models, and research on the unique philosophy, principles and practice of osteopathy whether or not the practitioner has full medical license.

SUMMARY AND CONCLUSION

Osteopathic medicine is based on a philosophy, and a system of logic for medical diagnosis and care, with rich roots found back to Hippocrates and before, and in the history of every known traditional medical practice. Andrew Taylor Still, MD, DO, a pioneer physician in Kansas and Missouri, developed the basic tenets of osteopathy and elaborated on them in his writings, which were adopted by the ASO (now Andrew Taylor Still University/ Kirksville College of Osteopathic Medicine).

The development of scientifically validated, efficacious medicines aided in the evolution of classical osteopathic philosophy to its current form, contemporary osteopathic medical philosophy. The work of Irvin Korr, PhD, a medical physiologist, further elaborated and explained osteopathic theory in the mid-twentieth century. Korr personally benefited from—and in addition to his basic science research, elaborated on—the preventive care and healthful practices promoted by the original philosophy.

Osteopathic philosophy uses a holistic approach to begin the evaluation of the patient, continuing with a reductionistic approach to focus on aspects of anatomical and physiological dysfunction. One goal of this system of logic is for the osteopathic physician to remember throughout diagnosis and treatment that he or she is working with and for a fellow human being, even as the physician uses tests that focus on the smallest microscopic details of that person. No cell or system in the body is seen as acting in isolation, and the importance of structure and function at each level is always kept in mind. Central to this philosophy is a tremendous respect for the innate capacity of the human being to heal. The physician works with the patient's physiological and psychological processes to obtain an optimal level of homeostasis and function.

OMT, the hallmark of osteopathic treatment as developed by Still, is used in patient care either alone or in conjunction with medicines and surgery, as appropriate.

OMT is recognized as having beneficial effects not only in treating pain and restricted motion, but also in decreasing physiological stress and assisting the body's self-healing mechanisms.

The application of contemporary osteopathic medical philosophy varies from physician to physician and, outside of the United States, from country to country.

As the osteopathic profession has evolved both within and outside the United States, it has changed significantly. The original osteopaths practiced in a distinctive manner very different from that of the allopathic physicians at the end of the nineteenth century. Still developed the osteopathic approach because the medications of his time were ineffective and toxic, based on tradition or conjecture rather than research. His important contribution to medicine was the idea that by adjusting (normalizing) anatomical functional abnormality, a physician could enhance natural physiological function; that by enhancing the delivery and clearance of blood, lymphatic fluid, and neurotrophic elements, a physician could promote delivery of endogenous substances; and that these endogenous substances were able to do more than the medicines of his time to normalize physiology, eliminate illness, and reestablish health. His development and teaching of OMT were designed not only to accomplish this goal, but also to eliminate pain and improve biomechanical (physiologic) function in body systems other than the neuromusculoskeletal system, such as the respiratory system.

American osteopathic physicians continued to address the full medical, obstetric, and surgical care of patients. Each succeeding generation of DOs adopted the use of researched medications and decreased the use of OMT for anything but neuromusculoskeletal complaints, so that at the present time, a significant number of American DOs do not use the manipulative skills at all that they learned in osteopathic medical school. Internationally, osteopathy developed in a manner that did not incorporate surgery, obstetrics, or the use of medication. This form of osteopathy continues to rely on endogenous substances for treatment, and the presenting complaints of its patients are generally neuromusculoskeletal pain or movement problems.

The twentieth century saw the development of scientifically researched, efficacious medications sometimes with fewer but still significant accompanying side effects. As these medications became the standard of allopathic care, they were also adopted by osteopathic physicians. Increasing numbers of osteopathic medical students were attracted to the profession, not by the difference that OMT could make in patient outcomes but by the availability of the full scope of medical and surgical possibilities and a full license to practice as they saw fit. The osteopathic medical profession in the United States has thus ceased to have a distinct identification in the mind of much of the American public, and many patients are unaware that their doctors came from a different tradition. This evolution has followed a standard sociological pattern in which an offshoot of a main group initially diverges, makes a contribution by developing an idea or skill that fills a vacuum not addressed by the main group, then reconverges with the mainstream as changes in both groups make them more similar. As the osteopathic physicians evolved, so did the allopathic physicians. Both sets of licensed physicians practice very differently than their predecessors, relying on research and progress unforeseen in Still's time, and in today's medical milieu, practice cooperatively.

Other factors affecting the evolution of osteopathic medicine have included student recruitment demographics, postgraduate training trends, advances in technology, increasing government control, and medical economic factors. The development of a specialty in osteopathic neuromusculoskeletal medicine, as well as widespread dispersion of osteopathic treatment methods through a number of health care professions, has helped to meet patients' perceived medical needs that remain poorly addressed by today's standard medical education and practice.

In the twenty-first century, American osteopathic medical physicians and international osteopaths have become reacquainted and have begun cooperative efforts in areas of common interest, while recognizing the distinctive scopes of practice in different countries.

References

American Association of Colleges of Osteopathic Medicine: *Osteopathic Medical College Information Book, 2014 Entering Class*, Chevy Chase, MD, 2013, The Association.

Baltazar GA, Betler MP, Akella K, et al: Effect of osteopathic manipulative treatment on incidence of postoperative ileus and hospital stay in general surgery, *J Amer Osteopath Assoc* 113:204–209, 2013.

Crow WT, Gorodinsky L: Does osteopathic manipulative treatment (OMT) improves outcomes in patients who develop postoperative ileus: a retrospective review, *Intern J Osteopath Med* 12:32–37, 2009.

Fraix M, Gordon A, Graham V, et al: Use of the SMART Balance Master to Quantify the Effects of Osteopathic Manipulative Treatment in Patients with Dizziness, *J Am Osteopath Assoc* 113(5):394–403, 2013.

Gleick J: *Chaos*, New York, 1987, Viking/Penguin.

Hildreth A: *The lengthening shadow of Dr. Andrew Taylor Still*, Paw Paw, Mich, 1942, privately published.

Holmes OW: *Medical essays, 1842–1882*, Boston, 1892, Houghton Mifflin.

Licciardone J, Minotti D, Gatchel R, et al: Osteopathic manual treatment and ultrasound therapy for chronic low back pain: a randomized controlled trial, *Ann Fam Med* 11(2):l22–l29, 2013.

Lopez D, King HH, Knebl JA, et al: Effects of comprehensive osteopathic manipulative treatment on balance in elderly patients: a pilot study, *J Am Osteopath Assoc* 111:382–388, 2011.

Noll DR, Degenhardt BF, Morley TF, et al: Efficacy of osteopathic manipulation as an adjunctive treatment for hospitalized patients with pneumonia in the elderly: a randomized controlled trial, *Osteopath Med Prim Care* 4:2, 2010.

Schiowitz S: Facilitated positional release. In Ward RC, Jerome JA, Jones JM, editors: *Foundations of osteopathic medicine*, Philadelphia, 1997, Lippincott Williams & Wilkins.

Singer C, Underwood EA: *A short history of medicine*, ed 2, New York, 1962, Oxford University Press.

Still AT: *Autobiography of Andrew T. Still*, Kirksville, Mo, 1897, The Author.

Still AT: *Osteopathy, research, and practice*, Kirksville, Mo, 1910, The Author.

Still AT: *The philosophy and mechanical principles of osteopathy*, Kirksville, Mo, 1902, The Author.

Trowbridge C: *Andrew Taylor Still*, Kirksville, Mo, 1991, Thomas Jefferson University Press.

Van Buskirk RL: A manipulative technique of Andrew Taylor Still as reported to Charles Hazzard, DO, in 1905, *J Am Osteopath Assoc* 96(10):597, 1996.

Sage sayings of Still. In Webster GV, editor: *Year book of the AOA*, Los Angeles, 1935, Wetzel Publishing.

Yurvati AH, Carnes MS, Clearfield MB, Stoll ST, McConathy WJ: Hemodynamic Effects of Osteopathic Manipulative Treatment Immediately After Coronary Artery Bypass Graft Surgery, *J Am Osteopath Assoc* 105:475–481, 2005.

Suggested Readings

American Association of Colleges of Osteopathic Medicine: *Glossary of Osteopathic Terminology*, Chevy Chase, MD, 2011, The Association.

American Osteopathic Association: *Yearbook and directory of osteopathic physicians*, Chicago, 2000, The Association.

Northup GW: *Osteopathic medicine: an American reformation*, ed 2, Chicago, 1966, American Osteopathic Association.

CHAPTER 19

CHIROPRACTIC

DANIEL REDWOOD

Born in the American Midwest in the late nineteenth century, chiropractic has evolved and matured toward mainstream status while largely preserving its essential principles. The contemporary chiropractic profession is in the unique position of having scaled many walls of the health care establishment (with licensure, an increasingly strong scientific research base, widespread insurance coverage, and 20 million patients per year in the United States), while at the same time maintaining strong roots in the complementary and alternative medicine (CAM) community, with a philosophy that emphasizes healing without drugs.

Chiropractic is the third largest independent health profession in the Western world, following conventional (allopathic) medicine and dentistry. Its practitioners are "portal of entry" providers, licensed for both diagnosis and treatment. Unlike dentistry, podiatry, and optometry, chiropractic practice is limited not by anatomical region but by procedure. The chiropractor's scope of practice excludes surgery and the prescription of pharmaceuticals; its centerpiece is the manual adjustment or manipulation of the spine.

The United States is now home to approximately 70,000 of the world's 100,000 chiropractors (Chapman-Smith, 2000). Chiropractors are licensed throughout the English-speaking world and in an increasing number of other nations (see Box 19-1). Rigorous educational standards are supervised by government-recognized accrediting agencies, including the Council on Chiropractic Education (CCE) in the United States. After fulfilling college science prerequisites analogous to those required to enter medical or osteopathic schools, chiropractic students must complete a chiropractic school program lasting 4 academic years, which includes a wide range of courses in anatomy, physiology, pathology, and diagnosis, as well as spinal adjusting, physical therapy, rehabilitation, public health, prevention, health promotion, and nutrition.

At least 90% of chiropractic patients present with neuromusculoskeletal conditions, principally back pain, neck pain, and headaches, the conditions for which spinal manipulation (also known as spinal adjustment, spinal manual therapy, or SMT) is most effective. As described later in this chapter, chiropractic researchers have sought to define further the role of SMT in the management of various musculoskeletal conditions, as well as to evaluate its effectiveness for visceral organ disorders, including hypertension, infantile colic, otitis media, dysmenorrhea, and asthma.

HISTORICAL ROOTS, EVOLUTIONARY PROCESS

PRECURSORS IN WESTERN TRADITIONS

Spinal manipulation has been practiced for millennia in cultures throughout the world. Chiropractic's forebears have included prominent figures in the history of medicine.

Hippocrates was an early practitioner of spinal manipulation (Withington, 1959), and according to some scholars, he used manipulation "not only to reposition vertebrae, but also thereby to cure a wide variety of dysfunctions" (Leach, 1994). Galen was a Greek-born Roman physician who lived in the second century AD, whose approach to

BOX 19-1 *Legal Status of Chiropractic by Country*

African region	Eastern Mediterranean region	European region	Latin American region	North American region
Botswana[a]	Cyprus[a]	Belgium[a]	Argentina[b]	Bahamas[a]
Ethiopia[b]	Egypt[b]	Croatia[b]	Bolivia[a]	Barbados[a]
Ghana[b]	Iran[a]	Denmark[a]	Brazil[b]	Belize[b]
Kenya[b]	Israel[a]	Estonia[b]	Chile[b]	Bermuda[b]
Lesotho[a]	Jordan[b]	Finland[a]	Colombia[b]	British Virgin Islands[b]
Mauritius[b]	Lebanon[b]	France[a]	Costa Rica[a]	Canada[a]
Namibia[a]	Libya[b]	Germany[b]	Ecuador[b]	Cayman Islands[a]
Nigeria[a]	Morocco[c]	Greece[c]	Guatemala[a]	Jamaica[b]
South Africa[a]	Qatar[a]	Hungary[c]	Honduras[b]	Leeward Islands[a]
Swaziland[a]	Saudi Arabia[a]	Iceland[a]	Mexico[a]	Puerto Rico[a]
Zimbabwe[a]	Syria[c]	Ireland[b]	Panama[a]	Trinidad & Tobago[b]
	Turkey[c]	Italy[a]	Peru[b]	Turks & Caicos[a]
Asian region	United Arab Emirates[a]	Liechtenstein[a]	Venezuela[b]	United States[a]
China[c]		Luxembourg[b]		US Virgin Islands[b]
Hong Kong–SAR		Malta[a]		
China[a]		Netherlands[b]		**Pacific region**
Indonesia[c]		Norway[a]		Australia[a]
Japan[b]		Portugal[a]		Fiji[b]
Malaysia[b]		Russian Federation[b]		Guam[a]
Philippines[a]		Serbia[a]		New Caledonia[a]
Singapore[b]		Slovakia[b]		New Zealand[a]
South Korea[d]		Spain[c]		Papua New Guinea[b]
Taiwan[d]		Sweden[a]		Tahiti[a]
Thailand[a]		Switzerland[a]		
Vietnam[c]		United Kingdom[a]		

[a]Legal pursuant to legislation to accept and regulate chiropractic practice.
[b]Legal pursuant to general law.
[c]Legal status unclear, but de facto recognition.
[d]Legal status unclear and risk of prosecution.
Source: World Federation of Chiropractic. Reproduced with permission. http://www.wfc.org/website/index.php?option=com_content&view=article&id=123&Itemid=139&lang=en (accessed November 5, 2013).

healing set a recognized standard in Western medicine for 1500 years after his death. He also used spinal manipulation and reported the successful resolution of a patient's hand weakness and numbness through manipulation of the seventh cervical vertebra (Lomax, 1975).

As Europe entered the Middle Ages, these healing traditions had been preserved in the learning centers of the Middle East by the ascendant Arabic civilization. This body of knowledge returned to Europe, and the preserved works of Hippocrates and Galen, together with new insights from Avicenna (Ib'n Sina) and Unani medicine (see Chapter 32), helped form the foundations of Renaissance medicine. Ambroise Paré, sometimes called the "father of surgery," used manipulation to treat French vineyard workers in the sixteenth century (Lomax, 1975; Paré, 1968).

In the centuries that followed, to the beginning of the modern era, manipulative techniques were passed down from generation to generation within families. These "bonesetting" methods, transmitted not only from father to son but often from mother to daughter, played an important role in the history of nonmedical healing in

Great Britain, and similar methods are common in the folk medicine of many nations (Bennett, 1981).

During the nineteenth century, the new United States became a vibrant center of natural healing theory and practice. Two manipulation-based healing arts, osteopathy and chiropractic, trace their origins to that era. Both began in the American Midwest.

BEGINNINGS OF A NEW PROFESSION

Daniel David Palmer, a self-educated "magnetic" or "mesmeric" healer in the Mississippi River town of Davenport, Iowa, founded the chiropractic profession in 1895 with two fundamental premises: (1) vertebral subluxation (which he defined as spinal misalignment causing abnormal nerve transmission) is the primary cause of virtually all disease; and (2) chiropractic adjustment (manual manipulation of the subluxated vertebra) is its cure (Palmer, 1910). This "one cause–one cure" philosophy played a central role in chiropractic history, first as a guiding principle, then later as a historical remnant, providing a target for the slings and arrows of organized medicine (Figure 19-1).

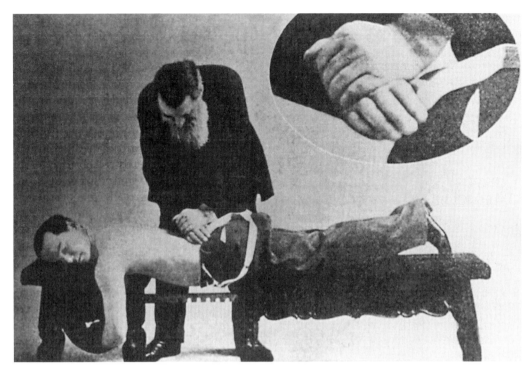

Figure 19-1 Daniel David Palmer, the founder of chiropractic, adjusting a patient (circa 1906). (Courtesy Palmer College of Chiropractic.)

Although few if any contemporary chiropractors would endorse such a simplistic and all-encompassing formulation, it nonetheless remains true that subluxation (now commonly defined as spinal joint dysfunctions or segmental dysfunctions) and adjustment remain central to chiropractic practice. Chiropractors may do much more, but it is their ability to evaluate and adjust the spine with great expertise that has allowed the chiropractic art to survive for over a century under a barrage of medical opposition, some of it justified, most of it not.

The one cause–one cure adherents among the early chiropractors had two major political effects on the development of the profession. First, their deep faith in the truth of their message, combined with the positive results of chiropractic adjustments, created a strong and steadily growing activist constituency of chiropractic patients and supporters. In their zeal, they generated a grassroots movement that ensured the survival of the profession through stormy years in the first half of the twentieth century. Civil disobedience was an integral part of the early development of the chiropractic profession, as it would later become in the American civil rights movement. Hundreds, including the founder himself, went to jail, charged with practicing medicine without a license. Yet they persisted and ultimately prevailed, eventually winning licensure throughout North America and in many other nations.

Putting Down of Hands

That chiropractic would prove controversial was evident from its inception. In the first chiropractic adjustment, the patient sought treatment for deafness and attained results that greatly exceeded his expectations. Harvey Lillard, a deaf janitor in the building where Palmer had an office, came to him for help. Noting an apparent misalignment in the patient's spine, Palmer administered the first chiropractic adjustment, after which Lillard is reported to have been able to hear for the first time in nearly two decades.

Similar results were not forthcoming when other deaf people sought his assistance. There have been other reports through the years of hearing restored through spinal manipulation, including one by a Canadian orthopedist (Bourdillion, 1982), but these have been rare. The story of Lillard's dramatic recovery was often used to disparage chiropractic, with charges that such an event is impossible, because no spinal nerves supply the ear.

Current knowledge of neurophysiology provides a credible theoretical basis for this and other apparent visceral organ responses to chiropractic adjustments. The underlying physiological mechanism is the somatoautonomic (or somatovisceral) reflex. Chiropractors and osteopaths assert that signals initiated by spinal manipulation are transmitted through autonomic pathways to internal organs.

That such autonomic pathways exist is not in dispute, but whether manipulation can elicit such healing responses via these pathways remains unproven. In the case of Palmer's first adjustment, the relevant nerve pathway begins in the thoracic region, coursing up through the neck and into the cranium along sympathetic nerves that eventually lead to the blood vessels of the inner ear. Normal function of the hearing apparatus depends on an adequate blood supply, which in turn depends on a properly functioning sympathetic nerve supply.

A key question is unresolved: why are there sometimes dramatic positive somatovisceral responses to chiropractic adjustments, whereas most such cases appear to be nonresponsive?

Marked individual variations in response to virtually all CAM therapies remains a hallmark of these practices—an issue that has yet to be seriously addressed by these professions but about which there have been some recent advancements, as discussed in Chapters 3 and 10.

LEGACY OF CONTENTION WITH ALLOPATHIC MEDICINE

All nascent healing arts face serious challenges, particularly the need to maintain the enthusiasm generated by positive therapeutic results while clearly and consistently distinguishing among proven, probable, and speculative findings. Some of the harshest criticism of chiropractic has been in reaction to the tendency of some chiropractors to "globalize" (Gellert, 1994), making broad, overarching claims on the basis of limited, no matter how powerful, anecdotal evidence.

Whatever the validity of these medical critiques (some of which mirror intensive self-criticism within the chiropractic profession), the American medical establishment's policy on chiropractic has never been that of a disinterested group solely seeking to serve solely the public good. Its century-long campaign against chiropractic impeded chiropractic's advancement and at times posed a severe threat to its survival. Until recently, allopathic medical students were taught that chiropractic is harmful, or at best worthless, and they in turn inculcated these prejudices in their own patients.

That such a fiercely antichiropractic policy was pursued by the American Medical Association (AMA) is no longer in dispute. In 1990, the U.S. Supreme Court affirmed a lower court ruling in which the AMA was found liable for federal antitrust violations for having engaged in a conspiracy to "contain and eliminate" (the AMA's own words) the chiropractic profession (*Wilk v AMA*, 1990). The process that culminated in this landmark decision began in 1974 when a large packet of confidential AMA documents was provided anonymously to leaders of the American Chiropractic Association and International Chiropractors Association. As a result of the ensuing *Wilk v AMA* case, the AMA reversed its long-standing ban on interprofessional cooperation between medical doctors and chiropractors, agreed to publish the full findings of the court in the *Journal of the American Medical Association*, and paid an undisclosed sum, most of which was earmarked for chiropractic research.

This ruling has not completely reversed the effects of organized medicine's boycott, but is nonetheless a laudable milestone on the long road toward reconciliation. Although the swords of contention have not yet been beaten into plowshares of amity, the pace of progress has accelerated substantially in the years after the *Wilk* decision, as men

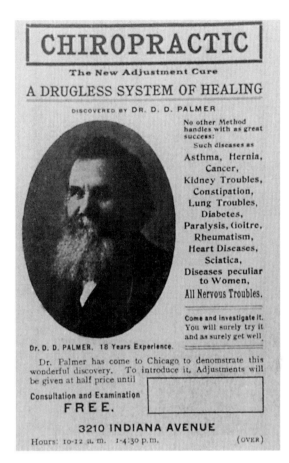

Figure 19-2 In this 1904 advertisement, Dr. Palmer touted chiropractic as a cure for virtually all human ailments. Such claims engendered great controversy. (Courtesy Palmer College of Chiropractic.)

and women of goodwill in both professions strive to inaugurate a new era in which their patients are the beneficiaries of their mutual cooperation (Figures 19-2 and 19-3).

INTERPROFESSIONAL COOPERATION

Historically, relations between the medical and chiropractic professions outside the United States were also less than cordial. Earlier than in the United States, however, collaboration developed between chiropractors and allopathic physicians. This cooperation has had particularly salutary effects in the research arena. Many of the key clinical trials that first established chiropractic's scientific credibility were conducted in Europe and Canada. Nearly all of the major universities in Canada now have endowed research chairs held by dual-degreed chiropractors (primarily DC-PhDs).

Gradually, the tide has turned in the United States as well. Research projects funded by the federal government (through the National Center for Complementary and Alternative Medicine, the Health Resources and Services Administration, the Agency for Health Care Quality, and the Department of Defense) have encouraged an atmosphere of growing medical-chiropractic cooperation.

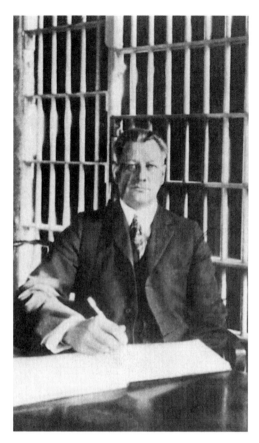

Figure 19-3 Dr. D.S. Tracy behind bars in Los Angeles. Hundreds of chiropractors served time in jail to secure the right to practice their healing art freely. (Courtesy Palmer College of Chiropractic.)

Multidisciplinary organizations such as the American Back Society, as well as "integrative" spine centers, back centers, and related clinical practices and facilities, also reflect a newfound common ground. The American Public Health Association, which previously had an explicitly antichiropractic policy, reversed course in the 1980s and now has a thriving Chiropractic Health Care section, which during the 2000s has presented landmark studies on the effectiveness of spinal manual therapy for low back pain, for example (Lawrence et al, 2008). The incorporation of chiropractic into the health care systems serving active duty members of the U.S. military, and military veterans through the Veterans Health Administration (VA), has provided an exceptional opportunity for interprofessional cooperation as well as a model for multidisciplinary team-based care. In 2013, the VA initiated postdoctoral residency training programs for doctors of chiropractic.

AHCPR GUIDELINES: HISTORIC BREAKTHROUGH

One of the breakthrough moments in chiropractic history was the 1994 publication of the Guidelines for Acute Lower Back Pain, developed for the Agency for Health Care Policy and Research (AHCPR) of the U.S. Department of

Health and Human Services by a blue-ribbon panel composed primarily of medical physicians and chaired by an orthopedic surgeon (2 of the 23 members were chiropractors); the Guidelines included a powerful endorsement of spinal manipulation (Bigos et al, 1994).

Based on an extensive literature review and consensus process, the AHCPR Guidelines concluded that spinal manipulation "hastens recovery" from acute low back pain (LBP) and recommended it either in combination with or as a replacement for nonsteroidal anti-inflammatory drugs (NSAIDs). At the same time, the panel rejected as unsubstantiated numerous methods (including bed rest, traction, and various other physical therapy and pharmaceutical modalities) that for many years constituted the foundation of conventional medicine's approach to acute LBP. The panel further endorsed the use of such self-care measures as exercise, ergonomic seating, and wearing low-heeled shoes. In addition, the panel cautioned against lumbar back surgery except in the most severe cases.

Perhaps most significantly, the AHCPR Guidelines stated that spinal manipulation offers both "symptomatic relief" and "functional improvement." Because none of the other recommended nonsurgical interventions offers both, one might reasonably infer that for patients with acute LBP who show none of the guideline's diagnostic "red flags" (e.g., fractures, tumors, infections, cauda equina syndrome), manipulation had become the treatment of choice.

The release of the AHCPR Guidelines was a landmark event. Since that time, standards for the treatment of LBP, the most prevalent musculoskeletal ailment in the United States and the most frequent cause of disability for persons under age 45, have assigned a pivotal role to spinal manipulation, of which over 90% is provided by chiropractors (Shekelle & Adams, 1991). This outcome provides a quintessential contemporary example of an "alternative" health care method achieving entry into the health care mainstream.

Assessment by government agencies in Canada (Manga et al, 1993), Great Britain (Rosen, 1994), Sweden (Commission on Alternative Medicine, 1987), Denmark (Danish Institute for Health Technology Assessment, 1999), Australia (Thompson, 1986), and New Zealand (Hasselberg, 1979) has brought similar approval of spinal manipulation for LBP.

Following investigations by the American College of Physicians (ACP) in Philadelphia (e.g., Micozzi, 1998), guidelines jointly issued in 2007 by the American College of Physicians (ACP) and the American Pain Society (APS) similarly recommended spinal manipulation based on its "proven benefits" for acute, subacute, and chronic LBP (Chou et al, 2007). The ACP-APS guidelines state that spinal manipulation is the only nonpharmacologic method with proven benefits for acute LBP, while also recognizing the benefits of both manipulation and other methods within the chiropractor's scope of practice for subacute and chronic LBP—intensive interdisciplinary rehabilitation, exercise therapy, acupuncture, massage therapy, and yoga. The ACP-APS low back pain guidelines have essentially replaced the AHCPR Guidelines, and are the most influential LBP guidelines worldwide.

With special funding from the U.S. Health Resources and Services Administration obtained by Sen. Tom Harkin (D-Iowa) through the Policy Institute for Integrative Medicine (Bethesda, Maryland), the Palmer College Chiropractic Research Consortium (Davenport, Iowa) of over a dozen chiropractic and medical schools also convened an expert consensus development panel to review nearly 1000 studies worldwide on the treatment of back pain and concurred with these findings, as reported to the American Public Health Association (Lawrence et al, 2008).

INTELLECTUAL FOUNDATIONS

The history of chiropractic, as with all healing arts, is largely one in which empirical process has preceded theoretical formulation. From the earliest days, practitioners have applied new treatment methods on an intuitive, empirical basis, noted that some appeared to be more effective than others, and then theorized on the basis of these clinical findings as to the underlying physiological mechanisms. The resultant body of chiropractic theory, philosophy, and practice draws from principles in the common domain shared by all natural healing arts. In addition, it contains unique chiropractic contributions to the cumulative sum and substance of health knowledge.

 Common Domain Principles

Fundamental principles of natural healing, which have been part of chiropractic from the beginning and are incorporated into the curricula at chiropractic training institutions, include the following:

1. Humans possess an innate healing potential, an "inner wisdom of the body."
2. Maximally accessing this healing system is the goal of the healing arts.
3. Addressing the cause of an illness should take precedence over suppressing its surface manifestations in most cases.
4. Pharmaceutical suppression of symptoms can sometimes compromise and diminish the body's ability to heal itself.
5. Natural, nonpharmaceutical measures (including chiropractic spinal adjustments) should generally be an approach of first resort, not last. This can be expressed concisely as "conservative care first."
6. A balanced, natural diet is crucial to good health.
7. Regular exercise is essential to proper bodily function.

These principles, endorsed and elucidated by chiropractors for more than a century, form the foundation of the emerging holistic health or wellness paradigm. ∾

 Core Chiropractic Principles

In addition to precepts shared with other natural healing arts such as acupuncture and naturopathy, core theoretical constructs that form the underpinning of chiropractic are as follows:

1. Structure and function exist in intimate relation with one another.
2. Structural distortions can cause functional abnormalities.
3. Vertebral subluxation (spinal joint dysfunction with neurologic effects) is a significant form of structural distortion and leads to a variety of functional abnormalities.
4. The nervous system occupies a central role in the restoration and maintenance of proper bodily function.
5. Subluxation influences bodily function primarily through neurologic means.
6. The chiropractic adjustment is a specific and definitive method for the reduction or correction of the vertebral subluxation. ∾

These chiropractic principles reveal something unexpected: although chiropractic is best known for its success in the relief of musculoskeletal pain, its basic axioms do not directly address the question of pain relief. Instead, they focus on the correction of structural and functional imbalances, which in some cases cause pain. This fundamental paradox—that a profession renowned for the relief of musculoskeletal pain does not define its basic purpose in those terms—has been a persistent and sometimes discordant theme in chiropractic history.

DIVERGENT INTERPRETATIONS: TRADITIONALISTS AND MODERNISTS

Historically, a dichotomy has existed within the chiropractic profession between what were once called "straights" and "mixers," although most chiropractors are part of a broad middle ground between the extremes. Central to this controversy is the degree to which chiropractic practice should focus on symptom relief. Traditionalist, "straight" chiropractors see their approach as being subluxation-based rather than symptom driven; they largely confine their role to analyzing the spine for subluxations, then manually adjusting the subluxated vertebrae. A minority within the profession, they generally reject the use of symptom-oriented ancillary therapies such as heat, electrical stimulation, and dietary supplementation. A few jurisdictions limit chiropractors to this circumscribed scope of practice.

With few dissenters, both groups agree that spinal adjusting is a paramount feature of chiropractic practice, and that advising patients on exercise, natural diet, and other aspects of evidence-based prevention (Redwood &

Globe, 2008) is appropriately within the chiropractor's scope. The chief philosophical difference between them is that whereas traditionalists seek to treat the cause and not the symptom (some even reject the term "treat" as excessively allopathic), broad-scope modernists seek to treat both the cause and the symptom. Although broad-scope chiropractors share their traditionalist colleagues' appreciation of spinal adjusting, they contend that patient care is sometimes enhanced by such adjuncts as electrical physical therapy modalities, hands-on muscle therapies, acupuncture, and nutritional regimens, including supplementation with vitamins, minerals, and herbs. Longstanding intraprofessional disagreements concerning the use of electrical therapies by chiropractors may be gradually overtaken by an emerging shift, in chiropractic and other professions that treat musculoskeletal pain, away from such passive therapies toward active care, exercise-based rehabilitation approaches.

THEORETICAL CONSTRUCTS AND PRACTICAL APPLICATIONS

BONE-OUT-OF-PLACE THEORY

Pioneer-era chiropractors, following Palmer's lead, assumed that their adjustments worked by moving misaligned vertebrae back into line, thereby relieving pressure caused by direct bony impingement on spinal nerves. The standard explanation given to patients was the analogy of stepping on a garden hose: if you step on the hose, the water cannot get through, and then if you lift your foot off the hose, the free flow of water is restored. Similarly, it was claimed that the chiropractic adjustment removes the pressure of bone on nerve, thus allowing free flow of nerve impulses.

Based on the information available at the time, such nineteenth-century concepts were considered plausible. Chiropractors were able to feel interruptions in the symmetry of the spinal column with their well-trained, experienced hands, as many times verified on x-ray examination. More often than not, when they adjusted the subluxated vertebra with manual pressure, patients reported significant functional improvements and healing effects.

Problems exist with this theory, however, as best illustrated by noting that, after an adjustment resulting in dramatic relief from headaches or sciatica, an x-ray study rarely shows any discernible change in spinal alignment. (The American Chiropractic Association Council on Diagnostic Imaging now considers such comparative x-ray films inappropriate because of the unnecessary radiation exposure.) Positive health changes have not consistently correlated with vertebral alignment and this issue has not been fully resolved. A 2007 randomized clinical trial, the first to demonstrate significant benefit from chiropractic in cases of hypertension, used a technique that places great reliance on x-ray analysis of upper cervical vertebral alignment (Bakris et al, 2007).

MOTION THEORY AND SEGMENTAL DYSFUNCTION

Alternative hypotheses have been proposed to replace the bone-out-of-place concept. Chief among these is the theory of intervertebral motion and segmental dysfunction (SDF), the dominant chiropractic model of the contemporary era. Advocated by a small minority of chiropractors for many decades, this model first achieved profession-wide attention among chiropractors in the 1980s and now has broad acceptance in chiropractic college curricula throughout the world. This theory also offers a coherent explanation of chiropractic and the vertebral subluxation complex (VSC) to be communicated in familiar terms to medical practitioners and researchers.

Motion theory contends that loss of proper spinal joint mobility, rather than positional misalignment, is the key factor in joint dysfunction. It posits that the subluxation always involves more than a single vertebra and that subluxation mechanics involve SDF, an interruption in the normal dynamic relationship between two articulating joint surfaces (Schafer & Faye, 1989).

Anatomically, the vertebral motor unit (or motion segment) consists of an anterior segment, with two vertebral bodies separated by an intervertebral disc, and a posterior segment, consisting of two adjacent articular facets, along with muscles, ligaments, blood vessels, and nerves, interfacing with one another. Restriction of joint motion, a common feature of the manipulable lesion or subluxation, is termed a fixation. Fixation-subluxations are the clinical entity most amenable to spinal manipulation.

L. John Faye, DC, a pioneer in moving the dynamic or motion model into the chiropractic mainstream, identifies a five-component model for the vertebral subluxation complex. In Faye's original formulation (Schafer & Faye, 1989), these are the neurologic, kinesiolgic, myologic, biochemical, and histologic components. Faye later amended his model to replace the final two components with inflammatory and stress components (seminar at Cleveland Chiropractic College–Kansas City, 2009).

Former college president and national spokesperson for the American Chiropractic Association, J.F. McAndrews, DC, an early advocate of motion theory and practice, described a visual model of spinal motion principles (Figure 19-4), as follows:

> View it as a mobile hanging from the ceiling, with many strings on which ornaments are suspended. As the mobile hangs there, it is in a state of dynamic equilibrium. Then, if you cut one of the strings, the whole mobile starts moving, because its balance has been upset. Eventually, it slows down and reaches a new state of dynamic equilibrium. But things have changed. It does not look the same. All those ornaments have shifted, in relation to the central axis and also in relation to each other.

The body's musculoskeletal system works in much the same way. If its normal balance is disrupted, it must compensate. Structural patterns will be altered to a greater or

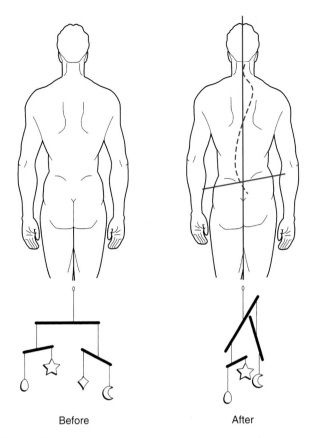

Before   **After**

Figure 19-4 Visual model of spinal motion principles comparing mobile hanging from ceiling to body's musculoskeletal system before and after imbalance is introduced.

lesser degree, depending on the nature and intensity of the forces that threw off the old pattern of balance (Chapter 16).

Leach (1994) cites a triad of signs classically accepted as evidence for the existence of SDF: (1) point tenderness or altered pain threshold to pressure in the adjacent paraspinal musculature or over the spinous process; (2) abnormal contraction or tension within the adjacent paraspinal musculature; and (3) loss of normal motion in one or more planes. Chiropractic education includes extensive training in the development of the psychomotor skills necessary to diagnose the VSC or SDF and to perform the manipulative maneuvers best suited to its correction.

Much more problematic than fixations are subluxations involving joint hypermobility, characterized by ligamentous laxity, frequently of traumatic etiology. Hypermobility may be clinically diagnosed by eliciting a repeated click when a joint is moved through its normal range of motion. Hypermobile joints should not be forcibly manipulated, because this can further increase the degree of hypermobility. However, nearby articulations that have become fixated to compensate for the hypermobile joint may require manipulation, and muscles in the area should be strengthened and toned to minimize the workload of the overstressed hypermobile joint.

The motion segment is the initial focus of chiropractic therapeutic intervention and is the site where the most direct and immediate effects of manipulation are likely to be noted. More far-reaching effects are possible, however, through neural facilitation.

SEGMENTAL FACILITATION

Segmental facilitation has been defined as a lowered threshold for firing in a spinal cord segment, caused by afferent bombardment of the dorsal horn associated with spinal lesions (Korr, 1976).

Once a segment has become facilitated, the effects can include local somatic pain or visceral organ dysfunction. Segmental facilitation is the dominant hypothesis proposed as the neurophysiological basis by which the VSC or SDF influences autonomic function.

Some models for the specific mechanisms of facilitation postulate that inflammation is a key factor (Dvorak, 1985; Gatterman & Goe, 1990; Mense, 1991), whereas others have proposed neurological models through which such facilitation could occur even in the absence of inflammation (Korr, 1975; Patterson & Steinmetz, 1986). When present, inflammation alters the local milieu of the nerve, causing chemical, thermal, and mechanical changes; inflammation surrounding a nerve is likely to compromise its function. Such aberrant nerve activity, researchers theorize, can disrupt the homeostatic mechanisms essential to normal somatic or visceral organ function.

A facilitated segment may result in either parasympathetic vagal dominance or excessive sympathetic output. As Leach (1994) concludes, "It appears that SDF is capable of initiating segmental facilitation and that certainly this is the most logical explanation for the use of [chiropractic] adjustment . . . for other than pain syndromes; certainly the segmental facilitation hypothesis is gaining greater acceptance and is based upon a large body of acceptable scientific research."

RATIONALE FOR CHIROPRACTIC ADJUSTMENT

INDICATIONS AND CONTRAINDICATIONS

The central focus of chiropractic practice is the analytical process for determining (1) when and where spinal manipulative therapy (SMT) is appropriate and (2) the type of adjustment most appropriate in a given situation.

Proposed algorithms for this process detail procedures whereby the chiropractor, after arriving at an overall diagnostic impression (not limited to the spine) and methodically ruling out pathologies that contraindicate SMT, proceeds to evaluate SDF in order to arrive at a specific chiropractic diagnosis (Leach, 1994). This diagnostic process takes into account subluxations that are present, along with other clinical entities (e.g., degeneration, disc involvement, carpal tunnel syndrome), which in certain cases require additional treatment besides SMT or affect the style of SMT that is appropriate.

For example, the presence of advanced degenerative joint disease would not render SMT inappropriate but would rule out forms of SMT that introduce substantial amounts of force into the arthritic joint. According to the Guidelines for Chiropractic Quality Assurance and Practice Parameters (Haldeman et al, 1993), the high-velocity low-amplitude (HVLA) thrust adjustment, the most common form of chiropractic SMT, is "absolutely contraindicated" in anatomical areas where the following occur:

- Malignancies
- Bone and joint infections
- Acute myelopathy or acute cauda equina syndrome
- Acute fractures and dislocations, or healed fractures and dislocations with signs of ligamentous rupture or instability
- Acute rheumatoid, rheumatoid-like, or nonspecific arthropathies, including ankylosing spondylitis characterized by episodes of acute inflammation, demineralization, and ligamentous laxity with anatomical subluxation or dislocation
- Active juvenile avascular necrosis
- Unstable os odontoideum

These guidelines also rate, in descending order of severity, conditions in the following categories: "relative to absolute contraindication," "relative contraindication," and "not a contraindication." Listing all conditions in each category is beyond the scope of this chapter. The key point is that chiropractic diagnosis is geared toward evaluating where each case falls on this spectrum, then proceeding with appropriate medical referral, chiropractic treatment, or concurrent care.

TYPES OF MANUAL INTERVENTIONS USED BY CHIROPRACTORS

The HVLA technique, also known as osseous adjustment, is performed by manually moving a joint to the end point of its normal range of motion (ROM), isolating it by local pressure on bony prominences, and then imparting a swift, specific, low-amplitude thrust. This thrust is frequently accompanied by a clicking sound indicating joint cavitation, as the joint moves into the "paraphysiological space" between normal ROM and the limits of its anatomical integrity. Properly applied, the adjustment usually involves little or no discomfort.

Other adjusting methods with wide application in the chiropractic profession include the following:

- High-velocity thrust with recoil
- Low-velocity thrust
- Flexion-distraction (originally an osteopathic technique for lumbar disc syndrome)
- Adjustment with mechanically assisted drop-piece tables
- Adjustment with compression-wave instruments
- Various specific light-touch techniques

Some of these procedures are "low-force" methods, developed to assist chiropractors in managing cases where standard HVLA adjustment is either contraindicated or judged to be undesirable by doctor or patient. A minority of chiropractors choose to use these low-force methods as the sole form of manual intervention. Nonadjustive manual measures are also employed by most chiropractors, generally to supplement rather than replace SMT, and include trigger-point therapy, joint mobilization, and massage (Figure 19-5).

CLINICAL SETTINGS AND METHODOLOGIE

MOVEMENTS TOWARD "INTEGRATION"

For most of their professional history, chiropractors have seen themselves and been seen by others as a dissenting wing of the Western healing arts. Until recently, chiropractors have practiced in almost all cases within the context of freestanding private practice. Similarly, chiropractic educational facilities have been private institutions, functioning almost entirely without public funding.

This outsider status is changing. Chiropractors now serve on the staffs of a small but growing number of hospitals and corporate health clinics. Moreover, as noted by the World Federation of Chiropractic in its 2012 report to the World Health Organization, "while most chiropractic schools in the United States are in private colleges, most of the newer schools internationally are within the national university system (e.g., Australia, Brazil, Canada, Chile, Denmark, Japan, South Korea, Malaysia, Mexico, South Africa, Spain, Switzerland, and the UK). In some of these programs, for example, at the University of Southern Denmark in Odense and the University of Zurich in Switzerland, chiropractic and medical students take the same basic science courses together for three years before entering separate programs for clinical training. . . . In 1990 there were only four recognized programs outside the USA, one each in Australia, Canada, South Africa, and the United Kingdom . . . there are now 41 programs in 16 countries. New schools are currently being planned in other countries in all world regions" (World Federation of Chiropractic, 2012).

Chiropractors have served in official capacities at the Olympic Games since 1980 and play an increasingly prominent role in the treatment of sports injuries. In 2007, Michael reed became the first chiropractor to serve as medical Director of the Performance Services Division of the United States Olympic Committee and was one of four chiropractors sent to Beijing to treat American athletes at the 2008 Olympic Games (Redwood, 2008). In 2010, for the first time, the two top medical officials of the U.S. Olympic Committee were chiropractors—Michael Reed and William Moreau, the USOC's director of clinics. Reed and Moreau rose to these positions as a result of having demonstrated world-class expertise in managing multidisciplinary sports medicine programs. In professional sports

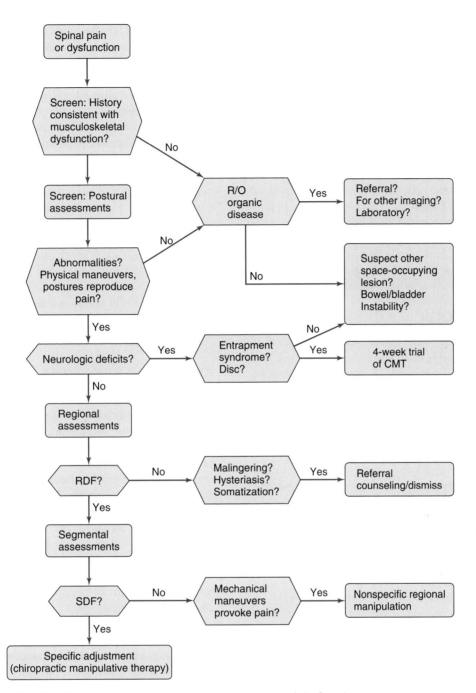

Figure 19-5 Proposed algorithm for the assessment of regional and segmental dysfunction.

at the major league level, virtually all teams now make chiropractic services available to their members.

In 1993, J.R. Cassidy became the first chiropractor to be named research director of a university hospital orthopedics department, at the University of Saskatchewan in Canada. In 1994, John Triano became the first member of the profession to join the staff of the Texas Back Institute, where he worked in the dual role of staff chiropractic physician and clinical research scientist. As noted earlier, perhaps the most promising developments in the mainstreaming of chiropractic is the recent (post-2000) inclusion of chiropractic in the health care systems serving

veterans and the active duty military personnel in the United States (Redwood & Globe, 2008).

Such developments bode well for the future but are still more the exception than the rule. Evolving outside the mainstream has been a struggle, although it has strengthened many practitioners committed to chiropractic. By far the most serious negative effect of chiropractic's peripheral status has been that the majority of patients who could benefit from chiropractic care have not received it, because referrals from allopathic physicians to chiropractors remain much rarer than referrals to other medical practitioners or physical therapists.

The most salient positive aspect of operating outside the establishment for so many years is that the creative impulses and capacities of individual chiropractors were encouraged rather than quashed. One of the greatest challenges currently facing the profession is developing uniform practice standards—the Guidelines for Chiropractic Quality Assurance and Practice Parameters (Haldeman et al, 1993) was an initial effort—while simultaneously maintaining the innovative atmosphere that has characterized the profession since its inception. Ongoing practice standards development continues under the auspices of the Council on Chiropractic Guidelines and Practice Parameters (www.ccgpp.org), formed in 1995 at the behest of the Congress of Chiropractic State Associations, with support from the American Chiropractic Association, International Chiropractors Association, Association of Chiropractic Colleges, and other organizations.

DIAGNOSTIC LOGIC

In the clinical setting, the chiropractic model demonstrates both similarities and differences compared with the standard medical approach. Foremost, chiropractors seek to evaluate individual symptoms in a broad context of health and body balance, not as isolated aberrations to be suppressed. This holistic viewpoint shares much with both ancient and emerging models elsewhere in the healing arts.

Chiropractors recognize the need for thorough evaluation of symptoms, and they are trained to take histories and perform physical examinations in a similar manner to that done at the typical medical office. However, the chiropractic paradigm does not hold the elimination of symptoms to be the sole or ultimate goal of treatment. Health is more than the absence of disease symptoms. The true goal is sustainable balance, a fact recognized by chiropractors and other holistically oriented health practitioners.

Chiropractors are trained in state-of-the-art diagnostic techniques, and chiropractic examination procedures overlap significantly with those used by orthodox medical physicians. However, chiropractors evaluate the information gleaned from these methods from a perspective that places greater emphasis on the intricate structural and functional interplay between different parts of the body.

CHIROPRACTIC AND MEDICAL APPROACHES TO PAIN

In widespread experience, conventional medical physicians engage in symptom suppression much more than chiropractors do and also more frequently assume that the site of a pain is also the site of its cause. Thus, knee pain is generally assumed to be a knee problem, shoulder pain is assumed to be a shoulder problem, and so forth. This pain-centered diagnostic logic frequently leads to increasingly sophisticated and invasive, but misdirected, diagnostic and therapeutic procedures. For example, if physical examination of the knee fails to define the problem clearly, the knee is radiographed. If the x-ray film fails to offer adequate clarification, magnetic resonance imaging (MRI) of the knee is performed, and in some cases an invasive surgical procedure follows.

As with their allopathic colleagues, chiropractors use diagnostic tools such as radiography and MRI. The point here is not to criticize these useful technologies but to present an alternative diagnostic model. Chiropractors are familiar with patients in whom this entire high-tech diagnostic scenario, as in the previous knee example, is played out, after which the knee problem is discovered to be a compensation for a mechanical disorder in the lower back, a common condition that too often remains outside the medical diagnostic loop.

If the lower back is mechanically dysfunctional and in need of spinal adjustment, this can often place unusual stress on one or both knees. In these patients, medical physicians can and often do spend months or years medicating the knee symptoms or performing surgery, never addressing the source of the problem.

REGIONAL AND WHOLE-BODY CONTEXT: NEUROLOGY AND BIOMECHANICS

The chiropractic approach to musculoskeletal pain involves evaluating the site of pain in a regional and whole-body context. Although shoulder, elbow, and wrist problems can be caused by injuries or pathologies in these areas, pain in and around each of the shoulder, elbow, and wrist joints can also have as its source segmental dysfunction in the cervical spine. Similarly, symptoms in the hip, knee, and ankle can also originate at the site of the pain, but in many cases the source lies in the lumbar spine or sacroiliac joints. Besides pain, other neurologically mediated symptoms (e.g., paresthesia) can have a similar etiology. The need to consider this chain of causation is built into the core of chiropractic training.

Chiropractors since Palmer have intentionally refrained from assuming that the site of a symptom is the site of its cause. They assume instead that the source of the pain should be sought along the path of the nerves leading to and from the site of the symptoms. Thus, pain in the knee might come from the knee itself, but tracing the nerve pathways between the knee and the spine reveals possible areas of causation in and around the hip, in the deep muscles of the buttocks or pelvis, in the sacroiliac joints, or in the lumbar spine.

Furthermore, if segmental joint dysfunction does exist, for example, at the fourth and fifth lumbar levels, it might have its primary source at L4–5, or it might represent a compensation for another subluxation elsewhere in the spine, perhaps in the lower or middle thoracic vertebrae or in a mechanical dysfunction of the muscles and joints of the feet. Such an integrative, whole-body approach to structure and function is of great value.

For patients whose presentation includes visceral organ symptoms, chiropractic diagnostic logic includes (once contraindications to manipulation have been ruled out) evaluation of the spine, with particular attention to spinal levels providing autonomic nerve supply to the involved area, as well as consideration of possible nutritional, environmental, and psychological factors.

CRITERIA FOR REFERRAL TO MEDICAL PHYSICIANS

Chiropractic practice standards mandate timely referral to an medical physician for diagnosis and treatment for conditions beyond the chiropractor's domain, or when a reasonable trial of chiropractic care (current standards in most cases limit this to about one month) fails to bring satisfactory results (Haldeman et al, 1993; Baker et al, 2012).

In addition, chiropractors frequently seek second opinions in less dramatic cases if chiropractic treatment, though helpful, fails to bring full resolution. Referrals from chiropractors to neurologists, neurosurgeons, orthopedic surgeons, internists, and other medical specialists are common. Referrals to complementary practitioners such as acupuncturists, massage therapists, and naturopaths also occur when appropriate, in areas where such practitioners are available.

ETHICS OF REFERRAL

The medical profession has long had a clearly defined set of ethics for intraprofessional referral: a report is sent to the referring physician, and the patient remains the patient of the referring physician. In the era before *Wilk v AMA*, when the medical establishment prohibited collegial relations with chiropractors, physicians receiving referrals from chiropractors frequently failed to extend such professional courtesies to them. This now occurs far more rarely. In addition, the fast-moving adoption of electronic health records (EHR) throughout the health care system in the United States and other nations facilitates proper communication, speeding the day when difficulties in accessing records will be a relic of the past.

RESEARCH

For years, chiropractors were attacked for offering only anecdotal evidence in support of their methods. Since the early 1990s, only those ignorant of the scientific literature can still make such claims. As summarized by Bronfort et al (2010) in their comprehensive UK Evidence Report, there are now over 100 randomized trials of manual manipulation, virtually all of which were conducted after the mid-1970s. A substantial majority are low back pain studies, most of which found manipulation to be more effective than the methods to which it was compared. The current literature also contains a substantial number of studies on neck pain and headaches, along with a smaller number on musculoskeletal conditions of the extremities and nonmusculoskeletal conditions.

UNIVERSITY OF COLORADO PROJECT

Contemporary chiropractic research began at the University of Colorado in the 1970s. First with grants from the International Chiropractors Association and later with added financial support from the American Chiropractic Association and the U.S. government, Chung Ha Suh and colleagues at the Biomechanics Department undertook a series of studies that provided an extensive body of chiropractic-related, basic science research.

Suh, the first American college professor willing to defy the AMA boycott to pursue chiropractic research, was a native of Korea, where he was not subjected to the same antichiropractic bias as the American health care academics of his era. In launching this research, he had to withstand intense pressure from powerful political forces within the American medical and academic establishments, which condemned chiropractic for lack of scientific underpinning while striving to prevent chiropractors from obtaining the funding and university connections necessary for the development of such a research base (*Wilk v AMA*, 1990).

The University of Colorado team pursued research in two major areas. First, Suh (1974) developed a computer model of the cervical spine that allowed a deeper understanding of spinal joint mechanics and their relationship to the chiropractic adjustment. The second area involved a range of studies on nerve compression and various aspects of neuron function (Kelly & Luttges, 1975; Luttges et al, 1976; MacGregor & Oliver, 1973; MacGregor et al, 1975; Sharpless, 1975; Simske & Schmeister, 1994; Triano & Luttges, 1982). Sharpless, for example, demonstrated that minuscule amounts of pressure (10 mm Hg) on a nerve root resulted in up to a 50% decrease in electrical transmission down the course of the nerve supplied by that root.

LOW BACK PAIN

A substantial body of research has addressed the effectiveness of SMT in the treatment of LBP. As referenced earlier, consensus panels evaluating the data have consistently placed spinal manipulation on the short list of recommended procedures for LBP.

The use of spinal manipulation as a treatment for acute, subacute, and chronic low back pain received the rating "A: Supported by good evidence from relevant studies" from the Council on Chiropractic Guidelines and Practice Parameters" (Lawrence et al, 2008; Globe et al, 2008). Moreover, current joint guidelines from the ACP and the APS, noted earlier, endorsed manipulation for both chronic and acute low back pain (Chou et al, 2007).

Evidence for Manual Methods: A Basis for Referral to Chiropractors

Because a primary care physician's decision about whether and where to refer LBP patients hinges on which treatments are expected to yield the most satisfactory outcomes, a summary of studies on spinal manipulation for LBP may aid the decision-making process.

In an influential trial with more than 700 patients, British orthopedic surgeon T.W. Meade compared chiropractic manipulation with standard hospital outpatient treatment for LBP, which consisted of physical therapy and wearing a corset (Meade et al, 1990, 1995). He concluded, "For patients with low back pain in whom manipulation is not contraindicated, chiropractic almost certainly confers worthwhile, long-term benefit in comparison to hospital outpatient management." He described the applicability of these findings for primary care physicians as follows:

> Our trial showed that chiropractic is a very effective treatment, more effective than conventional hospital outpatient treatment for low back pain, particularly in patients who had back pain in the past and who [developed] severe problems. So, in other words, it is most effective in precisely the group of patients that you would like to be able to treat. One of the unexpected findings was that the treatment difference—the benefit of chiropractic over hospital treatment—actually persists for the whole of that three-year period [of the study] . . . the treatment that the chiropractors gives does something that results in a very long-term benefit. (Meade, 1992)

Meade's study was the first large randomized clinical trial to demonstrate substantial short- and long-term benefits from chiropractic care. Because it dealt with both acute LBP patients and chronic LBP patients, Meade's data support the use of SMT for both populations.

Besides Meade et al (1990, 1995), an impressive prospective study of LBP was performed at the University of Saskatchewan Hospital orthopedics department by Kirkaldy-Willis, a world-renowned orthopedic surgeon, and Cassidy, the chiropractor who later became the department's research director (Kirkaldy-Willis & Cassidy, 1985). The approximately 300 subjects in this study were "totally disabled" by LBP, with pain present for an average of 7 years. All had gone through extensive, unsuccessful medical treatment before participating as research subjects. After 2 to 3 weeks of daily chiropractic adjustments, more than 80% of the patients without spinal stenosis had good to excellent results, reporting substantially decreased pain and increased mobility. After chiropractic treatment, more than 70% were improved to the point of having no work restrictions. Follow-up a year later demonstrated that the changes were long-lasting. Even those with a narrowed spinal canal, a particularly difficult subset, showed a notable response. More than half of the patients improved, and about one in five was pain free and on the job 7 months after treatment.

In a randomized trial of 209 patients, Triano et al (1995) compared SMT to education programs for chronic LBP, which they defined as pain lasting 7 weeks or longer, or more than six episodes in 12 months. These investigators found greater improvement in pain and activity tolerance in the SMT group, noting that "immediate benefit from pain relief continued to accrue after manipulation, even for the last encounter at the end of the 2-week treatment interval." They concluded, "There appears to be

clinical value to treatment according to a defined plan using manipulation even in low back pain exceeding 7 weeks duration."

The UK Back Pain Exercise and Manipulation study (UK BEAM, 2004a, 2004b) was a large randomized trial, with over 1300 patients. As noted earlier, a previous study by orthopedic surgeon Thomas Meade and colleagues, also published in *British Medical Journal* (Meade et al, 1990, 1995), had a dramatic impact in the United Kingdom and beyond, because it showed that chiropractic care brought better outcomes for low back pain patients than standard medical care.

However, one key criticism of Meade's landmark study was that the medical care group was treated within National Health Service facilities while the chiropractic group was treated in private practice settings. To the consternation of many chiropractors and other manual manipulation practitioners, concern was quite vocal from certain conventional medicine advocates that this may have compromised Meade's findings, by creating higher expectations of success among the patients randomized to chiropractic care in his study. The UK BEAM study was partly aimed at answering the questions raised by those skeptical of Meade's positive evaluation of chiropractic care.

UK BEAM brought a remarkable and unprecedented collaboration among chiropractors, physical therapists and osteopaths (the scope of osteopathic practice in the United Kingdom is closer to that of chiropractors in the United States than to osteopaths in the United States). In the UK, spinal manipulation is within the scope of practice of these three disciplines.

The investigators set out to replicate some of the other essentials of Meade's research approach by pragmatically comparing manual therapy and other treatment approaches. To address the concern raised by Meade's critics, they arranged for some spinal manipulation patients to receive care in private practices while others were treated in National Health Service settings, and divided the medical care group similarly.

The UK BEAM treatment package (Brealey et al, 2003) agreed to by representatives of the professional associations representing chiropractors, osteopaths, and physiotherapists took as its foundation the evidence-based recommendation that patients should have early access to physical treatments and should return to normal activities as soon as possible. The interdisciplinary planning group also strongly recommended that the spinal manipulation arm of the trial should *not* involve the use of manipulation in isolation, but should include "care that reflected the holistic nature of their approaches." Moreover, they urged that practitioners be permitted to exclude from manipulative treatment patients found at their assessment to be unsuitable candidates for manipulation.

The patients were randomized into one of the following groups: (1) exercise classes; (2) spinal manipulation; or (3) spinal manipulation followed by exercises. The manipulation group was divided in two, with care delivered either at a private practice or an NHS facility. Members of all groups also received "usual care" from a medical physician, based on UK national guidelines and consisting of advice to continue normal activities and avoid bed rest, along with provision of *The Back Book*.

Both manipulation (delivered by chiropractors, osteopaths and physiotherapists) and manipulation plus exercise produced statistically significant gains at 3 and 12 months. The exercise-only group had statistically significant improvements at 3 months but not at 12 months. Also, for those who had already received manipulation for 6 weeks, the addition of exercise starting at that point appeared to help less than for those who had not previously had manipulation. Importantly, in terms of defusing the objections to Meade's earlier study, there were no significant differences between manipulation delivered in NHS or private locations.

As a follow-up to UK BEAM, a smaller study by Wilkey et al (2008) featured a head-to-head comparison of chiropractic care (pragmatically defined to allow all procedures the participating chiropractors would normally employ) versus medical care in the British National Health Service Hospital's pain clinic (defined in similar pragmatic terms). The chiropractic and pain clinic groups started at baseline with similar levels of pain, though the chiropractic group was on average a decade older than the pain clinic group and chiropractic subjects had endured their pain for a mean of 3 years longer (7.34 vs. 4.04 years) than the pain clinic group.

Nevertheless, improvement in pain intensity at week 8 was 1.8 points greater (on a 0 to 10 scale) for the chiropractic group than for the pain clinic group, a dramatic difference. Disability scores (which measure the impact of pain on daily activities) measured with the Roland Morris Disability Questionnaire also demonstrated a far larger benefit from chiropractic care, with a greater than fivefold difference in the degree of improvement. These data measured effects through the end of the 8-week treatment period. Shortly after publication of Wilkey et al's study, the British National Health Service began to cover spinal manipulation for low back pain.

In the first randomized controlled trial of chiropractic care for older adults, and one of the first to compare different methods of chiropractic adjustment to each other and to conservative medical care, Hondras et al (2009) evaluated the effects of these three approaches for 240 people with subacute and chronic low back pain. High-velocity and low-velocity chiropractic techniques (combined with standardized exercise recommendations) resulted in similar levels of improvement, with both chiropractic methods substantially outperforming the medical care group, who received the same exercise instructions along with pain medication.

A multidisciplinary team at the National Spine Center in Canada (Bishop et al, 2010) compared guidelines-based care (including chiropractic spinal manipulation) vs. usual care by family practice medical physicians for acute low back pain, defined as 16 weeks or less in duration. They found that guidelines-based care was far more effective and also found, alarmingly, that typical medical care was poorly adherent to guidelines, with 78% of medical patients receiving prescriptions for narcotics (e.g.,Tylenol 3 with Codeine), which are not guideline endorsed. This result so alarmed the editors of *Spine Journal* that they included a "grey box" "Evidence and Methods" commentary with Bishop et al's article, imploring medical physicians to adhere more closely to evidence-based guidelines, with regard to their excessive prescription of opioids and passive modalities, as well as their reluctance to recommend spinal manipulation and exercise.

Preventing Acute Cases from Becoming Chronic

Because the prognosis for patients with acute LBP is better than for those with chronic pain, high priority must be accorded to preventing acute cases from becoming chronic. However, a key factor leads physicians to minimize this concern: conventional wisdom that 90% of LBP resolves on its own within a short time. Findings published in a landmark *British Medical Journal* study (Croft et al, 1998) called for urgent reassessment of the assumption that most LBP patients seen by primary care physicians attain resolution of their complaints. Contrary to prevailing assumptions, Croft and colleagues found that at 3-month and 12-month follow-up, only 21% and 25%, respectively, had completely recovered in terms of pain and disability. However, only 8% continued to consult their physician for longer than 3 months. In other words, the oft-quoted 90% figure actually applied to the number of patients who stopped seeing their physicians, not the number who recovered from their back pain. Their dissatisfaction with conventional medical care was also reminiscent of Cherkin's earlier work (Cherkin & MacCornack, 1989; Cherkin et al, 1991). Croft et al (1998) stated the following:

> We should stop characterizing low back pain in terms of a multiplicity of acute problems, most of which get better, and a small number of chronic long-term problems. Low back pain should be viewed as a chronic problem with an untidy pattern of grumbling symptoms and periods of relative freedom from pain and disability interspersed with acute episodes, exacerbations and recurrences. This takes account of two consistent observations about low back pain: firstly, a previous episode of low back pain is the strongest risk factor for a new episode, and, secondly, by the age of 30 years almost half the population will have experienced a substantial episode of low back pain. These figures simply do not fit with claims that 90 percent of episodes of low back pain end in complete recovery.

The patients in Croft's study were not referred for manual manipulation, and most developed chronic LBP. Based on the AHCPR Guidelines, which emphasize the functionally restorative qualities of SMT, it seems reasonable to expect that early chiropractic adjustments could have prevented this progression in many patients. Recall that follow-up in both the Meade (1 year and 3 years) and the Kirkaldy-Willis (1 year) studies showed that the beneficial effect of manipulation was sustained for extended periods (Kirkaldy-Willis & Cassidy, 1985; Meade et al, 1990, 1995). The decision not to refer patients to chiropractors may mean that many LBP patients will develop long-standing problems that could have been avoided.

Benefits of SMT for Low Back Pain Patients with Leg Pain

Differential diagnosis is crucial for cases in which LBP radiates into the leg. Specifically, motor, sensory, and reflex testing should be used to screen for signs of radiculopathy and cauda equina syndrome. Such factors play a central role in determining which patients should be referred directly for surgical consultation and which should be referred for manual manipulation.

A growing body of evidence indicates that in even in cases in which radicular signs such as muscle weakness or decreased reflex response are present, chiropractic can yield beneficial results. In a series of 424 consecutive cases, Cox and Feller (1994) reported that 83% of 331 lumbar disc syndrome patients completing care (13% of whom had previous low back surgeries) had good to excellent results. ("Excellent" was defined as >90% relief of pain and return to work with no further care required, and "good" as 75% relief of pain, return to work with periodic manipulation or analgesia required.) There was a median of 11 treatments and 27 days to attain maximal improvement.

BenEliyahu (1996) followed 27 patients receiving chiropractic care for cervical and lumbar disc herniations, the majority being lumbar cases. Pretreatment and posttreatment MRI studies were performed: 80% of the patients had a good clinical outcome, and 63% of the posttreatment MRI studies showed herniations either reduced in size or completely resorbed.

In a study of 14 patients with lumbar disc herniation, Cassidy et al (1993) reported that all but one obtained significant clinical improvement and relief of pain after a 2- to 3-week regimen of daily side-posture manipulation of the lumbar spine, directed toward improving spinal mobility. All received computed tomography (CT) scans before and 3 months after treatment. In most patients the CT appearance of the disc herniation remained unchanged after successful treatment, although five showed a small decrease in the size of the herniation, and one patient showed a large decrease.

Santilli et al (2006) assessed the short- and long-term effects of spinal manipulation and simulated manipulation on acute back pain and sciatica with disc protrusion, in a randomized trial with 102 ambulatory patients with acute lumbar disc syndrome verified with clinical findings and MRI. Treatments were given 5 days per week by experienced chiropractors using a rapid thrust technique. The number of treatment sessions depended on the level of pain relief achieved, up to a maximum of 20 sessions. Manipulations appeared more effective on the basis of the percentage of pain-free cases (local pain, 28% vs. 6%; radiating pain, 55% vs. 20%).

McMorland et al (2010) compared the spinal manipulation vs. microdiskectomy in patients with sciatica secondary to lumbar disc herniation (LDH) in 40 patients who met participating neurosurgeons' inclusion criteria for surgery (having failed at least 3 months of nonoperative management including treatment with analgesics, lifestyle modification, physiotherapy, massage therapy, and/or acupuncture). Patients were randomized to either surgical microdiskectomy or standardized chiropractic spinal manipulation. Crossover to the alternate treatment was allowed after 3 months. Sixty percent of patients with sciatica who had failed other medical management benefited from spinal manipulation to the same degree as those who underwent surgical intervention. Of the other 40%, subsequent surgical intervention conferred an excellent outcome, countering the hypothesis that a course of manipulation may be harmful by causing a delay in surgery. The authors (a chiropractor and three neurosurgeons) concluded that patients with symptomatic LDH failing medical management should consider spinal manipulation followed by surgery if warranted.

Evidence of this kind, combined with its own cost-benefit analyses, led the University of Pittsburgh Medical Center to institute a policy under which patients with chronic low back pain must be treated with a 3-month course of care including both chiropractic and physical therapy, before any spine surgery is approved (Redwood, 2013).

Maintenance Spinal Manipulation

Senna and Machaly (2011) performed a prospective single-blinded randomized trial to assess the effectiveness of SMT for the management of chronic nonspecific LBP and to determine the effectiveness of maintenance SMT in long-term reduction of pain and disability levels associated with chronic low back conditions after an initial phase of treatments. Sixty patients with chronic, nonspecific LBP lasting at least 6 months were randomized to receive either: (1) 12 treatments of sham SMT over a 1-month period; (2) 12 treatments, consisting of SMT over a 1-month period, but no treatments for the subsequent 9 months; or (3) 12 treatments over a 1-month period, along with "maintenance spinal manipulation" every 2 weeks for the following 9 months. Patients in second and third groups experienced significantly lower pain and disability scores than first group at the end of 1 month. Only the third group that received maintenance manipulation during the follow-up period showed more improvement in pain and disability scores at the 10-month evaluation. In the nonmaintained SMT group, however, the mean pain and disability scores returned to levels close to their pretreatment levels.

Cifuentes and his team at the Center for Disability Research at the Liberty Mutual Research Institute for Safety explored the effectiveness of various approaches—from medicine, physical therapy, and chiropractic—for the prevention of injury recurrence when "health maintenance care" is provided to workers who have returned to their jobs after a work-related low back injury (Cifuentes et al, 2011). The authors define health maintenance care as "a clinical intervention approach thought to prevent recurrent episodes of LBP . . . it blends the public health concepts of secondary prevention (treatment and prevention of recurrences) with tertiary prevention (obtaining the best health condition while having an incurable disease). Health maintenance care can include providing advice, information, counseling and specific physical procedures. Health maintenance care is predominantly and explicitly recommended by DCs, although some physical therapists also advocate health maintenance procedures to prevent recurrences."

After controlling for demographics and severity, patients treated by DCs were significantly less likely to have a disabling recurrence than those treated by medical doctors or physical therapists. Because chiropractic care fared best, its hazard ratio (HR) was used as the reference point (1.0). In comparison, the HR was 1.6 for MDs and 2.0 for physiotherapists. However, the HR for those not receiving any health maintenance care after they returned to work was 1.2, which was described as similar to the HR for chiropractic in terms of statistical significance.

Cost Effectiveness of Spinal Manipulation for Low Back Pain

A retrospective claims analysis of 85,000 low back pain patients insured by Tennessee Blue Cross/Blue Shield found that those initiating care with chiropractors had 40% lower treatment costs for low back pain episodes than those initiating care with medical physicians. When severity was factored in, those who initiated care with chiropractors had 20% lower costs (Liliedahl et al, 2010).

A systematic review of guideline-endorsed treatments for low back pain found that spinal manipulation was cost effective for patients with subacute or chronic LBP but that there was insufficient evidence for the cost effectiveness of spinal manipulation for acute LBP (Lin et al, 2011). In contrast, the epidemiologist authors of this study reported that they could find "no evidence" on cost effectiveness of medications for low back pain.

A systematic review found spinal manipulation was cost effective for neck and back pain, used either alone or combined with other therapies (Michaleff et al, 2012).

A prospective cohort study of Washington state workers found that 1.5% of workers who saw a chiropractor first for work-related back pain review later had surgery, compared to 42.7% of those who first saw a surgeon. This was for cases equivalent in severity (Keeney et al, 2013).

NECK PAIN

Neck pain is the second most common reason patients seek chiropractic care. Although chiropractic care can be helpful to individuals with acute or chronic neck pain, at this time the research from randomized trials on spinal manipulation is equivocal, which is unfortunately true for all other neck pain treatments as well. In stark contrast to the strong evidence on low back pain, neck pain is a disorder for which no single method can be said to have strong research support at this time.

World Health Organization Bone and Joint Decade Report (2008)

By far the most comprehensive recent evaluation of all neck pain therapies was that performed by the Bone and Joint Decade 2000-2010 Task Force on Neck Pain and Its Associated Disorders (Haldeman et al, 2008; Hurwitz et al, 2008). The panel concluded, "Our best evidence synthesis suggests that therapies involving manual therapy and exercise are more effective than alternative strategies for patients with neck pain; this was also true of therapies which include educational interventions addressing self-efficacy." Because chiropractors consistently include exercise advice and share relevant self-care educational materials with patients as part of overall care (Jamison, 2002), chiropractic management of neck pain substantially embodies the full range of noninvasive therapeutic approaches recommended by the Bone and Joint Decade Task Force.

Neck Pain Research: Key Studies

A team of Dutch researchers led by Koes et al (1993) studied patients with persistent back and neck complaints. In a randomized trial, they were treated with either manual therapy (spinal manipulation and mobilization), physiotherapy (exercises, massage, electrotherapy, ultrasound, shortwave diathermy), treatment by the general practitioner (analgesics, posture advice, home exercise, and bed rest), or a placebo treatment consisting of detuned shortwave diathermy and detuned ultrasound. For neck and back complaints together, improvements in severity of the main complaint were larger with manipulative therapy than physiotherapy; for neck complaints only, the mean improvement in the main complaint as shown by the visual analog scale was slightly better for manipulative rather than physical therapy. Both manual therapy and physiotherapy (both of which are part of the chiropractor's scope of practice) were superior to medical care and placebo. In this study, the placebo yielded results superior to medical care.

In a randomized clinical trial, Palmgren et al (2006) found that a group of chronic neck pain patients who received 15 to 25 chiropractic treatments over a 5-week period had significantly lower pain scores and greater head repositioning accuracy than another group with the same condition given a similar examination but no treatment. Chiropractic care included high- and low-velocity techniques, myofascial release, and spine-stabilizing exercises. The researchers concluded that chiropractic care could be effective in reducing pain originating in the cervical spine—as well as enhancing proprioceptive sensibility (movement and position sense).

Bronfort et al (2012), at Northwestern University of Health Sciences (NWUHS), hypothesized that "SMT is more effective than medication or home exercise with advice (HEA) for acute and subacute neck pain." In a randomized trial, they did find that neck pain patients receiving spinal manipulation achieved significantly more pain relief than those receiving medication. However, they also found that a group that received a few instructional sessions of home exercise advice achieved results that were, for all practical purposes, equal to the manipulation group.

Regarding adverse side effects, Bronfort's group reported that although "the frequency of reported side effects was similar among the three groups (41% to 58%), the nature of the side effects differed, with participants in the SMT and HEA groups reporting predominantly musculoskeletal events and those in the medication group reporting side effects that were more systemic in nature. Of note, participants in the medication group reported higher levels of medication use after the intervention." Also worth noting is that the medication group reported the most side effects and the manipulation group reported the least.

A second neck pain study from a team at NWUHS (Evans et al, 2012) looked at chronic neck pain, in contrast to the Bronfort et al study that focused on acute and subacute neck pain. The chronic neck pain project compared two different exercise regimens: "high-dose" supervised exercise and "low-dose" home exercise. In addition, they divided the high-dose exercise group in half, with one subgroup also receiving chiropractic spinal manipulation while the other was treated solely with intensive exercise. Unlike the Bronfort et al trial, there was no additional group randomized to receive medication as a primary treatment.

In the Evans et al trial, all groups showed improvement, with the two supervised strengthening groups improving significantly more than the home exercise group. However, "no significant differences were found between supervised exercise with or without spinal manipulation, suggesting that spinal manipulation confers little additional benefit." The authors appropriately note that this finding "differs from the conclusion of the Task Force on Neck Pain and Its Associated Disorders and systematic reviews (Kay et al, 2005; Gross et al, 2007), which found an advantage for exercise combined with manual therapy for chronic neck pain." They added, "Importantly, our study was not designed to assess the effect of spinal manipulation alone. A recent Cochrane systematic review has found limited evidence to support spinal manipulation alone for the short-term relief of chronic neck pain."

HEADACHES

In a practice guideline for chiropractic care of adults with headaches, Bryans et al (2011) provide a systematic review of the relevant literature. Based on the 21 articles that met their inclusion criteria, they found that spinal manipulation and multimodal multidisciplinary interventions including massage are recommended for management of patients with episodic or chronic migraine. They reported that the literature does not support spinal manipulation for the management of episodic tension-type headache and that a recommendation cannot be made for or against the use of spinal manipulation for patients with chronic tension-type headache. Instead, they found that low-load craniocervical mobilization may be beneficial for longer term management of patients with episodic or chronic tension-type headaches. For cervicogenic headache, spinal manipulation is recommended, and joint mobilization or deep neck flexor exercises may improve symptoms.

Overall, Bryans and colleagues concluded that "evidence suggests that chiropractic care, including spinal manipulation, improves migraine and cervicogenic headaches. The type, frequency, dosage, and duration of treatment(s) should be based on guideline recommendations, clinical experience, and findings. Evidence for the use of spinal manipulation as an isolated intervention for patients with tension-type headache remains equivocal."

Probably the most noteworthy chiropractic research on headaches to emerge from the United States is the work on headaches conducted by Boline et al (1995), in which chiropractic was shown to be more effective than the tricyclic antidepressant amitriptyline for long-term relief of headache pain.

During the treatment phase of the trial, pain relief among those treated with medication was comparable to the SMT group. Revealingly, however, the chiropractic patients maintained their levels of improvement after treatment was discontinued, whereas those taking medication returned to pretreatment status an average of 4 weeks after its discontinuation. This strongly implies that although medication suppressed the symptoms, chiropractic addressed the problem at a more causal level.

A subsequent trial by this group of investigators employing a similar protocol for patients with migraine headaches demonstrated that migraines were similarly responsive to chiropractic, and that adding amitriptyline to chiropractic treatment conferred no additional benefit (Nelson et al, 1998).

EXTREMITY CONDITIONS

Chiropractors' focus on the spine is enhanced through attention to the role of the extremities (arms and legs). Since the earliest days of the profession, doctors of chiropractic have adjusted extremity joints. In some cases, this is to address local problems at, for example, the ankle, knee, or shoulder, and in other cases to influence the overall balance of the body, including the spine. Causation runs in both directions—spinal adjustments can influence the extremities, and extremity manipulation can influence the spine.

Two comprehensive reviews have evaluated the status of extremity manipulation research, which is currently much less extensive than research on manipulation of the spine.

Brantingham et al (2009), part of an expert panel appointed by the Scientific Commission of the Council on Chiropractic Guidelines and Practice Parameters, reviewed all available research on lower extremity conditions and found fair evidence for manipulative therapy of the knee and/or full kinetic chain, and of the ankle and/or foot, combined with multimodal or exercise therapy for knee osteoarthritis, patellofemoral pain syndrome, and ankle inversion sprain. They found limited evidence for manipulative therapy of the ankle and/or foot combined with multimodal or exercise therapy for foot conditions such as plantar fasciitis, metatarsalgia, and hallux limitus/rigidus.

Bronfort et al (2010), in their comprehensive UK Evidence Report, included a review of research on manual therapies for upper and lower extremity problems. For lower extremity conditions, they reached conclusions quite similar to the Brantingham review. For upper extremity conditions (which were not included in the Brantingham review), Bronfort's group found moderate evidence supporting the addition of manipulation or joint mobilization to usual medical care for shoulder girdle pain; inconclusive evidence in a favorable direction on manipulation/ mobilization for rotator cuff pain; moderate evidence that long-term benefits from elbow mobilization with exercise exceed those from corticosteroid injections; and inconclusive evidence in a favorable direction for manipulation and mobilization in the treatment of carpal tunnel syndrome.

Specific trials on manual methods for extremity (arm and leg) conditions are as follows.

Shoulder

In a study from the Netherlands published in *British Medical Journal*, Winters et al (1997) found that for "shoulder girdle" pain, manipulation was superior to physical therapy, whereas for "synovial" pain at the shoulder's ball-and-socket joint, corticosteroid injections were the most effective approach. Another Dutch study by Bergman et al (2004) found that adding manipulative therapy to usual medical care yielded superior outcomes in patients with shoulder dysfunction and pain. And in a study from the United States published in *Journal of the American Chiropractic Association*, Munday and colleagues conducted a randomized, single-blinded, placebo-controlled clinical trial on shoulder impingement syndrome, in which one group received shoulder adjustments and the other a placebo (detuned ultrasound). Participants were treated 8 times over 3 weeks, resulting in a significant pain reduction for the group receiving chiropractic care (Munday et al, 2007).

Hip

The one major study on hip manipulation was conducted by Hoeksma and colleagues, who compared hip manipulation and mobilization to an exercise program. Patients were treated once a week for 9 weeks. Success rates (perceived improvement) after 5 weeks were 81% in the manual therapy group and 50% in the exercise group. Patients in the manual therapy group had significantly better outcomes on pain, stiffness, hip function, and ROM. Effects of manual therapy on the improvement of pain, hip function, and ROM endured after 29 weeks (Hoeksma et al, 2004).

Knee

At a military medical center in Texas, Deyle and colleagues compared a program of manual therapy (applied to the knee as well as to the lumbar spine, hip, and ankle as required), plus standardized knee exercises to a placebo involving subtherapeutic ultrasound applied to the knee. Clinically and statistically significant improvements in 6-minute walk distance and WOMAC score (for osteoarthritis symptoms) at 4 and 8 weeks were seen in the treatment group but not the placebo group. By 8 weeks, average 6-minute walk distances had improved by 13.1%, and WOMAC scores had improved by 55.8%. At 1 year, patients in the treatment group had clinically and statistically significant gains over baseline WOMAC scores and walking distance; 20% of patients in the placebo group and 5% of patients in the treatment group had undergone knee surgery. The researchers concluded that "a combination of manual physical therapy and supervised exercise yields functional benefits for patients with osteoarthritis of the knee and may delay or prevent the need for surgical intervention" (Deyle et al, 2000).

Deyle and colleagues' large study on knee osteoarthritis compared a home-based physical therapy regimen with a clinic-based program that included both supervised exercise and manual therapy (Deyle et al, 2005). These investigators concluded that a home exercise program was effective for patients with osteoarthritis of the knee and that clinical visits with manual therapy and supervised exercise increased the benefit.

Ankle

Pellow and Brantingham (2001) performed the first chiropractic trial on ankle inversion sprains, comparing results of an ankle mortise separation adjustment to a placebo intervention of detuned ultrasound. Patients received eight treatment sessions over 4 weeks. The researchers found that "although both groups showed improvement, statistically significant differences in favor of the adjustment group were noted with respect to reduction in pain, increased ankle ROM, and ankle function."

Standard treatment for ankle sprains is based on the RICE (rest, ice, compression and elevation) protocol. Green et al (2001) found that adding mobilization to RICE was more effective than RICE alone for decreasing pain and increasing ankle mobility. Patients were treated every second day for 2 weeks or until discharge criteria were met. The experimental group had greater improvement in range of movement before and after each of the first three treatment sessions. The experimental group also had greater increases in stride speed during the first and third treatment sessions.

SOMATOVISCERAL DISORDERS

Although the bulk of chiropractic research still focuses on musculoskeletal disorders, some investigators have studied the effects of SMT for somatovisceral disorders. There is currently no visceral disorder for which more than one randomized trial has shown a benefit from spinal manipulation. A systematic review by Hawk et al (2007) summarizes the literature on chiropractic treatment of nonmusculoskeletal disorders, applying both conventional methods of analysis and a whole systems perspective.

Infantile Colic

A randomized trial by chiropractic and medical investigators at University of Southern Denmark showed chiropractic spinal manipulation to be more effective for treating infantile colic than dimethicone, an antifoaming agent for the gastrointestinal (GI) tract (Wiberg et al, 1999). An estimated 22.5% of newborns suffer from colic, a condition marked by prolonged, intense, high-pitched crying. Numerous studies have explored a possible GI etiology, but the cause of colic has long remained a mystery.

The mean daily hours of colic in the chiropractic group were reduced by 66% on day 12, which is virtually identical to the 67% reduction in a previous prospective trial. In contrast, the dimethicone group showed a 38% reduction.

The Danish study on infantile colic is the first randomized controlled trial to demonstrate effectiveness of chiropractic manipulation for a disorder generally considered nonmusculoskeletal. Addressing this issue, the authors conclude that their data lead to two possible interpretations: "Either spinal manipulation is effective in the treatment of the visceral disorder infantile colic or infantile colic is, in fact, a musculoskeletal disorder" (Wiberg et al, 1999).

A contrasting view is provided by a study performed under the auspices of a university pediatrics department in Norway (Olafsdottir et al, 2001). In this study, 86 infants were randomly assigned to chiropractic care or placebo (held for 10 minutes by nurse, rather than given 10-minute visit with chiropractor). In the chiropractic group, adjustments were administered by light fingertip pressure. Both groups experienced substantial decreases in crying, the primary outcome measure; 70% of the chiropractic group improved versus 60% of those held by nurses. However, no statistically significant differences were found between the two groups in terms of the number of hours of crying, or as measured on a five-point improvement scale (from "getting worse" to "completely well"). The researchers concluded that "chiropractic spinal manipulation is no more effective than placebo in the treatment of infantile colic." This conclusion raises a significant methodological issue regarding the role of control or placebo interventions in chiropractic and other nonpharmacologic research, described later in this chapter.

Hypertension

In a recent example of medical-chiropractic collaboration, Marshall Dickholtz, a Chicago chiropractor, and George Bakris, a medical hypertension specialist at the University of Chicago and director of the Rush University Hypertension Center, published a study in which upper cervical chiropractic adjustments led to sustained improvement in chronic hypertension patients, "similar to that seen by giving two different anti-hypertensive agents simultaneously" (Bakris et al, 2007). The subjects in the chiropractic treatment group showed an average drop of 17 mm Hg in systolic and 8 mm Hg in diastolic blood pressure. Of particular note was the fact that all subjects were taken off their hypertension medications prior to the study, and 85% of the patients in the chiropractic treatment group required only one adjustment to yield these benefits through the full 8 weeks of the study.

Other Visceral Disorders

A pilot study by Fallon, a New York pediatric chiropractor, evaluating chiropractic treatment for children with *otitis media* demonstrated improved outcomes compared to the natural course of the illness. Using both parental reports and tympanography with a cohort of more than 400 patients, data suggest a positive role for spinal and cranial manipulation in the management of this challenging condition (Fallon, 1997; Fallon & Edelman, 1998).

Two small controlled clinical trials evaluating the effects of chiropractic manipulation for *primary dysmenorrhea* showed encouraging results, with both pain relief and changes in certain prostaglandin levels noted (Kokjohn et al, 1992; Thomasen et al, 1979). However, a much larger randomized trial concluded that there was no significant benefit from manipulation (Hondras et al, 1999). The validity of this larger trial's comparison group intervention has been criticized (Hawk et al, 2007) on methodologic grounds.

METHODOLOGICAL CHALLENGES IN CHIROPRACTIC RESEARCH

Two challenging methodologic issues in chiropractic research are:

1. What constitutes a genuine control or placebo intervention?
2. How can practitioners properly interpret data collected in trials that compare active and control treatments?

These questions apply not only to chiropractic, but also to a broad range of procedures, particularly nonpharmaceutical modalities such as massage, acupuncture, physical therapy, and surgery. Depending on how one defines the placebo, the same set of research data can be interpreted as supporting or refuting the value of the therapeutic method under study (Redwood, 1999).

WHAT CONSTITUTES AN APPROPRIATE PLACEBO?

Two widely publicized studies illustrate the potential difficulties of defining the placebo or control too broadly. In their research on children with mild to moderate asthma, Balon et al (1998) randomly assigned individuals to either active manipulation or simulated manipulation groups. Both groups experienced substantial improvement in symptoms and quality of life, reduction in the use of beta-agonist medication, and statistically insignificant increases in peak expiratory flow. Because these two groups did not differ significantly in regard to these improvements, however, the researchers concluded that "chiropractic spinal manipulation provided no benefit."

If the simulated manipulation had no therapeutic effect, this is a reasonable conclusion, but a closer reading of the article's text reveals the following:

> For simulated treatment, the subject lay prone while soft tissue massage and gentle palpation were applied to the spine, paraspinal muscles and shoulders. A distraction maneuver was performed by turning the patient's head from one side to the other while alternately palpating the ankles and feet. The subject was positioned on one side, a nondirectional push, or impulse, was applied to the gluteal region, and the procedure was repeated with the patient positioned on the other side; then the subject was placed in the prone position, and a similar procedure was applied bilaterally to the scapulae. The subject was then placed supine, with the head rotated slightly to each side, and an impulse applied to the external occipital protuberance. Low-amplitude, low-velocity impulses were applied in all these nontherapeutic contacts, with adequate joint slack so that no joint opening or cavitation occurred. Hence, the comparison of treatments was between active spinal manipulation as routinely applied by chiropractors and hands-on procedures without adjustments or manipulation. (Balon et al, 1998)

The validity of this study's conclusion hinges entirely on the assumption that these procedures are therapeutically inert. The following questions may be helpful in evaluating this claim:

1. Would massage therapists view these hands-on procedures as "nontherapeutic"?
2. Would acupuncturists or practitioners of Shiatsu concur that direct manual pressure on multiple areas rich in acupuncture points is so inconsequential as to allow its use as a "placebo"?
3. Perhaps most significantly for this study on chiropractic, would the average chiropractor agree that these pressures, impulses, and stretches are an appropriate placebo, particularly in light of the fact that they overlap with certain "low-force" chiropractic adjustments and mobilization procedures?

The authors of the study address these concerns as follows: "We are unaware of published evidence that suggests that positioning, palpation, gentle soft tissue therapy, or impulses to the musculature adjacent to the spine influence the course of asthma" (Balon et al, 1998). A reasonable alternative interpretation of this study's results, however, is that various forms of hands-on therapy, including joint manipulation and various forms of movement, mobilization, and soft tissue massage, appear to have a mildly beneficial effect for asthmatic patients (Redwood, 1999).

ACTIVE CONTROLS

Another study that raises similar questions involves manipulation for episodic tension-type headache (ETTH) (Bove & Nilsson, 1998). Patients were randomized into two

groups; one received soft tissue therapy (deep friction massage) plus spinal manipulation, and the other (the "active control" group) received soft tissue therapy plus application of a low-power laser to the neck. All treatments were applied by one chiropractor. Both groups had significantly fewer headaches and decreased their use of analgesic medications. As in the asthma study, differences between the two groups did not reach statistical significance. Thus the authors concluded that "as an isolated intervention, spinal manipulation does not seem to have a positive effect on tension-type headache."

Unlike the asthma study (Balon et al, 1998), Bove and Nilsson's carefully worded conclusion is justified by their data. But would it not have been more informative to affirm an equally accurate conclusion—that hands-on therapy, whether massage or manipulation, plus massage demonstrated significant benefits? Shortly after his paper's publication, Bove noted in a message to an Internet discussion group, "Our study asked one question [whether manipulation as an isolated intervention is effective for ETTH] and delivered one answer, a hallmark of good science. . . . We stressed that chiropractors do more than manipulation, and that chiropractic treatment has been shown to be somewhat beneficial for ETTH and very beneficial for cervicogenic headache. The message was that people should go to chiropractors with their headaches, for diagnosis and management."

The mass media's reporting on Bove and Nilsson's headache study provides a telling illustration of why defining the placebo or control correctly is more than an academic curiosity. Media reports on this study put forth a message quite different than Bove's nuanced analysis, with headlines concluding that chiropractic does not help headaches. Reports on the asthma study were similar. Moreover, future Medline searches will include the authors' tersely stated negative conclusions, with no mention of any controversy surrounding their interpretation.

The best way to avoid such confusion in the future is to emphasize increased usage of other valid methodologies, particularly direct comparisons of CAM procedures and standard medical care. Some comparative studies have shown manipulation to be equal or superior to conventional medical procedures, with fewer side effects (Boline et al, 1995; Meade et al, 1990, 1995; Nelson et al, 1998; Wiberg et al, 1999; Winters et al, 1997). If fairly constructed, such studies will yield data that allow health practitioners and the general public to place CAM procedures in proper context. Comparing chiropractic and other nonpharmaceutical procedures to highly questionable placebos confuses the issue and delays the advent of a "level playing field."

SAFETY OF SPINAL MANIPULATION

All health care interventions entail risk, which is best evaluated in relation to other common treatments for similar conditions (i.e., adjustment/manipulation vs.

anti-inflammatory medications for neck pain). Medications with a safety profile comparable to that of spinal manipulation are considered quite safe. Although minor, temporary soreness after a chiropractic treatment is not unusual, major adverse events resulting from chiropractic treatment are few and infrequent. As a result, chiropractic malpractice insurance premiums are substantially lower than those for medical and osteopathic physicians.

RESEARCH ON STROKE

The potential reaction to chiropractic treatment that has raised the greatest concern is vertebrobasilar accident (VBA), or stroke, following cervical spine manipulation. Stroke following manipulation occurs so rarely that it is virtually impossible to study other than on a retrospective basis, because the cohort necessary for a prospective study would involve hundreds of thousands of patients, at a minimum. Statistical correlation does not equal causation. Moreover, when such correlation is based on events involving numbers of stroke patients in single digits interspersed among millions of chiropractic visits, conclusions about direct causation not possible.

Lauretti (2003) provided a summary of chiropractic safety issues based on the information available several years ago, putting forth the following key points:

> Every reliable published study estimating the incidence of stroke from cervical adjustment/manipulation agrees that the risk is less than 1 to 3 incidents per 1 million treatments and approximately 1 incident per 100,000 patients.
>
> Haldeman and colleagues (2001) found the rate of stroke to be 1 in 8.06 million office visits, 1 in 5.85 million cervical adjustment/manipulations, 1 in 1430 chiropractic practice years, and 1 in 48 chiropractic practice careers.
>
> NSAIDs, which are also widely used for neck pain and headaches, have a much less desirable safety record than manipulation.

Since that time, relevant analysis of an unusually large database in Canada has been completed. The two most important and revealing studies exploring the possible relationship between chiropractic and stroke were based on retrospective reviews of hospital records in the province of Ontario.

Rothwell et al (2001) reviewed all records from 1993 to 1998 and found a total of 582 vertebrobasilar accident cases. Each was age and sex matched to four controls from the Ontario population with no history of stroke at the event date. Public health insurance billing records were used to document utilization of chiropractic services during the year prior to VBA onset. Because health care in Canada is publicly funded, this data is presumed to be comprehensive.

Slightly more than 90% of the entire cohort (525 of 582 cases) had no chiropractic visits in the year preceding their VBA. Of the 57 individuals with VBAs who did visit a chiropractor in the 365 days preceding the VBA (out of 50 million chiropractic visits during the 5-year period studied), 27 are thought to have had cervical manipulation. Of these, 4 individuals visited a chiropractor on the day immediately preceding the VBA, 5 in the previous 2 to 7 days, 3 in the previous 8 to 30 days, and 15 in the previous 31 to 365 days.

Compared to the controls, there was an increased association of VBA among patients who saw a chiropractor 1 to 8 days prior to the VBA event, but a decreased association of CVA among patients who saw a chiropractor 8 to 30 days before the event. Parsing their data for age-related differences, Rothwell et al found no positive association between recent chiropractic visits and VBAs in patients over age 45. However, patients under age 45 were five times more likely to have visited a chiropractor within the week prior to the VBA and five times more likely to have had three or more visits with a cervical diagnosis in the month preceding the VBA.

"Despite the popularity of chiropractic therapy," the authors wrote in their conclusion, "the association with stroke is exceedingly difficult to study. Even in this population-based study the small number of events was problematic. Of the 582 VBA cases, only 9 had a cervical manipulation within one week of their VBA. Focusing on only those aged <45 reduced our cases by 81%; of these, only 6 had cervical manipulation within 1 week of their VBA." Regarding incidence, they add, "Our analysis indicates that, for every 100,000 persons aged <45 years receiving chiropractic, approximately 1.3 cases of VBA attributable to chiropractic would be observed within 1 week of their manipulation." Recognizing that such a temporal relationship does not imply causation, Rothwell et al "caution that such rate estimates can easily be overemphasized . . . this study design does not permit us to estimate the number of cases that are truly the result of trauma sustained during manipulation."

Several years later, Cassidy et al (2008) completed a review of the same records evaluated by Rothwell's group and extended the time period covered in the review by 3 years. They performed additional analyses to determine whether patients who had seen a chiropractor were more likely to have had a stroke than patients who had seen a medical physician. This question, which had not been part of the earlier Rothwell et al (2001) review, was crucial because patients in the early stages of stroke commonly experience symptoms (headache, neck pain) that may lead them to consult either a chiropractor or a medical doctor. Cassidy et al (2008) found that it was no more likely for a stroke patient to have seen a chiropractor than a primary care medical physician. The authors concluded, "The increased risks of VBA stroke associated with chiropractic and PCP visits is likely due to patients with headache and neck pain from VBA dissection seeking care before their stroke. We found no evidence of excess risk of VBA stroke associated chiropractic care compared to primary care."

CHIROPRACTIC IN THE HEALTH CARE SYSTEM

The greatest issue facing chiropractic in its first century was survival: whether it would remain a separate and distinct healing art, succumb to the substantial forces against it, or be subsumed into allopathic medicine. The question of survival has been resolved.

A key question for the next generation remains: How can chiropractic best be integrated into the mainstream health care delivery system so that chiropractic services are readily available to all who can benefit from their application? A corollary follows as well: As with other "complementary/alternative" medical practices (see Chapter 3), how can such integration be achieved without diluting chiropractic principles and practice to the point where chiropractic becomes a weak shadow of its former self? How then can the desired integration be achieved for the benefit of many millions of current and future patients?

To answer this question in a manner satisfactory to chiropractors, conventional physicians, and the general public, a mutually agreed framework based on common goals is essential. A common purpose does exist in that all parties presume to create the most effective, efficient health care system possible for the greatest number of people. A framework for implementation also exists, at least in theory, based on the "level playing field" concept, which embodies a synthesis of two principles, democracy and hierarchy, coexisting in dynamic harmony.

The democracy of science is one in which equal opportunity is enjoyed by all, and all hypotheses are "innocent until proven guilty." Blind prejudice on the part of allopathic physicians, chiropractors, or anyone else has no place in this environment. All methods, whether presently considered conventional or alternative, must prove themselves effective and cost effective, and they must also demonstrate minimal iatrogenic effects. Approaches presently enjoying the imprimatur of the mainstream medical establishment should not be exempt from this scrutiny.

Hierarchy also has a place on the level playing field, as long as it is based on demonstrable skills and proven methods. Hierarchy in this sense does not imply a "control and domination" model. This idea is a lateral conception of hierarchy rather than a vertical one, a relationship among equals where precedence is based on quality, which in turn is determined through adherence to agreed-upon standards.

To continue the integration of chiropractic into the mainstream, there is a continuing need to broaden lines of communication between the chiropractic and medical professions, on a one-to-one basis and in small and large groups, with the goal of offering to all patients the gift of their practitioners' cooperation. Each side must learn to recognize its own strengths and weaknesses, as well as the strengths and weaknesses of the other. No one has all the answers, and humility befits our common role as seekers after truth.

The future need not mirror the worst aspects of the past. It is incumbent on all health care providers, as well as wholly consonant with their role as healers, that practitioners heal not only sickness but old rifts among themselves. They now have an unprecedented opportunity to do so.

References

Baker GA, Farabaugh RJ, Augat TJ, Hawk C: Algorithms for the Chiropractic Management of Acute and Chronic Spine-Related Pain, *Topics in Integrative Healthcare* 3(4):2012. http://www.tihcij.com/Articles/Algorithms-for-the-Chiropractic-Management-of-Acute-and-Chronic-Spine-Related-Pain.aspx?id=0000381. Accessed 9/4/13.

Bakris G, Dickholtz M Sr, Meyer PM, et al: Atlas vertebra realignment and achievement of arterial pressure goal in hypertensive patients: a pilot study, *J Hum Hypertens* 21:347–352, 2007.

Balon J, Aker PD, Crowther ER, et al: A comparison of active and simulated chiropractic manipulation as adjunctive treatment for childhood asthma, *N Engl J Med* 339(15):1013–1020, 1998.

BenEliyahu DJ: Magnetic resonance imaging and clinical follow-up: study of 27 patients receiving chiropractic care for cervical and lumbar disc herniations, *J Manipulative Physiol Ther* 19(9):597–606, 1996.

Bennett GM: *The art of the bonesetter*, Isleworth, 1981, Tamor Pierston.

Bergman GJ, Winters JC, Groenier KH, et al: Manipulative therapy in addition to usual medical care for patients with shoulder dysfunction and pain: a randomized, controlled trial, *Ann Intern Med* 141(6):432–439, 2004.

Bigos S, Bowyer O, Braen G: *Acute lower back pain in adults*. Clinical Practice Guideline, Quick Reference Guide No 14, AHCPR Pub No 95-0643, Rockville, MD, 1994, US Department of Health and Human Services, Public Health Service, Agency for Health Care Policy and Research.

Bishop PB, Quon JA, Fisher CG, Dvorak MFS: The Chiropractic Hospital-based Interventions Research Outcomes (CHIRO) Study: a randomized controlled trial on the effectiveness of clinical practice guidelines in the medical and chiropractic management of patients with acute mechanical low back pain, *Spine J* 10(12):1055–1064, 2010.

Boline PD, Kassak K, Bronfort G, et al: Spinal manipulation vs. amitriptyline for the treatment of chronic tension-type headaches: a randomized clinical trial, *J Manipulative Physiol Ther* 18(3):148–154, 1995.

Bourdillion JF: *Spinal manipulation*, ed 3, East Norwalk, Conn, 1982, Appleton-Century-Crofts.

Bove G, Nilsson N: Spinal manipulation in the treatment of episodic tension-type headache: a randomized controlled trial, *JAMA* 280(18):1576–1579, 1998.

Brantingham JW, Globe G, Pollard H, et al: Manipulative therapy for lower extremity conditions: expansion of literature review, *J Manipulative Physiol Ther* 32(1):53–71, 2009.

Brealey S, Burton K, Coulton S, et al: UK Back pain Exercise And Manipulation (UK BEAM) trial–national randomised trial of physical treatments for back pain in primary care: objectives, design and interventions [ISRCTN32683578], *BMC Health Serv Res* 3(1):16, 2003.

Bronfort G, Haas M, Evans R, et al: Effectiveness of manual therapies: the UK evidence report, *Chiropr Osteopath* 18(1):3, 2010.

Bronfort G, Evans R, Anderson AV, et al: Spinal manipulation, medication, or home exercise with advice for acute and subacute neck pain, *Ann Intern Med* 156(1 Part 1):1–10, 2012.

Bryans R, Descarreaux M, Duranleau M, et al: Evidence-based guidelines for the chiropractic treatment of adults with headache, *J Manipul Physiolog Ther* 34(5):274–289, 2011.

Cassidy JD, Thiel HW, Kirkaldy-Willis WH: Side posture manipulation for lumbar intervertebral disk herniation, *J Manipulative Physiol Ther* 16(2):96–103, 1993.

Cassidy JD, Boyle E, Cote P, et al: Risk of vertebral-basilar stroke and chiropractic care: results of a population-based case-control and case-crossover study, *Spine* 33(4 Suppl):S176–S183, 2008.

Chapman-Smith DA: *The chiropractic profession*, West Des Moines, Iowa, 2000, NCMIC Group.

Cherkin D, Deyo RA, Berg AO: Evaluation of a physician education intervention to improve primary care for low back pain. I. Impact on physicians, *Spine* 16(10):1168–1172, 1991.

Cherkin DC, MacCornack FA: Patient evaluations of low back pain care from family physicians and chiropractors, *West J Med* 150(3):351–355, 1989.

Chou R, Qaseem A, Snow V, et al: Diagnosis and treatment of low back pain: a joint clinical practice guideline from the American College of Physicians and the American Pain Society, *Ann Intern Med* 147(7):478–491, 2007.

Cifuentes M, Willetts J, Wasiak R: Health maintenance care in work-related low back pain and its association with disability recurrence, *J Occup Environ Med* 53(4):396–404, 2011.

Commission on Alternative Medicine, Social Departementete: Legitimization for vissa kiropraktorer, *Stockholm* 12:13–16, 1987.

Cox JM, Feller JA: Chiropractic treatment of low back pain: a multicenter descriptive analysis of presentation and outcome in 424 consecutive cases, *J Neuromusculoskel Syst* 2:178–190, 1994.

Croft PR, Macfarlane GJ, Papageorgiou AC, et al: Outcome of low back pain in general practice: a prospective study, *BMJ* 316(7141):1356–1359, 1998.

Danish Institute for Health Technology Assessment: Low-back pain: frequency, management, and prevention from an HTA perspective, *Danish Health Tech Assess* 1(1), 1999.

Deyle GD, Henderson NE, Matekel RL, et al: Effectiveness of manual physical therapy and exercise in osteoarthritis of the knee. A randomized, controlled trial, *Ann Intern Med* 132(3):173–181, 2000.

Deyle GD, Allison SC, Matekel RL, et al: Physical therapy treatment effectiveness for osteoarthritis of the knee: a randomized comparison of supervised clinical exercise and manual therapy procedures versus a home exercise program, *Phys Ther* 85(12):1301–1317, 2005.

Dvorak J: Neurological and biomechanical aspects of pain. In Buerger AA, Greenman PE, editors: *Approaches to the validation of spinal manipulation*, Springfield, Ill, 1985, Charles C Thomas, pp 241–266.

Evans R, Bronfort G, Schulz C, et al: Supervised exercise with and without spinal manipulation performs similarly and better than home exercise for chronic neck pain: a randomized controlled trial, *Spine* 37(11):903–914, 2012.

Fallon J: The role of the chiropractic adjustment in the care and treatment of 332 children with otitis media, *J Clin Chiropr Pediatr* 2(2):167–183, 1997.

Fallon J, Edelman MJ: Chiropractic care of 401 children with otitis media: a pilot study, *Altern Ther Health Med* 4(2):93, 1998.

Gatterman MI, Goe DR: Muscle and myofascial pain syndromes. In Gatterman MI, editor: *Chiropractic management of spine related disorders*, Baltimore, 1990, Williams & Wilkins, pp 285–329.

Gellert G: Global explanations and the credibility problem of alternative medicine, *Adv Mind Body Med* 10(4):60–67, 1994.

Globe GA, Morris CE, Whalen WM, et al: Chiropractic management of low back disorders: report from a consensus process, *J Manipulative Physiol Ther* 31(9):651–658, 2008.

Green T, Refshauge K, Crosbie J, Adams R: A randomized controlled trial of a passive accessory joint mobilization on acute ankle inversion sprains, *Phys Ther* 81(4):984–994, 2001.

Gross AR, Goldsmith C, Hoving JL, et al: Conservative management of mechanical neck disorders: a systematic review, *J Rheumatol* 34(5):1083–1102, 2007.

Haldeman S, Carey P, Townsend M, Papadopoulos C: Arterial dissections following cervical manipulation: the chiropractic experience, *Can Med Assoc J* 165:905, 2001.

Haldeman S, Chapman-Smith D, Peterson DM, editors: Guidelines for chiropractic quality assurance and practice parameters. In *Proceedings of the Mercy Center Consensus Conference*, Gaithersburg, Md, 1993, Aspen.

Haldeman S, Carroll L, Cassidy JD, et al: The Bone and Joint Decade 2000–2010 Task Force on Neck Pain and Its Associated Disorders: executive summary, *Spine* 33(4 Suppl):S5–S7, 2008.

Hasselberg PD: *Chiropractic in New Zealand: report of a commission of inquiry*, Wellington, NZ, 1979, Government Printer.

Hawk C, Khorsan R, Lisi AJ, et al: Chiropractic care for nonmusculoskeletal conditions: a systematic review with implications for whole systems research, *J Altern Complement Med* 13(5):491–512, 2007.

Hoeksma HL, Dekker J, Ronday HK, et al: Comparison of manual therapy and exercise therapy in osteoarthritis of the hip: a randomized clinical trial, *Arthritis Rheum* 51(5):722–729, 2004.

Hondras MA, Long CR, Brennan PC: Spinal manipulative therapy versus a low force mimic maneuver for women with primary dysmenorrhea: a randomized, observer-blinded, clinical trial, *Pain* 81(1–2):105–114, 1999.

Hondras MA, Long CR, Cao Y, et al: A randomized controlled trial comparing 2 types of spinal manipulation and minimal conservative medical care for adults 55 years and older with subacute or chronic low back pain, *J Manipulative Physiol Ther* 32(5):330–343, 2009.

Hurwitz EL, Carragee EJ, van der Velde G, et al: Treatment of neck pain: noninvasive interventions: results of the Bone and Joint Decade 2000–2010 Task Force on Neck Pain and Its Associated Disorders, *Spine* 33(4 Suppl):S123–S152, 2008.

Jamison JR: Health information and promotion in chiropractic clinics, *J Manip Physiol Ther* 25:240–245, 2002.

Kay TM, Gross A, Goldsmith C, et al: Exercises for mechanical neck disorders, *Cochrane Reviews* (3):CD004250, 2005.

Keeney BJ, Fulton-Kehoe D, Turner JA, et al: Early predictors of lumbar spine surgery after occupational back injury: results from a prospective study of workers in Washington State, *Spine* 38(11):953–964, 2013.

Kelly PT, Luttges MW: Electrophoretic separation of nervous system proteins on exponential gradient polyacrylamide gels, *J Neurochem* 24:1077–1079, 1975.

Kirkaldy-Willis W, Cassidy J: Spinal manipulation in the treatment of low back pain, *Can Fam Physician* 31:535–540, 1985.

Koes BW, Bouter LM, van Mameren H, et al: A randomized clinical trial of manual therapy and physiotherapy for persistent back and neck complaints: subgroup analysis and relationship between outcome measures, *J Manip Physiol Ther* 16(4):211–219, 1993.

Kokjohn K, Schmid DM, Triano JJ, Brennan PC: The effect of spinal manipulation on pain and prostaglandin levels in women with primary dysmenorrhea, *J Manip Physiol Ther* 15(5):279–285, 1992.

Korr IM: Proprioceptors and the behavior of lesioned segments. In Stark EH, editor: *Osteopathic medicine*, Acton, Mass, 1975, Publication Sciences Group, pp 183–199.

Korr IM: The spinal cord as organizer of disease processes: some preliminary perspectives, *J Am Osteopath Assoc* 76:89–99, 1976.

Lauretti WJ: Comparative safety of chiropractic. In Redwood D, Cleveland CS III, editors: *Fundamentals of chiropractic*, St Louis, 2003, Mosby, p 561.

Lawrence DJ, Meeker W, Branson R, et al: Chiropractic management of low back pain and low back-related leg complaints: a literature synthesis, *J Manip Physiol Ther* 31(9):659–674, 2008.

Leach RA: *The chiropractic theories: principles and clinical applications*, ed 3, Baltimore, 1994, Williams & Wilkins.

Liliedahl RL, Finch MD, Axene DV, Goertz CM: Cost of care for common back pain conditions initiated with chiropractic doctor vs medical doctor/doctor of osteopathy as first physician: experience of one Tennessee-based general health insurer, *J Manip Physiol Ther* 33(9):640–643, 2010.

Lin CW, Haas M, Maher CG, et al: Cost-effectiveness of guideline-endorsed treatments for low back pain: a systematic review, *Eur Spine J* 20(7):1024–1038, 2011.

Lomax E: Manipulative therapy: a historical perspective from ancient times to the modern era. In Goldstein M, editor: *The research status of spinal manipulation: 1975*, Washington, DC, 1975, US Government Printing Office, pp 11–17.

Luttges MW, Kelly PT, Gerren RA: Degenerative changes in mouse sciatic nerves: electrophoretic and electrophysiological characterizations, *Exp Neurol* 50:706–733, 1976.

MacGregor RJ, Oliver RM: A general-purpose electronic model for arbitrary configurations of neurons, *J Theor Biol* 38:527–538, 1973.

MacGregor RJ, Sharpless SK, Luttges MW: A pressure vessel model for nerve compression, *J Neurol Sci* 24:299–304, 1975.

Manga P: *The effectiveness and cost-effectiveness of chiropractic management of low-back pain*, Richmond Hill, VA, 1993, Kenilworth.

McMorland G, Suter E, Casha S, et al: Manipulation or microdiskectomy for sciatica? A prospective randomized clinical study, *J Manipulative Physiol Ther* 33(8):576–584, 2010.

Meade TW: Interview on Canadian Broadcast Corporation. In *Chiropractic: a review of current research*, Arlington, VA, 1992, Foundation for Chiropractic Education and Research.

Meade TW, Dyer S, Browne W, Frank AO: Randomised comparison of chiropractic and hospital outpatient management for low back pain: results from extended follow up, *BMJ* 311(7001):349–351, 1995.

Meade TW, Dyer S, Browne W, et al: Low back pain of mechanical origin: randomised comparison of chiropractic and hospital outpatient treatment, *BMJ* 300(6737):1431–1437, 1990.

Mense S: Considerations concerning the neurobiological basis of muscle pain, *Can J Physiol Pharmacol* 69:610–616, 1991.

Michaleff ZA, Lin CW, Maher CG, van Tulder MW: Spinal manipulation epidemiology: systematic review of cost effectiveness studies, *J Electromyogr Kinesiol* 22(5):655–662, 2012.

Micozzi MS: Complementary Medicine: What Is Appropriate? Who will Provide It? *Ann Int Med* 129:65–66, 1998.

Munday S, Jones A, Brantingham J, et al: A randomized, single-blinded, placebo-controlled clinical trial to evaluate the effi-cacy of chiropractic shoulder girdle adjustment in the treatment of shoulder impingement syndrome, *J Amer Chiropr Assoc* 44(6):6–15, 2007.

Nelson CF, Bronfort G, Evans R, et al: The efficacy of spinal manipulation, amitriptyline and the combination of both therapies for the prophylaxis of migraine headache, *J Manip Physiol Ther* 21(8):511–519, 1998.

Olafsdottir E, Forshei S, Fluge G, Markestad T: Randomised controlled trial of infantile colic treated with chiropractic spinal manipulation, *Arch Dis Child* 84:138, 2001.

Palmer DD: *Textbook of the science, art, and philosophy of chiropractic*, Portland, Ore, 1910, Portland Printing House.

Palmgren PJ, Sandstrom PJ, Lundqvist FJ, Heikkila H: Improvement after chiropractic care in cervicocephalic kinesthetic sensibility and subjective pain intensity in patients with non-traumatic chronic neck pain, *J Manipulative Physiol Ther* 29(2):100–106, 2006.

Paré A: *The collected works of Ambroise Paré*, New York, 1968, Milford House.

Patterson MM, Steinmetz JE: Long-lasting alterations of spinal reflexes: a potential basis for somatic dysfunction, *Man Med* 2:38–42, 1986.

Pellow JE, Brantingham JW: The efficacy of adjusting the ankle in the treatment of subacute and chronic grade I and grade II ankle inversion sprains, *J Manipulative Physiol Ther* 24(1):17–24, 2001.

Redwood D: Same data, different interpretation, *J Altern Complement Med* 5(1):89–91, 1999.

Redwood D: Olympic Chiropractor: Interview with Michael Reed,. DC, DACSP, *Health Insights Today* 1(4):2008a. http://www.healthinsightstoday.com/articles/v1i4/olympicchiro_p1.html.

Redwood D: Chiropractic at National Naval Medical Center, *Health Insights Today* 1(1):2008b. http://www.healthinsightstoday.com/articles/v1i1/naval.html.

Redwood D, Globe G: Prevention and health promotion by chiropractors, *Am J Lifestyle Med* 2(6):537–545, 2008.

Redwood D: DC Receives Federal Grant to Study Nonsurgical Alternatives to Surgery for Spinal Stenosis: Interview with Michael Schneider, DC, PhD, *Health Insights Today* 6(2):2013. http://www.cleveland.edu/media/cms_page_media/811/MichaelSchneiderInterview.pdf. Accessed 9/4/13.

Rosen M: *Back pain: report of a clinical standards advisory group committee on back pain*, London, 1994, HMSO.

Rothwell DM, Bondy SJ, Williams I: Chiropractic manipulation and stroke: a population-based case-control study, *Stroke* 32:1054–1060, 2001.

Santilli V, Beghi E, Finucci S: Chiropractic manipulation in the treatment of acute back pain and sciatica with disc protrusion: a randomized double-blind clinical trial of active and simulated spinal manipulations, *Spine J* 6(2):131–137, 2006.

Schafer RC, Faye LJ: *Motion palpation and chiropractic technique*, Huntington Beach, Calif, 1989, Motion Palpation Institute.

Senna MK, Machaly SA: Does maintained spinal manipulation therapy for chronic nonspecific low back pain result in better long-term outcome? *Spine* 36(18):1427–1437, 2011.

Sharpless S: Susceptibility of spinal roots to compression block. In Goldstein M, editor: *The research status of spinal manipulation: 1975*, Washington, DC, 1975, US Government Printing Office, pp 155–161.

Shekelle PG, Adams AH: *The appropriateness of spinal manipulation for low-back pain: project overview and literature review*.

Report No R-4025/1-CCR/FCER, Santa Monica, Calif, 1991, RAND.

Simske SJ, Schmeister TA: An experimental model for combined neural, muscular, and skeletal degeneration, *J Neuromusculoskel Syst* 2:116–123, 1994.

Suh CH: The fundamentals of computer aided x-ray analysis of the spine, *J Biomech* 7:161–169, 1974.

Thomasen PR, Fisher BL, Carpenter PA, Fike GL: Effectiveness of spinal manipulative therapy in treatment of primary dysmenorrhea: a pilot study, *J Manip Physiol Ther* 2:140–145, 1979.

Thompson CJ: *Second report: Medicare Benefits Review Committee*, Canberra, Canada, 1986, Commonwealth Government Printer.

Triano JJ, Luttges MW: Nerve irritation: a possible model of sciatic neuritis, *Spine* 7:129–136, 1982.

Triano JJ, McGregor M, Hondras MA, Brennan PC: Manipulative therapy versus education programs in chronic low back pain, *Spine* 20:948–955, 1995.

UK BEAM Trial Team: United Kingdom back pain exercise and manipulation (UK BEAM) randomised trial: effectiveness of physical treatments for back pain in primary care, *BMJ* 329(7479):1377, 2004a.

UK BEAM Trial Team: United Kingdom back pain exercise and manipulation (UK BEAM) randomised trial: cost effectiveness of physical treatments for back pain in primary care, *BMJ* 329(7479):1381, 2004b.

Wiberg JM, Nordsteen J, Nilsson N: The short-term effect of spinal manipulation in the treatment of infantile colic: a randomized controlled clinical trial with a blinded observer, *J Manip Physiol Ther* 22(8):517–522, 1999.

Wilk v AMA, 895 F2D 352 Cert den, 112.2 ED 2D 524, 1990.

Wilkey A, Gregory M, Byfield D, McCarthy PW: A comparison between chiropractic management and pain clinic management for chronic low-back pain in a National Health Service outpatient clinic, *J Altern Complement Med* 14(5):465–473, 2008.

Winters JC, Sobel JS, Groenier KH, et al: Comparison of physiotherapy, manipulation, and corticosteroid injection for treating shoulder complaints in general practice: randomised, single blind study, *BMJ* 314(7090):1320–1325, 1997.

Withington ET: *Hippocrates* (vol 3), Cambridge, Mass, 1959, Harvard University Press.

World Federation of Chiropractic: The Current Status of the Chiropractic Profession: Report to the World Health Organization from the World Federation of Chiropractic. 2012. http://www.wfc.org/website/images/wfc/WHO_Submission-Final_Jan2013.pdf. Accessed 9/4/13.

Suggested Readings

Brennan PC, Kokjohn K, Kaltinger CJ, et al: Enhanced phagocytic cell respiratory burst induced by spinal manipulation: potential role of substance P, *J Manipulative Physiol Ther* 14(7):399–408, 1991.

Cherkin DC, Deyo RA, Wheeler K, Ciol MA: Physician views about treating low back pain: the results of a national survey, *Spine* 20(1):1–9, 1995.

Coulter I, Hurwitz EL, Adams AH, et al: *The appropriateness of spinal manipulation and mobilization of the cervical spine: literature review, indications and ratings by a multidisciplinary expert panel*. Monograph No DRU-982-1-CCR, Santa Monica, Calif, 1995, RAND.

Illingworth RS: Infantile colic revisited, *Arch Dis Child* 60:981–985, 1985.

Lucassen PL, Assendelft WJ, Gubbels JW, et al: Effectiveness of treatments for infantile colic: a systematic review, *BMJ* 316:1563–1569, 1998.

Meeker WC, Haldeman S: Chiropractic: a profession at the crossroads of mainstream and alternative medicine, *Ann Intern Med* 136(3):216–227, 2002.

Rosner AL: Musculoskeletal disorders research. In Redwood D, Cleveland CS III, editors: *Fundamentals of chiropractic*, St Louis, 2003, Mosby, p 465.

Van Tulder MW, Koes BW, Bouter LM: Conservative treatment of acute and chronic nonspecific low back pain: a systematic review of randomized controlled trials of the most common interventions, *Spine* 22:2128–2156, 1997.

Von Kuster T: *Chiropractic health care: a national study of cost of education, service, utilization, number of practicing doctors of chiropractic and other key policy issues*, Washington, DC, 1980, Foundation for the Advancement of Chiropractic Tenets and Science.

Resources

American Chiropractic Association
1701 Clarendon Blvd
Arlington, VA 22209
Phone: 703-276-8800
E-mail: AmerChiro@aol.com
Website: www.amerchiro.org

World Federation of Chiropractic
3080 Yonge St, Suite 5065
Toronto, Ontario, M4N3N1, Canada
Phone: 416-484-9978
E-mail: worldfed@sympatico.ca
Website: www.wfc.org

International Chiropractors Association
1110 North Glebe Rd, Suite 1000
Arlington, VA 22201
Phone: 703-528-5000
E-mail: chiro@erols.com
Website: www.chiropractic.org

Canadian Chiropractic Association
1396 Eglinton Ave West
Toronto, Ontario, M6C2E4, Canada
Phone: 416-781-5656
E-mail: www.inforamp.net/~ccachiro
Website: www.ccachiro.org

National Board of Chiropractic Examiners
901 54th Ave
Greeley, CO 80634
Phone: 970-356-9100
E-mail: nbce@nbce.org
Website: www.nbce.org

Council on Chiropractic Education
8049 N. 85th Way
Scottsdale, AZ 85258

Phone: 480-443-8877
E-mail: cce@cce-usa.org
Website: www.cce-usa.org

Council on Chiropractic Education International
8049 North 85th Way
Scottsdale, AZ 85282-4321
Phone: 480-922-8763

Fax: 480-922-8767
E-mail: ccei@cceintl.org
Website: www.cceintl.org

Other Informative Websites

Dynamic Chiropractic: www.chiroweb.com
Health Insights Today: www.cleveland.edu/hit
The Chiropractic Resource Organization: www.chiro.org

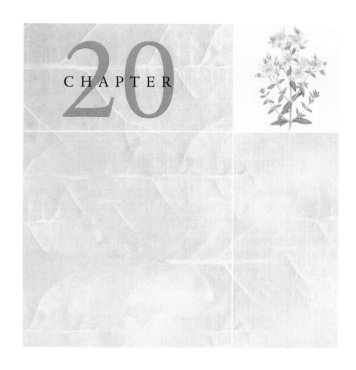

CHAPTER

20

REFLEXOLOGY

DONALD A. BISSON

Reflexology is a focused pressure technique, usually directed at the feet or hands. It is based on the premise that there are zones and reflexes in different parts of the body that correspond to all parts, glands, and organs, as well as systems, of the body (Wilson, 2012). Stimulation of these reflex areas helps the body to correct, strengthen, and reinforce itself by returning to a state of homeostasis. In Asian countries, some reflexologists also use electrical or mechanical devices. However, these approaches have been discouraged in North America.

One of the oldest documentations of the premise of reflexology can be found in an ancient Egyptian papyrus depicting medical practitioners treating the hands and feet of their patients in approximately 2500 BC (Issel, 1990). William H. Fitzgerald, MD (1872-1942), is credited with being a founder of modern reflexology (Marquardt, 2000). His studies brought about the development and practice of reflexology in the United States.

Dr. Fitzgerald's studies found that application of pressure to various locations on the body deadened sensation in definite areas and relieved pain. These findings led to the development of zone therapy. In the early years, Dr. Fitzgerald worked mainly on the hands. Later, the feet became very popular as a site for treatment. In his book on zone therapy in 1917, Dr. Fitzgerald wrote about working on the palmar surface of the hand for any pains in the back of the body, and working on the dorsal aspect of the hands and fingers for any problems on the anterior (front) part of the body. Dr. Fitzgerald claimed to have relieved pain in a patient by applying pressure to the patient's hands and feet (Fitzgerald & Bowers, 1917).

Joe Shelby Riley, MD, was taught zone therapy by Dr. Fitzgerald. He developed the techniques out to finer points,

making the first detailed diagrams and drawings of the reflex points located on the feet and hands (Riley, 1924).

While working with Dr. Riley in the 1930s, Eunice Ingham, a nurse and physical therapist, became a staunch supporter of helping people help themselves with the use of reflexology. She shared her techniques and knowledge with many, and, in 1938, published the first of three books on reflexology (Ingham, 1938). After her passing in 1974, her nephew, Dwight Byers, continued to teach her work in the United States (Byers, 2001).

THEORY

As noted earlier, reflexology is based on the premise that there are zones and reflexes in different parts of the body that correspond to all parts, glands, and organs of the entire body. Manipulating specific reflexes removes stress, activating a parasympathetic response to enable the blockages to be released by a physiological change in the body. With stress removed and circulation enhanced, the body is allowed to return to a normal state of homeostasis.

CONVENTIONAL ZONE THEORY

Conventional zone theory (CZT) is the foundation of hand and foot reflexology. An understanding of CZT and its relations to the body is essential to understand reflexology and its applications (Kunz & Kunz, 1987).

Zones are a system for organizing relations among various parts, glands, and organs of the body, and the reflexes. There are 10 equal longitudinal or vertical zones running the length of the body from the tips of the toes and the tips of the fingers to the top of the head. From the dividing center line of the body, there are five zones on the right side of the body and five zones on the left side. These zones are numbered 1 to 5 from the medial side (inside) to the lateral side (outside). Each finger and toe falls into one of the five zones; for example, the left thumb is in the same zone as the left big toe, zone 1.

The reflexes are considered to pass all the way through the body within the same zones. The same reflex, for example, can be found on the front and also on the back of the body, and on the top and on the bottom of the hand or foot. This is the three-dimensional aspect of the zones.

Reflexology zones are not to be confused with acupuncture or acupressure meridians, which is the basis of ear and facial "reflexology" currently popular.

Pressure applied to any part of a zone will affect the entire zone. Every part, gland, or organ of the body represented in a particular zone can be stimulated by working any reflex in that same zone. This concept is the foundation of zone theory and reflexology.

In addition to the longitudinal zones of CZT, reflexology also uses the transverse zones (horizontal zones) on the body and feet or hands. The purpose is to help fix the image of the body by mapping it onto the hands or feet in proper perspective and location. Four transverse zone lines are commonly used: transverse pelvic line, transverse waistline, transverse diaphragm line, and transverse neck line. These transverse zone lines create five areas: pelvic area, lower abdominal area, upper abdominal area, thoracic area, and head area.

INTERNAL ORGANS AND THE THREE-DIMENSIONAL BODY

It is important to remember that internal organs lay on top of, over, behind, between, and against each other in every possible configuration. The reflexes on the hands and feet, corresponding to the parts, organs, and glands, overlap as well. For example, the kidney reflexes on the foot chart (Figure 20-1A) or hand chart (Figure 20-1B) overlap with many other reflexes, just as the kidneys overlap other organs and parts of the body when viewed from the back or the front.

EXCEPTION TO THE ZONE THEORY

The basic concept of CZT is that the right foot or hand represents the right side of the body, and the left foot or hand, the left side. However, in the central nervous system, the right half of the brain controls the left side of the body and vice versa. In any disorders that affect the brain or the central nervous system, a reflexologist will emphasize the reflexes or areas of the disorder on the opposite hand or foot. For example, the brain reflexes will be worked on the left foot or hand for strokes that caused paralysis on the right side of the body. This approach matches the neuroanatomical organization of the left brain to the right side of the body, and the right brain to the left side of the body.

ZONE-RELATED REFERRAL

It is a common assumption that the hands and feet are the only areas to which reflexology can be applied. However, there are reflexes throughout the 10 zones of the body, and they may present unlikely relations within these zones (Kunz & Kunz, 1987). For example, there is a zonal relationship between the eyes and the kidneys, because both lie in the same zone. Working the kidney reflexes can affect the eyes.

If there is a physical injury on the foot, the area should be avoided and should not be worked. Alternate parts of the body in the same zones may be worked instead. For example, the arm is a reflection of the leg, the hand of the foot, the wrist of the ankle, and so forth. If any part of the arm is injured, the corresponding part of the leg can be worked and vice versa. Common problems, such as varicose veins and phlebitis in the legs, can be helped by working the same general areas on the arms.

This approach can be used to find other referral areas by identifying the zone(s) in which an injury has occurred and tracing it to the referral area. Tenderness in the referral area will usually help the reflexologist find it.

Referral areas can give insights into problem areas by showing the relationships to the areas in the same zone(s) that may be at the root of the problem. For example, a shoulder problem may be caused by a hip problem, because the shoulder lies in the same zone as the hip.

NEGATIVE FEEDBACK LOOP

A reflexology session usually begins on the right foot or hand and finishes on the left foot or hand. In addition, the reflexes on both feet and hands are worked from the base of the foot or hand up to the top, with the toes or fingers worked last.

To aid the body's self-regulation, a highly complex and integrated communication control system or network is required. This type of network is called a "feedback control loop." Different networks in the body control diverse functions such as blood carbon dioxide levels, temperature, and heart and respiratory rates. Homeostatic control mechanisms are categorized as negative or positive feedback loops. Many of the important and numerous homeostatic control mechanisms are negative feedback loops.

Negative feedback loops (Figure 20-2) are stabilizing mechanisms; that is, they maintain homeostasis of blood carbon dioxide concentration. As blood carbon dioxide increases, the respiration rate increases to permit carbon dioxide to exit the body in increased amounts through expired air. Without this homeostatic mechanism, body carbon dioxide levels would rapidly rise to toxic levels, and death would result.

The blood circulation loop is from the left side of the body to the right side—fresh oxygenated blood enters the aorta from the left ventricle of the heart and travels to the body, and venous blood with carbon dioxide enters the

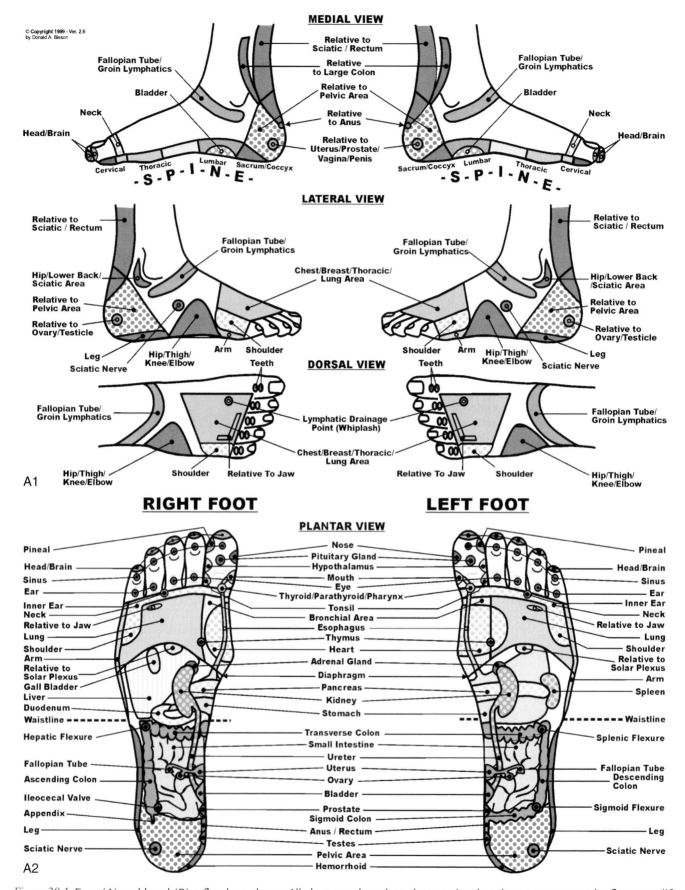

Figure 20-1 Foot (A) and hand (B) reflexology charts. All charts are based on the premise that there are zones and reflexes on different parts of the body that correspond to and are relative to all parts, glands, and organs, as well as systems, of the entire body. Reflexologists do not diagnose, prescribe, or treat specific conditions. Reflexologists do not work in opposition to the medical or other fields, but complement and enhance them. (Copyright © Donald A. Bisson, 2010, Version 2.6.)

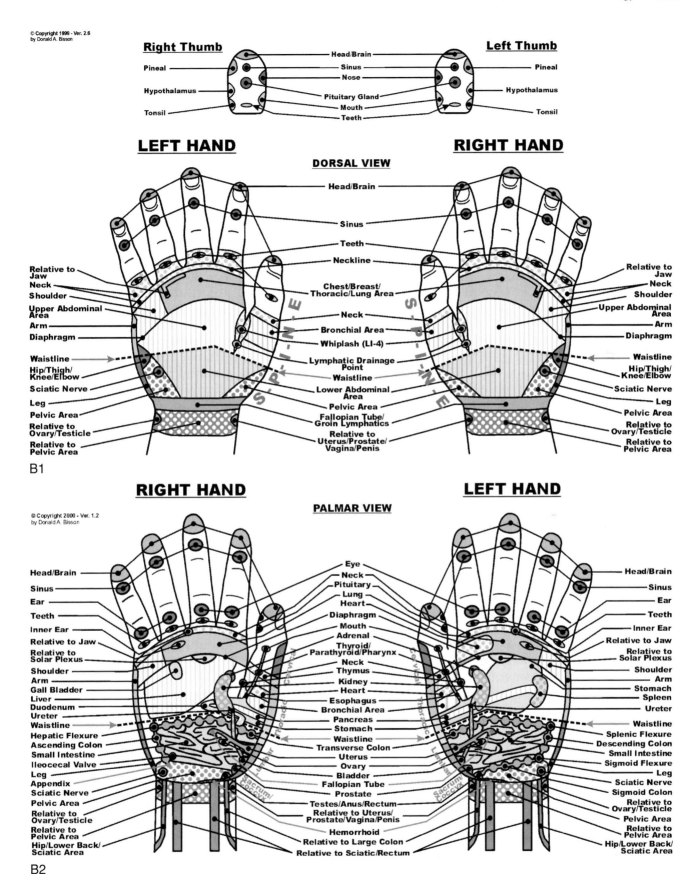

Figure 20-1, cont'd

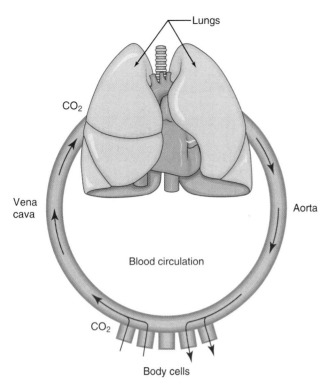

Figure 20-2 Homeostasis negative feedback loop.

vena cava on the right side of the heart. By beginning a reflexology session on the right foot or hand, the reflexologist is helping to boost the loop by pushing venous or deoxygenated blood into the heart and lungs so that fresh oxygenated blood will be available to the body cells. The same rationale applies to the direction that the reflexologist works on the foot or hand—from the bottom of the foot upward, to bolster the homeostatic loop.

BENEFITS AND SCOPE

Reflexology demonstrates four main benefits: (1) it promotes relaxation with the removal of stress; (2) it enhances circulation; (3) it assists the body to normalize the metabolism naturally; and (4) it complements all other healing modalities.

When the reflexes are stimulated, the body's natural electrical energy works along the nervous system to clear any blockages in the corresponding zones.

A reflexology session seems to break up deposits (felt as a sandy or gritty area under the skin), which may interfere with the flow of the body's electrical energy in the nervous system.

Reflexologists do not diagnose medical conditions unless qualified to do so. The only diagnosis made is that of a tender reflex. A reflexologist will refer to other qualified health care practitioners when the services required are outside the reflexologist's scope of practice.

Similarly, reflexologists do not prescribe medications unless qualified to do so. The therapeutic intervention is limited to working the reflexes.

In randomized controlled trials, reflexology has been found to be effective in reducing pain in women with severe premenstrual symptoms (Oleson & Flocco, 1993) and in patients with migraine and tension headaches (Launso et al, 1999). It has also demonstrated benefit in alleviating motor, sensory, and urinary symptoms in patients with multiple sclerosis (Siev-Ner et al, 2003). Recent systematic reviews on the efficacy of reflexology in cancer patients found positive improvements in anxiety and pain (Andersen & Hodgson, 2007; Solà et al, 2004; Stephenson & Dalton, 2003).

Reflexology is a useful complementary or alternative therapy to decrease anxiety and pain in patients with cancer (Lacey, 2002).

In a systematic review of randomized clinical trials (RCTs) on reflexology, Ernst et al (2011) assessed the results of the RCTs and methodological criteria used to develop the studies. This review points to the essential problem that the methodological quality of reflexology RCTs is often limited at least by this limited approach (see Chapter 3). Of the 23 studies that met their particular inclusion criteria, they reported, "Eight RCTs suggested that reflexology is effective for the following conditions: diabetes, premenstrual syndrome, cancer, multiple sclerosis, symptomatic idiopathic detrusor over-activity and dementia . . ." Despite their own findings on effectiveness in eight studies that met their own criteria, these particular authors remain unconvinced of the reliability of the research on reflexology (as they often remain regarding CAM in general) as it pertains to medical conditions. They make the point that flawed research designs, according to their criteria, should be corrected prior to clinical trials in order for the results of studies to be more useful.

ADVERSE EFFECTS

The adverse effects of reflexology are minor and may include fatigue (increase in parasympathetic activity), headache, nausea, increased perspiration, and diarrhea.

CREDENTIALING AND TRAINING

No formal or standardized credentialing exists for reflexology in North America. Certification is provided by certain educational institutions specializing in this training. A patient should look for a therapist who is certified and/or registered as a qualified reflexologist by a reputable organization.

There are many schools of reflexology that can provide adequate training, ranging from 100 to 1000 hours of instruction. The interested individual should look for a school that is established and, if possible, recognized by a local governing body.

In the United States and Canada, there are regulations for practicing reflexology, and individual states and provinces (though not all) have their own sets of educational or licensing requirements.

SUMMARY

Reflexology is a form of manipulative therapy that has been used successfully to treat various disorders and to provide pain management. There are many conditions for which reflexology can assist in healing, especially in pain management, as confirmed by recent studies and publications.

It is believed by reflexologists that reflexology impacts the autonomic nervous system, balancing the parasympathetic nervous system and the sympathetic nervous system (Hughes et al, 2011), the two subdivisions of the autonomic nervous system that exert opposite effects on the end organs, to maintain or restore homeostasis (Crane, 1997). Many of the benefits of reflexology come from the relief of tension and stress (Andersen & Hodgson, 2007; Stephenson & Dalton, 2003). As with many alternative medical approaches, good scientific studies to confirm the benefits of reflexology are relatively sparse, and more research is required. Reflexology does appear to relieve stress, which in turn could reduce or minimize physical symptoms (Stephenson & Dalton, 2003). Reflexology can be used as an adjunct to proven therapies in the treatment of disease. The profession and application of reflexology would benefit from being better regulated and standardized.

References

Andersen SG, Hodgson NA: Reflexology with nursing home residents: a case vignette, *Internet J Geriatr Gerontol* 3(2):2007. http://www.ispub.com/ostia/index.php?xmlFilePath=journals/ijgg/vol3n2/reflexology.xml.

Byers D: *Better health with foot reflexology: the original Ingham Method®*, Revised ed, St Petersburg, FL, 2001, Ingham Publishing.

Crane B: *Reflexology: the definitive practitioner's manual*, Shaftesbury, England, 1997, Element.

Fitzgerald WH, Bowers EF: *Zone therapy, relieving pain at home*, Columbus, Ohio, 1917, IW Long.

Ernst E, Posadzki P, Lee MS: Reflexology: an update of a systematic review of randomized clinical trials, *Maturitas* 68(2):116–120, 2011.

Hughes CM, Krirsnakriengkrai S, Kumar S, McDonough SM: *The effect of reflexology on the autonomic nervous system in healthy adults: a feasibility study*, 2011, School of Health Sciences, University of Ulster, Northern Ireland, United Kingdom. Available at: http://mycoignofvantage.files.wordpress.com/2012/08/reflexology-and-the-autonomic-nervous-system.pdf.

Ingham E: *Stories the feet can tell*, St. Petersburg, FL, 1938, Ingham Publishers.

Issel C: *Reflexology: art, science and history*, Sacramento, CA, 1990, New Frontier.

Kunz K, Kunz B: *The complete guide to foot reflexology*, Englewood Cliffs, NJ, 1987, Prentice-Hall.

Lacey MD: The effects of foot massage and reflexology on decreasing anxiety, pain, and nausea in patients with cancer, *Clin J Oncol Nurs* 6(3):183, 2002.

Launso L, Brendstrup E, Arnberg S: An exploratory study of reflexological treatment for headache, *Altern Ther Health Med* 5(3):57, 1999.

Marquardt H: *Reflexotherapy of the feet*, Stuttgart, Germany, 2000, Georg Thieme Verlag.

Oleson T, Flocco W: Randomized controlled study of premenstrual symptoms treated with ear, hand and foot reflexology, *Obstet Gynecol* 82(6):906, 1993.

Riley JS: *Zone reflex*, Santa Cruz, Calif, 1924, Daglish Health Food Service (reprinted 1942).

Siev-Ner I, Gamus D, Lerner Geva L, et al: Reflexology treatment relieves symptoms of multiple sclerosis: a randomized controlled study, *Mult Scler* 9(4):356, 2003.

Solà I, Thompson E, Subirana M, et al: Non-invasive interventions for improving well-being and quality of life in patients with lung cancer, *Cochrane Database Syst Rev* (4):CD004282, 2004.

Stephenson N, Dalton JA: Using reflexology for pain management: a review, *J Holist Nurs* 21:179, 2003.

Wilson E: Reflexology. In DeLany J: *3D Anatomy for massage and manual therapies*, London, 2012, Primal Pictures.

Suggested Readings

Bisson DA: *N101 foot reflexology course*, New Liskeard, Canada, 2010, Ontario College of Reflexology.

Bisson DA: *N201 hand reflexology course*, New Liskeard, Canada, 2010, Ontario College of Reflexology.

CHAPTER 21

YOGA

JULIE K. STAPLES

The Sanskrit word *yoga* comes from the root *yug*, meaning "to join together" or "union" (as in modern English use of the word "yoke"). There are different interpretations of the nature of this union, but one interpretation is that of a spiritual union. It represents a method by which an individual's consciousness becomes united with what may be considered the Infinite Consciousness, the Divine Consciousness, or the Reality underlying the universe (Prabhavananda & Isherwood, 1981). Yoga as practiced in the West in modern times often has less emphasis on spiritual union and more emphasis on simply performing physical yoga postures, and perhaps meditation, for physical and emotional well-being. However, yoga is a multifaceted, meditative, and devotional practice with a history rich in texts and literature teaching the various dimensions discussed in this chapter.

Archeological evidence has linked the beginning of yoga to the Indus Valley Civilization which ended about 1500 BC and now comprises present day India and Pakistan (Khalsa & Gould, 2012) (see also Chapters 31 and 35). The dates of each of the yogic philosophical eras vary depending on the source of the information and, in general, are quite conjectural. As a guide though, the timing of the epochs is outlined below (Bhajan, 2003a; Feuerstein, 2001e). The philosophical eras and creation of yogic literature are located as early as the Pre-Vedic Age, from about 6500–4500 BC. The Vedic Age is considered 4500–2500 BC and includes the composition of the four *Vedas* (books of knowledge), the sacred literature of Hinduism. The Brahmanical Age was from 2500 to 1500 BC. The literature created in this latter era was the *Brahmana*, literature on rites rituals and behaviors of the priesthood, and *Aranyakas*, ritual texts for aesthetics, or "forest dwellers."

The Upanishadic Age was from 1500 to 1000 BC. The name is taken from the creation of the *Upanishads* during this era. The word *Upanishad* literally means to "sit near, and be meditative," and reflects the transmission of knowledge from the teacher to the student (Bhajan, 2003a). The Pre-Classical Age was from 1000 to 100 BC. During this time, the *Mahabharata* epic was created. The *Bhagavad-Gita* is part of the *Mahabharata* and is one of the important pillars in the history of yoga. Next was the Classical Age, from 100 BC to AD 500. It was during the Classical Age that the *Yoga Sutra* of Patanjali was composed. The *Yoga Sutra* is "a systematic treatise concerned with defining the most important elements of Yoga theory and practice" (Feuerstein, 2001a) (see a more detailed description in the next section of this chapter). The Puranic Age was from AD 500 to 1300. The *Puranas* were created during this time and contain philosophical, mythological, and ritual knowledge. The Sectarian Age from 1300 to 1700 included the *bhakti* movement of religious devotionalism. The Modern Age began round 1700. During this age there was the growing political presence of European nations in India and, beginning at about the same time, exchange and spread of Hindu wisdom and tradition, later including yoga, to the West (see Chapter 7). During early periods, Hindu wisdom and tradition had also spread eastward throughout South and Southeast Asia (historically known as "Further India"; see Chapters 35 and 36).

PHILOSOPHY OF YOGA

PATANJALI'S *YOGA SUTRA*

Of the literature arising from the eras outlined above, Patanjali's *Yoga Sutra* is one of the most definitive works on yoga and remains widely studied in modern times. It provides an overview of the goals, philosophy, and structure of a yoga and meditation practice. *Sutra* means "thread" and the *Yoga Sutra* contains aphorisms that provide a thread that strings together ideas and thoughts related to yoga. The *Yoga Sutra* consists of 195 *sutra*s that are presented in four *padas*, or chapters: 1. *Samadhi-pada*, chapter on Ecstasy (Higher States of Awareness); 2. *Sadhana pada*, chapter on the Path of Realization; 3. *Vibhuta-pada*, chapter on the Powers; and 4. *Kaivaly-pada*, chapter on Liberation. The second aphorism in the first chapter defines yoga by stating in Sanskrit, *"Yogash chitta-vritti-nirodhah."* Translations include "Yoga is the restriction of the whirls of consciousness" (Feuerstein, 2001a) and "Yoga is that by which we still the fluctuations of the mind" (Keller, 2012). While the aphorisms seem simple on the surface, there are many books written on the translation and meaning of these basic teachings.

In second and third chapters, Patanjali sets forth the eight limbs of yoga, also known as *ashtanga* (*ashta* = eight; *anga* = limbs). (Not to be confused with the *style* of yoga called Ashtanga, which is widely practiced in the West.) The eight limbs are as follows (Feuerstein, 2001b; Keller, 2012):
1. Discipline (*Yama*)

    There are five *Yamas* related to moral discipline and ethics: Non-harming or non-violence (*Ahimsa*), Truthfulness (*Satya*), Non-stealing (*Asteya*), Continence (*Brahmacarya*), and Non-possessiveness (*Aparigraha*).
2. Restraint (*Niyama*)

    There are also five *Niyama*s related to self-restraint and internal observances: Purity (*Shauca*), Contentment (*Samtosha*), Austerity (*Tapas*), Study (*Svadhyana*), and Surrender and devotion to God (*Ishvara-Pranidhana*).
3. Posture (*Asana*)
4. Breath Control (*Pranayama*)
5. Sense—Withdrawal (*Pratyahara*)
6. Concentration (*Dharana*)
7. Meditation (*Dhyana*)
8. Ecstasy (*Samadhi*)

The first two limbs, *Yama* and *Niyama*, provide the guidance to create the proper external interactions and internal environment in preparation for, and as part of, the path of self-transcendence. The third limb, *Asana*, takes the process into the body. The fourth limb, *Pranayama*, is the regulation of the life force *Prana* (explained below) by controlling the breath. Control of the breath combined with the practice of physical postures leads to withdraw of the senses to external stimuli, which is the fifth limb, *Pratyahara*. The process of sensory inhibition creates the setting for concentration, *Dharana*, the sixth limb. *Dharana* involves focus on a single object, which may be attention to a particular part of the body, a mantra, or an object of devotion (such as a deity). As *Dharana* is steadily practiced, it becomes meditation, or *Dhyana*, the seventh limb of the eightfold path. During meditation, the mind is still, there is a peaceful disposition, and attention is paid to inner awareness. Ultimately the final limb may be reached, which is *Samadhi*.

This state is difficult to describe because it is so different from everyday life. According to the translation and interpretation of the aphorism, it involves merging with the point of focus so that what remains is only pure awareness (Keller, 2012).

BRANCHES (SCHOOLS) OF YOGA

During the time the *Upanishads* were recorded, and beyond, the tradition and teachings of yoga were passed down from teacher to student in oral tradition by word of mouth. As time progressed, new teachings were added, and others were left out or changed. The result was the formation of schools or branches of yoga representing distinct traditions (Feuerstein, 2001c). Despite the diversity among the schools, they all have the same common goal. In his book *The Yoga Tradition*, Georg Feuerstein described the schools of yoga as spokes on a wheel, where the rim symbolizes the *Yamas* and *Niyamas* and the hub is the single center, self-transcendence (*Samadhi*), as common goal and result of the practices set forth by the different branches (Figure 21-1).

Hatha Yoga is a branch of yoga focused on developing the body's potential to prepare for self-transcendence. It can be considered a system to purify the body. It is the most explicitly physical, and, perhaps not surprising, is the branch of yoga most widely practiced in the West. However, Western practitioners of *Hatha Yoga* do not always adhere to the ethical principles or spiritual goals of this yoga, and in some cases it is used solely for the purposes of physical fitness and social interactions. There are many styles of *Hatha Yoga* as discussed in the next section of this chapter.

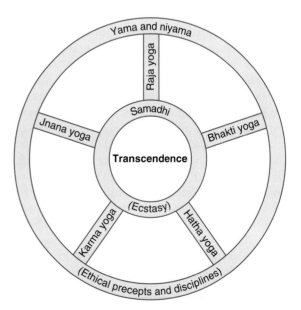

Figure 21-1 The schools of yoga. (Adapted with permission from Feuerstein G: The wheel of yoga. *In The Yoga Tradition: Its History, Literature, Philosophy, and Practice*, Prescott, AZ, 2001, Hohm Press.)

Raja Yoga is a branch of yoga involving adherence to the eightfold path described by Patanjali in the *Yoga Sutra,* with the main practice being meditation. *Raja* means "royal." This name may reflect a belief that *Raja Yoga* is superior to *Hatha Yoga* because traditionally it called for a monastic life needing years of practice and meditation to master. It is also possible that this path is known by this name because it was practiced by kings (Feuerstein, 2001c).

Bhakti means "devotion," and *Bhakti Yoga* is the path of devotion and commitment to the love of the Divine as the Beloved (Bhajan, 2003c; Feuerstein, 2001c). This devotion can take place as worship in song, ritual action, or meditation. The final moment of transcendence is when the practitioner merges with the Divine in a state of pure love.

Jnana (*Gyana*) means "knowledge" or "wisdom," and *Jnana Yoga* is the path of wisdom associated with discerning the Real without the subconscious clouding the clarity (Bhajan, 2003c; Feuerstein, 2001c). This path involves deep exploration, contemplation, or study to achieve direct knowledge of the Divine and eliminating what is illusion.

Karma Yoga is the Yoga of Action. *Karma Yoga* is based on the teachings of the *Bhagavad-Gita,* which describes an inner attitude to the actions of daily living. The action is selfless activity that transcends the ego and is a means to merger with the Divine (Feuerstein, 2001c; Miryala et al, 2011).

ENERGY ANATOMY

NADIS

Western anatomy is classified into distinct organ systems, whereas yogic anatomy is based on a completely different concept of subtle energy (see Chapter 14). The idea of life force is found in many traditions, and in the yogic tradition it is called *Prana*. *Prana* was described in the *Vedas* and elaborated in the *Upanishads.* The information presented in this section is discussed as it is set forth in the yogic literature. *Prana* moves through the human body through energy channels known as *nadis*. There are 72,000 *nadis* mentioned in yogic texts with three main pathways, which are the *ida,* the *pingala,* and the *sushumna.* The *sushumna* is known as the central channel. It begins at the base of the spine and ends at the top of the head. The *ida* and *pingala* also begin at the base of the spine, the *ida* on the left and the *pingala* on the right. Because these *nadis* are subtle energy channels and are not physical structures, the exact path of the channels is described in different ways in modern interpretations of the yogic texts. The most common description is that the *ida* and *pingala* wind around the *sushumna* like a helix, crossing at the *chakras* (described below) and that the *ida* ends at the left nostril and the *pingala* ends at the right nostril. Another description is that the *ida* and *pingala* terminate at the sixth *chakra* (*ajna*) between the eyebrows but are connected to the left and right nostrils. The qualities of the *ida* and *pingala* as well as their role in *pranayama,* breath practices controlling the flow of *Prana,* are discussed in the next section.

VAYUS

Prana is considered the life force, and this life force is in constant movement. This movement, in turn, has an organization. In the human body, this organization means that *Prana* (with a capital "P") is divided into different "frequencies" or types of motion within different areas of the body. These subdivisions of *Prana* are known as the *vayus* and are taught in the *Upanishads.* The description of the *vayus* and their relation to regular bodily functions is as follows (Bhajan, 2003d; Keller, 2013).

The first *vayu* is *prana* with a lowercase "p." The physical location of this *vayu* is between the base of the heart and the neck in the thoracic area. It is linked to the function of the lungs and inspiration. The motion of *prana* is the expansion of the lungs to bring about inhalation, thereby receiving the essential energy, *Prana,* contained air that is breathed. The experience is expansive and stimulating.

The second *vayu* is *apana.* The physical location is below the navel, and it governs all functions related to elimination. This includes the voiding of urine, passage of stools, elimination of menstrual blood, ejaculation of semen, and delivery of the fetus. The experience of *apana* is grounding, calming, and rooted.

The third *vayu* is *samana.* The physical location is between the heart and the navel, that is, between the space of *prana* and *apana.* It is linked to digestion and assimilation. Strong *samana* also aids in discrimination and emotional clarity.

The fourth *vayu* is *udana.* The physical location is in the larynx and upward into the head. *Udana* throws the air up and out. It is the upward force of exhalation that powers speech and expression. It is also involved in the energy of expelling through vomiting. Strong *udana* allows the power to project and create with speech and one's words.

The fifth *vayu* is *vyana.* *Vyana* pervades the entire body and fascia. It governs the overall coordination of movement and muscles and joints throughout the body. When it is strong, there is a sense of interconnectedness and flow.

The *vayu*s also have a function in *pranayama* and meditation. But before describing these teachings from the yogic texts, it is necessary to introduce a few more concepts on yogic anatomy and techniques because all of these are integrated into the final description on the energy of self-transformation or enlightenment. The next element of yogic anatomy is the *chakras.*

CHAKRAS

The word *chakra* means "wheel." *Chakras* are energy centers or energy vortices, which are part of the yogic subtle energy system located along the *sushumna* (Figure 21-2). Like the *nadis,* the *chakras* are not physical structures but they do correspond to the location of various organ or glandular systems or nerve plexuses in Western anatomy. In yogic texts, the *chakras* are referred to metaphorically as lotuses, and each *chakra* has a certain number of petals, increasing in number from the bottom to the top of the spine

4. *Anahata*: located at the heart and corresponds to the cardiac plexus and the heart, lungs, and thymus gland. It is associated with the element air and is related to the qualities of compassion, kindness, forgiveness, and love.
5. *Vishuddha*: located at the throat and corresponds to the laryngeal plexus and the trachea, throat, and thyroid gland. It is associated with the element ether and is the center for truth, language, knowledge, and the ability to communicate effectively.
6. *Ajna*: located in the brain between the eyes and corresponds to the cavernous plexus and the pituitary gland. It also known as the "third eye" and is related to the qualities of intuition, concentration, and determination.
7. *Sahasrara*: located at the crown of the head and corresponds to the pineal gland. It is associated with unity, spiritual elevation, and enlightenment.

LOCKS (*BANDHAS*) AND *MUDRAS*

While not strictly part of yogic anatomy, the description of *bandhas* is included here because they direct the flow of *prana* and *apana* as described below. They are techniques known as "muscle locks," or muscular contractions that are consciously or intentionally applied to certain body areas. These techniques can be used with certain *asanas* or in conjunction with *pranayama*. There are three main *bandhas*: *Jalandhar bandha* (neck lock), *Uddiyana bandha* (diaphragm lock), and *Mulabandha* (root lock). Descriptions of the locks are provided to explain the concepts. However, it is best to learn these locks by observing demonstrations of their performance and practicing under the detailed guidance of a yoga teacher.

Neck lock is achieved by lifting the chest and sternum upward while stretching the chin toward the back of the neck. For the diaphragm lock, the abdominal region is pulled upward and toward the spine. Diaphragm lock is never performed on a full stomach and is only performed with the breath fully exhaled. The root lock is done by contracting the muscles around the anal sphincter, the sex organs, and the lower abdominal muscles. When all three locks are applied together, it is known as *Maha bandha* (the great lock) or *Traya bandha* (triple lock).

Mudras, or "seals," also guide energy flow. They involve particular positions of the hands that cultivate a corresponding state of mind. There are many *mudras* described and used in different yoga traditions (Feuerstein, 2001d). One of the most common is *gyan mudra* (seal of knowledge). In *gyan mudra* the thumb touches the tip of the index finger while the other three fingers remain straight and touching each other. This hand position is said to stimulate knowledge and to give receptivity and calmness. It is often used during meditation.

ENERGY FLOW

One of the yogic teachings on how higher states of consciousness may be reached is through the movement of

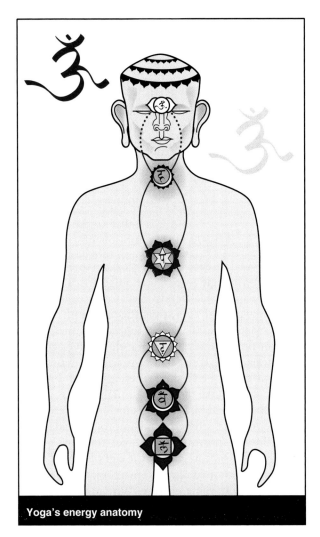

Yoga's energy anatomy

Figure 21-2 Symbolic representation of the yogic nadi and chakra model.

(Sturgess, 1997b). A summary of the *chakras*, their location, qualities, and corresponding elements is as follows (Bhajan, 2003e, Sturgess, 1997b):
1. *Muladhara*: located at the perineum and corresponds to the coccygeal nerve plexus and the organs of elimination. It is associated with the element earth and survival instincts and is related to the qualities of being grounded, centered, secure, loyal, and stable.
2. *Svadhisthana*: located at the genitals and corresponds to the sacral plexus and the reproductive organs, kidneys, and bladder. It is associated with the element water and related to the qualities of patience, creativity, and responsible relationships.
3. *Manipura*: located at the navel point and corresponds to the solar plexus and the liver, gallbladder, spleen, small intestines, stomach, pancreas, and adrenal glands. It is associated with the element fire, and it is the center of personal power and commitment. It is related to the qualities include self-esteem, identity, and judgment.

energy along the *sushumna* to the *sahasrara* (Crown) *chakra*. As the energy moves upward, the *chakras* become balanced and the pituitary and pineal glands are activated. The energy being raised is called *Kundalini* energy, and it is considered to be the fundamental energy of consciousness that lies dormant at the base of the spine. The concepts of yogic anatomy—the *nadis*, *vayu*s, and *chakras*—are involved this process as are the physical techniques of *pranayama*, meditation, mantra, *asnana*, and the *bandhas*.

The first components are the *prana* and *apana vayu*s. Inhalation involves the *prana vayu*, while the exhalation involves the *apana vayu*. These two *vayu*s work in opposition: *prana* moves upwards and *apana* moves downwards. Note that this description refers to the flow of the energy and not the movement of the breath, because the breath paradoxically is moving in the opposite direction as the energy flow (Keller, 2013). The balance of the *prana* and *apana vayu*s during *pranayama* takes place in the *samana vayu*, which is located in between these two *vayu*s. It is at this point that the energies begin to merge by reversing their directions. Through inhalation and retention, *prana* is directed down to the *manipura* (Navel) *chakra*. This creates a tremendous heat, not in regard to temperature, but what is described as a "white" heat.

Through breath control and mental direction these integrative energies can descend from the Navel *chakra* to the *muladhara* (Root) *chakra*, where they stimulate the *Kundalini* energy. Then through the power of the breath, along with various postures and the *bandhas*, the energy channels can be cleared of any "blockages" so that the energy may flow along the *sushumna*. Because the *udana vayu* is power behind speech, mantra vocalization is also one of the techniques that may be used in this process of clearing the energy channels. In order to raise the *Kundalini* energy, the pressure of the root lock can bring the energy to the Navel *chakra*. Application of the diaphragm lock will bring the energy up to the *vishuddha* (Throat) *chakra*, where it can then be brought up to the pituitary and pineal gland by using the neck lock. When the pituitary and pineal gland are stimulated, the gate to the Crown *chakra* opens (Bhajan, 2003d). Finally, *vyana vayu* may provide the experience of union with the all-pervasive consciousness (Keller, 2013).

These concepts are rather abstract to the Western way of thinking, but they present a general representation how self-transcendence, *Samadhi*, or enlightenment is achieved. The following section focuses on the physical practices used to channel the flow and to balance the energy. It also presents the Western science that supports some of the mechanisms described in the yogic texts.

ELEMENTS OF PHYSICAL YOGA PRACTICE

As mentioned above, Hatha yoga is the most widely practiced branch of yoga in the West. There are, in turn, many styles within Hatha yoga itself, including Anada, Ashtanga, Bikram, Integral, Iyengar, Kripalu, Kundalini, Sivananda, Viniyoga, and Vinyasa. These styles range from vigorous to gentle, with varying degrees of emphasis on the precision of the postures. Some styles still maintain a stronger emphasis on psychological and spiritual growth. Brief descriptions of these styles, as well as their developers and centers, are provided on the *Yoga Journal* website (Yoga Journal Editors, 2013a) and in the book *Your Brain on Yoga* (Khalsa & Gould, 2012). Although some styles may place more emphasis on one element of yoga or another, the elements of an authentic Hatha yoga practice include physical postures, breathing techniques, deep relaxation, and meditation.

POSTURES (*ASANAS*)

There are several categories of physical postures performed in yoga. They include seated, standing, twisting, and arm balance postures; backbends and forward bends; side stretches; inversions; core-strengthening; and restorative postures (McCall, 2007; Yoga Journal Editors, 2013b). Most of the physical postures are labeled with original Sanskrit names and are consistent as practiced across the different yoga styles. Performing these postures provides a systematic way to take the body through various ranges of motion. Obvious physical benefits include increasing flexibility and muscle strength and improving balance and posture. Specific postures also direct the flow of *prana*, and *apana* and *asanas* are part of the eight limbs of yoga on the path to self-transcendence. Therefore, taken as a comprehensive system, these postures have more far-reaching benefits according to the yogic tradition than simply increasing flexibility and strength.

CONTROL OF *PRANA* THROUGH BREATHING PRACTICES (*PRANAYAMA*)

As described above, *Prana* is the life force in the yogic anatomy. *Pranayama* is the control of the movement of *Prana* through the use of breathing techniques. There are many kinds of yogic breathing techniques, each with specific effects.

Long Deep Breathing

One of the simplest techniques is long deep breathing. This breath utilizes the full vital capacity of the lungs: inhaling and (1) letting the belly expand and the air move into the lower portion of the lungs, then (2) expanding the chest to fill the middle part of the lungs, and (3) finally, lifting the chest to fill the upper part of the lungs. The exhale is done in reverse order: releasing the air from the top, then middle, then bottom of the lungs. One of the benefits of long deep breathing is that it is calming and relaxing as accompanied by an increase in parasympathetic nervous system dominance (see Chapter 8). This type of *pranayama* is commonly performed during the practice of yoga. Beneficial effects on lung physiology can carry over even when the practitioner returns to breathing normally, as demonstrated in a study on the chemoreflex response.

Chemoreflex receptors trigger breathing and chemoreflex sensitivity is often increased in individuals with chronic heart failure, resulting in dyspnea and reduced tolerance to exercise. Therefore, decreasing chemoreflex sensitivity is beneficial for these patients. To determine the role of long deep breathing and yoga practice on the chemoreflex response, yoga practitioners were compared to non-yoga practitioners. Long deep breathing (6 breaths per minute) decreased chemoreflex sensitivity in *both* yoga practitioners and non-practitioners. But only yoga practitioners appeared to have a longer term benefit in that chemoreflex sensitivity remained lower even during spontaneous breathing or breathing at 15 breaths per minute (Spicuzza et al, 2000). Yoga practitioners had a baseline of decreased chemoreflex sensitivity that persisted even when not actually performing long deep breathing.

Individual Nostril Breathing/Alternate Nostril Breathing

Individual nostril breathing stimulates the *ida* and *pingala* energy channels and has effects related to the qualities of these channels. The *ida* is associated with the "moon energy." It has cooling and receptive characteristics and is associated with calmness, sensitivity, empathy, and synthesis. The *pingala* is associated with the "sun energy." It has warming and projective characteristics and is associated with vigor, alertness, will-power, concentration, and a readiness for action. As mentioned earlier, the *ida* and *pingala* are subtle energy structures and have no currently detectible physical structures in the human body. However, they resemble the characteristics of the sympathetic and parasympathetic nervous systems, or the "yin" (moon, etc.) and "yang" (sun, etc.) phases in Chinese cosmology (Chapter 28) and constitutional medicine (see Chapter 31). Because the *ida* ends at the left nostril, breathing through the left nostril is a calming breath. Left nostril breathing may result in a reduction of sympathetic activity as demonstrated by an increase in volar galvanic skin resistance (Telles et al, 1994). Because the *pingala* ends at the right nostril, breathing through the right nostril is an energizing breath that also improves alertness and focus. Right nostril breathing has been shown to stimulate the sympathetic nervous system as measured by increased heart rate and peripheral vasoconstriction, resulting in decreased digit pulse volume (Shannahoff-Khalsa & Kenney, 1993; Telles et al, 1996).

Another regulated yoga breathing technique is alternate nostril breathing that can be performed by inhaling through the left, exhaling through the right, then inhaling through the right, exhaling through the left (*Nadi Shodhana*). As part of a more advanced practice, certain breath retentions and breath ratios are added. According to yogic theory, alternate nostril breathing is said to purify the *ida* and *pingala* and to balance the right and left hemispheres of the brain.

From the yogic perspective, breathing through the right nostril stimulates the left side of the brain, and breathing through the left nostril stimulates the right side of the brain. Research studies support these effects of individual nostril breathing. There is a natural nasal cycle related to relative congestion/decongestion of the nasal passages, which in turn results in more predominant airflow in one nostril versus the other at a given point in time. The nasal mucosae are densely innervated with autonomic fibers, and it is the autonomic nervous system that regulates the congestion/decongestion. Sympathetic dominance in one nostril produces vasoconstriction and decongestion, allowing for greater airflow. Simultaneous parasympathetic dominance occurs in the contralateral nostril, resulting in vasodilation and congestion, which restricts airflow. The hypothalamus is thought to be responsible for regulating the nasal cycle. The length of the cycle varies and may be from 25 minutes to 8 hours. But, in general, the average cycle lasts approximately 1.5 to 4 hours and takes place 24 hours per day.

The natural nasal cycle has been shown to have a direct relationship to the cerebral hemispheric activity as measured by electroencephalogram (EEG) (Werntz et al, 1983). During the portion of the nasal cycle when airflow is predominantly through the right nostril, EEG activity is greater in the left hemisphere; and when airflow is predominantly through the left nostril, the EEG activity was greater in the right hemisphere. By performing forced nostril breathing through one nostril at a time, the ability to shift the contralateral dominance in hemispheric activity was measured. In this study, participants were asked to close off the more open nostril and breathe through the opposite, more closed nostril, and then alternate sides for 11 to 20 minutes. As predicted, while breathing through the right nostril, the EEG amplitude in the left hemisphere is enhanced; then, upon changing to the left nostril, the enhanced EEG activity switches to the right hemisphere (Werntz et al, 1987).

Another study was done to assess whether there is any change observed in functional activities among the two cerebral hemispheres when forced nostril breathing is applied (Shannahoff-Khalsa et al, 1991). Verbal and spatial tests were administered before and after breathing though the right nostril, the left nostril, and both nostrils for 30 minutes. The results showed that right nostril breathing results in higher verbal scores; left nostril breathing results in higher spatial test scores; there were no significant changes while breathing through both nostrils. The greatest improvements were observed in the groups with the forced nostril breathing through the nostril that was initially dominant. These studies suggest that the nasal cycle and alternating cerebral dominance are closely correlated; and by using forced nostril yogic breathing techniques, it is possible to influence cognitive performance. A proposed mechanism for these findings is that decreased cognitive performance is related to decreased cerebral blood flow caused by vasoconstriction of the cerebral blood vessels. Because the majority of autonomic nerve fibers travel ipsilaterally and do not cross over (Saper et al, 1976), enhanced sympathetic activity on one side of the body would result in increased airflow in that nostril, and decreased cerebral blood flow with diminished cognitive function in the ipsilateral hemisphere (Shannahoff-Khalsa et al, 1991).

The nasal cycle is also a marker for various physiological states, and one theory is that the hypothalamus not only regulates the nasal cycle but also regulates the coupled ultradian rhythms of the other body systems, including the neuroendocrine, cardiovascular, and immune systems (Shannahoff-Khalsa et al, 1996). There is a resting phase and activity phase of these cycles, originally proposed as the "basic rest-activity cycle" (BRAC). Because of the association of the *ida* and *pingala* to the right and left nostrils and the nasal cycle in being tied to multiple body rhythms, the resting phase may be the equivalent of the *ida* and the activity phase may be the equivalent of the *pingala* (Shannahoff-Khalsa, 2007).

Fast Breathing

Depending on the style of yoga practiced, different types of fast breathing may also be incorporated. These types of breathing include *Bhastrika*, Breath of Fire, and *Kapalabhati*. Both *Bhastrika* (bellows) and Breath of Fire comprise breathing with rapid and forceful inhalation and exhalation through the nose. Both breaths are stimulating, raising vital energy levels, increasing alertness, and, according to yogic teachings, both balance the nervous system. Breath of Fire is less forceful than *Bhastrika*. In *Kapalabhati* the inhalation is long and mild and the exhalation is forceful and rapid. *Kapalabhati* can be done at either slow speeds of 60 exhales per minute or at fast speeds of 240 exhales per minute (Sturgess, 1997a). *Kapalabhati* is considered a cleansing breath.

Other Breathing Techniques

The long deep breathing, alternate nostril breathing, and fast breathing techniques represent main types of *Pranayama*. There are also additional breathing techniques observed to have specific benefits. Some brief explanations and examples include a common breath known as *Ujjayi Pranayama*. During *Ujjayi* breath the glottis, above the trachea, or airway, is partially closed and the breath becomes audible to produce a balancing and calming effect. *Sitali Pranayama* is another type of breath that has a cooling effect on the body. It is performed with the tongue sticking out (like panting) and curled, and inhaling through the curled tongue. *Bhramari Pranayama* (humming bee breath), a breath that calms the mind, is performed by closing off the ears with the fingers and making a high pitched humming sound on the exhale.

MEDITATION

Meditation is the seventh of the eight limbs of the path of self-transcendence set forth in the Patanjali's *Yoga Sutra*. Here, meditation is known as *dhyana* and is a component of most modern yoga practices. The sixth limb, concentration, or *dharana*, "holding of the mind in a motionless state," is considered an early step in meditation. "One-

pointedness" of attention (*ekagrata*) has been described as the mechanism of concentration, and "one flowingness" (*ekatanata*) has been described as the mechanism of meditation (Feuerstein, 2001b). Modern definitions of meditation include Focused Attention (FA) and Open Monitoring (OM) (Lutz et al, 2008). FA meditation involves voluntary focusing of attention on a chosen object and may be comparable to the concentration aspect of *dharana*, whereas OM meditation involves being attentive in each moment to anything that occurs in the experience without focusing on any explicit object (this might remind you of the Western adaption of Mindfulness; see Chapters 7 and 10).

Although it can be difficult to completely define the *dhyana* state, OM meditation may be equivalent to or contain the core qualities of *dhyana*. The concentration aspect of yoga is an integrated part of both the *asanas* and the *pranayama* practices. The meditation aspect of yoga may also be achieved while holding a posture, or doing a breathing exercise, or it may be done as a separate component, usually following the performance of the *asanas*.

FA and OM meditations, which may be an element of yoga practice, have been shown to stimulate different areas of the brain. FA has been shown to activate the dorsal anterior cingulate cortex involved in conflict monitoring. OM meditation has been shown to activate the orbital inferior frontal gyrus, the medial anterior prefrontal cortex, and the rostral anterior cingulate cortex, which are all involved in self-referential processing (Manna et al, 2010). The amount of meditation experience also influences the pattern of activation. Activation was measured during FA meditation in multiple brain regions implicated in monitoring, attention orienting, and engaging attention (Brefczynski-Lewis et al, 2007). Experienced meditators showed a peak of rapid activation of these regions compared to non-meditators. The most experienced meditators returned to a below-baseline state, whereas less experienced meditators maintained an increased state of activation following the initial peak. These results suggest that the experienced meditators may have a less cognitively active mental state, requiring reduced meditative effort, compared to less experienced meditators. Finally, the patterns of brain activity in monks during OM meditation represented their ordinary resting brain state, whereas there was a great contrast in activity between the FA and the OM meditation states among the same individuals (Manna et al, 2010). These results suggest that the open monitoring state for experienced meditators may become a more sustained way of being even in daily life.

From an Eastern perspective, one of the results of meditation and certain yoga styles, such as *Kundalini* yoga (with an emphasis on bringing energy up the *sushumna*), is the stimulation of the pineal gland. Note that although the pineal gland is often called the "vestigial third eye" embryologically, this differs somewhat from the nomenclature used in chakra system, where the "third eye" is considered to be the *ajna chakra* associated with the pituitary gland. The pineal gland produces the hormone melatonin, which has many functions, including: regulation of the sleep–wake cycle, modulating reproductive development, influencing mood, and regulating hunger and satiety. Melatonin is also a powerful antioxidant and has immune-enhancing activity, which may, in turn, ameliorate the stress response (Wisneski & Anderson, 2009). In order to determine the effect of yoga and meditation on the production of melatonin, melatonin levels were measured before and after a 3-month yoga program consisting of *asanas, pranayama,* and meditation of chanting "OM" (Harinath et al, 2004). The night-time production of melatonin was significantly increased following the yoga program compared to a control group performing physical exercises and playing games in place of the yoga and meditation. Improved well-being was also significantly correlated with increased melatonin levels. Given the regulation of melatonin on several body systems and functions and its role as an antioxidant, increased melatonin production may result in some of the health benefits of yoga and meditation (see Table 21-1). The association of the pineal gland with the *sahasrara chakra* and the relationship of this *chakra* to the quality of enlightenment allows for speculation of how activation of this area may be extrapolated to the path of achieving enlightenment according to yogic tradition.

Mantra

Mantra is used during meditation in several yoga styles. The reasons why the use of mantra contributes to a meditative effect are not fully understood. One mechanism may be due to the rhythm of the chant, which results in slowing down the breath. In a study comparing the physiological effects of chanting while using either a yogic mantra or the *Ave Maria* recited in Latin, the spectrum of changes in respiration, diastolic blood pressure, and microcerebral blood flow velocity were all nearly identical in both forms. These patterns, in turn, were in contrast to patterns measured during spontaneous breathing (Bernardi et al, 2001) (see also Chapters 9 and 10).

One effect of the mantras was that the breath was slowed to about 6 breaths per minute. Because breathing at 6 breaths per minute had effects on respiratory variability and baroreflex (blood pressure) sensitivity similar to those of the mantras, the slowing of the breath as a result of the chanting may have been responsible for the observed effects. According to the yogic tradition, the effects of mantra are thought to also be due to the meaning of the words that are chanted, and to the vibration of the sound that is generated by annunciating the words. One theory postulates that the pronunciation of certain mantras causes the stimulation of the 84 meridian points on the roof of the mouth: 32 pairs of points are located along the inside of the teeth, and 20 more points are located in a U shape on the central part of the palate. The tongue moves and touches, and vibrations stimulate, these points when chanting, which is then thought to stimulate the hypothalamus gland (Bhajan, 2003b). Meridian points on the roof of the mouth are also recognized in Chinese medicine.

However, no research has been done to date to test the theory of the stimulation of these points using mantra.

YOGA THERAPY AND HEALTH BENEFITS

Whereas yoga historically is known as a path to spiritual enlightenment, the physical and mental benefits of yoga are becoming widely recognized. Yoga is being incorporated in places such as cancer centers throughout the United States as well as in institutions such as the Department of Veterans Affairs (VA), which incorporates yoga in its post-traumatic stress disorder (PTSD) treatment programs (Libby et al, 2012). Yoga therapy, as a professional practice, is in a relatively early stage in the United States. The International Association of Yoga Therapists (IYTA) published Educational Standards for the Training of Yoga Therapists in 2012 and is beginning the process of accrediting yoga therapy programs that meet these standards. However, yoga therapy is not new, and the clinical application of yoga as a therapeutic intervention first began in 1918 at the Yoga Institute at Versova in Mumbai, India (Khalsa, 2004). The Kaivalyadhama Yoga Institute in Lonavala, Maharashtra, India, under Swami Kuvalayananda, was established a few years later (Khalsa, 2004). Kuvalayananda began the first research on the psychophysiological effects of yoga in the 1920s and published the first yoga specialty journal in 1924, called *Yoga Mimamsa.* Yoga research has since spread to the United States, and there are now studies supporting the use of yoga for various physical and mental diseases and disorders. Table 21-1 shows a list of the most widely researched health conditions categorized according to body system.

According the conclusions of the review articles and meta-analyses cited in Table 21-1, the health conditions with the strongest research evidence for the benefits of yoga include heart disease and hypertension. It is noted, however, that most of the studies on heart disease involved a more "holistic" approach that also included a dietary modification and an exercise program in addition to a yoga component. Conditions that are likely to be benefitted by yoga based on reasonably strong research evidence include: back pain, chronic pain, diabetes, depression, fibromyalgia, osteoarthritis, and rheumatoid arthritis. Studies of yoga with cancer patients have shown improvements in quality of life, sleep, anxiety, depression, perceived stress, and psychological distress. In women with breast cancer, yoga practice has also resulted in improved quality of life as well as function, social, spiritual, and emotional well-being. Short-term positive psychological effects of yoga have also been measured for women in menopause. For a variety of illnesses involving fatigue, yoga has been most beneficial for fatigue related to cancer or cancer treatment. Positive results have been reported for yoga using anxiety as an outcome measure in a variety of health conditions (Sharma et al, 2013; Sharma & Haider, 2013), but the use of yoga for anxiety disorders per se has not been widely studied.

TABLE 21-1 *Most Widely Studied Health Conditions Showing Benefit Using Yoga Interventions*

Body system and health condition	Meta-Analyses/Reviews/Summaries[a]
Circulatory	
Heart disease	1 Review (Raub, 2002)
Hypertension	1 Meta-analysis (Hagins et al, 2013)
	1 Systematic review (Innes et al, 2005)
	2 Reviews (Okonta, 2012; Raub, 2002)
Endocrine	
Diabetes	3 Systematic reviews (Aljasir et al, 2010; Innes et al, 2005; Innes & Vincent, 2007)
Immune	
Rheumatoid arthritis	1 Meta-analysis (Ward et al, 2013)
	2 Reviews (Haaz & Bartlett, 2011; Cramer et al, 2013c)
Muscular	
Back pain	2 Meta-analysis (Cramer et al, 2013a; Ward et al, 2013)
	1 Systematic review (Posadzki & Ernst, 2011b)
	2 Reviews (Hill, 2013; Kelly, 2009)
Nervous	
Anxiety (and anxiety disorders including post-traumatic stress disorder)	1 Systematic review (Kirkwood et al, 2005)
	1 Review (Telles et al, 2012)
	1 Summary (Saeed et al, 2010)
Depression	1 Meta-analysis (Cramer et al, 2013b)
	1 Systematic review (Balasubramaniam et al, 2012)
	2 Reviews (Pilkington et al, 2005; Uebelacker et al, 2010)
	1 Summary (Saeed et al, 2010)
Reproductive	
Breast cancer	2 Meta-analyses (Zhang et al, 2012; Cramer et al, 2012a)
	1 Systematic review (Harder et al, 2012)
	1 Review (Levine & Balk, 2012)
Menopausal symptoms	1 Meta-analysis (Cramer et al, 2012b)
	1 Systematic review (Lee et al, 2009)
Respiratory	
Asthma	1 Systematic review (Posadzki & Ernst, 2011a)
	1 Review (Raub, 2002)
Skeletal	
Osteoarthritis	1 Meta-analysis (Ward et al, 2013)
	3 Reviews (Haaz & Bartlett, 2011; Raub, 2002; Cramer et al, 2013c)
Multiple Systems	
Cancer	2 Meta-analyses (Buffart et al, 2012; Lin et al, 2011)
	1 Systematic reviews (Sharma et al, 2013)
	2 Reviews (Bower et al, 2005; Smith & Pukall, 2009)
Fatigue	1 Meta-analysis (Boehm et al, 2012)
Fibromyalgia	1 Meta-analysis (Ward et al, 2013)
	1 Systematic review (Cramer et al, 2013c)
Chronic pain	1 Meta-analysis (Bussing et al, 2012)
	1 Systematic review (Posadzki et al, 2011c)

[a]Adapted from Table 1 from Bussing & Michalsen (2012), with updates.

However, there has been recent interest in the use of yoga for one particular anxiety disorder, PTSD, and several research studies are being performed. The results of one pilot study provides evidence that yoga may be helpful for reducing the hyperarousal symptoms of PTSD and for improving sleep quality (Staples et al, 2013). Finally, research on asthma to date has shown mixed results on the effectiveness of yoga for symptom improvement, and further studies are needed.

There are several proposed mechanisms on how yoga may benefit health. Stress is an underlying factor in many diseases and disorders (see Chapter 10). The cost to the body for maintaining stability and coping in the presence of chronic stress is termed allostatic load (Streeter et al, 2012; Taylor et al, 2010). One recent theory on the benefits of yoga is that it reduces allostatic load and restores optimal homeostasis (Streeter et al, 2012). Stress is associated with decreased activity of the neurotransmitter gamma amino-butyric acid (GABA) and just 1 hour of yoga practice increased thalamic GABA levels compared to 1 hour of reading (Streeter et al, 2007). Increased GABA production by yoga may be a mechanism for benefiting conditions such as major depressive disorder, PTSD, and chronic pain, which are characterized by low GABA activity.

Oxidative stress has also been linked to several diseases, such as heart disease, cancer, rheumatoid arthritis, hypertension, Alzheimer's disease, and Parkinson's disease (Martarelli et al, 2011). Increased oxidative stress also leads to increased inflammation and the production of proinflammatory cytokines, which also play a role in most of the diseases above in addition to osteoporosis and diabetes (Kiecolt-Glaser et al, 2010). Yoga, including yogic breathing practices, have been shown to increase antioxidant formation (Martarelli et al, 2011; Sharma et al, 2003; Sinha et al, 2007) and decrease the production of proinflammatory cytokines (Kiecolt-Glaser et al, 2010), suggesting that these may be other mechanisms by which yoga helps protect against disease. Other possible mechanisms by which yoga may improve health include increasing melatonin production, decreasing cortisol levels, decreasing sympathetic activity and increasing parasympathetic activity, and regulating the hypothalamic-pituitary-adrenal axis (McCall, 2013).

SUMMARY

Although the origin of yoga is located thousands of years ago, during the last century yogic techniques have been studied from a scientific perspective. The ancient yogic teachings were based on empirical observation and experience. It is likely that the understanding of the mechanisms of yoga were fostered by an enhanced sense of awareness as a result of the yoga practice itself. Many of the yogic teachings, especially those related to energy anatomy, may seem unusual and incomprehensible to the Western way of viewing the body and its systems. However, science and technology have begun to validate the teachings of the yogic texts. If the elements of yoga are viewed and practiced only for the purpose of improving health, yoga is a useful adjunct to Western medicine because it helps alleviate some of the underlying contributors of many diseases. However, yoga is likely to have the most powerful and comprehensive effects when studied and practiced as a complete system for health and spiritual growth in light of the interconnection of the body and the spirit.

References

Aljasir B, Bryson M, Al-Shehri B: Yoga Practice for the management of type II diabetes mellitus in adults: a systematic review, *Evid Based Complement Alternat Med* 7(4):399, 2010.

Balasubramaniam M, Telles S, Doraiswamy PM: Yoga on our minds: a systematic review of yoga for neuropsychiatric disorders, *Front Psychiatry* 3:117, 2012.

Bernardi L, Sleight P, Bandinelli G, et al: Effect of rosary prayer and yoga mantras on autonomic cardiovascular rhythms: comparative study, *BMJ* 323(7327):1446, 2001.

Bhajan Y: A brief history of yoga and Patanjali's sutras. In *The Aquarian teacher*, Santa Cruz, NM, 2003a, Kundalini Research Institute.

Bhajan Y: Sound and mantra. In *The Aquarian teacher*, Santa Cruz, NM, 2003b, Kundalini Research Institute.

Bhajan Y: The varieties of yoga. In *The Aquarian teacher*, Santa Cruz, NM, 2003c, Kundalini Research Institute.

Bhajan Y: Yogic anatomy-prana, vayus, nadis, the Kundalini and the navel point. In *The Aquarian teacher*, Santa Cruz, NM, 2003d, Kundalini Research Institute.

Bhajan Y: Yogic anatomy-the chakras. In *The Aquarian teacher*, Santa Cruz, NM, 2003e, Kundalini Research Institute.

Boehm K, Ostermann T, Milazzo S, Bussing A: Effects of yoga interventions on fatigue: a meta-analysis, *Evid Based Complement Alternat Med*, Article ID 124703, 2012.

Bower JE, Woolery A, Sternlieb B, Garet D: Yoga for cancer patients and survivors, *Cancer Control* 12(3):165, 2005.

Brefczynski-Lewis JA, Lutz A, Schaefer HS, et al: Neural correlates of attentional expertise in long-term meditation practitioners, *Proc Natl Acad Sci U S A* 104(27):11483, 2007.

Buffart LM, van Uffelen JG, Riphagen II, et al: Physical and psychosocial benefits of yoga in cancer patients and survivors, a systematic review and meta-analysis of randomized controlled trials, *BMC Cancer* 12:559, 2012.

Bussing A, Michalsen A, Khalsa SB, et al: Effects of yoga on mental and physical health: a short summary of reviews, *Evid Based Complement Alternat Med*, Article ID 165410, 2012.

Bussing A, Ostermann T, Lüdtke R, et al: Effects of yoga interventions on pain and pain-associated disability: a meta-analysis, *J Pain* 13(1):1, 2012.

Cramer H, Lange S, Klose P, et al: Yoga for breast cancer patients and survivors: a systematic review and meta-analysis, *BMC Cancer* 12:412, 2012a.

Cramer H, Lauche R, Haller H, Dobos G: A systematic review and meta-analysis of yoga for low back pain, *Clin J Pain* 29(5):450, 2013a.

Cramer H, Lauche R, Langhorst J, Dobos G: Effectiveness of yoga for menopausal symptoms: a systematic review and meta-analysis of randomized controlled trials, *Evid Based Complement Alternat Med*, Article ID 863905, 2012b.

Cramer H, Lauche R, Langhorst J, Dobos G: Yoga for depresson: a systematic review and meta-analysis, *Depress Anxiety*, 30(11): 1068–83, 2013b.

Cramer H, Lauche R, Langhorst J, Dobos G: Yoga for rheumatic diseases: a systematic review, *Rheumatology (Oxford)*, 52(11): 2025–30, 2013c.

Feuerstein G: The history and literature of Patanjala-Yoga. In *The yoga tradition: its history, literature, philosophy, and practice*, Prescott, AZ, 2001a, Hohm Press.

Feuerstein G: The philosophy and practice of Patanjala-Yoga. In *The yoga tradition: its history, literature, philosophy, and practice*, Prescott, AZ, 2001b, Hohm Press.

Feuerstein G: The wheel of yoga. In *The yoga tradition: its history, literature, philosophy, and practice*, Prescott, AZ, 2001c, Hohm Press.

Feuerstein G: *The yoga tradition: it's history literature philosophy and practice*, Prescott, AZ, 2001d, Hohm Press.

Feuerstein G: Yoga and other Hindu traditions. In *The yoga tradition: its history, literature, philosophy and practice*, Prescott, AZ, 2001e, Hohm Press.

Haaz S, Bartlett SJ: Yoga for arthritis: a scoping review, *Rheum Dis Clin North Am* 37(1):33, 2011.

Hagins M, States R, Selfe T, Innes K: Effectiveness of yoga for hypertension: systematic review and meta-analysis, *Evid Based Complement Alternat Med*, Article ID 649836, 2013.

Harder H, Parlour L, Jenkins V: Randomised controlled trials of yoga interventions for women with breast cancer: a systematic literature review, *Support Care Cancer* 20(12):3055, 2012.

Harinath K, Malhotra AS, Pal K, et al: Effects of Hatha yoga and Omkar meditation on cardiorespiratory performance, psychologic profile, and melatonin secretion, *J Altern Complement Med* 10(2):261, 2004.

Hill C: Is yoga an effective treatment in the management of patients with chronic low back pain compared with other care modalities—a systematic review, *J Complement Integr Med* 10(1):1, 2013.

Innes KE, Vincent HK: The influence of yoga-based programs on risk profiles in adults with type 2 diabetes mellitus: a systematic review, *Evid Based Complement Alternat Med* 4(4):469, 2007.

Innes KE, Bourguignon C, Taylor AG: Risk indices associated with the insulin resistance syndrome, cardiovascular disease, and possible protection with yoga: a systematic review, *J Am Board Fam Pract* 18(6):491, 2005.

Keller D: *Heart of the yogi: the philosophical world of Hatha yoga*, 2012, DoYoga Productions.

Keller D: Healing the prana body: the role of the five vayus in Hatha yoga and Ayurveda, *Session* 1:2013, Yoga U Online.

Kelly Z: Is yoga an effective treatment for low back pain: a research review, *Int J Yoga Therap* 19:103, 2009.

Khalsa SB: Yoga as a therapeutic intervention: a bibliometric analysis of published research studies, *Indian J Physiol Pharmacol* 48(3):269, 2004.

Khalsa SBS, Gould J: *Your brain on yoga*, New York, 2012, RosettaBooks.

Kiecolt-Glaser JK, Christian L, Preston H, et al: Stress, inflammation, and yoga practice, *Psychosom Med* 72(2):113, 2010.

Kirkwood G, Rampes H, Tuffrey V, et al: Yoga for anxiety: a systematic review of the research evidence, *Br J Sports Med* 39(12):884, 2005.

Lee MS, Kim JI, Ha JY, et al: Yoga for menopausal symptoms: a systematic review, *Menopause* 16(3):602, 2009.

Levine AS, Balk JL: Yoga and quality-of-life improvement in patients with breast cancer: a literature review, *Int J Yoga Therap* 22:95, 2012.

Libby DJ, Reddy F, Pilver CE, et al: The use of yoga in specialized VA PTSD treatment programs, *Int J Yoga Therap* (22):79, 2012.

Lin KY, Hu YT, Chang KJ, et al: Effects of yoga on psychological health, quality of life, and physical health of patients with cancer: a meta-analysis, *Evid Based Complement Alternat Med*, Article ID 659876, 2011.

Lutz A, Slagter HA, Dunne JD, et al: Attention regulation and monitoring in meditation, *Trends Cogn Sci* 12(4):163, 2008.

Manna A, Raffone A, Perrucci MG, et al: Neural correlates of focused attention and cognitive monitoring in meditation, *Brain Res Bull* 82(1-2):46, 2010.

Martarelli D, Cocchioni M, Scuri S, et al: Diaphragmatic breathing reduces exercise-induced oxidative stress, *Evid Based Complement Alternat Med* Article ID 932430, 2011.

McCall MC: How might yoga work? An overview of potential underlying mechanisms, *J Yoga Phys Ther* 3(1):130, 2013.

McCall T: Yoga as medicine. In *Yoga as Medicine*, New York, 2007, Bantam Dell.

Miryala R, Micozzi M, Vlahos C, et al: Yoga. In Micozzi M, editor: *Fundamentals of Complementary and Alternative Medicine*, ed 4, St. Louis, MO, 2011, Saunders Elsevier.

Okonta NR: Does yoga therapy reduce blood pressure in patients with hypertension?: an integrative review, *Holist Nurs Pract* 26(3):137, 2012.

Pilkington K, Kirkwood G, Rampes H, Richardson J: Yoga for depression: the research evidence, *J Affect Disord* 89:13, 2005.

Posadzki P, Ernst E: Yoga for asthma? A systematic review of randomized clinical trials, *J Asthma* 48(6):632, 2011a.

Posadzki P, Ernst E: Yoga for low back pain: a systematic review of randomized clinical trials, *Clin Rheumatol* 30(9):1257, 2011b.

Posadzki P, Ernst E, Terry R, Lee MS: Is yoga effective for pain? A systematic review of randomized clinical trials, *Complement Ther Med* 19(5):281, 2011c.

Prabhavananda S, Isherwood C: Yoga and its aims. In *How to know God: the yoga aphorisms of Patanjali*, Hollywood, CA, 1981, The Vendata Society of Southern California, pp 15–94.

Raub JA: Psychophysiologic effects of Hatha Yoga on musculoskeletal and cardiopulmonary function: a literature review, *J Altern Complement Med* 8(6):797, 2002.

Saeed SA, Antonacci DJ, Bloch RM: Exercise, yoga, and meditation for depressive and anxiety disorders, *Am Fam Physician* 81(8):981, 2010.

Saper CB, Loewy AD, Swanson LW, Cowan WM: Direct hypothalamo-autonomic connections, *Brain Res* 117(2):305, 1976.

Shannahoff-Khalsa DS, Kennedy B: The effects of unilateral forced nostril breathing on the heart, *Int J Neurosci* 73(1–2):47, 1993.

Shannahoff-Khalsa DS, Boyle MR, Buebel ME: The effects of unilateral forced nostril breathing on cognition, *Int J Neurosci* 57 (3–4):239, 1991.

Shannahoff-Khalsa DS, Kennedy B, Yates FE, et al: Ultradian rhythms of autonomic, cardiovascular, and neuroendocrine systems are related in humans, *Am J Physiol* 270(4 Pt 2):R873–R887, 1996.

Shannahoff-Khalsa DS: Yogic insights into mind-body medicine and healing. In *Kundalini yoga meditation: techniques specific for psychiatric disorders, couples therapy, and personal growth*, New York, 2007, W.W. Norton & Company.

Sharma H, Sen S, Singh A, et al: Sudarshan Kriya practitioners exhibit better antioxidant status and lower blood lactate levels, *Biol Psychol* 63(3):281, 2003.

Sharma M, Haider T: Yoga as an alternative and complementary therapy for patients suffering from anxiety: a systematic review, *J Evid Based Complementary Altern Med* 18(1):15, 2013.

Sharma M, Haider T, Knowlden AP: Yoga as an alternative and complementary treatment for cancer: a systematic review, *J Altern Complement Med* 19(11):870–5, 2013.

Sinha S, Singh SN, Monga YP, Ray US: Improvement of glutathione and total antioxidant status with yoga, *J Altern Complement Med* 13(10):1085, 2007.

Smith KB, Pukall CF: An evidence-based review of yoga as a complementary intervention for patients with cancer, *Psychooncology* 18(5):465, 2009.

Spicuzza L, Gabutti A, Porta C, et al: Yoga and chemoreflex response to hypoxia and hypercapnia, *Lancet* 356(9240):1495, 2000.

Staples JK, Hamilton MF, Uddo M: A yoga program for the symptoms of post-traumatic stress disorder in Veterans, *Mil Med* 178(8):854, 2013.

Streeter CC, Gerbarg PL, Saper RB, et al: Effects of yoga on the autonomic nervous system, gamma-aminobutyric-acid, and allostasis in epilepsy, depression, and post-traumatic stress disorder, *Med Hypotheses* 78(5):571, 2012.

Streeter CC, Jensen JE, Perlmutter RM, et al: Yoga Asana sessions increase brain GABA levels: a pilot study, *J Altern Complement Med* 13(4):419, 2007.

Sturgess S: Pranayama. In *The yoga book: a practical guide to self-realization*, Rockport, MA, 1997a, Element Books Limited.

Sturgess S: The subtle bodies and the chakras. In *The yoga book: a practical guide to self-realization*, Rockport, MA, 1997b, Element Books Limited.

Taylor AG, Goehler LE, Galper DI, et al: Top-down and bottom-up mechanisms in mind-body medicine: development of an integrative framework for psychophysiological research, *Explore (NY)* 6(1):29, 2010.

Telles S, Nagarathna R, Nagendra HR: Breathing through a particular nostril can alter metabolism and autonomic activities, *Indian J Physiol Pharmacol* 38(2):133, 1994.

Telles S, Nagarathna R, Nagendra HR: Physiological measures of right nostril breathing, *J Altern Complement Med* 2(4):479, 1996.

Telles S, Singh N, Balkrishna A: Managing mental health disorders resulting from trauma through yoga: a review, *Depress Res Treat*, Article ID 401513, 2012.

Uebelacker LA, Epstein-Lubow G, Gaudiano BA, et al: Hatha yoga for depression: critical review of the evidence for efficacy, plausible mechanisms of action, and directions for future research, *J Psychiatr Pract* 16(1):22, 2010.

Ward L, Stebbings S, Cherkin D, Baxter GD: Yoga for functional ability, pain and psychosocial outcomes in musculoskeletal conditions: a systematic review and meta-analysis, *Musculoskeletal Care* 11(4):203–17, 2013.

Werntz DA, Bickford RG, Bloom FE, et al: Alternating cerebral hemispheric activity and the lateralization of autonomic nervous function, *Hum Neurobiol* 2(1):39, 1983.

Werntz DA, Bickford RG, Bloom FE, Shannahoff-Khalsa D: Selective hemispheric stimulation by unilateral forced nostril breathing, *Hum Neurobiol* 6(3):165, 1987.

Wisneski LA, Anderson L: *The scientific basis of integrative medicine*, ed 2, Boca Raton, FL, 2009, CRC Press.

Yoga Journal Editors: Which yoga is right for you? Retrieved 8-31-2013a, from http://www.yogajournal.com/basics/2353

Yoga Journal Editors: Yoga poses. Retrieved 8-31-2013b, from http://www.yogajournal.com/poses/finder/browse_categories

Zhang J, Yang KH, Tian JH, Wang CM: Effects of yoga on psychologic function and quality of life in women with breast cancer: a meta-analysis of randomized controlled trials, *J Altern Complement Med* 18(11):994, 2012.

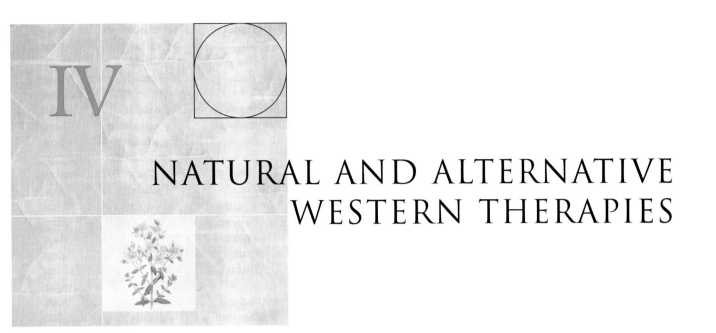

NATURAL AND ALTERNATIVE WESTERN THERAPIES

Section IV describes the background, context, and clinical approaches of selected alternative therapeutic disciplines and systems as developed through European and American history. This section describes individual approaches as suggested from contemporary Western research, both within and beyond the biomedical paradigm. Where these systems and approaches can be understood in light of the contemporary biomedical paradigm, this view is examined; where they cannot be understood in these terms, this paradox is addressed. When and how these medical systems are embedded in the natural curative environment is clarified, as well as when and how they are embedded in technology. In each case, these medical practices are presented as products of history that make sense in terms of that history.

Selected therapies from each of these disciplines and systems are also found as modalities (a small subset or group of therapies from one discipline or system contained within another discipline or system) (Benjamin et al, 2007) within the discipline of naturopathic medicine.

For example, homeopathy is a highly systematized method of healing that utilizes the principle of "use likes to treat likes" practiced by licensed physicians, naturopathic physicians, and other health care professionals throughout the world. Within integrative medical and naturopathic practice, homeopathy may be found practiced as a modality (more narrowly) or as a full discipline or system (comprehensively), with postgraduate training and credentialing. Two states specifically license homeopathic medical doctors. Naturopathic physicians are licensed within their scope of practice to provide homeopathic therapies. In the United States, homeopathic medicines are protected by federal law, and most are available over the counter. The greatest challenge that homeopathy may pose to conventional medicine and science is the common use of extremely diluted medicinal substances.

Naturopathic medicine itself is both a distinct, organized system of practice, as well as a real example in contemporary practice of "eclectic" (in prior editions, the editor has called it "neoeclectic") medicine that makes an authentic effort to fundamentally integrate different therapeutic approaches together. NM provides an authentic example of the integration of "CAM therapies" in distinction to the issues that beset what is called "integrative medicine" by the mainstream medical community today (see Chapter 3). Simultaneously, NM embraces the elements of what has commonly been called "nature cure" as well as specific alternative therapeutic traditions and practices that make use of one or more curative technologies.

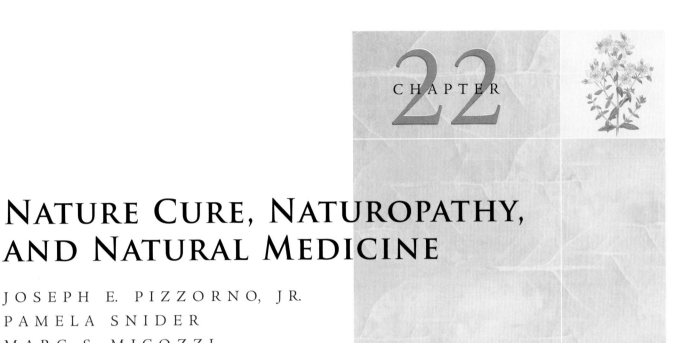

NATURE CURE, NATUROPATHY, AND NATURAL MEDICINE

JOSEPH E. PIZZORNO, JR.
PAMELA SNIDER
MARC S. MICOZZI

> The doctor of the future will give no medicine, but will interest his patient in the care of the human frame, in diet and in the cause and prevention of disease.
>
> —Thomas Edison

Thomas Edison's insightful prediction is proving true today, as natural medicine finds itself in the midst of an unprecedented explosion into mainstream health care. Consumers are spending more annually out of pocket for alternative medicine than for conventional care. In particular, naturopathic medicine is emerging as *the authentic model for integrative primary health care*. Natural medicine is undergoing a powerful resurgence, growing from estimates of only 200 to 500 naturopathic physicians and one naturopathic college extant in North America in 1977, to approximately 7000 licensed NDs and eight accredited naturopathic colleges and universities in the United States and Canada today. With its unique integration of vitalistic, scientific, academic, and clinical training in medicine, as well as incorporation of many specific alternative medical modalities and treatments, the naturopathic medical model is a potent contributing factor to this potential health care revolution.

HISTORY OF "REGULAR" MEDICINE AND NATUROPATHIC MEDICINE*

"REGULAR" MEDICINE

Conventional, or "regular," medicine (as it was historically known during the eighteenth and nineteenth centuries in

distinction to all the viable "alternatives") and natural medicine have shaped and helped to define each other throughout history, often in reaction to each other. Perhaps nothing had as much historic influence on naturopathic medicine as did the rise of regular medicine during the nineteenth and early twentieth centuries. Much as naturopathic doctors today may trace some of their roots to Hippocrates, regular physicians also generally consider his view of health and disease to have contributed to the basis of today's medicine. A primary reason was rejection of supernatural or divine forces as the cause of illness, which facilitated transition to a more physiological and *rational* approach to health and wellness. However, in contrast to naturopathic medicine, for which it is a core belief, regular medicine has come to reject Hippocrates' equally important concept of the "physis," or healing power of nature, a principle that may have done more to define and shape naturopathic medicine than anything else.

Of course regular medicine has made many technological leaps since the time of Hippocrates, particularly during the last century. Many aspects of today's education, scientific understanding, and therapeutic modalities would be unrecognizable to an MD only 125 years ago. We have also seen an unprecedented explosion in the size and role of the health care system in the United States, with over 780,000 MDs practicing as of the year 2013 (Accenture Physician Alignment Survey, 2012; American Medical Association, n.d.), and $2.1 trillion spent on health care in 2006 (Catlin, 2008).

By comparison, in the year 1800 there were only 200 graduates of the elite medical schools in the United States, along with 300 immigrants with European diplomas (Kaptchuk & Eisenberg, 2001). The consistent thread that ties these "regular" doctors of the past to those practicing today may be a philosophy of allegiance to the principles of

*The authors express their appreciation to George Cody, whose chapter "History of Naturopathic Medicine" in *Textbook of Natural Medicine* (JE Pizzorno and MT Murray, editors, St. Louis, 2004, Elsevier), provided a basis for much of this section.

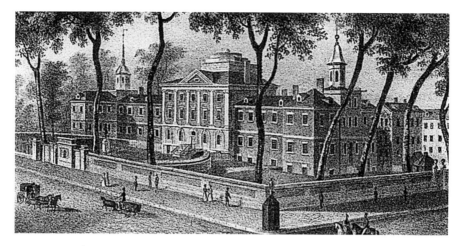

Figure 22-1 Pennsylvania Hospital, the nation's first hospital, founded in 1752. (Courtesy the Pennsylvania Hospital, Philadelphia, PA.)

scientific materialism and adoption of a basic biomedical orientation to illness, but coupled with disregard for the body's innate healing capacity and rejection of a "vitalistic" orientation (see Chapters 3 and 6).

In the European countries from which formal American medical education was derived, medicine first became institutionalized in the twelfth and thirteenth centuries, following a low ebb during the Dark Ages of AD 500 to 1050. In the 1050s, the Spanish Reconquista took back the historic citadel of Toledo from the Moors and rediscovered centuries of knowledge about medicines, foods, and related technologies.

Sarleno, Italy, was one of the earliest centers of medical training, followed by universities in Paris and England, where some of the first hospitals were built (Cruse, 1999). Although a graduate from Oxford in the 1500s had received up to 14 years of university education, very poor training was offered in the practice of medicine and patient care (Magee, 2004). By the time the European Enlightenment of the seventeenth and eighteenth centuries arrived at the far reaches of Europe in Scotland, it had become a mature intellectual movement emphasizing observation (empiricism) and reason (rationality). The Scottish Enlightenment of the late eighteenth century produced advancements in thinking about the role of economics (Adam Smith, *The Wealth of Nations,* 1776) and law (David Hume) in human society, as well as the roots of the Industrial Revolution with the application of the steam engine (James Watt) based on principles used for the steam distillation of scotch whiskey. Of course, an enlightened, rational approach to the rights of man and the ordering of human society influenced the American Revolution of 1776 (see Chapter 1) as well as the French Revolution of 1793.

The "rational medicine" movement was embodied in the school of medicine at the University of Edinburgh, Scotland, from whence Drs. William Hutchison and John Morgan came to establish the first school of medicine in the United States in 1767 at the College of Philadelphia

(now the University of Pennsylvania), by charter of British colonial governor of Pennsylvania Thomas Penn. This development followed the establishment of the first hospital in the nation by Benjamin Franklin and Dr. Thomas Bond during the prior decade in 1752 (Figure 22-1).

In general, however, in the 1700s little had yet improved—regular doctors had limited diagnostic ability, and aside from feeling the pulse, inspecting the tongue, and examining the urine and stool, physicians did not touch their patients and often did not even see them (Magee, 2004). There were no consistent or commonly accepted theories to explain the cause(s) of illness, nor could the modalities used to treat them be agreed upon. As a result, the medical landscape in the 1800s remained very diverse.

This situation was not inconsistent with the enlightened political climate at the time, however. Like today, the cultural values of the early nineteenth century greatly influenced the practice of medicine. In the era of "Jeffersonian" agrarian democracy and "Jacksonian democracy" of the common man, by the 1820s, American society had begun to reject any form of "elitism," and the "elites" often included physicians, in large part because regular doctors were mostly available only to the wealthy in society. Much of the public harbored a fervent anti-intellectualism coupled with belief in the tenet of economic freedom. As a consequence, laws controlling medical practice were viewed by the public as a form of class legislation; a general belief that citizens should have the right to choose their own medical care was combined with a distrust of the motives of "regular physicians" (Ober, 1997). Medical licensing became effectively irrelevant. For most of early America's Colonial and Federal periods, anyone could practice medicine, without a license, regardless of qualification or training. This situation can be likened to the traditional British "common law" system. This law also influenced the early practice of medicine and health care in Australia and is still influential in health care practice in the UK and Australia today (Newman Turner, 2011).

By 1850, all but two states in the United States had removed medical licensing statutes from the books (Whorton, 2002). Numerous conflicting claims of efficacy were made by a variety of practitioners, and an intense and heated competition often left patients confused by and dissatisfied with their experience with all types of physicians. The result has been described as both "medical anarchy" (Ober, 1997) and "a war zone" (Kaptchuk & Eisenberg, 2001). Because regular medicine was often ineffective and frequently toxic, many patients and physicians defected to other "alternatives." This situation was particularly relevant to experiences dealing with epidemics of infectious diseases that periodically afflicted large proportions of the population during the 1700s and early 1800s (see Chapters 1 and 40), with successive attacks of yellow fever, typhoid fever, typhus, and cholera. The aggressive therapies of the regular early American physicians such as Benjamin Rush were called heroic (see below) but had the general effect of weakening the patient. During the yellow fever epidemics of the 1790s in the then-new nation's capital in Philadelphia (what was described as "a melancholy scene of devastation"), there was much debate and dissension over using the heroic approach ("British") vs. a more conservative, supportive therapy that focused on building the host's reserves and defenses ("French" style) that emphasized "la terrain" or host factors (as microbial causes were as yet unknown). The failure of regular medicine and the toxic drug treatments of the time led patients and doctors in droves to emerging alternatives, such as homeopathic medicine, and various forms of natural medicine during the early 1800s.

In 1847, partially in response, and after prior attempts, a group of regular physicians founded an organization to serve as the unifying body for orthodox medical practitioners, the American Medical Association (AMA), initially under Nathaniel Chapman in Philadelphia. Physicians who belonged to the AMA considered themselves regular practitioners and adhered to therapeutics termed *heroic medicine* (Rutkow & Rutkow, 2004). It was their treatments that may have most distinguished these regular doctors to their patients, because they often consisted of bleeding and blistering in addition to administering harsh concoctions to induce vomiting and purging, treatments that at the time were considered state of the art.

The motivation behind such harsh treatments was a commitment to a scientific materialist medical theory and a move away from empirically based medicine. Also, because regular doctors did not share belief in the concept of the healing power of nature (the *vis medicatrix naturae*), they felt that a physician's duty was to provide active, "heroic" intervention. Because the majority of patients recovered notwithstanding their treatments, this reality had the ironic effect of encouraging both regular doctors' belief in heroic treatments and irregulars' belief in the inborn capacity for self-healing, despite the further injuries caused by many regular treatments. Much like physicians today are pressured to provide an active treatment that may sometimes be unnecessary (such as prescribing an antibiotic for a viral infection), regular doctors of the 1800s also felt pressure to give the heroic treatments for which they were known. As James Whorton (2002) writes, "it was only natural for MDs to close ranks and cling more tightly to that tradition as a badge of professional identity, making depletive therapy the core of their self-image as medical orthodoxy."

Although the AMA initially held no legal authority, like the multiplying medical specialty associations of today, it began a major push during the second half of the nineteenth century to create legislation and standards of medical education and competency. This process culminated in 1910 with the publication of *Medical Education in the United States and Canada,* compiled by Abraham Flexner (Figure 22-2), also known as the Flexner Report. It has been described as "a bombshell that rattled medical and political forces throughout the country" (Petrina, 2008). It criticized the medical education of its era as a loose and poorly structured apprenticeship system that generally lacked any defined standards or goals beyond commercialism (Ober, 1997). In some of his specific accounts, Flexner described medical institutions as "utterly wretched . . . without a redeeming feature" and as "a hopeless affair" (Whorton, 2002). Many of the regular medical institutions were rated poorly, and most of the irregular schools fared the worst. After this report, nearly half of the medical schools in the country closed, and by 1930 the remaining schools had 4-year programs of rigorous "scientific medicine."

Following the Flexner Report, a tremendous restructuring of medical education and practice occurred. The remaining medical schools experienced enormous growth: in 1910 a leading school might have had a budget of

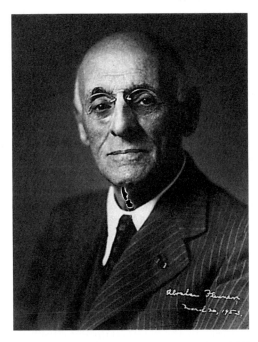

Figure 22-2 Abraham Flexner. (Courtesy National Library of Medicine, Bethesda, MD.)

$100,000; by 1965 it was $20 million, and by 1990 it would have been $200 million or more (Ludmerer, 1999). Faculty were now called upon to engage in original research, and students not only studied a curriculum with a heavy emphasis on science, but also engaged in active learning by participating in real clinical work with responsibility for patients. Hospitals became the locus for clinical instruction. As scientific discovery began to accelerate, these higher educational standards helped to bridge the gap between what was known and what was put into practice, and more stringent licensing and independent testing provided a greater degree of confidence in the competence of the nation's doctors. During this same time period, the suppression and decline of alternative schools of health care occurred, as both public and political pressure increased.

The post–World War II era was one of undeniable and astonishing achievements by scientific medicine, which coincided with great strides in public health, sanitation, and living conditions. As understanding of basic clinical science has grown, the biomedical model has continued to evolve, and so has the capacity to make accurate and precise biomedical diagnoses and interventions. Today's conventional biomedical physician faces new challenges, however, and some of the deficiencies of "regular" medicine in the past have reared their heads once again, particularly with respect to the toxicity and danger of so many contemporary medical treatments and procedures.

In an era of emerging medical homes, accountable care organizations, a downturn in payments to physicians, and the rising rate of behaviorally related chronic diseases, it has become increasingly difficult for physicians to spend quality time with patients or to focus on preventative medicine, and the treatment and prevention of chronic disease has suffered. A 2012 survey conducted by Accenture found that "increasingly private practice doctors have sacrificed their independence to seek employment . . . as independent physicians have dropped from 57 percent in 2000 to 39 percent in 2012." By the end of 2013, Accenture estimates the market will be composed of only 36 percent of independent physicians. Physicians surveyed cited rising business costs and expenses (87%) and the prevalence of managed care organizations (61%) as the top two reasons for leaving independent practice (Accenture Physician Alignment Survey, 2012).

Also, physicians must be vigilant against the constant and insidious efforts of the pharmaceutical industry to corrupt medical science, education, and practice for commercial gain. In addition, the increase in specialization and the decline of primary care is a growing problem that shows no sign of slowing, with estimates of primary care physician shortages predicted of up to 100,000 by 2025 (NY Times, 2012). A survey completed at Harvard in 2013 found that over the prior three decades, only 10% of new drugs approved by the FDA had greater effectiveness, but that 50% had a worse safety record , compared to the older drugs they were meant to replace (Light et al, 2013).

Today's regular doctors are also not easily defined—they have been referred to as "mainstream," "orthodox," "conventional," "allopathic," "scientific," "biomedical," and "authoritarian," all of which have their own positive and negative connotations (see Chapter 3). None is universally accepted or accurate as individual MDs are more and more either engaged in or becoming receptive to developing new "integrative" and holistic models of health care (Berkenwald, 1998; Kaptchuk & Eisenberg, 2001; Consortium of Academic Health Centers for Integrative Medicine, 2013; American Holistic Medical Association, 2013; American Board of Integrative and Holistic Medicine, 2013). It is also increasingly being recognized that although regular doctors have presented themselves as the "scientific" branch of medicine throughout recent history, the mantle of science cannot be claimed or exclusively worn by any one discipline or field of medicine, and integration of various medical specialties and philosophies, and collaboration among them, benefits all patients (Goldblatt et al, 2013; Weeks et al, 2010; Freshman et al, 2010).

A pluralistic health care setting is re-emerging. Optimally, it will value the organization, structure, and science-based approach of regular medicine, along with qualities regular medicine has typically been lacking, including patient-centered and individualized care that reaffirms the importance of the relationship between practitioner and patient, the recognition and support of innate healing systems, and a broadening of the scientific approach to allow for the evaluation and incorporation of traditional and natural medicines and systems into current health care delivery in a way that makes use of all appropriate therapeutic approaches, health care professionals, and disciplines (CAHCIM, 2013). "We find ourselves," John Weeks, the editor of *The Integrator*, wrote recently, "in an era beyond the polarization of alternative medicine and conventional medicine," with "an opportunity to become a seamless part of an integrated system that might rightfully be called, simply, *health care*" (Weeks, n.d.). What works will no longer be considered mainstream, or alternative, but simply good medicine (Micozzi, 1998).

EMERGENCE OF NATUROPATHIC MEDICINE PROPER

Although naturopathic medicine traces its philosophical roots to many traditional world medicines, its body of knowledge derives from a rich heritage of writings and practices of Western and non-Western nature doctors since Hippocrates (circa 400 BC). Modern naturopathic medicine grew out of healing systems of the eighteenth and nineteenth centuries. The term *naturopathy* was coined in 1895 by Dr. John Scheel of New York City to describe his method of health care. However, earlier forerunners of these concepts already existed in the history of natural healing, both in America and in the Austro-Germanic European core. Naturopathy became a formal profession in the United States, and in other countries after its creation by Benedict Lust in 1896.

Over the centuries, natural medicine and conventional medicine have alternately diverged and converged, shaping each other, often in reaction to each other. During the past hundred years the naturopathic profession progressed through several fairly distinct phases, as follows:

1. Latter part of the nineteenth century: *The founding by Benedict Lust.* Origin in the Germanic hydrotherapy and nature cure traditions, and diverse systems.
2. 1900 to 1917: *The formative years.* Convergence of the American dietetic, hygienic, nature cure, physical culture, spinal manipulation, mental, spiritual and emotional healing, Thomsonian/eclectic, and homeopathic systems.
3. 1918 to 1937: *The halcyon days.* During a period of great public interest and support, the philosophical basis and scope of naturopathic therapies diversified to encompass botanical, homeopathic, and environmental medicine.
4. 1938 to 1970: *Suppression and decline.* Growing political and social dominance of the AMA, lack of internal political unity, and lack of unifying standards, combined with the American love affair with technology and the emergence of "miracle" drugs and effective modern surgical techniques perfected in two world wars, resulted in legal and economic suppression, decline in enrollments, closure of schools, and decrease in the number of practicing naturopathic physicians.
5. 1971 to present: *Re-emergence of naturopathic medicine.* Reawakened awareness in the American public of the importance of health promotion and prevention of disease, concern for the environment, and the establishment of modern, accredited, physician-level training reignited public interest in naturopathic medicine, which resulted in rapid resurgence. Current projections predict a continuing increase in the number of licensed naturopathic physicians through 2025 and beyond.

Cooper and Stoflet reported in 1996 that the per capita supply of alternative medicine clinicians (chiropractors, naturopaths, and practitioners of Oriental medicine) would grow by 88% between 1994 and 2010, while allopathic physician supply would grow by 16%. . . . "The total number of naturopathy graduates would double over the five years from 1996-2001. The total number of naturopathic physicians will triple" (Cooper & Stoflet, 1996). This trend has borne out as the profession increased from (estimated) 200 to 500 licensed naturopathic physicians in 1977 (United States and Canada) to nearly 7000 in 2013.

FOUNDING OF NATUROPATHY

Naturopathy, as a generally used term, began with the teachings and concepts of Benedict Lust. In 1892, at age 23, Lust came from Germany as a disciple of Father Sebastian Kneipp (the greatest practitioner of hydrotherapy) to bring Kneipp's hydrotherapy practices to America. Exposure in

the United States to a wide range of practitioners and practices of natural healing arts broadened Lust's perspective, and after a decade of study, in 1902 he purchased the term *naturopathy* from Scheel of New York City (who coined the term in 1895) to describe the eclectic compilation of doctrines of natural healing that he envisioned was to be the future of natural medicine. Naturopathy, or "nature cure," was defined by Lust as both a way of life and a concept of healing that used various natural means (selected from various systems and disciplines) of treating human infirmities and disease states. The earliest therapies associated with the term involved a combination of American hygienics and Austro-Germanic nature cure dietetics, botanical medicines, and hydrotherapy.

In January 1902, Lust, who had been publishing *The Kneipp Water Cure Monthly* and its German-language counterpart in New York since 1896, changed the name of the journal to *The Naturopathic and Herald of Health* and began promoting a new way of thinking of health care with the following editorial:

> We believe in strong, pure, beautiful bodies . . . of radiating health. We want every man, woman and child in this great land to know and embody and feel the truths of right living that mean conscious mastery. We plead for the renouncing of poisons from the coffee, white flour, glucose, lard, and like venom of the American table to patent medicines, tobacco, liquor and the other inevitable recourse of perverted appetite. We long for the time when an eight-hour day may enable every worker to stop existing long enough to live; when the spirit of universal brotherhood shall animate business and society and the church; when every American may have a little cottage of his own, and a bit of ground where he may combine Aero-therapy, Heliotherapy, Geotherapy, Aristophagy and nature's other forces with home and peace and happiness and things forbidden to flat-dwellers; when people may stop doing and thinking and being for others and be for themselves; when true love and divine marriage and prenatal culture and controlled parenthood may fill this world with germ-gods instead of humanized animals.

In a word, naturopathy stands for the reconciling, harmonizing, and unifying of nature, humanity, and God.

Fundamentally therapeutic because men need healing; elementarily educational because men need teaching; ultimately inspirational because men need empowering.

Benedict Lust

According to his published personal history, Lust had a debilitating condition in his late teens while growing up in Michelbach, Baden, Germany, and had been sent by his father to undergo the Kneipp cure at Woerishofen. He stayed there from mid-1890 to early 1892. Not only was he "cured" of his condition, but he became a protégé of Father Kneipp. He emigrated to America to proselytize the principles of the Kneipp water cure (Figure 22-3).

By making contact in New York with other German Americans who were also becoming aware of the Kneipp principles, Lust participated in the founding of the first

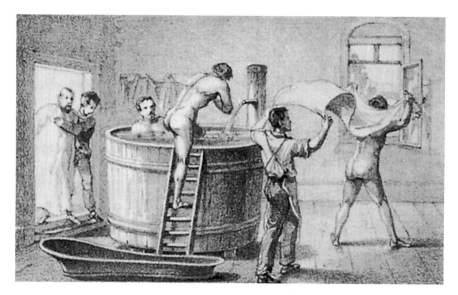

Figure 22-3 Curative baths, one form of hydrotherapy, were a popular form of natural healing in the late nineteenth century. (Courtesy Wellcome Institute Library, London.)

"Kneipp Society," which was organized in Jersey City, New Jersey, in 1896. Subsequently, through Lust's organization and contacts, Kneipp societies were also founded in Brooklyn, Boston, Chicago, Cleveland, Denver, Cincinnati, Philadelphia, Columbus, Buffalo, Rochester, New Haven, San Francisco, the state of New Mexico, and Mineola on Long Island. The members of these organizations were provided with copies of the *Kneipp Blatter* and a companion English publication Lust began to put out called *The Kneipp Water Cure Monthly*. In 1895, Lust opened the Kneipp Water Cure Institute on 59th Street in New York City.

Father Kneipp died in Germany, at Woerishofen, on June 17, 1897. With his passing, Lust was no longer bound strictly to the principles of the Kneipp water cure. He had begun to associate earlier with other German American physicians, principally Dr. Hugo R. Wendel (a German-trained "Naturarzt"), who began, in 1897, to practice in New York and New Jersey as a licensed osteopathic physician. Lust entered the Universal Osteopathic College of New York in 1896 and became licensed as an osteopathic physician in 1898.

Once he was licensed to practice as a health care physician in his own right, Lust began the transition toward the concept of "naturopathy." Between 1898 and 1902, when he adopted the term *naturopath*, Lust acquired a chiropractic education and he changed the name of his Kneipp Store (which he had opened in 1895) to "Health Food Store" (the first facility to use that name and concept in the United States). The store specialized in providing organically grown foods and the materials necessary for drugless cures. He also founded the New York School of Massage (in 1896) and the American School of Chiropractic.

In 1902, when he purchased and began using the term *naturopathy* and calling himself a "naturopath," Lust, in addition to operating his New York School of Massage and

American School of Chiropractic, issuing his various publications, and running his Health Food Store, began to operate the American School of Naturopathy. All these activities were carried out at the same 59th Street address. By 1907, Lust's enterprises had grown sufficiently large that he moved them to a 55-room building. It housed the Naturopathic Institute, Clinic, and Hospital; the American School of Naturopathy and American School of Chiropractic; the establishment now called the Original Health Food Store; Lust's publishing enterprises; and the New York School of Massage. The operation remained in this four-story building, roughly twice the size of the original facility, from 1907 to 1915.

From 1912 through 1914, Lust took a sabbatical from his operations to further his own education. By this time he had founded his large, estate-like sanitarium at Butler, New Jersey, known as *Yungborn* after the German sanitarium operation of Adoph Just. In 1912, he began attending the Homeopathic Medical College in New York, which granted him a degree in homeopathic medicine in 1913 and a degree in eclectic medicine in 1914. In early 1914, Lust traveled to Florida and obtained an MD's license on the basis of his graduation from the Homeopathic Medical College.

From 1902, when he began to use the term *naturopathy*, until 1918, Lust replaced the Kneipp societies with the Naturopathic Society of America. Then in December 1919, the Naturopathic Society of America was formally dissolved because of insolvency, and Lust founded the American Naturopathic Association (ANA). Thereafter, the association was incorporated in some additional 18 states. Lust claimed at one time to have 40,000 practitioners practicing naturopathy. In 1918, as part of his effort to dissolve the Naturopathic Society of America (an operation into which he invested a great deal of his funds and resources in an attempt to organize a naturopathic profession) and

BOX 22-1 *Definitions: Nature Cure, Naturopathy, Naturopathic Medicine, Natural Medicine*

Naturopathy, or *"nature cure,"* was defined by Lust as both a way of life and a concept of healing that used various natural means (selected from various systems and disciplines) of treating human infirmities and disease states. The earliest therapies associated with the term involved a combination of American hygienics and Austro-Germanic nature cure dietetics, botanical medicines, and hydrotherapy (*Benedict Lust, Nature Doctors*).

Naturopathic medicine is a distinct system of primary health care—an art, science, philosophy, and practice of diagnosis, treatment, and prevention of illness.

· Naturopathic physicians seek to restore and maintain optimum health in their patients by emphasizing nature's inherent self-healing process, the *vis medicatrix naturae.*

· Methods used are consistent with these principles and are chosen upon the basis of patient individuality.

· Naturopathic physicians are primary health care practitioners, whose diverse techniques include modem and traditional scientific and empirical methods.

The following principles are the foundation for the practice of naturopathic medicine (American Association of Naturopathic Physicians et al, 1989).

From *Nature Doctors* Intro: By Friedhelm Kirchfeld and Wade Boyle, 1994, pg. 1

Nature cure was a system for treating disease with natural agents such as water, air, diet, herbs, and sunshine that developed in nineteenth-century Europe.

Naturopathy was the combination of nature cure and homeopathy, spinal manipulation, and other natural therapies, which were developed in early twentieth-century America.

Naturopathic medicine is the application of the principles of naturopathy within the context of modern scientific knowledge that has evolved throughout the last half of this century.

The term *nature doctor* has been used to describe the practitioners of these permutations of nature-based medicine.

AANP

Naturopathic medicine is a distinct method of primary health care—an art, science, philosophy, and practice of diagnosis, treatment, and prevention of illness. Naturopathic physicians seek to restore and maintain optimum health in their patients by emphasizing nature's inherent self-healing process, the *vis medicatrix naturae.* This is accomplished through education and the rational use of natural therapeutics (AANP et al, 1989).

Naturopathy is a distinct type of primary care medicine that blends age-old healing traditions with scientific advances and current research. It is guided by a unique set of principles that recognize the body's innate healing capacity, emphasize disease prevention, and encourage individual responsibility to obtain optimal health. The naturopathic physician (ND) strives to thoroughly understand each patient's condition, and views symptoms as the body's means of communicating an underlying imbalance. Treatments address the patient's underlying condition, rather than individual presenting symptoms. Modalities utilized by NDs include diet and clinical nutrition, behavioral change, hydrotherapy, homeopathy, botanical medicine, physical medicine, pharmaceuticals, and minor surgery (Fleming & Gutknecht, 2010).

replace it with the American Naturopathic Association, Lust published the first *Yearbook of Drugless Therapy.* Annual supplements were published in either *The Naturopath and the Herald of Health* or its companion publication, *Nature's Path* (which began publication in 1925), with which *The Naturopath* at one time merged. *The Naturopath and Herald of Health,* sometimes printed with the two phrases reversed, was published from 1902 through 1927, and from 1934 until after Lust's death in 1945.

In 1922, Lust published the "Proclamation for the 26th Annual Convention of the N.Y. and N.J. State Societies of Naturopaths, Accredited Sections of The American Naturopathic Association," announcing the six major and five minor modalities of naturopathic medicine. The ANA's major modalities were: "*atmospheric* cure, the *light* cure, the *water* cure, the *diet* cure, the *earth* (clay) cure, the *work* cure, and the *mind* cure." ANA's minor modalities were mechanotherapy, psychotherapy, physiotherapy, phytotherapy, and biochemistry (Lust, 1922). Natural living, or living in accordance with natural law, underpinned all naturopathic use of various modalities and therapies.

Naturopathic medicine was founded by an MD in 1896 as an "integrative' medicine discipline, whose approach

founder Benedict Lust, MD, called "Therapeutic Universalism" (Whorton 2003). Today's naturopathic profession continues the integrative tradition in its self-definition: "Diagnostic and therapeutic methods are selected from various sources and systems and will continue to evolve with the progress of knowledge" (American Association of Naturopathic Physicians, 2013).

Benedict Lust's principles of health are found in the introduction to the first volume of the *Universal Naturopathic Directory and Buyer's Guide,* a portion of which is reproduced in Box 22-1. Although the terminology is almost a century old, the concepts and integrative therapeutic universalism model Lust proposed have provided a powerful foundation that has endured despite over a century of active political suppression by the dominant school of medicine.

SCHOOLS OF THOUGHT: PHILOSOPHICAL BASIS OF NATUROPATHY

Because of the integrative, synthetic, and eclectic nature of naturopathic medicine, its history can be considered complex among healing arts, which is explained in the relatively large portion of this chapter devoted to this subject.

The following discussion is divided into distinct schools of thought, although it is somewhat arbitrary, because those who founded and practiced these arts (especially the Americans) were often trained in, influenced by, and practiced several therapeutic systems or modalities.

Centuries earlier, traditionally vitalistic Tibetan medicine developed an integrative approach by gathering medical scholars from various systems together, drawing from the best of their systems (Gyatso, 2010) in Asia (see Chapter 30). It was Benedict Lust who wove the many threads in Western and European cultures and schools of thought together into a unified professional practice. This development arguably makes naturopathic medicine the *first* Western system of full-scope *integrative* natural medicine based on the *vis medicatrix naturae*. When hailing the advent of so-called "integrative medicine" in the twenty-first century (see Chapter 3), we do well, as always, to remember this history and to recognize current reality.

Organized around the principle of the human capacity for healing (self-healing), naturopathic medicine has discriminately integrated diverse therapeutic systems and modalities into a cohesive framework. It acknowledges the biomedical model of health and illness, but also supports the whole person, including the psychological, social, and spiritual aspects of wellness. It has consistently promoted a patient-centered relationship, as well as collaboration with other health care professionals and disciplines, and today is poised as a useful, in-depth, *authentic model for integrative medicine.*

Although it draws from the eclectic tradition (see later), it does not do so randomly or indiscriminately. Rather, core principles, such as the *vis medicatrix naturae*, vital or life force, and its theory concerning the process and laws of health and healing guide its flexible but coherent structure, allowing it to navigate, perhaps uniquely, today's medical world, and the nature of health, illness, and healing in unique ways.

The following presents the formative schools of Western thought in natural healing and some of their leading adherents. Although the therapies differ, the philosophical thread of health promotion and supporting the body's own healing processes as inherent drive to health runs through them all. These threads are derived from centuries of medical observation and scholarship, both Western and non-Western, concerning the self-healing process.

After a brief overview of Hippocrates' seminal contribution to the foundations of natural medicine, the basic themes are presented: healthful living; natural diet; detoxification; exercise, mechanotherapy, and physical therapy; mental, emotional, and spiritual healing; and natural therapeutic agents. Hippocrates and centuries of nature doctors' writings remain empirically rich repositories of observations for future research.

Hippocratic School

During prehistoric times, there is evidence that people believed that disease was caused by magic or supernatural forces, such as devils or angry gods (see Chapter 34). Hippocrates, breaking with this superstitious belief, became the first naturalistic doctor recorded in the Western tradition. (A similar break occurred in ancient China in the Eastern tradition; see Chapters 28 and 34.) Hippocrates regarded the body as a "whole" and instructed his students to prescribe only beneficial treatments and refrain from causing harm or hurt.

Hippocratic practitioners assumed that everything in nature had a rational basis; therefore the physician's role was to understand and follow the laws of the intelligible universe. They viewed disease as an effect and looked for its cause in natural phenomena: air, water, food, and so forth (see also Chapter 26). His classical treatise "On Airs, Waters and Places" is exemplary. They first used the term *physis* to represent the *vis medicatrix naturae,* or "healing power of nature," as denoting the body's ability and drive to heal itself. One of the central tenets is that "there is an *order* to the process of healing which requires certain things to be done before other things to maximize the effectiveness of the therapeutics" (Zeff, 1997).

The "step order" used by Tibetan medicine is also an example of the representation of this tenet in traditional world medicines (see Chapter 30). Hippocrates recognized this "healing order" in his understanding of the concept of "coction." In today's terms and in naturopathic theory, coction is the inflammatory response as a key process in disease development, fever, and eventual healing (Zeff et al, 2013).

Hydrotherapy

The earliest philosophical origins of naturopathy were clearly in the German hydrotherapy movement: the use of hot and cold water for the maintenance of health and the treatment of disease. One of the oldest known therapies, water was used therapeutically by the Romans and Greeks. Hydrotherapy began its modern history with the publication of *The History of Cold Bathing* in 1697 by Sir John Floyer. Probably the strongest impetus for its use subsequently developed in Central Europe, where it was advocated by such well-known hydropaths as Priessnitz, Schroth, and Father Kneipp. They popularized specific water treatments that quickly became the vogue in Europe during the nineteenth century.

Vinzenz Priessnitz (1799–1851), of Graefenberg, Silesia, was a pioneer natural healer. He was prosecuted by the medical authorities of his day and was actually convicted of using witchcraft because he cured his patients by the use of water, air, diet, and exercise. He took his patients back to nature—to the woods, the streams, the open fields—treated them with nature's own forces, and fed them on natural foods. His cured patients numbered in the thousands, and his fame spread over Europe. *Father Sebastian Kneipp* (1821–1897) became the most famous of the European hydropaths, with Pope Leo XIII and Ferdinand of Austria (whom he had walking barefoot in new-fallen snow for the purposes of hardening his constitution) among his many famous patients. He standardized the practice of hydrotherapy and organized it into a system that was widely emulated through the establishment of health spas or "sanitariums."

Although the first such sanitarium in this country, the Kneipp and Nature Cure Sanitarium, was opened in Newark, New Jersey, in 1891, resort to health spas in early America was also practiced. During the colonial period, healing waters became known to leading Americans, including founding fathers Washington and Jefferson, who took healing cures at Berkely Springs, Virginia (now West Virginia). A resort in Bedford, Pennsylvania, became popular at Bedford Springs, with seven different natural water sources. When the Pennsylvania Railroad put its "Main Line" through the region during the 1850s, thousands were able to visit to take the cure, including President James Buchanan (1856–1860), who used it as a summer White House. Often, healing springs became known to European settlers from Native American traditions, such as the spring at Emmitsburg, Maryland, today a Catholic shrine located 15 miles south of Gettysburg.

Perhaps the best-known American hydropath was J.H. Kellogg, a medical doctor who approached hydrotherapy scientifically and performed many experiments trying to understand the physiological effects of hot and cold water. In 1900, he published *Rational Hydrotherapy,* which is still considered a definitive treatise on the physiological and therapeutic effects of water, along with an extensive discussion of hydrotherapeutic techniques. Drs. O.J. Carroll, Harold Dick, Robert V. Carroll, and John Bastyr, among others, brought the use of hydrotherapy techniques forward into modern naturopathic practice.

Nature Cure

Natural living, consumption of a vegetarian diet, and the use of light and air formed the basis of the nature cure movement founded by *Dr. Arnold Rickli* (1823–1926). In 1848, he established at Veldes Krain, Austria, the first institution of light and air cure or, as it was called in Europe, the *atmospheric cure*. He was an ardent disciple of the vegetarian diet and the founder, and for more than 50 years the president, of the National Austrian Vegetarian Association. In 1891, *Louis Kuhne* (ca. 1823–1907) wrote the *New Science of Healing,* which presented the basic principles of "drugless methods." *Dr. Henry Lahman* (ca. 1823–1907), who founded the largest nature cure institution in the world at Weisser Hirsch, near Dresden, Saxony, constructed the first appliances for the administration of electric light treatment and baths. He was the author of several books on diet, nature cure, and heliotherapy. *Professor F.E. Bilz* (1823–1903) authored the first natural medicine encyclopedia, *The Natural Method of Healing,* which was translated into a dozen languages, and in German alone ran into 150 editions.

Nature cure became popular in America through the efforts of *Henry Lindlahr,* MD, ND, of Chicago, Illinois. Originally a rising businessman in Chicago with all the bad habits of those in the Gay Nineties era, he became chronically ill while only in his thirties. After receiving no relief from the orthodox practitioners of his day, he learned of nature cure, which improved his health. Subsequently, he went to Germany to stay in a sanitarium to be cured and to learn nature cure. He went back to Chicago and earned his degrees from the Homeopathic/Eclectic College of Illinois. In 1903, he opened a sanitarium in Elmhurst, Illinois; established Lindlahr's Health Food Store; and shortly thereafter founded the Lindlahr College of Natural Therapeutics. In 1908, he began to publish *Nature Cure Magazine* and began publishing his six-volume series of *Philosophy of Natural Therapeutics.* Volume One: *The Philosophy of the Unity of Disease and Cure Through Nature Cure* (1913) is considered a seminal work in naturopathic theory, laying the groundwork for a coherent theory of illness, health, and healing, drawing concepts from diverse disciplines and a systematic approach to naturopathic treatment and diagnosis. Lindlahr ultimately presented the most coherent naturopathic theory extant at the time, summarized in his *Catechism of Naturopathy,* which presented a five-part therapeutic progression (Lindlahr, 1914b).

One of the chief advantages of training in the early 1900s was the marvelous inpatient facilities that flourished during this time. These facilities provided in-depth training in clinical nature cure and natural hygiene in inpatient settings. Nature cure and natural hygiene are still at the core of naturopathic medicine's fundamental principles and approach to health care, health promotion, and disease prevention.

The Hygienic System

Another forerunner of American naturopathy, the "hygienic" school, amalgamated the hydrotherapy and nature cure movements with vegetarianism. It originated as a lay movement of the nineteenth century and had its genesis in the popular teachings of *Sylvester Graham* and *William Alcott.* Graham began preaching the doctrines of temperance and hygiene in 1830, and in 1839 he published *Lectures on the Science of Human Life,* two hefty volumes that prescribed healthy dietary habits. He emphasized a moderate lifestyle, a flesh-free diet, and bran bread as an alternative to bolted or white bread (graham cracker). The earliest medical physician to have a significant impact on the hygienic movement and the later philosophical growth of naturopathy was *Russell Trall,* MD. According to Whorton (1982) in his *Crusaders for Fitness,*

> The exemplar of the physical educator-hydropath was Russell Thatcher Trall. Still another physician who had lost his faith in regular therapy, Trall opened the second water cure establishment in America, in New York City in 1844. Immediately, he combined the full Priessnitzian armamentarium of baths with regulation of diet, air, exercise and sleep. He would eventually open and or direct any number of other hydropathic institutions around the country, as well as edit the *Water Cure Journal,* the *Hydropathic Review,* and a temperance journal. He authored several books, including popular sex manuals which perpetuated Graham-like concepts into the 1890's, sold

Graham crackers and physiology texts at his New York office, was a charter member (and officer) of the American Vegetarian Society, presided over a short-lived World Health Association, and so on.

Trall established the first school of natural healing arts in this country to have a 4-year curriculum (anticipating the later 4-year curriculum of John Shaw Billings for the new Johns Hopkins School of Medicine in the 1880s) and the authorization to confer the degree of MD. It was founded in 1852 as a "Hydropathic and Physiological School" and was chartered by the New York State Legislature in 1857 under the name New York Hygio-Therapeutic College.

Trall eventually published more than 25 books on the subjects of physiology, hydropathy, hygiene, vegetarianism, and temperance, among many others. The most valuable and enduring of these was his 1851 *Hydropathic Encyclopedia,* a volume of nearly 1000 pages that covered the theory and practice of hydropathy and the philosophy and treatment of diseases advanced by older schools of medicine. The encyclopedia sold more than 40,000 copies.

Martin Luther Holbrook expanded on the work of Graham, Alcott, and Trall and, working with an awareness of the European concepts developed by Priessnitz and Kneipp, laid further groundwork for the concepts later advanced by Lust, Lindlahr, and others. According to Whorton (1982), Holbrook proposed the following:

> For disease to result, the latter had to provide a suitable culture medium, had to be susceptible. As yet, most physicians were still so excited at having discovered the causative agents of infection that they were paying less than adequate notice to the host. Radical hygienists, however, were bent just as far in the other direction. They were inclined to see bacteria as merely impotent organisms that throve only in individuals whose hygienic carelessness had made their body compost heaps. Tuberculosis is contagious, Holbrook acknowledged, but "the degree of vital resistance is the real element of protection. When there is no preparation of the soil by heredity, predisposition or lowered health standard, the individual is amply guarded against the attack." A theory favored by many others was that germs were the effect of disease rather than its cause; tissues corrupted by poor hygiene offered microbes, all harmless, an environment in which they could thrive.

The orthodox hygienists of the progressive years were equally enthused by the recent progress of nutrition, of course, and exploited it for their own naturopathic doctors, but their utilization of science hardly stopped with dietetics. Medical bacteriology was another area of remarkable discovery, bacteriologists having provided, in the short space of the last quarter of the nineteenth century, an understanding, at long last, of the nature of infection. This new science's implications for hygienic ideology were profound—when Holbrook locked horns with female fashion, for example, he did not attack the bulky, ground-length skirts still in style with the crude Grahamite objection that the skirt was too heavy. Rather he forced a gasp from his readers with an account of watching a smartly dressed lady unwittingly drag her skirt "over some virulent, revolting looking sputum, which some unfortunate consumptive had expectorated."

Trall and Holbrook both advanced the idea that physicians should teach the maintenance of health rather than simply provide a last resort in times of health crisis. Besides providing a strong editorial voice denouncing the evils of tobacco and drugs, they strongly advanced the value of vegetarianism, bathing and exercise, dietetics and nutrition, along with personal hygiene.

John Harvey Kellogg, MD, another medically trained doctor who turned to more nutritionally based natural healing concepts, also greatly influenced Lust. Kellogg was renowned through his connection, beginning in 1876, with the Battle Creek Sanitarium, which was founded in the 1860s as a Seventh Day Adventist institution designed to perpetuate the Grahamite philosophies. Kellogg, born in 1852, was a "sickly child" who, at age 14, after reading the works of Graham, converted to vegetarianism. At the age of 20, he studied for a term at Trall's Hygio-Therapeutic College and then earned a medical degree at New York's Bellevue Medical School. He maintained an affiliation with the regular schools of medicine during his lifetime, more because of his practice of surgery than because of his beliefs in that area of health care (Figure 22-4).

Kellogg designated his concepts, which were basically the hygienic system of healthful living, as "biologic living." Kellogg expounded vegetarianism, attacked sexual misconduct and the evils of alcohol, and was a prolific writer

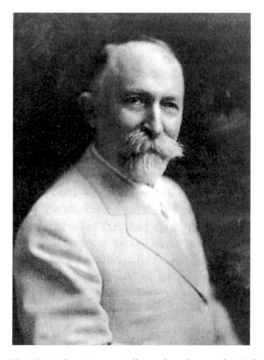

Figure 22-4 Dr. John Harvey Kellogg, brother to the Kellogg of breakfast cereal fame and a physical culture movement proponent. (Courtesy Historical Society of Battle Creek, Battle Creek, MI.)

through the late nineteenth and early twentieth centuries. He produced a popular periodical, *Good Health,* which continued in existence until 1955. When Kellogg died in 1943 at age 91, he had had more than 300,000 patients through the Battle Creek Sanitarium, including many celebrities, and the "San" became nationally known.

Kellogg was also extremely interested in hydrotherapy. In the 1890s he established a laboratory at the San to study the clinical applications of hydrotherapy. This led to his writing of *Rational Hydrotherapy* in 1902. The preface espoused a philosophy of drugless healing that came to be one of the bases of the hydrotherapy school of medical thought in early twentieth century America. Herbert Shelton, leader and founder of the profession of natural hygiene, wrote extensively on the theory and practice of natural hygiene, from the basis of his observation that "Perhaps the greatest want of our age is a correct knowledge of the physiology of our being and the laws that govern life, health and disease" (Shelton, 1968).

INFLUENCE ON PUBLIC HEALTH

It is a little-known fact that most of our current and accepted public hygiene practices, which are responsible for the majority of the advances in health and longevity during the twentieth century, were brought into societal use by the early hygienic reformers. Before their efforts, ignorance or neglect of these basic physiological safety measures was rampant. The hygienists had a great influence on decreasing morbidity and mortality and increasing life span, as well as on the adoption of public sanitation. Orthodox medicine is typically credited with these advances.

Currently, certified professional Natural Hygienists are advocates of the highest standards of training and supervised clinical fasting and participate in the training of naturopathic physicians. Naturopathic medicine uses the precepts of natural hygiene in re-establishing the basis of health, the first step in the therapeutic order.

Autotoxicity and Autointoxication

Lust was also greatly influenced by the writings of *John H. Tilden,* MD (who published between 1915 and 1925). Tilden became disenchanted with orthodox medicine and began to rely heavily on dietetics and nutrition, formulating his theories of "autointoxication" (the effect of fecal matter remaining too long in the digestive process) and "toxemia." He provided the natural health care literature with a 200-plus-page dissertation entitled *Constipation,* with a whole chapter devoted to the evils of not responding "when nature called." These concepts are reflected today in mainstream medicine by the newfound concern with the microbiome and probiotics.

Elie Metchnikoff (director of the prestigious Pasteur Institute and winner of the 1908 Nobel Prize for his contribution to immunology) and Kellogg wrote prolifically on the theory of autointoxication. Kellogg, in particular, believed that humans, in the process of digesting meat, produced a variety of intestinal toxins that contributed to autointoxication. As a result, Kellogg widely advocated that people return to a more healthy natural state by allowing the naturally designed use of the colon. He believed that the average modern colon was devitalized by the combination of a low-fiber diet, sedentary living, the custom of sitting rather than squatting to defecate, and the modern civilized habit of ignoring "nature's call" out of an undue concern for politeness.

Although the concept of toxemia is not a part of the body of knowledge taught in conventional medical schools, all naturopathic students are presented with this concept and its scientific basis and research support. Some of that presentation relies on outdated materials, such as the naturopathic texts of 75 and 100 years ago (e.g., Lindlahr, Tilden). However, modern research and textbooks are beginning to investigate this phenomenon. Drasar and Hill's *Human Intestinal Flora* (1974) demonstrates some of the biochemical pathways involved in the generation of metabolic toxins in the gut through dysbiotic bacterial action on poorly digested food (Zeff, 1997), and these mechanisms have been investigated in terms of causation of colon cancer and breast cancer (Micozzi, 1989).

In the last 30 years, our understanding of the concept of toxemia has been significantly updated by practitioners in the newly emerging field of *functional medicine,* a health care approach that focuses attention on biochemical individuality, metabolic balance, ecological context, and unique personal experience in the dynamics of health. Maldigestion, malabsorption, and abnormal gut flora and ecology are often found to be primary contributing factors not only to gastrointestinal disorders but also to a wide variety of chronic systemic illnesses. Laboratory assessment tools have been developed that are capable of evaluating the status of many organs, including the gastrointestinal tract. These cutting-edge diagnostic tools provide physicians with an analysis of numerous functional parameters of the individual's digestion and absorption and precisely pinpoint what in the colonic environment is imbalanced, thus promoting dysbiosis (Jones, 2005). In the most current naturopathic textbook, the *Textbook of Natural Medicine* (Pizzorno & Murray, 2013), seven chapters cover this important topic.

Thomsonianism

In 1822, *Samuel Thomson* published his *New Guide to Health,* a compilation of his personal view of medical theory and American Indian herbal and medical botanical lore. Thomson espoused the belief that disease had one general cause—derangement of the vital fluids by "cold" influences on the human body—and that disease therefore had one general remedy—animal warmth or "heat." The name of the complaint depended on the part of the body that was affected. Unlike the conventional American "heroic" medical tradition that advocated bloodletting, leeching, and the substantial use of mineral-based purgatives such as antimony and mercury, Thomson believed that minerals

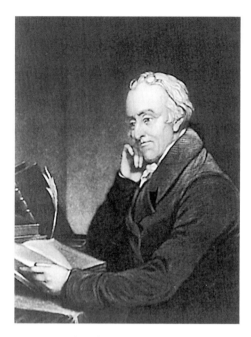

Figure 22-5 Samuel Thomson (1769–1843). (Courtesy National Library of Medicine, Bethesda, MD.)

were sources of "cold" because they come from the ground and that vegetation, which grew toward the sun, represented "heat" (Figure 22-5).

Thomson's view was that individuals could self-treat if they had an adequate understanding of his philosophy *and* a copy of *New Guide to Health*. The right to sell "family franchises" for use of the Thomsonian method of healing was the basis of a profound lay movement between 1822 and Thomson's death in 1843. Thomson adamantly believed that no professional medical class should exist and that democratic medicine was best practiced by laypersons within a Thomsonian "family" unit. By 1839 Thomson claimed to have sold some 100,000 of these family franchises, called "friendly botanic societies."

Despite his criticism of the early medical movement for its heroic tendencies, Thomson's medical theories were heroic in their own fashion. Although he did not advocate bloodletting or heavy metal poisoning and leeching, botanical purgatives—particularly *Lobelia inflata* (Indian tobacco)—were a substantial part of the therapy.

Eclectic School of Medicine

Some of the doctors practicing the Thomsonian method, called *botanics,* decided to separate themselves from the popular, lay movement and develop a more physiologically sound basis of therapy. They established a broader range of therapeutic applications of botanical medicines and founded a medical college in Cincinnati. These Thomsonian doctors were later absorbed into the "eclectic school," which originated with Wooster Beach of New York.

Wooster Beach, from a well-established New England family, started his medical studies at an early age, apprenticing under an old German herbal doctor, Jacob Tidd, until Tidd died. Beach then enrolled in the Barclay Street

Medical University in New York. After opening his own practice in New York, Beach set out to win over fellow members of the New York Medical Society (into which he had been warmly introduced by the screening committee) to his point of view that heroic medicine was inherently dangerous and should be reduced to the gentler theories of herbal medicine. He was summarily ostracized from the medical society.

He soon founded his own school in New York, calling the clinic and educational facility the United States Infirmary. Because of political pressure from the medical society, however, he was unable to obtain charter authority to issue legitimate diplomas. He then located a financially ailing but legally chartered school, Worthington College, in Worthington, Ohio. There he opened a full-scale medical college, creating the eclectic school of medical theory based on the European, Native American, and American traditions. The most enduring eclectic herbal textbook is *King's American Dispensary* by *Harvey Wickes Felter* and *John Uri Lloyd*. Published in 1898, this comprehensive two-volume, 2500-page treatise provided the definitive work describing the identification, preparation, pharmacognosy, history of use, and clinical application of more than 1000 botanical medicines. The eclectic herbal lore formed an integral core of the therapeutic armamentarium of the naturopathic doctor (ND).

Homeopathic Medicine

Homeopathy, the creation of an early German physician, *Samuel Hahnemann* (1755–1843), had four central doctrines: (1) that like cures like (the "law of similars"); (2) that the effect of a medication could be heightened by its administration in minute doses (the more diluted the dose, the greater the "dynamic" effect); (3) that nearly all diseases were the result of a suppressed itch, or "psora"; and (4) healing proceeds from within outward, above downward, from more vital to less vital organs, and in the reverse order of the appearance of symptoms (pathobiography), known as Hering's rules.

Hahneman's *The Organon of Medicine,* the seminal text on homeopathic theory and method, was published from the first edition in 1810 (*The Organon of the Healing Art* [*Organon der rationellen Heilkunde*]) to the sixth edition, posthumously, in 1921. Homeopathic theory significantly influenced Lindlahr's *Nature Cure,* and later scholars on naturopathic theory, integrating such concepts as the vital force and others.

Originally, most U.S. homeopaths were converted orthodox medical doctors, or *allopaths* (a term coined by Hahnemann), disappointed in the counterproductive effects of regular medicine, especially in dealing with infectious disease epidemics (see above). The high rate of conversion helped make this particular medical profession the archenemy of the rising orthodox medical profession. The first American homeopathic medical school was founded in 1848 in Philadelphia; the last purely homeopathic medical school, based in Philadelphia, survived into the early 1930s. After the original homeopathic medical school moved to a larger building in Philadelphia, it then became the home of the first women's medical school in the United States. The homeopathic school eventually adopted biomedicine during the early twentieth century, and the two schools were to eventually be merged during the 1990s, and is today named for Hahnemann. Two contributors to this textbook are on the faculty there.

Manipulative Therapies: Osteopathy and Chiropractic

In Missouri, *Andrew Taylor Still,* originally trained as an orthodox practitioner, founded the school of medical thought known as *osteopathy.* He conceived a system of healing that emphasized the primary importance of the structural integrity of the body, especially as it affects the vascular system, in the maintenance of health. In 1892, he opened the American School of Osteopathy in Kirksville, Missouri.

In 1895, Daniel David Palmer, originally a magnetic healer from Davenport, Iowa, performed the first spinal manipulation, which gave rise to the school he termed *chiropractic.* His philosophy was similar to Still's except for a greater emphasis on the importance of proper neurological function. He formally published his findings in 1910, after having founded a chiropractic school in Davenport, Iowa (see Chapters 18 and 19).

Less well known is "zone therapy," originated by *Joe Shelby Riley,* DC, a chiropractor based in Washington, D.C. In zone therapy, pressure to and manipulation of the fingers and tongue and percussion of the spinal column were applied according to the relation of points on these structures to certain zones of the body (Chapter 20).

Christian Science and the Role of Belief and Spirituality

Christian Science, formulated by *Mary Baker Eddy* in 1879, after the teachings of Phineas Quimby, comprises a profound belief in the role of systematic religious study (which led to the widespread Christian Science Reading Rooms), spirituality, and prayer in the treatment of disease. In 1875, she published *Science and Health with Key to the Scriptures,* the definitive textbook for the study of Christian Science (Chapter 6).

Lust was also influenced by the works of *Sidney Weltmer,* the founder of "suggestive therapeutics." Weltmer's work dealt specifically with the psychological process of desiring to be healthy. The theory behind Professor Weltmer's work was that, whether it was the mind or the body that first lost its grip on health, the two were inseparably related in a cybernetic "vicious cycle." When the problem originated in the body, the mind nonetheless lost its ability and desire to overcome the disease because the patient "felt sick" and consequently slid further into the diseased state. Alternatively, if the mind first lost its ability and desire to "be healthy" and some physical infirmity followed, the patient was susceptible to being overcome by disease (see Chapter 6).

Henry Lindlahr addressed spiritual origins of illness, the spiritual nature of the human being (the tri-fold nature of man), and spiritual aspects of healing and therapeutics in *Nature Cure* (Lindlahr, 1914a).

Physical Culture

Bernarr Mcfadden, a close friend of Lust's, founded the "physical culture" school of health and healing, also known as *physcultopathy.* This school of healing gave birth across the United States to gymnasiums where exercise programs were designed and taught to allow individual men and women to establish and maintain optimal physical health.

Although so strongly based on common sense and observation, many theories exist to explain the rapid dissolution of these diverse healing arts. The practitioners at one time made up more than 25% of all U.S. health care practitioners in the early part of the twentieth century. Low ratings in the infamous Flexner Report (which ranked all these schools of medical thought among the lowest), allopathic medicine's anointing of itself with the blessing "scientific," and the growing political sophistication of the AMA clearly played significant roles. Of course, the acceptance of the germ theory of disease and development of effective antibiotics for the first time provided a strong rationale for the new, "scientific," regular medicine.

All the natural healing systems and modalities were ultimately unified in the field of naturopathic medicine because they shared one common tenet: respect for and inquiry into the self-healing process and what is necessary to establish and maintain health.

HALCYON DAYS

In the early 1920s, the "health fad" movement was reaching its peak in terms of public awareness and interest. Conventions were held throughout the United States, one of which was attended by several members of Congress, culminating in full legalization of naturopathy as a healing art in the District of Columbia. One physician serving in the U.S. Senate, Royal Copeland, was a homeopath and worked for the creation of the national homeopathic formulary in the 1930s. Not only were the conventions well attended by professionals, but the public also flocked to them, with more than 10,000 attending the 1924 convention in Los Angeles.

During the 1920s and up until 1937, naturopathy was in its most popular phase. Although the institutions of the orthodox school had gained ascendancy, before 1937 the medical profession had no relatively safe and effective solutions to the problems of human disease.

During the 1920s, *Gaylord Hauser,* later to become the health food guru of Hollywood, came to Lust as a seriously ill young man. Lust, through application of the nature cure, removed Hauser's afflictions and was rewarded by Hauser's lifelong devotion. His regular columns in *Nature's Path* became widely read among the Hollywood celebrity crowd with its growing influence on the popular imagination.

The naturopathic journals of the 1920s and 1930s provide much valuable insight into the prevention of disease and the promotion of health. Much of the dietary advice focused on correcting poor eating habits, including the lack of fiber in the diet and an overreliance on red meat as a protein source. Finally, in the 1990s, we began to hear the pronouncements of the orthodox profession, the National Institutes of Health (NIH) and the National Cancer Institute, after billions of dollars spent on research in the flagging "war on cancer," that the early assertions of the naturopaths that such dietary habits would lead to degenerative diseases, including colon cancer and other cancers, are true (e.g., Micozzi et al, 1989).

The December 1928 issue of *Nature's Path* contained the first American publication of the work of *Herman J. DeWolff*, a Dutch epidemiologist. DeWolff was one of the first researchers to assert, on the basis of studies of the incidence of cancer in the Netherlands, that there was a correlation between exposure to petrochemicals and various types of cancerous conditions. He contended that the use of chemical fertilizers and their application in some soils (principally clay) led to their remaining in vegetables after they had arrived at the market and were purchased for consumption. It was almost 50 years before orthodox medicine began to see the wisdom of such assertions. As late as 1980, two British epidemiologists in an influential analysis on population attributable risks minimized the contribution of environmental and chemical pollutants, consumer products, processed foods, and additives, finding that most cancer risk is due to personal lifestyle, diet, body composition, physical activity, alcohol and tobacco consumption, sun exposure, etc. (Doll & Peto, 1981). In the ensuing decades, multiple studies have had difficulties being able to demonstrate that "lifestyle" factors explain all the large increases in cancer during the past century.

SUPPRESSION AND DECLINE

In 1937, the popularity of naturopathy began to decline. The change came, as both Thomas and Campion note in their works, with the era of "miracle medicine." Lust recognized this, and his editorializing became, if anything, even more strident. From the introduction of sulfa drugs in 1937 to the release of the Salk vaccine in 1955, the post–World War II American public became accustomed to annual developments of "miracle" vaccines for prevention and antibiotics for cures. The naturopathic profession adhered to its vitalistic philosophy and a full range of practice but was poorly unified at this time on standards and other issues, making the profession vulnerable to inter-guild competition.

Lust died in September 1945 in residence at the Yungborn facility in Butler, New Jersey, preparing to attend the 49th Annual Congress of his American Naturopathic Association. Although a healthy, vigorous man, he had seriously damaged his lungs the previous year saving patients when a wing of his facility caught fire; he never fully recovered. On August 30, 1945, writing for the official program

of that Congress, held in October 1945 just after his death, he noted his concerns for the future. He was especially frustrated with the success of the medical profession in blocking the efforts of naturopaths to establish state licensing laws to establish appropriate practice rights for NDs and also protect the public from the "pretenders" (i.e., those who chose to call themselves naturopaths without ever bothering to undergo formal training). As Lust (1945) stated:

> Now let us see the type of men and women who are the Naturopaths of today. Many of them are fine, upstanding individuals, believing fully in the effectiveness of their chosen profession—willing to give their all for the sake of alleviating human suffering and ready to fight for their rights to the last ditch. More power to them! But there are others who claim to be Naturopaths who are woeful misfits. Yes, and there are outright fakers and cheats masking as Naturopaths. That is the fate of any science—any profession—which the unjust laws have placed beyond the pale. Where there is no official recognition and regulation, you will find the plotters, the thieves, the charlatans operating on the same basis as the conscientious practitioners. And these riff-raff opportunists bring the whole art into disrepute. Frankly, such conditions cannot be remedied until suitable safeguards are erected by law, or by the profession itself, around the practice of Naturopathy. That will come in time.

In the mid-1920s, *Morris Fishbein* had come onto the scene as editor of the *Journal of the American Medical Association (JAMA)*. Fishbein took on a personal vendetta against what he characterized as "quackery" (see Chapter 19). Lust, among others, including Mcfadden, became Fishbein's epitomes of quackery. He proved to be particularly effective politically and in the media.

The public infatuation with new technology, the introduction of "miracle medicine," World War II's stimulation of the development of surgery and procedural medicine, the Flexner Report, the growing political sophistication of the AMA under the leadership of Fishbein, intraprofession squabbles, and the death of Lust in 1945 all combined to instigate the decline of naturopathic medicine and natural healing in the United States. In addition, these years, called the years of *the great fear* in David Caute's book of the same name, were also the years of the Cold War, during which it became politically unorthodox to be considered "un-American."

U.S. courts began to take the view that naturopaths were not truly doctors because they espoused doctrines from "the dark ages of medicine" (something American medicine had supposedly come out of in 1937) and that drugless healers were intended by law to operate without "drugs" (which came to be defined as anything a physician would prescribe for a patient to ingest or apply externally for any medical purpose). The persistent lack of uniform standards, lack of insurance coverage, lost court battles, a splintered profession, and a hostile legislative perspective progressively restricted practice until the core naturopathic therapies became essentially illegal and practices financially nonviable.

Although it was under considerable public pressure in those years, the American Naturopathic Association undertook some of its most scholarly work, coordinating all the systems of naturopathy under commission. This resulted in the publication of a formal textbook, *Basic Naturopathy* (Spitler, 1948), and a significant work compiling all the known theories of botanical medicine, *Naturae Medicina* (Kuts-Cheraux, 1953). Naturopathic medicine began fragmenting when Lust's American Naturopathic Association was succeeded by six different splinter organizations in the mid-1950s.

By the early 1970s, the profession's educational institutions had dwindled to only one: the National College of Naturopathic Medicine, with branches in Seattle and Portland, Oregon.

RE-EMERGENCE

The combination of the counterculture years of the late 1960s, the public's growing awareness of the importance of nutrition and the environment, and awareness of "holism" became powerful and persistent social forces (see Chapters 1, 3, and 7). America's disenchantment with organized institutional medicine began after the miracle cure era faded and it became apparent that orthodox medicine has significant limitations and is prohibitively dangerous and expensive. Antibiotic "magic bullets" for infections became "friendly fire" with the rapid emergence of intractable multiple antibiotic-resistant strains of bacteria. The pharmaceutical breakthroughs of the "golden age" were largely replaced by "blockbuster" drugs to be taken by millions of "patients" without diseases, but only putative "risk factors" for medical conditions, many of which are simply medicalized versions of normal life experiences.

All of these difficult developments resulted in the emergence of new respect for alternative medicine in general and in the rejuvenation of naturopathic medicine. At this time, a new generation of students was attracted to the philosophical precepts of the profession. They brought with them an appreciation for the appropriate use of science, modern college education, and matching expectations for quality education. Meeting these students was a small but deeply committed community of elder naturopathic physicians and teachers, pivotal in keeping the profession (barely) alive. These elders mentored this new generation clinically and professionally, supporting them in rebuilding and advancing, naturopathic medicine.

Dr. John Bastyr (1912–1995) and his firm, efficient, professional leadership inspired science- and research-based training in natural medicine to begin to reach toward its full potential. Dr. Bastyr, whose vision was of "naturopathy's empirical successes documented and proven by scientific methods," was "himself a prototype for the modern naturopathic doctor, who culls the latest findings from the scientific literature, applies them in ways consistent with naturopathic principles, and verifies the results with appro-

priate studies." Bastyr also saw "a tremendous expansion in both allopathic and naturopathic medical knowledge, and he played a major role in making sure the best of both were integrated into naturopathic medical education" (Kirchfeld & Boyle, 1994).

In response to the growth in public interest during the late 1970s, naturopathic colleges were established in Arizona (Arizona College of Naturopathic Medicine, 1978), Oregon (American College of Naturopathic Medicine, 1980), and California (Pacific College of Naturopathic Medicine, 1979). None of these three survived. In 1978, the John Bastyr College of Naturopathic Medicine (later renamed Bastyr University) was formed in Seattle by founding president Joseph E. Pizzorno, ND (one of the authors of this chapter), Lester E. Griffith, ND, William Mitchell, ND, and Sheila Quinn to teach and develop what Pizzorno termed "science-based natural medicine."

They believed that for the naturopathic profession to move back into the mainstream, it needed to establish accredited institutions, perform credible research, and establish itself as an integral part of the health care system. Bastyr University not only survived but thrived, and it became the first naturopathic college ever to become regionally accredited. In 1978, the Ontario College of Naturopathic Medicine was founded by Ken Dunk, ND, Gordon Smith, ND, Eric Srubb, ND, and John LaPlante, ND, later becoming Canadian College of Naturopathic Medicine, now a thriving college and research center north of Toronto, Ontario. In 1993, Michael Cronin, ND, Kyle Cronin, ND, and Konrad Kail, ND, founded the Southwest College of Naturopathic Medicine and Health Science in Scottsdale, Arizona "primarily due to the wide scope of practice available to naturopathic physicians under ND licensing in Arizona and the growing demand for naturopathic education, especially in the southwest" (http://www.scnm.edu/about/history-founders).

In 1997, the University of Bridgeport, with the leadership of James Sensenig, ND, founded the University of Bridgeport College of Naturopathic Medicine, meeting the growing demand for a naturopathic college in the northeastern states. In 1999, Boucher Institute of Naturopathic Medicine was founded in Vancouver, BC, by a small group of visionaries on the principles of "inclusion, integration, integrity, respect, academic freedom, self-responsibility and innovation . . . to educate a different kind of physician—one who commits to the ongoing practice of self-reflection and personal growth, who has a passionate belief in the efficacy of naturopathic medicine and a commitment to leading our world toward sustainable health principles intrinsic to the mission of modern naturopathc institutions."

Later, during the mid-2000s, National University of Health Sciences (re)opened its naturopathic medicine program under the leadership of president Jim Winterstein, DC, and assistant dean Fraser Smith, ND, in Lombard, Illinois, the home of Henry Lindlahr's original inpatient facility, building a strong science-based curriculum on well-integrated naturopathic principles. In 2012, Bastyr University opened a branch campus in San Diego under the leadership of President Dan Church, PhD, and Vice President Moira Fitzpatrick, ND, PhD, welcomed by the community in an environment ripe for Bastyr's partnership in collaborative and integrative health care.

With eight credible colleges, a rapidly growing research community, an appreciation of the appropriate application of science to natural medicine education, growing enrollments, and diverse and growing opportunities for clinical practice, naturopathic medicine is now a leading voice in the growing integrative health care and health care reform movements in North America today.

RECENT INFLUENCES

A tremendous amount of research providing scientific support for the principles of naturopathic medicine has been conducted at mainstream research centers and increasingly at naturopathic medical schools. In fact, conventional biomedicine is turning more to the use of naturopathic methods in the search for effective prescriptions for diseases that are currently intractable and expensive to treat (Werbach, 1996; Pizzorno & Katzinger, 2012; Pizzorno & Murray, 2013). It is now well established that nutritional factors are of major importance in the pathogenesis of both atherosclerosis and cancer, the two leading causes of death in Western countries. Studies validating the importance of nutritional factors in the pathogenesis of many other diseases continue to be published. Much of the research now documenting the scientific foundations of naturopathic medicine practices and principles can be found in *Textbook of Natural Medicine* (Pizzorno & Murray, 2013). This 200-plus-chapter work contains more than 7500 citations to the peer-reviewed scientific literature documenting the efficacy of many natural medicine therapies.

Naturopaths were astute clinical observers and a century ago recognized many of the concepts that are now gaining popularity and are being supported by scientific data. However, the scientific tools of the time were inadequate to assess the validity of their concepts. In addition, as a group in the early years of the profession's formation, they seemed to have little inclination for the application of laboratory research, especially because "science" was the bludgeon used by the AMA to suppress the profession. This situation has changed.

In the past few decades, a considerable amount of research has now provided the scientific documentation of many of the concepts of naturopathic medicine, and the new breed of scientifically trained naturopathic physician is using this research to continue development of the profession, as naturopathic colleges foster a growing array of research studies, research institutes, and research training for naturopathic physicians. In 2002–2004, NCCAM funded *The Future and Foundations of Naturopathic Medical Science: The Naturopathic Medical Research Agenda* (Standish et al, 2004) through naturopathic colleges, external re-

search scientists, and the American Association of Naturopathic Physicians. The following sections describe a few of the most important trends.

Therapeutic Nutrition

Since 1929, when Christiaan Eijkman and Sir Frederick Hopkins shared the Nobel Prize in medicine and physiology for the discovery of vitamins, the role of these trace substances in clinical nutrition has been the subject of considerable scientific investigation. The discovery that metabolic systems depend on essential nutrients provided the naturopathic profession with great insights into why an organically grown, whole-foods diet is so important for health. Formulation of the concept of "biochemical individuality" by nutritional biochemist Roger Williams in 1955 further developed these ideas and provided great insights into the unique nutritional needs of each individual. This knowledge led to ways to correct inborn errors of metabolism and even prevent and treat specific diseases through the use of nutrient-rich foods or large doses of specific nutrients. Linus Pauling, PhD, the two-time Nobel Prize winner, and Abrahm Hoffer, MD, PhD, originated the concept of "orthomolecular medicine" and provided further theoretical substantiation for the use of nutrients as therapeutic agents (see also Chapter 26).

Functional Medicine

In 1990, Jeff Bland, PhD, coined the term *functional medicine* to describe a putatively science-based development of therapeutic nutrition for the prevention of illness, promotion of health, and treatment of disease. Focusing on biochemical individuality, metabolic balance, and the ecological context, functional medicine practitioners avail themselves of recently developed laboratory tests to pinpoint imbalances in an individual's biochemistry that are thought to cause a cascade of biological triggers, paving the way to suboptimal function, chronic illness, and degenerative disease. A broad range of functional laboratory assessment tools in the areas of digestion (gastrointestinal system), nutrition, detoxification and oxidative stress, immunology and allergy, production and regulation of hormones (endocrinology), and the heart and blood vessels (cardiovascular system) provide physicians with a basis to recommend nutritional interventions specific to the individual's needs and to monitor their efficacy. Evidence assembled in the functional medicine literature is integral to naturopathic training, forming the basis for therapies in the "strengthening systems" aspect of the naturopathic therapeutic order. Two modern textbooks have been published to codify this "systems" medicine: Jones et al's (2005) *Textbook of Functional Medicine* and Pizzorno and Katzinger's (2012) *Clinical Pathophysiology, A Functional Perspective*.

Environmental Medicine and Clinical Ecology

Although recognition of the clinical impact of environmental toxicity and endogenous toxicity has existed since the earliest days of naturopathy, it was not until the environmental movement and the seminal work of Rachel Carson and others that a scientific basis was established. Clinical research and the development of laboratory methods for assessing toxic load provided objective tools that have greatly increased the sophistication of clinical practice. Clinical and laboratory methods were developed for the assessment of idiosyncratic reactions to environmental factors and food sensitivities (see Chapter 26).

Spirituality, Health, and Medicine

Naturopathic medicine's philosophy of treating the whole person and enhancing the individual's inherent healing ability is closely aligned with its mission of integrating spirituality into the healing process. Scientific evidence is growing on the part spirituality can play in healing (see Chapter 11). René Descartes has been accused of separating mind from body back in the seventeenth century. Medical science has since attempted to explain disease independently of mind, due to external agents such as germs, environmental agents, or more recently in terms of wayward genes. At present, however, the evidence on the link between mind and body is not just clinical observation but biochemical fact (see Chapters 8, 9, and 10).

An explosion of research in the new and rapidly expanding field of psychoneuroimmunology is revealing physical evidence of the mind–body connection that is changing our understanding of disease (see Chapter 8). Scientists no longer question *whether* but rather *how* our minds have an impact on our health, and the implications of the connections uncovered in only the last 20 years are extraordinary.

In his book *Healing Words* (1993)—and several other works—Larry Dossey, MD, pulls together what he describes as "one of the best kept secrets in medical science": the extensive experimental evidence for the beneficial effects of prayer. Dossey (1993) reviews studies that provide evidence for a positive effect of prayer on not only humans but mice, chicks, enzymes, fungi, yeast, bacteria, and cells of various sorts (see Chapter 14). He emphasizes, "We cannot dismiss these outcomes as being due to suggestion or placebo effects, since these so-called lower forms of life do not think in any conventional sense and are presumably not susceptible to suggestion" (Pizzorno & Murray, 1985–1995). Dossey's most recent book, *One Mind*, engages in-depth discussion of the science of connection and "entanglement" (see Chapter 14), an important advance integral to the discussion of spiritual aspects of health and health care, illness and healing.

Contemporary Laboratory Methods

Another significant influence has been the development of laboratory methods for the objective assessment of nutritional status, metabolic dysfunction, digestive function, bowel flora, endogenous and exogenous toxic load, liver detoxification and other system functions, and genomics. Each of these has provided ever more precise tools for accurate assessment of patient health status and effective application of naturopathic principles.

Genomics and Epigenetics

One of the most heralded recent advances is genomic testing, the ability to evaluate each individual's template for creating the biochemical enzymes of life, and recognition of epigenetic modulation of genetic manifestation. Assessment of a person's genome is now providing a level of objective evaluation of biochemical individuality never before available, greatly strengthening the naturopathic doctor's ability to practice truly personalized medicine. The ability to assess each individual's unique nutrient needs as well as susceptibilities to environmental toxins promises to change fundamentally the practice of medicine (Pizzorno, 2003).

Despite the huge public and private investment in human genome science, we have yet to witness the development of safe and effective "gene therapies" from the burgeoning biotech industry. Instead, genetic science is revealing how natural and nutritional approaches actually work in the body, much beyond theories of their actions as "anti-oxidants," for example. Recent research has revealed how vitamin D, for example, regulates genetic expression, turning "on" and "off" multiple genes that are key in metabolic processes and physiologic responses, explaining the multiple benefits of adequate vitamin D in human health studies (see Chapter 26). In addition, recent research by Benson et al (see Chapter 10) at Harvard has demonstrated that "mind–body" approaches like relaxation therapies also influence gene expression, producing healthful physiologic states.

The new era in gene science appears to be validating and explaining how natural and nutritional medicine actually works at the cellular, genetic, and molecular levels that have been the almost-exclusive focus of all biomedical research for the past half-century.

CONCLUSION

During the last several years, as America's staggering health care debt accumulates together with an aging population and increases in chronic diseases, the core, traditional naturopathic principles are surfacing widely as central to creating an effective health care system.

Current medical education inculcates many of the dominant values of modern medicine: reductionism, specialization, mechanistic models of disease, and faith in a definitive cure (see Chapter 1). What is needed is a model of care that addresses the whole person and integrates care for the person's entire constellation of comorbidities. Nothing short of a fundamental redesign of primary care systems is required (Grumbach, 2003).

Over a century ago, the founders of organized, naturopathic medicine were among those who predicted that a medical system that treats the symptoms of disease rather the reversing the underlying causes would result in an ever increasing burden of chronic disease. Their understanding has proven prophetic. In light of its emphasis on therapeutic order (see Chapter 3) and its neo-eclectic approach to including a wide-range of safe and effective CAM treatment modalities, contemporary naturopathic medicine stands poised to provide an authentic model for truly "integrative medicine," as discussed further in the next chapter.

References

Accenture Physician Alignment Survey: Accenture News Release: More U.S. Doctors Leaving Private Practice Due to Rising Costs and Technology Mandates, Accenture Report Finds, 2012. http://newsroom.accenture.com/news/more-us-doctors-leaving-private-practice-due-to-rising-costs-and-technology-mandates-accenture-report-finds.htm.

American Association of Naturopathic Physicians: Naturopathic Medicine an "Answer for the Country," States Health Care Leader, http://www.naturopathic.org/content.asp?admin=Y&contentid=669. Accessed: May 20, 2013.

American Association of Naturopathic Physicians: Co-Chairs Snider P & Zeff J: Select Committee on the Definition of Naturopathic Medicine: *Definition of naturopathic medicine position paper*, Rippling River, OR, 1989, House of Delegates. www.naturopathic.org. Accessed: Oct 1, 2013.

American Board of Integrative and Holistic Medicine. http://www.abihm.org (Accessed: October 1, 2013)

American Holistic Medical Association. http://www.holisticmedicine.org/content.asp?pl=1&sl=16&contentid=16 (Accessed October 1, 2013)

Berkenwald A: In the name of medicine, *Ann Intern Med* 128:246, 1998.

Catlin A: *Health Aff* 27:14–29, 2008.

Consortium of Academic Health Centers for Integrative Medicine. http://www.imconsortium.org/ 2013.

Cooper R, Stoflet S: Trends in the education and practice of alternative medicine clinicians, *Health Aff* 15(3):226, 1996.

Cruse JM: History of medicine: the metamorphosis of scientific medicine in the ever-present past, *Am J Med Sci* 318(3):171, 1999.

Doll R, Peto R: *The causes of cancer*, 1981, Oxford University Press.

Dossey L: *Healing words*, San Francisco, 1993, Harper San Francisco.

Fleming SA, Gutknecht NC: Naturopathy and the primary care practice, *Prim Care* 37:119–136, 2010.

Freshman B, Rubio L, Chassiokas Y: *Collaboration across the disciplines in health care*, Sudbury, MA, 2010, Jones and Bartlett Publishers.

Goldblatt E, Snider P, Weeks J, editors: *Clinicians and educators desk reference on the licensed complementary and alternative healthcare professions*, ed 2, 2013, Academic Consortium for Complementary and Alternative Health Care (ACCAHC). www.accahc.org.

Grumbach K: Chronic illness, comorbidities, and the need for medical generalism, *Ann Fam Med* 1:4, 2003.

Gyatso DS: *Mirror of Beryl: a historical introduction to Tibetan medicine*, Boston, 2010, Wisdom Publications, pp 2–6.

Jones D: *Textbook of functional medicine*, 2005, Institute for Functional Medicine.

Kaptchuk T, Eisenberg DM: Varieties of healing. 1: medical pluralism in the United States, *Ann Intern Med* 135:189, 2001.

Kirchfield F, Boyle W: *Nature doctors*, Portland, Ore/East Palestine, Ohio, 1994, Medicina Biological/Buckeye Naturopathic Press, p 311.

Kuts-Cheraux AW: *Naturae medicina*, Des Moines, Iowa, 1953, ANPSA.

Light DW, Lexchin J, Darrow JJ: Institutional corruption of pharmaceuticals and the myth of safe and effective drugs, *J Law Med Ethics* 41(3):590–600, 2013.

Lindlahr H: *Nature cure*, Chicago, 1914a, The Nature Cure Publishing Company.

Lindlahr H: *Philosophy of natural therapeutics*, vols I, II, and III, Dietetics, Maidstone, England, 1914b, Maidstone Osteopathic.

Ludmerer K: *Time to heal: American medical education from the turn of the century to the era of managed care*, New York, 1999, Oxford University Press.

Lust B: *Program*, 1945. 49th Congress of American Naturopathy Association.

Magee R: Medical practice and medical education 1500-2001: an overview, *ANZ J Surg* 74(4):272, 2004.

Micozzi MS, Carter CL, Albanes D, et al: Bowel function and breast cancer in US women, *Am J Public Health* 79(1):73–75, 1989.

Micozzi MS: Complementary medicine: what is appropriate? Who will provide it? *Ann Intern Med* 129:65–66, 1998.

Newman Turner R: *Naturopathic medicine around the world*, May 2011. Presentation Bastyr University.

New York Times, April 2012.

Ober KP: The pre-Flexnerian reports: Mark Twain's criticism of medicine in the United States, *Ann Intern Med* 126(2):157, 1997.

Petrina S: Medical liberty: drugless healers confront allopathic doctors 1910–1931, *J Med Humanit* 29(4):205, 2008.

Pizzorno J: Editorial, *Integr Med Clinician J* 2:4, 2003.

Pizzorno J, Katzinger J: *Clinical pathophysiology, a functional perspective*, 2012, Mind Publishing.

Pizzorno JE, Murray MT, editors: *Textbook of natural medicine*, ed 4, St. Louis, 2013, Churchill Livingstone Elsevier.

Pizzorno JE, Murray MT: *A textbook of natural medicine*, Seattle, 1985-1995, John Bastyr College Publications.

Rutkow LW, Rutkow IM: Homeopaths, surgery, and the Civil War: Edward C. Franklin and the struggle to achieve medical pluralism in the Union army, *Arch Surg* 139(7):785, 2004.

Shelton HM: *Natural hygiene, man's pristine way of life*, Texas, 1968, Dr. Shelton's Health School.

Spitler HR: *Basic naturopathy*, Des Moines, Iowa, 1948, American Naturopathic Association.

Standish L, Snider P, Calabrese C, NMRA Core Team: The future and foundations of naturopathic medical science, *Report to NIHCCAM on Naturopathic Medical Research Agenda (NMRA)*, 2004.

Weeks J: The Integrator Blog, n.d., available at: http://theintegratorblog.com/index.php?option=com_frontpage&Itemid=1.

Weeks J, Goldblatt L, Snider P: Complementary, alternative, and integrative healthcare perspectives. In Freshman B, Rubino L, Chassiokas Y, editors: *Collaboration across the disciplines in health care*, Sudbury, MA, 2010, Jones and Bartlett Publishers.

Werbach M: *The American Holistic Health Association complete guide to alternative medicine*, New York, 1996, Werner Books, pp 118, 123.

Whorton J: *Crusaders for fitness*, Princeton, NJ, 1982, Princeton University Press.

Whorton J: *Nature cures: the history of alternative medicine in America*, New York, 2002, Oxford University Press.

Whorton J: Benedict Lust, naturopathy, & the theory of therapeutic universalism, *Iron Game History* 2(8):2003.

Zeff J: The process of healing: a unifying theory of naturopathic medicine, *J Naturopath Med* 7(1):122, 1997.

Zeff J, Snider P, Myers S, DeGrandpre Z: The hierarchy of healing: the therapeutic order—a unifying theory of naturopathic medicine. In Pizzorno J, Murray M, editors: *Textbook of natural medicine*, ed 4, 2013, Elsevier.

Suggested Readings

American Association of Naturopathic Physicians: Co-Chairs Snider P & Zeff J: Select Committee on the Defintion of Naturopathic Medicine: *Definition of naturopathic medicine position paper*, Rippling River, OR, 1989, House of Delegates. www.naturopathic.org. Accessed: Oct 1, 2013.

American Medical Association: Physicians in the United States and possessions by selected characteristics, n.d., available at: http://www.ama-assn.org/ama1/pub/upload/images/373/internettable.gif.

Beasley JD, Swift JJ: *The Kellogg report: the impact of nutrition, environment and lifestyle on the health of Americans*, Annandale-on-Hudson, NY, 1989, Institute of Health Policy and Practice, the Bard College Center.

Benjamin H: *Everybody's guide to nature cure*, ed 7, England, 1981, Thorsons.

Benjamin PJ, Phillips R, Warren D, et al: Response to a proposal for an integrative medicine curriculum, *J Altern Complement Med* 13(9):1021–1033, 2007.

Bilz FE: *The natural method of healing*, vols 1 and 2, New York, 1898, International News.

Brown D: *Quarterly Review of Natural Medicine*, Seattle, 1994, NPRC.

Coulter H: *Divided legacy*, vol II, Washington, DC, 1973, Wehawken Books.

Dejarnette MB: *Technic and practice of bloodless surgery*, Nebraska City, NE, 1939, private publication.

Eddy MB: *Science and health with key to the scriptures*, 1875.

Felter HW, Lloyd JU: *King's American dispensary*, 1898.

Filden JH: *Impaired health (its cause and cure)*, ed 2, Denver, 1921, private publication.

Garlic has to smell bad to do some good, *Fam Pract News* 22:31, 1992.

Graham RL: *Hydro-hygiene*, New York, 1923, Thompson-Barlow.

Griggs B: *Green pharmacy*, London, 1981, Jill, Norman, & Hobhouse.

Hofoss D, Hjort P: The relationship between action and research in health policy, *Soc Sci Med [A]* 15(3 Pt 2):371, 1981.

Johnson AC: *Principles and practice of drugless therapeutics*, Los Angeles, 1946, Chir Ed Extension Bureau.

Jones D: *Functional medicine application to disorders of gene expression*, Hawaii, 1998. *Paper presented at the Fifth International Symposium on Functional Medicine.*

Kellogg JF: *Rational hydrotherapy*, Battle Creek, Mich, 1901, p 1902.

Kellogg JH: *New dietetics*, Battle Creek, Mich, 1923, Modern Medical Publishing.

Kuhne L: *Neo-naturopathy (new science of healing)*, Butler, NJ, 1918, Lust Publishers (translated by B Lust).

Lindlahr H: *Philosophy, practice, and dietetics of natural therapeutics*, vols I and II, Maidstone, England, 1914-1919, Maidstone Osteopathic.

Lust B: Editorial, *The naturopathic and herald of health* 1896.

Lust B: *Universal directory of naturopathy*, Butler, NJ, 1918, Lust Publishers.

Lust B: *Universal naturopathic directory and buyer's guide*, Butler, NJ, 1918, Lust Publications.

Lust B: "Proclamation," *The Naturopath and the Herald of Health*, vol XXVII, #, New York, 1922, Benedict Lust Publishing, pp 583–584.

Mcfadden B: *Building of vital power*, New Jersey, 1904, Physical Culture Publishing.

McKeown T: *The role of medicine: dream, mirage, or nemesis?*, London, 1976, Nuffield Provincial Hospitals Trust.

Murray MT: *Natural alternatives to over-the-counter and prescription drugs*, New York, 1994, William Morrow.

Murray MT, Pizzorno JE: *Encyclopedia of natural medicine*, Rocklin, CA, 1991, Prima.

Petkov V: Plants with hypotensive, antiatheromatous and coronary dilating action, *Am J Chin Med* 7:197, 1979.

Pizzorno J: *Total wellness*, Rocklin, CA, 1998, Prima, p 14.

Pizzorno J, Murray M: *Textbook of naturopathic medicine*, New York, 1999, Elsevier.

Richter JT: *Nature—the healer*, Los Angeles, 1949, private publication.

Riley JS: *Zone reflex*, Washington, DC, 1924, Publications of Health Research.

Shelton H: *Natural hygiene, man's pristine way of life*, San Antonio, TX, 1968, Dr Shelton's Health School, p 8.

Snider P, Zeff J: *Select Committee on Definition of Naturopathic Medicine report*, House of Delegates, Portland, OR, 1988, 1989, American Association of Naturopathic Physicians.

St. Anthony's Business Report on Alternative and Complementary Medicine, May 1997, p 5.

St. Anthony's Business Report on Alternative and Complementary Medicine, July 1998, pp 6–7.

St. Anthony's Business Report on Alternative and Complementary Medicine, August 1998, pp 4–5.

Starr P: *Social transformation of American medicine*, New York, 1983, Basic Books.

Trall RT: *Hydropathic encyclopedia*, vol 3 vols, New York, 1880, SR Wells.

Weltmer E: *Practice of suggestive therapeutics*, Nevada, MO, 1913, Weltmer Institute.

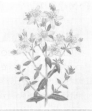

Contemporary Naturopathic Medicine

JOSEPH E. PIZZORNO, JR.
PAMELA SNIDER

Although in many ways, modern medicine resembles a science, it continues to be criticized for its lack of unifying theories, and for this reason alone its claim to being a science has remained suspect.

—BLOIS (1988)

What physicians think medicine is profoundly shapes what they do, how they behave in doing it, and the reasons they use to justify that behavior.... Whether conscious of it or not, every physician has an answer to what he thinks medicine is, with real consequences for all whom he attends.... The outcome is hardly trivial.... It dictates, after all, how we approach patients [and] how we make clinical judgments.

—PELLEGRINO (1979)

Medical philosophy comprises the underlying premises on which a healthcare system is based. Once a system is acknowledged, it is subject to debate. In naturopathic medicine, the philosophical debate is a valuable, ongoing process which helps the understanding that disease evolves in an orderly and truth-revealing fashion.

—BRADLEY (1985)

Naturopathic medicine developed from its basis in nature cure. Founded by Benedict Lust as the health care discipline of naturopathy (Box 23-1), today this same discipline in continuity is now known as naturopathic medicine. Early naturopathy and today's naturopathic medicine (NM) continue to *integrate*, as the hallmark of its approach, diverse therapies and concepts from various natural medicine disciplines and systems into a distinct system of health care. This integrative feature, together with its focus on therapeutic order, makes naturopathic medicine unique among today's systems of natural medicines. Most of complementary and alternative medicine (CAM) is "natural" in the broadest sense (see Chapter 1). The generic term *natural medicines* can be seen as applying to all CAM, including traditional ethnomedical and indigenous world medicines, together with other health care fields that espouse relations to natural principles of healing, health, and living.

Following Chapter 22, this chapter on naturopathic medicine broadly articulates (and reiterates, synthesizes, and expands), in naturopathic medicine's own terms, the common principles of all "natural medicine" in the context of the unifying theory and framework of naturopathic medicine. These principles can also be seen to underpin the so-called CAM and the traditional world medicine systems of today's global health care system. These principles provide one of the features, together with *therapeutic order*, that makes NM so appropriate as a model for authentic "integrative medicine."

This chapter continues to expand the discussion of naturopathic medicine, with an emphasis on areas that apply directly to contemporary practice as a model for integration. The reader is encouraged to recognize that both chapters can be taken to represent the profession, with the first underscoring the common threads and origins between naturopathic medicine and other disciplines in this section and textbook, a basis of its integrative approach.

In the editor's view, considering what is and is not available in practice today, contemporary NM best and most

BOX 23-1 *Principles, Aim, and Program of the Nature Cure System*

Since the earliest ages, medical science has been of all sciences the most unscientific. Its professors, with few exceptions, have sought to cure disease by the magic of pills and potions and poisons that attacked the ailment with the idea of suppressing the symptoms instead of attacking the real cause of the ailment.

Medical science has always believed in the superstition that the use of chemical substances that are harmful and destructive to human life will prove an efficient substitute for the violation of laws, and in this way encourages the belief that a man may go the limit in self-indulgences that weaken and destroy his physical system, and then hope to be absolved from his physical ailments by swallowing a few pills, or submitting to an injection of a serum or vaccine, that are supposed to act as vicarious redeemers of the physical organism and counteract life-long practices that are poisonous and wholly destructive to the patient's well-being.

The policy of expediency is at the basis of medical drug healing. It is along the lines of self-indulgence, indifference, ignorance, and lack of self-control that drug medicine lives, moves, and has its being.

The natural system for curing disease is based on a return to nature in regulating the diet, breathing, exercising, bathing, and the employment of various forces to eliminate the poisonous products in the system, and so raise the vitality of the patient to a proper standard of health.

Official medicine has, in all ages, simply attacked the symptoms of disease without paying any attention to the causes thereof, but natural healing is concerned far more with removing the causes of disease than merely curing its symptoms. This is the glory of this new school of medicine that it cures by removing the causes of the ailment, and is the only rational method of practicing medicine. It begins its cures by avoiding the uses of drugs, and hence is styled the system of drugless healing.

The program of naturopathic cure

1. ELIMINATION OF EVIL HABITS, or the weeds of life, such as overeating, alcoholic drinks, drugs, the use of tea, coffee, and cocoa that contain poisons, meat eating, improper hours of living, waste of vital forces, lowered vitality, sexual and social aberrations, worry, etc.
2. CORRECTIVE HABITS. Correct breathing, correct exercise, right mental attitude. Moderation in the pursuit of health and wealth.
3. NEW PRINCIPLES OF LIVING. Proper fasting, selection of food, hydropathy, light and air baths, mud baths, osteopathy, chiropractic and other forms of mechanotherapy, mineral salts obtained in organic form, electropathy, heliopathy, steam or Turkish baths, sitz baths, etc.

Natural healing is the most desirable factor in the regeneration of the race. It is a return to nature in methods of living and treatment. It makes use of the elementary forces of nature, of chemical selection of foods that will constitute a correct medical diet. The diet of civilized man is devitalized, is poor in essential organic salts. The fact that foods are cooked in so many ways and are salted, spiced, sweetened, and otherwise made attractive to the palate induces people to overeat, and overeating does more harm than underfeeding. High protein food and lazy habits are the cause of cancer, Bright's disease, rheumatism, and the poisons of autointoxication.

There is really but one healing force in existence and that is Nature herself, which means the inherent restorative power of the organism to overcome disease. Now the question is: can this power be appropriated and guided more readily by extrinsic or intrinsic methods? That is to say, is it more amenable to combat disease by irritating drugs, vaccines, and serums employed by superstitious moderns, or by the bland intrinsic congenial forces of Natural Therapeutics that are employed by this new school of medicine, that is naturopathy, which is the only orthodox school of medicine? Are not these natural forces much more orthodox than the artificial resources of the druggist?

(From Lust B: Principles of health, vol 1, Universal naturopathic directory and buyer's guide, Butler, NJ, 1918, Lust Publications.)

---

consciously incorporates many of these viable natural healing traditions in an authentic model of integration. Although it is also the editor's view that the health professions and the public are best served by respecting and retaining plurality and choice among specific, individual authentic CAM traditions and systems, NM is presently alone in providing authentic, effective integration. Naturopathy and NM are presented in this two-part approach to help illustrate the trajectory of this point. Set apart as they are, these chapters overarch and provide a capstone for this section of the book (as re-organized for fifth edition), and act as a keystone in the middle for the arch of the larger themes of the whole book.

PRINCIPLES

Naturopathic medicine is a distinct system of health-oriented medicine that stresses promotion of health, prevention of disease, patient education, and self-responsibility. However, naturopathic medicine symbolizes more than simply a health care system; it is a way of life and being in the world. Unlike most other health care systems, naturopathy is not identified with any one particular therapy, but rather is a way of thinking about life, health, disease, and the world. It is defined not by the therapies it uses but by the philosophical principles that guide the practitioner.

Seven powerful concepts provide the foundation that defines naturopathic medicine and create a unique group of professionals practicing a form of medicine that fundamentally changes the way we think of health care. In 1989, the American Association of Naturopathic Physicians unanimously approved the definition of *naturopathic medicine,* updating and reconfirming in modern terms its core principles as a professional consensus. "The definition and principles of practice provide a steady point of reference for this debate, for our evolving understanding of health and disease, and for all of our decision making processes as a profession" (Snider et al, 1989).

The seven core principles of naturopathic medicine are as follows, with "wellness and health promotion" emerging into the forefront of the scholarly discussion of naturopathic clinical theory:
1. The healing power of nature (*vis medicatrix naturae*)
2. First do no harm (*primum non nocere*)
3. Find the cause (*tolle causam*)
4. Treat the whole person (*holism*)
5. Preventive medicine
6. Wellness and health promotion (emerging principle)
7. Doctor as teacher (*docere*).

THE HEALING POWER OF NATURE (*VIS MEDICATRIX NATURAE*)

Belief in the ability of the body to heal itself—the *vis medicatrix naturae* (the healing power of nature)—if given the proper opportunity, and the importance of living within the laws of nature, is the foundation of naturopathic medicine. Although the term *naturopathy* was coined in the late nineteenth century, its philosophical roots can be traced back to Hippocrates and derive from a common wellspring in traditional world medicines: belief in the healing power of nature.

Medicine has long grappled with the question of the existence of the *vis medicatrix naturae*. As Neuberger stated, "The problem of the healing power of nature is a great, perhaps the greatest of all problems which has occupied the physician for thousands of years. Indeed, the aims and limits of therapeutics are determined by its solution." The fundamental reality of the *vis medicatrix naturae* was a basic tenet of the Hippocratic school of medicine, and "every important medical author since has had to take a position for or against it" (Neuberger, 1932).

When standard medicine soundly rejected the principle of the *vis medicatrix naturae* at the turn of the twentieth century, nature doctors, including naturopathic physicians in the United States from 1896 on, diverged from conventional, twentieth-century medicine. Naturopathic physicians recognized the clinical importance of the inherent self-healing process, embraced it as their core academic and clinical principle, and developed an entire system of medical practice, training, and research based on it and on related principles of clinical medicine.

Naturopathic medicine is therefore "vitalistic" in its approach (i.e., life is viewed as more than just the sum of biochemical processes), and the body is believed to have an innate intelligence or process (the *vis medicatrix naturae*), which is always striving toward health. Vitalism maintains that the symptoms accompanying disease are not typically caused by the morbific agent (e.g., bacteria); rather, they are the result of the organism's intrinsic response or reaction to the agent and the organism's attempt to defend and heal itself (Lindlahr, 1914a, Neuberger, 1932). Symptoms are part of a constructive phenomenon that is the best "choice" the organism can make, given the circumstances. In this construct, the physician's role is to understand and aid the body's efforts, not to take over or manipulate the functions of the body, unless the self-healing process has become weak or insufficient.

Although the context and life force of naturopathic medicine is its vitalistic core, both vitalistic and mechanistic approaches are applicable to modern naturopathic medicine. Vitalism has re-emerged in current terms in the energy medicine and body–mind–spirit dialogue, and scientific exploration of consciousness, placebo and nocebo, spontaneous healing, emergence, resilience, prayer, intention and healing, entanglement, the effect of consciousness on epigenetic expression, systems biology, and systems theory. Matter, mind, energy, and spirit are each part of nature and therefore are part of medicine that observes, respects, and works with nature. Much of modern biomedicine and related research is based on the application of the theory of mechanism (defined in *Webster's Dictionary* as the "theory that everything in the universe is produced by matter in motion; materialism") in a highly reductionist, single-agent, pathology-based, disease care model. Applied in a vitalist context, mechanistic and reductionist interventions provide useful techniques and tools to naturopathic physicians. The unifying theory of naturopathic medicine, as discussed later, provides clinical guidance for integrating both approaches.

FIRST DO NO HARM (*PRIMUM NON NOCERE*)

Naturopathic physicians prefer noninvasive treatments that minimize the risks of harmful side effects. They are trained to use the lowest-force and lowest-risk preventive, diagnostic, therapeutic, and co-management strategies. They are trained to know which patients they can safely treat and which ones they need to refer to other health care practitioners. Naturopathic physicians follow three precepts to avoid harming the patient:
1. Naturopathic physicians use methods and medicinal substances that minimize the risk of harmful effects and apply the least possible force or intervention necessary to diagnose illness and restore health.
2. When possible, the suppression of symptoms is avoided because suppression generally interferes with the healing process.

3. Naturopathic physicians respect and work with the *vis medicatrix naturae* in diagnosis, treatment, and counseling because, if this self-healing process is not respected, the patient may be harmed.

FIND THE CAUSE (*TOLLE CAUSAM*)

Every illness has an underlying cause or causes, often in aspects of the lifestyle, diet, or habits of the individual. A naturopathic physician is trained to find and remove the underlying cause(s) of disease. The therapeutic order helps the physician remove them in the correct "healing order" for the body (see later discussion). As the new science of psychoneuroimmunology is explicitly demonstrating, the body is a seamless web with a multiplicity of brain–immune system–gut–liver connections (see Chapter 8). Not surprisingly, chronic disease typically involves a number of systems, with the most prominent or acute symptoms being those chronologically last in appearance. As the healing process progresses and these symptoms are alleviated, further symptoms then resurface that must then be addressed to restore health. To paraphrase Sid Bakder, MD, on the "tack rules": "If you're sitting on a tack, it takes a lot of aspirin to feel better. If you're sitting on two tacks, removing one does not necessarily lead to a 50% improvement or reduction in symptoms."

TREAT THE WHOLE PERSON (*HOLISM*)

As noted previously, health or disease comes from a complex interaction of mental, emotional, spiritual, physical, dietary, genetic, environmental, lifestyle, and other factors. Naturopathic physicians treat the whole person, taking all these factors into account. Naturopathically, the body is viewed as a whole. Naturopathy is often called a *holistic medicine* in reference to the term *holism,* coined by philosopher Jan Christian Smuts in 1926 to describe the *gestalt* of a system as greater than the sum of its parts (see Chapter 2). A change in one part causes a change in every part; therefore the study of one part must be integrated into the whole, including the community and biosphere.

Naturopathic medicine asserts that one cannot be healthy in an unhealthy environment, and it is committed to the creation of a world in which humanity may thrive. In contrast to the high degree of specialization in the present medical system, which reflects a mechanistic orientation to single organs, the holistic model relegates specialists to an ancillary role. Emphasis is placed on the physical, emotional, social, and spiritual integration of the whole person, including awareness of the impact of the environment on health.

PREVENTIVE MEDICINE

The naturopathic approach to health care helps prevent disease and keeps minor illnesses from developing into more serious or chronic degenerative diseases. Patients are taught the principles for living a healthful life, and by following these principles, they can prevent major illness. Health is viewed as more than just the absence of disease; it is considered a dynamic state that enables a person to thrive in, or adapt to, a wide range of environments and stresses. Health and disease are points on a continuum, with death at one end and optimal function at the other. The naturopathic physician believes that a person who goes through life living an unhealthful lifestyle will drift away from optimal function and move relentlessly toward progressively greater dysfunction. Genotype, constitution, maternal influences, and environmental factors all influence individual susceptibility to deterioration, and the organs and physiological systems affected. Box 23-2 lists these and other determinants of health addressed by the naturopathic physician in both treatment and prevention.

BOX 23-2 *Determinants of Health and Other Factors in Naturopathic Preventive Medicine*

Determinants of health

Inborn

- Genetic makeup (genotype)
- Constitution (determines susceptibility)
- Intrauterine/congenital factors
- Maternal exposures
  - Drugs
  - Toxins
  - Viruses
  - Psychoemotional influences
- Maternal and paternal genetic influences
- Maternal nutrition
- Maternal lifestyle

Disturbances

- Illnesses: pathobiography
- Medical intervention (or lack of)
- Physical and emotional exposures, stresses, and trauma
- Toxic and harmful substances

Hygienic/Lifestyle Factors

- Nutrition
- Rest
- Exercise
- Psychoemotional health
- Spiritual health
- Community
- Culture
- Socioeconomic factors
- Fresh air
- Light
- Exposure to nature
- Clean water
- Unadulterated food
- Loving and being loved
- Meaningful work

The virulence of morbific agents or insults also plays a central role in disturbance, causing decreasing function and ultimately serious disease.

In our society, while our expected life span at birth has increased, our health span has not and neither has our health expectancy at age 65. We are living longer but as disabled individuals (Pizzorno, 2013). Although such deterioration is accepted by our society as the normal expectation of aging, it is not common in animals in the wild or among those fortunate peoples who live in an optimal environment (i.e., no pollution, low stress, regular exercise, and abundant natural, nutritious food).

In the naturopathic model, death is inevitable; progressive disability is not. This belief underscores a fundamental difference in philosophy and expectation between the conventional and naturopathic models of health and disease. In contrast to the disease treatment focus of allopathic medicine, the health promotion focus of naturopathic medicine emphasizes the means of maximizing health span.

WELLNESS AND HEALTH PROMOTION (EMERGING PRINCIPLE)

Establishing and maintaining optimal health and balance is a central clinical goal. Wellness and health promotion go beyond prevention. This principle refers to a proactive state of being healthy, characterized by positive emotion, thought, intention, and action. Wellness is inherent in everyone, no matter what disease is being experienced. The recognition, experience, and support of wellness through health promotion by the physician and patient will more quickly heal a given disease than treatment of the disease alone. The modern availability of genomic testing provides powerful tools for optimization of health (see Chapter 22).

DOCTOR AS TEACHER (*DOCERE*)

The original meaning of the word *docere* is "teacher." A principal objective of naturopathic medicine is to educate the patient and emphasize self-responsibility for health. Naturopathic doctors also recognize the therapeutic potential of the physician–patient relationship. The patient is engaged and respected as an ally and a member of her or his own health care team. Adequate time is spent with patients to diagnose, treat, and educate them thoroughly (see Chapters 1 and 2).

CONTEMPORARY PRACTICE

Currently naturopathic physicians are licensed primary care providers (in several states in the United States) of integrative natural medicine and are also recognized for their clinical expertise and effectiveness in preventive medicine and health promotion. NDs are trained as family physicians, regardless of elective postdoctoral training or clinical emphasis. This position is supported by the American Association of Naturopathic Physicians (American Association of Naturopathic Physicians, 1989) and the Naturopathic Academy of Primary Care Physicians (NAPCP, 2013). This requirement is intentional and consistent with naturopathic principles of practice. NDs are trained to assess causes and develop treatment plans from a systems perspective and with systems skills on the basis of naturopathic principles and, specifically, the principle of "treating the whole person," as follows:

> Naturopathy, in fact, is typically *meta-systematic*. . . . The organism [is] always seen in the context of its physical and social environment. . . . Beyond this, naturopathy ultimately might even be considered *cross-paradigmatic,* touching inevitably on the economics, politics, history, and sociology of the various healing alternatives, ultimately penetrating to the contrasting philosophies underlying naturopathy and allopathy. Naturopathy results from a guiding philosophy at odds with the dominant mechanistic philosophy undergirding Western industrialized society. Allopathy, in contrast, is clearly derived from these same premises. Or in Eisler's terms, naturopathy embraces a *partnership* model of relationship, while allopathy falls within the *dominator* model. . . . [T]his partnership/dominator model extends not only to the treatment process but to the healer/patient relationship itself. (Funk, 1995)

NDs may also practice as specialists, after postdoctoral training, in botanical medicine, homeopathy, nutritional medicine, physical medicine, acupuncture, Ayurvedic medicine, Oriental and Chinese herbal medicine, counseling and health psychology, spirituality and healing, applied behavioral sciences, or midwifery. Some NDs choose to focus their practice on population groups such as children, the elderly, or women, or in clinical areas such as cardiology, gastroenterology, immunology, or environmental medicine. These diverse practices are consistent with the eclectic origins of naturopathic medicine and are part of its strength. The whole person primary care foundation of naturopathic primary training makes the naturopathic specialist a nonreductionist, holistically skilled clinician while emphasizing a specific clinical area.

In addition to NDs with these specialties, at one end of the spectrum are practitioners who adhere to the nature cure tradition and focus clinically only on diet, detoxification, lifestyle modification, hydrotherapy, counseling, and other self-healing modalities. At the other end are those whose practices appear to be similar to the average conventional primary medical practice, with the only apparent difference being the use of pharmaceutical-grade botanical medicines and directed nutrient therapies, instead of synthetic drugs.

However, fundamental to all styles of naturopathic practice is a common philosophy and principles of health and disease: the unifying theory in the hierarchy of therapeutics, or the therapeutic order described in the following section. In 2006, Patricia Herman, ND, PhD, found that despite these differences, in a population of NDs practicing in Washington and Connecticut, 70% of office visits focused on lifestyle and behavioral modification, naturopathic health determinants, and therapies addressing *vis medicatrix naturae* (Herman et al, 2006), levels one and two of the naturopathic therapeutic order. The therapeutic order is derived from all of the principles and guides the choice of therapeutic interventions.

UNIFYING THEORY: HEALING POWER OF NATURE AND THERAPEUTIC ORDER

In facilitating the process of healing, the naturopathic physician seeks to use those therapies and strategies that are most efficient and that have the least potential to harm the patient. The concept of "harm" includes suppression or exhaustion of natural healing processes, including inflammation and fever. These precepts, coupled to an understanding of the process of healing, result in a therapeutic hierarchy. This hierarchy (or *therapeutic order*) is a natural consequence of how the organism heals. *Therapeutic modalities are applied in a rational order*, determined by the nature of the healing process. The natural order of appropriate therapeutic intervention is as follows:

1. Re-establish the basis for health:
   - Remove obstacles to healing.
   - Establish a healthy environment.
   - Address inborn susceptibility.
2. Stimulate the *vis medicatrix naturae*.
3. Tonify and nourish weakened systems.
4. Correct deficiencies in structural integrity.
5. Prescribe specific substances and modalities for specific conditions and biochemical pathways (e.g., botanicals, nutrients, acupuncture, homeopathy, hydrotherapy, counseling).
6. Prescribe pharmaceutical substances.
7. Use radiation, chemotherapy, and surgery.

This appropriate therapeutic order proceeds from least to most force. All modalities can be found at various steps, depending on their application. The spiritual aspect of the patient's health is considered to begin with step 1 (Zeff, 1997; steps 5 through 7 added by Snider, 1998; Zeff et al, 2013).

The concepts expressed in the therapeutic order are derived from the writings of Hippocrates and those of medical scholars since Hippocrates, concerning the function and activation of the self-healing process. Dr. Jared Zeff expresses these concepts as the hierarchy of therapeutics in his article "The Process of Healing: A Unifying Theory of Naturopathic Medicine" (Zeff, 1997). These concepts are further explored, refined, and developed in *The Textbook of Natural Medicine,* third edition (Pizzorno & Murray, 2013), in a chapter written by Zeff, Snider, Myers, and De Grandpre entitled "A Hierarchy of Healing: The Therapeutic Order—A Unifying Theory of Naturopathic Medicine" (Zeff et al, 2013).

The philosophy represented in the therapeutic order does not determine what modalities are good or bad. Rather, it provides a clinical framework for all approaches and modalities, used in an order consistent with that of the natural self-healing process. It respects the origins of disease and the applications of care and intervention necessary for health and healing with the least intervention.

The therapeutic order exemplifies the concept of using the least force, one of the key tenets of the naturopathic principle "Do no harm." The therapeutic order schematically directs the ND's therapeutic choices so that they are implemented in an efficient order rather than in a "shotgun" approach. This common philosophy and theory both distinguishes the field of naturopathic medicine and enables it to consider and incorporate new therapies.

Naturopathic medicine's philosophical approach to health promotion and restoration requires that practitioners possess a broad range of diagnostic and therapeutic skills and accounts for the eclectic interests of the naturopathic profession. Obviously, at times the body needs more than just supportive help. The goal of the ND in such situations is first to use the lowest-force and lowest-risk clinical strategies (i.e., the least invasive intervention that will have the most effective therapeutic outcome) and, when necessary, to co-manage or refer to specialists and other health care professionals.

Because the goal of the ND is to restore normal body function rather than to apply a particular therapy, virtually every natural medicine therapy may be used. In addition, to fulfill their role as primary care family physicians, NDs may also administer vaccines and use therapies such as office surgery and prescription drugs when less invasive options have been exhausted or found inappropriate. In the restoration of health, prescription drugs and surgery are a last resort but are used when necessary. As Kirschner and Brinkman (1988) noted, "The use of petroleum byproducts and the removal of body parts is a poor first line of defense against disease."

Naturopathic medical school curricula are continually revised in light of these principles. Curriculum integration is built on the science-based educational structure already in place in these colleges. Basic science, ND, and non-ND physician faculty are trained in naturopathic philosophy and principles and the therapeutic order as core assumptions that invite scholarly inquiry. Discussion and inquiry concerning the philosophy and theory are stimulated and supported in interdisciplinary faculty teams. The fruits of these endeavors are brought into the classroom to enhance students' critical thinking concerning clinical values and assumptions. Naturopathic research on these principles themselves is a widely embraced priority for the naturopathic profession. In 2004, the Naturopathic Medical Research Agenda identified three key hypotheses as central to the future and the foundations of naturopathic medical research. The third hypothesis states: "The scientific exploration of naturopathic medical practices and principles will yield important insights into the nature of health and healing" (Standish et al, 2004). The *Foundations of Naturopathic Medicine Project* was charged in the Naturopathic Medical Research Agenda (NMRA) report with operationalizing naturopathic concepts and principles for naturopathic research on Hypothesis Three (www.foundationsproject.com; Standish et al, 2004).

DIAGNOSIS

In the naturopathic medicine program at Bastyr University, for example, the principles just discussed and the therapeutic order are translated into a series of questions that drive curriculum development and case analysis and provide guidance to students learning the art and science of naturopathic medicine. These and other naturopathic case analysis and management questions (see next section) are integrated with conventional SOAP (*s*ubjective, *o*bjective, *a*ssessment, *p*lan) algorithms as the process of naturopathic case analysis and management, the clinical application of philosophy to patient care. For example, although a conventional pathological diagnosis is made through the use of physical, laboratory, and radiologic procedures, it is done in the context of understanding the underlying causes of the pathology and the obstacles to recovery.

CASE ANALYSIS AND MANAGEMENT

I.   The Healing Power of Nature (*vis medicatrix naturae*)
1. What is the level of the disease process? What is the direction of the disease process? What is the purpose of the disease process?
2. How is the healing power of nature supported in the case? What therapeutic interventions allow/respect, palliate, facilitate, or augment the self-healing process? How does the therapeutic intervention do this?
3. Is the person in balance with nature?
4. What is being in balance with nature?
5. Is this person in balance with his or her environment?
6. How are you assessing the healing powers of this individual?
7. What is the prognosis for this individual?
8. What is the patient's metaphor for healing? What moves or will move this patient toward healing or recovery?
9. How does the patient see himself or herself healing (the patient process)?
   - Are people helping him or her?
   - Is he or she doing it on his or her own?
   - How long will it take?
   - Is the doctor doing the healing?
   - Is the patient doing the healing?
   - Are the doctor and patient working together?
   - What else is important in this patient's healing process?
10. What is the pathobiography of the patient's illness: exposure, suppression, susceptibility, inception?

II. First Do No Harm (*primum non nocere*)
1. What is the potential for harm with this particular treatment plan?
2. Are you doing no harm? How?
3. How are you avoiding suppression? Is suppression necessary? Why?
4. What is the appropriate course of action? Is it waiting?
5. What is the appropriate level and force of intervention? Why? How is the least force applied?
6. Identify the appropriate treatment:
   - Level of therapeutic order
   - Modality/substance
   - Dosage
   - Frequency
   - Duration (justify the timing of the treatment in terms of short- and long-term management)
7. Are there any obstacles to the patient's recovery? Explain.
8. What referral or co-management strategies are required to ensure the patient's optimal outcome?

III. Find the Cause (*tolle causam*)
1. What level of healing are you aiming toward (i.e., suppression, palliation, cure)?
2. Where and/or what are the limiting factors in this person's life (concept: health is freedom from limitations)?
3. Where is the center of this person's disease (i.e., physical, mental, emotional, spiritual)?
4. What are the causative factors contributing to this patient's condition or state? What is the central cause or etiology? What are other contributing causes? Of these causative factors, which are avoidable or preventable?

IV. Treat the Whole Person (holism)
1. How are you working holistically?
2. Can you see the person beyond the disease?
3. What aspects of the person are you addressing?
4. What aspects of the person are you not addressing?
5. Would a referral to another health care practitioner assist you in working holistically? When? To whom? If not, why not?
6. What are the patient's goals and expectations in relation to his or her health and treatments?
7. What are your goals and expectations for the patient? What are the differences between yours and the patient's? How are they similar?
8. How will the treatment plan help the patient take more responsibility for his or her health and healing?
9. Are you empowering the patient? How?
10. What is the vitality level of this patient?
11. Identify cultural, community, and environmental issues and concerns that need to be included in the assessment.

12. What family/psychological/spiritual/social systems issues need to be included in the assessment?

V. Preventive Medicine
   1. What is being done or planned in regard to prevention?
   2. "Doctor" means "teacher"—what are you teaching this person about his or her health?
   3. Have you done a risk factor assessment for this patient? Have all preprimary, primary, secondary, and tertiary interventions and education relevant to life span or gender been identified and addressed?
   4. Does this patient do regular health screening self-examinations?

VI. Wellness and Health Promotion (emerging principle)
   1. What is being done to cultivate wellness?
   2. How are you contributing to optimal health in this individual?
   3. How can you contribute to optimal health in this individual?
   4. What are the patient's goals and expectations in relationship to his or her own wellness (e.g., creativity, energy, enjoyment, health, balance)?
   5. How can these goals be achieved? Are the expectations realistic?
   6. How can achievement of these goals be measured?
   7. Once these goals are achieved, how can the patient maintain an optimal level of wellness?
   8. Are you stimulating wellness or treating disease, or both?
   9. Is the patient demonstrating positive emotion, thought, and action? If not, why not?
   10. Can the patient recall or imagine a state of wellness?
   11. Is the patient able to participate in his or her own process toward a state of wellness?

VII. Doctor as Teacher (*docere*)
   1. What type of patient education are you providing? Assess wellness issues and prevention issues for this person. Identify educational needs of this patient regarding (a) therapeutic goals, (b) prevention, and (c) wellness.
   2. How can you determine the level of the patient's responsibility?
   3. In what ways do you cultivate and enhance your role as teacher?
   4. How have you listened to and respected the patient?
   5. In what ways are you engaging the patient's vital force and vitality through the physician-patient relationship, and a healing presence?
   6. How are you as physician providing an environment of integrity, respect, compassion, love and safety?

THERAPEUTIC MODALITIES

Naturopathic medicine is a vitalist system of health care that uses natural medicines and interventionist therapies as needed. Natural medicines and therapies, when properly used, generally have low invasiveness and rarely cause suppression or side effects. When used properly, they generally support the body's healing mechanisms rather than taking over the body's processes. The ND knows when, why, and with what patient more invasive therapies are needed based on the therapeutic order and appropriate diagnostic measures. The ND also recognizes that the use of natural, low-force therapies; lifestyle changes; and early functional diagnosis and treatment of nonspecific conditions is a form of preprimary prevention. This approach offers one viable solution for cost containment in primary health care. In addition, the ND recognizes when more conventional drugs (and other interventions) are in the patient's best interest and how to use these interventions safely with natural medicines.

Traditional health care disciplines such as traditional Chinese medicine (TCM), Unani medicine, and homeopathic medicine each have a philosophy, principles of practice, and clinical theory that form a system for diagnosis, treatment, and case management. A philosophy of medicine is, in essence, the rational investigation of the truth and principles of that medicine. The principles of practice form an outline of or guidelines to the main precepts or fundamental tenets of a system of medicine. Clinical theory provides a system of rules or principles explaining that medicine and applying that system to the patient by means of diagnosis, treatment, and management. The specific substances and techniques, as well as when, why, and to whom they are applied and for how long, depend on the system. Modalities (e.g., botanical medicine, physical medicine) are not systems but rather therapeutic approaches used within these systems. One modality may be used by many systems but in different ways.

The importance of systems is that the efficacy, safety, and efficiency of diagnostic and treatment approaches depend as much on the system as on the effects of the substance on physiology or biochemical pathways. This is exemplified by data in the TCM Work Force Survey conducted by the Department of Human Services in Victoria, New South Wales, and Queensland, Australia. In this study, Bensoussan and Myers (1996) assessed adverse events and length of TCM training for practitioners, as follows:

> The number of adverse events reported were compared to the length of TCM training undertaken by the practitioner. It appears from these findings that shorter periods of training in TCM (less than one year) carry an adverse event rate double that of practitioners who have studied for four years or more. . . . These practitioners were asked to respond to two questions regarding the theoretical frameworks they used to guide their TCM practice. TCM philosophy is adopted more readily as the basis for practice by primary

TCM practitioners than by allied health practitioners using TCM as part of their practice. In answer to the question, "Do you rely more predominantly on a TCM philosophy and theoretical framework for making your diagnosis and guiding your acupuncture or Chinese herbal medicine treatments?" 90% of primary TCM practitioners answered yes in contrast to 24% of nonprimary practitioners.

Nonprimary practitioners were typically educated for less than 1 year and were medical doctors.

It is the system used by each of these disciplines that makes it a uniquely effective field of medicine rather than a vague compendium of CAM modalities. Techniques from many systems are used in naturopathic medicine because of its primary care integrative approach and strong philosophical orientation.

Clinical nutrition, or the use of diet as a therapy, serves as the therapeutic foundation of naturopathic medicine. A rapidly increasing body of knowledge supports the use of whole foods, fasting, natural hygiene, and nutritional supplements in the maintenance of health and treatment of disease. Nutritional deficiencies are rampant with frank deficits commonly occurring in B vitamins and vitamin D, as well as suboptimal levels of several other vitamins and minerals. These deficiencies are arguably one of the primary causes of diseases and premature aging. Looking at just one nutrient, vitamin D, over half the population is deficient. This deficiency has serious health consequences, not just increased osteoporosis but less obvious problems like a 2.5-fold increase in progression to dementia (Llewellyn et al, 2009) and gives credence to the old "atmospheric" treatment concept (see Chapter 6).

Adding to the problem of common nutritional deficiencies is the recognition of unique nutritional requirements caused by biochemical individuality. This factor has provided a theoretical and practical basis for the appropriate use of high-dose vitamin therapy in certain circumstances for some patients. Controlled fasting is also used clinically.

Botanical medicines are also important. Plants have been used as medicines since antiquity. The technology now exists to understand the physiological activities of herbs, and a tremendous amount of research worldwide, especially in Europe, is demonstrating clinical efficacy. Botanical medicines are used for both vitalistic and pharmacological actions. Pharmacological effects and contraindications, as well as synergetic, energetic, and dilutional uses, are fundamental knowledge in naturopathic medicine (see Chapters 5 and 24). Today, thousands of studies have documented the efficacy of botanical medicines in the promotion of health and treatment of disease (see Chapter 24).

Homeopathic medicine derives etymologically from the Greek words *homeos,* meaning "similar," and *pathos,* meaning "disease." Homeopathy is a system of medicine that treats a patient and his or her condition with a dilute, potentiated agent, or drug, that will produce the same symptoms as the disease when given to a healthy individ-

ual, the fundamental principle being that *like cures like.* This principle was actually first recognized by Hippocrates, who noticed that herbs and other substances given in small doses tended to cure the same symptoms they produced when given in toxic doses. Prescriptions are based on the totality of all the patient's symptoms and matched to "provings" of homeopathic medicines. Provings are symptoms produced in healthy people who are unaware of the specific remedy they have received. Large numbers of people are tested and these symptoms documented. The symptoms are then added to toxicology, symptomatology, and data from cured cases to form the homeopathic *materia medica.* Homeopathic medicines are derived from a variety of plant, mineral, and chemical substances and are prepared according to the specifications of the *Homeopathic Pharmacopoeia of the United States.* Approximately 100 clinical studies have demonstrated the clinical efficacy of homeopathic therapies. "In late 2011, the Swiss Government's report on homeopathic medicine represented the most comprehensive evaluation of homeopathic medicine ever written by a government and was just published in book form in English (Bornhöft & Matthiessen, 2011). This breakthrough report affirmed that homeopathic treatment is both effective and cost effective and that homeopathic treatment should be reimbursed by Switzerland's national health insurance program" (Ullman, 2012).

Traditional Chinese medicine can be compared to naturopathic medicine to the extent that it is a system with principles corollary to working with the self-healing process. According to Bensoussan and Myers (1996):

> TCM shares some common ideas with other forms of complementary medicine, including belief in a strong inter-relationship between the environment and bodily function and an understanding of illness as starting with an imbalance of energy.... The TCM diagnostic process is... particularly holistic in nature [again similar to that in naturopathic medicine] and is usually contrasted to a reductionistic approach in Western medicine. Western medicine often defines disease at an organ level of dysfunction and is increasingly reliant on laboratory findings. In contrast, TCM defines disease as a whole person disturbance.

Quiang Cao, ND, LAc, Bastyr University, explains as follows:

> TCM never treats just the symptom, but the individual's whole constitution and environmental conditions; all are considered in a holistic context. The symptom signals constitutional excess or deficiency. The goal is not just to alleviate the symptom but to balance yin and yang, hot and cold, excess and deficiency, internally and externally.

Acupuncture is an ancient Chinese system of medicine involving the stimulation of certain specific points on the body to enhance the flow of vital energy (qi) along pathways called *meridians.* Acupuncture points can be stimulated by the insertion and withdrawing of needles, the application of heat (moxibustion), massage, laser, electrical means, or a combination of these methods. Traditional Chinese acupuncture implies use of a very specific acupuncture technique and knowledge of the Oriental system of medicine, including yin-yang, the five elements, acupuncture points and meridians, and a method of diagnosis and differentiation of syndromes quite different from that of Western medicine. Although most research in this country has focused on its use for the pain relief and the treatment of addictions, it is a complete system of medicine effective for management of many diseases (see Chapter 29).

Hydrotherapy is the use of water in any of its forms (e.g., hot, cold, ice, steam) and with any method of application (e.g., sitz bath, douche, spa and hot tub, whirlpool, sauna, shower, immersion bath, pack, poultice, foot bath, fomentation, wrap, colonic irrigation) in the maintenance of health or treatment of disease. It is one of the most ancient methods of treatment and has been part of naturopathic medicine since its inception. Nature doctors, before and since Sebastian Kneipp, have used hydrotherapy as a central part of clinical practice. Hydrotherapy has been used to treat disease and injury by many different cultures, including the Egyptians, Assyrians, Persians, Greeks, Hebrews, Hindus, and Chinese. Its most sophisticated applications were developed in eighteenth-century Germany. Naturopathic physicians today use hydrotherapy to stimulate and support healing, to detoxify, and to strengthen immune function in many chronic and acute conditions.

Physical medicine refers to the therapeutic use of touch, heat, cold, electricity, and sound. This includes the use of physical therapy equipment such as ultrasound, diathermy, and other electromagnetic energy devices; therapeutic exercise; massage; massage energy, joint mobilization (manipulative), and immobilization techniques; and hydrotherapy. In the therapeutic order, correction of deficiencies in structural integrity is a key factor; the hands-on approach of naturopathic physicians through physical medicine is unique in primary care.

Detoxification, the recognition and correction of endogenous and exogenous toxicity, is an important theme in naturopathic medicine. Liver and bowel detoxification, elimination of environmental toxins, correction of the metabolic dysfunction(s) that causes the buildup of non-end-product metabolites—all are important ways of decreasing toxic load. Of particular importance is recognition of the huge variation in exposure to environmental and self-toxins as well as ability to detoxify. For example, exposure to persistent organic pollutants is a stronger predictor of diabetes risk than obesity or lack of exercise (Lee, 2006). This is further aggravated by the surprising 1000-fold variation in human ability to detoxify chemical exposure (Wilkinson, 2005).

Spiritual and emotional toxicity are also recognized as important factors influencing health.

Spirituality and health measures are central to naturopathic practice and are based on the individual patient's beliefs and spiritual orientation; put simply, what moves the patient toward life and a higher purpose than himself or herself. Because total health also includes spiritual health, naturopathic physicians encourage individuals to pursue their personal spiritual development. As a plethora of studies in the newly emerging field of psychoneuroimmunology have demonstrated, particularly those examining both the placebo and the nocebo effect, the body is not a mere collection of organs, but rather a body, mind, and spirit in which the mind–spirit part of the equation marshals tremendous forces promoting health or disease.

Counseling, health psychology, and *lifestyle modification techniques* are essential modalities for the naturopathic physician. An ND is a holistic physician formally trained in mental, emotional, and family counseling. Various treatment modalities include hypnosis and guided imagery, counseling techniques, correction of underlying organic factors, and family systems therapy.

THERAPEUTIC APPROACH

RESPECT NATURE

We are natural organisms, with our genomes evolved and expressed in the natural world. The patterns and processes inherent in nature are inherent in us. We exist as a part of complex patterns of matter, energy, and spirit. Nature doctors have observed the natural processes of these patterns in health and disease and have determined that there is an inherent drive toward health that lives within the patterns and processes of nature.

The drive is not perfect. At times, when unguided, unassisted, or unstopped, the drive goes astray, causing preventable harm or even death; the healing intention becomes pathology. The ND is trained to know, respect, and work with this drive and to know when to wait and do nothing, act preventively, assist, amplify, palliate, intervene, manipulate, control, or even suppress, using the principle of the least force. The challenge of twenty-first-century medicine is to support the beneficial effects of this drive and come to a sophisticated application of the least-force principle in mainstream health care. This will prevent the last 20 years of life from being those of debility from chronic, degenerative disease for the average American and extend the health span throughout the life span.

Because the total organism is involved in the healing attempt, the most effective approach to care must consider the whole person. In addition to physical and laboratory findings, important consideration is given to the patient's mental, emotional, and spiritual attitude; lifestyle; diet; heredity; environment; and family and community life. Careful attention to each person's unique individuality and susceptibility to disease is critical to the proper evaluation and treatment of any health problem.

Naturopathic physicians believe that most disease is the direct result of the ignorance and violation of "natural living laws" (Lust, 1918) or the laws of nature concerning health and healing (Lindlahr, 1914b; Shelton, 1968; Spitler, 1948; Snider et al, 2014). These rules are summarized as consuming natural, unrefined, organically grown foods; ensuring adequate amounts of exercise and rest; living a moderately paced lifestyle; having constructive and creative thoughts and emotions; avoiding environmental toxins; and maintaining proper elimination. During illness, it is also important to control these areas to remove as many unnecessary stresses as possible and to optimize the chances that the organism's healing attempt will be successful. Therefore, fundamental to naturopathic practice is patient education and responsibility, lifestyle modification, preventive medicine, and wellness promotion.

NATUROPATHIC APPROACHES TO DISEASE

The therapeutic approach of the ND is therefore basically twofold: to help patients heal themselves and to use the opportunity to guide and educate the patient in developing a more healthful lifestyle. Many supposedly incurable conditions respond very well to naturopathic approaches. However, at times a more interventionist approach is needed acutely—which can be provided by the naturopathic doctor or referral to an appropriate colleague.

A typical first office visit to an ND takes 1 hour. The goal is to learn as much as possible about the patient using thorough history taking and review of systems, physical examination, laboratory tests, radiology, and other standard diagnostic procedures. Also, the patient's diet, environment, toxic load, exercise, stress, and other aspects of lifestyle are evaluated, and laboratory tests are used to determine physiological function. Once a good understanding of the patient's health and disease status is established (making a diagnosis of a disease is only one part of this process), the ND and patient work together to establish a treatment and health promotion program.

Although every effort is made to treat the whole person and not just his or her disease, the limits of a short description necessitate discussing typical naturopathic therapies for specific conditions in a simplified, disease-oriented manner. The following sections provide examples of how the person's health can be improved through naturopathic approaches, resulting in alleviation of the disease.

Cervical Dysplasia

The primary traditional medical approach to treating cervical dysplasia, a precancerous condition of the uterine cervix, is surgical resection. Nothing is done to treat the underlying causes. The typical naturopathic treatment would include the following:

1. *Education.* The patient should be educated about factors that increase the risk of cervical cancer, such as smoking >10 cigarettes/day (risk = 3.0), multiple sex partners (risk = 3.5), deficient beta-carotene (<5,000 IU/d) consumption (risk = 2.8), and deficient vitamin C (<30 mg/d) intake (risk = 6.7) (Hudson, 2013).

2. *Prevention.* Because 67% of patients with cervical cancer are deficient in one or more nutrients (Orr et al, 1985) and the level of serum β-carotene (critical for prevention of cancer of cells such as those in the cervix) is only half that of healthy women (Dawson et al, 1984), the woman's nutritional status should be optimized in general (through diet, especially by increasing intake of fruits and vegetables) and with regard to those nutrients known to be deficient (often as a result of oral contraceptive use) in women with cervical dysplasia and the deficiencies of which may promote cellular abnormalities (Tomita et al, 2009).

3. *Treatment.* The vaginal depletion pack (a traditional mixture of botanical medicines placed against the cervix) would be used to promote sloughing of the abnormal cells. Nutritional supplementation has been shown to lower the risk of cervical intraepithelial neoplasia by two- to threefold (Hwang et al, 2010).

The advantages of this approach are that (1) the causes of the cervical dysplasia have been identified and resolved, so the problem should not recur; (2) no surgery is used, thus no scar tissue is formed; and (3) the cost, particularly considering that many women with cervical dysplasia have recurrences when treated with standard surgery, is reasonable. More important, however, is that the woman's health has been improved, and other conditions that could have been caused by the identified nutritional deficiencies have now been prevented.

Migraine Headache

The standard medical treatment for migraine headache is primarily to use drugs to relieve symptoms, a costly and recurrent practice. Nothing is done to address the underlying causes. In contrast, the naturopath recognizes that most migraine headaches are due to food allergies, and abnormal prostaglandin metabolism caused by nutritional abnormalities results in excessive platelet aggregation. The approach is straightforward, as follows:

1. Identify and avoid the allergenic foods, because 70% or more of patients have migraines in reaction to foods to which they are intolerant (Natero et al, 1989; Hernandez et al, 2007).

2. Supplement with magnesium, because migraine patients have significantly lowered serum and salivary magnesium levels, which are even lower during an attack (Sarchielli et al, 1992). In one study, 42% of 32 patients with an acute migraine had low serum magnesium levels (Mauskop, 1993). In another report, magnesium levels in the brain, as measured by nuclear magnetic resonance spectroscopy, were significantly lower in patients during an acute migraine than in healthy individuals (Weaver, 1990). Several studies have shown the importance of magnesium in reversing the causes of migraine (Johnson, 2001).

3. Re-establish normal prostaglandin balance by decreasing consumption of animal fats (high in platelet-aggregating arachidonic acid) and supplementing with essential fatty acids such as fish oils (Woodcock et al, 1984). Omega-3 supplementation has proved effective in adolescents with migraine (Harel et al, 2002).

4. Supplement with riboflavin. "Forty-nine individuals with recurrent migraines were given 400 mg/day of the B-vitamin riboflavin for at least 3 months. The average number of migraine attacks fell by 67% and migraine severity improved by 68%" (Gaby, 1998).

Hypertension

Patients with so-called idiopathic, or essential, hypertension can be treated very effectively if they are willing to make the necessary lifestyle changes, as follows:

1. *Diet.* Numerous studies have shown that excessive dietary salt in conjunction with inadequate dietary potassium is a major contributor to hypertension (Fries, 1976; Khaw & Barrett-Connor, 1984; Meneely & Battarbee, 1976). Further, dietary deficiencies in calcium (Belizan et al, 1983; McCarron et al, 1982), magnesium (Dyckner & Wester, 1983; Resnick et al, 1989), essential fatty acids (Rao et al, 1981; Vergroesen et al, 1978), and vitamin C (Yoshioka et al, 1981) all contribute to increased blood pressure. Also, increased consumption of sugar (Hodges & Rebello, 1983), caffeine (Lang et al, 1983), and alcohol (Gruchow et al, 1985) are all associated with hypertension. Many studies have shown the antihypertensive effects of increasing consumption of fruits and vegetables, key to the dietary recommendations of NDs for over a hundred years (John et al, 2002).

2. *Lifestyle.* Smoking (Kershbaum et al, 1968), obesity (Havlik et al, 1983), stress (Ford, 1982), and a sedentary lifestyle are all known to contribute to the development of high blood pressure.

3. *Environment.* Exposure to heavy metals such as lead (Pruess, 1992) and cadmium (Glauser et al, 1976) increase blood pressure.

4. *Botanical medicine.* Many herbal medicines are used when necessary for the patient's safety initially to lower his or her blood pressure rapidly until the slower, but more curative, dietary, and lifestyle treatments can have their effects. Included are such age-old favorites as garlic (*Allium sativa*) and mistletoe (*Viscum album*).

The causes of high blood pressure are known, but they are generally unheeded.

Lifestyle modification is crucial to the successful implementation of naturopathic techniques—health does not come from a doctor, pills, or surgery, but rather from patients' own efforts to take proper care of themselves. Unfortunately, our society expends considerable resources to induce disease-promoting habits. Although it is relatively easy to tell a patient to stop smoking, get more exercise, and reduce his or her stress, such lifestyle changes are difficult in the context of peer, habit, and commercial pressure. The ND is specifically trained to assist the patient in making the needed changes. This involves many aspects: helping the patient acknowledge the need; setting realistic, progressive goals; identifying and working through barriers; establishing a support group of family and friends or of others with similar problems; identifying the stimuli that reinforce the unhealthy behavior; and giving the patient positive reinforcement for his or her gains.

ACCOUNTABILITY

Acceptance of a profession typically is seen to derive from sanctions associated with educational institutions, professional associations and licensing boards.
—ORZACK (1998)

It is extremely important to realize that the establishment of standards and especially credentialing standards is critical for the public to know . . . whatever the discipline is.
—LEVENDUSKI (1991)

Naturopathic medicine in the early part of the twentieth century was a unique natural practice, clinically effective, and powerfully vitalistic. It suffered because it had not reached maturity in terms of professional unification, scientific research, and other recognizable standards of public accountability. These goals have finally been achieved during the two decades of 1978 to 2000.

Naturopathic medicine has responded to the need to *integrate* the best that conventional and natural medicine have to offer, and to address the issues of public safety, efficacy, and affordability through the following mechanisms:

- Fully accredited naturopathic medical training (regional and professional)
- Standardized evidence -based naturopathic medical education
- Broad-scope licensing laws
- Nationally standardized licensing examinations
- Professional standards of practice and peer review
- Credentialing and quality improvement plans
- Documentation of scientific research and efficacy, development of institutional research centers

These mechanisms are well-accepted for public accountability in all forms of licensed health care. Naturopathic medicine's credibility has resulted in part from these important achievements by a unified profession.

SCOPE OF PRACTICE, LICENSING, AND ORGANIZATION

NDs practice as primary care providers. They see patients of all ages, from all walks of life, with every known disease. They make a conventional Western diagnosis using standard diagnostic procedures, such as physical examination, laboratory tests, and radiological examination. However, they also make a functional *pathophysiological diagnosis* using physical and laboratory procedures to assess nutritional status, metabolic function, and toxic load. In addition, considerable time is spent assessing the patient's mental, emotional, social, and spiritual status.

Therapeutically, NDs eclectically use virtually every known natural therapy: dietetics, therapeutic nutrition, botanical medicine (primarily European, Native American, Chinese, and Ayurvedic), physical therapy, spinal manipulation, lifestyle counseling, exercise therapy, homeopathic medicine, acupuncture, psychological and family counseling, hydrotherapy, and clinical fasting and detoxification. In addition, according to state law, NDs may perform office surgery, administer vaccinations, and prescribe a defined range of pharmaceutical drugs. Because NDs are an integral part of the health care system, they meet public health requirements and work within a referral network of specialists, CAM, public health workers, and integrative health provider in much the same way as a family practice medical doctor does. This network includes the range of conventional and nonconventional providers.

NDs (or NMDs) are licensed and regulated in the United States in 17 states (Alaska, Arizona, California, Colorado, Connecticut, Hawaii, Idaho, Kansas, Maine, Minnesota, Montana, New Hampshire, Oregon, South Dakota, Utah, Vermont, and Washington), the District of Columbia, and the two U.S. territories of Puerto Rico and the Virgin Islands. NDs have a legal right to practice in Minnesota. Because no licensing standards exist in this state and NDs also practice in other states without government approval, individuals with little or no formal education are still able to proclaim themselves NDs, to the significant detriment of the public and the profession. The American Association of Naturopathic Physicians (AANP, Washington, DC) assists consumers in identifying qualified NDs (http://www.naturopathic.org).

The scope of naturopathic practice is stipulated by state law. Legislation typically allows standard diagnostic privileges. Therapeutic scope is more varied, ranging from only natural therapies to vaccinations, a range of prescriptive rights, and office surgery. In addition, some states allow the practice of natural childbirth. Many states identify NDs as primary caregivers in their statutes. As of 2013, Vermont, Washington, and Oregon provide coverage for naturopathic primary care through medical homes, state primary care loan forgiveness programs for underserved communities, and Medicaid coverage for ND services (Bettenburg et al, 2013).

In addition to the Council on Naturopathic Medical Education (CNME), two key organizations provide leadership and standardization for the naturopathic profession. The AANP, founded in 1985 by James Sensenig, ND, and others, was established to provide consistent educational and practice standards for the profession and a unified voice for public relations and political activity. Most licensed NDs in the United States are AANP members. The Naturopathic Physicians Licensing Examination (NPLEx) was founded under the auspices of the AANP in 1986 by Ed Hoffman-Smith, PhD, ND, to establish a nationally recognized standardized test for licensing. NPLEx is recognized by all states licensing NDs. All states licensing NDs and all states in the process of attaining licensure have state professional naturopathic associations. The Alliance for State Licensing is an ongoing state licensure effort.

MEANINGFUL INTEGRATION

The American public has increasingly turned to alternative practitioners in search of healing for a variety of conditions not ameliorated by conventional medical practices. Such common conditions include otitis media, cardiovascular disease, depression, chronic fatigue syndrome, gastrointestinal disorders, chemical sensitivities, recurrent infectious diseases, rheumatoid arthritis, general loss of vitality and wellness, and many other chronic and acute conditions.

> Unquestionably, the health care system is undergoing profound change.... Many... current aspects of health care have resulted from a period of rapid change in the early part of this century. We are returning to a period of rapid change.... What is less certain is exactly where that change will lead. The task... is to identify and understand the forces of change and describe these forces so that [we] can make [our] decisions more wisely. (Bezold, 1986)

Since the publication of the first edition of this textbook, naturopathic colleges have doubled from four to eight in North America. The number of licensed naturopathic physicians was approximately 1500 and has grown to nearly 7000. Naturopathic physicians are engaged in state, local and federal health care policy, from the AMP CPT Coding Committee, to the White House Commission on CAM Policy, the Institute of Medicine, CMS Medicare Coverage Advisory Committee, the American College of Preventive Medicine, the U.S. Health Resources Services Administration, the NIH National Center for Complementary and Alternative Medicine, Cancer Treatment and Wellness Centers of America. They work with county boards of health, public hospital boards, state and federal health policy committees, faculty appointments at medical colleges, and in medical research initiatives, integrative, business and hospital practice settings, and public and community health. Naturopathic physicians play leading roles in the founding and advancement of the Integrative Healthcare Policy Consortium (IHPC) and the Academic Consortium for Complementary and Alternative Health Care (ACCAHC), which respectively, in collaboration with other integrative disciplines, had had an impact on the Affordable Care Act's (2010) "non-discrimination provisions," which are now being attacked by a posse of seven private medical specialty societies. Naturopathic physicians are working on key academic initiatives, including a significant presence within the IOM's Global Advances in Health Care Innovation initiative, widely considered the 100-year follow-up to the Flexner Report.

INTEGRATIVE STEPS

Naturopathic medicine has accomplished important steps in integrating into mainstream delivery systems.

Reimbursement: "Every Category of Provider" Law, Medicaid Coverage, Loan Forgiveness, Inclusion in Medical Homes, and Non-Discrimination

In 1993, during health care reform in Washington State, the "every category of provider" law was passed. This law mandated that insurance companies include access to every category of licensed provider in all types of plans in insurance systems for the treatment of all conditions covered in the basic health plan. Then Washington State Insurance Commissioner Deborah Senn, who vigorously enforced this law, formed the Clinician Working Group on the Integration of Complementary and Alternative Medicine, bringing together medical directors, plan representatives, and conventional and CAM providers to identify issues and solutions to integration barriers in insurance systems. This step has been important in increasing consumers' access to the health care providers of their choice, including licensed CAM professionals, as well as providing a solution focus to valid integration challenges.

Other reimbursement initiatives have also been successful. NDs throughout the United States are being integrated as primary care providers and specialists in traditional and managed care systems. The Pacific Northwest has emerged as a testing ground or model for integration because of the legislative and regulatory environment in the region. Washington, Oregon, and Vermont today authorize payment to NDs participating in primary care medical homes, Medicaid, and state loan forgiveness programs (Bettenburg et al, 2013). In 2007, Vermont passed a law mandating insurance coverage for naturopathic physicians, including Medicaid. In 2010, the Affordable Care Act passed containing the landmark Section 2706 on non-discrimination, modeled after Washington State's Every Category Law (ECL). The ECL and Section 2706 mandate non-discrimination for every type of licensed provider across all of the United States (IHPC, 2011).

Health Professional Loan Repayment and Scholarship Programs: Oregon and Washington

In 1995, Washington State's Department of Health made naturopathic physicians eligible for student loan repayment in the state's Health Professional Loan Repayment and Scholarship Program. Grants are awarded for student scholarships and student loan reimbursement to health care providers qualified and willing to provide health care in underserved areas or underserved populations. Numerous naturopathic physician grants for loan repayment have been awarded since 1995. In 2010, the Oregon State legislature, in collaboration with the Oregon Association of Naturopathic Physicians and National College of Naturopathic Medicine (NCNM), passed a new law including ND's in Oregon's primary care rural health care loan forgiveness program.

King County, Washington, Natural Medicine Clinic

No conventional model or infrastructure now exists in mainstream medicine for the systematic delivery of care that integrates natural and conventional providers. This integrative model is fundamental to naturopathic medicine. The King County Natural Medicine Clinic in Kent, Washington, is the first publicly funded integrative care clinic in the United States and has been a collaboration between Bastyr University and Community Health Centers of King County with funding provided by the Seattle King County Department of Public Health. This project forms an unprecedented union between three health forms: conventional medicine, natural medicine, and public health. The clinic has successfully applied a co-management model by using an interdisciplinary health care team co-led by naturopathic physicians and medical doctors, including nurse practitioners, acupuncturists, and dietitians. The clinic serves the medically underserved. The trend for naturopathic physicians to work in public and community health centers has grown dramatically since this initial model, with over 70 locations in North America associated with naturopathic colleges, particularly Bastyr University, NCNM, SCNM, and Canadian College of Naturopathic Medicine (CCNM), which have demonstrated significant commitment to community and public health partnerships.

The Centers for Disease Control and Prevention and independent investigators have studied the provider-to-provider interactions and their effect on health care, patient satisfaction, and cost effectiveness. Other studies have compared results from natural and conventional therapies on specific conditions treated using this model.

CO-MANAGEMENT AND INTEGRATIVE HEALTH CARE

In *The Emerging Integrative Care Model,* Milliman and Donovan (1996) describe co-management as follows:

> Naturopathic medical [co-management] is the practice of medicine by a naturopathic physician (ND) in concert with other care givers (ND, MD, DO, LAc, DC, etc.) wherein each care giver operates:
> - In communication with others, according to established convention
> - Within his licensed scope of practice and acknowledged domain of expertise
> - With respect for the other care giver's autonomy, but with recognition of the ultimate responsibility and, therefore, authority of the patient's primary care giver (PCP)
> - With respect for the other care giver's expertise, but with recognition of the ultimate responsibility and, therefore, final authority of the informed patient's choices and decisions.

Co-management presents an opportunity to educate other providers to naturopathic medicine as well as a chance to learn from them and expand one's information base and diagnostic and therapeutic potential. Most important, however, it greatly increases the therapeutic choices and quality of care to patients, often resulting in more supportive and less invasive therapies (minimizing iatrogenic diseases), while promoting healthier lifestyles and overall reduction in health care dollars spent. The ACCAHC has developed and published competencies for Interprofessional Education (Goldblatt et al, 2013), and published the second edition of the ACCAHC *Clinicians' and Educators' Desk Reference* (Goldblatt et al, 2013) as a tool to support a team care environment for all providers in the integrative spectrum.

RESIDENCY TRAINING

Utah is the first state to require a 1-year residency for naturopathic licensure. Residency opportunities for NDs are growing rapidly through sites established by the naturopathic colleges. Cancer Treatment Centers of America offers a growing number of residencies and staff positions to naturopathic physicians. All naturopathic colleges offer a growing number of residencies, now above 60, throughout the United States. Residencies are supported by the Naturopathic Post Graduate Residency Institute, individual practitioners, and through standards adopted by the CNME. All naturopathic colleges also offer on-site residencies.

HOSPITALS AND HOSPITAL NETWORKS

A number of hospitals across the United States continue to employ NDs as part of their physician staff in both inpatient and outpatient settings. Examples of the types of treatment centers established over the last 10 years are the following:

- HealthEast Healing Center, a clinic that is part of a larger "hospitals plus provider networks delivery system," employs MDs, an ND, an acupuncturist, and body workers, using a "learning organization" model (*St. Anthony's Business Report on Alternative and Complementary Medicine,* 1997).
- The Alternative and Complementary Medical Program at St. Elizabeth's Hospital in Massachusetts has a credentialed ND on staff. "The hospital is a teaching center for Tufts University Medical School" (*St. Anthony's Business Report on Alternative and Complementary Medicine,* 1998a).
- Centura Health (CH), the largest health care system in Colorado, is composed of an association of Catholic and Adventist hospitals. CH owns preferred provider organization Sloans Lake Managed Care. NDs are credentialed along with ND homeopaths and many other CAM providers in this hospital-based network (*St. Anthony's Business Report on Alternative and Complementary Medicine,* 1998b).
- American Complementary Care Network has recently placed two NDs in key positions: medical director of naturopathic medicine and chair of quality improvement (Alternative Medicine Integration and Coverage, 1998). Other networks, such as Wisconsin-based CAM Solutions and Seattle-based Alternare, have integrated ND-credentialed medical directors on staff.

When health systems, insurers, and health maintenance organizations decide to cover alternative medicine, NDs are sought out in states with licensure. Even in states without naturopathic licensure, health systems and managed care organizations exploring integration have come to understand and value the depth of training of naturopathic physicians (Weeks, personal communication, 1998).

EDUCATION

> The trend of modern medical research and practice in our great colleges and endowed research institutes is almost entirely along combative lines, while the individual, progressive physician learns to work more and more along preventive lines.
>
> —LINDLAHR (1914a)

The education of the ND is extensive and incorporates much of the diversity that typifies the natural health care movement. The training program has important similarities to conventional medical education (science based, identical basic sciences, intensive clinical diagnostic sciences), with the primary differences being in the therapeutic sciences, enhanced clinical sciences, clinical theory, and integrative case management. Naturopathic training places the pathology-based training of conventional physicians into the context of the broader naturopathic assessment and management model inclusive of nature, mind, body, and spirit in health care. To be eligible to enroll, prospective students must first successfully complete a conventional premedicine program that typically requires a college degree in a biological science. The naturopathic curriculum then takes an additional 4 years to complete. Residency opportunities are increasing rapidly throughout the United States, at all naturopathic colleges. As noted previously, residency is now required for licensure in the state of Utah.

The first 2 years concentrate on the standard human biological sciences, basic diagnostic sciences, and introduction to the various treatment modalities. The conventional basic medical sciences include anatomy, human dissection, histology, physiology, biochemistry, pathology, microbiology, immunology and infectious diseases, public health, pharmacology, and biostatistics. The development of diagnostic skills is initiated with courses in physical diagnosis, laboratory diagnosis, and clinical assessment. The program also covers natural medicine subjects such as environmental health, pharmacognosy (pharmacology of herbal medicines), botanical medicine, naturopathic philosophy and case management, Chinese medicine, Ayurvedic medicine, homeopathic medicine, spinal manipulation, nutrition, physiotherapy, hydrotherapy, physician well-being, counseling and health psychology, and spirituality and health.

The second 2 years are oriented toward the clinical sciences of diagnosis and treatment while natural medicine subjects continue. Not only are the standard diagnostic techniques of physical, laboratory, and radiological examination taught, but what makes the diagnostic training unique is its emphasis on *preventive* diagnosis, such as diet analysis, recognition of the early physical signs of nutritional deficiencies, laboratory methods for assessing physiological dysfunction before it progresses to cellular pathology and end-stage disease, assessment and treatment of lifestyle and spiritual factors, and methods of assessing toxic load and liver detoxification efficacy. The natural therapies, such as nutrition, botanical medicines, homeopathy, acupuncture, natural childbirth, hydrotherapy, fasting, physical therapy, exercise therapy, counseling, and lifestyle modification, are studied extensively. Courses in naturopathic case analysis and management integrate naturopathic philosophy into conventional algorithms using the therapeutic order.

Third- and fourth-year students also work in outpatient clinics, where they see patients first as observers and later as primary caregivers under the supervision of licensed NDs. A fundamental change occurring throughout naturopathic curricula is the integration of "integrated" or "problem based" curricular models, with less desk time and more hands-on learning, with clinical training beginning in year one. The AANMC CCACO recently passed an advanced set of learning objectives to more comprehensively integrate conceptual applications throughout the curricula, strengthening the "heart" of naturopathic medicine.

As previously mentioned, six federally accredited naturopathic schools currently exist in the United States [Bastyr University (BU], Bastyr University California [BUC] National College of Naturopathic Medicine [NCNM], the Southwest College of Naturopathic Medicine and Health Sciences [SCNM], the University of Bridgeport College of Naturopathic Medicine [UBCNM], National University of Health Sciences [NUHS]), and two in Canada (the Canadian College of Naturopathic Medicine [CCNM] and the Boucher Institute of Naturopathic Medicine).

The oldest institution is NCNM, which was established in 1965 in Portland, Oregon. "NCNM had its beginnings in the early 1950s, in response to the termination of the naturopathic program at Western States Chiropractic College. Members of the profession from Oregon, Washington and British Columbia planned the founding of the College and in May 1956, in Portland, Oregon, Drs. Charles Stone, W. Martin Bleything and Frank Spaulding executed the Articles of Incorporation of the National College of Naturopathic Medicine. After 50 years, in July 2006, NCNM changed its name to National College of Natural Medicine to be reflective of its two core programs and inclusive of its growing new programs" (http:\\www.ncnm.edu).

The largest institution and first to receive academic accreditation is Bastyr University, established in Seattle, Washington, in 1978. Over the years, Bastyr has broadened its mission also to include accredited degree and certificate programs in nutrition, exercise and wellness physiology, acupuncture and Chinese medicine, midwifery, herbal medicine, health psychology, exercise, Ayurvedic medicine, and spirituality and health. SCNM, established in 1993, has developed an active research department and a renowned environmental medicine program. The UBCNM, established in 1997, is the most recent addition; UBCNM recently launched the Center of Excellence in Generative Medicine, under the direction of Peter D'Adamo, ND.

Like its counterparts in the United States, CCNM in Toronto, Ontario, has a rapidly increasing enrollment. Naturopathic education is accredited by the CNME, recognized by the U.S. Department of Education. The CNME has granted accreditation to the naturopathic medicine programs at NCNM, Bastyr, SCNM, NUHS, Boucher, CCNM, and UBCNM. Bastyr and NCNM also have institutional accreditation by the Northwest Commission on Colleges and Universities, SCNM has institutional accreditation by the Higher Learning Commission of the North Central Association of Colleges and Schools, and UBCNM has institutional accreditation by the New England Association of Schools and Colleges. All states licensing naturopathic physicians recognize the CNME as the official accrediting agency for naturopathic medicine. The offices of the CNME are located in Portland, Oregon.

RESEARCH

Science clearly is an essential condition of a right decision.

—PELLEGRINO (1979)

However, clinical decisions cannot be solely dependent on science, when, with the best of efforts and with billions of public and private dollars spent, medical research has yielded twenty percent (and in some narrow areas up to fifty percent) of medical procedures and practices as scientifically proven and efficacious.

—OFFICE OF TECHNOLOGY ASSESSMENT (1978)

There is a paucity of theories of medicine.... The theory of medicine has lagged seriously behind theories of other sciences... any unitary theory of medicine which identifies it exclusively with science is doomed to failure.

—PELLEGRINO (1979)

The primary intellectual problem facing medicine today is that the information base of medicine is so poor. For a profession with a 2,000 year history which is responsible in the United States for 250 million lives and spends over $600 billion a year, we are astonishingly ignorant. We simply do not know the consequences of a large proportion of medical activities. The... task is to change our mind set about what constitutes an acceptable source of knowledge in medicine.

—EDDY (1993)

The relationship between scientific research and the study of the healing power of nature, a traditionally vitalistic principle, is important. The scientific method is a well-accepted approach to communicating what we learn about medicine's mysteries to others; however, it has been limited in its development by conventional medicine's approach to research. Orthodox biomedical research appears to turn on the premise that the universe functions without *telos* or purpose. Connections are mechanistic. Clinical investigation is directed toward pharmaceutical disease management based on a single-agent, placebo-controlled, double-blind crossover trial.

What distinguishes naturopathic medicine's clinical research from that of *biomedicine* (a term coined to refer to the currently dominant school of medicine) is not the presence or lack of science. It is a collective confidence in the perception of a vital force or life force. The arguments then follow. What is it? What exactly does it do and how? As Dr. John Bastyr noted in an interview in August 1989, "We all have an innate ability to understand that there is a moving force in us, that does not necessarily need to be understood mechanistically." Future scientific work and naturopathic medical research on this principle is bound by the shared perception that (1) there is a pattern in health and disease; (2) there is order in the healing process, and (3) order is based on the life force, which is self-organized, intelligent, and intelligible. Within this paradigm, we can research the life force.

Confirming and challenging clinical perceptions and even disproving core assumptions is fundamental to naturopathic medicine's core values. Scientific methods must be challenged to find new approaches to test large quantities and types of clinical data, outcomes, and systems from naturopathic practices. So far, the reality of the healing power of nature (*vis medicatrix naturae*) has not been proved or disproved by the single-agent double-blind study. New models (e.g., outcomes research, field- and practice-based research, multifactorial models) provide fruitful methods for researching the validity of nonconventional medicine and offer new opportunities for research on conventional practices. The U.S. Patient Protection and Affordable Care Act (2010) established the landmark Patient Centered Outcomes Research Institute (PCORI), whose purpose is to conduct outcomes research and ultimately to compare outcomes and effectiveness across various practices, including whole practices, bringing research in integrative and CAM disciplines and input from the integrative health care community.

Until recently, original research at naturopathic institutions has been quite limited. The profession has relied on its clinical traditions and the worldwide published scientific research, as follows:

> Research in whole practices [is] only recently gaining interest with the development of methodologies in practice-based and outcomes research. There is a lack of research in whole practices like naturopathy, Oriental medicine, or Ayurveda compared to conventional practice whether in a particular disease or in overall health outcomes [until recently]. Biomedical research methods which are considered gold-standard by the scientific community have been typically developed to provide reliable data on a single therapeutic intervention for a specific Western disease entity. The requirements of these research methods distort naturopathic practice and may render it apparently less effective than it may actually be. The measures may not take account of residual benefits in a patient's other health problems nor on future health and health care utilization.
>
> Compounding the methodological difficulties of research in this medical variant, there are structural obstacles as well. Distinct from the situation in conventional medicine, there is only the beginning of a research infrastructure at the profession's academic centers. Practitioners expert in naturopathic medicine and the individualization of treatment are typically not trained in rigorous comparative trials. Even if the infrastructure and training were in place, sources of funding remain few and small, and most funding agencies make their decisions on the basis of biomedical theories which naturopathy may directly challenge. When research is done on aspects of naturopathic treatment, more studies are done on substances rather than procedures or lifestyle changes. Without the economic incentives which favor the in-depth study of patentable drugs, trials in naturopathic therapeutics, often derived from a long history of human use, are smaller and with fewer replications. Many practices present special methodological or ethical problems for control, randomization, blinding, etc., perhaps making it impossible to perform a study as rigorous as some might wish. Nevertheless, there are numerous studies which yield indications of the effectiveness of individual treatments. (Calabrese et al, 1997)

As mentioned earlier, a comprehensive compilation of the scientific documentation of naturopathic philosophy and therapies can be found in *A Textbook of Natural Medicine*, coauthored and edited by Joseph Pizzorno, ND, and Michael Murray, ND. First published in 1985, the textbook was, until 1998, in a loose-leaf, two-volume set, published by Bastyr University Publications and updated regularly. The third edition (2006, Churchill Livingstone/Elsevier Health Sciences, publisher of this textbook) consists of more than 200 chapters and references more than 7500 citations from the peer-reviewed scientific literature.

Research has emerged (2009 to 2012) in the area of whole practice research in naturopathic medicine. Results are encouraging and hold promise for further evaluating the cost and effectiveness outcomes of naturopathic practice.

Finally, the Foundations of Naturopathic Medicine Project (Snider et al, 2014) [partially in response to the Future and Foundations of Naturopathic Medicine: The NMRA (Standish et al, 2004)] is close to publication of its textbook on the core concepts of naturopathic medicine and its traditional models. This long-planned text is modernized and operationalized to support academic advances, clinical practice, and to encourage research on naturopathic concepts, naturopathic practice, and the theoretical constructs of naturopathic medicine, in addition to naturopathic therapies.

The NMRA, as mentioned earlier, identified three hypotheses, including Hypothesis Three: "The scientific exploration of naturopathic medical practices and principles will yield important, even perhaps revolutionary, insights into the nature of health and healing" (Standish et al, 2004). "The NMRA identified three elements... necessary for such naturopathic 'discovery' research. The first is clear operational definitions of concepts such as the *vis medicatrix naturae* (the 'vital force,' 'healing power of nature,' etc.)". A primary question is: "How does the naturopathic physician work with nature to restore health?" These concepts are being rigorously explored and codified.

In the past 30 years, Bastyr University, NCNM, SCNM, NUHS, and CCNM have developed active research departments and Institutes, which has resulted in expanding publication of original research in both alternative and mainstream peer-reviewed journals. In 1994, Bastyr University was awarded a 3-year, $840,000 grant by the NIH Office of Alternative and Complementary Medicine to establish a research center to study alternative therapies for human immunodeficiency virus infection and acquired immunodeficiency syndrome (HIV/AIDS). The results of this review were presented in a textbook by Standish and Calabrese (2000).

Of particular importance has been the approval and funding by the federal government's National Center for Complementary and Alternative Medicine of numerous research studies as well as fellowships and postdoctoral study positions at the naturopathic institutions. The result has been a growing number of naturopathic physicians with strong research training and credentials.

The Helfgott Research Institute (NCNM), CCNM's advances in whole practice research, Bastyr's Integrative Oncology Research Center, the Naturopathic Physicians Research Institute, and growing peer-reviewed publications are evidence of a growing research emphasis in the field.

NATUROPATHIC MEDICINE IN THE HEALTHCARE SYSTEM

> We could have a significant and immediate impact on costly health care problems if the complementary and alternative medicine disciplines and interventions were widely available.
>
> —DOSSEY & SWYERS (1992)

The most pervasive and silently accepted crisis in America today is the ill health of our people. We must change our fundamental approach from a traditional disease-driven model to one that deals with the problem of improving people's health. The healthcare system of the future will value healthcare expenditures that improve health as much as those that treat disease.

> —JOSEPH E. PIZZORNO, ND, PRESIDENT, BASTYR UNIVERSITY, 1978–2000, PRESIDENT EMERITUS, BASTYR UNIVERSITY, 2003

Naturopathic medicine is enabling patients to regain their health as NDs effectively co-manage and integrate care with pertinent providers, to their patients' and the public's benefit. Today's ND, an extensively trained and state-licensed family physician, is equipped with a broad range of conventional and unconventional diagnostic and therapeutic skills. This modern ND considers himself or herself an integral part of the health care system and takes a full share of responsibility for common public health issues. NDs are healers and scientists, primary and specialty care givers, policy makers, and teachers and are active in industry and environmental issues.

The scientific tools now exist to assess and appreciate many aspects of naturopathic medicine's approach to health and healing. Conventional medical organizations that spoke out strongly against naturopathic medicine in the past now often endorse techniques such as lifestyle modification, stress reduction, exercise, consumption of a high-fiber diet rich in whole foods, other dietary measures, supplemental nutrients, and toxin reduction.

These changes in perspective signal the paradigm shift that is occurring in medicine. Emerging knowledge, ever-increasing burden of chronic disease in all age groups, high health care costs, and unmet health care needs continue to force this shift in perspective into changes in our current health care system. What was once rejected is now becoming generally accepted as effective. In many situations, it is now recognized that naturopathic understanding and approaches offer benefit over many orthodox practices. In the future, more concepts and practices of naturopathic medicine will undoubtedly be assessed and integrated into mainstream health care.

Historically, emerging bodies of knowledge in health care have formed into schools of thought and professions (with standards) as the public's need for their services increased. Naturopathic medicine's re-emergence is no accident or anomaly. Naturopathic medicine has followed the developmental stages that health care professions typically undergo while becoming accountable to the public. Access has increased with increasing research, conceptual unity, and standards.

These models, concepts, and standards in emerging CAM fields, including naturopathic medicine, hold answers to issues in health care, its delivery, and the health care system that are as significant as the interventions. With accreditation, licensure, reimbursement, ongoing research, modern publications of textbooks and books for the public, and widespread public acceptance, the naturopathic clinical model is reaching professional maturity today.

Mainstream health care leaders today recognize naturopathic medicine as an essential part of the present transformation in health care, a transformation which is no longer a luxury but a critical necessity, at a time where naturopathic medicine is becoming increasingly accessible through a growing and skilled workforce across the world.

Tracy Gaudet, MD, director of the Veterans Health Administration's Office of Patient Centered Care and Cultural Transformation, characterized naturopathic medicine as "a huge answer for the country, for practice, for patients" that is available "at a pivotal transformational moment" in health care. Naturopathic physicians understand that health care in the United States needs to fundamentally change, reflecting the fact that they are "pioneers" who have been practicing integrative medicine "all along." "The need is clear," she said, "through the simple fact is that the US spends far more per capita on health care than any other nation, yet life expectancy in the US is essentially the same as it is for Cuba" (American Association of Naturopathic Physicians, 2013).

As naturopathic medicine joins forces with policy makers, the public, and other integrative, holistic, public health, CAM, and traditional world medicine professions, practitioners, scientists, and leaders, naturopathic medicine is hopeful that together, we will "change the therapeutic order of our nation," deepen public investment in health, wellness, and healing, and create a healthier world.

Chapter 22 and this chapter presented the field of naturopathic medicine today as a whole. The reader is encouraged to read both chapters—one is not a complete picture without the other. The modern relevance of naturopathic medicine's historical identity, roots, traditional theory, and practices are dynamically alive in the profession of modern naturopathic medicine today, as it rebuilds a profession which almost died and whose transmission of knowledge was significantly constrained until a turning point that came in living memory, 35 years ago. The value and richness of naturopathic medicine's traditional body of knowledge cannot be adequately presented in these two chapters alone. The profession moves forward as an integrative, vitalist, broad-scope discipline built upon the foundations of nature cure, in harmony with natural medicines around the world. In addition, naturopathic medicine is strengthening, redefining, and advancing its traditional concepts and practices through the lens of modern research and frontier scientific discovery to bring in the best of biomedical understanding as well.

References

American Association of Naturopathic Physicians: *Naturopathic Medicine an "Answer for the Country," States Health Care Leader, May 20, 2013. http://www.naturopathic.org/content.asp?admin=Y&contentid=669.*

American Association of Naturopathic Physicians, Washington, DC, 1989. http://www.naturopathic.org/

Belizan J, Villar J, Pineda O, et al: Reduction of blood pressure with calcium supplementation in young adults, *JAMA* 249: 1161, 1983.

Bensoussan A, Myers S: *Towards a safer choice: the practice of traditional Chinese medicine in Australia*, Macarthur, Australia, 1996, University of Western Sydney, Faculty of Health, pp 20, 82, 109.

Bettenburg R, Milliman B, Pimentel B, et al: Naturopathic Medicine. In Weeks J, Goldstein M, editors: *Meeting the Nation's Primary Care Needs*, 2013, Global Advances in Health and Medicine. www.accahc.org. In press.

Bezold C: Health trends and scenarios: implications for the health care professions, *Am Ent Inst Stud Health Policy* 449:77, 1986.

Blois M: Medicine and the nature of vertical reasoning, *N Engl J Med* 318(13):847, 1988.

Bradley R: Philosophy of naturopathic medicine. In *Textbook of natural medicine*, Seattle, 1985, John Bastyr College Publications.

Bornhoft G, Matthiessen PF: *Homeopathy in Healthcare: Effectiveness, Appropriateness, Safety, Costs*, Goslar, Germany, 2011, Springer.

Calabrese C, Breed C, Ruhland J: *The effectiveness of naturopathic medicine in disease conditions*. Paper presented at State of the Science in Naturopathic Medicine, Annual Convention of the American Association of Naturopathic Physicians, 1997.

Dawson E, Nosovitch J, Hannigan E: Serum vitamin and selenium changes in cervical dysplasia, *Fed Proc* 46:612, 1984.

Dossey L, Swyers J: *Alternative medicine expanding medical horizons*, Washington, DC, 1992, US Government Printing Office.

Dyckner T, Wester O: Effect of magnesium on blood pressure, *BMJ* 286:1847, 1983.

Eddy D: Decisions without information, *HMO Pract* 5(2):58, 1993.

Ford MR: Biofeedback treatment for headaches, Raynaud's disease, essential hypertension, and irritable bowel syndrome: a review of the long-term follow-up literature, *Biofeedback Self Regul* 7(4):521–536, 1982.

Fries E: Salt, volume and the prevention of hypertension, *Circulation* 53:589, 1976.

Funk J: Naturopathic and allopathic healing: a developmental comparison, *Townsend Lett Doctors Patients* 50, October 1995.

Gaby A: *Commentary on migraine*, 1998.

Glauser S, Bello C, Gauser E: Blood-cadmium levels in normotensive and untreated hypertensive humans, *Lancet* 1:717, 1976.

Goldblatt E, Snider P, Weeks J, et al, editors: *Clinicians' and Educators' Desk Reference on the Licensed Complementary and Alternative Healthcare Professions*, ed 2, 2013, Academic Consortium for Complementary and Alternative Health Care (ACCAHC). www.accahc.org.

Gruchow HW, Sobocinski MS, Barboriak JJ: Alcohol, nutrient intake, and hypertension in US adults, *JAMA* 253:1567, 1985.

Harel Z, Gascon G, Riggs S, et al: Supplementation with omega-3 polyunsaturated fatty acids in the management of recurrent migraines in adolescents, *J Adolesc Health* 31:154, 2002.

Havlik R, Hubert H, Fabsitz R, Feinleib M: Weight and hypertension, *Ann Intern Med* 98:855, 1983.

Herman PM, Sherman KJ, Erro JH, et al: A Method for Describing and Evaluating Naturopathic Whole Practice, *Altern Ther Health Med* 12(4):20–28, 2006.

Hernandez CMA, Pinto ME, Montiel HLH: Food allergy mediated by IgG antibodies associated with migraine in adults, *Rev Alerg Mex* 54(5):162–168, 2007.

Hodges R, Rebello T: Carbohydrates and blood pressure, *Ann Intern Med* 98:838, 1983.

Hudson T: Cervical Dysplasia. In Pizzorno JE, Murray MT, editors: *Textbook of Natural Medicine*, ed 4, 2013, Elsevier.

Hwang J, Kim M, Lee J: Dietary supplements reduce the risk of cervical intraepithelial neoplasia, *Int J Gyn Cancer* 20(3):398-403, 2010.

(IHPC) Integrative Healthcare Policy Consortium, 2011. http://www.ihpc.org

John JH, Ziebland S, Yudkin P, et al: Effects of fruit and vegetable consumption on plasma antioxidant concentrations and blood pressure: a randomised controlled trial, *Lancet* 359:1969, 2002.

Johnson S: The multifaceted and widespread pathology of magnesium deficiency, *Med Hypotheses* 56:163, 2001.

Kershbaum A, Pappajohn D, Bellet S, et al: Effect of smoking and nicotine on adrenocortical secretion, *JAMA* 203:113, 1968.

Khaw KT, Barrett-Connor E: Dietary potassium and blood pressure in a population, *Am J Clin Nutr* 39:963, 1984.

Kirschner R, Brinkman R: American Association of Naturopathic Medicine Conference, Select Committee on Definition of Naturopathic Medicine, Billings, Mont, 1988.

Lang T, Degoulet P, Aime F, et al: Relationship between coffee drinking and blood pressure: analysis of 6,321 subjects in the Paris region, *Am J Cardiol* 52:1238, 1983.

Lee DH: A strong dose-response relation between serum concentrations of persistent organic pollutants and diabetes: results from the National Health and Examination Survey 1999-2002, *Diabetes Care* 2006.

Levenduski P: National Advisory Committee on Accreditation and Institutional Eligibility (Council on Naturopathic Medical Education hearing). In *Testimony to US Department of Education*, Washington, DC, 1991.

Lindlahr H: *Nature cure*, Chicago, 1914a, The Nature Cure Publishing Company.

Lindlahr H: Philosophy of natural therapeutics. In *Dietetics*, vol I, II, and III, Maidstone, England, 1914b, Maidstone Osteopathic.

Llewellyn DJ, Langa K, Lang I: Serum 25-Hydroxyvitamin D Concentration and Cognitive Impairment, *J Geriatr Psychiatry Neurol* 2009.

Lust B: *Universal naturopathic directory and buyer's guide*, Butler, NJ, 1918, Lust Publications.

Mauskop A: Deficiency in serum ionized magnesium but not total magnesium in patients with migraines, *Headache* 33(3):135, 1993.

McCarron D, Morris C, Cole C: Dietary calcium in human hypertension, *Science* 217:267, 1982.

Meneely G, Battarbee HD: High sodium–low potassium environment and hypertension, *Am J Cardiol* 38:768, 1976.

Milliman B, Donovan P: Naturopathic medical co-management. In *The emerging integrative care model: the best of naturopathic medicine anthology*, Tucson, 1996, Southwest College Press.

NAPCP (Naturopathic Academy of Primary Care Physicians). http://www.ndprimarycare.org/about.html. Accessed October 1, 2013.

Natero G, et al: Dietary migraine: fact or fiction? *Headache* 29:315, 1989.

Neuberger M: The doctrine of the healing power of nature throughout the course of time, *J Am Inst Homeopath* 25:861, 1932. (Translated by LJ Boyd).

Office of Technology Assessment, Washington, DC, 1978, US Department of Commerce, National Technical Information Service.

Orr J, Wilson K, Bodiford C, et al: Nutritional status of patients with untreated cervical cancer. II. Vitamin assessment, *Am J Obstet Gynecol* 151:632, 1985.

Orzack L: Professions and world trade diplomacy: national systems and international authority. In Olgiati V, Orzack LH, Saks M, editors: *Professions, identity, and order in comparative perspective*, Oñati, Spain, 1998, The International Institute for the Sociology of Law.

Pellegrino E: Medicine, science, art: an old controversy revisited, *Man Med* 4:43, 1979.

Pizzorno JE, Murray MT: *Textbook of Natural Medicine*, ed 4, 2013, Elsevier.

Pruess HG: Overview of lead toxicity in early life: effects on intellect loss and hypertension, *J Am Coll Nutr* 11:608, 1992.

Rao R, Rao U, Srikantia S: Effect of polyunsaturated vegetable oils on blood pressure in essential hypertension, *Clin Exp Hyperten* 3:27, 1981.

Resnick LM, Gupta RK, Laragh JH: Intracellular free magnesium in erythrocytes of essential hypertension: relationship to blood pressure and serum divalent cations, *Proc Natl Acad Sci U S A* 81:6511, 1989.

Sarchielli P, et al: Serum and salivary magnesium levels in migraine and tension-type headaches: results in a group of adult patients, *Cephalgia* 12:21, 1992.

Shelton, Herbert M: *Natural Hygiene, Man's Pristine Way of Life*. Published 1968; Dr. Shelton's Health School.

Snider P, Zeff J: Select Committee on Definition of Naturopathic Medicine report, House of Delegates, Portland, Ore, 1989, American Association of Naturopathic Physicians.

Snider P, Pizzorno J: Diversity of the Vis Medicatrix Naturae. In Snider P, Zeff J, Pizzorno J, et al, editors: *Foundations of Naturopathic Medicine—The Healing Power of Nature*, 2014, Elsevier. in press.

Spitler HR: *Basic naturopathy*, Des Moines, Iowa, 1948, American Naturopathic Association.

St. Anthony's Business Report on Alternative and Complementary Medicine, May 1997, p 5.

St. Anthony's Business Report on Alternative and Complementary Medicine, July 1998a, pp 6-7.

St. Anthony's Business Report on Alternative and Complementary Medicine, August 1998b, pp 4-5.

Standish L, Calabrese C: *Complementary & Alternative Therapies in HIV/AIDS*, London and New York, 2000, Churchill Livingstone.

Standish L, Snider P, Calabrese C, NMRA Core Team: *The future and foundations of naturopathic medical science, Report to NIHCCAM on Naturopathic Medical Research Agenda (NMRA)*, 2004.

Tomita L, Filho A, Costa M, et al: Diet and serum micronutrients in relation to cervical neoplasia and cancer among low-income Brazilian women, *Int J Cancer* 126:703-714, 2009.

Ullman D: Huffington Post 2/15/2012, http://www.huffingtonpost.com/dana-ullman/homeopathic-medicine-_b_1258607.html.

Vergroesen A, Fleischman A, Comberg H, et al: The influence of increased dietary linoleate on essential hypertension in man, *Acta Biol Med Germ Band* 37:879, 1978.

Weaver K: Magnesium and migraine, *Headache* 30(3):168, 1990.

Wilkinson GR: Drug metabolism and variability among patients in drug response, *N Engl J Med* 2005.

Woodcock BE, Smith E, Lambert WH, et al: Beneficial effect of fish oil on blood viscosity in peripheral vascular disease, *BMJ* 288:592, 1984.

Yoshioka M, Matsushita T, Chuman Y: Inverse association of serum ascorbic acid level and blood pressure or rate of hypertension in male adults aged 30–39 years, *Int J Vitam Nutr Res* 54:343, 1981.

Zeff J, Snider P, Myers SP: A Heirarchy of Healing: The Therapeutic Order: A Unifying Theory of Naturopathic Medicine. In Pizzorno JE, Murray MT, editors: *The Textbook of Natural Medicine*, ed 4, St. Louis, MO, 2013, Elsevier, pp 18–33.

Zeff J: The process of healing: a unifying theory of naturopathic medicine, *J Naturopath Med* 7(1):122, 1997.

Suggested Reading

American Association of Naturopathic Physicians, Snider P, Zeff J: Co-Chairs: Select Committee on the Definition of Naturopathic Medicine, *Definition of naturopathic medicine position paper* 1989. www.naturopathic.org. Accessed Oct 1, 2013. House of Delegates. Rippling River, OR.

ETHNOBOTANY AND WESTERN HERBALISM

MARC S. MICOZZI
LISA MESEROLE

Plants have been used by humans for food, medicine, clothing, dyes, and tools, as well as in religious rituals, since before recorded history. From more than 60,000 years ago, archaeologists uncovered evidence of pollen from plants that had been placed in Neanderthal cave burials found in Shanidar, in modern-day Iraq (Solecki & Shanidar, 1975). Indeed, the art of herbal medicine probably predates *Homo sapiens* in prehistory. In ancient history, catalogues of remedies in pharmacopeias date back 5000 years (Inamdar et al, 2008). No continent, island, climate, or geography that is home to human culture lacks a formal tradition of incorporating local flora into daily and ceremonial life as a means of enhancing health and well-being. Prehistoric plant life was a predominant part of the earth's environment, as the habitat to which *Homo sapiens* adapted. Plant ecology continues to help maintain the oceans, continents, and atmosphere today (see Chapter 27). It is only recently that many Western health care providers have begun to recognize and remember the number of modern remedies that had their origin in herbal medicine.

Herbal products have gained increasing popularity during the last quarter-century. This movement has been partially motivated by dissatisfaction with the mainstream health care system, distrust of modern drug development, desire for more natural approaches, and the growing tendency for self-care. When questioned, approximately one-quarter of adults reported using an herbal remedy to treat a medical condition within the past year (Bent & Ko, 2004). The most common herbal remedies used include ginkgo, garlic, St. John's wort, soy, kava, echinacea, and saw palmetto (Bent, 2008). Ginkgo and soy (also a food) are part of the tradition of Chinese medicine (see Chapter 28). Echinacea (purple coneflower) and saw palmetto are

part of Native North American traditions (Chapter 37), St. John's wort is a European folk remedy approved under historic usage in Germany and elsewhere, and garlic is a Eurasian food and remedy that has long gone "global." The global market for herbal products was over $60 billion annually in 2007 (Inamdar et al, 2008) and now exceeds $100 billion.

DEFINITIONS

Although herbal remedies have their origins in ethnomedical traditions that are discussed elsewhere in the book (Sections 5 and 6), herbalism (especially Western herbalism) is a term for the contemporary, eclectic study and use of herbal remedies that have come down to us historically from around the world and are known to contemporary practice and usage. This scope may not account for as-yet undiscovered remedies in still relatively unexplored regions of the globe, such as the Amazon and parts of Africa where there have not been historical traditions of making written records of effective remedies (see Chapter 34).

Herbalism is today's study and practice of using plant material for food, medicine, and health promotion. This field includes not only treatment of disease but also enhancement of quality of life, both physically and spiritually. A fundamental principle of herbalism is to promote preventive care and guided, simple treatment for the general population. An *herbalist*, or *herbal practitioner*, is someone who has undertaken specific study and supervised practical training to achieve competence in treating patients. Herbal medicines are also recommended by physicians in the practice of integrative medicine and by other practitioners within the pharmacopeia of their traditions.

There is also an eclectic practice of herbal medicine in Europe and North America that draws on herbs from many healing traditions and has been called *Western herbalism.*

A plant classified in usage as an "herb" botanically may be an angiosperm (i.e., a flowering plant), shrub, tree, moss, lichen, fern, algae, seaweed, or fungus. The herbalist may use the entire plant or just the flowers, fruits, leaves, twigs, bark, roots, rhizomes, seeds, or exudates (e.g., tapped and purified maple syrup), or a combination of parts. Botanical science specifically defines an *herb* as a nonwoody, low-growing plant, but herbalists use the entire plant kingdom. In many "herbal" traditions, nonplants, including animal parts (organs, bone, tissue), insects, animal and insect secretions and venoms, worm castings, shells, rocks, metals, minerals, and gemstones, are used as healing agents (all of which may be more inclusively considered as *materia medica*). These examples are recorded in ancient and contemporary materiae medicae and formal manuscripts of healing agents with their indications and uses. Egyptian, Chinese, Tibetan, European, American, and other worldwide materiae medicae provide important references for herbal practitioners. This chapter addresses only plant herbal agents.

Herbalism may be a misleading term because it implies that a single hidden "root," so to speak, gives rise to the diverse ways in which all human cultures across the millennia have used plants for food, medicine, and ritual. The use of herbs by the peoples of the Americas, Europe, Africa, the Middle and Far East, the Pacific Islands, and other regions is specific to each ecosystem, society, and paradigm, as demonstrated in the forthcoming chapters of this text. For example, contemporary Western scientists have been restricted until recently by the Western mechanistic premises of biology and physics (see Chapter 1).

Although there is no single, worldwide system of herbalism, herbal traditions share certain themes (Box 24-1).

 "Herb" and Other Words

Herb as a word has an ancient pedigree, originating with the Latin word *herba*, which refers to green crops and grasses and could also mean the same as meant by *herb* today (*Oxford English Dictionary*, or *OED*). The word entered English through Old French following the Norman Conquest of 1066. The English use of "herb" in the sense of a plant whose stem does not become woody and persistent but remains more or less soft and succulent, dying down to the ground (or entirely) after

BOX 24-1 *Common Themes of Herbalism*

- Optimization of health and wellness
- Emphasis on the whole person. This includes body, mind, and soul; past, present, and future; and community
- Emphasis on the individual
- Emphasis on the community. The illness or recovery of a member might influence the community itself, beyond emotional group empathy.
- Attention to finding and treating the root cause of a problem, not only the manifestations and symptoms. However, as with most healers and medicine suppliers, even if the cause remains unidentified or untreatable, symptomatic treatment is offered.
- Application of the principle of duality between both the healing and the life-threatening forces of nature. The fundamental assumption of this principle is that natural law is greater than the will of the individual or community, and that healing requires the healer, the patient, and the community be in alignment with natural forces.
- Belief in the reality of the unmeasurable and abstract. Although dual, the abstract and physical worlds are inseparable. An herbalist as healer devotes himself or herself to maintaining balance and communication between the visible and invisible. This goal might be accomplished through connecting with spirituality or by adjusting activities to natural cycles (e.g., in Tibetan

medicine, blending a formula during a specific season, moon phase, or auspicious date).
- Premise of recycling. Nature is inherently circular and repetitive; generally sequential, but not predominantly linear; and predictable, but seldom certain. This leads to the common traditional practice of offering an object or prayer in return for healing plants and for addressing requests for healing to both the physical and the spiritual world.
- Openness to exchange of knowledge. Most traditions incorporate new medicinal plants and new herbal uses and preparations that have been learned about through trade or travel.
- Regulation of the herbalist's practice through local accountability to his or her community. Success and prestige arise primarily from professional reputation that grows by word of mouth, not from image, business acumen, or material wealth (see Chapter 5).
- Humility generated from the healer's recognition of his or her own limits and skills. Because reputation generally depends on treatment efficacy and community standing, an herbalist would be reluctant to take on a case without reasonable confidence that he or she could succeed. Complex or incurable cases would be referred to another kind of practitioner, or the patient would be advised that no treatment was available other than palliation of suffering.

"Herb" and Other Words—cont'd

flowering, can be traced to the thirteenth century. In the thirteenth century, it was also understood that an "herb" (with variant spellings, e.g., "erbe") is a plant whose leaves and stems (and sometimes roots) could be used as food or medicine, or for scent (perfume) or flavor (spice).

Herbarium, in the sense of a collection of dried plants, has its origins in the eighteenth century. A source for the association of "herbarium" with the medicinal properties of plants is provided by the idea of drying plants for study, which originated with a professor in sixteenth-century Italy who also held a chair in "simples," in which he studied medicinal and other plants.

Herbalist has shifted meaning. Originally (in the sixteenth century) an "herbalist" was one versed in the knowledge of herbs and plants—a collector of and/or writer about plants, more what is meant by "botanist" today. (Thus, many early books about native flora were simply called "Herbals" during the seventeenth and eighteenth centuries). Usually, however, "herbalist" is now used to refer to early writers about plants, as well as persons who use alternative medical therapy, although the *OED* does not mention this usage.

Herbal, meaning a book containing names and descriptions of herbs (or other plants in general) that provides properties and virtues, came into use in the early sixteenth century just at the time of early European "discovery" and description of plants of the Americas (see Chapter 1). "Herbal," meaning belonging to, consisting of, or made from herbs, has its origins in the early seventeenth century.

Early botanical gardens started in Renaissance Italy. These arrangements should properly be called "physic gardens," because they were used to help educate medical students, that is, to teach people—in this case medical students—about medicinal plants. Physic gardens appeared in England in the sixteenth century, in private hands. The Oxford Physic Garden began in 1621, and the Chelsea Physic Garden was begun in 1673 by the Society of Apothecaries. The Oxford Physic Garden became the Botanic Garden in 1840, an important and representative change. There was no real difference between a "physic garden" and a "botanic garden," because botany versus the study of the medicinal properties of plants were not then distinct fields. William Turner (1510–1568) was a physician, was the author of an herbal, and is considered the father of English botany. For Turner, taxonomy (systematics) was not separate from pharmacology in the study of plants.

Although the process was gradual, by the nineteenth century the study of plants for their own sake—botany—was a clearly separate field. Pharmacopeias and botanical atlases grew in scientific importance even as the need for herbals waned.

There are clear ways to classify types of gardens. In the 1790s, Dr. Benjamin Rush called for the establishment of a "botanic garden" at the College of Physicians of Philadelphia. In Rush's time this would have meant a garden to study the properties of plants, in this case, medicinal properties. Rush suggested that the garden could also actually provide a source of medical preparations, as well as a place to grow both Native American and European plants that provided "folk remedies," which might otherwise be lost as Europeans settled North America. Although it was not the only purpose of Rush's garden, study was a component, and research lies at the heart of any botanical garden's purpose. (Botanical gardens are not limited strictly to taxonomy.)

Therefore, *medical botany* would be the study of the medicinal properties of plants, for example, chemical analysis to find new medically important compounds. A *medical botanical garden* would be the source of plants for studying their medical properties.

A *medicinal herb garden* would be a place that has examples of plants, from which samples could be taken to make medicinal preparations. Also, the garden would contain only herbaceous plants, not plants with woody stems and branches.

(Acknowledgment to Charles Griefenstein, American Philosophical Society, Philadelphia.) ∾

CLASSIFICATIONS OF HERBALISTS

Each cultural or medical system has different types of herbal practitioners, all consistent with its paradigm. However, most paradigms identify professional herbalists, lay herbalists, plant gatherers, and medicine makers. (Professional and lay herbalists often collect their own plants ["wild crafting"] and prepare their own medicines.)

PROFESSIONAL HERBALIST

A professional herbalist undergoes formalized training or a long apprenticeship in plant and medicinal studies or, alternatively, in plant and spiritual or healing studies. This knowledge includes extensive familiarity with specific plants, which involves their identification, habitat, harvesting criteria, preparation, storage, therapeutic indications, contraindications, and dosing. A professional herbalist is not necessarily the primary health practitioner (Iwu, 1993).

As with acupuncture and Chinese medicine (see Chapter 3), a professional herbalist might follow a family tradition or might be selected at a young age as being endowed with the potential for mastering the use of plants as healing aids. In Europe and the United States, this group includes officially trained medical herbalists, clinical herbalists, licensed naturopathic doctors specializing in botanical medicine, licensed acupuncturists with training in Chinese herbal medicine, licensed Ayurvedic doctors,

Native American herbalists and shamans, Latin American curanderos, and other lineage-recognized or culturally recognized professional herbalists. All of these topics are addressed specifically in forthcoming chapters.

A shaman from Madagascar who—although never acknowledged or compensated for his contribution—first revealed the usefulness of *Caranthas roseus*, the periwinkle plant from which vinblastine and vincristine were developed in the West for treatment of certain cancers. This shaman exemplified the spirit and expertise of a professional healer and herbalist. Furthermore, the herbal practitioner's familiarity with each medicinal plant or herbal formula usually is often greater than is the medical practitioner's familiarity with each individual pharmaceutical. This permits the herbalist to select precisely a particular plant or formula for each *individual* patient, rather than relying on the "one size fits all" approach of the standard dosage form of a drug. Three different patients with a chief complaint of headache would likely each receive a different herbal prescription. The approach that an herbalist uses to determine which herbs to prescribe is distinct from that used by a conventional Western physician to prescribe a pharmaceutical.

LAY HERBALIST

A lay herbalist has a broad knowledge of plants useful for health problems but does not have extensive training in medicinals nor spiritual diagnosis and management. He or she may even be an herb vendor with a sensitivity to the needs and desires of the marketplace, whose livelihood has been passed down as a family business. Evaluation of medicinal plant quality, strength, uses, and dose is included in the lay herbalist's domain. A traditional European herbalist who uses specific herbal treatments for certain skin or stomach symptoms is an example.

PLANT GATHERER, PLANT GROWER, AND MEDICINE MAKER

Plant gatherers, plant growers, and medicine makers might consider themselves herbalists; actually, they are to the practicing herbalist what the contemporary pharmacist is to the clinical physician. In Chinese medicine, there is one specialist who produces and collects plants, one who processes and stores plants, and a clinical herbalist/doctor who prescribes the medicines (see Chapter 28). In some systems, preparing and handling medicines is considered a spiritual privilege and responsibility. Therefore, certain herbal medicines are prepared only by the herbalist or healer or by a designated assistant.

HERBS AND MEDICINAL PLANTS

Physicians in the United States studied and relied on plant drugs as primary medicines through the 1930s almost everywhere, and in many places until after World War II (see Chapter 1). Until then, medical and pharmacy schools taught basic plant taxonomy and pharmacognosy and medicinal plant therapeutics. The term *drug* derives from an ancient word for *root*, and the roots and rhizomes of many medicinal plants continue to provide alkaloids, steroidal saponins, and many active constituents that remain clinically useful today. The *United States Pharmacopeia* listed 636 herbal entries in 1870; only 58 were listed in the 1990 edition (Boyle, 1991). Although some plants were dropped because they were found to be not potent or not safe, the majority of clinically useful plants were replaced with pharmaceuticals, which generated profits from patented drugs and contributed to the standardization and industrialization to "one size fits all" medicine.

CHARACTERISTICS AND COMPOSITION

In many traditional systems the characteristics of a medicinal plant are emphasized without attention to its composition, because techniques and equipment for plant analysis are relatively new compared to historical usage of the plant.

Preanalytical, chemical knowledge of medicinal and food plants is derived from direct perception through the five senses; from the herbalist's attentive, empirical observation of plants' effects on animals and humans; and, in some traditions, from sacred teachings and "sixth sense" intuition.

More recently, attention is being paid to standardizing the product, that is, to providing a consistent, measured amount of product per unit dose, and one ingredient is selected as the marker, usually the presumed active ingredient. Although research may reveal different or additional active ingredients, for convenience the designated constituent will usually remain the accepted marker. Over the years, more and more sophisticated methods of analysis to detect the marker have been developed, including such techniques as high-performance liquid chromatography and dioxide array detection. Perhaps a disadvantage to identifying, categorizing, and researching molecular constituents from plants is the risk of equating the plant's therapeutic efficacy to its composition. Analysis is reductionist in paradigm, and data cannot exist beyond the limits of the technology (and available funding to apply it) or the paradigm from which it arises (Cheng et al, 2008).

Food, medicinal, and healing plants may contain digestible fiber (carbohydrates and hemicellulose) and indigestible fiber (cellulose and lignins), nutritives (calories, vitamins, minerals, trace elements, amino acids, essential fatty acids), water, and inert and active constituents.

When a Western paradigm is followed, plant constituents can be classified according to their morphology, source plant taxonomy, therapeutic (pharmacological) applications, or chemical constituents (Tyler et al, 1988) (Box 24-2).

PHYSIOLOGICAL ACTIVITIES

Activities and corresponding indications for the use of plants are, again, paradigm specific (see the sidebar

BOX 24-2 *Classic Organization of the Active Chemical Constituents in Plants*

1. *Carbohydrates:* sugars, starches, aldehydes, gums, and pectins
2. *Glycosides:* cardiac glycosides in *Digitalis purpurea* leaf, anthraquinone glycosides in *Aloe* species latex, and rhubarb (*Rheum officinale*) root and rhizome, flavinol glycosides (rutin and hesperidin, used to reduce capillary bleeding), and other glycoside types
3. *Tannins:* present in coffee and tea
4. *Lipids:* fixed oils and waxes
5. *Volatile oils:* essential oils such as peppermint and eucalyptus
6. *Resins*
7. *Steroids:* including the steroidal saponins from Mexican yam (*Diocorea* species), the original source of early oral contraceptives
8. *Alkaloids:* atropine from *Atropa belladonna,* quinine from cinchona, morphine from *Papaver somniferum*
9. *Peptide hormones*
10. *Enzymes:* bromelain from pineapple

"Influences on Plant Activities and Their Therapeutic Properties"). In the United States alone, opinions vary regarding a particular plant's full spectrum of physiological action because of the complex nature of plants and their uses.

 Influences on Plant Activities and Their Therapeutic Properties

· Specific plant species, variety, and sometimes the individual plant itself
· Habitat, including latitude, longitude, exposure, humidity, rainfall, sun, shade, wind, temperature and daily and seasonal variation, soil composition, soil microorganisms, insects, birds, animals, companion plants, pests, plant diseases, and interaction with humans (damage, cultivation, harvesting, and pollution)
· Composition and constituents (presence of active and inert ingredients)
· How and when the plant is collected, stored, processed; how the herb is dispensed and dosed
· Presence of adulterants, pests, or plant disease
· The prescriber; many traditional systems in Africa and Asia ascribe the ability to potentiate the plant's healing properties only to initiated healers or shamans
· The patient's health status, disease, age, and receptivity to healing
· The symbolic or cultural significance of the plant
· The placebo effect ❧

A sample of some classic herb categories based on plant actions—often associated with identifiable nutritives or active constituents—are adaptogens (balance body systems), anticatarrhals (eliminate mucus), carminatives (antigas), demulcents (reduce inflammation), galactogogues (promote breast milk production), nervines (reduce stress), and tonics (promote optimal organ function).

These examples illustrate a few of the many actions ascribed to herbs viewed from the classic Western paradigm. Often, contemporary research explains the constituents, mechanisms of action, and clinical responses that justify traditional uses. Occasionally, some plants are found to be inactive or ineffective or to contain potential toxins, which results in their discontinuance or necessitates special methods of preparation and dosing. As with most current prescription medications, some strong herbs must be dosed carefully to render them safe and effective.

There are other limitations to the direct association of active constituents with in vivo and clinical medicinal actions. Many times the active compounds remain unidentified, or the physiological response to the medicinal part of the whole plant is distinct from the actions of the individual active constituents (e.g., *Valeriana, Echinacea*). In addition, ingredients that appear inert are sometimes later found to be active when a more accurate or precise mechanism of action or bioassay associated with the plant's effects is discovered.

When a nonreductionist paradigm is used, plant composition alone offers an incomplete explanation of the full scope of the properties and actions of food and healing plants. Traditional herbalists, nineteenth-century vitalists (see Chapter 6), naturopathic doctors (see Chapters 22, 23), and many contemporary medical doctors and practitioners share a belief in a "life force" that is yet to be fully understood. Many herbalists hold that healing energy is inherent to plants; it is this energy ("vibrational energy" in some herbal systems), in addition to nutritive or chemical constituents, that promotes healing. Shamans, traditional healers, and alchemists use their skills, knowledge, and power to instill certain plants with special healing properties, in this view.

HERBAL THERAPEUTICS

Different cultural paradigms use plants for healing in a manner founded on each paradigm's premises (Box 24-3). Ethnobotanical perspectives reveal that there may be three levels of effects in the types of physiologic responses engendered by a given plant: (1) a direct pharmacological effect based upon the presence of an "active ingredient" that would be classified as a "drug" in biomedicine; (2) nonspecific physiologic effects such as the effects of methyl xanthines in coffee, tea, or cacao that have strong physiological effects on the body but without a specific "drug" action (nonetheless, the patient is aware of tangible effects); and (3) symbolic effects in that cultural significance (or folklore) imbued in a plant recruits beliefs that could be called "placebo" effects (Micozzi, 1983). Of course, given

BOX 24-3 *Herbal Practices*

Herbal practitioners in the United States may rely primarily on one of the following, or a combination:

1. *The plant's pharmacological actions:* in some cases enhanced by specific processing and extractive solvents and techniques or formulation of plant medicines into standardized extract products to concentrate and guarantee unit doses of active constituents
2. *Individual plant pharmacokinetics:* best preserved by using single, whole plants or their extracts
3. *Synergistic formulating:* blending of a number of medicinal plants together to achieve specific therapeutic effects unachievable by using a single herb alone
4. *Nutritional value:* as when *Urtica repens,* or nettles, is recommended as a tea rich in absorbable iron
5. *Energetics:* vibrational energy, as for example with Bach flower remedies, and various flower essences

the complex phytochemical consitutuents, as well as historical usage, any or all of these kinds of effects may be present simultaneously.

Herbal medicines can be delivered in many forms. Some plants are best when used fresh but are seldom marketed fresh because they are highly perishable, and improper storage will affect quality. Dried, whole, or chopped herbs can be prepared either as *infusions* (steeped as tea) or *decoctions* (simmered over low heat). Typically, flowers, leaves, and powdered herbs are infused (e.g., chamomile or peppermint), whereas fruits, seeds, barks, and roots require decocting (e.g., rose hips, cinnamon bark, licorice root). Many fresh and dried herbs can be tinctured as medicines extracted and preserved in alcohol. Some plants are suited to acetracts (vinegar extracts), whereas others are active and well preserved as syrups, glycerites (in vegetable glycerine), or miels (in honey). Powdered or freeze-dried herbs are available in bulk and as tablets, troches, pastes, and capsules. Fluid and solid extracts—strong concentrates (four to six times the crude herb strength)—and fresh plant juices preserved in approximately 25% alcohol (as with the fresh plant *Echinacea succus*), as well as the crude juice extract of Aloe vera, are other forms.

Nonoral delivery forms include herbal pessaries, suppositories, creams, ointments, gels, liniments, oils, distilled waters, washes, enemas, baths, poultices, compresses, moxa, snuffs, steams, and inhaled smokes and aromatics (volatile oils). For example, in traditional Native American practices, smoking of the dried tobacco plant has ceremonial symbolic properties, whereas the rolled leaf may be inserted as a suppository for medicinal purposes. The predominant plant delivery forms vary among different herbal traditions. Tinctures are widely used in Britain and the United States; tablets of standardized extracts of certain herbs (e.g., *Ginkgo biloba*) are popular in Germany and the United States; decoctions are common in Tibetan, Chinese, and African traditions; therapeutic oils are used topically and internally in Ayurvedic treatments; and teas, smokes, and compresses are used in the Native American tradition.

Capsules and tablets are the most common delivery system today. Gelatin or vegetable-based capsules are filled with powdered dried herbs. Tablets are powdered herbs compressed into a solid pill, often with a variety of inert ingredients as fillers.

Herbs are supplied in a variety of sizes and strengths, so it is important to read the label carefully. The label also usually gives an average suggested dose as a guideline, based on research and clinical use. It is recommend to start at the low end, watch for a response (including unwanted effects) and adjust the dose accordingly.

Safety

Side effects of drugs can be serious or fatal; the worst is death by overdose. According to one report, overdoses are associated with an annual rate of 30 deaths per 1 million prescriptions of antidepressants. On the other hand, to quote Norman Farnsworth, PhD, professor of pharmacognosy at the University of Illinois, Chicago, "Based on published reports, side effects or toxic reactions associated with herbal medicines in any form are rare. . . . In fact, of all classes of substances . . . to cause toxicities of sufficient magnitude to be reported in the United States, plants are the least problematic."

Herbal products are often considered safe because they are "natural" products (Kuruvilla, 2002). Nonetheless, the quality of products may be affected by species differences, seasonal variations, environmental factors, collection methods, transport and storage, manufacturing practices, or contamination with foreign plant material, toxins, heavy metals, or environmental pollutants. One must also remember that any substance that has biological activity has the potential to cause adverse effects. Dangerous and lethal side effects related to direct toxic effects, allergic reactions, effects from contaminants, and interaction with drugs or other herbs have been reported (Chan, 2003; Dobos et al, 2005; Hu et al, 2005; Izzo & Ernest, 2001).

Groups have assembled to look at special circumstances of herb use in the context of dental procedures, in the perioperative period, and with concurrent use of particular prescribed drugs. Some cautions identified through these inquiries include the following herbs:

- Bromelain, cayenne, chamomile, and feverfew interact with aspirin.
- Aloe latex, ephedra, ginseng, and licorice interact with corticosteroids.
- Kava, St. John's wort, and valerian interact with central nervous system depressants; chamomile, horse chestnut, and fenugreek enhance the risk of bleeding.
- Ginseng can produce hypoglycemia.
- Ephedra may lead to cardiovascular instability (Abebe, 2002, 2003; Ang-Lee et al, 2001; Bent, 2008; Izzo & Ernest, 2001; Micozzi & Pribitkin, 2009).

Quality control is essential, with assurance that the product contains ingredients and quantities as labeled, and without such contaminants as bacteria, molds, or pesticides. Selection of plant material based on quality, standardization of methods of preparation, and enforcement of regulations regarding labeling improve the quality and safety of herbal preparations as therapeutic agents.

In traditional medicine systems, herbs are prepared to obtain the most active ingredient for use in the specific preparation discovered to be most effective for the particular herb and tailored to the unique characteristics of the patient (Khalsa, 2007).

In 2004, Europe enacted legislation designed to improve the protection of public health by setting up a registration scheme for manufactured traditional herbal medicines. The evidence of 30 years of traditional use was relied upon to establish a European list of herbal substances that includes indication, strength, dosing recommendations, and route of administration. The list was compiled by the Committee on Herbal Medicinal Products at the European Medicines Agency (Routledge, 2008). The European Agency for the Evaluation of Medicinal Products has drafted test procedures and acceptance criteria for herbal drug preparations (Rousseaux & Schachter, 2003).

In Australia, the Therapeutic Goods Administration created a Complementary Medicines Evaluation Committee to address the issue of regulation of herbal products (Rousseaux & Schachter, 2003).

In the United States, trade and professional organizations such as the American Herbal Products Association set standards including good agricultural practice, good laboratory practice, good supply practice, good manufacturing practice, and standard operating procedures that can help control environmental factors that may contribute to contamination (Chan, 2003; Fong, 2002; Routledge, 2008). Most herbal products in the United States are regulated as "dietary supplements." In 1994, the U.S. Dietary Supplement Health and Education Act (DSHEA) set new guidelines with regard to quality, labeling, packaging, and marketing of supplements. It also sparked a surge of interest in herbal products. DSHEA allows manufacturers to make "statements of nutritional support for conventional vitamins and minerals." Because herbs are not nutritional in the conventional sense, DSHEA allows manufacturers to make only what are called "structure and function claims," but no therapeutic or prevention claims regardless of what has been provided by research evidence. Thus a label can claim that St. John's wort "optimizes mood," but it cannot call it a "natural antidepressant," which would be a therapeutic claim. Despite all the emphasis on producing scientific evidence for the efficacy of any medical treatment, here is a glaring exception where a blind bureaucratic regulation takes precedence over any and all scientific investigation and evidence.

The next time someone tries to convince you that all biomedical practice is based only on science, this circumstance is one clear example to the contrary (among others).

General Guidelines for the Use of Herbal Medicines

1. The clinician should take a careful history of the patient's use of herbs and other supplements.
2. An accurate medical diagnosis must be made before herbs are used for symptomatic treatment.
3. Natural is not necessarily safe; attention should be paid to quality of product, dosage, and potential adverse effects, including interactions.
4. Herbal treatments should, for the most part, be avoided during pregnancy (and contemplated pregnancy) and lactation.
5. Herbal use by children should be done with care, using the appropriate dosage based on weight.
6. Adverse effects should be recorded, and the dosage reduced or the product discontinued. It can be carefully restarted to ascertain whether or not it is the source of the problem. ∾

The regulatory authority of the U.S. Food and Drug Administration (FDA) over herbs is frequently misrepresented as "absent," including by former FDA commissioner Jane Henney herself (in that case), as testified in hearings to the U.S. House of Representatives Committee on Government Reform in 2001. Nonetheless, the health care system must rely on vigilance by the medical profession and voluntary compliance by industry to safeguard patients against adverse reactions. Although legislative efforts are periodically made to alter the regulatory environment, changes are not anticipated in DSHEA, which regulates herbs as dietary supplements, not as drugs, despite persistent efforts by Sen. Dick Durbin (D-IL). Senator Orrin Hatch (R-Utah), co-chair of the Congressional Caucus on Complementary and Alternative Medicine and Dietary Supplements, has documented the unprecedented involvement of a coalition of citizens and commercial groups in the passage of this bill (Hatch, 2002). It is likely that better information and education of consumers and health professionals will help to achieve what more regulation cannot achieve (see the sidebar "Legislative and Regulatory Environment for Herbal Medicines").

Legislative and Regulatory Environment for Herbal Medicines

Under the U.S. Dietary Supplement Health and Education Act (DSHEA) of 1994, as amended 1998, the U.S. Food and Drug Administration (FDA) presently has power to regulate herbal remedies and dietary supplements in the following ways:

Continued

Legislative and Regulatory Environment for Herbal Medicines—cont'd

1. Institute "good manufacturing practices" (GMPs), including practices addressing identity, potency, cleanliness, and stability (although the FDA did not promulgate GMPs until 13 years after passage of DSHEA, long after the science-based sector of industry had implemented and/or exceeded anticipated GMPs).
2. Refer for criminal action the sale of toxic or unsanitary products.
3. Obtain injunction against the sale of products making false claims.
4. Seize products that pose an unreasonable risk of illness and injury.
5. Sue any company making a claim that a product "cures" or "treats" disease (regardless of scientific investigations, evidence and peer-reviewed publications).
6. Stop sale of an entire class of products if they pose an imminent health hazard.
7. Stop products from being marketed if the FDA does not receive sufficient safety data in advance (under "generally recognized as safe" [GRAS] provisions). ∾

Further abuses involving herbal products adulterated with therapeutic drugs and contaminants (especially a problem with imports from overseas, particularly China) are a serious safety issue. Many times the adulteration is inadvertent, but sometimes undeclared prescription drugs may be fraudulently added, allegedly for medicinal purposes (Chan, 2003). Consumers, health professionals, and responsible elements of the U.S. natural products industry all suffer when irresponsibly adulterated products are imported from abroad. The National Institutes of Health (NIH) Office of Alternative Medicine clinical trial investigating the Chinese herbal formulation PC-SPES for prostate cancer was undermined by the unwitting use of adulterated herbs, which may be one result of the lack of background in relevant fields of science and practice endemic to that office (see Chapter 3). Some natural products from China have even been contaminated with chloramphenicol (Micozzi, 2007), which may cause fatal bone marrow aplasia.

Improvements in manufacturing and marketing standards in much of the natural products industry are required for effective integrative medical practice (Fong, 2002), and health professionals must learn to discern the hallmarks of high-quality, science-based manufacturers versus marketing companies.

PREGNANCY AND BREASTFEEDING

Most of the deleterious effects of natural products on the unborn baby are likely related to hormonal effects and drug interactions rather than to direct teratogenicity. Many herbs have not been approved for use by pregnant and nursing women in the guidelines of the German Commission E, a regulatory agency in some ways comparable to the U.S. FDA. Commission E has published a collection of reports based on safety and efficacy data on more than 200 herbs that are available in English translation (Blumenthal et al, 2000).

CHILDREN

Herbs may often be a treatment of choice for children. Despite relative paucity of modern research, centuries of use have shown many products to be safe when dosed appropriately according to children's weight, although there is a general bias in medicine against using CAM treatments in children that many may consider "experimental" despite centuries of use.

Although concerns exist about safety, efficacy, and appropriate dosing in the pediatric population, families do offer herbs to their children. A group in Canada interviewed 1804 families who came to an emergency department. They found that 20% of the families used natural health products concurrently with drugs. A quarter of those paired agents had the potential to cause interactions (Goldman et al, 2008).

Another study was conducted at an emergency department at Emory University in Atlanta, Georgia. Over a 3-month period, 142 families with children aged 3 weeks to 18 years were interviewed. Of the 45% of caregivers who reported giving their children herbal products, 53% had given one type and 27% had given three or more types in the previous year. The most common therapies were aloe, echinacea, and sweet oil. The most dangerous combination reported was ephedra given concomitantly with albuterol for asthma. Seventy-seven percent of the caregivers did not suspect potential side effects. Only two-thirds of the families anticipated interactions with other herbal products or with medications (Lanski et al, 2003).

AGING

Considering the phenomenon of polypharmacy in elderly persons and problems of impaired metabolism and clearance, herbs may offer an alternative to drugs. On the other hand, the practitioner also must be aware of herb–drug interactions. St. John's wort can be very useful for managing depression in the elderly patient, berberine or ginkgo for cognitive decline, and kava for sedation, without the adverse effects of the benzodiazepines. These herbs can be used in combination with each other as well.

GENERAL CONSIDERATIONS

Health care providers have a responsibility to act as informed intermediaries for patients and families seeking information about the use of herbal products and must consider issues of quality, safety, and efficacy which the average patient may not be able to do on their own.

The role of herbalism in contemporary Western society is not to serve as a substitute for genuine pharmaceutical advances but to provide access to an ancient paradigm that is less mechanistic and more holistic and humane in scope and that, if responsibly reclaimed and integrated, can greatly benefit future health care worldwide. This perspective is illustrated in the following statement by Paiakan, a contemporary Kayapo Indian leader.

> I am trying to save the knowledge that the forest and this planet are alive, to give it back to you who have lost the understanding. (Odum, 1971)

Changes in the practice of medicine are causing a shift to increasing self-care with many patients demanding, and some health policy guidelines mandating, more benign, less invasive treatments. More and more patients prefer to take personal control over their health, such as through the use of herbal remedies not only for therapeutic benefit, but also for prevention of disease. Herbal remedies are commonly used by patients with chronic medical conditions such as cancer, liver disease, immunodeficiencies, asthma, and rheumatologic disorders (Inamdar et al, 2008). It is critical that practicing clinicians (and, in turn, patients) be made aware of the indications, actions, and drug interactions of herbal remedies.

The World Health Organization (WHO) estimates that 80% of the world's population relies on herbal medicine. Meanwhile, the use of herbs in the United States is expanding rapidly; herbal products are readily found in most pharmacies and supermarkets. Initially, when estimates were first being made, from 1990 to 1997, the use of complementary and alternative medicine rose from 34% to 42% among those surveyed, and herbal use quadrupled from 3% to 12% (Eisenberg et al, 1998). The growth of complementary and alternative medicine and the use of dietary supplements have continued apace in the years since then (see Chapter 3).

Importantly, these rapid changes have occurred because of popular demand. The public has discovered that natural medicines often provide a safe, effective, and economical alternative, and research is increasingly validating these findings. Many of those who use herbal and vitamin products fail to inform their physicians. Either they assume that "natural" products are harmless and not worth mentioning, or they fear telling health professionals who may be skeptical about their use. Health professionals, however, are beginning to familiarize themselves with the subject. Aside from the advantages of natural products, herb–drug interactions are perceived to be a growing concern: almost one in five prescription drug users were also using supplements (Eisenberg et al, 1998).

Reliance on the appropriate use of nutrients and herbs is a critical and fundamental component of many integrative medical practices. Presently in the United States, these natural products are widely available. Unlike for pharmaceuticals, information about the health effects cannot be provided on the product label or with the product as a product insert.

As observed by WHO, herbs are essentially "people's medicine." In many parts of the world, traditional systems of herbalism generally make little distinction between food and medicinal plants, and local accessibility of food, spices, and therapeutic herbs generally is assumed in traditional agrarian, nonindustrialized societies. Before the mid-twentieth century, most people everywhere generally had closer personal contact with food and medicinal plants.

A restoration of the personal and symbolic relationship to food and medicinal plants could be linked with contemporary scientific knowledge of herbal applications. Appropriate self-care could be encouraged with public education, access to consultation with professional herbalists and physicians, and access to fresh herbs and high-quality, processed herbal medicines when needed. This improved patient involvement in the self-care of the body and its signals might then improve the use of professional medical care.

Many herbalists consider the patient's direct involvement in his or her own healing and the summoning of the patient's intellectual, emotional, physical, and spiritual attention to the process as critical. Partly for this reason, and because of traditional herbalism's emphasis on "right relationship," social context, and self-responsibility, many herbal practitioners deliberately prescribe elaborate rather than convenient herbal therapies. For example, on returning home to Ghana, a merchant developed an infected leg ulcer. Instead of being supplied an herbal medicine by the herbalist, he was directed to the nearby live plant source (a local tree bark). He collected and prepared the antimicrobial and vulnery poultice and applied it daily until his wound healed.

Although self-collection and medicine preparation are generally impractical in the United States today (although see sidebar on American ginseng "sangers"), self-involvement in the healing process is possible in many ways and parallels the complex lifestyle changes now routinely recommended to patients with chronic ailments such as cardiovascular disease and diabetes.

There is increasing availability of credible third-party research on the efficacy of herbal and nutritional ingredients, as well as recognition by the medical profession of the importance of dietary supplementation for optimal health and for the prevention and management of many medical conditions. A landmark article in *Journal of the American Medical Association*, in July 2002, made clear the many clinical benefits and indications for dietary supplementation. It is incumbent on practitioners of integrative medicine to maintain a medical standard of information and practice about herbal and nutritional ingredients. One approach to this requirement is to develop and maintain capability for clinic-based or hospital-based formularies of appropriate, effective, and high-quality herbs and nutrients.

The current regulatory environment is coupled with the reality that much of the natural products industry still does not operate to medical and scientific standards, that many irresponsible marketing claims are made, and that many medical and scientific professionals are not knowledgeable about the science behind herbal and nutritional medicine (see Appendix to this chapter).

For practitioners new to the medicinal use of herbs, dose selection can be confusing. This volatile mix produces much confusion and misinformation on both sides, documented periodically by such august sources as the *New England Journal of Medicine*. Medical professionals are often largely on their own in trying to understand the proper indications, ingredients, and dosages for the appropriate scientific use of herbal and nutritional remedies, and consumers can only look to practitioners for guidance.

New information technologies are being brought on line to provide distributors, consumers, and practitioners fair and accurate information about the appropriate use of dietary supplements. The authors do not, however, recommend any one particular website alone nor advise using websites without confirmation by a knowledgeable practitioner (although some are mentioned at the end of this chapter).

In any case, to adequately guide patients, it is essential to obtain a complete drug and herbal history from the patient using an open and nonjudgmental approach.

RESEARCH

Although there is a relatively extensive contemporary literature on medicinal and healing plants, much of it exists outside the United States and often in languages other than English. In addition, there is little consistency in standard research designs and protocols among various countries.

Over the years, the National Center for Complementary and Alternative Medicine (NCCAM) funded the following centers for botanical research:

- Botanicals Research Center for Age Related Diseases (Indiana)
- Botanical Research Center: Metabolic Syndrome (Louisiana)
- Center for Botanical Dietary Supplements Research in Women's Health (Illinois)
- Center for Botanical Immunomodulators (New York)
- Center for Botanical Lipids (North Carolina)
- Center for Research on Botanical Dietary Supplements (Iowa).

More information regarding this research can be obtained by visiting the NCCAM website and clicking on the links.

The need for more research on food, spice, and medicinal plants remains, especially with regard to their potential use in functional complaints, syndromes and conditions not well recognized or treated by conventional Western medicine. The challenge is to conduct the research in a holistic context. This goal requires creative design and funding of research that is unlikely to provide high-profit returns to a single source.

Many medicinal plants eliminated from the *United States Pharmacopeia* over the years were dropped because contemporary research documentation of their efficacy was lacking, not because they were proved to be ineffective (although some plants proved less useful clinically than some newly developed drugs).

Retaining a holistic context in medicinal plant research also involves addressing differences in paradigm. Involving traditional herbalists as research design consultants would protect against inadvertently eliminating a critical element of the paradigm within which the herb is used. In the past, plant collection for research has sometimes proved an environmental threat (habitats, species, or traditional knowledge was lost or threatened). A holistic approach to contemporary plant collection and research must be implemented to conserve the traditional knowledge and ecology of the source plant and to avoid transgression of intellectual property rights, destruction of the plant habitat, or an imbalance of economic or intellectual returns to the source habitat and community.

Simple, well-documented analysis and outcome-based research of crude and whole plant medicines are still needed to determine their greatest potential applications and benefit to human health. Increasing contemporary research on medicinal plants is critical, but the importance of also documenting, respecting, and incorporating the empirical knowledge of healing plants cannot be overemphasized (see Appendix). Information gleaned from research should be linked with empirical knowledge (usually derived from hundreds of years of human use across many generations and ethnic groups), along with contemporary clinical reporting from patients and practitioners on tolerance and efficacy. Thus the sensible approach must be far more broad and inclusive than provided by the limitations of so-called evidence-based medicine (see Chapter 3). Then herbal therapeutics and preventive protocols can be better targeted to enhance the health of future generations.

ECONOMIC ISSUES

The modern era has brought many advantages in human health and sanitation, but one potential disadvantage of economic and occupational specialization is the loss of contact with the source of plant medicines. The marketplace has become multileveled, so the consumer usually has no direct or personal relationship with the herb producer. Sometimes, because of costs of production, taxes, and marketing, the packaged herbal product costs 20 times the price of the crude herb. There are undeniable advantages to certain prepackaged or concentrated herbal products, but two disadvantages are accountability and economic access. If the sale of fresh or bulk crude herbs is abandoned in the marketplace for the sale of less perishable and higher-return products, the patient has access to only highly processed products, and the cash-poor patient loses access altogether. This dilemma is particularly ironic in the case of medicinal plants; most traditional systems considered healing plants a gift of nature and access to them a basic human right.

State governments have developed a traditional role in regulating medical practice and in supporting medical education. The federal government maintains a unique and critical role in stimulating and supporting medical research, regulating medical products and devices, protecting the public health, and helping build health care infrastructure, and it is now paying approximately one-third the costs of health care in America.

Policy makers at the state and federal levels should become more knowledgeable about the needs and opportunities related to integrative medicine. The bipartisan Congressional Caucus on Complementary and Alternative Medicine and Dietary Supplements was organized for this purpose (see above). The Integrative Healthcare Policy Consortium, Policy Institute for Integrative Medicine, and other groups in former years had worked with members of the Caucus and other elected representatives to broaden and deepen federal support for appropriate analyses and programs in integrative medicine. Because many (but not all) legislators have finally confronted the need for budgetary restraints, for the foreseeable future, we are unlikely to see improvements in this area.

It is also unlikely that the current regulatory legislation governing dietary supplements (DSHEA of 1994, as amended in 1998) will be changed. Although the miniscule funding for NCCAM had increased commensurate with the multiyear doubling of the overall NIH budget over the period 1995–2005, that era is over. It remains critical that other federal agencies charged with programs related to health resources and services, primary care, health professions training and workforce development, consumer education, health services research, and other areas be brought to bear on the important challenge and opportunity to realize true cost savings and meaningful health care reform by taking rational approaches to providing access to safe, effective and cost-effective available services (see Chapter 3).

Integrative medicine has an important role that requires further articulation in current congressional actions on medical liability insurance reform and the national patient safety and quality assurance initiative. Public support together with private innovation has been the hallmark for medical advancement in the twentieth century and should continue to be the case for integrative medicine in the twenty-first century.

SUMMARY

Herbalism clearly offers potential benefit for the treatment of disease as well as promotion of wellness. Going forward, efforts should focus on more standardization of quality control, development of official compendia that encompasses the content of the various pharmacopeias currently available, clear and honest communication and sharing of information, and more inclusive research regarding safety and efficacy in all populations.

Assimilation of New Herbs into Ancient Pharmacopeia

The ancient pharmacopeia continues to grow with assimilation of herbs from global geographic regions. The Chinese pharmacopeia has its origins in the semi-mythical emperor Shen Nong, who compiled it approximately 3000 years ago. He was also known as the "Divine Husbandman," showing the association between cultivation of medicinal plants with agriculture and animal domestication. This pharmacopeia has expanded from hundreds to thousands of entries over the centuries.

For example, when Chinese laborers were employed by the Union Pacific Railroad for the construction of the western-half of the U.S. transcontinental railroad completed in 1869, they encountered North American herbs (many already known by then to European physicians as Native American remedies). The 3000-year-old Chinese pharmacopeia was quickly expanded to make room for these new discoveries.

Thus, the potent American ginseng was added alongside Siberian ginseng and Chinese ginseng. The properties of American ginseng were already highly valued by Native Americans and had quickly become known to the European settlers. It had become an important economic product, driving many literally into the mountains of Appalachia to collect it. The desire for ginseng helped stimulate exploration and eventually western expansion. The famous early-American frontier hero Daniel Boone (America's own version of a semi-mythical figure) made his start exploring the early western frontier of the Appalachians as a "sanger," gathering the valuable herb in the hills and hollows where it could be found (what today would be called "wild crafting.")

References

Abebe W: Herbal medication: potential for adverse interactions with analgesic drugs, *J Clin Pharm Ther* 27(6):391, 2002.

Abebe W: An overview of herbal supplement utilization with particular emphasis on possible interactions with dental drugs and oral manifestations, *J Dent Hyg* 77(1):37, 2003.

Ang-Lee MK, Moss J, Yuan CS: Herbal medicines and perioperative care, *JAMA* 286(2):208, 2001.

Bauchner H, Fontanarosa PH: Restoring Confidence in the Pharmaceutical Industry. *JAMA* 309(6):607–609, 2013. doi:10.1001/jama.2013.58.

Behnke K, Jensen GS, Graubaum HJ, Gruenwald J: *Hypericum perforatum* versus fluoxetine in the treatment of mild to moderate depression, *Adv Ther* 19(1):43–52, 2002.

Bent S: Herbal medicine in the United States: review of efficacy, safety, and regulation: grand rounds at University of California, San Francisco Medical Center, *J Gen Intern Med* 23(6):854, 2008. [Epub April 16, 2008].

Bent S, Ko R: Commonly used herbal medicines in the United States: a review, *Am J Med* 116(7):478, 2004.

Blumenthal M, Goldberg A, Brinckmann J: *Herbal medicine: expanded Commission E monographs*, Newton, Mass, 2000, Integrative Medicine Communications.

Boyle W: *Official herbs in the United States pharmacopoeias: 1820–1990*, East Palestine, Ohio, 1991, Buckeye Naturopathic Press.

Chan K: Some aspects of toxic contaminants in herbal medicines, *Chemosphere* 52(9):1361, 2003.

Cheng X, Wang D, Jiang L, et al: Simultaneous determination of eight bioactive alkaloids in *Corydalis saxicola* by high-performance liquid chromatography coupled with diode array detection, *Phytochem Anal* 19(5):420, 2008.

Dobos GJ, Tan L, Cohen MH, et al: Are national quality standards for traditional Chinese herbal medicine sufficient? Current governmental regulations for traditional Chinese herbal medicine in certain Western countries and China as the Eastern origin country, *Complement Ther Med* 13(3):183, 2005.

Eisenberg DM, Davis RB, Ettner SL, et al: Trends in alternative medicine use in the United States, 1990–1997: results of a follow-up national survey, *JAMA* 280(18):1569, 1998.

Fong HH: Integration of herbal medicine into modern medicine practices: issues and prospects, *Integr Cancer Ther* 1(3):287, discussion 293, 2002.

Goldman RD, Rogovik AL, Lai D, Vohra S: Potential interactions of drug–natural health products and natural health products–natural health products among children, *J Pediatr* 152(4):521, 2008. [Epub November 7, 2007].

Hatch O: *Square peg: confessions of a citizen senator*, New York, 2002, Basic Books, pp 81–95.

Hu Z, Yang X, Ho PC, et al: Herbal-drug interactions: a literature review, *Drugs* 65(9):1239, 2005.

Inamdar N, Edalat S, Kotwal V, et al: Herbal drugs in milieu of modern drugs, *Int J Green Pharm* 2(1):2, 2008.

Iwu MM: *Handbook of African medicinal plants*, Boca Raton, Fla, 1993, CRC Press, pp 343–349.

Izzo AA, Ernest E: Interactions between herbal medicines and prescribed drugs: a systematic review, *Drugs* 61(15):2163, 2001.

Khalsa KP: Preparing botanical medicines, *J Herb Pharmacother* 7(3–4):267, 2007.

Kuruvilla A: Herbal formulations as pharmacotherapeutic agents, *Indian J Exp Biol* 40(1):7, 2002.

Lanski SL, Greenwald M, Perkins A, et al: Herbal therapy use in pediatric emergency department population: expect the unexpected, *Pediatrics* 111(5 Pt 1):981, 2003.

Micozzi MS: Traditional ethnomedical resources: Three levels of effect among traditional ethnomedical resources, *Hum Organ: J Soc Appl Anthropol* 1983.

Micozzi MS: *Complementary and integrative medicine in cancer care and prevention*, New York, 2007, Springer.

Micozzi MS, Pribitkin E: *Skin medicine: Dermatology for the clinician,* 2009.

Odum H: *Environment, power and society*, New York, 1971, John Wiley & Sons, p 8.

Rousseaux CG, Schachter H: Regulatory issues concerning the safety, efficacy and quality of herbal remedies, *Birth Defects Res B Dev Reprod Toxicol* 68(6):505, 2003.

Routledge PA: The European Herbal Medicines Directive: could it have saved the lives of Romeo and Juliet?, *Drug Saf* 31(5):416, 2008.

Shelton RC, Keller MB, Gelenberg A, et al: Effectiveness of St John's wort in major depression: a randomized controlled trial, *JAMA* 285(15):1978–1986, 2001.

Solecki RS, Shanidar IV: a Neanderthal flower burial in northern Iraq, *Science* 190:880, 1975.

Tyler VE, Brady LR, Robbers JE: *Pharmacognosy*, Philadelphia, 1988, Lea & Febiger.

Suggested Readings

Astin JA: Why patients use alternative medicine: results of a national study, *JAMA* 279(19):1548, 1998.

Bausell RB, Lee WL, Berman BM: Demographic and health-related correlates to visits to complementary and alternative medical providers, *Med Care* 39(2):190, 2001.

Bensky D, Gamble A: *Chinese herbal medicine materia medica*, Seattle, 1986, Eastland Press, pp 34–35.

Berman BM: The Cochrane Collaboration and evidence-based complementary medicine, *J Altern Complement Med* 3(2):191, 1997.

Bisset NG, Wichtl M, editors: *Herbal drugs and phytopharmaceuticals: a handbook for practice on a scientific basis*, Boca Raton, Fla, 1994, CRC Press, pp 273–275.

Bourin M, Bougerol T, Guitton B, et al: A combination of plant extracts in the treatment of outpatients with adjustment disorder with anxious mood: controlled study versus placebo, *Fundam Clin Pharmacol* 11(2):127, 1997.

Cott JM: In vitro receptor binding and enzyme inhibition by *Hypericum perforatum* extract, *Pharmacopsychiatry* 30(Suppl II): 108, 1997.

Davies LP, Drew CA, Duffield P, et al: Kava pyrones and resin: studies on GABAA, GABAB and benzodiazepine binding sites in rodent brain, *Pharmacol Toxicol* 71(2):120, 1992.

DeFeudis FV: *Ginkgo biloba extract (Egb 761): pharmacological activities and clinical applications*, Paris, 1991, Elsevier.

DeSmet PA: Herbal remedies, *N Engl J Med* 347:2046, 2002.

Donden Y: *Health through balance: an introduction to Tibetan medicine*, Ithaca, NY, 1986, Snow Lion Publications.

Dorn M: Efficacy and tolerability of Baldrian versus oxazepam in non-organic and non-psychiatric insomniacs: a randomised, double-blind, clinical, comparative study, *Forsch Komplementarmed Klass Naturheilkd* 7(2):79, 2000.

Druss BG, Rosenheck RA: Association between use of unconventional therapies and conventional medical services, *JAMA* 282(7):651, 1999.

Eisenberg DM, Kessler RC, Foster C, et al: Unconventional medicine in the United States: prevalence, costs, and patterns of use, *N Engl J Med* 328(4):246, 1993.

European Scientific Cooperative on Phytotherapy: *Monographs on the medicinal use of plants*, Exeter, England, 1997, The Cooperative.

Fairfield KM, Fletcher RH: Vitamins for chronic disease prevention in adults: scientific evidence, *JAMA* 287:3116, 2002.

Farnsworth NR, Bunyapraphatsara N: *Thai medicinal plants recommended for primary health care systems*, Bangkok, 1992, Medicinal Plant Information Center.

Fletcher RH, Fairfield KM: Vitamins for chronic disease prevention in adults: clinical applications, *JAMA* 287:3127, 2002.

Fontana RJ, Lown KS, Paine MF, et al: Effects of a chargrilled meat diet on expression of CYP3A, CYP1A, and P-glycoprotein levels in healthy volunteers, *Gastroenterology* 117(1):89, 1999.

Fugh-Berman A, Cott JM: Dietary supplements and natural products as psychotherapeutic agents, *Psychosom Med* 61:712, 1999.

Garrett BJ, Cheeke PR, Miranda CL, et al: Consumption of poisonous plants by rats, *Toxicol Lett* 10:183, 1982.

Gomez-Beioz A, Chavez N: The botanica as a culturally appropriate health care option for Latinos, *J Altern Complement Med* 7(5):537, 2001.

Gruenwald J, Skrabal J: Kava ban highly questionable: a brief summary of the main scientific findings presented in the "In depth investigation on European Union member states market restrictions on kava products," *Sem Integrative Med* 1(4):199, 2003.

Hoffmann DL: *The herb user's guide: the basic skills of medical herbalism*, Wellingborough, England, 1987, Thorsons.

Johne A, Brockmoller J, Bauer S, et al: Pharmacokinetic interaction of digoxin with an herbal extract from St. John's wort (*Hypericum perforatum*), *Clin Pharmacol Ther* 66(4):338, 1999.

Junius MM: *The practical handbook of plant alchemy*, Rochester, NY, 1993, Healing Arts Press.

Kessler RC, Davis RB, Foster DF, et al: Long-term trends in the use of complementary and alternative medical therapies in the United States, *Ann Intern Med* 135(4):262, 2001.

Kinzler E, Kromer J, Lehmann E: Wirksamkeit eines Kava-Spezial-Extraktes bei Patienten mit Angst: Spannungs-und Erregungszustanden nicht-psychotischer Genese, *Arzneim Forsch/Drug Res* 41:584, 1991.

Landes P: Market report, *HerbalGram* 42:64, 1998.

Landmark Healthcare: *I. The Landmark Report II on HMOs and Alternative Care. II*, 1999, Landmark Healthcare.

Linde K, Ramirez G, Mulrow CD, et al: St. John's wort for depression: an overview and meta-analysis of randomized clinical trials, *BMJ* 313:253, 1996.

Maurer A, Johne A, Bauer S, et al: Interaction of St. John's wort extract with phenprocoumon, *Eur J Clin Pharmacol* 55(3):A22, 1999.

McGuffin M, Hobbs C, Upton R, et al: *Botanical safety handbook*, Boca Raton, Fla, 1997, CRC Press, p 105.

Micozzi MS: Complementary medicine: what is appropriate? Who will provide it?, *Ann Intern Med* 129:65, 1998.

Micozzi MS: Culture, society and the return of complementary medicine, *Med Anthropol Q* 2002.

Müller WE, Rolli M, Schäfer C, et al: Effects of *Hypericum* extract (LI 160) in biochemical models of antidepressant activity, *Pharmacopsychiatry* 30(Suppl II):102, 1997.

Newall CA, Anderson LA, Phillipson JD: *Herbal medicines: a guide for health-care professionals*, London, 1996, Pharmaceutical Press, pp 239–240.

Ohnishi A, Matsuo H, Yamada S, et al: Effect of furanocoumarin derivatives in grapefruit juice on the uptake of vinblastine by Caco-2 cells and on the activity of cytochrome P450 3A4, *Br J Pharmacol* 130(6):1369, 2000.

Ortiz BI, Shields KM, Clauson KA, et al: Complementary and alternative medicine use among Hispanics in the United States, *Ann Pharmacother* 41(6):994, 2007. [Epub May 15, 2007].

Piscitelli SC, Burstein AH, Chaitt D, et al: Indinavir concentrations and St. John's wort, *Lancet* 355(9203):547, 2000.

Ruschitzka F, Meier PJ, Turina M, et al: Acute heart transplant rejection due to Saint John's wort, *Lancet* 355(9203):548, 2000.

Santos MS, Ferreira F, Faro C, et al: The amount of GABA present in aqueous extracts of valerian is sufficient to account for [3H] GABA release in synaptosomes, *Planta Med* 60(5):475, 1994.

Schelosky L, Raffauf C, Jendroska K, et al: Letter to the editor, *J Neurol Neurosurg Psychiatry* 45:639, 1995.

Scudder JM: *Specific diagnosis: a study of disease with special reference to the administration of remedies*, Cincinnati, 1874, Wilstach, Baldwin.

Shelton RC, Keller MB, Gelenberg A, et al: Effectiveness of St. John's wort in major depression: a randomized controlled trial, *JAMA* 285(15):1978, 2001.

Stetter C: *The secret medicine of the pharaohs: ancient Egyptian healing*, Chicago, 1993, Edition Q.

Suzuki D, Knudtson P: *Wisdom of the elders: sacred native stories of nature*, New York, 1992, Bantam Books.

Upton R, Graff A, Williamson E, et al: American herbal pharmacopoeia and therapeutic compendium on St. John's wort (*Hypericum perforatum*): quality control, analytical and therapeutic monograph, *Herbal Gram* 40(Suppl):1, 1997.

Upton R, Graff A, Williamson E, et al: *American herbal pharmacopoeia and therapeutic compendium on valerian root: analytical, quality control, and therapeutic monograph*, Santa Cruz, Calif, 1999, AHP.

Vorbach EU: Efficacy and tolerability of St. John's wort extract LI 160 vs. imipramine in patients with severe depressive episodes according to ICD-10, *Pharmacopsychiatry* 30(Suppl 2):81, 1997.

Woelk H, Kapoula O, Lehrl S, et al: Behandlung von Angst-Patienten, *Z Allgemeinmed* 69:271, 1993.

Wolfman C, Viola H, Paladini A, et al: Possible anxiolytic effects of chrysin, a central benzodiazepine receptor ligand isolated from *Passiflora coerulea*, *Pharmacol Biochem Behav* 47(1):1, 1994.

Wood M: *Seven herbs: plants as teachers*, Berkeley, Calif, 1986, North Atlantic Books.

Wooton J, Sparber A: Surveys of complementary and alternative medicine usage: review of general population trends and specific populations, *Semin Integrat Med* 1(1):2003.

Yue Q-Y, Bergquist C, Gerdén B: Safety of St. John's wort (*Hypericum perforatum*), *Lancet* 355:576, 2000.

Zenk SN, Shaver JL, Peragaiio N, et al: Use of herbal therapies among midlife Mexican women, *Health Care Women Int* 22(6): 585, 2001.

Websites

Alternative Medicine Foundation, Inc: http://www.HerbMed.org

American Botanical Council: http://www.herbalgram.org

Herb Research Foundation: http://www.herbs.org

The National Center for Complementary and Alternative Medicine: http://nccam.nih.gov

The Natural Pharmacist

Natural Product Research Consultants (NPRC): http://www.nprcdb.com

APPENDIX: MAINSTREAM RESEARCH ON HERBAL REMEDIES

Marc S. Micozzi and Claire M. Cassidy

There are fundamental problems with the manner in which much contemporary research is conducted when mainstream scientists, epidemiologists, statisticians, disease-researchers, and clinicians attempt studies on diet, nutrition, and herbal medicines and dietary supplements. In recent decades, biomedical scientists have been turned loose to conduct clinical research on complementary and alternative medicine (CAM) with access to unprecedented levels of funding, state-of-the-art technologies, and new patient populations. But they often lack even rudimentary knowledge about CAM practices and usage of herbal remedies and their medical model contexts, which would be known to any reader of this text. Such studies may fail to ask relevant research questions—that is, questions phrased in such a way as to reflect the medical model of the practice they want to study.

Applying biomedical model questions to the assessment of nonbiomedical practices makes no more sense than playing football by the rules of baseball. If unable to ask relevant questions, they cannot design research with any reasonable level of model fit validity. The resulting "data" are often unrecognizable and unacceptable to CAM practitioners. With these points in mind, let us examine studies on four common herbal remedies—ginkgo biloba, St. John's wort, kava kava, and ephedra. Dietary supplements provide dramatic examples because as treatments they can be given in a pill with a simple placebo control, like drugs, using the controlled clinical methods that have been developed uniquely for drugs. Therefore, we do not have to address here many of the limitations of the controlled clinical trial that emerge for studying various other CAM treatments (for example, acupuncture; see Chapter 3). Thus, it should be relatively straightforward to design appropriation experiments, right? Read on.

These herbs are presently regulated as dietary supplements in the United States. Well-publicized, controversial studies of each of these herbs have been conducted that illustrate some of the challenges faced in conducting contemporary research on historically established herbal remedies.

Ginkgo biloba is a well-established treatment for cognitive impairment and dementia. As of 25 years ago, over 40 studies had already been performed showing these benefits, which were documented in a meta-analysis, at the time new research was undertaken. Since then, there have been several clinical trials that substantiated the use of ginkgo for this purpose. Gingko has other uses as well. From year to year, it has been the most popular herbal remedy in Europe and the United States.

Although prior evidence, and responsible use of gingko, shows benefits for the treatment of cognitive impairment and dementia, a well-publicized study involving healthy volunteers *without* cognitive impairment was published in the *Journal of the American Medical Association (JAMA)* in August 2002. The 6-week psychological study predictably showed that gingko did not improve memory in elderly adults *without* cognitive impairment. The study was conducted at an undergraduate college by academic PhD psychologists and their undergraduate students—the results

did not emanate from clinical researchers at an academic medical center, and were not surprising given the existing body of clinical research on the *appropriate* use of gingko. Nonetheless, the results were treated as a major news event by the public media. Experts contended that the study, which tested one brand of gingko of unknown potency, has flaws. This "news" illustrates two major biases in such research. Credence is given to sources that would never be given a second glance if the research had been on "mainstream" medical treatments. Second, there is a much greater propensity to publish and report negative findings than positive findings on alternative remedies (see section on so-called evidence-based medicine in Chapter 3).

By the spring of 2003, this study and the publicity surrounding it were raising many questions. A high-level conference for the functional foods and dietary supplements industry, sponsored by Hoffmann-La Roche, Pfizer, and others, addressed the topic on March 6, 2003. A question was posed: the federal government is presently supporting research on dietary supplements, but what is the reward for that investment and are these studies asking the right questions about traditional herbal medicines?

As interest in research on traditional remedies grows, researchers will have access to new populations and powerful research capabilities and methodologies. Knowledge of the traditional and appropriate use of herbal remedies, and their applications in integrative medicine, is an important part of the equation.

Studies conducted on *St. John's wort* (SJW, *Hypericum perforatum*) illustrate the difficulties of studying traditional herbal remedies in new populations. St. John's wort had an established utility (over 30 studies) in the treatment of mild to moderate depression. In April 2001, Shelton et al published a study in *JAMA* entitled "Randomized Controlled Trial of St. John's Wort in Major Depression." The new study selected 200 patients with *severe* depression, whereas SJW is not recommended for treatment of severe depression, or for hospitalized patients or patients undergoing active psychiatric treatment. This study confirmed the findings of prior studies that adverse side effects of SJW were low, especially compared with those of antidepressants, but also claimed that STW was ineffective for the study population.

The Shelton article was published in April; by May physicians, researchers, and leading authorities in the psychiatric community responded. The most common theme of the rebuttals centered on the actual foundation of the study. Shelton et al were using their study to openly refute many of the earlier, landmark studies based on *mild to moderate* depression, but the Shelton study had actually enrolled only patients with *severe* depression.

Further, it was disclosed at the Annual Meeting of the American Psychiatric Association that 43 of the 200 participants of the study dropped out early; Shelton had reported only 28 drop-outs. After being called to question by his peers, Shelton disclosed (July 2001, in his response to rebuttal letters) that the drop-out rate had been adjusted to 33. How accurate was record keeping? Was it 28, 33, or 43? In addition, in his response letter, Shelton stated, "We did note the possibility of a sampling bias in our article."

Two physicians at the Council for Responsible Nutrition in Washington, D.C., found additional flaws in the Shelton et al study and went so far as to say that the authors may have acted unethically according to the World Medical Association Declaration of Helsinki by exposing 200 patients known to be suffering from severe depression both to a placebo and to an herbal extract that the researchers themselves did not believe worked even for mild forms of depression. This behavior clearly fails to comply with item 19 of the Helsinki Declaration, which states, "Medical research is only justified if there is a reasonable likelihood that the populations in which the research is carried out stand to benefit from the results of the research."

As evidenced by Shelton's clear and express repudiation of preceding studies on the effects of SJW, he clearly held no belief that there was a reasonable likelihood that the study group would benefit in any way from the study. Yet he subjected these patients to the study.

In addition to the ethics issue, two physicians in the Department of Epidemiology and Social Medicine at the Albert Einstein College of Medicine in New York called the authors' math into question. Although Shelton et al claimed an 80% power to detect their response rate, Dr. Cohen and Dr. Marantz stated that "Shelton and associates only had a power of 46% to find a statistically significant difference."

Another group of physicians in similar positions at leading psychiatric institutions ran Shelton's numbers and found similar discrepancies. They offered a notable suggestion that would have put Shelton et al back on the ethical side of the fence: To remove the discrepancies between placebo and St. John's wort why did they not add a third arm to their research—an antidepressant drug—to assess its effects on severe depression? At least this way, they would have been able to maintain some level of belief that the study would benefit some patients on whom they were experimenting—thus staying within the Helsinki Declaration of medical research ethics.

In summary, this study of SJW on severely depressed patients (1) ignored historic usage, and rejected a considerable prior research base; (2) used faulty statistics; (3) did not report drop-outs accurately; and (4) created ethical problems by exposing severely depressed patients to "no therapy" (placebo) or to an intervention *that the researchers did not themselves credit,* thus creating nocebo effects and significant ethical problems. What can be done? First, design appropriate research, and conduct it properly. Second, in the present case, create a conclusion that reads something like, "The efficacy of St. John's wort in patients with mild to moderate depression *was not evaluated,*" and perhaps, though the study was inappropriate for the population, add, "We confirmed that St. John's wort was not effective for treatment of major depression."

Writing about this study in *Advances in Therapy* in February 2002, Behnke et al noted that the *JAMA* study selected patients from psychiatric institutions who had suffered from major depression for more than 10 years and whose current depressive disorder had lasted for 2.5 years before they entered the study, and that the severity of disease and the study population were not appropriately selected for the SJW treatment. Behnke et al also showed SJW to be 80% as effective as drug therapy for mild to moderate depression, and to be safe.

Another study reported in *JAMA* in April 2002 found that neither SJW *nor* drug therapy produced effects that were significantly different from those for the placebo control—in other words, "no healing effect." This study enrolled patients with "moderately severe major depression." The dosages of both SJW and the drug varied for different patients. The authors' review identified several studies performed before 1996 that reported positive effects for SJW. They also cited five studies that showed SJW treatment to be comparable to drug therapy and four studies showing SJW to be superior to placebo conducted since 1996. The historically established use for SJW has been in the management of mild to moderate depression, not of severe depression, the treatment of which is likely to be in the hands of psychotherapists and psychiatrists. What was most interesting about this study is that that all study participants also received an average of 15 hours of intensive talk therapy with a highly skilled mental health professional. What the study really underlines is that neither a drug nor an herb is more effective than actually talking with a patient suffering from depression.

Kava kava (Piper methysticum) is well accepted under historical use for its actions as a muscle relaxant and sleep inducer (see Chapter 40). However, among anecdotal experiences of approximately 70 million users, kava kava was claimed, in an internal EU report titled "In-depth Investigation into [European Union] Members States Market Restrictions on Kava Products," to cause rare liver toxicity. Liver toxicity is not uncommon with many prescription and over-the-counter drugs, and there are hundreds of deaths due to liver failure each year form the routine use of over-the-counter acetaminophen, for example (see Chapter 3). Joerg Gruenwald, MD, demonstrated that the assignment of liver toxicity to the use of kava kava in the cases cited by the European Union study was highly questionable. This analysis led to the issue of whether kava kava, which is an effective treatment for anxiety, should be banned or whether, instead, a responsible approach to risk–benefit should be developed as with many other treatments potentially manifesting side effects. The case by case analysis by Gruenwald and colleagues at the Phytopharm Consulting Group in Berlin, Germany, found several alternative explanations for liver toxicity in those taking kava kava. Nonetheless, many retailers had voluntarily taken kava kava off the shelves in response to these claims. This result demonstrates the loss to the public of a potentially

Common Herbs in Integrative Medicine

Herb	Common Uses (Box A24-1)*	Activity
Aloe (*Aloe vera, Aloe barbadensis*)	**Burns and wound healing** **Constipation** Gastritis Ulcers Psoriasis	Antiinflammatory Antiseptic
Bilberry (*Vaccinium myrtillus*)	**Eye disorder** **Antidiarrheal** Circulatory disorders Diabetes	Antioxidant Collagen stabilizer Vasoprotective Astringent ↓ Platelet aggregation
Black cohosh (*Cimicifuga racemosa*)	**Menopause symptoms** **Menstrual problems** Rattlesnake bites	Probable SSRI-like effects Possible estrogenic activity Possible luteinizing hormone suppression
Cat's claw (*Uncaria tomentosa*)	**Arthritis** Cancer HIV Diverticulitis Herpes simplex and zoster	Immune stimulant Antiinflammatory Antimutagenic
Cayenne (*Capsicum annum*)	**Arthritis** **Muscle pain** **Neuralgia** Postmastectomy pain Psoriasis Diabetes Antiflatulent Diarrhea	Blocks substance P (pain peptide) ↓ Lipids ↓ Platelet aggregation
Chamomile (*Matricaria recutita,* *Matricaria chamomilla*)	**GI complaints** **Skin and mucous membrane problems** **Stress and anxiety** Wound healing	Antispasmodic effect Sedative effect Antiinflammatory Carminative
Chaste tree (*Vitex agnus-castus*)	**Menstrual problems** **Hyperprolactinemia** Acne Infertility	Hormonal modulator
Cranberry (*Vaccinium macrocarpon*)	**Urinary tract infections**	↓ Bacterial adherence to bladder endothelium
Dong quai (*Angelica sinensis*)	**Dysmenorrhea** **Other menstrual disorders** Menopause symptoms Allergies	Phytoestrogen Antimicrobial effects Smooth muscle relaxant IgE inhibition
Echinacea (*Echinacea* spp)	**Colds and flu** **Immunity** **Upper respiratory infections** **Urinary tract infections** Wound healing (topical) Recurrent candidal vaginitis	Immunostimulant ↑ Macrophage phagocytosis Stimulates lymphocyte activity Antiinflammatory Antimicrobial properties
Eleuthero (*Eleutherococcus senticosus*)	**Herpes type II** Fatigue **Athletic performance** Influenza complications	↑ Lymphocyte count Tonifying Immunomodulator Adaptogen

Adverse Effects and Contraindications	Doses†	Drug Interactions‡
Dermatitis GI upset (PO) Diarrhea Avoid in children and pregnancy. Avoid latex with inflammatory intestinal disease	Liberal application of gel topically No more than 1 qt of juice per day	Cardiac glycoside containing herbs and drugs Licorice Stimulant laxatives
May alter insulin requirements	Anthocyanosides (calculated as anthocyanidin): 20–40 mg tid *V. myrtillus* (25% extract): 80–160 mg tid Fresh berries: 55–115 g tid	Warfarin (at high doses of bilberry)
GI upset ↑ BP Avoid in pregnancy and lactation. Vertigo Rash Liver disease 250–500 mg	27-Deoxyacteine: 2 mg bid Powdered rhizome: 1–2 g Tincture (1:5): 4–6 ml Fluid extract (1:1): 3–4 ml (1 tsp) Solid (dry powder) extract: (4:1):	Hepatotoxic herbs and drugs
Avoid in pregnancy and lactation, autoimmune illness, MS, TB, and leukemia (awaiting bone marrow transplant). Avoid in children <3 years old. Headaches Dizziness Vomiting	Tea (1 g/250 ml): 1 cup tid Tincture: 1–2 ml tid Standardized dry extract: 20–60 mg qd	Avoid combining with hormone drugs, insulin, vaccines, iron, NSAIDs, and salicylates. Antihypertensives Cytochrome P450 substrates Chemotherapy Hyperimmune globulin IV thymic preparations
Eye irritation Burning, local and mucous membranes Gastritis Diarrhea (with internal use) Avoid in children <2 years old	Cream (0.025% or 0.075% capsaicin) topically qid	Warfarin: ↓ platelet aggregation with internal use MAOIs ACE inhibitors Aspirin Cocaine Antacids H₂ blockers Theophylline
Avoid if allergy to member of daisy family (Asteraceae; e.g., ragweed, asters, chrysanthemums). Contact dermatitis Urticaria Rash Headache GI upset Avoid in pregnancy and lactation Diarrhea May increase risk of kidney stones	Tea: 3–4 cups per day Capsules: 300–500 mg tid-qid Tincture: 4–6 ml tid Apply topically to affected area Solution (9 g in 100 ml): 40 gtts qam Dried extract: 4.2 mg qd Must take consistently for several months to see effect Prophylaxis: 90 ml qd Treatment: 360–960 ml qd Tincture 0.5–1 tsp tid	Caution if using with tranquilizers or CNS depressants (?) Warfarin Chemotherapy Cytochrome P450 substrates Metoclopramide (Reglan) Contraceptive agents Avoid with dopamine agonists Lansoprazole, omeprazole Warfarin Cytochrome P450 substrates
Photodermatitis Uterine stimulant Carcinogenic constituents Hypersensitivity Excess bleeding and fever Avoid with hormone-sensitive tumors	Dried root or rhizome: 1–2 g PO or IV tid Tincture (1:5): 3–5 ml tid Fluid extract (1:1): 0.5–2 ml tid	Warfarin Heparin Ticlopidine
Avoid in HIV/AIDS, autoimmune disease, collagen vascular disease, MS, and TB. Avoid if allergy to sunflower seeds or member of daisy family (Asteraceae) such as ragweed. (?) Avoid during pregnancy	Dried root (or as tea): 0.5–1 g Freeze-dried plant: 325–650 mg Juice of aerial portion of *E. purpurea* stabilized in 22% ethanol: 2–3 ml (0.5–0.75 tsp) Tincture (1:5): 2–4 ml (1–2 tsp) Solid (dry powdered) extract (6.5:1 or 3.5% echinacoside): 150–300 mg	Chemotherapy agents Cytochrome P450 substrates Immuno-suppressants
Diarrhea Sleep disturbance Anxiety Alters diabetes control Caution with cardiovascular disorders Avoid during antibiotic treatment of dysentery	Dried root: 2–4 g Tincture (1:5): 10–20 ml Fluid extract (1:1): 2–4 ml Solid (dry powdered) extract (20:1): 100–200 mg	Caution with antipsychotics, barbiturates, and sedatives Anticoagulants Chemotherapy agents Digoxin Hypoglycemics Kanamycin

Continued

Herb	Common Uses (Box A24-1)*	Activity
Ephedra (Ephedra sinensis, ma huang)	**Asthma** **Bronchitis** **Cough** **Decongestant** **Energy** **Weight loss** Diuretic	Sympathomimetic activating α and β_1/β_2 receptors CNS stimulant Stimulates uterine contractions
Evening primrose oil (Oenothera biennis)	**Fibrocystic breast** **Eczema** Diabetic neuropathy Psoriasis Breast pain Lactation	Source of GLA (gamma-linoleic acid)
Feverfew (Tanacetum parthenium)	**Migraine prophylaxis and treatment** Dizziness Tinnitus Dysmenorrhea	↓ Platelet aggregation Smooth muscle relaxant ↓ Prostaglandin synthesis and serotonin release from platelets and WBCs Antinociceptive Inhibits serotonin release
Flax seed (Linumus itatissimum)	**Hyperlipidemia** **Constipation** **Cardiovascular risk reduction** **Systemic lupus erythematosus** Breast cancer risk reduction Irritable bowel; inflammatory bowel disease	↓ Platelet aggregation Antiinflammatory
Garlic (Allium sativum)	**Hyperlipidemia** **Hypertension** Cancer prevention Antimicrobial Atherosclerosis	Inhibits platelet aggregation ↑ Fibrinolysis Antioxidant ↓ Systolic and diastolic blood pressure
Ginger (Zingiber officinale)	**Antiemetic** **Nausea** **Motion sickness** **Morning sickness** **Arthritis** Antiinflammatory Rheumatological	Stimulates intestinal tone and peristalsis Cholagogue Antiinflammatory Antioxidant Positive inotrope Inhibits platelet aggregation
Ginkgo biloba (Ginkgo biloba)	**Cerebrovascular insufficiency** **Peripheral vascular disease** **Vascular dementia** **Alzheimer's disease** **Memory** Vertigo Tinnitus Macular degeneration Depression PMS Diabetic neuropathy Raynaud's syndrome Retinopathy Glaucoma Sexual dysfunction associated with SSRIs	Membrane stabilizer Antiplatelet activating factor (PAF) Free radical scavenger Antioxidant ↑ Alpha brain waves ↓ Theta brain waves

Adverse Effects and Contraindications	Doses†	Drug Interactions‡

↑ BP, root
↓ BP, plant above ground
Anxiety, restlessness
Headaches
Irritability
Nausea, vomiting
Urinary obstruction with BPH
Addictive potential
Dysrhythmias
Alters diabetes control
Kidney stones
Glaucoma
Caution in heart disease, hypertension,
   diabetes, or thyroid disease
	Based on alkaloid content 1%-3%
	   12.5–25 mg bid-tid
	Crude herb 500–1000 mg tid
		Cardiac glycosides
		Halothane
		Guanethidine
		MAOIs
		Oxytocin
		Diabetic medication
		Dexamethasone
		Ergot derivatives
		Methylxanthines
		Reserpine
		Must be protected from the light

Headache
GI symptoms
Insomnia
May exacerbate temporal lobe epilepsy and
   schizophrenia
	Based on 8% GLA content 500–
	   2000 mg tid-qid
		Phenothiazines
		Tamoxifen
		Anesthetics
		Anticoagulants

Stop 2 weeks before major surgery.
Oral ulcers
GI upset
Rash
Rebound migraine
Nervousness
Avoid in pregnancy and lactation, or if allergy
   to sunflower seeds or member of daisy family
   (Asteraceae) such as ragweed.
	Depends on adequate level of
	   parthenolide (0.4%-0.66%)
	Freeze-dried, pulverized leaves:
	   25–50 mg bid
		Warfarin: ↓ platelet aggregation
		NSAIDs

Diarrhea Allergic reaction Caution with hormone-sensitive cancers Contraindicated with bowel obstruction	Capsule (1 g): 3–6 capsules qd Oil: 1–2 tbsp qd	Mucilage may affect absorption of oral drugs. Anticoagulants Antidiabetic drugs

Stop 2 weeks before major surgery
Heartburn
GI upset
Flatulence
Body/breath odor
↓ Blood glucose
	10 mg allicin or 4 g fresh garlic;
	   equivalent to 1–2 cloves/day
		May potentiate antithrombotic effect of
		   antiinflammatories, warfarin, and aspirin
		Saquinavir
		Cyclosporin
		Chlorzoxazone
		Dipyridamole
		Ticlopidine
		Cytochrome P450 substrates

Stop 2 weeks before major surgery. GI upset Caution if patient has gallstones	Dry powder ginger root: 1 g Extract (20% gingerol and shogaol): 100–200 mg tid	Warfarin: ↓ platelet aggregation Chemotherapy agents General anesthetics Heparin Antacids Antidiabetic drugs Antihypertensives Barbiturates H_2 blockers Proton pump inhibitors

Stop 2 weeks before major surgery
GI upset
Allergies (whole plant)
Spontaneous bleeding problems
Headaches
Skin rashes
Dizziness
Palpitations
Seizures
Avoid in pregnancy
	Based on standard extract 25% ginkgo
	   heterosides 40 mg tid up to 80 mg
	   bid-tid
	Use consistently for at least 12 weeks to
	   determine effectiveness
		Warfarin
		Aspirin (↓ platelet aggregation)
		MAOIs (↑ effect)
		Fluoxetin
		Glyburide
		Insulin
		Haloperidol
		Heparin
		Metformin
		Thiazide diuretics
		Ticlopidine
		Trazodone
		Buspirone
		Cytochrome P450 substrates

Continued

Common Herbs in Integrative Medicine—cont'd

Herb	Common Uses (Box A24-1)*	Activity
Ginseng *(Panax ginseng) (Ginseng radix) (Eleutherococcus senticosus)*	**Fatigue** **Weakness** **Energy** Immunity Mentation Diabetes Respiratory illnesses Libido Stress-induced GI ulcers Postoperative stress	Immune enhancement Prevention of platelet aggregation Tonic effect
Goldenseal *(Hidrastis canadensis)*	**Cold** **Immunity** Diarrhea Sore throat Ocular trachoma infections	Antimicrobial (often combined with echinacea) Immune stimulant Activates phagocytes
Grape seed extract *(Vitis vinifera)*	Atherosclerosis **Retinopathy** **Venous insufficiency** Hepatic protective Dental caries	Proanthocyanidins: powerful antioxidants Vascular renewal and stability Collagen support
Hawthorn *(Crataegus laeviagata)*	**Congestive heart failure** **Hypertension** **Angina** Cardiac function	Cardioactive glycosides Positive inotropic ACE inhibition Mild diuretic Collagen stabilizer Dilates coronary vessels ↓ Peripheral resistance ↓ Oxygen consumption
Horse chestnut *(Aesculus hippocastanum)*	**Venous insufficiency** **Varicose veins** **Nocturnal leg cramps** **Pruritus and swelling of legs** Topically for hemorrhoids, skin ulcers, varicose veins, sport injuries, trauma	Aescin component reduces lysosomal activity, improves venous tone, and inhibits capillary protein permeability. Diuretic
Kava *(Piper methysticum)*	Anxiety **Restlessness** **Insomnia** Anticonvulsant Oral anesthetic Depression Attention-deficit hyperactivity disorder	GABA receptor–like actions Limbic system modulation Inhibits voltage-dependent sodium channels in brain Skeletal muscle relaxant
Licorice *(Glycyrrhiza* spp)	Upper respiratory infection Oral and gastric ulcers Infection	Antiinflammatory Expectorant Antioxidant Demulcent Adrenocorticotropin

Adverse Effects and Contraindications	Doses†	Drug Interactions‡
Stop 2 weeks before major surgery. Agitation Insomnia (PM doses) BP Edema Hypertonia Caution with cardiac problems, diabetes, psychosis, and agitation	Based on ginsenoside content 4.5-6 g daily Root powder (5% ginsenoside): 100 mg qd-tid May use cyclically for 15-20 days, followed by 2-week interval without ginseng	Warfarin (↓ platelet aggregation) Corticosteroids (↑ side effects) Digoxin (↑ serum levels) MAOIs, hypoglycemics (↑ effects) Opioids, diuretics (↓ effect) Stimulants Antidiabetic drugs
Avoid in pregnancy, lactation, and diabetes (may lower glucose) Mouth irritation Digestive disorders Avoid in infants	Dried root or as infusion (tea): 2-4 g Tincture (1:5): 6-12 ml (1.5-3 tsp) Fluid extract (1:1): 2-4 ml (0.5-1 tsp) Solid (powdered dry) extract (4:1 or 8%-12% alkaloid content): 250-500 mg	Antihypertensives Cytochrome P450 substrates Antacids CNS depressants Heparin H_2 blockers Proton pump inhibitors
None known	25-250 mg bid	Tetracycline, doxycycline Warfarin
Hypotension GI distress Rash Arrhythmia Avoid in pregnancy	Berries or flowers (dried): 3-5 g or as infusion Tincture (1:5): 4-5 ml (alcohol may elicit pressor response in some individuals) Fluid extract (1:1): 1-2 ml Freeze-dried berries: 1-1.5 g Flower extract (standardized to contain 1.8% vitexin-4)	May potentiate effects of digitalis drugs Calcium channel blockers CNS depressants Nitrates
GI irritation ↓ gastric emptying Pruritus Nausea Standardized seed extracts are safe, but whole herb may be fatal. Avoid in pregnancy and lactation, liver disease, renal disease. May cross-react with latex allergy	Based on aescin 90-150 mg initially, followed by 35-70 mg qd	Anticoagulants Antidiabetic drugs
Dermatitis Sedation May impair reflexes and judgment for driving Avoid in pregnancy and lactation, depression, and Parkinson's disease. Contraindicated in endogenous depression Hepatotoxicity *Note:* kava is nonaddictive.	Anxiolytic dose: 45-70 mg kavalactones tid Sedative dose: 180-210 mg 1 hour before bedtime	Alcohol Benzodiazepines Barbiturates Anti-Parkinson's drugs Other psycho-pharmacological agents, general anesthetics Cytochrome P450 substrates
Avoid in pregnancy. Contraindicated in cholestatic liver disease, cirrhosis, hypertension, hypokalemia, and renal insufficiency	Powdered root: 1-2 g Fluid extract (1:1): 2-4 ml Solid (dry powdered) extract (4:1): 250-500 mg	Furosemide Estrogens Chorothiazide, metolazone Isoniazid Antihypertensives Insulin Risperidone Ibuprofen Digitalis glycosides Corticosteroids Cytochrome P450 substrates

Continued

Common Herbs in Integrative Medicine—cont'd

Herb	Common Uses (Box A24-1)*	Activity
Milk thistle *(Silybum marianum)*	**Cirrhosis** **Alcoholic and viral hepatitis** **Mushroom poisoning *(Amanita)*** **Other hepatotoxins**	Cell membrane stabilizer Stimulates ribosomal protein synthesis Free radical scavenger Antioxidant Contraindicated in liver disease Inhibits leukotriene formation Choleretic and lipotropic
Peppermint *(Mentha piperita)*	**Dyspepsia** **Irritable bowel syndrome** **Biliary dyskinesia** **Digestive aid** Myalgia Neuralgia Nasal decongestant Tension headache (topically)	Antispasmodic Cholagogue Menthol is active ingredient. Antibacterial Antiviral Stimulates gastric secretion Coolant ↓ Lower esophageal sphincter tone Carminative
Saw palmetto *(Serenoa repens)*	**Benign prostatic hyperplasia (stages I and II)** **Prostatitis**	Antiandrogenic (5α-reductase) Bladder muscle spasmolytic Antiinflammatory

St. John's wort *(Hypericum perforatum)*	**Depression: mild to moderate**
	Anxiety
	Insomnia
	Contusions
	First-degree burns
	Wound healing
	Antiinflammatory (topically)
	Myalgias
	Eczema
		Affects neurotransmitters serotonin,
		  dopamine, catecholamines, and possibly
		  MAOIs; reduction of interleukin-6
		Antiviral
		Antibacterial

Tea tree oil *(Melaleuca alternifolia)*	**Skin infections** **Acne** Mucosal and vaginal lesions Fungal infections (skin/nails)	Antibacterial Antiviral Antifungal
Valerian *(Valeriana officinalis)*	**Insomnia** **Anxiety**	GABA domain effects Improves latency and quality of sleep Improves slow-wave sleep

↑, Increased; ↓, decreased; *g,* gram(s); *GI,* gastrointestinal; *PO,* oral; *IV,* intravenous; *SSRI,* selective serotonin reuptake inhibitor; *BP,* blood pressure; *qd,* every day; *bid,* twice daily; *tid,* three times daily; *qid,* four times daily; *qam,* every morning; *HIV,* human immunodeficiency virus; *AIDS,* acquired immunodeficiency syndrome; *TB,* tuberculosis; *MS,* multiple sclerosis; *NSAIDs,* nonsteroidal antiinflammatory drugs; *MAOIs,* monoamine oxidase inhibitors; *ACE,* angiotensin-converting enzyme; *CNS,* central nervous system; *PMS,* premenstrual syndrome; *BPH,* benign prostatic hypertrophy; *IgE,* immunoglobulin E; *WBCs,* white blood cells; *GABA,* gamma-aminobutyric acid.

*The most frequent indications are shown in **boldface** type.

†Dosages vary by preparation. Consult sources listed or expert practitioner.

‡Drug-herb interactions: many interactions as cited are theoretical, based on mechanism of action, pharmacokinetics, or other preclinical data and have not been observed in patients. Although this type of data suggests caution, it may not contraindicate combined use. For in-depth detail on conteractions, consult the Natural Medicine Comprehensive Database, other sources listed, or an expert botanical medicine practitioner.

Adverse Effects and Contraindications	Doses†	Drug Interactions‡
GI upset Laxative effect Alcohol-based extracts Contraindicated in liver disease	Based on silymarin content 70–210 mg tid Silybin bound to phosphatidylcholine: 120–240 mg bid	Acetaminophen Butyrophenones Phenothiazines Indinavir Metronidazole Nitrous oxide Chemotherapy Clofibrate General anesthetics Haloperidol Cytochrome P450 substrates
Nonenteric dosage may worsen heartburn in esophageal reflux and hiatal hernia. Caution in pregnancy and in small children (choking from menthol) Allergic reactions Bradycardia Muscle tremor Dermatitis, skin rash Contraindicated in gallstones, achlorhydria, and liver damage	Infusion: 1–2 tsp dried leaves per 8 oz water Enteric-coated capsule (0.2 ml oil/capsule): 1–2 capsules tid Menthol 1.26–16% applied topically up to qid	Antacids Cisapride
GI side effects Diarrhea Avoid in pregnancy. Potential risk of aggravation of estrogen-sensitive tumors. Rule out advanced prostatic hypertrophy and prostate cancer	Crude berries: 10 g bid Liposterolic extract (standardized at 85%-95% fatty acids and sterols): 160 mg bid	Anticoagulants Contraceptives Estrogens
Avoid in pregnancy (? uterotonic). GI side effects Photodermatitis Allergy Fatigue Insomnia Headache Restlessness Avoid in bipolar disorder.	Dried flowers: 2–4 g tid Tincture (1:5): 3–6 ml tid Fluid extract (1:1): 1–2 ml tid Standardized fluid extract (0.14% hypericin: 1 mg hypericin/3 ml): 0.5–0.9 ml tid Standardized solid (dry powdered) extract (0.14% hypericin): 600 mg tid Standardized solid (dry powdered) extract (0.3% hypericin): 300 mg tid	Potential interaction with SSRIs, general anesthetics, and benzodiazepines Chemotherapy Cyclosporine Digoxin Indinavir Oral contraceptives Theophylline Trazadone *No longer contraindicated:* use with MAOIs, tyramine-containing compounds, 5-L-dopa, hydroxytryptophan
Contact dermatitis Allergic reaction Orally may cause significant toxicity; confusion and ataxia	Apply topically to affected area	None known
Overdose with temporary GI, chest, and CNS symptoms (?) Use in pregnancy and lactation Caution in children <12 years old Odor Cardiac disturbances *Note:* Valerian is not habit-forming.	Dried root (or as tea): 1–2 g Tincture (1:5): 4–6 ml (1–1.5 tsp) Fluid extract (1:1): 1–2 ml (0.5–1 tsp) Solid (dry powdered) extract (4:1): 250–500 mg Valerian extract (1%-1.5% valtrate or 0.5% valerenic acid): 150–300 mg	Avoid with benzodiazepines, barbiturates, general anesthetics, and alcohol. Cytochrome P450 substrates

BOX A24-1 *Common Uses for Top 20 Herbs*

1. Aloe: skin, gastritis
2. Black cohosh: menstrual symptoms, menopause
3. Dong quai: menstrual symptoms, menopause
4. Echinacea: colds, immunity
5. Ephedra: asthma, energy, weight loss (ma huang)
6. Evening primrose oil: eczema, psoriasis, premenstrual syndrome, breast pain
7. Feverfew: migraine
8. Garlic: cholesterol, hypertension
9. Ginger: nausea, arthritis
10. Ginkgo biloba: cerebrovascular insufficiency, memory
11. Ginseng: energy, immunity, mentation, libido
12. Goldenseal: immunity, colds
13. Hawthorn: cardiac function
14. Kava kava: anxiety
15. Milk thistle: liver disease
16. Peppermint: dyspepsia, irritable bowel syndrome
17. Saw palmetto: prostate problems
18. St. John's wort: depression, anxiety, insomnia
19. Tea tree oil: skin infections
20. Valerian: anxiety, insomnia

valuable, inexpensive product for reasons that are not scientifically sound.

Ephedra (*Ephedra sinensis*) has been used historically in the treatment of asthma and other breathing difficulties. More recently, millions began using it for weight loss, and it was also inappropriately used as a performance enhancer—in the latter case leading it to be listed on a number of autopsy reports as contributing to fatalities among otherwise healthy individuals.

Integrative medical research is problematic in many ways and is not likely to be able to supplant knowledge of historical use, which is an appropriate foundation for the practice of CAM as long recognized in Europe. The prospect of integrating herbal medicine into clinical practice has nothing to fear from good, properly conducted research. The challenge going forward is to avoid the kind of missteps and media misrepresentations seen in these studies of gingko biloba, St. John's wort, kava kava, and ephedra. Other questions about these herbs and others are addressed in Chapter 3.

Suggested Readings

Hypericum Depression Trial Study Group: Effect of Hypericum perforatum (St John's wort) in major depressive disorder: a randomized controlled trial. *JAMA* 287(14):1807, 2002. http://www.ncbi.nlm.nih.gov/pubmed/?term=JAMA+apr+2002+wort

Zhou L, Maviglia SM, Mahoney LM, et al: Supratherapeutic dosing of acetaminophen among hospitalized patients, *Arch Intern Med* 172(22):1721–1728, 2012.

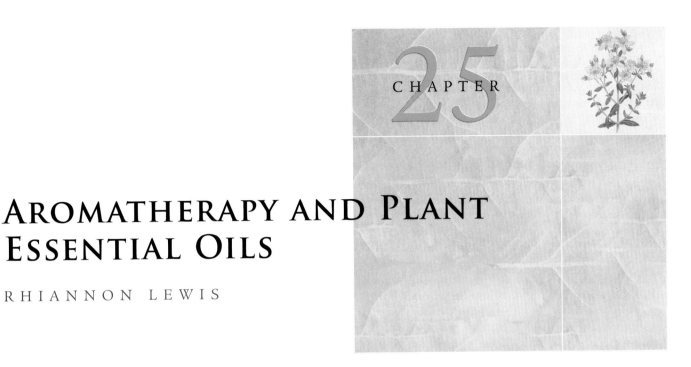

AROMATHERAPY AND PLANT ESSENTIAL OILS

R H I A N N O N   L E W I S

The versatile nature of essential oils leads to a wide range of potential uses, and their therapeutic value is being harnessed, evaluated, and appreciated in a number of health care settings worldwide. This chapter explores the use of essential oils and aromatherapy with particular reference to clinical relevance. By the end of the chapter, the reader will have a global overview of the potential of essential oils as therapeutic agents as well as an appreciation of the particular benefits and challenges of using these powerful substances in health environments.

Modern-day aromatherapy has origins spanning sacred and ritual use, perfumery, aesthetics, and medical applications, and these aspects continue to be relevant today when considering the psychophysiological benefits that essential oils bring to the therapeutic encounter. For a historical overview of the therapy, the reader can refer to specialist aromatherapy texts and articles that include accounts of the history and development of modern British aromatherapy by Bensouilah (2005) and Harris (2003) and the development of aromatherapy in the United States by Buckle (2003a, 2003b). This chapter focuses on the current situation and future potential of this versatile therapy.

THEORETICAL FOUNDATIONS

Aromatherapy may be defined as the selected use of essential oils and related products of plant origin with the general goal of improving health and well-being. The word *aromatherapie* was first used in 1937 by the French perfumer and chemist René Maurice Gattefossé (1881-1950), who, along with pioneers Jean Valnet (1920-1995) and Marguerite Maury (1895-1968), is largely credited with the modern revival of interest in the use of essential oils for therapeutic purposes.

In modern-day aromatherapy, the therapist uses these fragrant and active substances to affect the body-mind via a number of administration methods (external, inhalational, internal), usually in dilution and with a focus on a holistic approach to health in cooperation with the patient or client. The concept of the "individual prescription," as stressed by Maury in her seminal work *Secret of Life and Youth: Regeneration Through Essential Oils—A Modern Alchemy* (1964) (originally published in 1961 in French as *La capitale jeunesse*), remains key in contemporary aromatherapy practice.

Essential oils are the main active tools of aromatherapy. These highly concentrated and fragrant substances of plant origin have a complex chemical composition, the totality of which determines the essential oil's aroma and therapeutic potential. The concept of the "whole oil"—as opposed to one that has been rectified, concentrated by deterpenation, or otherwise chemically altered—is fundamental to most aromatherapists, who believe that there is an inherent synergy between the chemical components that needs to be preserved as much as possible. This concept does have some weight behind it, at least in terms of antimicrobial and anti-inflammatory effects, because a number of studies have demonstrated synergy between main active components and minor, less active components in an individual essential oil (Harris, 2002), similar to the observed synergic effects of herbal remedies taken internally.

Essential oils themselves are clearly defined by the industry that uses them. The International Organization for Standardization (ISO) defines them as follows:

Products obtained from natural raw materials by distillation with water or steam or from the epicarp of citrus fruits by a mechanical process or by dry distillation. The essential oil is subsequently separated from the aqueous phase by physical means.

This criterion sets essential oils apart from other plant extracts, such as those produced with solvents (e.g., hexane or supercritical fluid extraction), which can have quite different chemical compositions and organoleptic properties (Kotnik et al, 2007; Pourmortazavi & Hajimirsadeghi, 2007). These differences mean that the therapeutic effects of these two types of extracts cannot always be compared. Newer advanced technology, however, such as microwave hydrodiffusion with gravity, offers the potential for new extraction methods that yield products of composition similar to that obtained with distillation (Vian et al, 2008), while economizing on time and energy for extraction.

Although aromatherapists use predominantly essential oils as defined earlier, they may also use aromatic extracts (e.g., absolutes, resinoids, carbon dioxide extracts), because these products often have a fragrance that is very close to that of the original plant. These extracts are thus frequently used more to confer fragrance benefits than to produce specific physiological or pharmacological benefits.

Other related natural products at the aromatherapist's disposal include the following:

- Hydrolats (also known as hydrosols), fragrant waters that are the second product of distillation and are used predominantly for their therapeutic benefits in topical preparations.
- Fixed vegetable oils of varying origin and fatty acid composition chosen for their benefits for skin applications or simply as fatty vehicles for essential oil dilution and administration.
- Macerated or infused oils such as arnica, calendula, or St. John's wort incorporated into blends as active bases to complement essential oil efficacy.
- Creams, lotions, gels, and other bases, which are also used as required.

EVOLVING THERAPY

Over the past 25 years, as the use of essential oils has grown in popularity and potential, their versatility has led to different styles of aromatherapy, the main ones of which are shown in Figure 25-1. As can be seen, the aromatic medicine style is usually considered to be a branch of herbal medicine rather than purely associated with aromatherapy as it is most commonly perceived.

HOLISTIC AROMATHERAPY

Holistic aromatherapy usually combines essential oils with body massage (see Chapters 16 and 17), and this application remains the main form of aromatherapy as taught and practiced worldwide, with at least 6000 aromatherapists practicing in the United Kingdom alone (Walker & Budd, 2002). Characteristics of this form of aromatherapy include the following:

- Low doses (0.5% to 2.5%) of essential oils are blended into lipophilic bases such as vegetable oil or lotion and applied to the body with massage.
- The concept of the "individual prescription" with client participation in essential oil selection is regarded as an important part of the therapy process.
- Essential oils are usually blended together (between two and four essential oils), and the fragrance of the overall combination is a main consideration.
- More than one aromatherapy session is usually necessary, with between four and six sessions being the norm.
- A holistic approach is taken with thorough consultation and focus on balance to the body–mind.
- Self-care and home use of essential oils between therapy sessions is usually actively promoted.
- The main risks to the client relate to the methods of administration used; thus dermatitis (irritant, photocontact, or allergic) along with mucous membrane irritation are the key hazards.

The Holistic Aromatherapist

A profile of the average aromatherapist was compiled from a U.K.-based survey conducted by Osborn et al (2001). Obviously these trends are not necessarily representative of all countries where aromatherapy is practiced, but in the author's opinion they do reflect an international profile of holistic-style aromatherapists. Key profile points include the following:

- Most holistic aromatherapists are women.
- Most are middle aged.
- Most are from the middle to upper income bracket.
- Most also practice other complementary therapies, including reflexology, massage, Indian head massage, and energy therapies such as reiki.
- Most are in private practice, although aromatherapy might not be their main source of income.
- Most are working from home or providing domiciliary visits.
- Many also volunteer their aromatherapy services in the community (in rehabilitation centers, hospice settings, residential facilities).
- They liaise with and actively refer to other health care professionals.

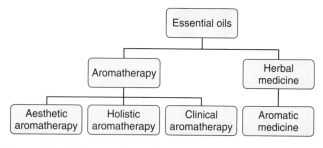

Figure 25-1 Different styles of aromatherapy.

MEDICAL AROMATHERAPY (AROMATIC MEDICINE)

As can be seen in Figure 25-1, aromatic medicine, or medical aromatherapy, has its origins in phytotherapy and largely arises, is taught, and is practiced in European countries such as Germany and France, where only licensed medical professionals are legally sanctioned to practice. This more intensive and often internal use of essential oils is being increasingly taught and practiced in other countries, such as the United Kingdom, where there may be greater freedom to practice by nonlicensed medical professionals such as herbalists, traditional Chinese medicine practitioners, and practitioners of aromatic medicine (usually qualified aromatherapists who have pursued supplementary training in this discipline). This style of aromatherapy is characterized by the following:

- Essential oils are prescribed to treat a range of predominantly physical disorders (e.g., infection, pain, inflammation, specific pathologies).
- Administration methods include topical, oral, sublingual, rectal, vaginal, and inhalational.
- Dosages vary widely according to requirements but are generally higher or more intensive than those employed in holistic aromatherapy.
- Essential oils and other active agents such as herbal tinctures might be used in combination, and they are usually administered by the patient himself or herself rather than by the practitioner.
- It is usually the pharmacological activity of the essential oils that determines their selection rather than aroma or psychophysiological effects.
- The overall formulation takes into account the chemistry of each active ingredient along with the pathologies concerned as the main considerations.
- Selection of essential oils is usually made by the practitioner with little patient participation.
- Risks to the client are mainly related to the administration methods employed, and thus dermatitis, mucous membrane irritation, and toxicity and drug–essential oil interactions are all possible.

The Medical Aromatherapist

A profile of the medical aromatherapist has not yet been determined, but because of the more allopathic approach, trends resemble those among orthodox practitioners, especially in terms of gender. Having worked closely with medical aromatherapists over a number of years, the author has the following observations.

- There is a larger representation of male practitioners than among holistic aromatherapists.
- Practitioners combine essential oil prescriptions with other orthodox care methods for diagnosis and treatment.
- They are more likely to combine prescriptions with alternative forms of medicine such as homeopathy, acupuncture, and herbal medicine.

- They are more likely to be in private practice than employed in a national health service.
- They are less likely to practice other therapies that involve direct care delivery such as massage.

CLINICAL AROMATHERAPY

When essential oils are integrated into medical environments to address particular patient challenges alongside mainstream care, the practice is often termed *clinical aromatherapy*. It effectively represents a merging of both holistic and medical styles that are adapted to individual needs. Although most interventions in medical environments still tend toward use of the lower-dose and external and inhalational methods, as in holistic aromatherapy, there is an increasing trend toward and acceptance of using more intensive interventions where necessary for particular clinical challenges, such as pain management, malodor control, wound care, oral care, and treatment of infection. This style of aromatherapy is characterized by the following:

- A holistic approach, especially with regard to well-being and anxiety reduction, remains a key feature of the clinical aromatherapist's role.
- Interventions are often brief and specifically focused (e.g., anxiety management, relief of nausea, oral care, wound care, pain relief).
- Most interventions involve topical (including buccal) application or inhalation. Ingestion or rectal administration is less frequent.
- Clinical aromatherapy is usually delivered by a trained practitioner as part of regular health care provision.
- Involvement of the caregiver or the patient's immediate family is often a key element in care provision.
- There is active liaison with other health professionals with the therapist often being part of the multidisciplinary care team.

The Clinical Aromatherapist

The development of essential oil use in the clinical environment was and remains largely nurse driven, although in many settings it is not a prerequisite that the practitioner be medically qualified (e.g., nurse, midwife); indeed, many aromatherapists working in hospitals and hospice settings are not nurses. They are often qualified therapists with good understanding of pathology and experience in their specialist areas. For example, before working in cancer care or hospice settings, aromatherapists often pursue supplementary training to prepare them specifically for this field that usually offers ongoing support through clinical supervision (Carter et al, 2009; Mackereth et al, 2009, 2010). A range of specialist texts and articles exist for clinical aromatherapy integration (Buckle, 2003a, 2003b; Dunning, 2007; Price et al, 2007; Smith & Kyle, 2008; Tavares, 2011; Tiran, 2000).

The clinical aromatherapist usually has undertaken training that prepares him/her to:

- Communicate effectively with other members of the health care team.

- Work confidently and safely with sick patients.
- Be familiar with research methodology.
- Be able to evaluate and measure the outcomes of his/her intervention.

As yet there has been no global survey of clinical aromatherapists, however, based on the author's experience in working and training in this style coupled with an exploratory survey of delegates at a recent U.K. conference (Carter et al, 2009), a typical profile becomes apparent:

- Most clinical aromatherapists are women.
- Many, but not all, have current or prior medical training in disciplines such as nursing, midwifery, physiotherapy, and occupational therapy.
- Many are able to use essential oils within their full or part-time employment as part of their role (e.g., nurse aromatherapists or midwife aromatherapists).
- Others are employed as aromatherapists in a specialized health sector such as midwifery, cancer care, or geriatric care.
- Many have education to a higher level (e.g., university).
- More aromatherapy research is conducted by or supported by clinical aromatherapists than by either holistic or medical aromatherapists.
- They are more likely to critically evaluate their work, conduct research, and document their findings in professional publications.

AESTHETIC AROMATHERAPY

Aesthetic aromatherapy has its origins in the Anglo-Saxon holistic style of aromatherapy in which pioneers of the art and science of aromatherapy such as Marguerite Maury and Micheline Arcier explored the cosmetic benefits of essential oils combined with the whole aromatherapy experience, including massage. Today, work in the research and development departments of many leading cosmetic companies has led to the inclusion of essential oils in cosmetic products as active agents, and research exists to confirm the role of essential oils in skin care. Because of proprietary interestes, results of cosmetic research conducted by leading companies are not widely diffused in the professional literature.

What has been published confirms the valuable role of essential oils in dermatology (Denda et al, 2000; Hosoi & Tsuchiya, 2000; Lee et al, 1999; Monges et al, 1994; Mori et al, 2002), and one specialist aromatherapy text now exists for this field (Bensouilah et al, 2006).

The surge in popularity of the health resort–spa movement has also led to aromatherapy treatments being offered for well-being and cosmetic benefit. Many therapists training for the spa setting receive rudimentary instruction in aromatherapy along with other spa techniques and often use preblended commercial products rather than providing individualized care. It is also now common for basic aromatherapy training to be included in aesthetician training programs.

Main styles of aromatherapy as detailed earlier can have significant variations and, depending on the country in

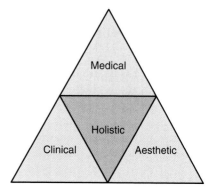

Figure 25-2 Interdependence of styles of aromatherapy.

which each method has evolved, differences in technique and application. For example, in the United Kingdom aromatherapy training and practice almost invariably includes massage. In the United States (due to massage licensing laws, which can vary among states), holistic aromatherapists often are not massage practitioners, working instead with custom blends of essential oils that are then promoted for use in self-care. In addition, the various aromatherapy styles show significant interdependence, with holistic care usually at the core of all the styles (Figure 25-2).

It is also apparent from the earlier discussion that the main styles of aromatherapy may have different training requirements; however, the reality is that, although training provision is well structured for holistic aromatherapy, with minimum standards already established in a number of countries, training in clinical and medical styles is less well recognized and standards are not consistent internationally. For example, in France, training in the medical aromatherapy style aimed at medical professionals is extremely variable in duration and content. In Australia, the establishment of national training standards and competencies for aromatic medicine as separate from aromatherapy; it is the first such move in the world, and it is anticipated that other countries will respond in a similar fashion in the future.

THERAPEUTIC POTENTIAL

There is a wealth of research to support the therapeutic value of essential oils, and in recent years this evidence has become increasingly disseminated and accessible in professional publications. The immense psychophysiological potential of essential oils is due to two or three factors.

1. Essential oils are fragrant substances. Thus they are able to impact the body–mind via the olfactory sense, with all its direct, deep-seated limbic and higher brain connections that influence, among other things, emotions, memory, desire, basic drive, and hormonal response. The olfactory neurons travel directly to the frontal portions of the brain. For these reasons, inhalation of essential oil fragrance is considered a key aspect of an aromatherapy treatment.

The capacity of fragrant substances to influence emotions and behavior has led to the field of aromachology as defined by the Sense of Smell Institute (formerly the Olfactory Research Fund; http://www.senseofsmell.org) in 1989. This field is dedicated to the study of measurable effects of the interrelationships between psychology and fragrance technology and is not restricted to essential oils and naturally derived aromatics. However, there is a significant overlap between aromachology and aromatherapy, with aromatherapists going a step further to seek physiological benefits of essential oils, either indirectly via the olfactory sense or more directly through their absorption and pharmacological activity. A recent systematic review addressing the psychophysiological effects (on mood, cognition, behavior, performance, physiology) of fragrant substances (Herz, 2009) confirms that they can significantly impact the body-mind via inhalation. Research is ongoing into how aromas can modulate mood, cognition, and behavior, with research regularly published by units such as the Brain Performance and Nutrition Research Centre at Nothumbria University, Newcastle (Moss et al, 2008, Moss et al, 2010; Neale et al, 2008).

Aromatherapists use these confirmed mood-enhancing benefits of fragrance to reduce stress and thereby improve general health and well-being. However, these effects are largely influenced by context, expectation, prior experience of the aroma, its concentration when presented, and perception of the fragrance as pleasant or unpleasant. Indeed, it may be possible that psychological effects can override the potential physiological properties of an essential oil (Moss et al, 2006; Robbins & Broughan, 2007). This may explain the inconsistencies that are sometimes found when attempts are made to measure the effects of individual essential oils on the body-mind (Neale et al, 2008). There is nevertheless supportive evidence for the positive and measurable effects of aromatherapy in relieving stress and anxiety and promoting well-being over a range of administration methods and evaluation tools (Atsumi & Tonosaki, 2007; Cooke & Ernst, 2000; Morris, 2008; Saeki, 2000).

2. Essential oils are pharmacologically active. Their chemical components are secondary metabolites produced by the plant predominantly for defensive purposes, and they are thus biologically active substances. Because of their lipophilic nature and small molecular size, many components of essential oils are able to penetrate the body irrespective of their route of administration and exert a pharmacological impact either locally (in the tissues surrounding their application site) or systemically (via the bloodstream). For these reasons, essential oils are often administered via different routes according to the needs of the individual.

The capacity of essential oil components to enter the bloodstream via different routes has been studied, at least for inhalation (Buchbauer et al, 1991; Jager et al, 1996; Stimpfl et al, 1995) and topical administration (Fewell et al, 2007; Fuchs et al, 1997; Jager et al, 1992), and pharmacological effects are confirmed via ingestion for a range of pathologies (Goerg & Spilker, 2003; Juergens et al, 2003;

Kehrl et al, 2004; Uehleke et al, 2012; Woelk & Schläfke, 2010) Because of the increased physical and metabolic barriers at the skin interface (stratum corneum, especially) compared with other routes of administration, this route is likely to result in extremely low (but non-negligible) amounts of active components' reaching the bloodstream.

Assuming therefore that some essential oil components are able to enter the tissues locally and/or enter the bloodstream, there are a number of pharmacological possibilities. The main actions are listed in Table 25-1.

TABLE 25-1 *Main Pharmacological Actions of Essential Oils*

Action	Research studies (not exhaustive)
Analgesic	Yip & Tam, 2008 (ginger and orange)
	Le Faou et al, 2005
	Greenway et al, 2003 (geranium)
Antibacterial	Cermelli et al, 2008
	Enshaieh et al, 2007
	Dryden et al, 2004
Antifungal	Soković et al, 2008
	Khosravi et al, 2008
	Jirovetz et al, 2007
Anti-inflammatory	Chao et al, 2008 (cinnamaldehyde)
	Lee et al, 2007
	Ghazanfari et al, 2006
Antioxidant	Singh et al, 2008
	Chung et al, 2007
	Zhang et al, 2006
Antiparasitic	Navarro et al, 2008
	Scanni et al, 2006
	Oladimeji et al, 2005
Antispasmodic	Goornemann et al, 2008
	Grigoleit et al, 2005
	Jahromi et al, 2003
Antiviral	Schnitzler et al, 2008
	Schnitzler et al, 2007
	Giraud-Robert, 2005
Carminative	Alexandrovich et al, 2003
	Goerg et al, 2003
Cicatrisant	Amanlou et al, 2007
	Orafidiya et al, 2005
	Orafidiya et al, 2003
Deodorizing	Warnke et al, 2006
	Mercier et al, 2005
	Sherry et al, 2003
Immune stimulating	Nam et al, 2008
	Serafino et al, 2008
	Mikhaeil et al, 2003
Mucolytic and expectorant	Fenu et al, 2008
	Kehrl et al, 2004
	Mattys et al, 2000
Rubefacient	Xu et al, 2006
	Hong et al, 1991
	Green et al, 1989
Sedative	Moss et al, 2006
	Lim et al, 2005
	Koo et al, 2003

In addition to the aforementioned fragrance and pharmacological factors, many aromatherapists would add the following third dimension to essential oil therapeutics.

3. *Essential oils are able to impact the individual at a subtle or vibrational level.* Many therapists refer to essential oils as the "life force" of the plant and believe that their vibrational energetic qualities are able to influence the individual on a subtle level. Thus practices that include different forms of energy medicine such as traditional Chinese and Ayurvedic medicines may use essential oils as part of their therapy and select these remedies according to energetic principles. A number of aromatherapy texts support these energetic approaches (Holmes, 2007, 2008; Miller & Miller, 1995; Mojay, 1996). Although it is as yet hard to find credible and reproducible evidence for the energetic-vibrational impact of essential oils, as has been previously seen, the impact of fragrance on the body–mind as well as the pharmacological activity of essential oils has been well studied. The vibrational energies of different flowering plants have been developed to offer their own forms of therapy, as with the Bach flower remedies, for example.

EVALUATION

The effectiveness of aromatherapy as assessed and reported in the literature is highly variable, ranging from single case study reports and evidence-based articles in professional publications to surveys of service provision, audits, and full-scale clinical trials. A review of the literature demonstrates that the last 20 years have witnessed an increase in both the number and quality of documented benefits of aromatherapy integration into the clinical environment. The challenge always remains of how to evaluate successfully the benefits of what is in fact a multifaceted therapy that typically combines fragrance (aroma) with touch (typically with massage), potential pharmacological activity (chemical components), individualized care, and positive client–therapist interaction. For these reasons it is not surprising that some still question the validity of many aromatherapy interventions (e.g., Cooke & Ernst, 2000; Lee et al, 2012). Wherever possible, this chapter reports on recent work and research and focuses mainly on human studies.

CLINICAL APPLICATIONS

Aromatherapy is increasingly integrated into a wide range of health care settings. These are summarized (not in order of prevalence) in Box 25-1.

To provide concrete examples of where and how aromatherapy is increasingly integrated, the following sections outline five of these clinical areas in more detail:

- Midwifery
- Cancer and palliative care
- Elder care
- Special needs
- Psychiatry

BOX 25-1 *Examples of Health Care Areas into Which Aromatherapy Is Being Integrated*

Cancer care	Postoperative care
Critical care	Preprocedural care
Drug rehabilitation	Prison and young
Elder care	offender units
HIV/AIDS care	Psychiatry
Midwifery	Rheumatology
Neurology	Special needs
Pain management	Sports rehabilitation
Palliative care	Therapy for staff and
Pediatrics	caregivers
Pneumology/ears,	Wound care
nose, and throat	

AIDS, Acquired immunodeficiency syndrome; *HIV,* human immunodeficiency virus.

MIDWIFERY

The holistic and clinical styles of aromatherapy have been used in pregnancy care and midwifery for many years, assisting the expectant mother predominantly in stress and anxiety management but also providing relief with common pregnancy-associated symptoms such as nausea, skin changes, altered sleep patterns, pain, and fatigue. In the labor environment, essential oils are most often administered by midwife aromatherapists, whereas preconception, antenatal, and postnatal aromatherapy care is often provided by nonmidwife aromatherapists and traditional birth attendants, or *doulas.*

The accidental or deliberate misuse of essential oils can pose a risk to the unborn child (Anderson et al, 1996; Weiss, 1973); however, so far no reports have been published of pregnancy-related risk when the holistic style of aromatherapy is used, although some have labelled aromatherapy provision by nonmidwives as "an accident waiting to happen" (Tiran, 1996). This issue of safety is a hotly debated topic in the midwifery field, and opinions differ as to what dosages should be employed and which essential oils are safe or hazardous in pregnancy. These discrepancies are due to lack of reporting of adverse effects, and thus risk assessment is based on prediction, speculation, and each practitioner's individual experience in this field. A few essential oil components such as sabinyl acetate have been confirmed as potentially hazardous to fetal development in animal studies (Pages et al, 1996); however, these components are not found in the essential oils commonly used in holistic aromatherapy.

Providing stress reduction during labor has multiple benefits for both mother and baby. These include less need for mechanical intervention and opioid analgesia, reduced use of epidural anesthesia, improved mobility during labor, and generally increased control over the labor process, all of which may contribute to a safer birthing process and a more alert baby (Bastard & Tiran, 2006;

Burns, 2005; Burns et al, 2000, 2007; Fanner, 2005; Simkin & Bolding, 2007).

In the postnatal period, benefits can also be seen, including improved psychological status, improved bonding, and increased coping skills (Antoniak, 2008; Imura et al, 2006; Meyer, 2005; Conrad & Adams, 2012).

CANCER AND PALLIATIVE CARE

Along with the favorable effects of aromatherapy in midwifery, its benefits in oncology and palliative care environments are increasingly well surveyed, documented, and researched. Aromatherapy and massage are the most popular complementary therapies for persons with cancer in the United Kingdom. A recent survey (Egan et al, 2012) reported the use of complementary therapies in cancer care within the U.K.'s National Health Service, based on an Internet search conducted in 2009. A total of 142 units were identified across England, Wales, Scotland, and Northern Ireland, providing 62 different therapies. Aromatherapy and reflexology were offered in approximately 60% of all settings.

The predominant style used in cancer and palliative care settings is holistic aromatherapy coupled with massage or light touch techniques, and the focus is mostly on anxiety reduction and promotion of well-being (Abel, 2000; Cawthorne & Carter, 2000; De Valois & Clarke, 2001; Dyer, 2004; Imanishi et al, 2009; Peace et al, 2002; Stringer, 2000; Wilkinson et al, 1999). With regard to improvement in well-being and reduction of anxiety and fatigue, research shows that aromatherapy can offer significant benefit, at least in the short term, to persons with cancer and to their families and/or caregivers (Curry et al, 2008; Wilkinson et al, 2007). A recent systematic review of complementary therapies for supportive and palliative care (Ernst, 2009) lends further weight to the role of aromatherapy and massage for improving well-being along with other therapies including such as music therapy, acupuncture, hypnotherapy and some herbal extracts for controlling symptoms. In some countries (e.g., the United Kingdom), clear guidelines have been established for the use of complementary therapies like aromatherapy in palliative care (Tavares, 2003) and a specialist text on integrating clinical aromatherapy in specialist palliative care has begun informing practice (Tavares, 2011).

A more recent development in oncology and palliative care is the increasing use of non–massage-associated clinical aromatherapy interventions with positive results for challenges such as nausea, fatigue, malodor, breathlessness, pain relief, wound management, skin care, and oral care (Dyer et al, 2008; Dyer et al, 2010; Hackman et al, 2012; Knevitt, 2004; Kohara et al, 2004; Louis & Kowalski, 2002; Maddocks-Jennings, 2007; Maddocks-Jennings et al, 2009; Mercier & Knevitt, 2005; Schwan, 2004; Stringer & Donald, 2010; Warnke et al, 2006), as well as specific aromatherapy massage interventions for challenges like constipation (Lai et al, 2011). These clinical interventions include the use of essential oils in the following:

- Foot baths
- Inhaler devices
- Nasal gels
- Airborne diffusers
- Airborne spritzers
- Topical preparations
- Wound dressings
- Mouth rinses

ELDER CARE

Aromatherapy is a well-established treatment in elder care in various countries, particularly in residential care environments. Nursing home physicians are generally in favor of using nonpharmacological interventions for management of behavioral disturbances associated with dementia, but their level of knowledge is variable; this may restrict patient access to therapies such as aromatherapy (Cohen-Mansfield & Jensen, 2008).

Benefits have been reported in working with individuals who have dementia or Alzheimer disease, including help in reducing agitation, modifying behavior, providing stimulation and social interaction, and assisting in orientation (Ballard et al, 2002; Holmes et al, 2002; MacMahon & Kermode, 1998; Smallwood et al, 2001), although a recent Cochrane systematic review confirms that more sound research evidence is required in this area (Thorgrimsen et al, 2003). In some cases of severe dementia, aromatherapy massage interventions might actually lead to an increase in agitation (Brooker et al, 1997).

Lavandula angustifolia (lavender) essential oil is one of the most commonly used essential oils for elderly populations (Bowles et al, 2005). The benefit of its inhalation in reducing dementia-related agitation in one Chinese crossover randomized trial has been confirmed (Lin et al, 2007) as well as a recent action research project from Norway (Johannessen, 2013). Another element of importance in this field is providing aromatherapy support for caregivers of persons with dementia, who themselves are subject to significant stress and decline in health (Henry, 2008).

Other benefits of aromatherapy in these settings include malodor control and potential reduction in need for medication (Berlie, 2008) as well as improvement in sleep patterns in the older patient (Cannard, 1996). A recent study demonstrates that aromatic stimuli such as those provided by essential oils—in this case *Piper nigrum* (black pepper) and *Lavandula angustifolia* (lavender)—may improve posture and balance in older persons (Freeman et al, 2009), who are more prone to falling. Aromatic stimuli such as black pepper and menthol can assist in improving the swallowing reflex (Ebihara et al, 2006a, 2006b).

Another aspect of aromatherapy care for this age group is the management of pain (especially chronic pain). Here there is evidence that aromatherapy can offer at least short-term assistance with pain management (Bensouilah, 2004; Bowles et al, 2005; Yip & Tam, 2008).

SPECIAL NEEDS

In the field of special needs, a number of aromatherapists work independently, and to the author's knowledge, few clinical trials have been conducted in this domain. Therapists work with a range of patients with special needs, such as deaf and deaf-blind individuals (Armstrong et al, 2000), individuals with autism (Ellwood, 2008), and those with other mental health and special needs (Durell, 2002; Greenwood, 2008). Recently, therapists have begun reporting on work with individuals affected by attention-deficit hyperactivity disorder (Friedmann, 2009). To date only one specialist text exists on aromatherapy for people with learning difficulties (Sanderson et al, 1991). Case reports, articles, and therapists' experience in the special needs environment demonstrate real benefits of using essential oils, some of which are the following:

- Promoting relaxation and well-being
- Aiding communication
- Reinforcing positive acceptance of touch
- Empowering the individual
- Improving mobility and posture
- Encouraging trust and confidence
- Helping with orientation in time and space

In most cases, therapy is given coupled with massage or other touch techniques and incorporates the use of other sensory stimuli. However, one crossover study examining four interventions (Snoezelen therapy, relaxation therapy, aromatherapy hand massage, and physical activity) did not find that the aromatherapy intervention was beneficial for improving alertness in individuals with profound learning disabilities (Lindsay et al, 1997).

MENTAL HEALTH

The benefits of fragrance on mood, cognition, and behavior are well established, and aromatherapy is used widely in the care of persons with affective disorders and mental health issues. Indeed, olfactory impairment is associated with depressive behavior and occurs in the early stages of several central nervous system and neuropsychiatric diseases, such as depression, Parkinson disease, schizophrenia, Alzheimer disease, and multiple sclerosis (Atanasova et al, 2008; Moscavitch et al, 2009).

Self-care with essential oils to improve mood and well-being is common in the general population, and persons with mild to moderate depression and anxiety disorders are more likely to seek complementary therapies such as aromatherapy than are those with severe depression (Hsu et al, 2008). In addition to benefiting from simple self-care measures such as lavender baths for reducing anxiety (Morris, 2008), residents in short-term psychiatric care facilities may also profit from aromatherapy under the guidance of a qualified therapist, as reported by Kyle (2008).

Aromatherapy offers many benefits to the individual with psychiatric illness, including the following:

- Establishing a sense of normalcy
- Improving self-esteem and well-being
- Encouraging self-care
- Increasing confidence and providing choice
- Raising mood
- Increasing social interaction
- Improving sleep

In psychiatry, the main benefits of essential oils come through their inhalation via diffusion or the use of scented products applied to the skin or added to baths, with massage conferring added psychophysiological benefit. Inhalation of a pleasantly perceived fragrance has confirmed benefits in humans in reducing symptoms of depression and improving general immune function (Komori et al, 1995). When coupled with other mind–body therapies such as counselling, relaxation therapy, or hypnotherapy (see Chapter 10), a form of "odor"-conditioned response can assist the person, particularly in the realm of stress and anxiety management. This application is well illustrated in the work of Spector et al (1993) on the use of odor cues to promote relaxation in the treatment of speech anxiety and in the work of Betts (2003) on reducing the incidence of epileptiform convulsions through association of fragrance with hypnosis.

In addition to these benefits, largely associated with the effects of a pleasant fragrance, there may also be pharmacological activity, which further increases sedative, anxiolytic, and mood-enhancing effects (Buchbauer et al, 1993). The degree of sedation achieved may be on a par with that produced by benzodiazepines or other hypnotic medications and indeed may assist with withdrawal from or reduction in dependence on these drugs (Hardy et al, 1995; Komori et al, 2006). Both traditional and scientific evidence exists supporting the use of *Lavandula angustifolia* (lavender) and *Melissa officinalis* (lemon balm) essential oils to benefit individuals with anxiety, depression, and psychotic disorders (Abuhamdah & Chazot, 2008; Huang et al, 2008). Based on the results of a number of clinical trials, lavender essential oil is now available commercially in capsule form as an oral medication suitable for treatment of mild to moderate anxiety disorders with effects comparable to that of a benxodiazepine, lorazepam (Uehleke et al, 2012; Woelk & Schläfke, 2010).

It can be seen from the foregoing discussion that aromatherapy is increasingly accepted and implemented alongside mainstream medical care for patients in a diverse range of settings. Many essential oils are used in therapy worldwide. The most common are listed in Box 25-2.

Potential benefits such as lowered perception of stress by staff and caregivers comprise another important area of aromatherapy provision (Curry et al, 2008; Pemberton & Turpin, 2008; Tysoe, 2000). Because of the multifaceted nature of the therapy, it can be challenging to measure outcomes effectively, but there is now increasingly sound qualitative and quantitative evidence to encourage its continued use in specialty areas such as elder care and cancer and palliative care. It is always essential, however, to link efficacy with safety, and issues of safe practice are of paramount importance.

BOX 25-2 *Twenty-Seven Essential Oils Commonly Used in Clinical Environments (Latin Name and Common Name)*

Boswellia carterii, frankincense	*Cupressus sempervirens*, cypress	*Origanum majorana*, sweet marjoram
Cananga odorata, ylang ylang	*Cymbopogon citratus*, lemongrass	
Chamaemelum nobile, Roman chamomile	*Cymbopogon martinii*, palmarosa	*Pelargonium × asperum*, geranium
	Eucalyptus radiata, eucalyptus	*Piper nigrum*, black pepper
Citrus aurantium var. *amara flos.*, neroli	*Lavandula angustifolia*, lavender	*Rosa damascena*, rose
	Lavandula latifolia, spike lavender	*Rosmarinus officinalis*, rosemary
Citrus aurantium var. *amara fol.*, petitgrain	*Matricaria recutita*, German chamomile	*Sabinyl acetate*, juniper
		Santalum album, sandalwood
Citrus bergamia, bergamot	*Melaleuca alternifolia*, tea tree	*Vetiveria zizanioides*, vetiver
Citrus paradisii, grapefruit	*Mentha citrata*, bergamot mint	*Zingiber officinale*, ginger
Citrus sinensis, sweet orange	*Mentha × piperita*, peppermint	

SAFETY

Essential oils, as concentrated active agents, have the capacity to cause harm if not used appropriately. Because of their widespread inclusion in foods, flavorings, fragrances, and cosmetics, many have been rigorously assessed for any potential hazards, and guidelines exist for safe levels of their inclusion in these products, such as the code of practice and guidelines established by the International Fragrance Association (http://www.ifraorg.org) and the "generally recognized as safe" (GRAS) status conferred by the Flavor and Extracts Manufacturers Association (http://www.femaflavor.org). However, these limits and guidelines are not always applicable or relevant to the way that essential oils are employed in aromatherapy, and thus further safety advice for this discipline is important. The recently updated and expanded edition of *Essential Oil Safety* (Tisserand & Young, 2014) is a welcome resource for practitioners.

Given the main routes of administration of essential oils, the predominant potential hazards are dermatitic reactions (allergic, irritant, and photocontact) and mucous membrane irritation. The risk of systemic toxicity is very low unless the essential oil is consumed or used in inappropriate concentrations on the skin.

RISKS

There have been very few documented cases of client harm as a result of essential oil use when administered or recommended by aromatherapists. However, reporting of adverse effects is not well coordinated. Currently there is no effective hazard/adverse reactions reporting system in place for aromatherapy.

Accidental or deliberate misuse of essential oils in the home environment is more widely reported and often involves children, who are generally more vulnerable to adverse effects (Beccara, 1995; Darben et al, 1998; Tibballs, 1995). Consistent abuse of airborne aromatics in the home environment can also lead to airborne contact dermatitis (Schaller & Korting, 1995) as well as skin allergy (Weiss & James, 1997). Occupational exposure can also lead to contact dermatitis reactions (Ackermann et al, 2009; Wakelin et al, 1998).

Anecdotal negative reporting regarding the use of professional aromatherapy in clinical environments includes instances in which clients or care staff find some aromas too harsh or strong, provoking headaches, malaise, nausea, or coughing, although such cases are extremely rare.

It is difficult to control for adverse incidents in the use of essential oils by the general public, who have easy access to these potent substances without the necessary safety information, support, and guidance. The role of the aromatherapist as educator, as with other health professionals, is of paramount importance.

RISK TO THE THERAPIST

There is increased exposure of aromatherapists to essential oils and related products, in terms of both dose and frequency of exposure. Thus, there is more reporting of risk to the therapist than of risk to the client, especially with regard to skin reactions such as allergic contact dermatitis, although sparsely documented. There are a number of case reports of aromatherapists (usually those who have been in practice for a number of years) becoming sensitized or allergic to the products that they consistently use over time (Bleasel et al, 2002; Boonchai et al, 2007; Selvaag et al, 1995). Many of these products have similar chemical composition. Once sensitization is established the therapist often reacts to not just one but several essential oils, which in some cases necessitate a change in career.

QUALITY

It has been known for a number of years that the presence of oxidized essential oil components increases the risk of contact allergy and skin irritation (Chang et al, 1997; Christensson et al, 2008, 2009; Wakelin et al, 1998). These include the oxidation products of very common and unstable components such as d-limonene and linalool. Thus, quality control is of utmost importance in terms of sourcing and storage of essential oils. An additional challenge for the therapist is to obtain fresh and high-quality essential oils that are fully identified with regard to their species, plant part origin, and precise chemical composition.

POTENTIAL CONFLICT WITH MEDICATIONS

Few documented drug–essential oil interactions have been reported in the literature, and most pertain to the internal consumption of essential oils rather than exposure via dermal application or inhalation. This situation is in contrast to the well-documented drug–herb interactions such as those involving *Hypericum perforatum, Panax ginseng, Gingko biloba,* and other herbs (see Chapter 24). As a result of lack of reporting, much of the information on risk of interactions between drugs and essential oils is speculative, with most research coming from animal studies rather than actual reporting of interactions in humans.

Many essential oil components have been found to be inducers or inhibitors of enzyme systems such as members of the cytochrome P-450 family and glutathione *S*-transferase (Ganzera et al, 2006; Jori et al, 1969; Lam & Zheng, 1991; Parke et al, 1974). There are pharmacokinetic differences and relatively low concentrations of doses of essential oils when they are inhaled or topically applied. The likelihood of drug–essential oil interaction is greatly reduced if traditional holistic aromatherapy interventions are used (unless the drug is also administered topically or inhaled).

When essential oils are taken orally on a regular basis, however, given their concentrated nature, the risk of interaction is possibly equal to or greater than that with ingested herbal medicines. As yet there is little reporting of this risk, which may relate to the fact that only relatively recently has there been upsurge in interest and use of ingestion as a means of administering essential oils. The aromatherapy profession needs to remain vigilant in this regard, because in some countries, ingestion of essential oils by the general public without support or professional supervision is increasingly promoted by essential oil companies, along with the universal assumption that natural products are safe alternatives to medical care.

Even when essential oils are administered via inhalation, there may be possible conflicts, such as between essential oils that contain 1,8-cineole (e.g., niaouli, eucalyptus) and certain drugs like barbiturates (Jori et al, 1970). This component has been shown to induce enzyme systems and thus drug detoxification.

As with all potential drug interactions, the risk is raised when the patient is prescribed drugs that have a low therapeutic index (toxic dose is not much higher than therapeutic dose), such as warfarin, barbiturates, and digoxin. With these medications, any small shift in serum levels can have significant consequences, and thus typically aromatherapists use lower doses of oils and work only with topical and inhaled formulations for patients taking these medications. They also need to be aware of the increased risk associated with certain essential oils containing potent components such as methyl salicylate (e.g., wintergreen) and eugenol (e.g., cloves), even when applied externally,

BOX 25-3 *Individuals Most at Risk for Essential Oil Hazard*

- Elderly
- Children and babies
- Pregnant women
- Individuals with skin diseases such as eczema
- Individuals with fragrance and cosmetic allergies
- Individuals with a history of allergy (including asthma, eczema)
- Individuals taking multiple medications, especially those with a low therapeutic index such as digoxin, warfarin, barbiturates
- Individuals with unstable medical conditions
- Individuals who have a history of an unstable psychiatric condition and who are taking psychotropic medications
- Individuals with significant renal or hepatic dysfunction

because of the higher risk of bleeding if the patient is taking anticoagulant therapy or has a clotting disorder (Joss & LeBlond, 2000; Srivastava et al, 1990).

When essential oils are administered via the skin, beware of potential conflict with topical drug preparations such as corticosteroids and transdermal drug delivery systems such as nicotine patches, hormone patches, and nausea medication patches.

INDIVIDUALS AT HIGHER RISK

As can be seen, the risk of harm from essential oils when used appropriately is extremely low. Certain individuals may be more at risk than others from essential oil hazards; these groups are listed in Box 25-3. Although aromatherapy is not contraindicated for these individuals, it is common for the aromatherapist to use extra caution with essential oil selection, dose, and route of administration to minimize risk.

FUTURE POTENTIAL

As can be seen, with the increase in research and publication of studies in professional journals that demonstrate the therapeutic benefits of essential oils in clinical settings, the future looks bright for continued integration into a range of medical settings, especially as training standards improve and specialist courses are developed for certain areas such as elder care, psychiatry, oncology, palliative care, and midwifery.

A significant (as yet relatively unimplemented) aspect of essential oil therapeutics is in infection control (prevention and treatment). Because the biological evolutionary role of essential oils is to protect the plant from predation, including by microorganisms, it is not surprising that they have antimicrobial activities. There is ever-increasing evidence that essential oils can exert significant antimicrobial effects via both direct contact (Jirovetz et al, 2007; Sherry et al, 2003) and airborne contact (Inouye, 2003; Inouye et al, 2001, 2003; Krist et al, 2006; Pibiri et al, 2006; Sato et al, 2007) and that they may offer antimicrobial solutions for multidrug-resistant organisms (Caelli et al, 2000; Dryden et al, 2004; Fadli et al, 2011; Opalchenova & Obreshkova, 2003; Purkayastha et al, 2012; Yap et al, 2013).

The natural presence of essential oils protects their host plants from microbial predation, and these oils may exert these same influences in clinical settings. This activity raises real possibilities for essential oils to offer direct solutions in clinical environments that typically have a high microbial load, in which patients are more likely to be prone to nosocomial infections that are resistant to antibiotic or antifungal therapy. A recent text dedicated entirely to fighting nosocomial multidrug antibiotic resistance with the synergic effects of herbal extracts and essential oils (edited by Rai & Kon, 2013) is undoubtedly an important and welcome step forward.

PUBLIC POLICY

The continued evolution of clinical aromatherapy is not without its challenges, as with other aspects of complementary and alternative medicine (CAM) and integrative medicine (see Chapter 3). The contemporary health economic situation within Europe and North America is resulting in financial constraints. Although, in fact, CAM therapies offer cost-effective solutions to the economic crisis in health care (see Chapter 3), they are also still subjected to fierce, usually unscientific, criticism and lobbying against "non-discrimination" in health care proposals by individuals, vested interests, and organizations who are anti–complementary therapies.

These developments have been associated with a noticeable drop in the number of establishments such as universities and colleges offering quality aromatherapy education within the United Kingdom, for example, and potentially in Australia in light of a recent firestorm of attacks. To similar effect, many charities, hospitals, and hospices that had previously guaranteed and financed placements of therapists in medical settings are cutting back on services. These cutbacks have implications for training, placement, and number of therapists employed as part integrative health care.

Although these limitations are not related to science, more auditing and research is being conducted to clearly demonstrate the value of clinical aromatherapy as a cost-effective intervention that improves health status.

In a cost-driven health care system with the financial constraints that exist in medical settings, departments of finance hold the purse strings at all levels. Choosing essential oil suppliers by cost alone, the result can be the sourcing of cheaper essential oils of poorer quality for therapy. This practice can ultimately be detrimental in terms of both reduced efficacy and increased risk to the client.

In addition, with the increase in the risk of litigation, certain constraints are put on the therapy that also can limit its potential use. One example is the use of airborne diffusion for effective disinfection in clinical environments. There is clear evidence demonstrating the potential of these active agents to provide airborne disinfection, significantly reducing microbial load, including that of multiresistant strains. This application simply replicates the obvious effects of essential oils among growing plants. However, the diffusion of essential oils in public areas such as waiting rooms or hospital wards is not widely practiced for fear of complaint or adverse reactions that may result in legal claims.

One other limiting factor is the perceived rise in "multiple chemical sensitivity syndromes" and the development of "fragrance-free" environments. Because essential oils are often viewed more as fragrances than as therapeutically active substances with potential benefit, their use in some hospitals has been withdrawn based on a poor understanding of the science.

It would help to have a clearer distinction between the main aromatherapy practice styles and greater public awareness of these styles. Currently public opinion of aromatherapy remains quite general, with little expectation as to its benefits other than providing a "feel good" therapy. Although the psychological benefits of aromatherapy can be readily appreciated through the well-being aspect of this pleasurable therapy, essential oils also offer demonstrated benefit in many specific ways.

References

Abel J: Complementary therapy at St. Luke's Hospice, Plymouth, *Complement Ther Nurs Midwifery* 6:116, 2000.

Abuhamdah S, Chazot P: Lemon balm and lavender herbal essential oils: old and new ways to treat emotional disorders? *Curr Anaesth Crit Care* 19:221, 2008.

Ackermann L, Aalto-Korte K, Jolanki R, et al: Occupational allergic contact dermatitis from cinnamon including one case from airborne exposure, *Contact Dermatitis* 60:96, 2009.

Alexandrovich I, Rakovitskaya O, Kolmo E, et al: The effect of fennel (*Foeniculum vulgare*) seed oil emulsion in infantile colic: a randomised, placebo-controlled study, *Altern Ther Health Med* 9:58, 2003.

Amanlou M, Babaee N, Saheb-Jamee M, et al: Efficacy of *Satureja khuzistanica* extract and its essential oil preparations in the management of recurrent aphthous stomatitis, *Daru* 15:231, 2007.

Anderson IB, Mulen WH, Meeker JE, et al: Pennyroyal toxicity: measurement of toxic metabolite levels in two cases and review of the literature, *Ann Intern Med* 124(8):726, 1996.

Antoniak P: Essential oil therapy with a client experiencing postpartum psychosis: a case study, *Int J Clin Aromather* 5(1):8, 2008.

Armstrong F, Heidingsfield V: Aromatherapy for deaf and deafblind people living in residential accommodation, *Complement Ther Nurs Midwifery* 6:180, 2000.

Atanasova B, Graux J, El Hage W, et al: Olfaction: a potential cognitive marker of psychiatric disorders, *Neurosci Biobehav Rev* 32:1315, 2008.

Atsumi T, Tonosaki K: Smelling lavender and rosemary increases free radical scavenging activity and decreases cortisol levels in saliva, *Psychiatr Res* 150(1):89, 2007.

Ballard CG, O'Brien JT, Reichelt K, et al: Aromatherapy as a safe and effective treatment for the management of agitation in severe dementia: the results of a double-blind, placebo-controlled trial with *Melissa*, *J Clin Psychiatr* 63(7):553, 2002.

Bastard J, Tiran D: Aromatherapy and massage for antenatal anxiety: its effect on the fetus, *Complement Ther Clin Pract* 12:48, 2006.

Beccara MAD: Melaleuca oil poisoning in a 17-month-old, *Vet Hum Toxicol* 37(6):557, 1995.

Bensouilah J: Pain management in the elderly, *Int J Aromather* 1(1):33, 2004.

Bensouilah J: The history and development of modern-British aromatherapy, *Int J Aromather* 15(2):134, 2005.

Bensouilah J, Buck P: *Aromadermatology: Aromatherapy in the treatment and care of common skin conditions*, Oxford, England, 2006, Radcliffe.

Berlie L: Using essential oils in a French elderly care facility, *Int J Clin Aromather* 5(1):26, 2008.

Betts T: Use of aromatherapy (with or without hypnosis) in the treatment of intractable epilepsy—a two-year follow-up study, *Seizure* 12:534, 2003.

Bleasel N, Tate B, Rademaker M: Allergic contact dermatitis following exposure to essential oils, *Australas J Dermatol* 43:211, 2002.

Boonchai W, Iamtharachai P, Sunthonpalin P: Occupational allergic contact dermatitis from essential oils in aromatherapists, *Contact Dermatitis* 56(3):181–182, 2007.

Bowles EJ, Cheras P, Stevens J, et al: A survey of aromatherapy practices in aged care facilities in Northern NSW, Australia, *Int J Aromather* 15:42, 2005.

Brooker DJR, Snape M, Johnson E, et al: Single case evaluation of the effects of aromatherapy and massage on disturbed behaviour in severe dementia, *Br J Clin Psychol* 36:287, 1997.

Buchbauer G, Jirovetz L, Jager W, et al: Aromatherapy: evidence for sedative effects of the essential oil of lavender after inhalation, *Z Naturforsc C* 46:1067, 1991.

Buchbauer G, Jirovetz L, Jager W, et al: Fragrance compounds and essential oils with sedative effects upon inhalation, *J Pharmaceut Sci* 82(6):660, 1993.

Buckle J: Aromatherapy in the USA, *Int J Aromather* 31(1):42, 2003a.

Buckle J: *Clinical aromatherapy: essential oils in practice*, ed 2, Edinburgh, 2003b, Churchill Livingstone.

Burns E: Aromatherapy in childbirth: helpful for mother—what about baby? *Int J Clin Aromather* 2(2):36, 2005.

Burns E, Blamey C, Ersser SJ, et al: The use of aromatherapy in intrapartum midwifery practice: an observational study, *Complement Ther Nurs Midwifery* 6(1):33, 2000.

Burns E, Zobbi V, Panzeri D, et al: Aromatherapy in childbirth: a pilot randomised controlled trial, *Br J Obstet Gynecol* 114:838, 2007.

Caelli M, Porteous J, Carson CF, et al: Tea tree oil as an alternative topical decolonization agent for methicillin-resistant *Staphylococcus aureus*, *J Hosp Infect* 46:236, 2000.

Cannard G: The effects of aromatherapy in promoting relaxation and stress reduction in a general hospital, *Complement Ther Nurs Midwifery* 2:38, 1996.

Carter A, Mackereth P, Tavares M, Donald G: Take me to a clinical Aromatherapist: An exploratory survey of delegates to the first Clinical Aromatherapy Conference, Manchester UK, *IJCA* 6(1):3–8, 2009.

Cawthorne A, Carter A: Aromatherapy and its application in cancer and palliative care, *Complement Ther Nurs Midwifery* 6:83, 2000.

Cermelli C, Fabio A, Fabio G, et al: Effect of eucalyptus essential oil on respiratory bacteria and viruses, *Curr Microbiol* 56:89, 2008.

Chang Y-C, Karlberg A-T, Maibach HI: Allergic contact dermatitis from oxidised *d*-limonene, *Contact Dermatitis* 37:308, 1997.

Chao LK, Hua K-F, Hsu H-Y, et al: Cinnamaldehyde inhibits pro-inflammatory cytokines secretion from monocytes/macrophages through suppression of intracellular signaling, *Food Chem Toxicol* 46:220, 2008.

Christensson JB, Forsstrom P, Wennberg A-M, et al: Air oxidation increases skin irritation from fragrance terpenes, *Contact Dermatitis* 60:32, 2009.

Christensson JB, Johansson S, Hagvall L, et al: Limonene hydroperoxide analogues differ in allergenic activity, *Contact Dermatitis* 59:344, 2008.

Chung MJ, Kang AY, Park SO, et al: The effect of essential oils of dietary wormwood (*Artemisia princeps*), with and without added vitamin E, on oxidative stress and some genes involved in cholesterol metabolism, *Food Chem Toxicol* 45:1400, 2007.

Cohen-Mansfield J, Jensen B: Nursing home physicians' knowledge of and attitudes toward nonpharmacological interventions for treatment of behavioural disturbances associated with dementia, *J Am Med Dir Assoc* 9:491, 2008.

Conrad P, Adams C: The effects of clinical aromatherapy for anxiety and depression in the high risk postpartum woman—A pilot study, *Complement Ther Clin Pract* 18(3):164–168, 2012.

Cooke B, Ernst E: Aromatherapy: a systematic review, *Br J Gen Pract* 50(455):493, 2000.

Curry SV, Donaghy K, Hughes CM: Aromatherapy massage for improving well-being of carers of patients with cancer: a pilot double-blind randomised controlled clinical trial, *Int J Clin Aromather* 5(2):9, 2008.

Darben T, Cominos B, Lee CT: Topical eucalyptus oil poisoning, *Australas J Dermatol* 39:265, 1998.

De Valois B, Clarke E: A retrospective assessment of 3 years of patient audit for an aromatherapy massage service for cancer patients, *Int J Aromather* 11(3):134, 2001.

Denda M, Tsuchiya T, Shoji K, et al: Odorant inhalation affects skin barrier homeostasis in mice and humans, *Br J Dermatol* 142:1007, 2000.

Dryden MS, Dailly S, Crouch M: A randomised, controlled trial of tea tree topical preparations versus a standard topical regimen for the clearance of MRSA colonization, *J Hosp Infect* 56:283, 2004.

Dunning T: *Essential oils in therapeutic care*, Melbourne, 2007, Australia Scholarly Publishing.

Durell S: An aromatherapy service for people with a learning disability, *Int J Aromather* 12(3):152, 2002.

Dyer J: The use of aromatherapy massage for the relief of pain in cancer patients, *Int J Clin Aromather* 1(1):8, 2004.

Dyer J, Ragsdale-Lowe M, McNeill S, et al: A snapshot survey of current practice: the use of aromasticks for symptom management, *Int J Clin Aromather* 5(2):17, 2008.

Dyer J, Ragsdale-Lowe M, Cardoso M, et al: The use of aromasticks for nausea in a cancer hospital, *IJCA* 7(2):3–6, 2010.

Ebihara T, Ebihara S, Maruyama M, et al: A randomised trial of olfactory stimulation using black pepper oil in older people with swallowing dysfunction, *J Am Geriatr Soc* 54:1401, 2006a.

Ebihara T, Ebihara S, Watando A, et al: Effects of menthol on the triggering of the swallowing reflex in elderly patients with dysphagia, *Br J Clin Pharmacol* 62(3):369, 2006b.

Egan B, Gage H, Hood J, et al: Availability of complementary and alternative medicine for people with cancer in the British National Health Service: Results of a national survey, *Complement Ther Clin Pract* 18(2):75–80, 2012.

Ellwood J: Aromatherapy and autism, *Int J Clin Aromather* 5(1):12, 2008.

Enshaieh S, Jooya A, Siadat AH, et al: The efficacy of 5% topical tea tree oil gel in mild to moderate acne vulgaris: a randomised, double-blind-placebo-controlled study, *Indian J Dermatol Venereol Leprol* 73:22, 2007.

Ernst E: Advice offered by practitioners of complementary/alternative medicine: an important ethical issue. *Eval Health Prof* 32(4):335–342, 2009. doi: 10.1177/0163278709346812.

Fadli M, Chevalier J, Saad A, et al: Essential oils from Moroccan plants as potential chemosensitisers restoring antibiotic activity in resistant Gram-negative bacteria, *Int J Antimicrob Agents* 3(4):325–330, 2011.

Fanner F: The use of aromatherapy for pain management through labour, *Int J Clin Aromather* 2(1):10, 2005.

Fenu G, Foddai M, Carai A, et al: Therapeutic properties of myrtle essential oil: an in vitro study on human nasal mucosa cells, *Int J Essent Oil Ther* 2:21, 2008.

Fewell F, McVicar R, Gransby R, et al: Blood concentration and uptake of d-limonene during aromatherapy massage with sweet orange oil: a pilot study, *Int J Essent Oil Ther* 1:97, 2007.

Freeman S, Ebihara E, Ebihara T, et al: Olfactory stimuli and enhanced postural stability in older adults, *Gait Posture* 29(4):658, 2009. [Epub March 14, 2009].

Friedmann TS: Attention deficit and hyperactivity disorder (ADHD), *Int J Clin Aromather* 6(2):33–36, 2009.

Fuchs N, Jager W, Lenhardt A, et al: Systemic absorption of topically applied carvone: influence of massage technique, *J Soc Cosmet Chem* 48:277, 1997.

Ganzera M, Scheider P, Stuppner H: Inhibitory effects of the essential oil of chamomile (*Matricaria recutita L.*) and its major constituents on human cytochrome P450 enzymes, *Life Sci* 78:856, 2006.

Ghazanfari G, Minaie B, Yasa N, et al: Biochemical and histopathological evidences for beneficial effects of *Satureja khuzestanica Jamzad* essential oil on the mouse model of inflammatory bowel diseases, *Toxicol Mech Methods* 16:365, 2006.

Giraud-Robert AM: The role of aromatherapy in the treatment of viral hepatitis, *Int J Aromather* 15:183, 2005.

Goerg KJ, Spilker T: Effect of peppermint oil and caraway oil on gastrointestinal motility in healthy volunteers: a pharmacodynamic study using simultaneous determination of gastric and gall-bladder emptying and orocaecal transit time, *Aliment Pharmacol Ther* 17:445, 2003.

Goornemann T, Nayal R, Pertz HH, et al: Antispasmodic activity of essential oil from *Lippia dulcis Trev*, *J Ethnopharmacol* 117:166, 2008.

Green BG, Flammer LJ: Methyl salicyclate as a cutaneous stimulus: a psychophysical analysis, *Somatosens Mot Res* 6:253, 1989.

Greenway FL, Frome BM, Engels TM, et al: Temporary relief of postherpetic neuralgia pain with topical geranium oil, *Am J Med* 115:586, 2003. (letter).

Greenwood B: Aromatherapy in the special needs environment: interview with Barb Greenwood, *Int J Clin Aromather* 5(1):41, 2008.

Grigoleit H-G, Grigoleit P: Pharmacology and preclinical pharmacokinetics of peppermint oil, *Phytomedicine* 12:612, 2005.

Hackman E, Mackereth P, Maycock P, et al: Expanding the use of aromasticks for surgical and day care patients, *International Journal of Clinical Aromatherapy* 8(1&2):10–15, 2012.

Hardy M, Kirk-Smith MD, Stretch DD: Replacement of drug treatment for insomnia by ambient odour, *Lancet* 346:701, 1995.

Harris R: Synergism in the essential oil world, *Int J Aromather* 12(4):179, 2002.

Harris R: Anglo-Saxon aromatherapy: its evolution and current situation, *Int J Aromather* 13(1):9, 2003.

Henry J: Working with dementia and stroke: interview with Jenny Henry, *Int J Clin Aromather* 5(2):42, 2008.

Herz RS: Aromatherapy facts and fictions: a scientific analysis of olfactory effects on mood, physiology and behaviour, *Int J Neurosci* 119:263, 2009.

Holmes C, Hopkins V, Hensford C, et al: Lavender oil as a treatment for agitated behaviour in severe dementia: a placebo controlled study, *Int J Geriatr Psychiatry* 17(4):305, 2002.

Holmes P: *The energetics of Western herbs*, ed 4, 2 vols, Boulder, Colo, 2007, Snow Lotus Press.

Holmes P: *Clinical aromatherapy*, Cotati, Calif, 2008, Tigerlily Press.

Hong C-Z, Sellock FG: Effects of topically applied counterirritant (Eucalyptamint) on cutaneous blood flow and on skin and muscle temperatures, *Am J Phys Med Rehabil* 70:29, 1991.

Hosoi J, Tsuchiya T: Regulation of cutaneous allergic reaction by odorant inhalation, *J Invest Dermatol* 114:541, 2000.

Hsu MC, Creedy D, Moyle W, et al: Use of complementary and alternative medicine among adult patients for depression in Taiwan, *J Affect Disord* 111:360, 2008.

Huang L, Abuhamdah S, Howes MJR, et al: Pharmacological profile of essential oils derived from *Lavandula angustifolia* and *Melissa officinalis* with anti-agitation properties: focus on ligand-gated channels, *J Pharm Pharmacol* 60:1515, 2008.

Imanishi J, Kuriyama H, Shigemori I, et al: Anxiolytic effect of aromatherapy massage in patients with breast cancer, *eCAM* 6(1):123–128, 2009.

Imura M, Misao H, Ushijima H: The psychological effects of aromatherapy-massage in healthy postpartum mothers, *J Midwifery Women's Health* 51:e21, 2006.

Inouye S: Laboratory evaluation of gaseous essential oils (part 1), *Int J Aromather* 13(2–3):95, 2003.

Inouye S, Abe S, Yamaguchi H, et al: Comparative study of antimicrobial and cytotoxic effects of selected essential oils by gaseous and solution contacts, *Int J Aromather* 13(1):33, 2003.

Inouye S, Takizawa T, Yamaguchi H: Antibacterial activities of essential oils and their major constituents against respiratory tract pathogens by gaseous contact, *J Antimicrob Chemother* 47:565, 2001.

Jager W, Buchbauer G, Jirovetz L, et al: Percutaneous absorption of lavender oil from a massage oil, *J Soc Cosmet Chem* 43:49, 1992.

Jager W, Nasel B, Nasel C, et al: Pharmokinetic studies of the fragrance compound 1,8-cineole in humans during inhalation, *Chem Senses* 21:477, 1996.

Jahromi BN, Tartifizadeh A, Khabnadideh S: Comparison of fennel and mefenamic acid for the treatment of primary dysmenorrhea, *Int J Gynecol Obstet* 80:153, 2003.

Jirovetz L, Wicek K, Buchbauer G, et al: Antifungal activity of various Lamiaceae essential oils rich in thymol and carvacrol against clinical isolates of pathogenic *Candida* species, *Int J Essent Oil Ther* 1(4):179, 2007.

Johannessen B: Nurses experience of aromatherapy use with dementia patients experiencing disturbed sleeppatterns. An action research project, *Complement Ther Clin Pract* (2013):2013. http://dx.doi.org/10.1016/j.ctcp.2013.01.003.

Jori A, Bianchetti A, Prestini PE: Effect of essential oils on drug metabolism, *Biochem Pharmacol* 18(9):2081, 1969.

Jori A, Blanchetti A, Prestini PE, et al: Effect of eucalyptol (1,8-cineole) on the metabolism of other drugs in rats and in man, *Euro J Pharmacol* 9:362, 1970.

Joss JD, LeBlond RF: Potentiation of warfarin anticoagulation associated with topical methylsalicylate, *Ann Pharmacother* 34:729, 2000.

Juergens UR, Dethlefsen U, Steinkamp G, et al: Anti-inflammatory activity of 1,8-cineole (eucalyptol) in bronchial asthma: a double blind placebo-controlled trial, *Resp Med* 97:250, 2003.

Kehrl W, Sonnemann U, Dethlefson U: Therapy for acute nonpurulent rhinosinusitis with cineole: results of a double-blind, randomised, placebo-controlled trial, *Laryngoscope* 114:738, 2004.

Khosravi AR, Eslami AR, Shokri H, et al: *Zataria multiflora* cream for the treatment of acute vaginal candidiasis, *Int J Gynecol Obstet* 101:201, 2008.

Knevitt A: Therapeutic aromatherapy in a palliative setting, *Int J Clin Aromather* 1(2):46, 2004.

Kohara H, Miyauchi T, Suehiro Y, et al: Combined modality treatment of aromatherapy, footsoak and reflexology relieves fatigue in patients with cancer, *J Palliat Med* 7(6):791, 2004.

Komori T, Fujiwara R, Tanida M, et al: Effects of citrus fragrance on immune function and depressive states, *Neurommunomodulation* 2:174, 1995.

Komori T, Matsumoto T, Yamamoto M, et al: Application of fragrance in discontinuing the long-term use of hypnotic benzodiazepines, *Int J Aromather* 16:3, 2006.

Koo BS, Park KS, Ha JH, et al: Inhibitory effects of the fragrance inhalation of essential oil from *Acorus gramineus* on central nervous system, *Biol Pharm Bull* 26:978, 2003.

Kotnik P, Skerget M, Knez Z: Supercritical fluid ectraction of chamomile flowerheads: comparison with conventional extraction, kinetics and scale up, *J Supercritical Fluids* 43:192, 2007.

Krist S, Halwachs L, Sallberger G, et al: Effects of scents on airborne microbes, part I: thymol, eugenol, transcinnamaldehyde and linalool, *Flav Fragr J* 22(1):44, 2006.

Kyle L: Aromatherapy report: the use of essential oils on an acute care psychiatric unit, *Int J Clin Aromather* 5(2):30, 2008.

Lai TKT, Cheung MC, Lo CK, et al: Effectiveness of aroma massage on advanced cancer patients with constipation: A pilot study, *Complement Ther Clin Pract* 17:37–43, 2011.

Lam LK, Zheng B: Effects of essential oils on glutathione S-transferase activity in mice, *J Agric Food Chem* 39:660, 1991.

Lee KK, Kim JH, Cho JJ, Choi JD: Inhibitory effects of 150 plant extracts on elastase activity and their anti-inflammatory effects, *Int J Cosmet Sci* 21(2):71–82, 1999.

Lee MS, Choi J, Posadzki P, Ernst E: Aromatherapy for health care: an overview of systematic reviews, *Maturitas* 71(3):257–260, 2012.

Lee Y-Y, Hung S-L, Pai S-F, et al: Eugenol suppressed the expression of lipopolysaccharide-induced proinflammatory mediators in human macrophages, *J Endodontics* 33:698, 2007.

Le Faou M, Beghe T, Bourguignon E, et al: The effects of the application of Dermasport plus Solution Cryo in physiotherapy, *Int J Aromather* 15:123, 2005.

Lim WC, Seo JM, Lee CI, et al: Stimulative and sedative effects of essential oils upon inhalation in mice, *Arch Pharm Res* 28:770, 2005.

Lin PW, Chan W, Ng BF, et al: Efficacy of aromatherapy (*Lavandula angustifolia*) as an intervention for agitated behaviour in Chinese older persons with dementia: a cross-over randomized trial, *Int J Geriatr Psychiatr* 22:405, 2007.

Lindsay WR, Pitcaithly D, Geelen N, et al: A comparison of the effects of four therapy procedures on concentration and responsiveness in people with profound learning disabilities, *J Intellect Disabil Res* 41:201, 1997.

Louis M, Kowalski SD: Use of aromatherapy with hospice patients to decrease pain, anxiety and depression and to promote an increased sense of well-being, *Am J Hosp Palliat Care* 19(6):381, 2002.

Mackereth P, Carter A, Parkin S, et al: Complementary Therapist's training and cancer care: a multi-site survey, *Eur J Oncol Nurs* 13:330–335, 2009.

Mackereth P, Parkin S, Donald G, Antcliffe N: Clinical supervision and complementary therapists: An exploration of the rewards and challenges of cancer care, *Complement Ther Clin Pract* 16(3):143–148, 2010.

MacMahon S, Kermode S: A clinical trial of the effect of aromatherapy on motivational behaviour in a dementia care setting using a single subject design, *Aust J Holist Nurs* 5(2):47, 1998.

Maddocks-Jennings W: Using essential oils for the care of the oropharyngeal area during radiotherapy and chemotherapy, *IJCA* 4(2):14–20, 2007.

Maddocks-Jennings W, Wilkinson JM, Cavanagh HM, Shillington D: Evaluating the effects of the essential oils Leptospermum scoparium (manuka) and Kunzea ericoides (kanuka) on radiotherapy induced mucositis: A randomized, placebo controlled feasibility study, *Eur J Oncol Nurs* 13:87–93, 2009.

Mattys H, de Mey C, Carls C, et al: Efficacy and tolerability of myrtol standardised in acute bronchitis: a multi-centre, randomised, double-blind, placebo-controlled parallel group clinical trial vs. cefuroxime and ambroxol, *Arzneimittelforschung* 50(8):700, 2000.

Mercier D, Knevitt A: Using topical aromatherapy for the management of fungating wounds in a palliative care unit, *J Wound Care* 14(10):497, 2005.

Meyer M: Aromatherapy in a Melbourne mother-baby unit, *Int J Clin Aromather* 2(1):33, 2005. (letter).

Mikhaeil BR, Maatooq GT, Badria FA, et al: Chemistry and immunomodulatory activity of frankincense oil, *Z Naturforsch C* 58:230, 2003.

Miller L, Miller B: *Ayurveda and aromatherapy: the earth essential guide to ancient wisdom and modern healing,* Twin Lakes, Wisc, 1995, Lotus Press.

Mojay G: *Aromatherapy for healing the spirit,* New York, 1996, Henry Holt.

Monges P, Joachim G, Bohor M, et al: Comparative in vivo study of the moisturising properties of three gels containing essential oils: mandarin, German chamomile, orange, *Nouv Dermatol* 13:470, 1994.

Mori M, Ikeda N, Kato Y, et al: Inhibition of elastase activity by essential oils in vitro, *J Cosmet Dermatol* 1:183, 2002.

Morris N: The effects of lavender (Lavandula angustifolia) essential oil baths on stress and anxiety, *Int J Clin Aromather* 5(1):3, 2008.

Moscavitch SD, Szyper-Kravitz M, Shoenfeld Y: Autoimmune pathology accounts for common manifestations in a wide range of neuro-psychiatric disorders: the olfactory and immune system relationship, *Clin Immunol* 130:235, 2009.

Moss L, Rouse M, Wesnes KA, Moss M: Differential Effects of the Aromas of Salvia Species on Memory and Mood, *Hum Psychopharmacol* 25:388–396, 2010.

Moss M, Hewitt S, Moss L, Wesnes K: Modulation of cognitive performance and mood by aromas of Peppermint and Ylang-Ylang, *Int J Neurosci* 118:59–77, 2008.

Moss M, Howarth R, Wilkinson L, et al: Expectancy and the aroma of Roman chamomile influence mood and cognition in healthy volunteers, *Int J Aromather* 16:63, 2006.

Nam S-Y, Chang M-H, Do J-S, et al: Essential oil of niaouli preferentially potentiates antigen-specific cellular immunity and cytokine production by macrophages, *Immunopharmacol Immunotoxicol* 30:459, 2008.

Navarro MC, Noguera MA, Romero MC, et al: Anisakis simplex s.l.: larvicidal activity of various monoterpenic derivatives of natural origin against L_3 larvae in vitro and in vivo, *Exper Parasitol* 120:295, 2008.

Neale L, Moss L, Moss M: Lavender aroma moderates endocrine response to an acute psychological stressor but does not impact on subjective measures of mood and demand, *Int J Clin Aromather* 5(2):3–8, 2008.

Oladimeji FA, Orafidiya LO, Ogunniyi TAB, et al: A comparative study of the scabicidal activities of formulations of essential oil of *Lippia multiflora Moldenke* and benzyl benzoate emulsion BP, *Int J Aromather* 15:87, 2005.

Opalchenova G, Obreshkova D: Comparative studies on the activity of basil—an essential oil from *Ocimum basilicum*—against multidrug resistant clinical isolates of the genera *Staphylococcus, Enterococcus* and *Pseudomonas* by using different test methods, *J Microbiol Methods* 54:105, 2003.

Orafidiya LO, Agbani EO, Abereoje B, et al: An investigation into the wound healing properties of essential oil of *Ocimum gratissimum Linn, J Wound Care* 12:331, 2003.

Orafidiya LO, Fakoya FA, Agbani EO, et al: Vascular permeability-increasing effect of the leaf essential oil of *Ocimum gratissimum Linn* as a mechanism for its wound healing property, *Afr J Tradit Complement Altern Med* 2:253, 2005.

Osborn CE, Barlas P, Baxter GD, et al: Aromatherapy: survey of common practice in the management of rheumatic disease symptoms, *Complement Ther Med* 9:62, 2001.

Pages N, Fournier G, Baduel C, et al: Sabinyl acetate, the main component of *Juniperus sabina L'Herit.* essential oil, is responsible for anti-implantation effect, *Phytother Res* 10(7):438, 1996.

Parke DV, Rahman KMQ, Walker R: Effect of linalol on hepatic drug-metabolising enzymes in the rat, *Biochem Soc Trans* 2:615, 1974.

Peace G, Manasse A: The Cavendish Centre for Integrated Cancer Care: assessment of patients' needs and responses, *Complement Ther Med* 10:33, 2002.

Pemberton E, Turpin PG: The effect of essential oils on work related stress in intensive care unit nurses, *Holist Nurs Pract* 22(2):97, 2008.

Pibiri M-C, Goel A, Vahekeni N, et al: Indoor air purification and ventilation system sanitation with essential oils, *Int J Aromather* 16:148, 2006.

Pourmortazavi SM, Hajimirsadeghi SS: Supercritical extraction in plant essential and volatile oil analysis, *J Chromatogr A* 1163:2, 2007.

Price S, Price L: *Aromatherapy for health professionals*, ed 3, Edinburgh, 2007, Churchill Livingstone.

Purkayastha S, Narain R, Dahiya P: Evaluation of antimicrobial and phytochemical screening of Fennel, Juniper and Kalonji essential oils against multidrug resistant clinical isolates, *Asian Pac J Trop Biomed* 2(3):S1625–S1629, 2012.

Rai M, Kon K, editors: *Fighting Multidrug Resistance with Herbal Extracts, Essential Oils and their Components*, 2013, Academic Press, Elsevier.

Robbins G, Broughan C: The effects of manipulating participant expectations of an essential oil on memory through verbal suggestion, *Int J Essent Oil Ther* 1:56, 2007.

Saeki Y: The effect of foot-bath with or without the essential oil of lavender on the autonomic nervous system: a randomised trial, *Complement Ther Med* 8(1):2, 2000.

Sanderson H, Harrison J, Price S: *Aromatherapy and massage for people with learning difficulties*, Birmingham, England, 1991, Hands On Publishing.

Sato K, Krist S, Buchbauer G: Antimicrobial effect of vapours of geraniol, (R)-(-)-linalol, terpineol, γ-terpinene and 1,8-cineole on airborne microbes using an airwasher, *Flav Fragr J* 22:435, 2007.

Scanni G, Bonifazi E: Efficacy of a single application of a new natural lice removal product: preliminary data, *Euro J Pediatr Dermatol* 16:231, 2006.

Schaller M, Korting HC: Allergic airborne contact dermatitis from essential oils used in aromatherapy, *Clin Exp Dermatol* 20(2):143, 1995.

Schnitzler P, Koch C, Reichling J: Susceptibility of drug-resistant clinical herpes simplex virus type 1 strains to essential oils of ginger, thyme, hyssop, and sandalwood, *Antimicrob Agents Chemother* 51:1859, 2007.

Schnitzler P, Schumacher A, Astani A, et al: *Melissa officinalis* oil affects infectivity of enveloped herpesviruses, *Phytomedicine* 15:734, 2008.

Schwan R: Integrative palliative aromatherapy care program at San Diego Hospice and Palliative Care, *Int J Clin Aromather* 1(2):5, 2004.

Selvaag E, Holm J-O, Thune P: Allergic contact dermatitis in an aromatherapist with multiple sensitisations to essential oils, *Contact Dermatitis* 33(5):354, 1995.

Serafino A, Vallebona P, Andreola F, et al: Stimulatory effect of eucalyptus essential oil on innate cell-mediated immune response, *BMC Immunol* 9:17, 2008.

Sherry E, Sivananthan S, Warnke P, et al: Topical phytochemicals used to salvage the gangrenous lower limbs of type I diabetic patients, *Diabetes Res Clin Pract* 62:65, 2003. (letter).

Simkin P, Bolding A: Update on nonpharmacologic approaches to relieve labor pain and prevent suffering, *J Midwifery Women's Health* 49(6):480, 2007.

Singh G, Kapoor IPS, Singh P, et al: Chemistry, antioxidant and antimicrobial investigations on essential oil and oleoresins of *Zingiber officinale, Food Chem Toxicol* 46:3295, 2008.

Smallwood J, Brown R, Coutler F, et al: Aromatherapy and behavior disturbances in dementia: a randomized controlled trial, *Int J Geriatr Psychiatry* 16(10):1010, 2001.

Smith MC, Kyle L: Holistic foundations of aromatherapy for nursing, *Holist Nurs Pract* 22(1):3, 2008.

Soković M, Glamoclíja J, Ćirić A, et al: Antifungal activity of the essential oil of *Thymus vulgaris L.* and thymol on experimentally induced dermatomycoses, *Drug Dev Ind Pharm* 34:1388, 2008.

Spector IP, Carey MP, Jorgensen RS, et al: Cue-controlled relaxation and "aromatherapy" in the treatment of speech anxiety, *Behav Cogn Psychother* 21:239, 1993.

Srivastava KC, Malhotra N: Acetyl eugenol, a component of oil of cloves (*Syzygium aromaticum L.*) inhibits aggregation and alters arachidonic acid metabolism in human blood platelets, *Prostaglandins Leukot Essent Fatty Acids* 42:73, 1990.

Stimpfl T, Nasel B, Nasel C, et al: Concentration of 1,8-cineole in human blood during prolonged inhalation, *Chem Senses* 20:349, 1995.

Stringer J: Massage and aromatherapy on a leukaemia unit, *Complement Ther Nurs Midwifery* 6:72, 2000.

Stringer J, Donald G: Aromasticks in cancer care: An innovation not to be sniffed at, *Complement Ther Clin Pract* 11(11):1222–1229, 2010.

Tavares M: National guidelines for the use of complementary therapies in supportive and palliative care, 2003, available at http://www.fih.org.uk.

Tavares M: Integrating aromatherapy in specialist palliative care: The use of essential oils for symptom management, 2011, available at www.clinicalaromapac.ca.

Thorgrimsen L, Spector A, Wiles A, et al: Aroma therapy for dementia, *Cochrane Database Syst Rev* (3):CD003150, 2003.

Tibballs J: Clinical effects and management of eucalyptus oil ingestion in infants and young children, *Med J Austral* 163:177, 1995.

Tiran D: Aromatherapy in midwifery: benefits and risks, *Complement Ther Med* 2:88, 1996.

Tiran D: *Clinical aromatherapy for pregnancy and childbirth*, ed 2, Edinburgh, 2000, Churchill Livingstone.

Tisserand R, Young R: *Essential Oil Safety*, ed 2, 2014, Churchill Livingstone.

Tysoe P: The effect on staff of essential oil burners in extended care settings, *Int J Nurs Pract* 6:110, 2000.

Uehleke B, Schaper S, Dienel A, et al: Phase II trial on the effects of Silexan in patients with neurasthenia, post-traumatic stress disorder or somatization disorder, *Phytomedicine* 19(8–9):665–671, 2012.

Vian MA, Fernandez X, Visinoni F, et al: Microwave hydrodiffusion and gravity, a new technique for extraction of essential oils, *J Chromatogr A* 1190:14, 2008.

Wakelin SH, McFadden JP, Leonard JN, et al: Allergic contact dermatitis from *d*-limonene in a laboratory technician, *Contact Dermatitis* 38:164, 1998.

Walker LA, Budd S: UK: the current state of regulation of complementary and alternative medicine, *Complement Ther Med* 10(1):8, 2002.

Warnke PH, Sherry E, Russo PAJ, et al: Antibacterial essential oils in malodorous cancer patients: clinical observations in 30 patients, *Phytomedicine* 13(7):463, 2006.

Weiss J: Camphorated oil intoxication during pregnancy, *Paediatr* 52:713, 1973.

Weiss RR, James WD: Allergic contact dermatitis from aromatherapy, *Am J Contact Dermat* 8(4):250, 1997.

Wilkinson S, Aldridge J, Salmon I, et al: An evaluation of aromatherapy massage in palliative care, *Palliat Med* 13:409, 1999.

Wilkinson SM, Love SB, Westcombe AM, et al: Effectiveness of aromatherapy massage in the management of anxiety and depression in patients with cancer: a multicenter randomized controlled trial, *J Clin Oncol* 25(5):532, 2007.

Woelk H, Schläfke S: A multi-center, double-blind, randomised study of the Lavender oil preparation Silexan in comparison to Lorazepam for generalized anxiety disorder, *Phytomedicine* 17(2):94–99, 2010.

Xu H, Delling M, Jun JC, et al: Oregano, thyme and clove-derived flavors and skin sensitisers activate specific TRP channels, *Nat Neurosci* 9:628, 2006.

Yip YB, Tam ACY: An experimental study on the effectiveness of massage with aromatic ginger and orange essential oil for moderate-to-severe knee pain among the elderly in Hong Kong, *Complement Ther Med* 16:131, 2008.

Yap PSX, Lim SHE, Hu CP, Yiap BC: Combination of essential oils and antibiotics reduce antibiotic resistance in plasmid-conferred multidrug resistant bacteria, *Phytomedicine* 20(8–9):710–713, 2013.

Zhang H, Chen F, Wang X, et al: Evaluation of antioxidant activity of parsley (*Petroselinum crispum*) essential oil and identification of its antioxidant constituents, *Food Res Int* 39:833, 2006.

Suggested Readings

Carter A, Mackereth P, Stringer J: Aromatherapy in Cancer Care; do aromatherapists in cancer care need specific training to do this work? *In Essence* 9:20–22, 2010.

Kayne S: Problems in the pharmacovigilance of herbal medicines in the UK highlighted, *Pharmaceut J* 276:543, 2006.

Maury M: *The secret of life and youth: regeneration through essential oils—a modern alchemy*, (translated by M Saville, reprinted in 1989, London, MacDonald). London, 1964.

Yap PSX, Lim SHE, Hu CP, Yiap BC: Combination of essential oils and antibiotics reduce antibiotic resistance in plasmid-conferred multidrug resistant bacteria, *Phytomedicine* 20(8–9):710–713, 2013.

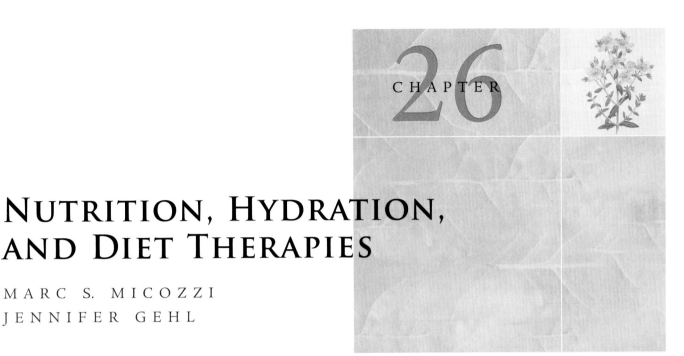

CHAPTER 26

NUTRITION, HYDRATION, AND DIET THERAPIES

MARC S. MICOZZI

JENNIFER GEHL

People eat food, not nutrients. When we rummage through the refrigerator for a snack or cruise the supermarket aisles trying to decide what to fix for dinner, our choices are much more likely to reflect cultural, social, and family patterns than to be based on the federal government's food pyramid and recommended daily allowances.

Food has powerful symbolic meaning and has played a key role in our religious and social rituals for thousands of years. From birthday cake to the bitter herbs of the Passover Seder to Thanksgiving turkey to communion wafers, food helps form our social bonds, express our spirituality, and define who we are. Rituals remain powerful even when we no longer recall their origins. For example, Christians worldwide celebrate Easter by eating colored eggs, although few could explain the religious connection with hard-boiled eggs (more having to do with the arrival of Spring).

Substances can have radically different meanings for different groups. For Muslims, Christian Scientists, and members of Alcoholics Anonymous, wine is strictly "taboo," whereas for Catholics, wine is part of a sacrament that is by definition "an outward sign instituted to give grace." Individuals also bring very different perspectives to the table. For some vegetarians, chicken soup represents cruelty to animals, whereas for many other people it recalls mom's tender care during childhood illnesses.

An intellectual understanding of what constitutes good nutrition may be no match for the powerful psychological, social, and spiritual forces that have been shaping human eating habits since the Stone Age.

EATING HABITS OF EARLY HUMANS

Humans are omnivores. We can eat almost every food found in nature, and with some few exceptions (e.g., wood, grass), we can extract nutrition from whatever food source we consume. For millions of years, our early ancestors roamed the forests and plains as hunter-gatherers. The hunters brought home very lean meat; wild game has only 4% to 6% body fat versus the 40% to 60% body fat found in modern domesticated animals. The gatherers collected plants that were high in fiber and complex carbohydrates and provided many necessary vitamins. These early humans obtained calcium from animal bones and cartilage, and other minerals from the soil that ultimately were present in wild plants and game.

Life could be a constant struggle to obtain enough fats and calories, and our ancestors developed a decided preference for foods that tasted rich in these needed nutrients. Among small, hunter-gatherer tribes, food was often allocated on the basis of social status, gender, and age, which provided it with significance beyond the satisfaction of hunger. When sedentary agriculture was developed 10,000 years ago, diets became more stable as sources of carbohydrate and calories (but could make it more difficult for larger populations to obtain sufficient protein, essential fats, and vitamins and minerals). Seasonal crops led to the occurrence of seasonal feasts, and famines, which added another layer of cultural meaning to food consumption.

Although even the earliest farmers sought to improve their crops genetically—for example, selecting and sowing the seeds of wheat that had stronger stalks and quicker, more uniform germination—the quality of food did not change much. Humans learned to use yeast (made from microbes, which had been present on the planet for millions of years) to produce bread, beer, and wine; other microbes were used to make cheese and yogurt. These microbes made certain plants and dairy products easier (and more enjoyable) to consume and digest, but humans were still eating the diet for which their digestive system and metabolism were designed: low in simple carbs and total calories with adequate amounts of essential fats, protein, complex carbohydrates, and fiber, with no refined sugar. Everything in the human diet remained completely natural—until modern times.

MODERN ERA: FOOLING MOTHER NATURE

Fast-forwarding to the twentieth century, we suddenly find a very different picture of food production and consumption. Early in the century, advances in biochemistry allowed scientists to isolate some of the active ingredients in food. In 1928, for example, it was discovered that limes, the British Navy's traditional method of preventing scurvy, worked by providing sailors with vitamin C. Unfortunately, although vitamin C supplements proved easier to store and dispense, they did not provide the full benefits of the fruit. Later research disclosed that citrus pulp also contains *bioflavonoids,* which are necessary for absorbing and processing vitamin C. Bioflavonoids also help maintain collagen and capillary walls and protect against infection and cancer. Scientists were discovering that replacing natural products with artificial ones did not always improve on the original.

This finding, however, did not stop scientists from trying to improve on nature. Currently, modern technology and agribusiness have "improved" crops by covering them with artificial chemicals, including pesticides, fungicides, ripening agents, and fumigants, all of which make them more efficient to grow, ship, and store. Genetic engineering is changing the biological structure of many plants, and the ecology of plantlife on the planet, in ways not yet fully understood. Some plants are irradiated (flooded with "harmless" radiation) to lengthen their shelf life. Others are "genetically modified" by genetic engineering, not selective breeding. Animals destined for the table are dosed with antibiotics to prevent disease and fatten them up, and with hormones to make them even more fat and juicy.

Once vegetables, fruit, milk, meat, and eggs leave the farm, they are often "processed" into "food products," such as canned soup and frozen dinners. Processed foods are generally high in artificial chemicals, fats, salt, and sugar; are lower in nutrients than fresh foods; and contain a host of chemicals to boost flavor, color, texture, and shelf life. Consider the following:

- Pounds of sugar the average American consumed per year in the nineteenth century: less than 10
- Pounds of sugar the average American consumes per year today: 150

Among the many artificial substances used in processed foods are such synthetic chemicals as aspartame, silicon dioxide, phenylalanine, tribasic calcium phosphate, benzoic sulfimide, and calcium silicate. The effects of all these chemicals on our bodies are not entirely known, but

saccharin, the first widely used artificial sweetener, was shown to cause cancer in laboratory animals. Saccharin was banned in Canada, while kept on the shelves in the United States. Meantime, another artificial sweetener, cyclamates, were banned in the United States but kept on the shelves in Canada. Does that give you a lot of confidence in the scientific basis of government regulatory decisions? Aspartame (e.g., NutraSweet™) is being studied for possible neurological effects. Large quantities of one of the chemicals present, methanol, have been shown to cause blindness, brain swelling, and inflammation of the pancreas and heart muscle.

In addition to all these pseudo-sugars, we now have "fake fats." Partially hydrogenated oil does not occur in nature but can be manufactured in the laboratory when liquid vegetable fats are turned into solids by pumping hydrogen into them. This process makes them more like tasty animal fats in texture and feel, but this unnatural substance has harmful effects on the cardiovascular system. In fact, partially hydrogenated fats have been associated with higher cancer rates, while saturated fats have yet to be proven as causes of cancer or heart disease. The FDA finally acted in 2013 to ban these wholly unnatural *trans*-fats from foods and the ban will take effect in 2016 after a lengthy comment and review period.

Trans fatty acids (TFAs) are formed when unsaturated fatty acids (the building blocks of fat) are deformed by certain heat or chemical treatments. These deformed fats are toxic. TFAs in the diet damage the regulatory machinery of the body, significantly compromising health. Despite these concerns, partially hydrogenated oils and TFAs have been used (until 2016) in a wide range of processed foods, including almost all margarines, mass-produced breads, convenience foods, and junk foods, as well as some baby foods. More generally, while substitutes are being found to replace TPAs, any processed food that needed TPAs in the first place does not belong in a healthy diet regardless of what else may be in it. These are not natural foods.

For a variety of reasons, including productivity, efficiency, convenience, profit, arrogance, and curiosity, we have found abundant ways to change the nature of our diets and the nature of the animals and plants that feed us. As a group, the U.S. population eats at the top of the food chain, consuming unprecedented amounts of meat, chicken, fish, dairy products, fat, salt, and sugar. We cover our food with artificial chemicals while it is grown, processed, preserved, and genetically altered in ways that have only recently been introduced on this planet.

AGRICULTURE AND FARMING

Even natural and local farming is being polluted with chemicals that the government stipulates is a requirement to maintain pH balance in the soil, for example. But in the process of adding chemicals and pesticides, the mineral content of the soil is being greatly depleted. Required naturally is a balance of phosphorus and potassium to provide high mineral content and naturally reduce insect infestations. Phosphorus helps provide the energy and nutritive quality of plants, whereas potassium facilitates maintaining the pH balance. Land grant colleges and agricultural government agents have told farmers they need more potassium to maintain pH. This has thrown off the phosphorus levels, reducing mineral content and allowing insect infestation, which then requires more chemicals. This vicious cycle has been repeated relentlessly since the 1940s, resulting in an 80% reduction of mineral content in soil and loss of nutritional content in plants.

Some research has focused on these factors in terms of the increase of cancer and other chronic diseases with respect to both the decline of nutrient content of foods as well as contamination by agricultural chemicals, illustrating the importance of relating individual organisms to a larger system. After millions of years of adaptation to the environment, during which the human body became perfectly adapted to drawing nutrition from the natural environment, we have suddenly introduced large quantities of new, artificial substances into our diets, hoping to improve on nature.

How have these "advances" affected our health? There might be a parallel regarding the use of chemicals to rid the soil from insect infestation, and the use of pharmaceuticals to treat disease in the body, when that disease may have been caused from chemically contaminated food in the first place. In contrast, traditional Chinese culture has provided a more balanced, natural approach to food and health from which we may learn and benefit. Compared to the West, until recently, the Chinese did not appear to suffer from high rates of obesity, diabetes, most cancers, heart disease, and other chronic diseases to the degree of populations in the West. By examining their cultural approach to food and health, perhaps we can learn how to mitigate diseases that are becoming increasingly common in Western populations.

EAST-WEST CULTURAL COMPARISON

Chinese foods and herbs have been recognized and utilized for medicinal purposes since antiquity. Three thousand years ago, the pharmacopeia of the semi-mythical Emperor Shen Nong ("The Divine Husbandman") began cataloguing and classifying the medicinal properties of plants. Two-thousand years ago, *The Yellow Emperor's Inner Classic of Internal Medicine* discusses therapeutic application of the five-phase theory to foods. Today it is not unusual to see a classroom kitchen in a traditional college of Chinese medicine. In larger Chinese cities, special restaurants prepare meals for specific medicinal purposes. (In the West, they would be shut down for practicing medicine without a license: and their menus would be seized by the FDA for making health claims—even when proven by 3000 years of historical evidence.)

The practices of this field are deeply rooted in the cultural traditions of China and that culture's beliefs concerning diet. They also stem from cultural beliefs regarding the body's relationship to its environment, correlation of the microcosm to the macrocosm, and the impact on health. For example, to the extent that we take care for the soil in which food is cultivated, that soil will produce foods rich in minerals and herbs that will heal disease. The Chinese see systematic correspondences between physiological processes and the cycles and seasons in nature. Therefore they take their cue from nature on how to bring disease-causing imbalances back into harmony. Rather than working against the natural cycles, they allow the cycles to support healing. Many of the foods that are used in medical therapy also are routinely prepared by families when seasons change, when illness strikes, to strengthen a woman after birth, to cause milk to fill the breasts of a new mother, and to nourish the elderly in their declining years.

The traditional Chinese *materia medica* includes minerals and animal products as well as herbs and plants. There are almost 6000 different substances recorded in the *Encyclopedia of Traditional Chinese Medicinal Substances* (*Zhong Yao Da Ci Dian*), published in 1977 by the Jiangsu College of New Medicine. This publication is actually a later entry in a long line of definitive discussions of *materia medica* that have been produced in China over the millennia.

The earliest known work is *The Divine Husbandman's Classic of the Materia Medica*, which was reconstructed by Tao Hong Jing (452–536 AD) based upon earlier sources attributed to the semi-mythical Shen-Nong. This text classified upper-, middle-, and lower-grade herbs, and discussed the tastes, temperatures, toxicities, and medicinal properties of 364 substances.

A Chinese "prescription" for medical purposes might consist of both constituents we would consider as medicinal herbs, as well as others we would more typically consider as foods. For example, the constituents and dosage of one formula for a diagnosis of "wind cold evil" are 9 g of ephedra, 6 g of cinnamon twig (*gui zhi*), 9 g of apricot kernel (*xing ren*), and 3 g of licorice (*gan cao*).

Ingredients in a traditional formula are identified as the ruler, minister, adjutant, and emissary, according to the governmental roles analogous to historical Chinese social organization (see Chapter 28). The ruler sets the therapeutic direction of the formula. In this case, the ruler of the formula is ephedra (traditional source of sympathomimetic ephedrine), which is acrid and warm; it promotes sweating, dispels cold, and resolves the surface. Cinnamon twig is the minister, working to assist the ruler in carrying out its objectives; in addition, cinnamon itself is said to warm the body (it drives glucose into muscle and tissues). Apricot kernel (containing minerals and a very minute dose of cyanide, stimulating breathing) is the adjutant, and so addresses the possible involvement of the lung and moderates the acrid flavor of the two other substances. Finally, licorice (effects renal filtration of the blood) is the emissary, serving both to render the action of the other herbs harmonious and to distribute them through the body.

The foregoing is a brief, simple example of Chinese diet-herbal therapy, which can be related to pharmacological properties, but is quite complex and capable of addressing an even broader range of conditions than is Chinese acupuncture. In terms of complexity and the diagnostic acumen required of the practitioner, it resembles the Western practice of internal medicine. Herbal therapy encompasses the external applications of herbs as well as internal doses taken in the form of powder, pills, pastes, or tinctures as well as traditional water decoctions.

FOODS, NUTRITION, AND DIET

It is part of conventional wisdom in the West that many useful technologies were developed in ancient China, including animal domestication, plant cultivation, and irrigation agriculture to nourish large numbers of people. However, it is not as readily accepted that the Chinese civilization also developed thousands of effective medicines from plants, and to a lesser extent, from animal and mineral sources. Just as plants are cultivated and prepared to produce nourishing foods, so are they for effective medicines. Further, the distinction between plants used as food versus medicines is not rigid, because foods themselves are considered a central part of health and healing.

FOUR SACRED GRAINS

The agricultural properties of plants were known from early times in China. The four sacred grains (barley, millet, rice, and wheat) are represented in early Chinese pictographs that emphasize the above-ground, grain-producing, nourishing portions of these plants. That barley, millet, and wheat, also known to the West, were important is evidenced by northern Chinese cuisine, for example. However, the ability of rice to withstand periodic flooding and grow partially underwater (as the Chinese waterways were being brought under control by massive state projects) gained it a prominent position throughout China. The ability of these grains to provide carbohydrates and calories to large, dense populations was an important factor in the rise of Chinese civilization.

Numbering the Diet and Counting for Tastes

Ancient Chinese wisdom calls for eating "the five cereals to nourish the vital qi of the five zhang organs, together with the five fruits, the five meats, and the five vegetables (*Su Wen*)." The center of the meal is grain, but a variety of foods should also be consumed.

The five foods within each of the categories also represent tastes. A satisfying meal should nourish the senses as well as the body. In the West, the foods with different tastes are taken in sequential order, so that at end of the meal, sweet taste buds still call for the stimulation of dessert. In Chinese and Asian cuisine the acrid, bitter, sweet, sour, and salty tastes can all be mixed together in each dish, providing a fully satisfying sensory experience:

· sweet—rice
· sour (astringent)—sesame
· salty—soybeans
· bitter—wheat
· pungent (*Ling shu*)—millet (broomcorn).

Missing from the Chinese diet is milk and there is effectively no dairy industry, probably associated with the high rate of lactose intolerance. However, it is arguable that humans are not designed to consume milk past infancy. In China, milk consumption is said to weaken the spleen creating conditions of excess phlegm such as asthma, fibroids, headaches, and nasal congestion. The association of milk with allergies and these related symptoms is well noted in Western biomedicine. ∾

However, these populations also require protein, as well as vitamins and minerals (the latter present in the unpolished husk of grains, such as brown rice and whole wheat, but removed by the milling processes that produce white rice, blanched wheat and bleached flour). Thus, we are familiar with the twentieth-century tragedy of famines in Asia, where children who were getting milled rice for calories suffered from protein deficiency (kwashiokor), or B vitamin deficiencies such as beri beri (thiamine) and pellagra (niacin). Protein is harder to come by in the plant kingdom but the botanical species know as legumes (the large family and varieties of beans) is relatively high in proteins. Proteins are made up of chains of nitrogen-containing amino acids. Legumes are able to obtain nitrogen from the soil to ultimately make amino acids and proteins due to the presence of nitrogen-fixing bacteria in their root nodules.

Thus, in addition to the four sacred grains producing carbohydrate, another Chinese plant of great agricultural importance and nutritional significance is the legume, soybean.

ADDING A FIFTH "GRAIN"

Unlike the Chinese characters for the four sacred grains, the character for soy emphasizes the lower part of the pictograph, or the portion of the plant that is underground. Another characteristic of legumes, like soy, together with the protein they produce, is the ability of their roots to host nitrogen-fixing bacteria.

These legume plants allow bacteria that pull nitrogen from the air to literally "take root" underground, feeding the plant and replenishing nitrogen into the soil. Soils rich in nitrogen do not require nitrogen fertilizers. Thus, this remarkable plant replenishes soils that become exhausted through intensive growing of grains. Furthermore, the ability to draw nitrogen from the atmosphere also allows leguminous plants to form the amino acids (nitrogen-based biochemicals) that, in turn, are the building blocks of protein. Rotating crops by planting soy in between seasons of cultivating grains helps the soil to remain productive. There is some evidence that ancient Chinese practiced this kind of "crop rotation."

As a food, however, the soybean's nutritious proteins come together with other constituents that are virtually indigestible (although they prevent animals and insects from predation as natural pesticides). These other substances include antitryptic factors that literally inhibit the digestive enzyme trypsin (and in severe poisonings can cause some symptoms like cystic fibrosis). Somehow, through historical trial and error, the Chinese learned to prepare the soy in various ways that eliminate the toxic poisons. For example, if soy is mixed with water, and then sea salt is added, or simply mixed with sea water, the calcium (chemical symbol Ca), magnesium (Mg) and other minerals in the sea salt combine with the soy proteins to form solids (technically a divalent cation protein precipitation, where minerals with two positive (2+) chemical charges, like Ca^{2+} and Mg^{2+}, combine with protein in water solution to form solids). These proteins precipitate from the water to form solids, leaving the toxic poisons behind in the water. When the water is squeezed out of the solid protein, as with the preparation of tofu, a nutritious food results. Another way to neutralize the poisons is to ferment the soy and add salts, creating the well-known soy sauce, which, when added to rice, forms a more nutritionally adequate meal of carbohydrate and protein.

DIET AS THERAPY

In addition to nourishment, diet can be used to prevent disease, promote longevity or help treat an existing condition. For disease treatment, diet is usually employed as an adjunct to acupuncture and/or herbal medicine. Dietary guidelines for disease are based upon the correspondences that apply in other areas of treatment. To soothe the liver qi and clear heat, the patient avoids liver-heating foods such as alcohol, coffee, cola, and red meat, so that these foods do not interfere with the treatments. The exclusion of certain foods is just as important as the prescription of others.

DIGESTION

Chinese medicine recognizes the role of a healthy digestive system in preventing and treating disease. The *Zang-Fu* organ system identified as the spleen and stomach correspond most closely to the functions of digestion and absorption in Western medicine. The strength of the spleen and the stomach are considered critical to prevention, treatment or recovery from essentially every condition, as they are responsible for taking in food and fluids, transforming them to qi and blood, and transporting them throughout the body. The importance of relationships between the organs is emphasized as we look at the role they play in terms of production, transformation and transportation of qi. Beginning with food consumption, the stomach breaks down the food, and its (earth element) pair, the spleen, then transforms it into blood and qi. Each organ relays energy in specific ways, much like members of a team. The spleen moves energy up to the lungs to "mist" the body, creating what eventually becomes nutritive qi for the organs and defensive qi that circulates just under the skin (the body's protective layer and first defense against pathogens). The lungs, through the expelling of respirated toxins (sneezing, coughing, etc.), are paired with the large intestine through the metal element responsible for elimination. Very often what presents as sinus and allergy problems are due to the stagnation of the large intestine's function to properly eliminate waste products from the body.

These concepts illustrate why digestion is central to Chinese medical beliefs regarding health and recovery from illness. From this example, we can begin to see the "domino effect" that each organ's role and function, as it relates to the transformation and transportation of qi, has on the rest of body. Besides the five-element pairing, each organ has an impact on other organs. In the foregoing example, the lungs, responsible for water (*yin*) regulation in the upper half of the body, also share a relationship with the kidneys, which regulate water in the lower half of the body. Outside of its (metal element) relationship with the lungs, the large intestine can produce a deleterious effect on all organs if toxins back up and leach into the blood stream.

In Chinese medicine, the *way* one eats is just as important for health as *what* one eats. Irregular eating times, eating in haste, and eating iced foods all weaken the function of the spleen and stomach. Importantly, the state of the spleen–stomach functions are crucial to every condition in Chinese medicine. In Western medicine, the state of digestion is considered only when it is the chief complaint rather than being considered in *all* medical conditions.

Chinese diet therapy emphasizes that only foods of good quality, properly prepared, are healthful. As an ancient tradition, it cannot directly address the problems of modern agricultural practices such the use of antibiotics, food processing, herbicides, hormones, pesticides, irradiation or genetic manipulation.

Likewise, ancient Chinese medicine does not consider terms such as nutrients or phytochemicals, although there is recognition that fresh foods (higher in nutrients) are preferable. Thus, locally grown foods are fresher and considered preferable. Further, food is a source of qi. The vitality, or life force, remaining in the food is the main consideration.

FOOD OR HERBAL MEDICINE?

The properties by which foods are considered are the same as those used for medicinal plants: five flavors, four natures, four directions, and channel propensity. There is a fine line between foods and herbs and they are often used together. Certainly, herbs which are considered as spices can be ingredients in preparation of foods for consumption. Plants contain biologically active constituents as a product of their adaptation and growth in the terrestrial environment where they compete for sustenance and against predation by animals, insects, fungi, and bacteria. In fact, the antibacterial properties of many spices, allowing the preservation of meats and other foods, made them very valuable during the period of Portuguese, Spanish, Dutch, French, and British exploration in Greater China and Southeast Asia (see Chapter 35) and were a prime motivator for establishing a European presence there. It is no accident that the Indonesian archipelago of Southeast Asia was long called the "Spice Islands."

In general, strictly herbal preparations are stronger than food preparations and are meant to be used only for short periods of time.

THE FIVE FLAVORS

As described in the highlighted section "Numbering the Diet and Counting for Tastes" on page 458, the five different tastes each have different actions in the body:

Sour (including astringent)
>   Retains and arrests loss of fluids (for diarrhea, sweat)
>   Generates fluids, promotes proper digestion
>   Hawthorne berries (cardioactive), lemons, apricots, cherries, grapefruit (also sweet)

Bitter
>   Drying and purging (for constipation, reflux, cough)
>   Bitter melon, dandelion greens

Sweet
>   Tonify and strengthen blood (for pain and spasms)
>   Chicken, eggs, fruits, mutton, root vegetables

Pungent
>   Expels pathogens and promotes qi and blood flow
>   Chilis, ginger, pepper, spring onions

Salty
>   Softens and resolves masses (goiter)
>   Kelp, seaweed (iodine)

FOUR NATURES, DIRECTIONS, AND CHANNEL PROPENSITY

The four *natures* of foods refer to the temperatures of cold, cool, warm and hot. The nature of the food is determined by its effect on the body. If it lowers a fever, it is considered cold. If it promotes blood circulation and warms the extremities, it is considered warm or hot.

Once food is digested it can have an impact on the *direction* of the flow of qi (ascending, descending, floating, and sinking):

- Ascending for diarrhea and organ prolapse
- Floating (dispersing) for common cold, promotes perspiration
- Sinking for constipation, high blood pressure, mania
- Descending for belching and indigestion, hiccups, nausea and vomiting.

The nature of disease is often characterized by "rebellious qi," that is, qi that is moving in the opposite direction of its natural flow. For example, the spleen, once it transforms the food, moves it up to the lungs. When rebellious qi occurs, energy moves down before being digested and one experiences diarrhea. Another example of qi moving opposite to natural flow is when women experience hot flashes or night sweats. Yin energy governs rest and night time, while yang governs waking and day time. When women experience a depletion of the yin energy due to menopause or illnesses that cause hormonal imbalance, yang overacts on yin and produces heat when the body should be cool and resting. But even hormonal imbalances have a direct connection to digestion by way of the spleen and liver. The spleen is responsible for the formation of blood, and the liver for the storing of blood when the body rests. If an imbalance in diet causes hormonal changes, the liver overacts on the spleen and can produce blood stagnation and/or other blood flow issues that disrupt the natural flow of blood and qi.

The *parts* of a plant food are also relevant. Flowers and leaves tend to move upward; fruits, roots and seeds tend to move downward. The propensity determines the organ channel to which a food is likely to travel. Most foods go to at least two channels. For example, lemons, pears and tangerines clear heat from the lung channel to stop coughs. Tangerines also go to the stomach channel to address loss of appetite and nausea. The flavor, nature and channel propensity of a food determines its medicinal value.

SEASONALITY

Just as time of day and circumstances for food preparation and consumption are important, so are the four seasons. Beyond the fact that different foods are available in different seasons (sweet potatoes and root vegetables in winter; watermelon and salad greens in summer), in Chinese medicine the seasons have a direct effect on the body, which in turn indicates different foods to be appropriate:

- **Spring**: warming; more sweet than sour foods, to nourish spleen qi when liver qi is strong
- **Summer**: hot; digestion slows, light foods to clear heat and generate fluids; more fruits and vegetables, less meat
- **Autumn**: cooling, avoid extremes of hot or cold; yang-qi diminishing (energy), yin-qi (substance) growing; foods moderate in nature
- **Winter**: cold; tonify and rebalance; yang-qi deficient, yin-qi in excess; beef, mutton, nourishing and invigorating diet

Living inside controlled environments works against the natural effects of the seasonal cycle. Excessive indoor cooling when temperatures should normally be hot in summer, and dry heating when temperatures should be cold in winter, require modifications: add some warming foods to a light summer diet of fruits and vegetables; tonify with moistening foods in winter. Geographic locations also influence seasonal climate. In hot, humid climates, "damp" disorders will be worse in later summer; while in hot, dry desert climates, "dry" disorders may worsen in autumn.

The aging process mirrors the seasons. In children (Spring), internal damp syndromes frequently lead to nasal congestion and running, asthma, and ear infections. Cold and moist foods such as dairy aggravate damp conditions and should be avoided in children. The elderly (Winter) have weakening digestive functions and should have small, frequent meals, well-cooked and easy to digest soups and stews. In pregnant women, fluids collect in certain channels, leaving others relatively dry, so drying foods such as spices and wines should be avoided.

Emotional states also have an effect on digestion. Stress hinders proper function of spleen and stomach and requires a diet that tonifies the spleen and is easy to digest. Anger and disappointment require a diet that soothes the liver qi.

PREPARATION

Healthy food preparation begins with selection based upon cleanliness, color intensity, texture and fragrance. A key is making food that is easy to digest while retaining its nourishing value and vitality, including cutting foods into proper shapes and sizes and using appropriate cooking methods and condiments. Classic Chinese cuisine accomplishes healthy cooking by quickly heating small pieces of foods, making them easy to digest while retaining nourishment by not overheating or overcooking. Steaming, braising, stir-frying, stewing, roasting and quick boiling are common methods as suited to particular foods.

Frequently added condiments include: cilantro, chili, garlic, ginger, mustard, pepper, and spring onions. A medicinal diet can be dispensed in the form of teas, decoctions, juices, wines, gruels (with rice and millet), soups, pancakes, candied fruits, and other forms.

The healthful properties of foods are maintained or enhanced through proper cultivation, selection, preparation, consumption and digestion. Each step in this process "from field to table," to spleen–stomach, is given attention by Chinese medicine. The properties of foods are similar to those ascribed to medicinal plants and other healthful influences on qi, blood and body.

Traditionally, careful attention is given to how foods are cultivated, how they are prepared, when they are eaten, and in what combinations. Loss of attention to these important factors in the modern Western diet has led to dietary constituents, habits and patterns that appear to be associated with increasing rates of chronic diseases.

DISEASES OF WESTERN AFFLUENCE AND DIET

In the West it is thought that many contemporary diseases are associated with diet and other lifestyle factors that accompanied rapid changes associated with "modernity," including relative affluence and leaving behind agrarian practices, physical labor, and local community activities.

One-third of the U.S. population is significantly overweight, and one-quarter of adult males, adult females, and children are considered obese. This development (now considered a "disease" by the American Medical Association and the Federal Government) is caused by a variety of factors, ranging from genetics to the introduction of the automobile (reducing the necessity to move around) and television (reducing the motivation to move around). A clear and direct correlation exists between excess food and total caloric consumption and excess body weight.

Research has shown an equally clear and direct connection between excessive body weight and some illnesses, including leading killers in the U.S.: cardiovascular disease and certain cancers. Today, 60 million Americans have cardiovascular disease, including high blood pressure, heart disease, and stroke. Annually, cardiovascular disease kills about 1 million Americans, more than 2600 a day, or one death every 33 seconds. Another 1.2 million people are diagnosed with cancer, and almost 600,000 die from it. Millions more suffer from other diseases related to diet: diabetes, gallbladder disease, respiratory disease, sleep apnea, gout, osteoporosis, and a host of other conditions.

For more than a century, the U.S. Department of Agriculture (USDA) has been trying to influence our eating habits by issuing dietary recommendations. It currently spends hundreds of millions of dollars per year educating the public about what we should and should not consume and in what quantities (USDA, 2010). That cost seems a great expenditure until we consider that America's food manufacturers spend that amount just promoting snacks and nuts; their total annual advertising budget is more than $10 billion, most of which is spent promoting highly processed, packaged foods. The fast-paced American lifestyle relies on these convenience foods and on restaurant and take-out fare. We now spend about 50% of our food dollars on away-from-home meals and snacks, most of which are higher in fat, salt, and sugar and lower in fiber and calcium than meals prepared at home—not to mention the larger, "oversized" portions that have become fashionable.

According to the USDA's *Healthy Eating Index,* some small improvements were made in the American diet at the end of the last century (Box 26-1). On a scale of 1 to 100, the average U.S. score rose from 61.5 in 1990 to 63.8 in 1995, but it still falls far short of the 80 or above that marks a good diet. Put another way, Americans are earning about a C− in healthy eating practices.

BOX 26-1 *American Eating Habits: 1900 to 1980*

Fresh fruit and vegetable consumption drops from 40% to 5% of the diet
Sugar consumption rises 50%
Beef consumption rises 50%
Fat and oil consumption rises 150%
Cheese consumption rises 400%
Margarine consumption rises 800%

WHAT ARE WE EATING?

Most Americans know (but do not necessarily act on) the basic facts: a healthy diet includes lots of fresh, unprocessed fruits, vegetables, and grains; modest amounts of protein and fat; and very little white bread, rice, sugar and salt. The question of precisely how much of each type of food we need, however, becomes more complicated.

All food provides energy, which is measured in units called *calories*. Nutritionists generally recommend daily intake of 1600 calories for older adults and sedentary women; 2200 calories for children, teenage girls, active women, and sedentary men; and 2800 calories for teenage boys, active men, and very active women. Calories are taken into our bodies as carbohydrates, proteins, and fats (which are known as *macronutrients,* or major constituents of diet). We also require vitamins and minerals (which are active in small amounts and thus are known as *micronutrients*) to process these nutrients and maintain body functions.

Nutritionists, physicians, research scientists, alternative practitioners, food manufacturers, and consumers hold differing views about what percentage of calories we should obtain from each macronutrient. People favoring a largely vegetarian, low-fat diet tend to recommend that we receive about 15% of our calories from protein, 60% from carbohydrates, and 25% from fats. Proponents of high-protein diets often advocate 30% protein, 40% carbohydrates, and 30% fats. The food pyramid, developed by the U.S. Department of Health and Human Services and USDA, whose job is to support agricultural commodities, suggests that we use fat "sparingly" and that our daily fare include two to three servings of dairy products; two to three servings of meat, poultry, fish, eggs, beans, and nuts; three to five servings of vegetables; two to four servings of fruit; and six to eleven servings of bread, cereal, rice, and pasta (Box 26-2).

Although these numbers may provide useful guidelines, they do not address one crucial factor: the *quality and quantity* of actual nutrients in each food category. The food pyramid, which recommends six to eleven servings of grain-based foods, fails to distinguish, for example, between the empty calories of frozen waffles, which are composed primarily of white sugar and white flour, and a bowl of whole-grain cereal. It encourages us to use fats "sparingly" but advocates two or three helpings of cheese and whole milk, which contain at least 8 g of fat per serving, plus up to three servings of meat, which can contain up to 26 g of

BOX 26-2 *The Changing Shape of U.S. Government Guidelines*

Over the years, the U.S. Department of Agriculture has revised its dietary recommendations in response to research findings and new concepts of nutrition.

1946 to 1958: The "Basic 7" Daily Food Guide

Leafy, green, and yellow vegetables: one or more servings
Citrus fruit, tomatoes, raw cabbage: one or more servings
Potatoes and other vegetables and fruits: two or more servings
Milk, cheese, ice cream: children, one to four cups of milk; adults, two or more cups
Meat, poultry, fish, eggs, dried peas, beans: one to two servings
Bread, cereal, flour: two or more servings
Butter and fortified margarine: two tablespoons

1958 to 1979: The Four Basic Food Groups (per day, for adults)

Milk group: two or more cups
Meat group: two or more servings
Vegetable and fruit group: four or more servings
Bread and cereal group: four or more servings

1979 to 2005 The Food Pyramid (per day)

Fats, oils, sweets: use sparingly
Milk, yogurt, cheese: three to five servings
Dried beans, nuts, seeds, eggs, meat: two to three servings
Vegetables: three to five servings
Fruits: two to four servings
Bread, cereal, rice, pasta: six to eleven servings

2005 MyPyramid

Customized based on personal characteristics
Personal plans available at http://www.mypyramid.gov

fat per serving. Is a Whopper® (40 g of fat) part of a healthy diet? Are Pop-Tarts® (20 g of white sugar) giving us the right kind of energy to start the day?

Clearly the numbers alone do not tell the whole story. All carbohydrates are not created equal, nor does everyone need the same amount of them, or of any given nutrient, in light of metabolic and nutritional individuality. "One-size-fits-all" works no better for diet and nutrition than it does for other health and medical treatments (Chapter 3). Our food needs are influenced by many factors, such as age, gender, body size, activity level, and reproductive status, and change over time. To determine what type of diet is best for our bodies at different stages of our lives, requires some understanding of how the nutrients in food enable our bodies to function.

CARBOHYDRATES

Carbohydrates (carbon, hydrogen and oxygen) provide large amounts of quick energy. We obtain carbohydrates from fruits, vegetables, beans, grains, and other plant materials, as well as from dairy products. Our bodies readily transform more complex carbohydrates into the simple carbohydrate *glucose* (blood sugar), which the body needs for fuel, and into *glycogen,* a form of sugar that can be stored in the liver and muscles until needed, then transformed into glucose. Fructose found in fruits is a simple carbohydrate that does not provide quite the quick energy of glucose. It's absorption is slower from the natural bio-matrix of fruit pulps and it appears to be metabolized differently (Stanhope et al, 2009). It's consumption does not appear to be associated with diabetes and metabolic syndrome in the same way as glucose and sucrose consumption.

There are two basic types of carbohydrates: simple and complex. *Simple* carbohydrates, or simple sugars, include white table sugar (sucrose), the sugar in fruit (fructose), and the sugar in milk (lactose). In *complex* carbohydrates, such as whole grains, beans, and vegetables, the sugar molecules are linked together in longer, more complicated chains, such as starches.

Both types of carbohydrates ultimately become blood sugar, but the simple sugar glucose is converted more quickly, elevating insulin levels and providing a "sugar rush" that quickly abates, often leading to feelings of tiredness. Fructose from fruits has a much more balanced effect on blood sugar and metabolism. Sucrose (cane sugar, table sugar, confectionary sugar) is a disaccharide of fructose and glucose that affects the body primarily like glucose itself.

Complex carbohydrates and fructose are absorbed and/or metabolized more slowly, providing a more sustained supply of energy. One complex carbohydrate has a different role: fiber is not absorbed into the body at all but helps with digestive and bowel function. One of the disadvantages of an overprocessed, highly refined, low-fiber diet is that foods tend to linger in the body, which can allow carcinogens (cancer-causing substances) to be more highly absorbed and/or produced by the body (see Chapters 22 and 23). The right fiber in the diet has been shown to reduce constipation, which decreases the risk of colon, breast, and other cancers; it also shrinks intestinal polyps (growths), which can lead to cancers. About 25 g of the right fiber a day is usually sufficient and occurs naturally in a diet that includes a good supply of complex carbohydrates, from whole grains, fruits and vegetables.

PROTEINS

Protein (carbon, hydrogen, oxygen and nitrogen) is essential for the growth, maintenance, and repair of every cell in the body and for the production of hormones, antibodies, and digestive enzymes. When we consume dietary protein, we break it down into amino acids, which are the building blocks we need to make our own proteins.

There are two types of dietary proteins: complete and incomplete. *Complete* proteins, which are found in meat, poultry, fish, eggs, dairy products, and soybeans, provide the full range of essential amino acids we need. *Incomplete* proteins, which include some but not all needed amino acids, are found in grains, beans, nuts, seeds, and leafy green vegetables. However, incomplete proteins can be combined to provide the full range of amino acids our bodies require. For example, brown rice served with beans, nuts, or seeds forms a whole protein source (like the classic beans and rice dishes in many traditional cuisines).

Protein forms muscle and other tissues, but is not stored in the body for ready use (not like glycogen is stored for energy), so we need to replenish our supply every day. Most Americans consume twice the protein they need. When more protein is taken in than the body can use, the excess carbon, hydrogen and oxygen is either burned off as energy or stored in the body as fat—and the excess nitrogen component is filtered through the kidney as urea and uric acid in the urine.

FATS

Fat is the most concentrated form of energy available in the diet (about 9 kcal of energy per gram; vs. 5 kcal per gram carbohydrate). It is necessary for growth and healthy function of all cells and tissues in the body. Babies and children need fat for brain development and adults for healthy central nervous system and peripheral nerve cells. As adults, many consume more than we need, which leads to weight gain and a national obsession about staying thin, especially for women. Conflicting cultural pressures and misdirection by government recommendations make it difficult to obtain a realistic picture of the right amounts and types of fat we need.

Our body's fats are made up of fatty acids, which come in three major types: saturated, polyunsaturated, and monounsaturated.

Saturated fatty acids come from meats (e.g., beef, lamb, veal, pork), egg yolks, dairy products (e.g., cream, whole milk), and a few plant products, including coconut oil and vegetable shortening. The liver turns saturated fat into cholesterol, which is used to make cell membranes, hormones, and vitamin D. Cholesterol in the diet is broken down through digestion and does not result in cholesterol in the blood nor correlate with serum cholesterol levels. Increased saturated fat consumption has been said to raise serum cholesterol levels, however. Despite misguided recommendations over many years, saturated fat consumption is not associated with increased risk of cardiovascular diseases (Hite et al, 2010; Ravnskov, 1998) and in fact omega-3 fats reduce the risk of heart disease and other chronic diseases (Lands, 2005). It is also questionable as to the actual role of cholesterol in cardiovascular diseases (Hite et al, 2010).

Cholesterol travels through the body in the form of lipoproteins. *Low-density lipoproteins* (LDLs, or "bad cholesterol") contain larger amounts of cholesterol, whereas *high-density lipoproteins* (HDLs, or "good cholesterol") carry relatively lesser amounts of cholesterol and help remove excess cholesterol from blood and tissues. If the LDL level is too high for the HDLs to clear away the excess cholesterol, it may be one factor contributing to forming plaque on the artery walls, which together with high blood pressure, and inflammation, may lead to heart disease. However, data from around the world indicated that lower cholesterol is actually associated with higher cancer and overall mortality rates (Hite et al, 2010).

Polyunsaturated fatty acids (PUFAs) are found in corn, soybean, safflower, and sunflower oils and some fish oils. PUFAs may actually help lower "bad" cholesterol levels, but they have a tendency to lower HDL levels as well, leaving the body less capable of removing the amounts of cholesterol that are present. PUFAs have been thought to pose a health risk if too many are used in the diet but their role in cardiovascular diseases is also questionable (Ravnskov, 1998).

Monounsaturated fatty acids are found in olive, peanut, canola, and other vegetable and nut oils. These fats actually reduce LDL level slightly and do not reduce HDL level, so they benefit the body when taken in moderation so as not to result in excess calories.

Many oils are actually a combination of these different types of fatty acids, but in general, one type predominates, which is how the oil is described on the food label.

Trans-fats are hydrogenated fats as described above, do not occur naturally and should be avoided in the diet. They are associated with marked increases in the risk of cardiovascular disease.

The Whole Truth About Whole Milk

Cow's milk can be an ideal food—it is for calves. When it comes to human infants, children, and adults, the cow's milk issue is cloudy. Cow's milk is three times higher in protein than is human breast milk. In fact, human breast milk has among the lowest levels of protein of any milk from mammals. Among different animal species, the higher the growth rate of infants of that species, the higher the protein content of that species' milk. Survival among the young of most species requires rapid rates of growth and maturation. This is not the case for human infants, who grow more slowly and mature over a longer time period.

Not only does cow's milk have higher total protein content, but the type of protein present is very different from that in human milk. Cow's milk is six times higher in casein protein (which has been shown to promote tumors in some laboratory animal experiments). Also, cow's milk is low in linoleic acid, which may be important for early human growth and health. For these reasons and more, cow's milk is not an ideal food for human infants and babies—breast milk is.

Among adults around the world, it is rare in most populations to consume whole milk in the diet. However, in some parts of the world, dairy animal domestication represents a renewable resource for converting plants and grasses from the environment (which are inedible for humans) into usable human food sources. Humans cannot digest or extract nutrients from many plants containing cellulose (grasses, woods). And, in fact, neither can cows—by themselves. However, ruminants like cows have multiple stomachs, which allow bacteria present in them to ferment cellulose so that it can be digested. In the cow, it is converted to meat and milk. Even termites rely on bacteria in their digestive tracts to digest cellulose from the wood they eat. The use of domesticated animals to graze on grasses allows humans to survive in relatively harsh, dry environments where there may not be enough other food to eat. Dairy animal domestication can be traced back approximately 10,000 years to parts of the world now called the Middle East, where the use of these animals allowed humans to survive in areas where they otherwise might not.

Human digestive problems can also be caused by milk consumption, however. Milk contains lactose, or milk sugar, which can only be digested by a special enzyme, lactase, that breaks down lactose. All infants are born with lactase to digest milk sugar. However, most adults in most populations lose the lactase enzyme when they get older (and no longer would normally be expected to drink milk). These adults are intolerant of milk because of the lactose, which they cannot digest. They experience indigestion, intestinal problems, and possible malnutrition due to malabsorption from drinking milk. In South Asia, the Middle East and the Mediterranean region, local cultures have developed processes that allow bacteria to break down lactose through fermentation. Thus, production of cheeses, yogurts, and other cultured dairy products allows people to eat dairy foods without getting the lactose in whole milk that causes digestive problems. In China and East Asia, there is no dairy production at all, and milk and milk products do not form any part of the diet. This circumstance raises a question: how do over 1 billion of the world's people get adequate calcium without any dairy foods? (see next section of this textbox)

Northern Europeans generally retain the lactase enzyme during adulthood, which allows them to digest milk and its lactose sugar without digestive problems. Whole milk (about 3.4% fat content) can be an important source of essential fat (and calories), as well as calcium, when consumed as a beverage in some populations. However, it is difficult for many Americans to avoid too much fat and calories (as well as carbs) in their foods, but to avoid drinking it in our beverages, there are no-fat and low-fat (1% and 2%) milks commonly available.

But what about calcium? Don't we need to drink milk to get calcium?

The Whole Truth About Whole Milk—cont'd

Milk as a Source of Calcium

Milk is a good source of calcium, and it becomes more difficult to obtain adequate calcium when bypassing all milk and dairy products (as in a strictly vegan diet). There is evidence to suggest that humans do not build bone by milk alone. Dairy-free diets are not necessarily deficient in calcium. Other sources of calcium in the diet include fish, and some vegetables, grains, and seeds. Over 1 billion people in China generally appear to get enough calcium in the diet, although, as noted earlier, there is no dairy industry or dairy consumption there. The Chinese refer to butter and cheese as "animal secretion" when they encounter it in the West. There are no words in Chinese for products that do not exist there. The Chinese also have high rates of lactose intolerance, which perhaps explains why a dairy industry never developed there. Perhaps the Chinese get enough calcium from eating bits of bone and sinew left behind in traditional preparations of meat and fish dishes. Bone is the best source of calcium of all, whether people eat the bones of sardines or when normally herbivorous animals consume bone. When deprived of calcium even cows (and other ruminants) will eat the bones of other animals (although they are normally herbivores).

Proper calcium nutrition is not only dependent on getting enough calcium in the diet but also having adequate vitamin D to absorb it from the gastrointestinal (GI) tract. Vitamin D must be activated by sunlight on the bare skin to be effective (see the highlighted section "The Light Cure and Vitamin D" in Chapter 15). Adequate calcium nutrition depends on the GI tract, liver, kidneys, bone, and skin cells. Vitamin D deficiency became a problem in many people when populations moved into dark urban centers during the Industrial Revolution over the last two centuries. People no longer got enough fresh vegetables (because they had left the farms) and they did not get enough sun because they were kept indoors or lived in dark urban "canyons." One result was high rates of rickets (vitamin D deficiency and bone deformity).

Plants naturally contain inactive vitamin D sources, which normally are eaten but then must be activated by sunlight in the skin cells. This inactive form is the kind of vitamin D naturally contained in cow's milk, which comes from plants eaten by the cow. Today, milk does contain artificially activated vitamin D that does not require conversion by sunlight in the skin. However, without enough consumption of calcium-containing foods and vegetables and without adequate exposure of the skin to sunlight, it is not possible for most people to get adequate amounts of vitamin D. Many experts observe that there is presently a worldwide insufficiency or outright deficiency of vitamin D when it comes to optimal levels for health (Holick, 2003).

Beyond the nutritional aspects of milk, cow's milk proteins may produce allergies in infants and children, which may threaten proper growth and be present for life. These infant allergies may have long-lasting effects on the immune systems. Many have noted an increase in adult allergies, which have been blamed on all manner of modern pollutants and allergens. One may well wonder whether a whole generation of infants raised on the "enlightened" practice of bottle feeding with cow's milk after WW II are now a generation of adults with lifelong allergies.

Twenty years ago, certified raw milk could be found contaminated with *Listeria*, a bacterium responsible for the deaths of infants and children and harm to pregnant women. Historically cows and cow's milk had been carriers of diseases, including tuberculosis. The reason milk required pasteurization is that it could be contaminated with dangerous bacteria. Some paleopathological research into the history of diseases shows that human tuberculosis may have originated with contact between humans and cows beginning 10,000 years ago.

Today the risks of chronic disease from excess consumption of fats and calories as present in whole milk are a greater danger than infectious contamination of raw milk. There are also risks to infants. Failure to breastfeed in infancy often leads to overnourished and overweight infants. Human infants given cow's milk are by definition overfed. This overfeeding during infancy may cause excess fat deposition and increase body mass. These problems may have long-term disease consequences.

Americans still drink more whole milk than other low-fat varieties such as skim. Substitute skim or low-fat milk for whole milk and learn to like it. Drinking liquid fat (whole milk) is an acquired taste in any case. ∾

VITAMINS

In 1913, American biochemist Elmer McCollum became the first scientist to isolate a vitamin. Further research revealed that this substance, which (in alphabetic order) became known as vitamin A, helps maintain skin, teeth, bones, hair, mucous membranes, and reproductive capacity. We can obtain vitamin A from cream, butter, egg yolks, cod liver oil, and some pre-vitamin A (alpha and beta-carotene) from some yellow-orange vegetables, or we can simply take a supplement containing vitamin A. The great vitamin debate for decades is that scientists have been arguing about whether supplements containing vitamins and minerals are a useful, even necessary, addition to the diet or whether we can and should obtain all the vitamins and minerals we need from the foods we eat.

No one disputes the need for vitamins, which enable us to make use of the energy and structural components stored in food to perform a variety of functions, ranging from maintaining the nervous system to forming red blood cells. There are two main categories of vitamins: fat soluble and water soluble. The *fat-soluble* vitamins, including A, D, E, and K, can be stored in the liver and in body fat for weeks or months, whereas *water-soluble* vitamins dissolve quickly in the bloodstream and are removed in urine or sweat. Because water-soluble vitamins cannot be stored, these vitamins need to be resupplied on a daily basis. The most essential water-soluble vitamins are B vitamins (B_1, B_2, B_6, B_{12}), folic acid, niacin, pantothenic acid, and biotin, and vitamin C. Humans are unique (together with guinea pigs) for being the only animals that do not make their own vitamin C.

There is some controversy about how much of each vitamin we need to stay healthy. The U.S. Food and Drug Administration issues guidelines based on the National Academy of Science's recommended daily allowances (often listed on supplement labels as RDAs). Some consider these numbers the minimum needed to maintain health, whereas others maintain that these amounts are not sufficient for optimal health as revealed by research.

Vitamin C Controversies

Vitamin C, one of the most popular and widely debated vitamins, provides a good example of these divergent views. The RDA for vitamin C is 60 mg/day, the amount found in a single orange. Consuming less than this amount compromises the immune system, bones, and skin and even the ability to reproduce. Researchers at the University of California at Berkeley and the USDA's Western Human Nutritional Research Center determined that without 60 mg of vitamin C per day, waste products of metabolism known as *free radicals* can damage DNA. This can lead to cancer, heart disease, and other illnesses in all of us. For would-be fathers, this means sperm may contain genetic mutations that can result in birth defects, genetic disease, and cancer in future children.

Since the amount of vitamin C in a single orange can prevent all that, what can larger amounts do?

Linus Pauling, winner of Nobel Prizes for Chemistry and for Peace, would have responded that megadoses of vitamin C can fight colds and boost the immune system. He consumed 300 times the recommended amount, about 18,000 mg every day. Because vitamin C is water soluble, he pointed out, any excess will wash out harmlessly in the urine. Some scientists argue that our physiology and metabolism may not be equipped to handle micronutrients at levels higher than could be found in nature. Many complementary and alternative medicine practitioners take the middle path, advocating 300 to 3000 mg of vitamin C per day.

Then there is the real controversy: are you better off eating oranges or taking vitamin C tablets? To some extent that depends on where you stand in the dosage debate; eating one orange a day is manageable, eating 300 is not. As we learned with limes, natural foods are complex arrangements of ingredients that tend to work best together rather than in isolation or synthesized form. We have identified a number of vitamins and their uses but may be far from understanding the full range of benefits we obtain from whole foods. Most physicians recommend receiving vitamins from a healthy diet. That is good advice, but in a nation earning a C– in nutrition, not very realistic. If your intake for the day consists of frozen waffles and coffee for breakfast, a hot dog with fries and cola for lunch, and pizza for dinner, you are probably going to miss a few nutrients. The most practical approach is to eat a balanced diet. Most daily, "multivitamin" supplements appear haphazard in their doses and ingredients and are often of poor quality by industry standards. Most people do not require the iron supplementation included in such standard formulations. Given the often poor nutritional quality of foods, and poor balance in our daily diets, dietary supplementation is best assured vitamin by vitamin.

Vitamin A

The medical world has been very vigilant about the possible toxicity of micronutrients while remaining reluctant to embrace the evidence that optimal levels of micronutrients to help prevent or treat diseases are higher than the well-established RDAs. Vitamin A is a particular example. Because it is a fat-soluble vitamin, excess intake is not readily eliminated, which leads to the possibility of toxicity. Today, although reports of hypervitaminosis A are rare, deficiency of vitamin A is common and can even be considered an epidemic in certain portions of the world population.

National data from the American Association of Poison Control Centers repeatedly fail to show even one death from vitamin A per year. Vitamin A is very safe. However, pregnancy is a special case in which prolonged intake of too much preformed oil-form vitamin A might be harmful to the fetus, even at relatively low levels (under 20,000 IU/day). Interestingly, you can get over 100,000 IU of vitamin A from eating only 7 oz of beef liver. Have you ever yet seen a pregnancy overdose warning on a supermarket package of liver?

In fact, lack of vitamin A, especially during pregnancy and in infancy, poses far greater risks. Deficiency of vitamin A in developing babies is known to cause birth defects, poor tooth enamel, a weakened immune system, and literally hundreds of thousands of cases of blindness per year worldwide. Those are reasons why developing countries safely give megadoses of vitamin A to newborns.

Vitamin A metabolism Vitamin A (retinol) functions as a constituent of visual pigments, allows for normal reproductive capacity in both males and females, and permits normal cellular growth and differentiation. Among micronutrients, only retinol and its chemical derivatives can serve all of these biological functions.

The fat-soluble substance essential for normal growth that we now call vitamin A was recognized in 1909 and named in 1920. Preformed vitamin A, or the aldehyde and alcohol forms and their esters, are found mainly in animal products, including milk, eggs, meat, and fish, and is not synthesized by plants. However, provitamin A, which includes β-carotene among several other carotenoids, is found in plant sources and cannot be synthesized either by humans or animals. Both forms are also commonly found in over-the-counter pharmaceutical compounds. For the most part, β-carotene is converted to vitamin A during absorption through the intestinal mucosa, where it and preformed vitamin A are transported in the plasma by lipoproteins. Vitamin A is then stored in the liver in fat cells.

Wolbach and Howe (1925) were the first investigators to discover a relation between vitamin A and neoplasia; that is, dietary deficiencies in rats led to "preneoplastic abnormalities," and restoration of vitamin A to their diet reversed the neoplastic process.

Many early studies, including that by Abels et al (1941) which associated vitamin A deficiency with human cancer, strongly supported the link between vitamin A and neoplastic disease. Recognition that vitamin A deficiency leads to abnormal growth of the skin and to preneoplastic changes spurred an initial rush to treat skin disorders with this new drug; however, early excitement was tempered because of toxic effects in many patients, especially liver toxicity.

Toxicity A hominid or prehuman skeleton of *Homo erectus* (approximately 100,000 years ago) discovered in Kenya exhibited the earliest pathologically documented changes consistent with chronic excessive intake of vitamin A, or hypervitaminosis A. The clinical effects of excessive intake of vitamin A were first reported over 100 years ago, many years before vitamin A itself had even been positively identified. These reports involved the ingestion of polar bear and seal livers (5–8 mg retinal per gram of liver) by Eskimos and Arctic explorers. Their acute symptoms included severe headaches, drowsiness, irritability, nausea, and vomiting. Twelve to 24 hours after ingestion, redness and loss of the skin of the face, trunk, palms, and soles developed. Seven to 10 days later, all symptoms resolved.

Subsequent clinical observations verified these major acute symptoms of hypervitaminosis A, which occur when the intake of vitamin A exceeds the capacity of the liver to remove and store it, and after ingestion of a dose of at least 350,000 IU of vitamin A by infants and 1,000,000 IU by adults. Minor acute side effects are more frequent and better described. They include dryness of skin and mucous membranes as well as ocular, gastrointestinal, and musculoskeletal complaints such as tenderness of long bones. Specific major chronic vitamin A toxicities include abnormalities of the following: embryological development, reproductive function, serum lipids, liver function, and the skeletal system. Minor chronic side effects resemble the minor acute toxicities described earlier but are more subtle (see Table 26-1).

Micronutrient interactions The principal micronutrients shown to interact with vitamin A are selenium, zinc, vitamins E and C, and iron. Selenium is an effective

TABLE 26-1 *Acute and Chronic, Major and Minor, Effects of Hypervitaminosis A*

	Minor	Major
Acute	Dryness of skin and mucous membranes Eye, gastrointestinal, muscle complaints Tenderness of long bones	Headache, drowsiness, irritability, nausea and vomiting Redness and loss of skin on the face, trunk, palms, soles
Chronic		Reproductive and embryological abnormalities Liver toxicity Serum lipid abnormalities Skeletal abnormalities

cancer-preventive agent in its own right, and its mechanism of action may be similar to that of vitamin A.

Several studies have indicated that interactions occur between zinc and vitamin A at many levels of cellular activity. Some human enzyme systems requiring zinc are directly and indirectly critical to vitamin A metabolism. Zinc reportedly influences the enzyme that catalyzes the conversion of retinaldehyde to retinoic acid. Indirectly, zinc may affect vitamin A through zinc-dependent enzymes, which may be involved in the synthesis of vitamin A carriers and cellular binding proteins.

Research suggests that interactions occur between both vitamins C and E and vitamin A. Some investigators believe that vitamin E has only a nonspecific, antioxidant role in its relationship with vitamin A. Vitamin E stabilizes cell membranes, and vitamin E deficiency shortens the survival time of red blood cells and accelerates the depletion rate of liver stores of vitamin A. Vitamin E provides vitamin A and carotenoids with protection from oxidation in mixed diets. This protection results in higher levels of liver vitamin A and, under certain circumstances, higher circulating vitamin A levels. Studies of vitamin E–deficient rats fed vitamin A indicate that vitamin E protects vitamin A at a cellular level as well. Vitamin E may also reduce vitamin A toxicity.

Vitamin A deficiency and excess appear to influence the liver's synthesis of vitamin C (ascorbic acid), and vitamin C apparently acts as an antioxidant for vitamin A. Some reports claim to demonstrate a direct association between vitamin A deficiency and vitamin C synthesis.

High levels of iron in the intestine may contribute to destruction of vitamin A active compounds. However, no data indicate that intake of high levels of inorganic iron causes vitamin A deficiency. Studies of human volunteers have revealed that vitamin A deficiency produces the gradual onset of anemia that responds to vitamin A but not to medicinal iron supplementation. Nutrition surveys commonly reveal an association between anemia and inadequate dietary vitamin A.

Epidemiological studies of children in developing countries showed a parallel increase in hemoglobin and serum iron levels with increasing blood levels of vitamin A. Experimental studies of the interaction between iron and vitamin A show that iron absorption is not altered by vitamin A deficiency and that vitamin A appears to help mobilize stored iron and incorporate it into red blood cells.

 Vitamin A: Cancer Cause or Cure ?

A few researchers have claimed that vitamin A, in test tube experiments, will push stem cells to change into cells that can build blood vessels. They contend that this activity may increase cancer through angiogenesis. When structures similar to blood vessels developed within the tumor masses grown in culture, the investigators concluded that vitamin A promotes carcinogenesis. However, an *in vitro* (test tube) experiment is far from clinical proof. Even the study authors admit that vitamin A is known to be necessary for embryonic development precisely because it helps to differentiate stem cells, pushing them to become normal tissue—which is fundamentally an "anticancer" activity.

There is an anticancer drug that specifically acts by blocking the breakdown of retinoic acid, derived from vitamin A. This approach has been found to be effective in treating animal models of human prostate cancer. Daily injections of the agent VN/14-1 resulted in up to a 50% decrease in tumor volume in mice implanted with human prostate cancer cells. No further tumor growth was seen during the 5-week study. It seems that when cancerous tumors have more vitamin A available, they shrink. Keeping more retinoic acid available within cancer cells redirects these cells back into their normal growth patterns, which includes programmed cell death. This potent agent causes cancer cells to differentiate, forcing them to turn back to a noncancerous state. Vitamin A seems to induce positive, healthy, cell changes. Vitamin A derivatives are already in wide use to fight skin cancer.

Sensational warnings and outright misstatements that natural vitamin A may "incite" cancer actually serve to excite newspaper readers and television viewers. Upon closer examination, a "vitamin promotes cancer" study often has the appearance of being conducted to prove an intended point. As the authors fuel fears about vitamin A, they also give away their goal, stating that these findings open a new door to drug development. New marketing avenues for the development of patentable vitamin A-like drugs are a commercial opportunity that the pharmaceutical industry has not overlooked.

A vitamin A derivative could protect against lung cancer development in former smokers, says another report. Significantly, the vitamin A derivative is used in combination with α-tocopherol (vitamin E) to reduce toxicity known to be associated with 13-*cis*-retinoic acid (the vitamin A derivative) therapy. This point illustrates why nutritional physicians do not use high doses of vitamin A by itself, but rather give it in conjunction with other important, synergistic nutrients. All nutrients are needed in a living body.

The following is an example: A study published in the *Journal of Nutritional Biochemistry* found that administering both vitamin A and vitamin C to cultured human breast cancer cells was more than three times as effective as administering either compound alone. The combination of the two vitamins inhibited proliferation by over 75% compared with untreated cells. The ability of retinoic acid (vitamin A) to inhibit tumor cell proliferation is well known, although its mechanism has not been defined. The authors suggested that the synergistic effect observed in this study was due to ascorbic acid's ability to slow the degradation of retinoic acid, thereby increasing vitamin A's cell proliferation inhibitory effects. Vitamin C helps vitamin A work even better.

Doctors' experience and clinical evidence both show that vitamin A helps prevent cancer, which has been known for a long time. The association of vitamin A and cancer was initially reported in 1926 when rats, fed a vitamin A–deficient diet, developed gastric carcinomas. The first investigation showing a relationship between vitamin A and human cancer was performed by Abels et al (1941), mentioned earlier, who found low plasma vitamin A levels in patients with gastrointestinal cancer.

Moon et al (1983, 1985) reported that daily supplemental doses of 25,000 IU of vitamin A prevented squamous cell carcinoma. Studies in animal models have shown that retinoids (including vitamin A) can act in the promotion-progression phase of carcinogenesis and block the development of invasive carcinoma at several epithelial sites, including the head and neck and lung. The Linus Pauling Institute states that studies in cell culture and animal models have documented the capacity for natural and synthetic retinoids to reduce carcinogenesis significantly in the skin, breast, liver, colon, prostate, and other sites.

There will always be those bent on believing that vitamins must be harmful somehow. For them, it only remains to set up some test tubes to try to prove it. Such has been done with other vitamins, perhaps most notably a famous experiment that claimed that vitamin C promoted cancer. The study, reported in *New Scientist*, September 22, 2001, was a prime example of sketchy science carelessly reported. The article would have readers uncritically extend the questionable findings of a highly artificial, electrical-current-vibrated quartz crystal test tube

Vitamin A: Cancer Cause or Cure ?—cont'd

study and conclude that 2000 mg of vitamin C can (somehow) do some sort of mischief to human DNA in real life. If 2000 mg of vitamin C was harmful, the entire animal kingdom would be dead. Our nearest primate relatives all eat well in excess of 2000 mg of vitamin C each day. And, pound for pound, most animals actually manufacture from 2000–10,000 mg of vitamin C daily, right inside their bodies. If such generous quantities of vitamin C were harmful, evolution would have had millions of years to select against it. The same is true for vitamin A.

The National Institutes of Health state that dietary intake studies suggest an association between diets rich in carotenoids and vitamin A and a lower risk of many types of cancer. A higher intake of green and yellow-orange vegetables or other food sources of carotenoids and/or vitamin A may decrease the risk of lung cancer. A study of over 82,000 people showed that high intakes of vitamin A reduce the risk of stomach cancer by one-half. Vitamin A appears to fight cancer by inhibiting the production of DNA in cancerous cells. It slows down tumor growth in established cancers and may keep leukemia cells from dividing. A derivative of the vitamin has been shown to kill CEM-C7 human T lymphoblastoid leukemia cells and P1798-C7 murine T lymphoma cells.

B Vitamins

B vitamins are water-soluble nutrients found in many foods, primarily animal-based products, such as red meat, poultry, eggs, fish, and dairy. They cannot be produced or stored by the body, and therefore must be consumed through the diet. They include B_1 (thiamine), B_2 (riboflavin), B_3 (nicotinic acid), B_6 (pyridoxine), and B_{12} (cobalamin), niacin, pantothenic acid and folate (folic acid). These nutrients contribute to a wide array of physiological functions, such as red blood cell production, nerve cell function, metabolism of carbohydrates and fats, energy production, and immune system function. Deficiency can occur from a poor diet or due to medical conditions that interfere with absorption of B vitamins from the gastrointestinal tract. Abnormalities in the stomach or small intestine can interfere with the biochemical "intrinsic factor" (IF), which must bind with B_{12} to be absorbed in the small intestine along with other nutrients.

B vitamin deficiency, particularly B_{12}, can contribute to several ailments, such as sore tongue or mouth, weight loss, pale skin, weak immunity, rapid heart rate, diarrhea, menstrual dysfunction, burning foot pain, pernicious anemia, and even tumor development. There are also specific diseases that cause B vitamin deficiency, such as autoimmune diseases, inflammatory bowel disease, and

multiple sclerosis. In the aging, deficiency is usually caused from malabsorption.

Significant data has shown that B vitamins play a role in cancer prevention. A study published in *Cancer Epidemiology Biomarkers & Prevention* in 2009 reported an association of low levels of B_6 (pyridoxine) in reducing colon cancer risk. An earlier study published in the *Annals of Internal Medicine* in 1998 had also shown a protective effect of dietary folate against the development of colon cancer. B vitamins also play a significant role in protecting the nervous system and spinal cord, including B_{12}, which is critical for the fatty myelin tissues that protect nerve and brain cells. B vitamins along with natural phytonutrients such as berberine, lutein and choline (L-α-glycerylphosphorylcholine or alpha-GPC) help maintain healthy brain function.

Vitamin C

Recent research indicates that vitamin C may contribute significantly to lowering blood pressure, maintaining muscle mass, and preventing cancer. Researchers at Johns Hopkins found sufficient evidence from research studies that a 500 mg daily dose of vitamin C can lower blood pressure by 5 mmHg. While it cannot take the place of medications, it may be a very useful supplement in the process of cutting back on the amount of medication one has to take, something each individual should consult a physician to do safely.

With regard to muscle mass, the entire musculoskeletal system accounts for about 85% of the body's weight, mass, and size. Vitamin C is a collagen-builder, and extremely important for the regeneration of every cell in the body, so it is not just for bones and joints. This nutrient is so important in so many ways that almost all animals make their own, as part of normal metabolism. In fact, all animals make their own vitamin C except for two—humans and guinea pigs. (This is one reason why guinea pigs originally became such an important laboratory model in scientific experiments.)

There has been more evidence on the potential health benefits of vitamin C than almost any other nutrient. And yet, the National Cancer Institute not only failed to conduct large-scale clinical trials on its cancer-preventing abilities, they went further to claim it had actually been "given a bad name" by two-time Nobel prize winner Linus Pauling's efforts to promote vitamin C's scientifically proven benefits for preventing everything from cancer to the common cold.

Vitamin D

The term vitamin D actually refers to a pair of biologically inactive precursors of a critical micronutrient. They are vitamin D_3, also known as cholecalciferol, and vitamin D_2, also known as ergocalciferol.

Cholecalciferol is produced in the skin by a photoreaction on exposure to ultraviolet B light from the sun (wavelength 290–320 nm). Ergocalciferol is produced in plants and enters the human diet through consumption of plant sources.

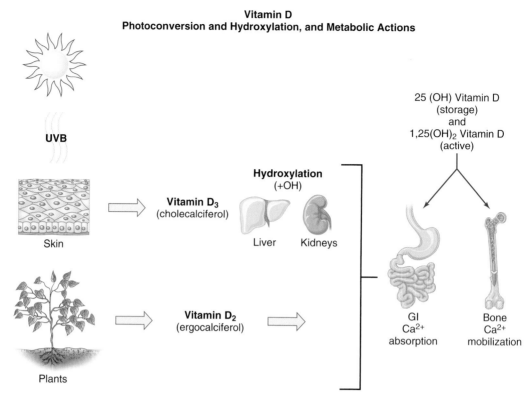

Vitamin D
Photoconversion and Hydroxylation, and Metabolic Actions

Figure 26-1 Sources and photoconversion of vitamin D. (Original artwork by Marc S. Micozzi, redrawn by Elsevier.)

Once present in the circulation, both D_2 and D_3 enter the liver and kidneys, where they are hydroxylated to form both 25-hydroxyvitamin D and 1,25-dihydroxyvitamin D. The former, 25-hydroxyvitamin D, is relatively inactive and represents the storage form of vitamin D. By contrast, 1,25-dihydroxyvitamin D is highly active metabolically, and its levels are tightly controlled. Vitamin D has many critical metabolic functions. There has been recent confusion in the literature regarding differences in relative abundance, availability and effects of vitamin D_2 and D_3, which have been reconciled by thoughtful investigation.

The major circulating form of vitamin D_3 in human blood is 25-hydroxyvitamin D_3, and therefore it is the form measured by physicians to evaluate vitamin D status in people worldwide. It takes a long time for this form to work on calcium absorption and mobilization, however, and it must be converted or metabolized to the more active 1,25-dihydroxyvitamin D for effectiveness in the body.

Knowledge of the role of vitamin D metabolic activity, its role in human health, and identification of the forms and metabolic pathways for vitamin D had been building for many decades but only became fully elucidated during the 1970s. Although nutrition is fundamental in human health, understanding of nutritional metabolism has generally lagged behind the pace of medical investigation and practice focusing on factors external to the host such as infectious microorganisms.

Versatility of vitamin D The first major functions of vitamin D to be recognized were: (1) enhancement of calcium absorption from the diet through the intestine; and (2) mobilization and reabsorption of calcium from bone, which represents the major store of calcium (or "calcium bank") in the body (see Figure 26-1) Calcium, in turn, is critical for cellular metabolism and membrane actions, enzymatic reactions, muscle function, skeletal structure, and a host of activities needed to sustain life and maintain homeostasis. Because vitamin D has long been recognized for its role in calcium metabolism, it has long been used to treat patients with renal failure and bone diseases. It also has an important role in the treatment of postmenopausal osteoporosis and the current epidemic of bone fractures in the elderly.

In 1979, however, DeLuca found that vitamin D is actually recognized by every tissue in the body (Holick, 2003). Every cell has receptors for vitamin D. Since then, vitamin D has been used to treat hyperproliferative skin diseases such as psoriasis.

In the immune system, the large white blood cell macrophages activate vitamin D. The activated vitamin D in turn causes macrophages to make a peptide that specifically kills infective agents such as tuberculosis mycobacteria. Vitamin D also has a role in helping prevent autoimmune diseases such as multiple sclerosis, rheumatoid arthritis, and diabetes type 1.

Vitamin D's activity in the kidney has long been recognized, and it has been found to affect the production of renin and angiotensin, the major regulators of blood pressure, in the kidney. There is a direct correlation between higher (further from the equator) latitudes (where both sunlight and vitamin D levels are lower) and higher blood pressure in both the northern and southern hemispheres of the earth. People at high latitudes with high blood pressure experience a return to normal blood pressure levels after exposure to ultraviolet B light in a tanning bed three times a week for 3 months and restoration of active vitamin D levels (and you thought it only worked if the sunlight was captured on a beach in the Bahamas!).

Multiple sclerosis also shows a marked association with higher latitudes worldwide, and there may be a similar protective role for vitamin D for this disease.

Vitamin D is also thought to have an important role in cancer (Albert et al, 2004; Holick, 2003). As early as the 1940s, it was noted that living at higher latitudes is associated with a higher incidence of several cancers (whereas only skin cancer specifically has a lower incidence at higher latitudes). Recent epidemiological observations have continued to bear out this association. A high frequency of sunbathing before age 20 was found to reduce the risk of non-Hodgkin lymphoma. And, although sun exposure is related to an increased incidence of malignant melanoma, it was also found to be associated with increased survival from melanoma in a recent study. In some of the sunniest spots on earth, both the Australian College of Dermatologists, the Cancer Council of Australia, and the New Zealand Bone and Mineral Society have concluded that a balance is required between avoiding an increased risk of skin cancer and achieving enough ultraviolet light exposure to maintain adequate vitamin D levels.

As in all things involving nutrition, achieving a balance is a good goal and guide for optimal health. It was thought that a balanced approach to this problem could be achieved through thoughtful dermatological screening for skin cancers. Thus, most skin cancers should be detected and treated early, because they are by definition visible on the surface of the skin, unlike cancers of other tissues, which begin growing hidden and undetected deep inside the body.

Dermatological intervention also took another, different direction, however. Rather than just focusing on early detection and treatment of skin cancer, dermatologists began fighting against the sun. That, in turn, has had profound effects on vitamin D nutrition and deficiency over the past 40 years.

Global Dimensions of D-ficiency

Essentially little or no active vitamin D is available from regular dietary sources. It is principally found in fish oils, sun-dried mushrooms, and fortified foods like milk and orange juice. However, many countries worldwide forbid the fortification of foods. There is potentially plenty of vitamin D in the food chain, because both phytoplankton and zooplankton exposed to sunlight make vitamin D. Wild-caught salmon, which feed on natural food sources, for example, have available vitamin D. However, farmed salmon fed food pellets with little nutritional value have only 10% of the vitamin D of wild fish. The "perfect storm" of photophobia, lack of exposure to sunlight, and insufficiency of available dietary vitamin D has led to a national and worldwide epidemic of vitamin D deficiency.

Estimates are that at least 30% and as much as 80% of the U.S. population is vitamin D deficient. In the United States, at latitudes north of Atlanta, the skin does not make (photoconvert) any vitamin D from November through March (i.e., essentially outside of daylight savings time; so although we shift the clock around, it does not salvage vitamin D synthesis). During this season the angle of the sun in the sky is too low to allow UVB light to penetrate the atmosphere, and it is absorbed by the ozone layer. Even in the late spring, summer, and early fall, most vitamin D is made between 10 am and 3 pm when UVB from the sun penetrates the atmosphere and reaches the earth's surface.

It might be expected that vitamin D deficiency would be a problem limited to northern latitudes.

In Bangor, Maine, among young girls 9 to 11 years old, nearly 50% were deficient at the end of winter and nearly 20% remained deficient at the end of summer. At Boston Children's Hospital, over 50% of adolescent girls and African American and Hispanic boys were found to be vitamin D deficient year round. In another study in Boston, 34% of whites, 40% of Hispanics, and 84% of African American adults over age 50 were found to be deficient.

Vitamin D deficiency is also a national problem, however. The U.S. Centers for Disease Control and Prevention completed a national survey at the end of winter and found that nearly 50% of African American women aged 15 to 49 years were deficient. These are women in the critical childbearing years. A growing fetus must receive adequate vitamin D from the mother, especially because breast milk does not provide adequate vitamin D. A study of pregnant women in Boston found that in 40 mother–infant pairs at the time of labor and delivery, over 75% of mothers and 80% of newborns were deficient. This observation was made despite the fact that pregnant women were instructed to take a prenatal vitamin that included 400 IU of vitamin D and to drink two glasses of milk per day.

Further, vitamin D deficiency is a global problem. Even in India, home to 1 billion of the earth's people, where

Continued

Global Dimensions of D-ficiency—cont'd

there is plenty of sun, 30% to 50% of children, 50% to 80% of adults, and 90% of physicians are deficient. In South Africa, vitamin D deficiency is also a problem even though Cape Town is situated at 34 degrees latitude.

Although there are many new bilateral and multilateral governmental and private efforts to export Western medical technology and pharmaceuticals to the Third World to combat infectious diseases such as acquired immunodeficiency syndrome (AIDS), there is no comparable effort to acknowledge and address the global dimensions of the vitamin D deficiency epidemic. The U.S. Congress and President just deemed it as a great achievement to give $40 billion in tax dollars to U.S. pharmaceutical companies to send expensive drug treatments for AIDS (a preventable disease) overseas. By contrast, addressing the vitamin D deficiency epidemic could be accomplished with much safer and less expensive nutritional supplements together with sunlight, the only source of energy that is still free (Holick, 2003).

Vitamin D Dose, Toxicity, and Formulation

It has been well established that giving 100 IU of vitamin D daily to children will prevent rickets (Table 26-2).

As with most of established thinking about recommended daily allowances (RDAs), the dosages are those that prevent the development of frank nutritional deficiencies and associated pathology. The idea of levels for optimal health does not enter the picture. Even the capricious RDA process raised the recommendation from 200 IU to 400 IU/day in 1997 (although technically it is not an "RDA" but an "AI," or adequate intake).

Currently, those more knowledgeable about human nutrition than the group involved in the outdated RDA/AI process recommend 1000 IU daily for both children and adults to maintain blood levels of 25-hydroxyvitamin D above 30 ng/mL. It is now recognized that each 100 IU of vitamin D ingested raises blood levels by only 1 ng/mL (Table 26-3).

Although a typical recommendation is in the range of 1000 to 2000 IU/day, it is reasonable to recommend up to 5000 IU/day.

It is not easy to become vitamin D intoxicated. Sunlight actually destroys any excess vitamin D that is made in the body, so it is not possible to become vitamin D intoxicated from too much sunlight alone. In a world in which dangerous and expensive drugs are doled out like candy, it is ironic to witness the degree of concern in the medical establishment over exposures to physiological levels of natural substances such as vitamins, and even sunlight!

Nonetheless, a medical lore has developed over the possible risks of excess vitamin D intake, although vitamin D intoxication is one of the most rare medical conditions in the world. If vitamin D were considered as a drug, it demonstrates a remarkably high therapeutic index of at least 300 for disease treatment (ratio of minimum toxic dose to dose given to treat rickets) and at least 20 for chronic disease prevention. If the patient has a chronic granulomatous disorder such as histoplasmosis, sarcoidosis, or tuberculosis, however, a vitamin D blood level above 30 ng/mL will cause hypercalcemia and hypercalciuria. Therefore, supplementation should be avoided in these cases.

Because the only pharmaceutical preparation of vitamin D is in 50,000 IU doses, one therapeutic regimen is 50,000 IU per week for 8 weeks to treat deficiency, with

TABLE 26-2 *The Evolving Picture of Vitamin D Daily Intake*

Daily intake	Associated effects
100 IU	Prevents rickets, frank nutritional deficiency disease
	Amount in one glass of milk or fortified orange juice
200 IU	"Adequate intake" per RDA pre-1997
400 IU	"Adequate intake" per RDA post-1997
	Reduces risk of rheumatoid arthritis in women by 50%
1000 IU	Reduces risk of cancer (breast, colorectal, ovarian, prostate) by 50%
2000 IU	Reduces risk of diabetes by 80%
	Reduces incidence of upper respiratory tract infections in the elderly by 90%
	Reduces PSA levels in men by 50%
30,000 IU	Minimum to develop toxicity over several months or years

PSA, Prostate-specific antigen; RDA, recommended daily allowance.

TABLE 26-3 *Blood Levels of Vitamin D (25-Hydroxyvitamin D)*

Level (ng/mL)	Associated intakes and effects
1	Amount blood level is raised by 100 IU intake
1–20	Deficiency
21–29	Insufficiency
30–150	Sufficiency, reached by 50,000 IU weekly for 8 weeks
50	Reduces risk of breast cancer by 50% (versus 20 ng/mL)
150–200	Onset of toxicity

Global Dimensions of D-ficiency—cont'd

50,000 IU every 2 weeks thereafter for maintenance of adequate vitamin D levels. Dietary supplements are also good choices for vitamin D.

Manufacturers often add 50% more vitamin D than is listed on the label to maintain potency during the shelf life of the product. Thus, a 1000-IU formulation that actually contains 1500 IU is still perfectly safe.

Despite the inadequacy of the RDA/AI process, there is ample evidence and clinical experience indicating that vitamin D blood levels and daily intakes should be much higher than they are, not only for prevention of bone diseases but to provide optimal health and help reduce the risk of many common chronic diseases, disorders, and medical conditions. Together with healthy sun exposure, vitamin D supplementation can be accomplished safely and effectively and should be a first-line consideration in any clinical practice and for the general population. ∾

Vitamin E (tocopherols and tocotrienols)

Natural vitamin E consists of four tocopherols and four tocotrienols. However, researchers generally test only one in isolation, either D-alpha-tocopherol or di-alpha-tocopherol acetate. They find no effect and make the claim that natural vitamin E also has no anticancer effect, providing an example of reductionist research that misleads the public. To be conducted accurately, the research should be done with mixed tocopherols and tocotrienols. Some studies have shown that alpha-tocopherol can neutralize the effects of certain cancer-causing compounds such as N-nitrosamines. It may also stimulate the release of antitumor factors from the immune system. Animal studies suggest that it can prevent some chemically induced cancers and may reduce the size of tumors. One study conducted on humans suggested a beneficial effect associated with the use of vitamin E in patients with superficial premalignant lesions in the mouth. In another laboratory study, vitamin E was found to inhibit the growth of breast cancer cells. Supplementation with alpha-tocopherol has been shown to reduce the side effects of patients undergoing radiation therapy for breast cancer.

MINERALS

Minerals are everywhere in nature and range from beneficial (calcium) to poisonous (arsenic). The minerals essential to human function include calcium, phosphorus, potassium, sodium (salt), chloride, and magnesium. In addition, we need a number of trace elements, including iron, zinc, selenium, manganese, copper, iodine, molybdenum, cobalt, chromium, and fluorine. As with vitamins, most physicians recommend obtaining minerals from a healthy diet, whereas many complementary and alternative medicine practitioners advocate supplements to ensure a regular supply. RDAs have been established for only six minerals—calcium, phosphorus, iron, magnesium, iodine, and zinc—and the calcium and iron guidelines are being seriously questioned.

Much current publicity surrounds the role of **calcium** in preventing osteoporosis, the brittle bones that come with age, especially for women. The National Academy of Science had raised the RDA for calcium from 800 mg to 1000 mg for nonpregnant women and from 1200 mg to 1500 mg for pregnant women. Although these steps were in the right direction, compliance remains doubtful. The old RDAs were not met by 68% of the total population; more significantly, they were not met by 84% of women between ages 35 and 50 and 87% of girls between 15 and 18 years of age. The standards have again been revised higher. With higher standards, these compliance percentages are slipping still lower. In addition to supplying cancer-fighting properties (Baron et al, 1999), calcium together with vitamin D appears important for the risk of many other chronic diseases.

Studies have long shown **selenium** to also reduce the risk of cancer, and diabetes as well. While getting too much selenium is a rare but significant possibility, staying within 400 mcg/day will avoid toxicity and aid in cancer and diabetes prevention.

The one mineral that medical professionals have been successful in promoting, **iron**, has turned out to be harmful in excess. Over many years, while expressing now-discredited concerns about putative dangers from most other supplements, the medical profession has advocated the use of iron supplements. Vital for the production of hemoglobin, which transports oxygen to the body's cells, iron is also necessary for many immune, growth, and enzyme functions. Lack of iron leads to anemia, especially in pregnant women, and to other conditions, including fatigue, fragile bones, and mental disorders. However, because iron is stored in the body, excesses can easily build up, causing the production of free radicals, which have been associated with cancer and heart disease. One of us (Micozzi) has conducted independent research with colleagues such as Nobel laureate Baruch Blumberg, MD, PhD (1925–2011; to whom this edition is partly dedicated), showing that excess iron can cause cancer. More often, overuse of iron supplements causes digestive discomforts and disorders. Dietary guidelines for iron are now being revised downward, and many multivitamin supplements are now available without iron.

Exactly how much of any nutrient is needed depends largely on the physical condition of the individual. Pregnant women, athletes, smokers, people with chronic illnesses, and those of various ages and lifestyles all have different dietary requirements. The one dietary requirement that is relatively consistent for all of us is the need for water.

HYDRATION: WATER, FLUID AND ELECTROLYTE BALANCE

The human body can survive up to 5 weeks without food but rarely lasts beyond a few days without water. Our bodies are almost 75% water, which is vital for every bodily process, including absorbing and digesting food, transporting nutrients throughout the body, and carrying out waste materials.

Water is naturally lost through sweat and elimination. Caffeine, Excess alcohol, and other intakes may act as diuretics, which increase urination and further deplete the body's reserves of liquids. To replace all this lost fluid, we need to drink up to eight glasses of water a day. Dry mouth, headache, and fatigue are often signs we are dehydrated. Exercise, massage, and other activities increase our need for water. When we are ill, additional fluids help flush toxins from the body and restore well-being.

Fluid and electrolyte balance is critical for good health and physical performance. The salinity of the blood and tissues matches the salinity of the oceans (much lower than today) at the time life is thought to have emerged from the sea into the terrestrial environment. Nearly all human cells use aquaporins, water channel proteins, in their cell membrane for metabolic processes. The content of water among the major organs demonstrates further the importance of water on health: brain (85%), lungs (80%), liver (73%), skin (71%), heart (77%), kidneys (80%), muscles (73%), blood (79%), bones (22%), and teeth (18%). Not only is adequate quantity of water consumption important to the body, but the quality of the water becomes important too. Referring back to holistic methods and relationships, does it serve us to continue separating our environment (soil and water) from our health?

A UNIQUE LIQUID

Water itself has some unique properties that has enabled life to exist on earth. Its properties also enabled physicians in ancient Greece and Rome and during the European Middle Ages to make sense of its role as one of the four humors in health (Chapter 1). Liquids generally freeze from the bottom up; as liquids cool, the colder molecules of the liquid (with lower kinetic energy) fall toward the bottom because they become more dense—and thus the liquid will become solid (freeze) from the bottom up. Water, to the contrary, has a distinctive molecular configuration.

As water cools the molecular configuration becomes more dense until it reaches approximately 4.0° F at which point a remarkable effect takes hold. The water molecules begin to lock into a molecular configuration that is less dense, and the molecules rise to the top as they freeze. So, water freezes from the top. In larger bodies of water, the frozen layer at the top then tends to trap any heat energy in the lower reaches, thus preventing the entire body of water from freezing. Imagine the implications for life on earth if bodies of water froze from the bottom up.

VIBRATIONAL ENERGY AND "MEMORY OF WATER"

In addition to this unique freezing process, water also demonstrates an ability to hold cellular memory through the process known as covalent bonding. The late Linus Pauling, who won the Nobel Prizes for Chemistry and for Peace, is responsible for bringing this theory of "Water Memory Transfer" to public awareness. Covalent bonding is the process of two atoms joining together to form a molecule. The electrons form an "orbit" that surrounds the water molecule. But in ionized water, one of the electrons is missing, which some consider allows unhealthy influences to accumulate (Suddath, 2005).

There are ways to influence the shape, health and energy of water crystals, one of which is vibration. An example of water crystalline transformation and memory can be seen in the work of Dr. Masaru Emoto, who studied the effects of words, music, and intention on water. First he froze the water into solid form, exposed it to positive and negative vibrations—words, music, or human-directed intention—and studied the crystal formations under a microscope. He discovered that the containers of water exposed to negative words or vibrations, such as "You fool," "You disgust me," etc., all had chaotic, unsymmetrical forms. The containers exposed to positive words, such as "Wisdom," "Harmony," and "Truth," took on vibrant, symmetrical forms, all unique, that resembled snowflakes. His work allows one to view the water during the course of its exposure, as it was captured on film, literally changing during the process. In one study, he used the music of Mozart, who himself was influenced by naturalistic conceptualizations such as the "music of the spheres" (see Chapter 1). In this experiment, the viewer can observe the water crystal "dancing" into symmetry while exposed to the music (Emoto, 2004).

THE FLUID OF THE BODY

Individual organisms rely on water to carry blood cells and nutrients to all parts of the body in the blood circulation, to bathe the tissue cells in extracellular fluid, to support the central nervous system through the cerebrospinal fluid, and to return excess body constituents to the circulation through the lymphatic vessels. It is one large, complex hydraulic system. Water is also the intracellular medium in which all cells carry out cellular metabolism, including cellular respiration which itself creates most of the water held within the cells.

Emoto's aforementioned work may be significant in light of the roles of water in the body and may potentially bear on the placebo effect (see Chapter 9). Because the body is composed of mostly water, and water responds in certain ways to vibration and intention, does the energy of therapeutic intervention work despite or because of the patient's and/or practitioner's beliefs? Or is water itself imbued with some kind of cellular memory or consciousness that responds to its environment? These are questions incumbent upon science to evaluate (see Chapter 14).

Can biomedical science continue to operate under the reductionist view of treating parts outside the context of a larger system? How does it serve the advancement of medicine? Can we be separated from our environment, from the quality of the soil in which our food grows, and the quality of the water that nourishes that soil, and our food and bodies? As in the case of soil in natural farming, pouring more chemicals into our waters to "purify" them does not seem realistic for good health, especially when there are natural ways allowing nature to purify water. ∾

CELLULAR HYDRATION

It is important to maintain both fluid and electrolyte levels for the body as a whole. The formation of urine occurs at a relatively constant rate to filter the blood and remove metabolic by-products to eliminate them from the body. Carbohydrate (glucose) from the diet is combined with oxygen from the air we breathe and broken down by a chemical combustion reaction ("burned") in the cells to produce energy (captured in the chemical bonds of ATP molecules), creating byproducts of carbon dioxide (which is carried back to the lungs in the blood and breathed out) and water which is retained in the cells. Some water vapor is ultimately breathed out and some water is eventually eliminated in urine. However, most of the water inside the cells is generated within the cells by this process of cellular respiration

Remarkably, this process of cellular respiration combines oxygen with carbohydrate to generate energy (stored in the chemical bonds of ATP) as well as carbon dioxide **and water**. Thereby, when properly nourished, *every cell generates its own water* in addition to energy. Water generated through cellular respiration is responsible for the majority of intracellular fluid. While external hydration is important for blood volume and extracellular fluid, nourishing the cell is the key factor for cellular hydration.

Cellular hydration is essentially a combustion reaction (like burning a fire) to produce energy which, in this case, is not primarily in the form of heat but is largely captured in the form of chemical bonds to be made available in cellular metabolism. The importance of using carbohydrate (carbon, hydrogen, *and* oxygen) as the source of energy, rather than hydrocarbons (carbon and hydrogen alone), is that the extra oxygen enables the by-products to be released in the form of carbon dioxide, relatively harmlessly transported to the lungs and exhaled, rather than the toxic carbon monoxide as in smoke inhalation from an actual fire.

Without understanding the molecular elements of the periodic chart, or cellular anatomy, the Persian-Arab physician *Ibn Sina* (Latin, Avicenna) pinpointed the essential nature of this cellular respiration process with creation of water in the cell by the cell itself (see Chapter 32; Amri et al, 2013).

Certain plant constituents such as ubiquinol (or coenzyme Q-10, obtained from foods and also manufactured by the body) and *Aspalathus linearis* (from South African red bush) appear to facilitate this cellular respiration process, generating hydration for the cells (Sanderson et al, 2014).

NITROGEN

Amino acids contain nitrogen as well as oxygen, carbon, and hydrogen, and are the building blocks of proteins. Likewise, nucleic acids contain nitrogen as well, and are the building blocks of DNA and RNA (the acids found in the nuclei of all cells in the body, except mature red blood cells). Organic nutrients containing nitrogen must be eliminated as metabolic by-products and excreted through the urine. The fate of proteins, purines, and pyrimidines (nucleic acids) is ultimately to become urea and uric acid in the urine. Buildup of uric acid in the blood leads to gout with deposits of uric acid crystals in joints and cartilage (such as in the earlobes). In kidney failure, nitrogen-containing metabolites build up in the blood to the point that they cause central nervous toxicity (renal encephalopathy).

WATER LOSS

In addition to elimination of fluid and electrolytes in the urine, there are continual insensible losses of water through respiration (the exhaled air carries out water vapor) as well as losses of both water and electrolytes through sweating. Humans, who are less hirsute mammals, have sweat glands throughout the skin of the body. Cooling by evaporation of water allows the surface of the body to reduce surface temperature. Hairier animals covered with fur cannot use this mechanism and rely on hyperpnea, or rapid panting, which allows blood in the tongue to be cooled by contact with air (like the old air-cooled engines of the Volkswagen Beetle) as well as fluid and heat loss through salivation. Smaller organisms, such as insects, have an open circulation system and air passes directly through the organism without the need for a circulatory system. When people sweat due to high ambient temperatures and/or high physical performance, it is important to replace both fluid and electrolytes.

Body water and electrolytes may also be lost by excretion of excessive fluids in the stool, as in diarrhea and dysentery (the latter implies loss of blood as well as water and electrolytes in the stool). In the case of cholera, the cholera bacteria produce a toxin that inhibits reabsorption of water from the intestinal contents by the cells lining the intestines. The result is massive fluid and electrolyte loss, which may result in death from dehydration within a few days. Diarrhea is still a very common cause of death in infants in developing countries, especially where nursing mothers are encouraged to use infant formula (made with contaminated water) instead of staying with the proven benefits of natural breastfeeding.

DIET AS THERAPY

Although most mainstream Western physicians receive little training in diet and nutrition and rarely consider it as a therapy, many other health practitioners consider diet, food, and nutrition a vital part of preventing and treating illness.

CHINESE MEDICINE

Since ancient times, as discussed earlier in this chapter, the Chinese have used food for medicinal purposes, and many contemporary medical schools include a classroom kitchen to train students in preparing beneficial foods. Families and some restaurants routinely prepare special dishes to meet the needs of people who are ill, elderly, pregnant, or lactating. Beneficial foods are identified and selected on the basis of such traditional Chinese medical concepts as the five-phase theory and yin and yang, two models for the dynamic processes governing the universe and human bodies. *Yin* is associated with the female principle, and its properties include cold, slowness, darkness, the interior, and deficiency. *Yang* is associated with the male principle; its properties include heat, light, speed, the exterior, and excess. A disease characterized by too much cold would be associated with yin, and a practitioner might prescribe foods and herbs that stimulate yang by enhancing heat or "scattering the cold" (see Chapter 28 and later section on macrobiotics).

AYURVEDA

Developed in ancient India, Ayurveda (Sanskrit for "the knowledge of long life") has always incorporated food into its holistic approach to health. In Ayurveda, three *doshas* (*vata, pitta,* and *kapha*) define the three basic mind-body or constitutional types. Each *dosha* finds certain foods and flavors beneficial, whereas others may be harmful if taken in too large a quantity. For instance, people whose dominant *dosha* is *vata,* which is responsible for the body's kinetic energy and associated with the element of air, may suffer from nervous energy and will be soothed by warm, moist, sweet foods and aggravated by pungent, bitter, raw foods. Following an appropriate *vata* diet can help people avoid or recover from a wide range of *vata* disorders, such as insomnia, constipation, anxiety, high blood pressure, and arthritis (see Chapter 31).

NATURE CURE AND NATUROPATHIC MEDICINE

A synthesis and refinement of nineteenth-century nature cures, naturopathic medicine considers a wholesome diet one of the cornerstones of good health, along with exercise, fresh air, adequate sleep, and low-stress lifestyle. Naturopathic physicians believe that the body has an innate tendency to heal itself and that nourishing food is necessary for the body's self-maintenance and repairs. Practitioners recommend a diet of whole (unprocessed) foods, especially fresh fruits and vegetables, which should be organic (free of chemicals and other additives) if possible. Fasting, including juice fasts, may be prescribed to rid the body of toxins. Early naturopaths started the first "health food stores" in America and developed many foods, such as graham crackers, that were revolutionary in their use of whole grains (see Chapters 22 and 23).

MACROBIOTICS

Loosely based on the traditional Chinese concepts of yin and yang, the macrobiotic diet was developed in the 1950s by George Osawa, a Japanese educator and philosopher. The name is derived from the Greek *makros* ("big" or "long") and *bios* ("life"), and its practitioners believe a long and healthy life can be achieved through a balanced diet and other beneficial practices. As do traditional Chinese physicians, macrobiotics advocates believe all foods have yin or yang properties. Yin foods, which are thought to be calming, include green vegetables, fruits, nuts, and honey. Yang foods, said to be strengthening, include meat, fish, eggs, and beans. Whole grains, which have balanced yin and yang, form the cornerstone of the diet. Too much yin food can leave a person feeling resentful and worried; an overly yang meal may generate feelings of aggressiveness. Eating the proper foods is held to help rebalance feelings and restore physical well-being. Unfortunately, for all the many decades of devotion to this diet, there has been relatively little research. Given the actual nutrient composition of this diet, and overreliance on grains (which have only been part of the human diet for 10,000 years), a physician might be reluctant to recommend such an extreme diet as balanced or optimal for the typical patient.

REVERSAL OF HEART DISEASE

Heart disease was considered irreversible until the 1980s, when cardiologist Dean Ornish proved that heart patients could restore heart health through diet, exercise, and stress management. Based on the Pritikin diet, Ornish's diet is very low in fat (probably too low at 15% of calories) and cholesterol, and is high (probably too high) in carbohydrates and fiber. It excludes almost all animal products except for skim milk and fat-free yogurt. An occasional glass of wine is permitted; smoking is not. In a rigorous week-long training session, participants are taught how to cook and eat according to Ornish's guidelines and are instructed in exercise, yoga, and meditation. When they go home, they are expected to continue the regimen indefinitely. This approach is not easy to maintain, but when the alternative is heart bypass surgery, possibly followed by another operation in 5 years, participants can sometimes be motivated; in 99% of cases, those who followed the regimen successfully reversed the course of their heart disease.

However, a low-fat diet does not improve lipoprotein profiles in men at increased risk of heart disease (Dreon et al, 1999). Many who question whether the Ornish diet composition itself is too low in fat and too high in carbs point to the benefits of social support and stress reduction to help account for the beneficial results.

VEGETARIAN AND VEGAN DIETS

A *vegetarian* does not eat meat, poultry, or fish but does eat eggs and dairy products. Research that showed an association of vegetarian diet with reduced risk of heart disease, high blood pressure, diabetes, osteoporosis, gallbladder disease, colon cancer, and other conditions, has recently been understand to be a result of other healthy practices among health-consicous vegetarians and not the diet composition itself. A *vegan* diet excludes all animal-based foods, including dairy products, eggs, and honey. Unless supplements are used, vegans risk real deficiencies of B vitamins, Vitamins A, D and E and many key mineral micronutrients. The vegan diet has been studied in the treatment of asthma, arthritis, high blood pressure, and angina.

RAW FOODS

In the late nineteenth century, Swiss physician Max Bircher-Benner developed a diet that contains 70% uncooked vegetables and fruits; the balance of the diet can include meat, dairy products, grains, nuts, and seeds. He believed that raw foods: (1) are more natural and appropriate for the human digestive system; (2) maintain their nutrients better than cooked food; and (3) prolong the life span.

Research shows that uncooked foods retain higher nutrient content as heat breaks down nutrients over time. However, heating also makes many foods much more digestible allowing the nutrient content to be better obtained by the body during digestion. Archaeological evidence shows humans have grown foods for only 10,000 years, while they have probably cooked foods for about 1,000,000 years; so it is probable that human nutrition is suited to the effects of cooking at least as well as it is suited to the results of agriculture.

DETOXIFICATION

Since ancient times, people have sought to eliminate toxins from the body by fasting and special diets, often in conjunction with other means, such as emetics and enemas. At present, many Americans are concerned about ridding their bodies of waste products that have accumulated because of poor digestion or sluggish elimination or that have resulted from environmental toxins. Practitioners recommend eating only raw fruits and vegetables and drinking large amounts of water; yogurt may also be included in the regimen (see also Chapters 22 and 23).

HIGH-PROTEIN DIET

In the 1970s, Robert Atkins (Atkins Center, n.d.) developed a diet based on the principle that sugar and refined carbohydrates increase the body's production of insulin, a hormone necessary for the transformation of carbohydrates to blood sugar and for passage of sugar from the blood into the tissues. Consumption of white bread, pasta, cereal, and other highly processed, low-fat foods causes insulin levels to spike. Once the carbohydrates are absorbed and high amounts of insulin are no longer needed, insulin levels drop sharply, which reduces energy and generates cravings for carbohydrate-laden snacks. Atkins developed a diet that severely restricts the intake of processed and refined carbohydrates and promotes instead a diet focusing on "nutrient-dense" foods—proteins, fats, and complex carbohydrates—supported by vitamins and other supplements (Atkins Center, n.d.). The Atkins diet has been demonstrated to be effective for short-term weight loss, but the long-term health effects are of concern to many, although it comes closer than many "fad" diets to approximating authentic human dietary intake.

THE "ZONE" DIET

Like Atkins, Barry Sears designed a diet that reduces the intake of processed foods and sugar to control insulin level. Sears's diet, which he calls "Zone Perfect" and most people know as "the Zone," uses food as a drug to keep insulin levels in the "therapeutic zone" 24 hours a day. According to Sears, every meal and snack should contain a set ratio of macronutrients: 30% protein, 40% carbohydrates, and 30% fats. Sears also suggests adding supplements, such as ω-3 fish oils and antioxidants, to enhance the Zone diet (Zone Perfect). This diet also had some characteristics of any "fad" diet, despite the selective reductionist scientific underpinnings, including a lot of hype and celebrity shenanigans. Fifteen years later, this diet appears to have "zoned out."

FOOD OR DRUG?

Sears and Atkins are not the only people using food's drug-like properties to affect the body. Scientists have long been aware that many fruits, vegetables, grains, and beans appear to reduce the risk of heart disease, cancer, and other conditions because they contain *antioxidants* (vitamins, minerals, and enzymes that protect cells from being damaged by oxidation). Now disease-fighting nutrients and constitutents in plants has been labeled as phytochemicals; also as commercial products, known as "nutraceuticals."

Phytochemicals are thought to fight cancer and other ailments by keeping disease-causing substances from effecting healthy cells and by removing toxins before they can cause harm. There are many thousands of phytochemicals—tomatoes alone contain 10,000 different kinds—each with a slightly different activity. Genistein, for example, which is found in soybeans, prevents the formation of the capillaries needed to nourish tumors. Indoles, which increase immune function, are found in members of the Brassica family such as broccoli and cauliflower. The bioflavonoids found in limes prevent certain cancer-causing hormones from attaching to the body's cells. Much as an earlier generation of scientists sought to identify and synthesize vitamins, today's researchers are working to isolate and manufacture phytochemicals that have not been considered micronutrients per se. However, it is unlikely that they will be able to reproduce the rich mix of beneficial substances found in a single tomato or a handful of broccoli sprouts. Two examples are popularized and commonly used as both foods *and* drugs, or remedies.

Garlic (*Allium sativum*) has been widely promoted as a remedy for colds, coughs, flu, chronic bronchitis, whooping cough, ringworm, asthma, intestinal worms, fever, and digestive, gallbladder, and liver disorders. Investigators have explored its use as a treatment for mild hypertension and hyperlipidemia. Heavy consumption may lead to lengthened clotting times, perioperative bleeding, and spontaneous hemorrhage. Numerous studies over a long period have documented garlic's irreversible inhibitory effect on platelet aggregation and fibrinolytic activity in humans.

Unlike many other herbal remedies, garlic is also a biologically active *food* with presumed medicinal properties, including possible anticancer effects. Clinical studies of garlic in humans address three areas: (1) effect on cardiovascular system-related disease and risk factors such as lipid levels, blood pressure, glucose level, atherosclerosis, and thrombosis; (2) protective associations with cancer; and (3) clinical adverse effects. There are multiple clinical studies with promising but conflicting results. There is high consumer usage of garlic as a health supplement.

Scant data, primarily from case-control studies, suggest that dietary garlic consumption is associated with decreased risk of laryngeal, gastric, colorectal, and endometrial cancer and adenomatous colorectal polyps. Single case-control studies suggest that dietary garlic consumption is not associated with breast or prostate cancer.

Cholesterol levels have been related to use of garlic as well. Thirty-seven randomized trials, all but one in adults, consistently showed that, compared with use of a placebo, use of various garlic preparations led to small, statistically significant reduction in total cholesterol at 1 month (range of average pooled reductions, 1.2–17.3 mg/dL). Garlic preparations studied included standardized dehydrated tablets, "aged garlic extract," oil macerates, distillates, raw garlic, and combination tablets. Statistically significant reduction in LDL levels (range, 0–13.5 mg/dL) and in triglyceride levels (range, 7.6–34.0 mg/dL) also were found. One multicenter trial involving 100 adults with hyperlipidemia found no difference in lipid outcomes at 3 months between persons who were given an antilipidemic agent and persons who were given a standardized dehydrated garlic preparation.

Garlic has a range of biological activities. Twenty-seven small, randomized, placebo-controlled trials, all but one in adults and of short duration, reported mixed but never large effects of various garlic preparations on blood pressure outcomes. Most studies did not find significant differences between persons randomly assigned to take garlic and those randomly assigned to take a placebo.

Adverse effects of oral ingestion of garlic are "smelly" breath and body odor. Other possible, but not proven,

adverse effects include flatulence, esophageal and abdominal pain, small intestinal obstruction, contact dermatitis, rhinitis, asthma, bleeding, and heart attack. How frequently adverse effects occur with oral ingestion of garlic as a food and whether they vary for particular garlic preparations have not been established. Adverse effects of inhaled garlic dust include allergic reactions such as asthma, rhinitis, urticaria, angioedema, and anaphylaxis. Adverse effects of topical exposure to raw garlic include contact dermatitis, skin blisters, and ulcerative lesions. Frequency of reactions to inhaled garlic dust or topical exposure to garlic has not been established. Whether adverse effects are specific to particular preparations, constituents, or dosages should be elucidated. In particular, adverse effects related to bleeding and interactions with other drugs such as aspirin and anticoagulants warrant further study.

Research questions on garlic include:
- Whether oral ingestion of garlic (fresh, cooked, or as supplements) compared with no garlic, other oral supplements, or drugs can lower lipid levels, blood pressure, glucose levels, and cardiovascular morbidity and mortality
- Whether garlic increases insulin sensitivity and antithrombotic activity
- Associations between garlic use and the occurrence of precancerous lesions, cancer, and cancer-related morbidity and mortality.

Ginger, like garlic, can be considered as both a popular ingredient in prepared foods and beverages, and as an effective medicinal plant remedy. Ginger has long been known and used for its antinausea effects and calming properties on the stomach—thus, the traditional popular beverages ginger ale and ginger beer. It is particularly useful for nausea associated with pregnancy and with chemotherapy, for which acupuncture is also a useful alternative therapy.

TEAS AND INFUSIONS

Oftentimes we do not need to eat the plant to obtain the benefits of phytochemicals. For example, brewing teas such as green tea can provide a natural mixture of antioxidants to be drunk as a beverage. The antioxidant profile of green tea (from Asia) has been studied extensively in terms of its anticancer effects. Research on individual constituents of green tea indicate that it may be necessary to drink up to 16 cups of typical green infusion to obtain the optimal health benefits. A newly popular red tea (from South Africa) has a similar profile of antioxidants, but without the caffeine, and also shows anticancer properties, as well promoting hydration (Sanderson et al, 2014).

FOOD ALLERGIES

Soybeans may contain nutrients and phytochemicals, but they are among the common foods that trigger allergies. Other major offenders include nuts (especially peanuts), dairy products, fish, shellfish, wheat, eggs, and food additives, especially preservatives and coloring agents.

An *allergy* occurs when the immune system reacts to an ordinary food as if it were a hostile invader, producing an antibody known as immunoglobin E. This antibody attaches itself to specialized immune cells known as mast cells, and when the offending food is encountered again, the antibody causes the mast cell to release chemicals that produce the allergic reaction. The result may be skin disorders (e.g., hives, eczema), respiratory conditions (e.g., allergic rhinitis, asthma), stomach problems (e.g., cramps, diarrhea), or headaches. In severe cases, people may develop anaphylactic shock, which causes collapse and possibly even death.

No one knows for certain what causes allergies to arise, but it is common for them to run in families, although each family member may have a different type. Some theorize a possible psychological component; on some deep level, allergy sufferers may view the world as inherently hostile being attacked by "allergens" from all sides.

START WITH THE USUAL SUSPECTS

The offending substance (known as an *allergen*) can often be identified by a simple skin prick test, in which one after another of the "usual suspects" is injected under the skin to see how the body responds. Another investigative technique is the radioallergosorbent test, in which blood is drawn, serum containing antibodies is extracted, and possible allergens are added to test for a reaction. Naturopaths favor an *elimination diet,* in which various foods are systematically removed from the menu for 2 weeks. When symptoms disappear, foods are reintroduced one by one until a reaction takes place, indicating which one is causing the allergy.

Herbalists often recommend that the elimination diet be accompanied by intake of immune boosters such as Echinacea (Chapter 24) and red clover, digestive aids (e.g., slippery elm, marshmallow, hops), and dandelion root to support liver function. Yoga practitioners can teach postures designed to aid digestion and overall well-being (see Chapter 21). Nutritionists with expertise in supplements advise taking vitamins and minerals, including zinc, selenium, vitamin C, magnesium, and manganese.

Homeopaths treat allergies with a form immunotherapy in which highly diluted amounts of the allergen are given with the aim of overcoming the reaction. This approach is similar to *desensitization,* in which people are exposed to minute but increasing amounts of the allergen until a higher level of tolerance is achieved. Enzymes have proved effective in treating some milk sugar allergies. For the majority of those with allergies, the most effective treatment is avoiding the allergen in question.

FUNCTIONAL FOODS

The American food industry is currently responding to the public's desire for healthier fare by creating a variety of products that, they claim, provide enhanced health benefits, such as lowering cholesterol and heightening mental abilities. Known as *functional foods,* these products include snacks, cereals, margarines, and salad dressings laced with calcium, vitamins, fiber, and such new constituents as DHA (docosahexaenoic acid), which is currently being used in Japanese schoolchildren and is said to improve concentration.

To achieve the benefits of functional foods, large quantities of them must be consumed. One margarine, for example, must be eaten three times a day for 2 weeks to lower cholesterol by 10%. To obtain their full allotment of vitamins from snack foods, toddlers must eat three and a half cookies a day. Often six times as expensive as standard fare (e.g., margarine retails for $17.22 a pound), these functional foods require a level of commitment many families are not prepared to make.

The greatest drawback to many functional foods is the flavor. As *New York Times* food critic William Grimes noted, one cholesterol-controlling apricot and orange cereal bar has the "texture of a rubber eraser, enlivened by a hideously artificial fruit flavor." He noted that a "sugar controller" for diabetic patients, a fudge brownie flavor nutrition bar, "chews like a plug of tobacco, minus the flavor, except for a hay-like aftertaste. The chocolate coating seems to be for color only. Nuts depicted on the wrapping fail to show up in the actual bar" (Grimes, 1999). In a taste test of 13 functional foods, five got a "thumb's up," including the bone-building Aviva Instant Hot Chocolate and Viactiv's caramel-flavored Calcium Plus D Soft Chews; the majority of products received a "thumb's down." Grimes addressed the "pleasure principle" as follows:

> All food is functional. That is why humans eat three times a day. But unlike animals and insects, they do not eat for function's sake alone. Somewhere in the tortured mental software that governs eating behavior, the pleasure principle lives in more or less uneasy proximity to the efficiency principle. We eat to live, but we also live to eat. (Grimes, 1999)

NUTRITION VERSUS NOURISHMENT

Food and emotions are very deeply linked in human beings for reasons far older than our current obsession with thinness. For centuries the human race was able to survive because we ate the things our tribes said were okay to eat. We avoided the poisonous berries and ate what our parents said was safe. Food has always been an essential part of the daily ritual of living, and the foods we were fed in childhood have left a very deep impression on us. At an unconscious and conscious level, they help us feel safe and cared for.

One of the reasons diets and food fads are so popular is that we are tribal beings who take our cues about what to eat from those around us. One of the reasons diets so often fail is that they conflict with much deeper cultural programming that comes from our family of origin. If generations of your relatives served beef brisket (or borscht or macaroni and cheese) for dinner every Sunday, that dish will forever be equated with family gatherings and feelings of belonging. However flawed they may be, our families usually present our strongest links to our past and to others; in a profound way, they represent safety and the sense of being at home.

Unfortunately, the eating patterns of the past do not always work well in the twenty-first century. The rib roast with gravy and buttered potatoes that once nourished our great grandparents on the farm may lead to a heart attack in someone whose most strenuous daily activity is booting up the computer. On the other hand, the food products our contemporary culture urges us to consume—loaded with fat, salt, sugar, artificial ingredients, and chemical additives and stripped of nutrients during processing—are equally unlikely to sustain us into a healthy and advanced old age. Taking a scientific, reductionist approach is not the answer either. Obsessing about every calorie and gram of fat on our plates can turn food into an enemy. Eating is one of the most vital ways we connect with our environment and with each other. Treating food as a hostile force is not good for our bodies, our souls, or our relationship with the world.

So, what is the key to healthy eating? Moderation and common sense are a good starting point. Once we understand our basic nutritional needs and which foods we would be wise to avoid when possible, we can move gradually into patterns of eating that provide us with a sense of physical well-being. However, unless we have a medical condition such as diabetes that requires strict dietary controls, healthy eating does not mean abandoning favorite foods forever. On occasion a piece of grandmother's fried chicken at a family gathering, an ice cream cone on a summer afternoon, or a mug of sugary cocoa after sledding is a necessary reminder that being alive is sometimes supposed to be fun and that sharing food with the people we love can be healthy for our hearts in ways not yet recognized by biomedical science. Food is rich in cultural, social, and personal meaning as well as nutrients, and all these elements are necessary for a balanced diet.

References

Abels JC, Gorham AT, Pack GT, Rhoads CP: Metabolic studies in patients cancer of the gastrointestinal tract: Plasma vitamin A levels, *J Clin Invest* 20:749, 1941.

Albert DM, Kumar A, Strugnell SA, et al: Effectiveness of vitamin D analogues in treating large tumors during prolonged use in murine retinoblastoma models, *Arch Ophthalmol* 122:1357–1362, 2004.

Amri H, Abu-Asab M, Micozzi MS: *Avicenna's medicine: a new translation of the 11ᵗʰ century canon with practical applications for integrative health care*, Rochester, VT, 2013, Healing Arts Press/ Inner Traditions.

Atkins Center: *The Atkins diet: a brief overview*, n.d. Available at: http://www.atkinscenter.com.

Baron JA, Beach M, Mandel JS, et al: Calcium supplements for the prevention of colorectal adenomas, *N Engl J Med* 342:1357–1362, 1999.

Dreon DM, Fernstrom HA, Williams PT, Krauss RM: A very low-fat diet is not associated with improved lipoprotein profiles in men with a predominance of large, low density lipoproteins, *Am J Clin Nutr* 69:411–418, 1999.

Emoto M: Healing with water, *L Altern Complement Med* 10(1):19–21, 2004.

Grimes W: But how do they taste? A food critic answers, *New York Times* 16, 1999.

Hite AH, Feinman RD, Guzman GE, et al: In the face of contradictory evidence: Report of the Dietary Guidelines for Americans Committee, *Nutrition* 26:915–924, 2010.

Holick MF: Vitamin D: a millennium perspective, *J Cell Biochem* 88:296, 2003.

Lands WE: Dietary fat and health: The evidence and the politics of prevention: Careful use of dietary fats can improve life and prevent disease, *Ann NY Sci* 1055:179–192, 2005.

Moon RC, McCormick DL, Mehta RG: Inhibition of carcinogenesis by retinoids, *Cancer Res* 43:2469, 1983.

Moon RC, Mehta RG, McCormick DL: Retinoids and Mammary Gland Differentiation. In Nugent J, Clark S, editors: *Retinoids, Differentiation and Disease*, London, 1985, Pittman, pp 156–167.

Ravnskov U: The questionable role of saturated and polyunsaturated fatty acids in cardiovascular diseases, *J Clin Epidemiol* 51:443–460, 1998.

Sanderson M, Mazibuko SE, Joubert E, et al: Effects of fermented rooibos (*Aspalathus linearis*) on adipocyte differentiation, *Phytomedicine* 21:109–117, 2014.

Stanhope KL, Schwarz JM, Keim NL, et al: Consuming fructose-sweetened, not glucose-sweetened, beverages, *J Clin Invest* 119:1322–1334, 2009.

Wolbach SB, Howe PR: Tissue changes following deprivations of fat soluble vitamin A, *J Exp Med* 42:753, 1925.

Dietary Guidelines for Americans, 2010. Center for Nutrition Policy and Promotion. Available at: http://www.cnpp.usda.gov/DGAs2010-PolicyDocument.htm

Suggested Readings

American Cancer Society: Statistics. Available at: http://www.cancer.org.

American Heart Association: Cardiovascular diseases. In *International classification of diseases*, ed 9, pp 390–459, 745–747. Available at: http://www.americanheart.org.

Ames BN: DNA damage from micronutrient deficiencies is likely to be a major cause of cancer, *Mutat Res* 475:7, 2001.

Annual reports of the American Association of Poison Control Centers' National Poisoning and Exposure Database (formerly known as the Toxic Exposure Surveillance System). AAPCC, 3201 New Mexico Avenue, Suite 330, Washington, DC 20016. Download any report from 1983 to 2006 at http://www.aapcc.org/dnn/NPDS/AnnualReports/tabid/125/Default.aspx free of charge. The "Vitamin" category is usually near the end of the report.

Appel LJ: Lifestyle modification as a means to prevent and treat high blood pressure, *J Am Soc Nephrol* 14:S99, 2003.

Appel LJ, Moore TJ, Obarzanek E, et al: A clinical trial of the effects of dietary patterns on blood pressure. DASH Collaborative Research Group, *N Engl J Med* 336:1117, 1997.

Balch JF, Balch PA: *Prescription for nutritional healing*, ed 2, New York, 1997, Avery Publishing Group, pp 8–9.

Basu S, Sengupta B, Paladhi PK: Single megadose vitamin A supplementation of Indian mothers and morbidity in breastfed young infants, *Postgrad Med J* 79(933):397, 2003.

Brett J: *How vitamin A works, 2006*. Available at: http://recipes.howstuffworks.com/vitamin-a.htm.

Calle EE, Rodriguez C, Walker-Thurmond K, et al: Overweight, obesity, and mortality from cancer in a prospectively studied cohort of US adults, *N Engl J Med* 348:2003, 1625.

Carter JP, Saxe GP, Newbold V, et al: Hypothesis: dietary management may improve survival from nutritionally linked cancers based on analysis of representative cases, *J Am Coll Nutr* 12:209, 1993.

Chan LN, Zhang S, Shao J, et al: N-(4-hydroxyphenyl)retinamide induces apoptosis in T lymphoma and T lymphoblastoid leukemia cells, *Leuk Lymphoma* 25(3–4):271, 1997.

Convit A, Wolf OT, Tarshish C, et al: Reduced glucose tolerance is associated with poor memory performance and hippocampal atrophy among normal elderly, *Proc Natl Acad Sci U S A* 100:2019, 2003.

Dietary supplement fact sheet: vitamin A and carotenoids. Available at: http://ods.od.nih.gov/factsheets/vitamina.asp

Drug slows prostate tumor growth by keeping vitamin A active: Findings from the AACR Centennial Conference on Translational Cancer Medicine: From Technology to Treatment, Singapore, November 4-8, 2007. Available at: http://www.aacr.org/home/public–media/aacr-press-releases/press-releases-2007.aspx?d=922.

Enig MG, et al: Dietary fat and cancer trends: a critique, *Fed Proc* 37:139, 1978.

Feldstein CA, Akopian M, Renauld A, et al: Insulin resistance and hypertension in postmenopausal women, *J Hum Hypertens* 16(Suppl 1):S145, 2002.

Ford ES, Giles WH, Dietz WH: Prevalence of the metabolic syndrome among US adults: findings from the third National Health and Nutrition Examination Survey, *JAMA* 287:356, 2002.

Foster GD, Wyatt HR, Hill JO, et al: A randomized trial of a low-carbohydrate diet for obesity, *N Engl J Med* 348:2082, 2003.

Giovannucci E: Tomatoes, tomato-based products, lycopene, and cancer: review of the epidemiologic literature, *J Natl Cancer Inst* 91:317, 1999.

Heilbronn LK, Ravussin E: Calorie restriction and aging: review of the literature and implications for studies in humans, *Am J Clin Nutr* 78:361, 2003.

Hildenbrand GL, Hildenbrand LC, Bradford K, et al: Five-year survival rates of melanoma patients treated by diet therapy after the manner of Gerson: a retrospective review, *Altern Ther Health Med* 1:29, 1995.

Hu FB, Willett WC: Optimal diets for prevention of coronary heart disease, *JAMA* 288:2569, 2002.

Jenkins DJ, Kendall CW, Marchie A, et al: Effects of a dietary portfolio of cholesterol-lowering foods vs lovastatin on serum lipids and C-reactive protein, *JAMA* 290:502, 2003.

Kalmijn S, Launer LJ, Ott A, et al: Dietary fat intake and the risk of incident dementia in the Rotterdam Study, *Ann Neurol* 42:776, 1997.

Larsson SC, Bergkvist L, Näslund I, et al: Vitamin A, retinol, and carotenoids and the risk of gastric cancer: a prospective cohort study, *Am J Clin Nutr* 85(2):497, 2007.

Le Bars PL: Magnitude of effect and special approach to Ginkgo biloba extract EGb 761 in cognitive disorders, *Pharmacopsychiatry* 36(Suppl 1):S44, 2003.

LeMarchand LL, White KK, Nomura A, et al: Plasma levels of B vitamins on colorectal cancer risk, *Cancer Epidemiol Biomarkers Prev* 18:2195–2201, 2009.

Li CI, Malone KE, Porter PL, et al: The relationship between alcohol use and risk of breast cancer by histology and hormone receptor status among women 65-79 years of age, *Cancer Epidemiol Biomarkers Prev* 12:1061, 2003.

Liu S, Manson JE, Buring JE, et al: Relation between a diet with a high glycemic load and plasma concentrations of high-sensitivity C-reactive protein in middle-aged women, *Am J Clin Nutr* 75:492, 2002.

Luchsinger JA, Tang MX, Shea S, et al: Antioxidant vitamin intake and risk of Alzheimer disease, *Arch Neurol* 60:203, 2003.

Luft FC, Weinberger MH: Heterogeneous responses to changes in dietary salt intake: the salt-sensitivity paradigm, *Am J Clin Nutr* 65:612S, 1997.

Messina MJ: Emerging evidence on the role of soy in reducing prostate cancer risk, *Nutr Rev* 61:117, 2003.

Morris MC, Evans DA, Bienias JL, et al: Consumption of fish and n-3 fatty acids and risk of incident Alzheimer disease, *Arch Neurol* 60:940, 2003.

Morrow DJ: A medicine chest or a grocery shelf?, *New York Times* 1, 1999.

Murray M, Birdsall T, Pizzorno JE, et al: *How to prevent and treat cancer with natural medicine*, New York, 2002, Riverhead Books.

Paolisso G, Sgambato S, Pizza G, et al: Improved insulin response and action by chronic magnesium administration in aged NIDDM subjects, *Diabetes Care* 12:265, 1989.

Pasternak RC: Report of the Adult Treatment Panel III: the 2001 National Cholesterol Education Program guidelines on the detection, evaluation and treatment of elevated cholesterol in adults, *Cardiol Clin* 21:393, 2003.

Rahmathullah L, Tielsch JM, Thulasiraj RD, et al: Impact of supplementing newborn infants with vitamin A on early infant mortality: community based randomized trial in southern India, *BMJ* 327(7409):254, 2003.

Reaven GM: Pathophysiology of insulin resistance in human disease, *Physiol Rev* 75:473, 1995.

Ridker PM, Buring JE, Cook NR, et al: C-reactive protein, the metabolic syndrome, and risk of incident cardiovascular events: an 8-year follow-up of 14 719 initially healthy American women, *Circulation* 107:391, 2003.

Robbins J, Malkmus G: *Food consumption in the USA, based on USDA statistics*. Available at: http://www.healthfree.com.

Sacks FM, Svetkey LP, Vollmer WM, et al: Effects on blood pressure of reduced dietary sodium and the Dietary Approaches to Stop Hypertension (DASH) diet. DASH-Sodium Collaborative Research Group, *N Engl J Med* 344:3, 2001.

Seshadri S, Beiser A, Selhub J, et al: Plasma homocysteine as a risk factor for dementia and Alzheimer's disease, *N Engl J Med* 346:476, 2002.

Stendig-Lindberg G, Tepper R, Leichter I: Trabecular bone density in a two year controlled trial of peroral magnesium in osteoporosis, *Magnes Res* 6:155, 1993.

Suddath R: Vibration, Energy, and Water, ExtraOrdinary Technology 3(4), 2005.

Tabet N, Mantle D, Walker Z, et al: Endogenous antioxidant activities in relation to concurrent vitamins A, C, and E intake in dementia, *Int Psychogeriatr* 14:7, 2002.

US Department of Agriculture: *Economic Research Service: Food consumption, prices and expenditures, 1970–1995*, Statistical Bulletin No 939, Washington, DC, 1997, The Author.

US Department of Agriculture, Economic Research Service: *Food consumption, prices and expenditures, 1970–97*, Statistical Bulletin No 965, Washington, DC, 1999, The Author. Available at: http://www.ers.usda.gov.

US Department of Agriculture, Economic Research Service: *America's eating habits: changes and consequences*, Agriculture Information Bulletin No 750, Washington, DC, 1999, The Author. Available at: http://www.ers.usda.gov.

US Department of Agriculture, Food and Nutrition Service: *USDA report encourages Americans to remember nutritional needs when eating out*, News Release No 0060.99, Alexandria, Va, 1999, The Author. Available at: http://www.ers.usda.gov.

Vitamin A, 2007. Available at: http://lpi.oregonstate.edu/infocenter/vitamins/vitaminA.

Vitamin A and C synergistically fight breast cancer cell growth, 2006. Available at: http://www.lef.org/whatshot/2006_05.htm.

See also Kim KN, Pie JE, Park JH, et al: Retinoic acid and ascorbic acid act synergistically in inhibiting human breast cancer cell proliferation, *J Nutr Biochem* 17(7):454, 2006. Epub November 15, 2005.

Vitamin A derivative could restore smokers' health, 2003. Available at: http://www.in-pharmatechnologist.com/news/ng.asp?id=26231-vitamin-a-derivative.

Vitamin A pushes breast cancer to form blood vessel cells, *Science Daily 2008*. Available at: http://www.sciencedaily.com/releases/2008/07/080715204719.htm.

Vitamin A/retinol, 2000. Available at: http://www.bccancer.bc.ca/PPI/UnconventionalTherapies/VitaminARetinol.htm.

Westman EC, Yancy WS, Edman JS, et al: Effect of 6-month adherence to a very low carbohydrate diet program, *Am J Med* 113:30, 2002.

Witteman JC, Grobbee DE, Derkx FH, et al: Reduction of blood pressure with oral magnesium supplementation in women with mild to moderate hypertension, *Am J Clin Nutr* 60:129, 1994.

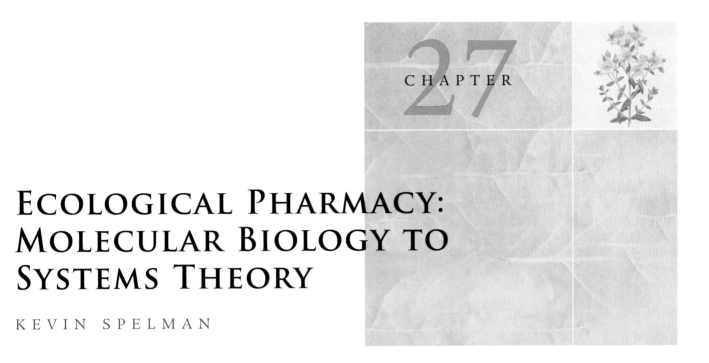

CHAPTER

ECOLOGICAL PHARMACY: MOLECULAR BIOLOGY TO SYSTEMS THEORY

KEVIN SPELMAN

First, the world of life, taken as a whole, forms a single system bound to the surface of the earth; a system whose elements, in whatever order of association they may be considered, are not simply thrown together and molded upon one another like grains of sand, but are organically interdependent like . . . molecules caught in a capillary surface.

—TEILHARD DE CHARDIN, 1943

In the middle of the last century, some years before the discovery of DNA, Erwin Schrödinger, in his classic 1944 book *What is Life?*, inspired a generation of scientists with his timeless philosophical question: "How can the events in space and time which take place within the spatial boundary of a living organism be accounted for by physics and chemistry?" (Schrödinger, 1944). To start at the microscopic, individual level, life (in the words of Schrödinger) depletes free energy and produces high entropy waste that maintains internal order.

Until recently, the approach in physics and chemistry has been that of reductionism, to study only the components of any given system. Biology has also given excessive authority to reductionism that collapses higher level accounts, such as social or behavioral events, into molecular ones (Rose, 1999). Influenced by such an approach, life may appear to be merely the sum of its chemical and physical parts. This view has come to dominate all sciences, including the medical sciences.

Contemporary science has overemphasized the reductionist model in its exploration of our world. Reductionism tends to attribute reality to component properties rather than the outcome that emerges from the interaction of the components (Kirchoff, 2002). And although reductionism is a powerful approach, the structure and func-

tional aspect of a system's components gives us little indication of the behavior of the corresponding networks (Buehler, 2003a,b). The properties of a system cannot be understood by accounting only for the properties of its components.

The medical sciences, and especially pharmacology, have fully embraced the reductionist construct, implying that human health can be reduced to the modulation of specific genes and proteins. The laboratory modeling has, until recently, limited observations to the interaction between one gene or protein with a single chemical. Such simplistic modeling has led to some life-saving drugs, but has also lead to pharmaceutical drugs (even when properly prescribed) being an embarrassing and unfortunate leading cause of death in the United States. A broader model accounting for evolution and biology's extraordinarily ability to adapt to the environment is suggested below.

GAIA THEORY: INTERDEPENDENCE OF ORGANISM AND ENVIRONMENT

Teilhard de Chardin, a visionary French Jesuit, paleontologist, biologist, and philosopher who was fascinated with evolution and its connection with spirituality, recognized the limitations of reductionism. De Chardin was involved with early archaeological investigations of Peking Man (and the first evidence of the use of fire from nearly one million years ago; but all the evidence mysteriously disappeared from a railroad car during the Japanese occupation of China in World War II). He insisted that life must be studied in its totality on a large scale as a single, unitary system. As he contemplated the Earth and its life forms in the 1940s, he suggested the term *geobiology* to embrace all life systems and their environment as a self-organizing whole (Galleni, 1995).

Within two decades of de Chardin's writing, a significant paradigm shift from the quantitative "clockworks" view to an exploration of the qualitative emergent view of self-organizing systems and even life itself, took place. A system's approach was starting to be supported in other sciences (Capra, 1996). For example, in Germany, Hermann Haken developed his nonlinear laser theory, and Manfred Eigen experimented on catalytic cycles; in the United States, Heinz von Foerster focused his interdisciplinary team on self-organization; in Belgium, Ilya Prigogine grasped the now-understood connections among nonequilibrium systems and nonlinearity; and in Chile, Humberto Maturana was postulating autopoiesis and life. In Denmark, Per Bak developed self-organizing principles relative to complexity or "chaos" theory (see Chapters 1 and 2).

These paradigms all converged on systems as a whole, coupled with Teilhard de Chardin's insistence that the Earth must be studied as a unity—together with both geological and biological points of view (Galleni, 1995)—perhaps led the British atmospheric chemist James Lovelock to one of the biggest revolutions in viewing our planet that perhaps we will ever know (Lovelock & Margulis, 1974).

Lovelock worked as a consultant to the U.S. National Aeronautics and Space Administration (NASA) in the early 1960s. NASA contracted Lovelock to aid in the quest to detect life on Mars. Lovelock, contemplating the chemistry of the atmosphere, found that an atmosphere that is out of chemical equilibrium was the signature of life on a planet. An atmosphere rich in oxygen and methane, for instance, demonstrates that organisms are responsible for the uneven mix. Earth has just that atmosphere (Lovelock, 1979). Through this investigation, Lovelock had a flash of insight one day: the planet Earth as a whole is a self-organizing system. He saw the unity of the biosphere—a global organism (Turney, 2005).

Just a few years later, the further study of these features of the Earth resulted in the idea that life vigorously regulated terrestrial conditions, a sort of "planetary homeostasis" (Turney, 2005). By observing the geological evidence and paleoclimatic evidence, Lovelock, influenced by ecology, physiology, cybernetics, and system analysis, hypothesized that the ocean's salinity, the gaseous atmospheric concentration, and the surface temperatures were maintained in narrow ranges by feedback loops of organisms responding to variations in their environments (Lovelock, 1979).

Lovelock postulated that the climate and chemical composition of the Earth's surface are kept in homeostasis at optimum levels by and for the biosphere (Lovelock & Watson, 1982). The notion was that the biosphere adaptively regulated the Earth (Lovelock & Margulis, 1974). In time, Lovelock (1995) saw self-organization as emerging from the ensemble of biota and environment. He saw the

flow of sunlight upon the planet and feedback systems from living organisms to automatically generate comfortable life conditions that synchronistically evolved with the needs of the organisms on the planet. He called this idea a living planet, the Gaia hypothesis. It is now called Gaia theory.

Collaboration with the Nobel Prize winner Lynn Margulis introduced autopoietic theory into Gaia science, presenting Earth as an autopoietic planet where the biosphere as a whole is autopoietic. Margulis suggests that planetary autopoiesis is the aggregate, emergent property of the many gas-trading, gene-exchanging, growing and evolving organisms in it (Margulis & Sagan, 2000).

A model as whole and beautiful as Gaia was predictable. Chemists and physicists probing matter were finding that nature did not consist of isolated components, but rather appeared as a complex web of relations among the various parts of a unified whole. As Heisenberg expressed decades before the Gaia hypothesis was formulated, "the world thus appears as a complicated tissue of events, in which connections of different kinds alternate or overlap or combine and thereby determine the texture of the whole" (Capra, 1982).

Life has existed on the Earth for over 3.8 billion years (Lenton, 2002). During this time, the Earth's surface has been subject to increasing solar luminosity declining volcanic and tectonic activity, and to such perturbations as massive asteroid impacts (Lovelock & Margulis, 1974; Watson & Lovelock, 1978; Lenton, 2002). For example, despite the fact that the heat of the sun has increased by 25% over the last 4 billion years, the Earth's surface temperature has remained relatively constant, creating an agreeable environment for life (Lovelock, 1987).

Gaia theory suggests that practically all metabolisms are intimately connected to the flow of chemical compounds (Lovelock, 1989). For instance the greenhouse gases of carbon dioxide, methane, and sulfur compounds can produce highly reflective clouds, thus affecting the temperature of the Earth's surface and, in turn, influencing the metabolism of life (due to temperature change) on the planet that again changes the flow of chemical compounds to the surface and atmosphere (Kleidon, 2004).

It seems that life affects the Earth's surface environment at a planetary level, significantly increasing the cycling of free energy, essential elements, and water, inducing extreme thermodynamic disequilibrium of the atmosphere and altering the chemistry of the atmosphere, oceans, land surface, and crust (Lovelock, 1987). In turn, the state of the environment influences life, creating feedback loops between life and its environment (Lenton, 2002). These circular processes are organized through feedback loops that are found in every living system. The unusual aspects of the Earth's hypothesized feedback loops is that they link together living and nonliving systems. For instance, Gaia theory weaves together plants, microorganisms, and animals with rocks, oceans, and the atmosphere (Capra, 1996).

In this construct, life and the environment evolve together as one system so that not only does the species that leaves the most progeny inherit the environment, but the environment that favors the most progeny is itself sustained (Kirchner, 2003). This life-enhancing interplay of environment and organism can be understood as an emergent property of evolution because life-enhancing effects would be favored by natural selection (Lenton, 1998). This concept—also radical—requires a rethinking of the neo-Darwinist view of evolution.

Lovelock deduced the following principles from his observations of the planet (Lovelock, 1989):

1. Life is a global phenomenon. There cannot be sparse life on a planet. It would be as unstable as half of a buffalo. Living organisms must regulate their planet; otherwise the inevitable forces of physical and chemical evolution would render it uninhabitable.
2. Gaia theory supplements Darwin's great vision. The evolution of the species needs to be considered hand in hand with the evolution of their environment. The two processes are closely linked as a single indivisible process. To say that the organism that leaves the most progeny succeeds is not enough. Success also depends upon coherent coupling between the evolution of the organism and the evolution of its material environment.
3. Finally, Gaia theory requires a mathematical model that accepts the nonlinearity of nature without being overwhelmed by the limitations imposed by the chaos of complex dynamics. The theory makes the seemingly irrelevant observations of ecological oscillations relevant (Lotka, 1925).

With these principles, Lovelock provides an analogy between the ability of a living organism and communication systems to maintain life and low entropy levels, mainly through a continuous energy leakage into the surroundings (Onori & Visconti, 2012).

At its simplest, the idea that the entire ensemble of living organisms in its interaction with the environment—the biosphere—can be considered a single system has become the basis for a whole series of unfolding programs of research (Turney, 2005).

Some 40 years after Lovelock's realization, a statement issued from a joint meeting in 2001 of the International Geosphere-Biosphere Programme, the International Human Dimensions Programme on Global Environmental Change, the World Climate Research Programme, and the International Biodiversity Programme in a meeting in Amsterdam to study our planet begins with: "The Earth System behaves as a single, self-regulating system comprised of physical, chemical, biological and human components." It seems the science of Gaia has become conventional wisdom (Turney, 2005).

Even some scientists who do not agree with Gaia theory acknowledge what Lovelock's vision has added to the study of Earth Sciences (Volk, 2002; Turney, 2005). The very term "Earth Science" exists because of Lovelock's work. Volk (2002), who does not embrace Gaia's implications, says,

"I was inspired by Lovelock's early writings to move into issues about the effects of life on a global scale that led to technical work I would not otherwise have accomplished ... Gaia became a way of thinking, a mantra to be mindful of the biggest scale." Many critics accept that it is essential to understand the Earth system as a unity, rather than as a set of disconnected components (Kirchner, 2003).

One of the issues is the defining feature of complex systems like Gaia, making it extremely difficult to analyze. The planet is not a well-designed machine, but a complex ensemble of life that constantly rebuilds itself within a range of variable parameters, like all living organisms. This creates a model impossible to analyze from a reductionist perspective (Kirchner, 2003).

Free and Barton (2007) point out that the overall prediction (i.e., that most real global biotic systems tend towards long-term stability) obviously cannot be tested. There are, however, some useful secondary predictions:

1. A coupled life–environment system shows better resistance and resilience than would the abiotic equivalent, and recovers faster from perturbation (has greater elasticity).
2. Small-scale biotic systems and those lacking efficient nutrient recycling and photosynthesis are less resistant and resilient than those of large scale and possessing these attributes.
3. Life–environment feedbacks should tend to stabilize the system on geological time scales.
4. As life and environment coevolve, the biosphere will tend towards greater stability and remain within tighter environmental bounds.
5. The stability of the biosphere should not depend on the presence of particular species or ecosystems, which can only have arisen by chance, and should be possible in a biosphere composed solely of microorganisms.

According to the more complex models of systems theory, Lovelock's proposal of very different and complex realities (like the biosphere and the inert environment) operating—in a unified and harmonious way—in the creation of a super-system may be both unexpected and provocative (Onori & Visconti, 2012). Another supportive model for Gaia theory comes from quantum mechanics from Byrne (2011). He recently identified entanglement as the most important discovery of quantum physics, in that it allows for the knowledge of everything there is to know about a composite system, without knowing everything about the individual constituents (see Chapter 14).

Yet a deeper reservation is that a living planet has all the hallmarks of scientific communities coming to grips with a major paradigm shift, a revolution in science (Kuhn, 1962). Whether or not one agrees with the enchanted vision of a biotic Earth, the issue is more than academic. Gaia theory stimulates us to draw together diverse lines of theory and experiment, investigate their connections, and query into whether they can be extended to the spatiotemporal scale of a closed system, the biosphere (Free & Barton, 2007). Given current concerns about anthropogenic perturbation of the biosphere, all relevant scientific disciplines should contribute to predicting its response. It is vital to comprehend how our planet functions and how it is likely to respond to immature fostering and guardianship (Lenton, 2002).

Capra (1996) points out that the conception of the universe as an interconnected web of relations is one of the major themes that recur throughout modern physics. The elucidation of the patterns and relationships between a system's components may provide models which provide a more accurate depiction of reality. He goes on to suggest that Gaia is a mere realization of this line of reasoning. Moreover, such a systems approach may provide a wider perspective to understanding the process of evolution, inviting us to recognize that humans belong to a process that is much more grand than the human species.

COHERENT COUPLING, EXPANDING THE COEVOLUTION CONSTRUCT, ADAPTATION TO THE ENVIRONMENT

Isolating the organism from its environment has been a fundamental tenet of studying biological processes. In almost all medical research laboratories around the world this practice is still followed in hopes of further insight into life processes. However, this may lead to incomplete conclusions. Maturana and Varela (1987) propose that due to organisms being inexorably interwoven with their environments, it is impossible to speak of environment and organism as separate entities. They presented this interrelationship as *structural coupling* (and later called coherent coupling) in the landmark book *The Tree of Knowledge*. They define coherent coupling as a history of recurrent interactions leading to the structural congruence between two (or more) systems (Maturana & Varela, 1987). In other words, autopoietic (self-organizing) unities, such as organisms and the environment, can undergo coupled histories of structural change due to their consistent and constant interactions. Coherent coupling recognizes the congruence between autopoietic systems (Maturana, 1975). This can include the system and its environment or systems affecting systems. In this paradigm, the environment is seen as a medium, which illustrates the interwoven nature between organism and environment. Development of the autopoietic systems involved thereby arises from transformations that each invokes in the other. This concept very much challenges the neo-Darwinist evolutionary theory, which in some authors' opinions drastically underestimates the effects and inseparability of the environment and organism (Thaler, 1994; Cairns, 1996; Scapini, 2001). Such interdependent relationship is considered unique and diachronic and is a defining principle of an organism and the environment (Scapini, 2001).

The construct of coherent coupling dictates that organism and environment are mutually enfolded in multiple

ways, and what constitutes the world of a given organism is enacted by that organism's history of coupling with its environment (Varela et al, 1991). Indeed, on a human level it is well accepted at this juncture that our interwoven nature with our environment provides constant perturbation requiring a systemic reorganization of physiologic functions (Schulkin, 2003) (see Chapter 2).

Whereas some researchers are realizing the profound relations the environment has with physiological function, especially in regard to health and disease, other researchers have taken it a step further. Cairns et al (1988) published a controversial paper some years ago, stating that mutations can be environmentally directed, supporting the historical "Lamarckian" view of biology. Following Cairns's work a few years later, Thaler (1994) came to the same conclusion, stating that the environment can invoke genotypic change and postulated that both the environment as well as the organism's *perception* of the environment can induce genetic engineering genes to rewrite themselves and thus, rewrite sections of DNA code. Cairns and Thaler are suggesting a complex engagement of organism and environment. What they perhaps did not yet know was that they provided Maturana and Varela with molecular evidence for their coherent coupling construct. This greatly challenged the prevalent Neo-Darwinist perspective that sees mutations as random events, not potentially adaptive, as suggested by Cairns and Thaler. Such an adaptive response, well beyond haphazard natural selection, infers a primary form of intelligence that had developed billions of years ago (Pechere, 2004).

The construct of coherent coupling provides the understanding of an autopoietic systems' ability to be extensively "shaped" by interactions with its environment over time, and vice versa. Many may see this construct as the fitting of a system to its environment, but that is not what is meant by coherent coupling. Rather, this construct denotes congruence between autopoietic systems and environment due to reciprocal changes. It is also important not to confuse this construct with coevolution, a subset of evolution that includes population genetics and theoretical ecology. Although coevolution accounts for species–species or species–environment interactions, it differs from the coherent coupling paradigm in that the species are still seen separately from their environment and surrounding species. Coevolution theory still follows the central dogma of biology: information flows from DNA to RNA, to protein and, by extension, to the cell and on to multicellular systems. Crick originally, purely arbitrarily, formulated this "dogma" as a negative hypothesis that states that information cannot flow from protein to DNA (Crick, 1970). What the doctrine of the central dogma of biology implies is that a cell's/organism's experience has no effect on the DNA sequence (Figure 27-1).

Maturana and Varela (1987) challenge the central dogma by implying that experience can have an effect on DNA. They point out that the confusion is seeing DNA as "uniquely responsible" instead of having an "essential

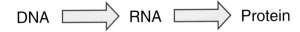

Figure 27-1 The central dogma of biology.

participation". Although the organisms and environment are recognized as autonomous in the coherent coupling model, they are also recognized as inseparably engaged in mutually affecting relationships. The result is ontogenic adaptation of the organism to its medium: "the changes of state of the organism correspond to the change of state of the medium" (Maturana, 1975). Thus organisms are seen as "shaped" due to historical recurrent interactions with their environment, just as the environment has been shaped by its interactions with the organism (see Chapter 2).

On a microcosmic scale, for instance, cellular membranes have coherently coupled with the abundance of sodium and calcium ions. This observation is made through the specialization of proteins in the membrane to allow for active transport and the inclusion of metabolic processes in which sodium and calcium participate. This fact implies that the genome adapted to the reoccurring experience of the membrane with sodium and/or calcium. On a macrocosmic scale, the paradigm of coherent coupling leads to an easy realization of the Gaia hypothesis wherein the planetary environment (e.g., temperature, ocean salinity and atmospheric gases) is modified by various species, and in turn, these species phenotypically and genotypically morph to the environment. It has been stated that all "evolution is coevolution" (Kauffman, 1995) and that all "development is co-development" (Gilbert, 2002). Thus, could it be that all evolution and all development is environmental coupling?

Ultimately interpreting Maturana and Varela's work results in the idea that the coupling of organisms with a high capacity for adaptation goes beyond response to the physicochemical dimension. The fluidity of morphological, physiological and psychological plasticity of an organism firmly embeds that organism with its surroundings, creating a dynamic response to recursive perturbations. Put simply, the phenotype depends to a significant degree on the environment, and this is a necessary condition for integrating the developing organism into its particular habitat (Gilbert, 2002).

COUPLING OF HUMANS WITH PHYTOCHEMISTRY: PLANT–HUMAN COALITIONS

The constant interwoven nature of organism and environment requires some sort of exchange of information to account for species plasticity. Markos (1995) defines this exchange that allows species to read their environment, thus integrating into Gaia, as "informational flow." The informational flow relevant to the discussion between plants and humans is, in its most basic form, chemistry–

molecular messaging—although there are likely many other cues that are important to plant-human coalitions (for example, botany of desire).

The secondary metabolites of plants are well known to modulate the relations—both positive (i.e., attractant) and negative (i.e., repellent)—among plants and their consumers. The presence of secondary compounds in plants provides information to other species, and due to a reiterative history of interactions, generates a mutually enfolding between plants and humans. Plants have always provided shelter, clothing, food and medicine for humans. In turn, humans (and animals) transport, seed, cultivate, and with metabolic waste, fertilize plants.

Higher primates have been evolving and have been exposed to plant chemistry for about 88 million years. The higher primates, considered to be omnivores, are nevertheless, herbivores as well. Over such an evolutionary time scale, all higher primates relied on the predictability of vegetative parts of plants as food sources (Johns, 1996). This circumstance includes *Homo sapiens*, with 5 million to 7 million years of exposure to phytochemistry. Of course, this exposure to various plant parts exposed the consumer to thousands of secondary metabolites. Estimates of the number of plants in the early human diet range from 80 to 220. Clearly, if *Homo sapiens* consumed such a regular number and volume of plant foods, they were exposed to a very high number of phytochemicals. A very conservative estimate would be in the range of 80,000 to 220,000, and quite likely much higher. Ames et al (1990) makes an estimate of the number of secondary metabolites in the current human diet taking into account only those secondary metabolites that are also known to function as natural pesticides. He observes that even with the great reduction in diversity and variety in the human diet compared to hunter-gatherer ancestors, the modern number of established natural pesticides in the diet is about 10,000 compounds. Thus, even now humans are constantly exposed to a great amount of "information" from plants.

If humans have coherently coupled with plants, then by default this means that plants have shaped humans through informational molecular exchange, and vice versa; humans have shaped plants by this means, as well as by conscious horticulture. This shaping, if the hypothesis is solid, should range from DNA to protein and include epigenetic activity. Epigenetic influences (through DNA methylation, chromatin remodeling, and microRNA-regulated transcriptional silencing) allow environmental inputs to shape human phenotype through alteration in gene expression. For instance, methyl-CpG-binding proteins and amino acids (such as methionine, cysteine, serine, and glycine) play a role in single-carbon metabolism (Niculescu & Zeisel, 2002; Valinluck et al, 2004), and key phytonutrients and phytochemicals (such as vitamins B6, folate, betaine, choline, selenium epigallocatechin-3-gallate, resveratrol, genistein, and curcumin) have also been shown to modulate epigenetic activity (Tammen et al, 2013). This author suggests that as further research

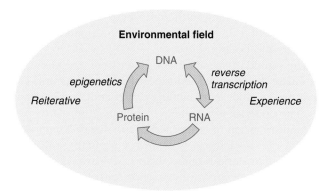

Figure 27-2 The central dogma of biology revised.

unfolds, epigenetic modulation through numerous phytochemicals will be recognized in the coming years as a key piece of an adaptive response, important in long-term human health.

It is easy to see that humans have shaped plants by looking at the cultivation of crops; the original species of any of the crop plants have changed drastically due to human intervention. It should also be obvious, although not quite as easy to recognize, that plants have shaped humans. One obvious, well-known example is the "shaping" of the cytochrome P450 (CYP 450) genes. This ancient superfamily of enzymes consists primarily of microsomal and mitochondrial proteins and in humans represents about 75 different CYP 450 genes (Danielson, 2002) (Figure 27-2).

Danielson (2002) points out that CYP 450 genes allow animals to generate a metabolic resistance to plant compounds designed to dissuade plant grazing, and conversely, to allow plants to generate new compounds to deter herbivory. He goes on to point out that these CYP 450 genes in plants and animals have been engaged in a cyclical process, generating novel compounds in plants and generating resistance in animals. Jackson (1991) discusses the observation that particular plant compounds (such as alkaloids, glycosides, phenolics, uncommon proteins, unusual free amino acids, steroids, essential oils, terpenes, and resins) are capable of altering the metabolism and potentially changing the biological fitness of humans as well as their domesticated animals, and even the obligate parasites of each species. She points out that detoxification of plant compounds represents an avenue of potentiating individual and group shifts in gastrointestinal function, structure, and endocrine metabolism. But this influence on physiology does not just stop with transient functional effects.

CYP 450 genes have an unusual ability to evolve rapidly, following a quick-paced, nonlinear time course (Nelson et al, 1993; Danielson, 2002). A large-scale expansion of the CYP 450 gene family is thought to have provided a cache of proteins from which novel isoforms provided adaptive strategies for metabolizing plant compounds. The resulting diversity in these genes is thought to be

due to the recurring exchange of molecular information among the secondary metabolites of plants and mammals needing new enzymes to detoxify these plant compounds (Gonzalez & Nebert, 1990). Therefore, the rich exposure of humans to phytochemistry ultimately promoted human biological variability affecting our genes (Gonzalez & Nebert, 1990; Jackson, 1991; Nelson et al, 1993). Was it haphazard mutations that lead to such abilities? Or were genotypic changes, as Cairns and Thaler's work suggest, environmentally directed?

Another example of coherent coupling between plants and humans are the steroid receptors. Specifically, the estrogen receptor is the original member of the steroid receptor family (Hawkins et al, 2000; Wu et al, 2003). The gene structure and ligand-binding properties of the classical estrogen receptor (ER-α) are known to have been highly conserved over 300 million years of vertebrate evolution. Thus, the binding of an estrogenic chemical to ER-α in fish, amphibians, reptiles, birds, and mammals (including humans) shows relatively little difference (Katzenellenbogen et al, 1979; Pakdel et al, 1989; White et al, 1994; Welshons et al, 2003). Orthodox thought of this protein as occurring only in vertebrates requires revision. The microbial organisms known as mycorrhiza, living on the roots of plants, have a receptor called NodD, which has a high amount of genetic homology with the human estrogen receptor. Plants also express an identical protein to the human 5α-reductase enzyme (Li et al, 1997; Fox, 2004). Steroids and flavonoids, produced by plants, bind these proteins (Gyorgypal & Kondorosi, 1991; Baker, 1992). Thus, molecules that have similar shape and electronegativity as the estrogens, such as select isoflavones, are utilized as a communication strategy between plants and fungi, for example (Gyorgypal & Kondorosi, 1991).

A perspective from an evolutionary context suggests that the communication strategy of plants pertains to us as well. Phytochemical messenger molecules used by symbiotic soil fungi can be sequestered by humans, bind to estrogen receptors, and thereby influence gene expression. In discussing that the NodD and the estrogen receptor share no common evolutionary ancestry, Fox (2004) attempts to explain this observation by invoking the construct of convergent evolution—that these different species have responded to similar environmental signals, via natural selection, with the same adaptive traits. However, this result leaves the homology between these proteins to mere chance. If we view this through the lens of the coherent coupling paradigm, it offers an example of interspecies plasticity in response to environmental context.

Through this lens, humans and plants would be seen to shape themselves to mutual signals. Wynne-Edwards (2001) postulates that plants chosen for domestication may have a higher occurrence of phytoestrogens. This could potentially enhance the ovulatory cycle in women, which might mean there are more humans to cultivate more crops—an arguable benefit for the particular plant species. Wynne-Edwards goes on to point out that humans

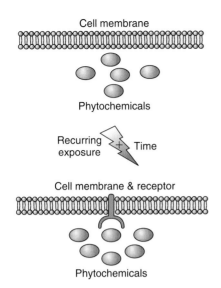

Figure 27-3 Coherent coupling between phytochemistry and eukaryotic cells.

have receptors in the nose and cheeks that bind native steroids and plant compounds, which in turn signal the brain. Studies have demonstrated that mammals will consume steroids in foods at some times and reject them at other times, depending on physiological and reproductive conditions (e.g., in pregnancy, rats will reject foods with steroids in them). Thus, true to the coherent coupling paradigm, there is a plasticity of response between animals and plants (Figure 27-3).

The effects of flavonoids, nonsteroidal secondary metabolites of plants, share key similarities in mycorrhiza and mammals. Flavonoids can regulate gene transcription in both groups. Moreover, some of these flavonoids can modulate the endocrine system and regulate mammalian physiology through activity on steroid receptors and prostaglandin synthesizing enzymes (Baker, 1995). In addition, humans express a protein, the 5α-reductase enzyme, that is homologous in sequence and identical in function (the reduction of steroid substrates) to a plant protein (Li et al, 1997; Fox, 2004). Hence, it should be of no surprise that plants have a long history of utilization in treating endocrine ailments; currently, phytochemistry is being explored for the regulation of human fertility. This leads Baker (1992) to suggest that flavonoids may have an evolutionary role in steroid hormone activity. It also provides an obvious example of informational exchange between plants and humans.

More recent work with a class of flavonoids known as isoflavones demonstrates intriguing epigenetic activity. Agouti mice, with their yellow coats and adult-onset obesity, diabetes, and tumor production, were protected from obesity by giving their mothers genistein at levels equivalent to a high soy diet. This phenotypic change correlated with methylation of the Avy locus (Dolinoy et al, 2006). In addition, supplementation of obese yellow agouti mice during pregnancy with methyl group donors (such as

betaine, choline, folic acid, and vitamin B_{12}) showed a reduction in the occurrence of obesity, diabetes and cancer, as well as altered coat color, in the offspring (Waterland & Jirtle, 2003).

That flavonoids are considered, conditionally, essential nutrients (Challem, 1999) adds to the intrigue. In other words, humans have "coupled" with these particular flavonoid "signals" to such a degree that they enhance our long-term health (Manthey & Buslig, 1998; Martinez-Valverde et al, 2000). One wonders how many other plant compounds, with regular consumption, enhance human health. As research on plant metabolites continues, it is increasingly apparent that many phytochemicals are at least favorable, if not necessary, to human health. Just considering the vitamins and minerals from plant origin makes it obvious that human physiological processes are dependent on the phytochemistry of plants. Moreover, the evolutionary history of humans ingesting plants with myriad phytochemicals suggests that the interface of multiple phytochemicals with mammalian physiology may be informative about pharmacology and induce an adaptive (hormetic) response to the environment (Vaiserman, 2011).

HORMESIS AND XENOHORMESIS— ADAPTATION TO THE PHYTOCHEMICAL ENVIRONMENT

There are a number of reasons that the complex chemistry inherent in ingestion of a plant acts differently than that of an isolated chemical. Of these reasons, pharmacokinetic potentiation, pharmacodynamic convergence, and hormesis/xenohormesis are the best known and the easiest to discuss in the existing framework of pharmacology. Although pharmacokinetic potentiation involves processes related to absorption, distribution, metabolism, and excretion (ADME), pharmacodynamic convergence involves modulation of multiple biochemical pathways, membrane dynamics, receptor-binding cooperativity, and shifts of the degrees of freedom of proteins (enzymes and receptors). Although both of these modes of activity are unique to the ingestion of chemical mixtures, they are commonly put under the rubric of synergy, even though they would ideally be discussed separately. The last mode, hormesis, is well established in the field of toxicology and is slowly encroaching into physiology and pharmacology. Regardless of the scientific discipline of origin, it is a useful construct for understanding how plant chemistry interfaces with living systems. Xenohormesis provides an overarching construct to embrace much of what has been previously discussed.

HORMESIS DEFINED

The term *hormesis* is derived from the Greek word *hormon,* meaning "to excite." In other words, on ingestion of a hormetin, physiological processes are stimulated. Simply put, hormesis is the paradoxical effect of a toxic chemical or radiation at low dose (Trewavas & Stewart, 2003).

TABLE 27-1 *Previous Terms Applied to the Hormesis Dose Response*

Compensatory response	Bell-shaped
Facilitation-inhibition	β-curve
Intermediate disturbance hypothesis	Bidirectional
Paradoxical dose responses	Biphasic
Reverse	J-shaped
Stimulatory-inhibitory	U-shaped
Subsidy-stress gradient	

Previous Laws Referring to Hormesis

Hebb Law
Yerkes-Dobson Law
Arndt-Schulz Law

From Calabrese EJ, Baldwin LA. Defining hormesis. *Hum Exp Toxicol* 2002;21:91–7, copyright ©2002 by Edward Arnold. Reprinted by permission of SAGE.

Stebbing (1982) defined hormesis as low-dose stimulation followed by higher-dose inhibition. A more complete definition by Calabrese and Baldwin (2002), who have spent the last few decades bringing hormesis back to the attention of physiologists and pharmacologists, is "an adaptive response characterized by biphasic dose responses of generally similar quantitative features with respect to amplitude and range of the stimulatory response that are either directly induced or the result of compensatory biological processes following an initial disruption in homeostasis." The idea behind hormesis is based on dose response; a beneficial physiological upregulation induced from small doses of a "toxin." Many terms have been used to describe this effect (Table 27-1), including the common biphasic dose response.

Calabrese and Baldwin point out that the hormesis dose-response phenomena has been labeled with diverse terminology and that there are also several biological "laws" referring to hormesis (see Table 27-1). Although this circumstance suggests that the phenomenon has repeatedly been "discovered" by different research groups, it is also an unfortunate comment on the lack of learning and conceptual integration across scientific disciplines.

The hormesis dose-response data suggest that there is a common regulatory strategy for biological resource allocation and a plasticity of regulatory processes dependent on environmental perturbations due to a long history of coherent coupling or coevolution with phytochemistry (Spelman, 2006).

HISTORY OF HORMESIS: POLITICALLY SUSPECT BUT SCIENTIFICALLY SOLID

As mentioned previously, the hormetic response is oriented toward dose-response effects of substance. Although Calabrese and coworkers have brought this construct back into acceptance in the sciences, it had long been recognized in ancient systems of pharmacology.

For example, in the 5000-year-old Ayurvedic and Siddha systems of India, there is a tenet that *everything*, even poisons, can be used as medicine if properly utilized (see Chapter 31). As such, very small amounts of heavy metals were used to rejuvenate the system in the weak, convalescing, and aging. In the sixteenth century, Paracelsus, a Swiss chemist, was known to use toxic substances with particular attention to dose (Wood, 1992; Gurib-Fakim, 2006). Although there is much skepticism about this therapy, it is written that his results were particularly positive (Wood, 1992). Nonetheless, Paracelsus' therapies included the use of heavy metals, such as mercury. Centuries later this usage led to the well-known term of "quack," derived from an old term for mercury, which was known as quicksilver (or *quacksalver*)—although ironically (or perhaps mercurially) mercury was actually a key "antibacterial" treatment of regular medicine in the preantibiotic era. Published research by the late 1800s had demonstrated that chemicals toxic to yeast could stimulate growth and respiration if used in lower doses (Calabrese et al, 1999).

By the 1920s a researcher committed a foible in the politics of science by associating the phenomena of hormesis with homeopathy (Calabrese, 2006). Considering that this association was only a few years after the Flexner Report (see Chapter 22), any association with homeopathy was like a death sentence to any scientific hypothesis, regardless of reproducible evidence. Although the Flexner Report had resulted in the needed elimination of many of the ineffective schools of medicine of the early twentieth century, it also, apparently by design, put on its "hit list" any school teaching a system of medicine besides allopathy. Not helping matters, there was also a paucity of explanations based on the biochemical understanding of hormesis at that time (Stebbing, 1982). However, laboratory observations of the hormesis phenomena continued unbiased in other parts of the world, such that a German journal, *Zell-Stimulations Forschungen*, was established to report hormetic effects (Calabrese et al, 1999). By 1943, the scientific method cut through the politics in the United States; researchers at the University of Idaho reproducibly observed the phenomena, calling it hormesis, unaware of its previous labels (Calabrese et al, 1999).

About 50 years later, a newsletter of original research, *Stimulation Newsletter*, lasted just over a decade, reporting the enhancement of plant growth and yield by exposure to low-dose radiation (Calabrese et al, 1999). By the 1980s in the United States, despite still lingering skepticism of the hormesis phenomena, a book providing a lengthy review of the research on radiation hormesis was published (Luckey, 1980). By the end of the twentieth century, through the work of the Calabrese group, a substantial database of dose-response studies demonstrating hormesis as common and reproducible, had caught the attention of physiologists and pharmacologists (Calabrese, 2006). Hormesis as a scientific principle is solid; but is it here to stay?

UTILITY OF HORMESIS: UNDERSTANDING HUMANS AND RELATIONS TO THE ENVIRONMENT

Hormesis is not just relevant to poisons such as heavy metals, synthetic pesticides, radiation and pollutants. Needed substances such as vitamins, minerals and oxygen are also toxic at excessive doses (Calabrese et al, 1999). Nor is this principle only observed with natural compounds such as listed in Box 27-1. This principle applies to endogenous compounds as well. Biosynthetic compounds moving through the human system, such as the adrenalines, adenosine, androgens, estrogens, nitric oxide, opioids, many peptides, and prostaglandins, all may have beneficial effects at low concentrations but detrimental effects at high concentrations (Calabrese, 2006). Some pharmaceuticals are also known to adhere to this principle. For example, low doses of antibiotics may actually enhance reproduction of pathogenic bacteria, whereas higher doses are toxic to these microbes (Calabrese et al, 1999). Probably the best known and most commonly consumed hormetin is alcohol. Ethanol, a chemical solvent, can clearly be toxic. However, at low doses ethanol as a biochemical metabolite is known to be beneficial to health and protective against cardiovascular diseases and some cancers.

Calabrese and Baldwin (2002) suggest the hormesis response provides a biological buffering response to protect against environmental and endogenous insults. The observation of this response in so many different organisms and cell types against such diverse chemical groups (and radiation) suggests a system-wide feedback response resulting in upregulation of many regulatory processes (Calabrese et al, 1999) and an evolutionary-wide biological strategy (Calabrese & Baldwin, 2002). By overcompensation to an initial disruption via an environmental stressor, an organism is protected against the possibility of further exposures (Calabrese et al, 1999).

The hormetic dose response seen in so many phytochemicals also suggests that the mode of activity for health enhancement by fruits, vegetables, and spices may be, at least partially, due to the evolutionary protective responses previously mentioned. Furthermore, it argues against a strictly "antioxidant" mode for the health benefits of plant-based foods, which has become a common assumption among many clinicians and researchers. Like exercise and caloric restriction, many phytochemicals may act as mild stressors to induce an adaptive response via upregulation of multiple genes inducing a protective effect (Calabrese, 2005; Mattson & Cheng, 2006).

At this juncture, some researchers thinking outside the box are applying the hormesis construct to grasp the relationship between the natural pesticides occurring in plants and human health. Many of the secondary compounds plants produce are antifeedants, antimicrobials, and insecticides for the plants' protection (Poitrineau et al, 2003). The well-respected researcher Bruce Ames points out that, of all the pesticides in the diet, those that are naturally produced by the plant itself or synthetic pesticides applied to the plant by farmers, 99.9% are naturally occurring (Ames et al, 1990). This becomes particularly relevant to human health in that many of these natural "pesticides" such as flavonoids (Baker, 1998) and coumarins (Zangerl & Berenbaum, 2004) are known to be beneficial to human health in multiple ways, including having anticancer activity and beneficial cardiovascular effects (Hoult et al, 1994; Knekt et al, 1996; Hollman & Katan, 1997; Lin et al, 2001; Nijveldt et al, 2001; Baba et al, 2002; Hamer & Steptoe, 2006). At low doses these compounds appear to activate adaptive cellular stress-response pathways (Mattson & Cheng, 2006). However, at high doses, many of these compounds can become carcinogens (Trewavas & Stewart, 2003).

Diets high in animal based-foods (to the exclusion of plant-based foods), and processed foods may lack the protective effect of diets high in phytochemicals (Johns, 1996). Ames and Gold (2000) point out that about 80% of U.S. and 75% of U.K. citizens eat insufficient fruit and vegetables to provide even minimal protection against cancer. After summarizing 200 epidemiological studies, Block et al (1992) reported that a phytochemical-rich diet from fruits and vegetables reduced cancer risks by about 50%. Knoops et al (2004) found that among individuals ages 70 to 90 years, adherence to a phytochemical-rich diet was associated with a more than 50% lower rate of all-cause and cause-specific mortality. Norris et al (2003) show that good health habits, one of which includes a phytochemical-rich diet, are associated with a 10- to 20-year delayed progression of morbidity. What might seem paradoxical to the casual observer, is that many phytochemicals, evolutionarily derived to protect plants from predators, are detrimental to health at higher doses. The exposure to secondary plant metabolites, many of which were naturally selected to protect plants against bacteria, insects, and herbivores, can be protective to human health. However, in excess doses, many of these natural microbicides and insecticides are toxic. In insufficient doses, human health may be compromised. At ideal doses, human health may be enhanced due to the hormesis principle and therefore be more resistant to disease processes and better able to respond to changing environmental circumstances (Johns, 1996).

Xenohormesis

Another well-known example of a hormetic process is exposure to low concentrations of certain phytochemicals. Unsurprisingly, organisms have evolved the ability to detect stress markers produced by other species in their habitats. Because the majority of life forms on the planet either feed on, or live in, close proximity to photosynthesizing organisms (photoautotrophs), there is a long-term evolutionary relationship between photoautotrophs (plants and photosynthetic bacteria) and heterotrophs (fungi and animals). Much of this relationship is based on the secondary metabolites from plants. Plants are known to synthesize compounds, such as stress markers, in response to environmental conditions. These phytochemicals, in turn, may be utilized by their surrounding heterotrophic neighbors as cues to impending environmental changes. Thus, when ingested or absorbed by coexisting life forms (such as bacteria, fungi, animals or humans), certain phytochemicals may provide a chemical signature of the state of the environment. In this way, organisms might prepare themselves in anticipation of potential adverse environmental conditions (Howitz & Sinclair, 2008; Menendez et al, 2013).

This interspecies hormesis is known as xenohormesis, the phenomenon in which an organism detects the chemical signals of another species regarding the state of the immediate environment or the availability of food (Menendez et al, 2013). The polyphenols are one example of phytochemical compounds carrying information about the immediate environment. This class of compounds includes the anthocyanidins, catchins, chalcones, flavanones, flavones, isoflavones, and tannins. Spelman and Duke (2006) suggest that the metabolic expense of generating such molecules would create a "chemical economy," an efficient and multiple use of one molecule. Indeed, these molecules are known to be multifunctional in that they are, all at once, antioxidants, antibiotics, fungicides, herbivory deterrents, and UV protection. However, they are also known to play a role as signaling molecules—carrying environmental information to heterotrophs. Stafford (1991) proposes that the original role of the polyphenols was as signaling molecules and that their other properties evolved later. Flavonoids do provide cues to plant development (Taylor & Grotewold, 2005) and it has also been proposed that flavonoids were the original steroid signaling molecules (Baker, 1992).

Accumulating evidence does suggest that mammals sense plant stress–signaling molecules. The mammal that could respond to molecules such as the polyphenols, would have an advantage over those competitors that could not interpret these environmental cues. A possible explanation for this phenomenon is based in evolutionary biology. Kushiro et al (2003) propose that the biosynthetic pathways for signaling compounds originated in a common ancestor of plants and animals. As the phyla diverged, the heterotrophs eventually lost their ability to *synthesize* polyphenols, but retained the ability to *respond* to these messenger molecules. The retention of the ability to respond to these molecular cues likely allowed for an anticipatory adaptation to environmental changes (Howitz & Sinclair, 2008).

At the least, recurring interactions between phytochemicals and heterotrophic proteins over an evolutionary time scale may have generated conditional requirements for some phytochemicals (Spelman et al, 2006). The consumers of these molecules have been shown to respond by inducing cellular defenses and resource conservation (Howitz et al, 2003). For example, it is well known that that the polyphenols butein, fisetin, and the very well-publicized resveratrol, extend the life span in fungi, nematodes, flies, fish, and mice (Westphal et al, 2007). In addition, the same concentrations of polyphenols that are required to extend life span in the laboratory (approximately 10 μM) are also detectable in the leaves and fruits of stressed plants (Howitz & Sinclair, 2008).

The xenohormesis hypothesis varies from the hormesis model. In xenohormesis, the stress occurs in one organism (inducing an upregulation of particular signaling molecules), whereas the coexisting species (which have evolved to sense the surrounding chemical ecology) are the beneficiaries (Howitz & Sinclair, 2008). In regard to the age-old process of adaptation to the environment, it is sensible to propose that absorbed phytochemicals carry information about the status of the environment and imminent changes in an animal's food supply. The evidence that stress-induced plant compounds upregulate pathways that provide stress resistance in animals/humans provides an evolutionary imperative for anticipatory adaptation. Plant consumers would sensibly have modes to perceive these chemical cues and react to them in ways that are beneficial.

The hormesis and the xenohormesis hypothesis are not mutually exclusive. Responses to absorbed toxins (hormesis) and the ability to respond to molecules of environmental origin as molecular signals (xenohormesis) were likely concurrent developments in evolution. Howitz and Sinclair (2008) point out that both responses are likely at play in animals' response to complex mixtures of phytochemicals.

Although xenohormetic compounds are often detrimental to smaller insects and microorganisms, the subtoxic levels at which humans consume them may result in moderate cellular stress responses. This could induce stress-response adaptation pathways, leading to increased expression of genes that encode cytoprotective proteins such as antioxidant enzymes, chaperones, growth factors, phase 2 detoxification enzymes, and mitochondrial proteins (Menendez et al, 2013).

This environmental coupling may have resulted in a conditional dependence on phytochemicals for the modulation of particular proteins as well. For example, the nucleotide-binding sites of protein kinases appear to bind the polyphenolic flavonoids and stilbenes with reasonable affinity. The evidence indicates that these polyphenols do not compete with the enzyme's nucleotide substrates, rather they bind elsewhere (Howitz et al, 2003; Gledhill et al, 2007). Molecules such as resveratrol and quercetin have been found to bind not to conserved domains, but to hydrophobic pockets (Gledhill et al, 2007). This observation may partially explain their ability to modulate multiple proteins. Howitz and Sinclair (2008) suggest that this property is consistent with these polyphenol-protein interactions being driven by selective pressures rather than coincidental binding—and also suggests that these interactions are likely potentiating with one another and with endogenous regulators.

There are also data that demonstrate that many of these compounds bind to the same binding pockets as endogenous regulators (Baker, 1992). Both types of interactions help substantiate the claimed observations of *synergy* so often cited for multi-component extracts from medicinal plants (Spelman et al, 2006). At the least, ingestion of the phytochemical mixtures in fruits, vegetables and herbs likely involve multiple interactions that go well beyond ligand binding and involve subtler molecular dynamics (see Molecular Models of Activity later in this chapter) (Spelman, 2005).

The xenohormesis hypothesis makes a number of predictions that rest squarely on organisms' relationship to coupling with their environments (Lamming et al, 2004; Howitz & Sinclair, 2008):

1. There is likely a substantial cache of medicinal molecules that are upregulated in stressed plants that can benefit the user.
2. Xenohormetic phytochemicals serve as messenger molecules by interacting with a variety of enzymes involved in regulating stress responses and survival.
3. These molecules should be relatively safe for human consumption.
4. There may be conserved domains in enzymes and receptors that do not interact with endogenous molecules.
5. Many phytochemicals, due to a history of recurrent interactions with heterotrophic proteins may have resulted in a structural congruence that potentiates the effects of endogenous regulatory molecules.

If the above predictions hold true, then xenohormesis may provide the philosophical underpinnings as to why many phytochemicals have been documented to enhance health parameters.

The xenohormesis hypothesis, when fully recognized, has implications for the foundations of pharmacology. Whereas classical pharmacology is based on high affinity and high selectivity, many physiologically active phytochemicals are known to function with broad specificity and low affinity (Ágoston et al, 2005). This reality creates a quandary for the pharmacological paradigm as many phytochemicals are known to affect multiple proteins. "Polyvalent" binding, whereby a small molecule binds to multiple proteins, is considered an inferior pharmacological strategy by pharmaceutical standards. However, it may well have been the original mode of upregulating defensive physiological responses, and it may well provide distinct pharmacological advantages based on evolutionary biology.

DANGER OF A SECOND REJECTION BY THE POLITICS OF SCIENCE

This argument is science based and a logical extension is that the use of food and medicinal plants for enhancement of health is biologically preferred to the use of isolated, synthetic drugs. Many critics of the beneficial health effects of plant-based foods and medicines claim there is not enough (a high enough "dose") of any one chemical present in plants to make them therapeutically useful (Spinella, 2002). Although this argument is consistent with medicinal plants sometimes being called "crude drugs," it also demonstrates a gross misunderstanding of the pharmacology of complex mixtures. Furthermore, it completely misses the hormesis phenomenon.

The argument that foods and medicinal plants are not effective for inducing physiological change because they are too dilute to have activity contradicts the entire hormesis database of studies demonstrating that minute doses of substances do have general and reproducible biological responses. At the same time, the hormesis principle should call into question the practice of concentrating an active constituent from a plant by standardization. Although we must be assured of the quality and identity of medicinal plant preparations, concentration of any one constituent in a medicinal plant preparation may, in some cases, breach the dose for beneficial activity and move toward a detrimental dose, particularly if the compound operates through a hormetic mode of activity. Nonetheless, understanding hormesis can help the allopathic community understand one of the possible modes of activity for medicinal plants. The hormesis principle was once dropped like a "hot potato" in the early part of the twentieth century because of the association with homeopathy. Will hormesis be shunned because of its ability to help explain observations on the health benefits of medicinal plants?

Viewing hormesis in an ecosystem context, hormetic responses measured by growth effects can turn out to be a result of altered competition between species. If a competitor, parasite, or disease of a species is more susceptible to a certain chemical than is the species itself, then the species will experience relief from a resource-demanding stress factor and hence increase growth at low concentrations of that chemical. This effect (also a basic principle behind the beneficial effect of pharmaceuticals such as penicillin on vertebrates) leads to the xenohormesis hypothesis.

ECOLOGICAL PHARMACY AND THE BASIS OF PHARMACOLOGY

The aforementioned evidence logically leads to a discussion on pharmacology; that is, how has adaptation to phytochemical exchange influenced the physiological processes of organisms consuming plants. A key point is that ingestion of plants, a process that has been going on for 300 million years for vertebrates, 88 million years for higher primates, and 7 million to 10 million years for humans, leads to exposure to an array of plant compounds in every swallowed mouthful. Never has the consumption of edible foodstuffs involved a single, isolated compound. This reality is of pharmacological significance. The current model in pharmacology attempts to induce physiological changes through the ingestion of one chemical at a time.

In an unspoken oversight of the medical sciences, the rationale for the approach of isolation and purification of active constituents from "crude drugs" has never actually been made explicit (Vickers, 2002). The general conclusion drawn from a century of research on active constituents from medicinal plants is that medicinal plants typically contain numerous active compounds (Singer & Underwood, 1962; Williamson, 2001; Gilbert & Alves, 2003; Spelman, 2005; Spelman et al, 2006). There is a key point regarding the economics around the use of food and medicinal plants for human health. Multiconstituent plant medicines were not forsaken because of research that demonstrated harmful or ineffective activity, but because they were too complex to study in their multiconstituent form (Vickers, 2002). Nevertheless, pharmacological modeling has used isolation as a fundamental tenet of inducing physiological shifts in humans. Unfortunately, this methodology is deficient in revealing the mode of activity of the bulk of food and medicinal plants as it neglects the concerted, synergic, additive and/or antagonist activities of multiconstituent remedies (Cech, 2003). Moreover, it grossly simplifies physiological processes to only those parameters possible to observe in reductionist models. Thus, fitting the biology to the method; rather than the method to the biology (see Chapters 1 and 3).

A pharmacological paradigm should be supported by a foundation of human adaptation to the informational input from plants. Physiological processes, down to the level of genes, have undergone a history of recurring biochemical interactions with complex phytochemistry that has led to the structural congruence of humans and plants. The previously discussed shifts in DNA, epigenetics, the homology of proteins, and the ligand–receptor relations among humans and plants are examples of "structural congruence." Human biology has integrated with that of plants so that multiple concurrent biochemical perturbations are ordinary. Reiterative exposure to minute doses of numerous plant metabolites provides constant stimuli for biological adaptation (Jackson, 1991). In turn, this adaptation has profound effects on human health.

Jackson (1991) aptly calls attention to system stability, writing that system diversity is proportional to system stability. Another way of expressing this relation in regard to human health is that the stability of health may be seen as a function of exposure to phytochemical diversity. Keith and Zimmerman (2004) suggest that many genes may require complementary action to modify disease processes. In other words, therapy could be more effective if pharmacological agents engaged with more than one biochemical

site. Quite likely, the majority of the multitude of plant constituents that ancient humans regularly consumed throughout evolutionary process had a positive effect on many of the health-modifying genes due to the millions of years of history of recurring exposure to multi-component phytochemical mixtures. Observations consistently indicate that people with a phytochemical-rich diet have a significantly improved health status over those with a diet low in phytochemicals (McCarty, 2004). To this author, it seems highly likely that many of the chronic health conditions observed in humans may actually be due to a dietary deficiency in phytochemistry. Minimally processed plant-based foods appear to be important in modulating physiological processes.

Keith and Zimmerman (2004) point out that there are an estimated 10,000 health-modifying genes. It is quite likely that phytochemicals interface with a large percentage of these genes. Unfortunately, the current number of pharmacological targets, approximately 300 to 400, is anemic as compared to the broad phytochemical-gene interfaces that occur in diets rich in plant-based foods.

A pharmacological model that accounts for millions of years of exposure to arrays of phytochemicals not only would recognize plants as inherent sources of medicines, but of a multi-target approach that single-chemical, stand-alone interventions cannot offer (Keith & Zimmermann, 2004). And it returns to the origins of pharmacology, where what humans regularly ingested, somewhere between 80 and 220 plants with an estimated 80,000 to 220,000 secondary metabolites, modified multiple physiological processes in a concerted manner. The understanding of the translational response of numerous proteins to multiple perturbations, such as provided through phytochemistry, holds promise for the fields of medicine and biology—not because it is new insight, but because it is an ancient process that shaped human physiology. Such a paradigm shift would also advance the understanding of biological molecular networks and open up further, more useful therapeutic strategies.

MOLECULAR MODELS OF ACTIVITY

CELLULAR MEMBRANE AND SIGNAL TRANSDUCTION

Cellular morphology is the result of nonlinear and dynamic molecular flux, especially related to the cell membrane. Although the membrane has been described as a system driven by thermodynamic equilibrium (Aon et al, 1996), it can also accurately seen as an emergent structure consisting of highly asymmetrical structures and phase transitions (Perillo, 2002).

Typically, mammalian cellular plasma membranes consist of about eight major classes of lipids (Simons & Vaz, 2004) that include embedded proteins in its bilipid structure. Signal transduction and the complex behavior of chemical reactions are coupled to the dynamics of membranes. Thus, the membrane has been closely scrutinized in hopes of further understanding cellular ability to receive, process, and respond to information. Unfortunately, there has been (and still is) an epistemological divide between the analysis of the complex behavior involved in biochemical events and the structural aspects of the membrane involved in signaling phenomena, especially in relation to signal transduction involving exogenous molecules (Perillo, 2002).

Until very recently, explanations of signal transduction were based on a linear model involving successive steps in the decoding process focused on compounds with high affinity and selectivity. However, the membrane is key in its interactions with the ensemble of phytochemicals to which early humans were consistently and constantly exposed. The membrane may also respond to compounds that do not exhibit high affinity and high selectivity to a particular receptor species. Ignoring these interactions may lead to erroneous conclusions in the basic cell sciences.

Significantly, systems properties of heterogeneous molecular ensembles could induce minute differences in the strength of attractive forces among molecules and increased degrees of freedom within a pharmacological system (Buehler, 2003a,b). Just as phase separations and self-assembly processes are systems properties of molecular ensembles, a phytochemical matrix interacting with another biological system requires a pharmacological systems approach (Spelman, 2005). The author proposes three modes of pharmacological activity for phytochemical matrices based on recently elucidated behaviors of the cell membrane; two involve the bilipid membrane and one is based on concerted activity. There are likely many more modes of activity not accounted in the below models.

Cooperative Binding by Receptors: Receptor Mosaics

Proteins form multimeric complexes capable of emergent functions (Agnati et al, 2005a). Thus the discovery of direct receptor–receptor interactions has profoundly shifted the understanding of receptor signal transduction. First, such interactions rigorously challenge the historical belief that the receptor is the minimal unit for drug recognition/activity. Second, the model that high-affinity, high-specificity compounds are superior ligands is also under review (Kenakin, 2004). The existence of various types of receptor mosaics (clusters of receptors functioning as a unit that demonstrate cooperative binding) suggests a plasticity of the steric conformation of receptors (Agnati et al, 2005b). In the receptor mosaic model, each receptor is seen as a subunit of a multimeric protein.

Recall the cooperative binding of oxygen to hemoglobin. After one oxygen molecule binds to hemoglobin, the affinity by the other binding pockets for oxygen increases. Thus, the likelihood of subsequent binding of oxygen molecules is increased.

Cooperativity is considered a mode of self-regulation by multimeric proteins (Koshland & Hamadani, 2002) and is hypothesized to be so for receptor systems as well (Agnati et al, 2005b). In receptor mosaics, the conformational change caused by the binding of the first ligand is transmitted to adjacent receptors with reciprocal contact to change the affinity for subsequent ligand binding. The change in affinity is due to the conformational change induced by the first bound ligand, which induces sequential changes of the multimeric protein's neighboring subunits. This change in protein conformation may make subsequent binding easier (positive cooperativity) or more difficult (negative cooperativity).

Because a phytochemical matrix consists of hundreds of compounds, including groups of constituents that vary slightly in their structure but are based on a common backbone (Yong & Loh, 2004), there may be both high-affinity ligands and lower affinity ligands for a given receptor. Once the high-affinity ligand binds to a species of receptor, other receptors, due to intramolecular transfer of the conformational change to the adjacent peptides, may be able to bind the lower affinity ligands and play a role in cellular messaging. Accordingly, the search for only high-affinity compounds in plants (and microbes) may miss lower affinity compounds that could bind within receptor mosaics due to cooperative binding. This is one possible molecular explanation of the synergy explanation so often invoked by phytotherapists to suggest that plant medicines and foods cannot be reduced to an "active" constituent. The receptor mosaic model also suggests that an expansion is needed of the traditional pharmacological methodology of searching for only high-affinity ligands within plant chemistry (Figure 27-4).

Shifts in Membrane Electronics and/or Shape: Nonspecific Membrane Interactions by Exogenous Molecules

Many components of signal transduction, such as receptors, are anchored in the plasma membrane and therefore are subject to the biochemical milieu of the plasma membrane. Of the four basic receptor signaling modes—gated ion channels, metabotropic receptors, receptor enzymes, and the steroid receptor—three are directly linked to plasma membrane processes. This lipid-rich, two-dimensional environment allows for hydrophobic interactions leading to alterations in component access, orientation and effective concentration (Weng et al, 1999). Hence, modulation of the molecular organization of the membrane may have an effect on signal transduction.

Many drugs are amphiphilic (hydrophobic) molecules and a common site of action for these compounds is the plasma membrane (Perillo, 2002). Among the amphiphilic compounds, many of the central nervous system depressants (Goodman et al, 2001) will, due to their molecular properties, self-aggregate into micelles (Hata et al, 2000; Kitagawa et al, 2004). Despite significant molecular investigation into modes of activity for some of the hydrophobic drugs (e.g. the local anesthetics) no specific receptors have been elucidated (Franks & Lieb, 1984; Schreier et al,

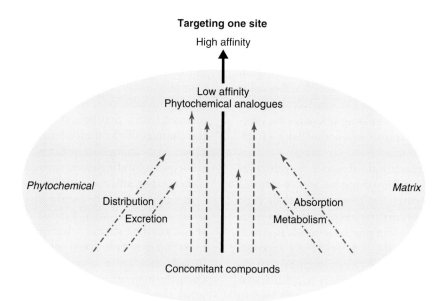

Figure 27-4 The current pharmacological model searches for only high-affinity and selectivity compounds, overlooking lower affinity compounds for receptor (and enzyme) binding. However, given the receptor mosaic model, the low-affinity compounds typically accompanying high-affinity compounds in plant extracts may cooperatively bind affecting signal transduction. Additionally, the concomitant compounds commonly improve pharmacokinetics (absorption, distribution, metabolism and excretion) of the low- to high-affinity compounds.

2000). Rather, these compounds demonstrate activity along the plasma membrane surface itself (Fernandez, 1980; Perillo, 2002; Kitagawa, et al, 2004).

Hydrophobic and amphiphilic compounds and the resulting micelles, may induce shape changes, membrane disruption, vesiculation, and solubilization (Schreier et al, 2000; Kitagawa et al, 2004). Consequently, exogenous molecules may generate membrane asymmetries resulting in membrane tensions (Garcia et al, 2000; Perillo & Garcia, 2001). As expected, given the thermodynamics of open systems far from equilibrium, the membrane perturbations due to curvature tensions and the flux of molecular movements from one monolayer to the other shift the resting state of the membrane and reorganize cellular shape (Perillo, 2002; McMahon & Gallop, 2005). Changes in the curvature of the membrane, as well as composition have demonstrated changes in function of the membrane when it interfaces with an exogenous molecule (Farge & Devaux, 1993; Mui et al, 1993; Garcia & Perillo, 2002; McMahon & Gallop, 2005). Given that protein conformation is dependent on molecular interactions, structural changes may also induce alterations in protein conformation (Simons & Vaz, 2004; Zimmerberg & Kozlov, 2006). This phenomenon could result in signal transduction (Groves & Kuriyan, 2010).

Notably, many of the secondary compounds of plants are amphiphilic or hydrophobic (e.g., hyperforin from St. John's wort and the curcuminoids in *Curucma longa*, alkylamides from *Echinacea* spp.) and would accordingly likely display similar behavior. Given the evolutionary history of plant ingestion by humans, membrane interactions by

"non-active" compounds in plants were likely routine. Consumption of a plant led to ingestion of "active" constituents *and* other phytochemicals that influence membrane dynamics. Consequently, with recognition of evolutionary precedent, the combination of compounds affecting the membrane and active compounds binding to receptors was part of routine physiology. This may be a partial explanation why many isolated plant constituents do not appear to function in the same way as when given in a whole plant extract.

Polyvalent Activity: Biochemical Convergence

The last two modes of activity were discussed in the realm of an isolated cell. However, signal transduction involves networks of cells, tissues and organs. Following the science of physics, molecular biology is slowly moving from the study of the components of signaling, to the context in which the signal participates. Study at the molecular level of components alone will not advance the understanding of when and why cells interact in their typically nonlinear, non-local, multiple-feedback loops (Maini, 2002).

Physiology does not run in linear, sequential processes one chemical at a time. Robust systems, like living organisms, are likely quite responsive to numerous but subtle chemical perturbations (Ágoston et al, 2005). Thus multisystem analysis will probably be found to be essential to understanding signaling networks (Plavec et al, 2004). Allowing for models that include multi-target and multipathway assaying could clearly elucidate the informational connectivity of networks. Aon et al (1996) refer to the network of interactions established between the dynamic subsystems through common intermediates or effectors (hormones and second messengers) as *dynamic coupling*.

It is well established that the overall combination of non-nutritive phytochemicals appears to be key in plants' positive effects on health, that the health-giving effects of plants are *not* always related to the nutrient content (McCarty, 2004), and that significant consumption of secondary compounds from plants play important roles in the prevention of chronic diseases (Liu, 2003). Whereas some constituents are interfacing with receptors and membranes, others are influencing pharmacokinetics. For example, concomitant compounds, frequently considered nonactive constituents, can affect absorption, distribution, metabolism, or excretion of other constituents, enhancing (or antagonizing) their bioavailability (Eder & Mehnert, 2000). Moreover, as the xenohormesis hypothesis suggests, many of the phytochemicals that have been removed from our foodstuffs and medicinal preparations may upregulate beneficial physiological processes.

Recognition of such subtle perturbation would eventually create the understanding of a disease-modifying molecular network and further pharmacological target potential. Monitoring of targets affected by polyvalent groups of compounds will almost certainly lead to the recognition of yet further biochemical webs. Moreover, as our knowledge of the range of perturbable sites improves, proteins expressed from mere "housekeeping" genes will likely be recognized as disease modifying. The outcome could be an expansion of the understanding of the disease-modifying gene network and further therapeutic targets (Keith & Zimmermann, 2004). Such perspective will likely lead to the acknowledgment that a multi-target perturbation, as happens with the consumption of minimally processed plant products, holds the potential for significantly more therapeutic activity than single-chemical, stand-alone interventions.

The ingestion of plants leads not only to the potential of multiple compounds interfacing with multiple targets, but also for single compounds, due to their broad specificity, to engage multiple targets. Generally, the pharmacological sciences consider these molecules "dirty" because of their lack of selectivity. Such molecules are thought to have more potential for generating adverse events because of "off-target" effects than does a highly selective chemical. However, dozens, if not hundreds, of multifunctional compounds are known natural products chemistry to be quite safe (Corson & Crews, 2007). For example, the well-known phytochemical group of the salicylates is known to interact with multiple proteins. The ubiquitous catechins, such as epigallocatechin-3-gallate, have demonstrated considerable chemopreventative activity via induction of apoptosis, inhibiting multidrug resistance pumps, promotion of cell cycle arrest, and inhibiting cyclooxygenase-2 (Khan et al, 2006). The curcuminoids are documented to engage over 60 molecular targets to protect against cancer and regulate the expression of inflammatory enzymes, cytokines, adhesion molecules, and cell survival proteins (Goel et al, 2008). The not uncommon resveratrol modulates the function of over two dozen enzymes and receptors, leading to protection against cancer, atherosclerosis, and diabetes while promoting endurance (Howitz & Sinclair, 2008).

Csermely et al (2005) have found, using network models of pharmacology, that the partial inhibition of multiple targets offered by a mixture of chemicals is often more efficient than the complete inhibition of a single target. For example, Wald and Law (2003) suggested that a combination of six drugs at subclinical doses—a baby aspirin, three blood pressure drugs (at half the standard dose), a statin, and 800 mcg of folic acid—could extend life by 11 years (Figure 27-5).

In addition, in a meta-analysis encompassing 56,000 patients with hypertension, Law et al (2003) concluded

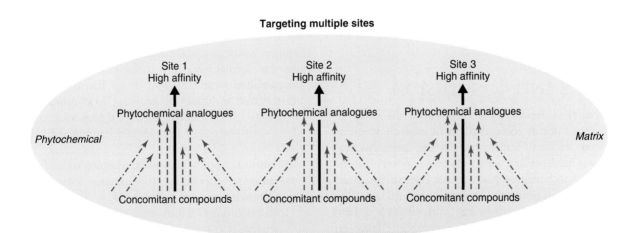

Targeting multiple sites

Figure 27-5 Physiology is a complex process that operates in a symphonic manner with multiple receptors, enzymes and genes being affected in any given second. When ingesting a plant extract or food, the phytochemistry triggers many sites concurrently that can then converge on a positive outcome.

that combinations of two or three drugs at half the standard doses delivered comparable therapeutic effects comparable to those of one or two full-dose antihypertension medications. Not surprisingly, the multiple low-dose drug combination was preferable due to the reduction in side effects. Clinicians have historically overcome single target insufficiency by using combination drug therapy such as seen in today's clinical protocols for HIV, tuberculosis, and cancer. Csermely et al (2005) propose that partial drug inhibition by multiple drugs could prove to be a superior pharmacological strategy to strong inhibition by one drug action at a single target. This is likely due to the need for complementary action on multiple targets to modify disease processes (Keith & Zimmermann, 2004).

When combinations of various pharmacological compounds are screened, the natural outcome will almost certainly necessitate further exploration of the connectivity of physiological pathways. Borisy et al (2003) discuss the unexpected but beneficial interactions that a systemic screening of combinations of small molecules reveals. They report, for example, that an antipsychotic agent coupled with an antiprotozoal drug demonstrates antineoplastic activity, and that a fungistatic compound coupled with an analgesic drug produces antifungal activity against resistant strains of *Candida albicans*. In these instances, however, these ensemble properties, if broken apart and studied in isolation, would have never been realized.

It appears that the ensemble properties of a chemical matrix are necessary for physiological and pharmacological effects, and that the purification process from whole plant to isolated compound is inadequate for the elucidation of pharmacological activity (Wagner, 1999; Wang et al, 2004). Moreover, the phytochemical matrix, rather than the phytochemical isolate, offers an opportunity for an enhanced perspective: the study of phytochemical matrices interfacing with mammalian systems, with the addition of improved technology, will almost certainly elucidate molecular networks that have been unseen with previous methodology. The medical sciences would do well to heed Exteberria (2004), who suggests that the properties of a unity cannot be accounted for by accounting for the properties of its components.

SUMMARY AND CONCLUSION

If Gaia theory is accurate, then it stresses the need for seeing humans not as the end-point of evolution, but as cells existing within a larger, grander life form. Medical scientists would do well to realize that we are part of something larger than ourselves. And as such, humans are interdependent on each other, the environment, and other life forms. We are a system within a system within a system, interdependently woven with an inseparable reliance on our planet.

Gaia theory also provides a global context in which to understand life and its adaptive brilliance and highlights the coupling of organism with its environment. This pertains to humans and their coupling with plants. While plants have provided shelter, clothing, food, and medicine, they have also shaped us, influencing our genome, epigenome, and proteome. Moreover, plants have xenohormetically provided environmental molecular messaging that has proven to be physiologically beneficial for humans.

Given that a large number of phytochemicals can directly or indirectly modulate gene expression, and that common phytochemicals appear to play a key role in signal transduction, it follows that the human genome is selected for multiple, concerted biochemical perturbations due to millions of years of recurrent interaction of mammalian genes with heterogeneous phytochemical matrices. The phytochemical intake for Paleolithic humans has been estimated to be at least eight times greater than that of modern humans (and is likely an order of magnitude higher). Many studies have consistently detected that an important association of chronic diseases with lower consumption of plant-based foods, which may be due to decreased intake of phytochemicals. Thus intake of fruits, vegetables, herbs and spices remain critically important in human health.

Our current models of physiology and pharmacology unfortunately still do not fully account for the importance of plants in the human diet. Nutrition and pharmacology are still focused on single constituents and do not recognize the complexity of human physiology interfacing with phytochemical matrices. The multiconstituent nature and ensemble of plant properties likely participate in emergent physiological behavior when ingested by humans. If the ensemble properties of a phytochemical chemical matrix are important for physiological and pharmacological effects, then the purification process from whole plant to isolated compound is inadequate for the elucidation of pharmacological activity of plant-based foods and medicines. Although isolation is methodologically convenient, and economically rewarding, it is not representative of real-time physiology or reflective of human evolution with millions of years of exposure to complex chemical matrices from plants. Pharmacology based on the affinity, selectivity, and acceptable toxicity of an isolated active constituent requires a serious update to match the current understanding of molecular biology. Although the reductionist model has provided some life-saving drugs, basing pharmacology on structure and function provides little indication of the behavior of the interacting biological networks. Even "nonactive" compounds in a phytochemical matrix likely play a role in biological networks.

Because biological systems are known to both adapt to environmental context and to reorganize in order to adapt, logical conclusions can be reached:

1. Pharmacological input that presents both high- and low-affinity compounds binding to receptor mosaics is important in signal transduction.
2. There are a multitude of plant compounds that can influence membrane dynamics, which is also likely important in signal transduction.

3. Phytochemical matrices act in a polyvalent manner by perturbing multiple sites.

Thus many phytochemicals act on multiple targets, functionally converging on therapeutic outcomes. Phytochemical matrices may provide an enhanced pharmacological efficiency as compared to isolated compounds. Moreover, the use of phytomedicines, as compared to isolated chemicals, appears to offer a reduced risk of adverse events in the treatment of many diseases.

It seems that the recognition of human evolutionary experience could not only guide the development of a framework for the anemic preventive medicine field, but lead to enhanced understanding of signal transduction for improved pharmacological therapeutics.

References

Agnati LF, Fuxe K, Ferre S: How receptor mosaics decode transmitter signals. Possible relevance of cooperativity, *Trends Biochem Sci* 30(4):188–193, 2005a.

Agnati LF, Guidolin D, Genedani S, et al: How proteins come together in the plasma membrane and function in macromolecular assemblies: focus on receptor mosaics, *J Mol Neurosci* 26(2–3):133–154, 2005b.

Ágoston V, Csermely P, Pongor S: Multiple, weak hits confuse complex systems: A transcriptional regulatory network as an example, *Phys Rev E* 71(5 Pt 1):1–8, 051909, 2005.

Ames BN, Gold LS: Paracelsus to parascience: the environmental cancer distraction, *Mutat Res* 447(1):3–13, 2000.

Ames BN, Profet M, Gold LS: Dietary pesticides (99.99% all natural), *Proc Natl Acad Sci U S A* 87:7777–7781, 1990.

Aon MA, Caceres A, Cortassa S: Heterogeneous distribution and organization of cytoskeletal proteins drive differential modulation of metabolic fluxes, *J Cell Biochem* 60(2):271–278, 1996.

Baba M, Jin Y, Mizuno A, et al: Studies on cancer chemoprevention by traditional folk medicines XXIV. Inhibitory effect of a coumarin derivative, 7-isopentenyloxycoumarin, against tumor-promotion, *Biol Pharm Bull* 25(2):244–246, 2002.

Baker ME: Evolution of regulation of steroid-mediated intercellular communication in vertebrates—insights from flavonoids, signals that mediate plant rhizobia symbiosis, *J Steroid Biochem Mol Biol* 41(3–8):301–308, 1992.

Baker ME: Endocrine activity of plant-derived compounds—an evolutionary perspective, *Proc Soc Exp Biol Med* 208(1):131–138, 1995.

Baker ME: Flavonoids as hormones. In Manthey JA, Buslig BS, editors: *Flavonoids in the living system*, vol 439, New York, 1998, Plenum Press, pp 249–264.

Block G, Patterson B, Subar A: Fruit, vegetables, and cancer prevention: a review of the epidemiological evidence, *Nutr Cancer* 18(1):1–29, 1992.

Borisy AA, Elliott PJ, Hurst NW, et al: Systematic discovery of multicomponent therapeutics, *Proc Natl Acad Sci U S A* 100(13):7977–7982, 2003.

Buehler LK: Beyond recognition: treating ligand-receptor recognition as a process rather than a structure is a first step toward developing rules of how a combination of hydrogen bonds, salt bridges and hydrophobic contact sites between a ligand and its receptor causes a conformational change in the receptor, *PharmaGenomics* 3(8):26–29, 2003a.

Buehler LK: What's in a structure? *PharmaGenomics* 3(5):20–21, 2003b.

Byrne P: Leonard Susskind: the bad boy of physics, *Sci Am* 305(1):80–83, 2011.

Cairns J, Overbaugh J, Miller S: The origin of mutants, *Nature* 335(6186):142–145, 1988.

Cairns RB: Aggression from a developmental perspective: genes, environments and interactions, *Ciba Found Symp* 194:45–56, discussion 57–60, 1996.

Calabrese E: Hormesis: A Key Concept in Toxicology. Biological concepts and techniques in toxicology: an integrated approach. Boca Raton, 2006, CRC Press.

Calabrese EJ: Cancer biology and hormesis: human tumor cell lines commonly display hormetic (biphasic) dose responses, *Crit Rev Toxicol* 35(6):463–582, 2005.

Calabrese EJ, Baldwin LA: Defining hormesis, *Hum Exp Toxicol* 21(2):91–97, 2002.

Calabrese EJ, Baldwin LA, Holland CD: Hormesis: a highly generalizable and reproducible phenomenon with important implications for risk assessment, *Risk Anal* 19(2):261–281, 1999.

Capra F: *The turning point*, New York, 1982, Bantam Books.

Capra F: *The web of life: a new scientific understanding of living systems*, New York, 1996, Anchor Books.

Cech NB: *Rigorous science for the study of holistic herbal medicine: Challenges, pitfalls, and the role of mass spectrometry. 226th ACS National Meeting*, New York, 2003, American Chemical Society.

Challem JJ: Toward a new definition of essential nutrients: is it now time for a third 'vitamin' paradigm? *Med Hypotheses* 52(5):417, 1999.

Corson TW, Crews CM: Molecular understanding and modern application of traditional medicines: triumphs and trials, *Cell* 130(5):769–774, 2007.

Crick F: Central Dogma Of Molecular Biology, *Nature* 227(5258):561–567, 1970.

Csermely P, Ágoston V, Pongor S: The efficiency of multi-target drugs: the network approach might help drug design, *Trends Pharmacol Sci* 26(4):178–182, 2005.

Danielson PB: The cytochrome P450 superfamily: biochemistry, evolution and drug metabolism in humans, *Curr Drug Metab* 3(6):561–597, 2002.

Dolinoy DC, Weidman JR, Waterland RA, et al: Maternal genistein alters coat color and protects Avy mouse offspring from obesity by modifying the fetal epigenome, *Environ Health Perspect* 114(4):567–572, 2006.

Eder M, Mehnert W: [Plant excipients-valuable pharmaceutical aids or superfluous ballast?] *Pharm Unserer Zeit* 29(6):377–384, 2000.

Exteberria A: Autopoiesis and natural drift: genetic information, reproduction, and evolution revisited, *Artif Life* 10(3):347–360, 2004.

Farge E, Devaux PF: Size-dependent response of liposomes to phospholipid transmembrane redistribution—from shape change to induced tension, *J Phys Chem* 97(12):2958–2961, 1993.

Fernandez MS: Formation of micelles and membrane action of the local anesthetic tetracaine hydrochloride, *Biochim Biophys Acta* 597(1):83–91, 1980.

Fox JE: Chemical communication threatened by endocrine-disrupting chemicals, *Environ Health Perspect* 112(6):648–653, 2004.

Franks NP, Lieb WR: Do general-anesthetics act by competitive-binding to specific receptors? *Nature* 310(5978):599–601, 1984.

Free A, Barton NH: Do evolution and ecology need the Gaia hypothesis? *Trends Eco Evol* 22(11):611–619, 2007.

Galleni L: How Does The Teilhardian vision of evolution compare with contemporary theories? *Zygon* 30(1):25–45, 1995.

Garcia DA, Perillo MA: Flunitrazepam-membrane non-specific binding and unbinding: two pathways with different energy barriers, *Biophys Chem* 95(2):157–164, 2002.

Garcia DA, Quiroga S, Perillo MA: Flunitrazepam partitioning into natural membranes increases surface curvature and alters cellular morphology, *Chem Biol Int* 129(3):263–277, 2000.

Gilbert B, Alves LF: Synergy in plant medicines, *Curr Med Chem* 10(1):13–20, 2003.

Gilbert SF: The genome in its ecological context: philosophical perspectives on interspecies epigenesis, *Ann N Y Acad Sci* 981:202–218, 2002.

Gledhill JR, Montgomery MG, Leslie AG, et al: Mechanism of inhibition of bovine F1-ATPase by resveratrol and related polyphenols, *Proc Natl Acad Sci U S A* 104(34):13632–13637, 2007.

Goel A, Kunnumakkara AB, Aggarwal BB: Curcumin as Curecumin: from kitchen to clinic, *Biochem Pharmacol* 75(4):787–809, 2008.

Gonzalez FJ, Nebert DW: Evolution of the P450-gene superfamily—animal plant warfare, molecular drive and human genetic-differences in drug oxidation, *Trends Genet* 6(6):182–186, 1990.

Goodman LS, Hardman JG, Limbird LE, et al: *Goodman & Gilman's the pharmacological basis of therapeutics*, New York, 2001, McGraw-Hill.

Groves JT, Kuriyan J: Molecular mechanisms in signal transduction at the membrane, *Nat Struct Mol Biol* 17(6):659–665, 2010.

Gurib-Fakim A: Medicinal plants: traditions of yesterday and drugs of tomorrow, *Mol Aspects Med* 27(1):1–93, 2006.

Gyorgypal Z, Kondorosi A: Homology of the ligand-binding regions of Rhizobium symbiotic regulatory protein NodD and vertebrate nuclear receptors, *Mol Gen Genet* 226(1–2):337–340, 1991.

Hamer M, Steptoe A: Influence of specific nutrients on progression of atherosclerosis, vascular function, haemostasis and inflammation in coronary heart disease patients: a systematic review, *Br J Nutr* 95(5):849–859, 2006.

Hata T, Matsuki H, Kaneshina S: Effect of local anesthetics on the bilayer membrane of dipalmitoylphosphatidylcholine: interdigitation of lipid bilayer and vesicle-micelle transition, *Biophys Chem* 87(1):25–36, 2000.

Hawkins MB, Thornton JW, Crews D, et al: Identification of a third distinct estrogen receptor and reclassification of estrogen receptors in teleosts, *PNAS* 97(20):10751–10756, 2000.

Hollman PC, Katan MB: Absorption, metabolism and health effects of dietary flavonoids in man, *Biomed Pharmacother* 51(8):305–310, 1997.

Hoult JR, Moroney MA, Paya M: Actions of flavonoids and coumarins on lipoxygenase and cyclooxygenase, *Methods Enzymol* 234:443–454, 1994.

Howitz KT, Bitterman KJ, Cohen HY, et al: Small molecule activators of sirtuins extend *Saccharomyces cerevisiae* lifespan, *Nature* 425(6954):191–196, 2003.

Howitz KT, Sinclair DA: Xenohormesis: sensing the chemical cues of other species, *Cell* 133(3):387–391, 2008.

Jackson FLC: Secondary compounds in plants (allelochemicals) as promoters of human biological variability, *Annu Rev Anthropol* 20:505–546, 1991.

Johns T: *The origins of human diet and medicine: chemical ecology*, Tucson, 1996, University of Arizona Press.

Katzenellenbogen BS, Katzenellenbogen JA, Mordecai D: Zearalenones: characterization of the estrogenic potencies and receptor interactions of a series of fungal beta-resorcylic acid lactones, *Endocrinology* 105(1):33–40, 1979.

Kauffman SA: *At home in the universe: the search for laws of self-organization and complexity*, New York, 1995, Oxford University Press.

Keith CT, Zimmermann GR: Multi-target lead discovery for networked systems, *Curr Drug Discov* 19–23, 2004.

Kenakin T: Principles: receptor theory in pharmacology, *Trends Pharmacol Sci* 25(4):186–192, 2004.

Khan N, Afaq F, Saleem M, et al: Targeting multiple signaling pathways by green tea polyphenol (-)-epigallocatechin-3-gallate, *Cancer Res* 66(5):2500–2505, 2006.

Kirchner JW: The Gaia hypothesis: conjectures and refutations, *Clim Change* 58:21–45, 2003.

Kirchoff BK: Aspects of a Goethan science: complexity and holism in science and art. In Rowland H, editor: *Goethe, chaos, and complexity*, Amsterdam, 2002, Offpring, pp 79–89.

Kitagawa N, Oda M, Totoko T: Possible mechanism of irreversible nerve injury caused by local anesthetics: detergent properties of local anesthetics and membrane disruption, *Anesthesiology* 100(4):962–967, 2004.

Kleidon A: Testing the effect of life on Earth's functioning: How Gaian is the Earth system? *Clim Change* 52:383–389, 2004.

Knekt P, Jarvinen R, Reunanen A, et al: Flavonoid intake and coronary mortality in Finland: a cohort study, *BMJ* 312(7029):478–481, 1996.

Knoops KT, de Groot LC, Kromhout D, et al: Mediterranean diet, lifestyle factors, and 10-year mortality in elderly European men and women: the HALE project, *JAMA* 292(12):1433–1439, 2004.

Koshland DE Jr, Hamadani K: Proteomics and models for enzyme cooperativity, *J Biol Chem* 277(49):46841–46844, 2002.

Kuhn TS: *The structure of scientific revolutions*, Chicago, 1962, University of Chicago Press.

Kushiro T, Nambara E, McCourt P: Hormone evolution: the key to signalling, *Nature* 422(6928):122, 2003.

Lamming DW, Wood JG, Sinclair DA, et al: Small molecules that regulate lifespan: evidence for xenohormesis, *Mol Microbiol* 53(4):1003–1009, 2004.

Law MR, Wald NJ, Morris JK, et al: Value of low dose combination treatment with blood pressure lowering drugs: analysis of 354 randomised trials, *BMJ* 326(7404):1427, 2003.

Lenton T: Testing Gaia: The effect of life on earth's habitability and regulation, *Clim Change* 52:409–422, 2002.

Lenton TM: Gaia and natural selection, *Nature* 394(6692):439–447, 1998.

Li JM, Biswas MG, Chao A, et al: Conservation of function between mammalian and plant steroid 5 alpha-reductases, *PNAS* 94(8):3554–3559, 1997.

Lin JK, Tsai SH: Antiinflammatory and antitumor effects of flavonoids and flavanoids, *Drugs Future* 26(2):145–152, 2001.

Liu RH: Health benefits of fruit and vegetables are from additive and synergistic combinations of phytochemicals, *Am J Clin Nutr* 78(3 Suppl):517S–520S, 2003.

Lotka AJ: *Elements of physical biology*, Baltimore, 1925, Williams & Wilkins.

Lovelock JE: *Gaia, a new look at life on earth*, Oxford; New York, 1979, Oxford University Press.

Lovelock JE: *Gaia: a new look at life on earth*. Oxford [Oxfordshire], New York, 1987, Oxford University Press.

Lovelock JE: Geophysiology, the science of gaia, *Rev Geophysics* 27(27):215-222, 1989.

Lovelock JE: New statements on the Gaia theory, *Microbiologia* 11(3):295-304, 1995.

Lovelock JE, Margulis L: Homeostatic tendencies of the earth's atmosphere, *Orig Life* 5(1):93-103, 1974.

Lovelock JE, Watson AJ: The regulation of carbon-dioxide and climate, *Planetary Space Sci* 30(8):795-802, 1982.

Luckey TD: *Hormesis with ionizing radiation*, Boca Raton, Fla, 1980, CRC Press.

Maini PK: Making sense of complex phenomena in biology. In Bock G, Goode J, editors: *'In silico' simulation of biological processes*, New York, 2002, John Wiley, p viii. 262 p.

Manthey JA, Buslig BS: *Flavonoids in the living system*, New York, 1998, Plenum Press.

Margulis L, Sagan D: *What is life?* Berkeley, 2000, University of California Press.

Markos A: The ontogeny of Gaia: the role of microorganisms in planetary information network, *J Theor Biol* 176(1):175-180, 1995.

Martinez-Valverde I, Periago MJ, Ros G: Nutritional importance of phenolic compounds in the diet], *Arch Latinoam Nutr* 50(1):5-18, 2000.

Mattson MP, Cheng AW: Neurohormetic phytochemicals: low-dose toxins that induce adaptive neuronal stress responses, *Trends Neurosci* 29(11):632-639, 2006.

Maturana H: The organization of the living: a theory of the living organization, *Int J Man Mach Stud* 7:313-332, 1975.

Maturana HR, Varela FJ: *The tree of knowledge: the biological roots of human understanding*, Boston, 1987, New Science Library. Distributed in the United States by Random House.

McCarty MF: Proposal for a dietary phytochemical index, *Med Hypotheses* 63(5):813-817, 2004.

McMahon HT, Gallop JL: Membrane curvature and mechanisms of dynamic cell membrane remodelling, *Nature* 438(7068):590-596, 2005.

Menendez JA, Joven J, Aragonès G, et al: Xenohormetic and anti-aging activity of secoiridoid polyphenols present in extra virgin olive oil: a new family of gerosuppressant agents, *Cell Cycle* 12(4):555-578, 2013.

Mui BLS, Cullis PR, Evans EA, et al: Osmotic properties of large unilamellar vesicles prepared by extrusion, *Biophys J* 64(2):443-453, 1993.

Nelson DR, Kamataki T, Waxman DJ, et al: The P450 superfamily—update on new sequences, gene-mapping, accession numbers, early trivial names of enzymes, and nomenclature, *DNA Cell Biol* 12(1):1-51, 1993.

Niculescu MD, Zeisel SH: Diet, methyl donors and DNA methylation: interactions between dietary folate, methionine and choline, *J Nutr* 132(8 Suppl):2333S-2335S, 2002.

Nijveldt RJ, van Nood E, can Hoorn DE, et al: Flavonoids: a review of probable mechanisms of action and potential applications, *Am J Clin Nutr* 74(4):418-425, 2001.

Norris JC, van der Laan MJ, Lane S, et al: Nonlinearity in demographic and behavioral determinants of morbidity, *Health Serv Res* 38(6 Pt 2):1791-1818, 2003.

Onori L, Visconti G: The GAIA theory: from Lovelock to Margulis. From a homeostatic to a cognitive autopoietic worldview, *Rend Lincei* 23(4):375-386, 2012.

Pakdel F, Le Guellec C, Vaillant C, et al: Identification and estrogen induction of two estrogen receptors (ER) messenger ribonucleic acids in the rainbow trout liver: sequence homology with other ERs, *Mol Endocrinol* 3(1):44-51, 1989.

Pechere JC: [How bacteria resist antibiotics: a primary form of collective intelligence?] *Bull Acad Natl Med* 188(8):1249-1256, 2004.

Perillo M: The drug-membrane interaction: its modulation at the supramolecular level. In Condat A, Baruzzi A, editors: *Recent Research Developments in Biophysical Chemistry C*, Kerala, 2002, Research Signpost.

Perillo MA, Garcia DA: Flunitrazepam induces geometrical changes at the lipid-water interface, *Colloids Surf B Biointerfaces* 20(1):63, 2001.

Plavec I, Sirenko O, Privat S, et al: Method for analyzing signaling networks in complex cellular systems, *Proc Natl Acad Sci U S A* 101(5):1223-1228, 2004.

Poitrineau K, Brown SP, Hochberg ME: Defence against multiple enemies, *J Evol Biol* 16(6):1319-1327, 2003.

Rose S: Precis of Lifelines: biology, freedom, determinism, *Behav Brain Sci* 22(5):871-921, 1999.

Scapini F: Environment and individual: a dialectic relationship, *Riv Biol* 94(2):293-303, 2001.

Schreier S, Malheiros SVP, de Paula E: Surface active drugs: self-association and interaction with membranes and surfactants. Physicochemical and biological aspects, *Biochim Biophys Acta* 1508(1-2):210-234, 2000.

Schrödinger E: *What is life? The physical aspect of the living cell*, Cambridge, 1944, The University Press; The Macmillan Company.

Schulkin J: Allostasis: a neural behavioral perspective, *Horm Behav* 43(1):21-27, discussion 28-30, 2003.

Simons K, Vaz WLC: Model systems, lipid rafts, and cell membranes, *Annu Rev Biophys Biomol Struct* 33:269-295, 2004.

Singer CJ, Underwood EA: *A short history of medicine*, Oxford, 1962, Clarendon Press.

Spelman K: Philosophy in phytopharmacology: Ockham's razor vs. synergy, *J Herb Pharmacother* 5(2):31-47, 2005.

Spelman K: Ecological pharmacology: humans and plants coherently couple through phytochemistry, *Unified Energetics* 2(5):40-45, 2006.

Spelman K, Duke JA: The synergy principle in plants, pathogens, insects, herbivores and humans. In Kaufman PB, editor: *Natural products from plants*, ed 2, Boca Raton, Fla, 2006, CRC Press, pp 475-501.

Spinella M: The importance of pharmacological synergy in psychoactive herbal medicines, *Altern Med Rev* 7(2):130-137, 2002.

Stafford HA: Flavonoid evolution: an enzymic approach, *Plant Physiol* 96(3):680-685, 1991.

Stebbing AR: Hormesis-the stimulation of growth by low levels of inhibitors, *Sci Total Environ* 22(3):213-234, 1982.

Tammen SA, Friso S, Choi SW: Epigenetics: the link between nature and nurture, *Mol Aspects Med* 34(4):753-764, 2013.

Taylor LP, Grotewold E: Flavonoids as developmental regulators, *Curr Opin Plant Biol* 8(3):317-323, 2005.

Thaler DS: The evolution of genetic intelligence, *Science* 264(5156):224-225, 1994.

Trewavas A, Stewart D: Paradoxical effects of chemicals in the diet on health, *Curr Opin Plant Biol* 6(2):185-190, 2003.

Turney J: Gaia: not nice enough, *Interdisc Sci Rev* 30(1):5–10, 2005.

Vaiserman AM: Hormesis and epigenetics: is there a link? *Ageing Res Rev* 10(4):413–421, 2011.

Valinluck V, Tsai HH, Rogstad DK, et al: Oxidative damage to methyl-CpG sequences inhibits the binding of the methyl-CpG binding domain (MBD) of methyl-CpG binding protein 2 (MeCP2), *Nucleic Acids Res* 32(14):4100–4108, 2004.

Varela FJ, Thompson E, Rosch E: *The embodied mind: cognitive science and human experience*, Cambridge, Mass, 1991, MIT Press.

Vickers A: Botanical medicines for the treatment of cancer: rationale, overview of current data, and methodological considerations for phase I and II trials, *Cancer Invest* 20(7–8):1069–1079, 2002.

Volk T: Toward a future for Gaia, *Clim Change* 52:423–430, 2002.

Wagner H: Phytomedicine research in Germany, *Environ Health Perspect* 107:779–781, 1999.

Wald NJ, Law MR: A strategy to reduce cardiovascular disease by more than 80%, *BMJ* 326(7404):1419, 2003.

Wang LG, Mencher SK, McCarron JP, et al: The biological basis for the use of an anti-androgen and a 5-alpha-reductase inhibitor in the treatment of recurrent prostate cancer: Case report and review, *Oncol Rep* 11(6):1325–1329, 2004.

Waterland RA, Jirtle RL: Transposable elements: targets for early nutritional effects on epigenetic gene regulation, *Mol Cell Biol* 23(15):5293–5300, 2003.

Watson A, Lovelock JE, Marguilis L: Methanogenesis, fires and the regulation of atmospheric oxygen, *Biosystems* 10(4):293–298, 1978.

Welshons WV, Thayer KA, Judy BM, et al: Large effects from small exposures. I. Mechanisms for endocrine-disrupting chemicals with estrogenic activity, *Environ Health Perspect* 111(8):994–1006, 2003.

Weng G, Bhalla US, Iyengar R: Complexity in biological signaling systems, *Science* 284(5411):92–96, 1999.

Westphal CH, Dipp MA, Guarente L: A therapeutic role for sirtuins in diseases of aging? *Trends Biochem Sci* 32(12):555–560, 2007.

White R, Jobling S, Hoare SA, et al: Environmentally persistent alkylphenolic compounds are estrogenic, *Endocrinology* %R 10.1210/en.135.1.175. 135(1):175–182, 1994.

Williamson EM: Synergy and other interactions in phytomedicines, *Phytomedicine* 8(5):401–409, 2001.

Wood M: *The magical staff: the vitalist tradition in Western medicine*, Berkeley, Calif, 1992, North Atlantic Books.

Wu KH, Tobias ML, Thornton JW, et al: Estrogen receptors in Xenopus: duplicate genes, splice variants, and tissue-specific expression, *Gen Comp Endocrinol* 133(1):38–49, 2003.

Wynne-Edwards KE: Evolutionary biology of plant defenses against herbivory and their predictive implications for endocrine disruptor susceptibility in vertebrates, *Environ Health Perspect* 109(5):443–448, 2001.

Yong EL, Loh YS: Herbal medicine, criteria for use in health and disease. In Packer L, Ong CN, Halliwell B, editors: *Herbal and traditional medicine: molecular aspects of health*, New York, 2004, Marcel Dekker, p 941.

Zangerl AR, Berenbaum MR: Genetic variation in primary metabolites of *Pastinaca sativa;* can herbivores act as selective agents? *J Chem Ecol* 30(10):1985–2002, 2004.

Zimmerberg J, Kozlov MM: How proteins produce cellular membrane curvature, *Nat Rev Mol Cell Biol* 7(1):9–19, 2006.

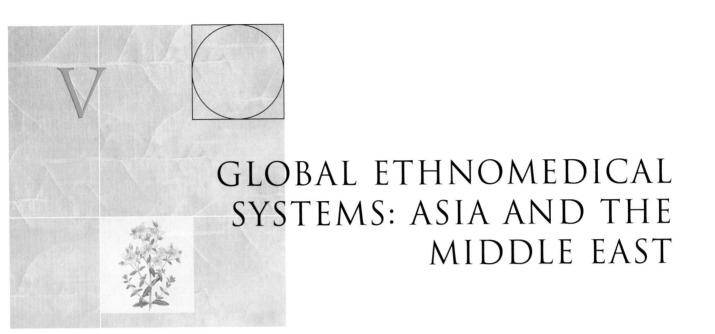

GLOBAL ETHNOMEDICAL SYSTEMS: ASIA AND THE MIDDLE EAST

Sections V and VI provide a survey of the fundamentals of global health traditions that form integrated systems of thought and practice, following from an explanation of their relevant worldviews. The sections are divided geographically into Asia and the Middle East (Section V) and Africa, the Americas, and Pacific (Section VI). While this book aims to present a unified body of the theories and practices of alternative and ethnomedicines, many healing traditions throughout the world are marked by significant heterogeneity, consistent with their historical evolution and their underlying philosophies.

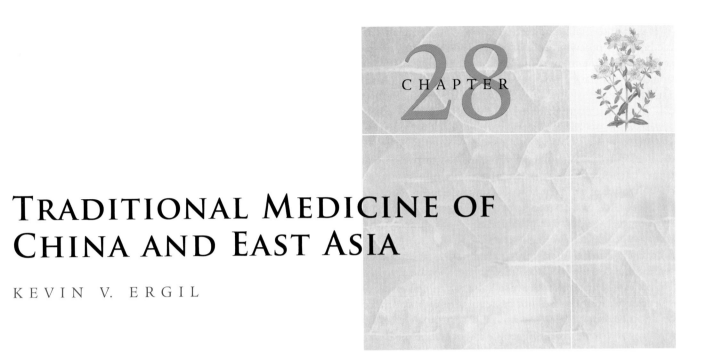

TRADITIONAL MEDICINE OF CHINA AND EAST ASIA

KEVIN V. ERGIL

CHINA'S TRADITIONAL MEDICINE IN CULTURAL PERSPECTIVE

Certain considerations are important to understanding ethnomedical systems in general and Chinese medicine in particular. Medicine is a human endeavor and as such is shaped by the considerations of the humans using and practicing it. These considerations sometimes have very little to do with curing disease in the most simple and efficient way and a great deal to do with economics, politics, and culture. Ideology, belief, and even simple ignorance have influenced the practice of medicine more than rationality. A medical historian or a physician might perceive medicine to be a steady march from ignorance to the light, but these are typically revisionist histories. Medicine is a human enterprise embedded in and intersected by myriad other human projects. Even the choice of how to conduct a medical procedure or what type of health care to choose may have more to do with habit or economics than with rationality or efficacy.

For example, take the case of a Chinese patient who chose traditional herbal medicine to manage painful and debilitating kidney stones. Although the treatment was ultimately efficacious, the patient's choice was not motivated by a desire for efficacy. Undergoing surgery would have meant that the patient would have been classified as an "invalid" on her work papers and therefore barred from advancement. A hospital in California closes its doors to the practice of acupuncture, even though acupuncturists in the state are licensed medical practitioners and their services are routinely requested by hospital patients. In each instance, considerations that are not directly linked to the rational and effective delivery of medical care influence medical choices.

Our own perspectives on medicine and our experience of our own medical systems provide us with ideas of what is normal or typical for medicine. We respond to aspects of a traditional system that correspond with our expectations. Americans accustomed to getting health care from Western, biomedically trained physicians in white coats may be satisfied with a licensed physician (MD) who has completed a six-week acupuncture course. At the same time, some Chinese-Americans still seek a traditional acupuncturist who may practice in Chinatown and be descended from six generations of acupuncturists. Both the "six-week wonders" in white coats and the sixth-generation traditional healers are able to deliver to effective care for many patients that meet their expectations (see Chapters 3, 5).

We might imagine Chinese herbal medicine to be a gentle therapy using nontoxic ingredients. Its use of highly toxic substances or drastic purgative therapies is easily overlooked. We know that many ethnomedical traditions have been intentionally or unintentionally "watered-down" (with the "hard" parts "edited out" so to speak) to be more acceptable to Western patients (see Chapter 3). It is unlikely, for example, that the traditional form of Tibetan therapeutic cautery applied with a hot iron (see Chapter 30) will elicit substantial interest as a form of alternative therapy. Naturalistic and rational elements of systems intrigue us. Unfamiliar or "magical" diagnostic and therapeutic modes cause us concern.

It is easy to make intellectual errors when dealing with medical systems. We forget that our own perspectives may prevent us from understanding the meaning and use of practices that have been developed within another culture. That failure to account for our own needs and biases also can lead to the overenthusiastic acceptance of ideas whose genesis and application we really do not understand.

If we want to avoid these errors, we must think about medical systems as being embedded in their respective cultures. Each system's structure and elements are vital to their practice in a particular cultural context. "Culture," in this sense, does not imply an all-embracing system of meaning subscribed to by all members of a community, country, or ethnicity. Culture is a complex network of signification; some elements might resonate only in a local sense, whereas other aspects have almost global relevance. This does not mean that the medical ideas and practices of one society cannot or will not be successfully appropriated by another, but rather that aspects of a system that are meaningful to one group of people might not be meaningful at all to another (see Chapter 5).

For example, neurasthenia *(sheng jin shuai ruo)* is an important syndrome in traditional Chinese medicine and Chinese psychiatry, even though this diagnosis has fallen into disrepute among Western psychiatrists and the condition is no longer classified as a disease entity in diagnostic manuals. Neurasthenia was an exceptionally popular diagnosis in the West in the nineteenth and early twentieth centuries during periods of extensive medical exchange between the United States and China and Japan. It was a term applied to "battle fatigue" among soldiers during and after the U.S. Civil War and World War I. Today we have "post-traumatic stress disorder" (PTSD) in the West.

The diagnosis of neurasthenia has continued to be clinically important in China because it fits well into certain traditional medical models and responds well to cultural and political concerns about mental illness (Kleinman, 1986). Americans and Europeans who encounter neurasthenia within the corpus of Chinese medicine now sometimes find it an unusual or obscure concept despite its relevance for Chinese medical practice.

Sometimes, on encountering a new idea, we choose to think about it in familiar terms. One example is the use of the word *energy* to express the idea of qi. An extension of this is the frequent translation of the term for the therapeutic method of draining evil influences from channels as "sedation." Neither energy nor sedation has much to do with the concepts that underlie qi and draining; however, these terms are more familiar to us and make Chinese medicine more accessible. Unfortunately, this practice can obscure the breadth of meaning in these terms (Wiseman et al, 1990). We try to make sense of the world from our position in it, historically as well as culturally. We tend to view history as progressing, as if by design, to a specific end. Events of the past, viewed from the perspective of the present, offer tempting opportunities for reinterpretation in relation to current experience.

For example, in the context of current perspectives on disease causation, Wu You Ke's statements in the *Wen Yi Lun (On Warm Epidemics)* written in 1642 that "miscellaneous qi" could cause epidemic disease and his concept of "one disease, one qi" (Wiseman, 1993) have led contemporary sources in China to suggest that, coming before the invention of the microscope, such an insight is quite remarkable (Wiseman et al, 1995). The idea that Wu You Ke's observation represented a precursor of germ theory is attractive to Chinese practitioners who are trying to find a place for traditional practices in an increasingly biomedicalized world. In fact, the concept of miscellaneous or pestilential qi has been used extensively in adapting traditional theory to the management of human immunodeficiency virus (HIV) infection. However, as Wiseman points out, it never was explored in relation to the causation of disease by microscopic organisms, nor was it ever conceived as a basis for such an exploration. Its relation to this concept is a retrospective interpretation.

The preceding points are generally relevant to almost any system or collection of medical practices. Some additional points are crucial to understanding the progression of medical thought in China. Although we tend to think that Chinese medicine has been practiced without significant change for millennia, this notion is simply not true. Chinese medicine has undergone significant change and development over the centuries. Ideas that once were important are now almost invisible, and ideas that had been left by the wayside for centuries again found favor in later times. Recent ideas have been relatively significant in the organization of the system. Changes in technology, for example, have broadened the clinical use of acupuncture and increased its safety. Ideas, substances, *material medica* (herbs), and medical practices have come to China from all over the world; some of them have become significant parts of traditional Chinese medicine, and some of them remain only as observations in ancient texts.

Within China itself, many competing ideas have existed side by side. Old theories have been rejected or discovered anew and accorded even more importance than they had at their conception. Some ideas found more fertile ground in other Asian countries, as with the transmission of acupuncture and Chinese herbal medicine to Japan, where particular aspects of the Chinese tradition were emphasized and adapted.

Historian and anthropologist Paul Unschuld (1985) critiques the perspective of Chinese medicine as a homogenous monolithic structure, as follows:

> Proponents of this view depict "Chinese Medicine" as an identifiable, coherent system, the contents of which they attempt to characterize. Such an approach is both ahistorical and selective. It focuses on but one of the many distinctly conceptualized systems of therapy in Chinese history, that is the medicine of systematic correspondence, and it neglects both the changing interpretations of basic paradigms offered by Chinese authors through the ages and the synchronic plurality of differing opinions and

ideas that existed for twenty centuries concerning even fundamental aspects of this therapy system such as pulse-diagnosis. (Unschuld, 1985:2)

This point is important, because it is extremely tempting to encounter medical systems with the expectation that they be possessed of an internal logic that reconciles all their aspects. Although many aspects of Chinese medicine can be applied with complete consistency, other aspects or concepts seem to be quite contradictory. This trait leads us to what has been probably the most important aspect of Chinese medicine throughout its history: *it is a medical tradition that never threw anything away*. Certain medical practices might have been relegated to the attic, but they were available if necessary.

A striking example is the work of Zhang Zhong Jing, whose system of diagnosis and therapy did not attract much attention during his lifetime but who became highly influential centuries after his death. Later, authors believed his theory to be incomplete and broadened its perspective, but his theories and these new theories that emerged in response to them are still important to the contemporary clinician. In the West an incomplete theory (that does not account for all of experimental observations) is rejected and disappears. In the history of Chinese medicine, theories, practices, and concepts may fade, but they do not entirely disappear. A new theory can exist beside the one that it sought to correct. Clinicians can choose to apply the perspective that they believe is most relevant. In this way, conflicting concepts of cause, systems of diagnosis, and treatment have continued to exist side by side.

Unschuld considers this one of the basic characteristics distinguishing traditional Chinese thought from modern Western science (Unschuld, 1985). It also is the aspect of Chinese medicine that is most challenging to Western students. The extent to which deductive reasoning and its necessary condition of "either this, or that, but not both" are pervasive in our society have made it difficult to approach a medical tradition that dispenses with what we view as a necessary precondition of valid human knowledge. Even European or American advocates of Chinese medical traditions sometimes err and insist that only certain theoretical perspectives or therapeutic methods are correct or authentic.

Years before Unschuld made his observations, Lin Yutang (1942) wrote that systematic metaphysics or epistemology were alien to traditional Chinese thought, as follows:

> The temperament for systematic philosophy simply wasn't there, and will not be there so long as the Chinese remain Chinese. They have too much sense for that. The sea of human life forever laps upon the shores of Chinese thought, and the arrogance and absurdities of the logician, the assumption that "I am exclusively right and you are exclusively wrong," are not Chinese faults, whatever other faults they may have.

The history of Chinese medical thought does include many individuals who thought that they were exclusively right. However, the breadth of traditional Chinese medical thought was sustained by an intellectual climate that retained all possible ideas for use and exploration. A given philosopher or clinician might reject an idea, but the idea itself would remain available for future use.

For example, during the Ming dynasty, Wu You Ke (ca. 1644) was the leading exponent of the "offensive precipitation sect" *(gong xia pai)* of physicians whose tenets included a distinctive set of ideas concerning the management of epidemic disease and a wholehearted rejection of many established ideas in Chinese medicine (Wong et al, 1985). He was subsequently viewed alternately as a contributor to Chinese medical thought, a proponent of a divergent and uninformed theory, and finally (as noted previously) as the intellectual antecedent of Koch, the discoverer of the tuberculosis bacillus. At no point were his ideas discarded.

Interestingly, in modern China, where the sheer volume of information and the nation's health care needs make it necessary to teach a standard curriculum to thousands of students each year, this tolerance for varying clinical perspectives continues. For example, certain herbal physicians are known as Minor *Bupleurum* Decoction *(xiao chai hu tang)* doctors because their prescriptions are organized around one formula from the *Treatise on Cold Damage (Shang Han Lun)*, an early text on diagnosis and herbal therapy written during the Han dynasty (206 BC–AD 220). On the other hand, herbal physicians may reject traditional formulas entirely and use only contemporary perspectives on the Chinese pharmacopeia to organize their prescriptions.

Some acupuncturists may have a clinical focus dedicated almost entirely to six acupuncture points and may use computed tomography scans to plan clinical interventions. At the same time, two floors down in the same hospital, physicians base their selection of acupuncture points on obscure and complex aspects of traditional calendrics and systems such as the "Magic Turtle."

Once it is understood that Chinese medicine is a large and varied tradition with many manifestations and philosophies, it is possible to begin its exploration.

DYNASTIC MEDICINE

Chinese medicine has an extensive history. As with most medical traditions, this history can be approached from several perspectives. There is the ancient mythology of Chinese medicine, which attributes the birth of medicine to the legendary emperors Fu Xi, Shen Nong, and Huang Di. There is the history that can be deduced from the careful study of available ancient texts and records, which indicate, for example, that there is no reference to acupuncture as a therapeutic method in any Chinese text before 90 BC, and that the oldest existing text to discuss medical practices resembling current Chinese medicine dates from the end of the third century BC (Unschuld, 1985). Finally, there are the more extravagant interpretations of archaeological evidence and textual materials that seek to establish the ancient character of certain Chinese medical practices. An example is the frequent assertion that the stone "needles" excavated at different times in various parts of China were remnants of ancient acupuncture (Chuang, 1982; Wang, 1986). This assertion is based on references to the ancient surgical application of sharp stones in texts from later periods and morphological similarities between the excavated stones and later metal needles. Characteristics of ancient and "pre-historic" Chinese medicine can be seen in continuity with shamanism in other cultures (see Chapter 34).

LEGENDARY AND SEMI-MYTHICAL ORIGINS

The origins of Chinese medicine are mythically linked to three legendary emperors: Fu Xi, Shen Nong, and Huang Di. Fu Xi, or the Ox Tamer (ca. 2953 BC), taught people how to domesticate animals and divined the *Ba Gua*, eight symbols that became the basis for the *I Ching (Yi Jing)*, or *Book of Changes.*

Shen Nong, or the Divine Husbandman, also known as the Fire Emperor, is said to have lived from 2838 to 2698 BC and is considered the founder of agriculture in China. He taught the Chinese people how to cultivate plants and raise livestock. He also is considered the originator of herbal medicine in China, having learned the therapeutic properties of herbs and substances by tasting them. Later authors would attribute their work to Shen Nong to indicate the antiquity and importance of their text. The *Divine Husbandman's Classic of the Materia Medica (Shen Nong Ben Cao Jing)* is a case in point. The text probably was written in AD 220 and reconstructed in AD 500 by Tao Hong Jing. Given that all historical evidence points to the ancient character of herbal medicine in China, it is appropriate that Shen Nong is considered its originator (Figure 28-1).

Huang Di, the Yellow Emperor (2698–2598 BC), is known as the originator of the traditional medicine of China. He also is seen as the "Father of the Chinese Nation." He is credited with teaching the Chinese how to make wooden houses, silk cloth, boats, carts, the bow and arrow, and ceramics, and introducing the art of writing. Legend has it that he gained his knowledge from visiting the immortals. Most important to this discussion is his work the *Yellow Emperor's Inner Classic (Huang Di Nei Jing)*, in which the traditional medicine of China is first expressed in a form that is familiar to us today. The text is divided into two books. *Simple Questions (Su Wen)* is concerned with medical theory, such as the principles of yin and yang, the five phases, and the effects of seasons. The *Spiritual Axis (Ling Shu)* deals predominantly with acupuncture and moxibustion. The texts are written as a series of dialogues between the emperor and his ministers. Qi Bo, the most famous among the ministers, is said to have tested the actions of drugs, cured people's sickness, and written books on medicine and therapeutics.

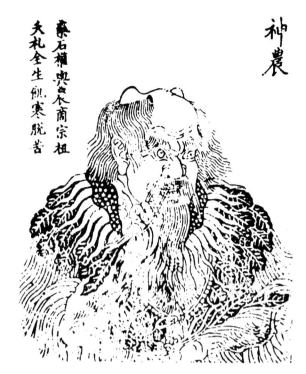

Figure 28-1 Image of Shen Nong.

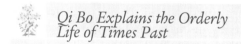
Qi Bo Explains the Orderly Life of Times Past

The first book of *Simple Questions* begins with the Yellow Emperor asking Qi Bo why people's life spans are now so short when in the past they lived close to a hundred years. Qi Bo explains that in the past people maintained an orderly life. "In ancient times those people who understood Dao patterned themselves upon the yin and the yang and they lived in harmony with the arts of divination" (Veith, 1972). ∾

It is generally agreed now that the *Yellow Emperor's Inner Classic* was first compiled around 200 to 100 BC. In terms of both legend and practice, it remains a text that is critical to Chinese medicine.

ANCIENT MEDICINE: 2205 TO 206 BC

Little is actually known about the practice of medicine in China before 200 BC. The Shang dynasty (1766–1121 BC) is the first dynasty of which there exists clear archaeological evidence. It appears likely that before the Shang, nomadic cultures were scattered across northern China. Interaction among these groups eventually led to the development of the Shang. This dynasty left the first traces of some form of therapeutic activity. In addition to developing the first Chinese scripts, the Shang had clearly defined social relations. There was a king and nobility, and perhaps most importantly, the people were no longer nomadic.

The Shang response to illness is documented by archaeological finds and writings from the succeeding Zhou dynasty (1122–221 BC). During this period, ideas developed that would be central to Chinese culture; specifically, a relationship between the living and the dead developed into a ritualized veneration of ancestors. Ancestors could be consulted concerning a variety of issues, including the cause of illness, through the use of oracle bones. Tortoise shells and the scapula of oxen were heated and rapidly cooled, which caused them to crack. The resulting patterns would be used for guidance in resolving questions. Often the question posed to the ancestors would be inscribed on the bone itself. Bones could be used for more than one divination. One tomb has yielded more than 100,000 oracle bones, displaying questions such as "Swelling of the abdomen. Is there a curse? Does the deceased Chin-wu desire something of the king?" (Unschuld, 1985). The ancestors were appropriately placated according to the response. Natural causes of illness also were encountered, but these appear to have been addressed through the intervention of ancestors as well.

The Zhou dynasty resulted from a political conflict with a group of Chinese-speaking descendants of the same Neolithic (New Stone Age) peoples who had settled to form the Shang. The defeat of the Shang established one of China's longest dynasties, as well as a pattern of governance that would characterize Chinese society—a central government working in relation to smaller principalities.

The Zhou continued the practices of the Shang rulers, consulting tortoise shell oracles with the aid of *wu*, or shamans. The *wu* acted as intermediaries between the living and the dead, played important ritual roles in court activities and with regard to the weather, and were called on to combat the demons who caused illness. During this period the shamanic activity of chasing evil spirits away from towns and homes with spears might have been transferred to the human body, and the practice of acupuncture emerged. Later accounts (eighth century AD) describe the needling techniques used by the physician Bian Qu (fifth century BC) to drive out demons. However, we have no clear evidence of this.

The Warring States period, toward the close of the Zhou, was marked by political strife and social upheaval. This era saw the emergence of two philosophers, Kong Fu Zi (Confucius) and Lao Zi (Lao Tzu), whose ideas about social and natural order were to have a lasting impact on Chinese culture. A similar trend occurred within medicine: the human body no longer was seen as subject only to the whims of spirits and demons, but as a part of nature and subject to discernible natural relationships. Those ideas were elaborated on during the Han dynasty. (see Chapter 334, Origins)

FLOWERING OF CHINESE MEDICINE: 206 BC TO AD 907

In 206 BC the empire was reunited under the Han. The Han (206 BC–AD 220) created a stable aristocratic social order, expanded geographically and economically, and spread Chinese political influence throughout Vietnam and Korea. The Chinese people currently refer to themselves as the Han. This dynasty presided over a period of great development for the Chinese, including the integration of the Confucian doctrine, elements of yin and yang, and the five-phase theory into the political picture. Textual evidence reveals the emergence of a medicine that is similar to current Chinese medicine.

The earliest texts available were recovered from three tombs dating to 168 BC that were excavated at Ma Wang Dui in Hunan province (Unschuld, 1985). These texts discuss magical and demonological concepts, as well as some ideas about yin and yang in relation to the body. The texts present an early concept of channels in the body, but in a less developed fashion than the later *Yellow Emperor's Inner Classic*. Ma Wang Dui texts mention moxibustion and the use of heated stones, but they do not speak about acupuncture or specific points on the body, which implies that the idea of acupuncture had not yet emerged.

A biography written by a contemporary in 90 BC describes Chun Yu Yi, the first physician known to record personal observations of clinical cases. Interestingly, he also was tried for malpractice because of his use of the apparently unfamiliar method of acupuncture to change the flow of qi (Unschuld, 1985).

The *Divine Husbandman's Classic of the Materia Medica*, mentioned earlier, appears during this era as well. This text is the first known formal presentation of individual medicinal substances, the first in a long line of such texts.

 Sun Si Miao Explains the Incurable Nature of Physicians

Finally, it is inappropriate to emphasize one's reputation, to belittle the rest of the physicians and to praise only one's own virtue. Indeed, in actual life someone who has accidentally healed a disease, then stalks around with his head raised, shows conceit and announces that no one in the entire world could measure up to him. In this respect all physicians are evidently incurable.

Quoted in Unschuld P: Medical ethics in Imperial China: a study in historical anthropology, *Berkeley, CA, 1979, University of California Press.*

The *Classic of Difficult Issues (Nan Jing)* was compiled sometime during the first or second century AD, although its authorship is attributed to the legendary physician Bian Qu. This text has had and continues to have a marked influence on the practice of Chinese medicine and, to an even greater extent, on the practice of Chinese medicine in Japan. It marks a drastic shift in medical thinking, systematically organizing the theory and practice of therapeutic acupuncture in terms of body structure, illness, diagnosis, and treatment. It is almost entirely devoid of magical elements. The author(s) of the *Classic of Difficult Issues* reconciled the contradictions of the *Inner Classic,* in addition to providing many new observations. Although it is thought to have been written as an independent text, the *Classic of Difficult Issues* met with so much resistance because of its radical organization that it became known as a commentary on the *Inner Classic.*

The texts *On Cold Damage* (Shang Han Lun) and the *Essential Prescription of the Golden Cabinet (Jin Gui Yao Lue)* were written in the second century AD by Zhang Zhong Jing, also known as Zhang Ji (AD 142–220). Chinese medical texts of this period were primarily philosophical, but as with the authors of the *Classic of Difficult Issues,* Zhang studied disease from a clinical standpoint, emphasizing the physical signs, symptoms, and course of disease; the method of treatment; and the action of the substances used. He was interested especially in fevers, because most of the people in his village died from fever epidemics (possibly typhoid). Although published during the Han dynasty, these texts remained relatively obscure until the Sung dynasty (after AD 960), when medical thinkers realized that the concepts of diagnosis and therapy presented reflected their own concerns. These texts enormously influenced the practice of herbal medicine in Japan. We will examine an herbal formula derived from *On Cold Damage* later in this chapter.

Hua Tuo (AD 110–207), acupuncturist, herbalist, and surgeon, is a near-legendary figure in Chinese medicine. Not only did he reportedly use acupuncture and herbs, his adaptation of animal postures is one of the early forms of qigong. He is said to have used the anesthetic properties of plants to render a patient insensible to pain, which enabled him to practice surgery successfully.

Despite Hua Tuo's reputation, his surgical innovations seem to have departed with him. Chinese medical history reveals the practice of a variety of minor surgical interventions for growths, hemorrhoids, and wound healing, but none of the significant abdominal surgeries attributed to Hua Tuo. The surgical castration used to produce eunuchs for the imperial court was medically significant, and there is textual evidence of Chinese exposure to the surgical practices developed in India for the treatment of cataracts, but these did not form surgical traditions per se.

Huang Fu Mi (AD 215–286) wrote the *Systematic Classic of Acupuncture (and Moxibustion) (Zhen Jiu Jia Yi Jing),* which exercised substantial influence over the acupuncture traditions of China, Korea, and Japan. This text presented and reorganized material from the *Inner Classic* and other earlier texts.

It is important to realize that the histories of individual physicians and the texts that have come down to us reflect the medicine of the literate elite of China more than the medical traditions of that nation as a whole. About 80% of the total population consisted of farmers, peasants, and farming villages. These people lived at a level of bare subsistence and worked extremely hard to stay there, entirely dependent on the soil and the weather. They were not exposed to formal education and typically were illiterate. Very little is known of what these people knew or thought at any particular time. Their traditions were regionally oriented and full of folk superstition, historical legend, and aspirations dominated by the hope of survival.

Some authors, especially compilers of *materia medica* texts, did explore the nonliterate traditions of the Chinese people, but the first systematic publication of this material did not occur until late in the Qing dynasty (1644–1911) (Unschuld, 1985). Folk herbal and medical traditions were most systematically explored under the guidance of the postrevolutionary government of China. Texts such as *The Barefoot Doctor's Manual* reflect the inclusion of this type of material in the 20th century.

In AD 220, after approximately 30 years of strife and religious rebellion by Daoist sects, the Han dynasty fell. After the Han there was another long period of division in China, although not as violent or as divisive as the Warring States period after the Zhou dynasty. In AD 589 the Sui dynasty reunified China and soon was succeeded by the Tang dynasty, considered by many to be the height of China's cultural development. The Tang dynasty spread China's influence as far as Mongolia, Vietnam, Central Asia, Korea, and Japan. During this period, both Buddhism and Daoism strongly influenced medical thought.

Sun Si Miao (AD 581–682), a famous physician of the period, was a prolific author and a productive Confucian scholar who was well versed in both Daoist and Buddhist practice. His works include *Thousand Ducat Prescriptions (Qian Jin Yao Fang),* a text on eye disorders, and the *Classic of Spells,* a guide to magic in medicine. The *Thousand Ducat Prescriptions* contains a section titled "On the Absolute Sincerity of Great Physicians" that established him as China's first known medical ethicist. He addresses the need for diligent scholarship, compassion toward the patient, and high moral standards in the physician, which remain pertinent and seem to speak directly to current medical issues.

LEARNED MEDICINE AND SYSTEMATIC THERAPEUTICS: AD 960 TO 1368

By the time of the Sung dynasty the practice of medicine had become more specialized, and efforts were made to integrate past insights systematically. The number of texts published during the period of this dynasty may have exceeded the number written during all the previous dynasties. In 1027, Wang Wei Yi oversaw the casting of two bronze figures that he designed to illustrate the location of acupuncture points. One of these was used in the Imperial Medical College. The bronzes were pierced at the location of the acupuncture points, covered with wax, and filled with water. When a student found the hole under the wax with a needle, water would drip out, indicating it to be the correct spot.

During the Sung dynasty, great advances occurred in herbal therapeutics, and several complete herbal texts with illustrations were published under imperial decree. Tastes and properties were assigned to herbs according to their yin or yang nature, and functions were assigned based on the herb's nature and its ability to treat specific symptoms. Efforts were made to systematize herbal therapeutics. The writings of Zhang Zhong Jing received great interest because of his systematic application of traditional theoretical principles to the use of herbal medicine. The revival of the *On Cold Damage* influenced medicine for the next several hundred years, because it sparked the development of warm-induced disease theory *(wen bing xue)* during the Ming dynasty.

During the Sung dynasty the education of physicians became more formal. The Imperial College, which had provided for the training of the emperor's physicians, was expanded. In 1076 the Imperial Medical College was founded, with an enrollment of 300 students. There were regional schools as well.

The Jin and Yuan dynasties saw the continuation of specialized medical thought and independent inquiry. Much of what we recognize as Chinese medicine today—and what we discuss in the section on fundamental concepts—stems from the Sung, Jin, and Yuan dynasties. Physicians of this period developed ideas involving the elaboration of therapeutic approaches on the basis of early theory. They espoused the application of five-phase theory in relation to seasonal influences, supplementing the body, purging the body to eliminate evil influences, and supplementing the yin.

MEDICINE IN MING AND QING DYNASTIES: AD 1368 TO 1911

During the Ming and Qing dynasties, or the Late Imperial Period, physicians continued to pursue lines of inquiry explored in preceding dynasties, such as the far-reaching naturalistic explorations of Li Shi Zhen (1518–1593). His *Grand Materia Medica (Ben Cao Gang Mu)* included discussions of 1892 substances and, among its topics, described the use of kelp and deer thyroid to treat goiter.

The exploration of more precise linkages between factors in disease causation and therapeutics continued, and a number of medical sects emerged. During a virulent epidemic that struck from 1641 to 1644, Wu You Ke (Xing) (1592–1672) used an unorthodox treatment method that was highly successful. His text, *Discussion of Warm Epidemics (Wen Yi Lun)*, explored the theoretical basis for his treatment with iodine.

Some authors consider the Ming dynasty to be the peak of the cultural expression of acupuncture and moxibustion in China (Qiu, 1993). This period saw the production of numerous texts on the subject. One of the most influential acupuncture texts, the *Great Compendium of Acupuncture and Moxibustion (Zhen Jiu Da Cheng)*, was written by Yang Ji Zhou toward the end of the Ming dynasty.

Intellectual trends of the Ming continued into the Qing dynasty. The *Discussion of Warm Disease (Wen Re Lun)* by Ye Tian Shi complemented Zhang Zhong Jing's method of diagnosing and treating diseases caused by cold with an equally systematic method of diagnosing and treating those caused by heat.

Political, economic, and social trends during the Qing dynasty exacerbated the isolation of the Manchu rulers of the time and exposed the Chinese to the power of Western knowledge, technology, and science. The broadening of cultural horizons and the broadening of medical inquiry combined to shake the classical underpinnings of Chinese medical thought. In 1822, the study of acupuncture was formally eliminated from the Imperial Medical College (Qiu, 1993).

By the close of the Qing dynasty in 1911, political and cultural institutions were in a state of decline. The scattered practitioners of traditional Chinese medicine found themselves increasingly under fire from the advocates of a new and modern China and a new and modern medicine.

The collapse of the Qing and the formation of the Republic laid traditional medicine open to the conquering influence of Western medicine. The Imperial College of Physicians was eliminated (Wong et al, 1985), and the Western-educated proponents of reform began to work toward the elimination of the traditional medicine of China and the establishment of Western medicine as the dominant medical system.

From 1914 through 1936 a series of encounters and clashes occurred over the regulation, establishment, or elimination of practitioners of Chinese medicine (Wong et al, 1985). The traditional medicine of China, or "medicine" *(yi)* as it had been known, came to be termed "Chinese medicine" *(zhong yi)*. Both nationalist and Marxist reformers intensely disliked Chinese medicine, a system that hearkened back to the ancients and whose use might keep China from modernizing.

SO-CALLED CHINESE MEDICINE

Initially the external threat reduced the internal spectrum of competing Chinese interpretations of the classics. The great diversity of individual efforts to reconcile insights from personal experience with the ancient theories of yin yang and the five phases, as well as with other older views about the structure of the body, disappeared behind the illusion of a so-called Chinese medicine *(chung-I [zhong yi])*, supposedly well defined and with theory easily converted into practice. This situation, in turn, has given rise to the historically misleading impression that these diverse elements, like the concepts and practices of Western medicine, constituted a unified, coherent system (Unschuld, 1985:250).

A critical feature of this new Chinese medicine was its rejection of practices that were manifestly "unscientific," represented in the creation of *zhong yi*. This disciplined form of medicine has emerged today as traditional Chinese medicine. (so-called TCM)

The aspects of the traditional medicine of China that were secured in *zhong yi* were later appropriated by the Chinese Marxists in an effort to build a strong medical infrastructure for substantial populations in the face of economic and technical limitations. Chairman Mao's declaration in 1958 that *"Chinese medicine is a great treasure house! We must uncover it and raise its standards!"* (Unschuld, 1985) inspired efforts to rehabilitate the traditional medicine of China and to "discover" a primitive dialectic within the theoretical underpinnings of the system. The *Revised Outline of Chinese Medicine* stated that "yin-yang and the five phases *(wu-hsing [wu xing])* are ancient Chinese philosophical ideas. They are spontaneous, naive materialist theories that also contain elementary dialectic ideas" (Sivin, 1987). Despite the "traditional" component of the medicine of China, Mao and the Communists saw the economically pragmatic aspect of its use and accordingly adopted and fostered it as an important medical system.

The development of Chinese medicine as a system parallel to Western medicine was already under way by the time of Mao's declaration. In 1956, four colleges of Chinese medicine were created, with many more to follow. At present, *zhong yi* exists as a parallel medical system, integrating necessary biomedical elements while retaining fidelity to the traditional concepts of Chinese medicine. Educational programs emphasize acupuncture and herbal medicine and range from an undergraduate technical certificate to doctoral programs. Most independent practitioners enter the field with a 5-year medical baccalaureate degree (MB/BS) that is earned after high school (Ergil, 1994). In this system, both inpatient and outpatient medical care is delivered from large, well-equipped hospitals, as well as private clinics and pharmacies.

FUNDAMENTAL CONCEPTS

YIN AND YANG

The philosophy of Chinese medicine begins with yin and yang. These two terms can be used to express the broadest philosophical concepts as well as the most focused perceptions of the natural world. Yin and yang express the idea of opposing but complementary phenomena that exist in a state of dynamic equilibrium. The most ancient expression of this idea seems to have been that of the shady and sunny sides of a hill (Unschuld, 1985:55; Wilhelm, 1967:297). The sunlit southern side was the yang, and the shaded northern side was the yin. The contrast between the bright and dark sides of a single hill portrayed the yang and the yin, respectively. If you imagine, for a moment, the different environments that exist on either side of this one hill, you can begin to get an idea of yin and yang. On the bright, sunny side, plants and animals that enjoy light are more prevalent, the air is drier, and the rocks are warm; on the dim, shaded side, the air seems moist and cool.

Yin and yang are always present simultaneously. The paired opposites observed in the world gave tangible

---

BOX 28-1 *Origins of Yin and Yang*

> Out of Tao, One is born;
> Out of One, Two;
> Out of Two, Three;
> Out of Three, the created universe.
> The created universe carries the yin at its back and the yang in front;
> Through the union of the pervading principles it reaches harmony.
> —Lao Zi

Quoted in Lin Y: Laotse, the book of Tao. In Lin Y, editor: *The wisdom of China and India,* New York, 1942, Modern Library.

---

expression to the otherwise uncontemplatable Dao of ancient Chinese thought (Box 28-1).

The *Book of Changes,* which sought to explore the myriad manifestations of yin and yang, expressed the idea as follows: "That which lets now the dark, now the light appear is tao" (Wilhelm, 1967).

The *Yellow Emperor's Inner Classic,* the oldest text to discuss the medical application of yin and yang in a comprehensive way (Unschuld, 1985:56), states that "yin and yang are the way of heaven and earth" (Wiseman et al, 1985). This text showed how yin and yang were to be used to correlate the body and other phenomena to the human experience of health and disease.

The Inner Classic on Yin and Yang

As to the yin and yang of the human body, the outer part is yang and the inner part is yin. As to the trunk, the back is yang and the abdomen is yin. As to the organs, the viscera are yin whereas the bowels are yang. The liver, heart, spleen, lung, and kidney are yin; the gallbladder, stomach, intestines, bladder, and triple burner are yang (Wiseman et al, 1993).

It is important to note that the preceding quote is taken from the translation of an important contemporary textbook of Chinese medicine. Many ideas expressed in the *Yellow Emperor's Inner Classic* are taught and applied routinely in the contemporary clinical practice of Chinese medicine.

Yin and yang were used to express ideas about both normal physiology and pathological processes. They were applied to the organization of phenomena in many ways, for example, to organize phenomena in terms of the emergence of its dominant yin or yang character. Summer was yang within yang, fall was yin within yang, winter was yin within yin, and spring was yang within yin. Thus the coldest, darkest, and most yin period was yin within yin, whereas spring, when the yang began to emerge from the yin, was yang within yin.

There is a distinctly ecological orientation to the worldview that is supported by yin and yang; each phenomenon is seen in relation to its surroundings, and it is expected that each phenomenon will exert an influence on its

TABLE 28-1 *Yang and Yin Correspondences*

Yang	Yin
Light	Dark
Heaven	Earth
Sun	Moon
Day	Night
Spring	Autumn
Summer	Winter
Hot	Cold
Male	Female
Fast	Slow
Up	Down
Outside	Inside
Fire	Water
Wood	Metal

surroundings that is balanced by an equal but opposing influence (Table 28-1). Just as the language of ecology is the language of interrelation and interdependence, the language of Chinese medicine is a language of interrelation and interdependence. The external landscape, or human environment, is understood to be in profound and dynamic relationship with the internal landscape, or human organism. This idea becomes clearer when we explore disease causation later.

The ancient Chinese understood humans to have a nature and structure inseparable from yin and yang and, as such, inseparable from the world around them—a structure that is to be understood by the same rules that guide us in understanding the world in which we live. Life on the shaded side of a mountain has characteristics that differ from those on the sunny side. Finally, the comprehension and adjustment of life in relation to yin and yang would support life itself. Thus it was said, "To follow (the laws of) yin and yang means life; to act contrary to (the laws of yin and yang) means death" (Unschuld, 1985).

Within the traditional medical community of contemporary China, there is debate over the actual nature of yin and yang. Some exponents of a more scientific, less traditional perspective on Chinese medicine want yin and yang to be used as concepts to organize phenomena. Others, who express a less modern perspective emphatically, state that yin and yang are actually tangible phenomena (Farquhar, 1987). Although it is probably easiest to think about yin and yang as descriptive terms that help the Chinese physician organize information, it should be remembered (especially in traditional pharmaceutics) that the yin and yang constituents of the body are actual things that can be reinforced by specific substances or actions.

A useful analogy for thinking about yin and yang in this way is that of a candle. If one considers the yin aspect of the candle to be the wax and the yang aspect to be the flame, one can see how the yin nourishes and supports the yang and how the yang consumes the yin and thus burns brightly. When the wax is gone, so is the flame. Yin and yang exist in dependence on each other.

THE FIVE PHASES

Another idea that has played a significant part in the development of some aspects of Chinese medicine is that of the five phases *(wu xing)*. The five phases are earth, metal, water, wood, and fire. In Chinese, *wu* means "five" and *xing* expresses the idea of movement, "to go." For a time the *wu xing* were translated as "the five elements." This elementary translation conveyed little of the dynamism of the Chinese concept, instead focusing on the apparent similarities between the *wu xing* and the elements of ancient Greco-Roman and European Medieval medicine (see Chapters 1, 2). This equivalence is an example of the translation problem in which we use the familiar to understand the new. However useful this method may be at first, it can lead to some confusion in the long run. *Wu xing* may include the implication of material elements, but in general, the five phases refer to a set of dynamic relations occurring among phenomena that are organized in terms of the five phases. This philosophy can cover almost every aspect of phenomena, from seasons to odors (Table 28-2).

QI AND THE ESSENTIAL SUBSTANCES OF THE BODY

Apart from the ideas of yin and yang and the five phases, no concept is more crucial to Chinese medicine than *qi*—the idea that the body is pervaded by subtle material and mobile influences that cause most physiological functions and maintain the health and vitality of the individual. This idea is not typical of biomedical thinking about the body. It is not unusual to see the concept of qi translated using the term *energy,* but this translation conceals its distinctly material attributes. Furthermore, although energy is defined as the capacity of a system to do work, the character of qi extends considerably further.

The Chinese character for qi is traditionally composed of two radicals; the radical that symbolizes breath or rising vapor is placed above the radical for rice (Figure 28-2). Qi is linked with the concept of "vapors arising from food" (Unschuld, 1985). Over time this concept broadened but never lost its distinctively material aspect. Unschuld favors the use of the phrase "finest matter influences" or "influences" to translate this concept. Some phenomena labeled as qi do not fit conventional definitions of substance or matter, which further confused the issue (Wiseman et al, 1995). For this reason, many authors prefer to leave the term *qi* untranslated.

The idea of qi is extremely broad, encompassing almost every variety of natural phenomena. Many different types of qi are in the body. In general, the features that distinguish each type derive from its source, location, and function. There is considerable room for debate in this area, and exploration of a wide range of materials can suggest different ideas about categories of qi. In general, qi has the

TABLE 28-2 *Correspondence of the Five Phases*

Category	Wood	Fire	Earth	Metal	Water
Viscus	Liver	Heart	Spleen	Lungs	Kidney
Bowel	Gallbladder	Small intestine	Stomach	Large intestine	Urinary bladder
Season	Spring	Summer	Late summer	Autumn	Winter
Time of day	Before sunrise	Forenoon	Afternoon	Late afternoon	Midnight
Climate	Wind	Heat	Damp	Dryness	Cold
Direction	East	South	Center	West	North
Development	Birth	Growth	Maturity	Withdrawal	Dormancy
Color	Cyan	Red	Yellow	White	Black
Taste	Sour	Bitter	Sweet	Pungent	Salty
Sense organ	Eyes	Tongue	Mouth	Nose	Ears
Odor	Goatish	Scorched	Fragrant	Raw fish	Putrid
Vocalization	Shouting	Laughing	Singing	Weeping	Sighing
Tissue	Sinews	Vessels	Flesh	Body hair	Bones
Mind	Anger	Joy	Thought	Sorrow	Fear

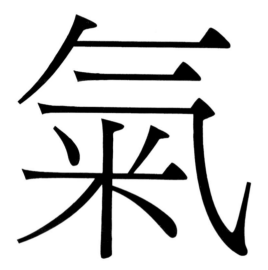

Figure 28-2 The character qi.

TABLE 28-3 *Five Types of Qi*

Type	Category	Function
Ying qi	Construction qi	Supports and nourishes the body
Wei qi	Defense qi	Protects and warms the body
Jing qi	Channel qi	Flows in the channels (felt during acupuncture)
Zang qi	Organ qi	Flows in the organs (physiological function of organs)
Zong qi	Ancestral qi	Responsible for respiration and circulation

functions of activation, warming, defense, transformation, and containment (Table 28-3).

The qi concept is important to many aspects of Chinese medicine. Organ qi and channel qi are influenced by acupuncture. In fact, one characteristic feature of acupuncture treatment is the sensation of obtaining the qi, or *de qi.* *Qigong* is a general term for the many systems of meditation, exercise, and therapeutics that are rooted in the concept of mobilizing and regulating the movement of qi in the body. Qi is sometimes compared with wind captured in a sail; we cannot observe the wind directly, but we can infer its presence as it fills the sail. In a similar fashion, the movements of the body and the movement of substances within the body are all signs of the action of qi.

In relation to qi, blood and fluids constitute the yin aspects of the body. *Blood* is produced by the construction qi, which in turn is derived from food and water. Blood nourishes the body. Blood is understood to have a slightly broader and less definite range of actions in Chinese

medicine than it does in biomedicine. Within the body, qi and blood are closely linked, because blood is considered to flow with qi and to be conveyed by it. This relationship often is expressed by the Chinese saying "Qi is the commander of blood and blood is the mother of qi," and some suggest that qi and blood are linked as a person and his or her shadow are linked.

Fluids are a general category of thin and viscous substances that serve to moisten and lubricate the body. Fluids can be conceptually separated into humor and liquid. *Humor* is thick and related to the body's organs; its functions include lubrication of the joints. *Liquid* is thin and is responsible for moistening the surface areas of the body, including the skin, eyes, and mouth.

ESSENCE AND SPIRIT

Qi, essence, and spirit make up the *three treasures* in Chinese medicine. In brief, essence is the gift of one's parents, and spirit is the gift of heaven. *Essence* is the most fundamental source of human physiological processes, the bodily reserves that support human life and that must be replenished by food and rest, and the actual reproductive substances of the body. *Spirit* is the alert and radiant aspect of human life. We encounter spirit in the luster of the eyes and face in healthy persons, as well as in their ability to think and respond appropriately to the world around them. The idea expressed by spirit, or *shen* in Chinese, encompasses consciousness and healthy mental and physical function.

The relation of the mind to the body in Chinese medicine does not include the notion of a distinct separation. It is understood that the psyche and soma interact with each other and that aspects of mental and emotional experience can have an impact on the body, and vice versa. In this sense, spirit is linked both to the health of the body and to the health of the mind. Similarly, aspects of human experience that are understood as predominantly mental in a biomedical frame of reference are linked to specific organs in Chinese medicine. For example, anger is related to the liver, obsessive thought to the spleen, and joy to the heart.

VISCERA AND BOWELS (*ZANG* AND *FU*)

The ancient Chinese understood human anatomy in ways not dissimilar from those of their European contemporaries, up to the seventeenth century. Chinese history includes cases of systematic dissection, but none of these reached the extensive explorations into the structure of the body that characterized European medicine by the fifteenth century. Instead, the Chinese medical perspective of the body, although rooted in familiar anatomical structures, represented a system in which organs serve as markers of associated physiological functions rather than actual physical structures.

The physician of Chinese medicine encounters a body in which 12 organs function. These organs are divided into the "viscera," which include six *zang* or solid organs, and the "bowels," which include six *fu* or hollow organs. These organs often are related to the physical structures that we associate with conventional biomedical anatomy. The six viscera are heart, lungs, liver, spleen, kidneys, and pericardium. The six bowels are the small intestine, large intestine, gallbladder, stomach, urinary bladder, and "triple burner" (*san jiao*). These organs have physiological functions that often are similar to those associated with them in biomedicine, but that also might be very different. The liver is said to store blood and to distribute it to the extremities as needed. The spleen is viewed as an organ of digestion. The Chinese understood the physical structure and location of most of the organs, but because systematic dissection was not extensively pursued, the close observation of physiological function was more often the basis of medical thought.

For example, circulation and elimination of fluids were observed and attributed to an organ that was said to have a name, but no form was established. This organ, the triple burner, is considered either the combined expression of the activity of other organs in the body or a group of spaces in the body. This example clearly expresses the idea that physiological function, rather than substance, establishes an organ in Chinese medicine. At the same time, the triple burner has always been surrounded by debate, because it does not have a clear anatomical structure.

The organs of viscera and bowel are paired in the yin and yang, or *interior-exterior relationship*. The heart is linked with the small intestine, the spleen with the stomach, and so on. Each viscus and each bowel has an associated channel that runs through the organ, through the organ with which it is paired, within the body, and across the body's surface, then connects with the channel of the related organ.

Historical evidence suggests that the idea of channels is more ancient than the idea of specific acupuncture points, as with the Chinese term *jingluo*, or channels (see Chapter 6). Although disagreement surrounds the location of specific points, research in the People's Republic of China recently led to the publication of a number of texts dedicated to resolving historical, philological, and anatomical questions about acupuncture points. At this time, 12 primary channels and 8 extraordinary vessels are understood to exist. The 12 channels are classically organized in terms of a sixfold yin-and-yang organizational scheme, although they can also be organized in terms of five-phase theory. Qi is understood to flow in these channels, making a rhythmical circuit.

Along the pathways of 14 of these channels (the 12 regular channels and 2 of the extraordinary channels) lie 361 specific points. In addition, a large number of "extra" points have been derived from clinical experience but are not traditionally considered part of the major channel systems. Beyond this, various individual elaborations of acupuncture theory suggest new points. There are also local microsystems of acupuncture points that have postulated numerous points on the ear, scalp, hand, foot, and other areas of the body.

Acupuncture points appear at many locations on the body. Most often they are located where a gentle and sensitive hand can detect a declivity (slope) with slight pressure on the skin surface. Points are located at the margins or bellies of muscles, between bones, and over distinctive bony features that can be detected through the skin. Methods used to locate points vary. In general, points are found by seeking anatomical landmarks, by proportionally measuring the body, and by using finger measurements; the first method is considered the most reliable. With time and clinical experience, some practitioners can be less formal in their approach to locating acupuncture points, but this topic interests even advanced practitioners. In Japan, clinicians gather regularly to hone their point location skills. In China, point location in relation to classical sources, anatomical study, and empirical evidence is an area of advanced study.

As with qi, the actual term and use of the Chinese expression that we translate as "point" is important. The character *xue*, which has been translated as "point," actually means "hole" in Chinese. A hole often is part of the clinician's subjective experience of the acupuncture point. Xue are holes in which the qi of the channels can be influenced by inserting a needle or by other means. Imagining the channel system as a vast subcutaneous waterway, with caves and springs punctuating its course as it flows to the surface, provides a concept of the holes similar to the way the Chinese thought of them for many centuries (Box 28-2).

Holes, or points along the channels, have been categorized and organized in myriad ways. One of the oldest and most well known is a system of categories based on the idea of *shu*, or transport points. This system of point categories applies exclusively to points on the forearm and lower leg, which embody the image of qi welling gently from a mountainous source at the fingertips and gradually gaining strength and depth as it reaches the seas located at the elbow and knee joints.

In reading the preceding brief discussion of the essential anatomy and physiology of Chinese medicine, it is important to remember that this anatomy forms a general reference for physiological function rather than an anatomy of direct links between discrete categories of tissue and specific physiological processes. A strength of Chinese medicine is that its theory allows for generalizations about complex physical processes, in addition to responding to signs and symptoms whose origins are obscure. Also, the distinction between mind and body is not present in Chinese medicine. Although Chinese physicians may display a disconcerting lack of interest in contemporary psychotherapy or its patients, they are quick to posit a link between affect and physiological process, in a manner that might intrigue a contemporary psychobiologist. Keeping this in mind, we can proceed to examine how illness manifests in the body.

CAUSES OF DISEASE

Ultimately, all illness results from an imbalance of yin and yang within the body manifesting as a disturbance of qi that leads to the disruption of physiological processes. Its expression as a pathological process displaying specific signs and symptoms depends on the location of the disturbance. Contemporary formal discussions on disease causation use the ideas of Chen Yen (1161–1174), who wrote *Prescriptions Elucidated on the Premise that All Pathological Symptoms Have Only Three Primary Causes (San Yin Qi Yi Bing Cheng Fang Lun)*, and an additional idea of Wu You Ke that each disease has its own qi.

The three categories of disease are organized in terms of external causes of disease, internal causes, and causes that are neither external nor internal (Wiseman et al, 1995) (Box 28-3). The first category includes six influences that are distinctly environmental: wind, cold, fire, dampness, summer heat, and dryness. When they cause disease, these six influences are known as *evils*. If the defense qi is not robust or the correct qi is not strong, or if the evil is powerful, the evil may enter the surface of the body and, under certain conditions, penetrate to the interior.

The nature of the evil and its impact on the body were understood through the observation of nature and the observation of the body in illness. The clinical meaning of the causes of disease does not lie, for the most part, in the expression of a distinct etiology, but in the manifestation of a specific set of clinical signs. In this sense, the biomedical distinction between etiology and diagnosis is somewhat blurred in Chinese medical theory.

For example, the evils of wind and cold often are implicated in the sudden onset of symptoms associated with the common cold: headache, pronounced aversion to cold, aching muscles and bones, fever, and a scratchy throat. Wind is expressed in the sudden onset of the symptoms and in their manifestation in the upper part of the body, and cold is displayed in the pronounced aversion to cold and the aching muscles and bones. Whether the patient had a specific encounter with a cold wind shortly before the onset of the symptoms is not particularly relevant. Although a patient may mention being outside on a chilly and windy day before the onset of a cold, such exposure could easily result in signs of wind heat as well; that is, a less marked aversion to cold, a distinctly sore throat, and a dry mouth. The six evils are not agents of specific etiology but agents of specific symptomatology. These ideas developed in a setting in which the possibility of investigating a bacterial or viral cause was nonexistent. Rather, careful observation of the body's response to disease provided the information necessary for treatment.

Each of the evils affects the body in a manner similar to its behavior in the environment. Images of these processes observed in nature and society were inscribed on the body to permit its processes to be readily understood. The human body stood between heaven and earth and was subject to all their influences in a relationship of continuity with its environment. Although these six evils are identified as environmental influences that attack the body's surface, it also is clearly understood they may occur within the body, causing internal disruption.

The second category of disease causation, "internal damage by the seven affects," refers to the way in which mental states can influence body processes. However, such a statement expresses a separation not implied in Chinese medicine. Each of the seven affects, or internal causes, can disturb the body if it is strongly or frequently expressed. As discussed earlier, each of the mental states—joy, anger, anxiety, thought, sorrow, fear, and fright—is related to a specific organ.

In the third category, nonexternal, noninternal causes encompass the causes of disease that do not result specifically from environmental influences or mental states. These include dietary irregularities, excessive sexual activity, taxation fatigue, trauma, and parasites. "Excessive sexual activity" suggests the possibility that too frequent emission of semen by the male can cause illness. This can occur because semen is directly related to the concept of essence, which is considered vital to the body's function and difficult to replace. This category also includes possible damage to the essence through excessive childbearing or bearing a child when the mother is too young or too old.

"Taxation fatigue" expresses the dangers of engaging in a variety of activities for a prolonged period. This category includes both the idea of overexertion and the idea of inactivity as possible causes of disease. All the concepts included within taxation fatigue reflect the essential thought of Chinese medicine that moderation is the key to health. Lying down for prolonged periods damages the qi, and prolonged standing damages the bones. From the moment that the Yellow Emperor asked Qi Bo why people now die before their time and received his answer, the images of balance, harmony, and moderation have informed Chinese medicine.

Each of the causes of disease, from prosaic causes such as dietary irregularities to exotic notions such as wind evil, disrupts the balance of yang and yin within the body and disrupts the free movement of qi. The next step is to determine the precise pattern of imbalance.

DIAGNOSTICS

Diagnostics in Chinese medicine is traditionally expressed within four categories: inspection, listening and smelling, inquiry, and palpation. The fundamental goal is to collect information that reflects the status of physiological processes, then to analyze this information to determine which impact a disorder has on that process.

The first of the four diagnostic methods, *inspection (wang)*, refers to the visual assessment of the patient, particularly the spirit, form and bearing, head and face, and substances excreted by the body. Inspection uses a large body of empirically derived information and theoretical considerations. The color, shape, markings, and coating of the tongue are inspected. For the patient attacked by wind and cold, the examiner would expect to see a moist tongue with a thin white coating, signaling the presence of cold. If heat were present, the examiner might expect a dry mouth and a red tongue. The observation of the spirit, which is considered very important in assessing the patient's prognosis, relies on assessing the overall appearance of the patient, especially the eyes, the complexion, and the quality of the patient's voice. Good spirit, even in the presence of serious illness, is thought to bode well for the patient.

The second aspect of diagnosis, *listening and smelling*, refers to listening to the quality of speech, breath, and other sounds, as well as being aware of the odors of breath, body, and excreta. As with each aspect of diagnosis, the five-phase theory can be incorporated into the assessment of the patient's condition. Each phase and each pair of viscus and bowel have a corresponding vocalization and smell.

The third aspect of diagnosis, *inquiry*, is the process of taking a comprehensive medical history. This process has been presented in many ways, but perhaps best known is the system of 10 questions described by Zhang Jie Bin in the Ming dynasty. The questions were presented as an outline of diagnostic inquiry and included querying the patient about sensations of hot and cold, perspiration, head and body, excreta, diet, chest, hearing, thirst, previous illnesses, and previous medications and their effects. For example, the examiner might expect the patient who has wind and cold symptoms to report an aversion to exposure to cold, headache, body aches, and an absence of thirst.

This step is considered critical to a good diagnosis. Although pulse diagnosis is sometimes regarded as a central feature of Chinese medicine and is rightly regarded as an art, it should not form the sole basis of a complete diagnosis, as follows:

The *Simple Questions* expresses the following idea: If, in conducting the examination, the practitioner neither inquires as to how and when the condition arose nor asks about the nature of the patient's complaint, about dietary irregularities, excesses of sleeping and waking, and poisoning, but instead proceeds immediately to take the pulse, he will not succeed in identifying the disease (Wiseman et al, 1995).

Contemporaries of Li Shi Zhen, the author of the *Pulse Studies of Bin Hu (Bin Hu Mai Xue)*, placed great emphasis on the pulse. Although considered an expert, he rejected the idea that one would place an unequal emphasis on any aspect of the diagnostic process.

Palpation (qie), the fourth diagnostic method, includes pulse examination, general palpation of the body, and palpation of the acupuncture points. *Pulse diagnosis* offers a range of approaches and can provide a remarkable amount of information about the patient's condition. The process of pulse diagnosis is carried out on the radial arteries of the left and right wrists. The patient may be seated or lying down and should be calm. The pulse is divided into three parts. The middle part is adjacent to the styloid process of

TABLE 28-4 *Pulse Positions*

| | Left | | Right | |
Position	Deep	Superficial	Deep	Superficial
Nanjing				
Inch	Heart	Small intestine	Lung	Large intestine
Bar	Liver	Gallbladder	Spleen	Stomach
Cubit	Kidney	Urinary bladder	Pericardium	Triple warmer
Contemporary Chinese Sources				
Inch	Heart		Lung	
Bar	Liver	Gallbladder	Spleen	Stomach
Cubit	Kidney	Urinary bladder	Kidney	Urinary bladder

the radius and is called the "bar" position; the "inch" is distal to it, and the "cubit" is proximal. The *inch position,* which is nearest the wrist, can indicate the status of the body above the diaphragm; the *bar position* indicates the status of the body between the diaphragm and the navel; and the *cubit position* indicates the area below the navel. Beyond this simple conceptual structure, each pulse position can be interpreted to determine the status of the organs and the channels.

Table 28-4 summarizes two models of what can be felt at each pulse position. The first chart is derived from the *Classic of Difficult Issues,* which first presented this type of pulse diagnosis in a systematic way, and the second chart shows a less elaborate, contemporary pattern. Some authors suggest that the pattern associated with the *Classic of Difficult Issues* is related more to the use of pulse diagnosis in the practice of acupuncture, whereas the later pattern is more relevant to the herbalist (Maciocia, 1989). Not all herbalists or acupuncturists make use of the pulse, but certain styles of acupuncture rely quite heavily on it. There are many possible approaches to the pulse, which makes it a rich area for the clinician and a vexing area for the biomedically oriented researcher (Birch, 1994).

The pulse allows the clinician to feel the quality of the qi and blood at different locations in the body. Table 28-5 provides a list of 29 pulse qualities and possible associations (Wiseman, 1993). Pulse qualities are organized on the basis of the size, rate, depth, force, and volume of the pulse. The overall quality of the pulse and the variations in quality at certain positions can become quite meaningful to the clinician after several years of close attention. For example, the patient afflicted with a wind cold evil might display a floating and tight pulse, signaling the presence of a cold evil on the surface of the body.

After carrying out the diagnostic process, the practitioner of Chinese medicine must make sense of the information derived. The practitioner constructs an appropriate image of the configuration of the disease so that it can be addressed by effective therapy. Central to this process is the concept of *pattern identification (bian zheng),* which involves gathering signs and symptoms through the diagnostic process and using traditional theory to understand their

impact on the fundamental substances of the body, the organs, and the channels. Many intellectual aspects of the diagnostic processes of Chinese medicine, especially when applied to the practice of herbal medicine, are as analytical as a biomedical clinical encounter. The physician must elicit signs and symptoms from the patient and then use them to understand the disruption of underlying physiological processes.

The first step of pattern identification is the localization of the disorder and the assessment of its essential nature, using the eight principles that are an expansion of yin and yang correspondences: yin, yang, cold, hot, interior, exterior, vacuity, and repletion.[a]

As with many other aspects of contemporary Chinese medicine, the *eight principles* originated in the Sung dynasty. Kou Zong Shi proposed a structure that organized disease into eight essentials: cold, hot, interior, exterior, vacuity, repletion, evil qi, and right qi (Bensky & Barolet, 1990). These were improved on in 1732, in the text *Awakening the Mind in Medical Studies (Yi Xue Xin Wu)* (Sivin, 1987). The original source was written, in the spirit of the times, to create a formal diagnostic structure for herbs that could be conceptually integrated with the ideas already in use for acupuncture. Today this formal structure is applied to both acupuncture and herbal medicine.

The patient with a wind cold evil had these symptoms: marked aversion to exposure to cold, headache, body aches, absence of thirst, a moist tongue with a thin white coating, and a floating and tight pulse. In terms of the eight principles, this would be an exterior, cold, repletion pattern. The principles of yin and yang would not directly apply.

What does this mean? The eight principles serve fundamentally to localize a condition. When Chinese physicians say that a condition is "external," they mean that it has not

---

[a]Although many authors continue to use the terms excess and deficiency to express the Chinese expressions shi and xu, I prefer Wiseman's "repletion" and "vacuity" as a translation. The use of "excess" simply is incorrect because of the existence of other Chinese terms that convey this idea exactly. "Deficiency" is problematic because it implies measurable quantity, which is not a consideration in the Chinese concept (Wiseman et al, 1990). Unschuld uses "depletion" and "repletion" instead.

TABLE 28-5 *Pulse Types*

	English	Chinese	General Association
1	Normal	*zheng chang mai*	Normal pulse
2	Floating	*fu mai*	Exterior condition
3	Deep	*chen mai*	Interior condition
4	Slow	*chi mai*	Cold and yang vacuity
5	Rapid	*shuo mai*	Heat
6	Surging	*hong mai*	Exuberant heat, hemorrhage
7	Faint	*wei mai*	Qi and blood vacuity desertion
8	Fine	*xi mai*	Blood and yin vacuity
9	Scattered	*san mai*	Dissipation of qi and blood, critical
10	Vacuous	*xu mai*	Vacuity
11	Replete	*shi mai*	Exuberant evil with right qi strong
12	Slippery	*hua mai*	Pregnancy, phlegm, abundant qi and blood
13	Rough	*se mai*	Blood stasis, vacuity of qi and blood
14	Long	*chang mai*	Often normal
15	Short	*duan mai*	Vacuity of qi and blood
16	String-like	*xian mai*	Liver disorders, severe pain
17	Hollow	*kou mai*	Blood loss
18	Tight	*jin mai*	Cold, pain
19	Moderate	*huan mai*	Slower than normal, not pathological
20	Drum skin	*ge mai*	Blood loss
21	Confined	*lao mai*	Cold, pain
22	Weak	*ruo mai*	Vacuity of qi and blood
23	Soggy	*ru mai*	Vacuity of qi and blood with dampness
24	Hidden	*fu mai*	Deep-lying internal cold
25	Stirred	*dong mai*	High fever, pregnancy
26	Rapid, irregular	*cu mai*	Debility of visceral qi or emotional distress
27	Slow, irregular	*jie mai*	Debility of visceral qi or emotional distress
28	Regularly intermittent	*dai mai*	Debility of visceral qi or emotional distress
29	Racing	*ji mai*	Heat, possible vacuity

Data from Wiseman N, Ellis A, Zmiewski P, et al: Fundamentals of Chinese medicine, Brookline, Mass, 1995, Paradigm.

yet penetrated beyond the skin and channels to the deeper parts of the body. In this case, a cold condition betrays itself through the body's expression of cold signs. To say a condition is "replete" is to say that the evil attacking the body is strong, or that the body itself is strong.

Assessment according to the eight principles is typically the first step in developing a clear pattern identification, especially if the patient has organ involvement. The eight principles are the application of a yin and yang–based theoretical structure.

A single biomedical disease entity can be associated with several Chinese diagnostic patterns (Box 28-4). For example, viral hepatitis is associated with at least six distinct diagnostic patterns, and lower urinary tract infection might be related to one of four patterns (Ergil, 1995a, 1995b). Each of these patterns would be treated in different ways, according to the saying "One disease, different treatments." The patient whose clinical pattern is wind cold has the common cold and a headache, but the same disease could manifest in other patterns.

Also, many different diseases may be captured within one pattern, thus the saying "Different diseases, one treatment." One contemporary text lists such diverse entities as

BOX 28-4 *Types of Diagnostic Patterns*

· Eight principles
· Six evils
· Qi and blood and fluids
· Five phases
· Channel patterns
· Viscera and bowels
· Triple burner
· Six channels
· Four levels

nephritis, dysfunctional uterine bleeding, pyelonephritis, and rheumatic heart disease under the diagnostic pattern of "disharmony between the heart and kidney" (Huang et al, 1993:79).

This comparatively precise diagnostic linkage begins to be broadly appreciated in the historical trends of the Sung, Jin, and Yuan dynasties. The six-channel pattern identification proposed by Zhang Zhong Jing is one of many patterns currently used. The patient who has encountered a wind cold evil would, under Zhang Jong Jing's system, be categorized as having *tai yang* disease. There is considerable room for overlap within the available methods of pattern identification.

THERAPEUTIC CONCEPTS

Once a diagnosis has been determined and, when relevant, a pattern has been differentiated, therapy begins. Therapeutics in Chinese medicine is fundamentally allopathic; that is, it addresses the pathological condition with opposing measures, as follows:

> Cold is treated with heat, heat is treated with cold, vacuity is treated by supplementation, and repletion is treated by drainage (*Inner Classic* in Wiseman et al, 1985).

Within the realm of acupuncture, moxibustion, and herbal medicine, three fundamental principles of therapy are understood: (1) treating disease from its root; (2) eliminating evil influences and supporting the right; and (3) restoring the balance of yin and yang. These refer to approaches that are appropriate to the patient's condition. It would be appropriate to eliminate the cold evil and support the right qi of the patient with a wind cold pattern. In a patient with symptoms that reflect a complex underlying pattern, the physician might attempt to treat the root of the patient's condition. For example, functional uterine bleeding caused by a disharmony of the heart and kidney would be addressed primarily by harmonizing the heart and kidney; treating the root of the condition would adjust its symptoms. Treatment methods vary widely; Box 28-5 provides the simplest expression of their organization.

THERAPEUTIC METHODS

This section introduces the therapeutic methods of acupuncture and moxibustion (see Chapter 29), and discusses cupping and bleeding, Chinese massage, qi cultivation, Chinese herbal medicine, and dietetics.

ACUPUNCTURE AND MOXIBUSTION

Although acupuncture and moxibustion can be used independently, they are so deeply interrelated in Chinese medicine that the term for this therapy is *zhen jiu*, meaning "needle moxibustion." To capture the distinctively com-

posite character of this phrase, some authors translate the expression as "acumoxa therapy." This close linkage is based on the ancient origins of these methods, and moxibustion apparently was the form of therapy first applied to the channels and holes to treat problems on or within the body. Both acupuncture and moxibustion are used to provide a discrete stimulus to points that lie along channel pathways or to other appropriate sites.

Points may be chosen on the basis of the actual trajectory of the channel on which the points lie. For example, *Union Valley* is considered an important point for the head and face because it lies on the pathway of the large intestine channel, which traverses that area of the body. Similarly, points on the lower extremity that lie on the urinary bladder channel, which traverses the entire back, often are used for treatment of back pain (Figure 28-3).

Points also are often selected entirely on the basis of their sensitivity to palpation or based on a variation in texture perceived by the practitioner. Often a number of

BOX 28-5 *Methods of Treatment*

- Diaphoresis
- Clearing
- Ejection
- Precipitation
- Harmonization
- Warming
- Supplementation
- Dispersion
- Orifice opening
- Securing astriction
- Settling and absorption

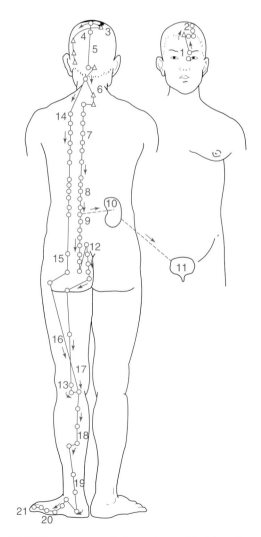

Figure 28-3 The course of the urinary bladder channel of the foot tai yang. (Modified from Qiu ML: Chinese acupuncture and moxibustion, Edinburgh, 1993, Churchill Livingstone, p 103.)

suitable acupuncture points in a specific area may be assessed to determine which would be most suitable for needling. In some cases, points that do not lie on specific channels or form part of the collection of recognized extra points can be identified by their tenderness. These points are known as *ah shi*, or "Ouch, that's it," points and are an important part of clinical acupuncture's traditional history and contemporary practice.

With many acupuncture points from which to choose, and multiple methods on which to base that choice, it is not surprising that many clinicians focus on a few specific methods or a particular collection of points. Some clinicians restrict their approach so that they can focus on adjusting the application of treatment.

A detailed discussion of acupuncture as a therapeutic method can be found in Chapter 29.

Moxibustion *(Jiu Fa)*

Moxibustion *(jiu)* refers to the burning of the dried and powdered leaves of *Artemisia vulgaris (ai ye),* either on or in proximity to the skin, to affect the movement of qi in the channel, locally or at a distance. *A. vulgaris* is said to be acrid and bitter and, when used as moxa, to have the ability to warm and enter the channels. References to moxa appear in early materials, such as the texts recovered from the excavated tombs at Ma Wang Dui (Unschuld, 1985). These texts discuss a number of therapeutic methods, including moxibustion, but do not mention acupuncture. The *Treatise on Moxibustion of the Eleven Vessels of Yin and Yang (Yin Yang Shi Yi Mai Jiu Jing)* describes the application of moxa to treat illness by performing moxibustion on the channels (Auteroche et al, 1992).

Moxibustion can be applied to the body in many ways: directly, indirectly, using the pole method, and using the warm needle method. *Direct moxibustion* involves burning a small amount of moxa, about the size of a grain of rice, directly on the skin. Depending on the desired effect, larger or smaller pieces of moxa can be used, and the moxa fluff can be allowed to burn directly to the skin, causing a blister or a scar, or it can be removed before it has burnt down to the skin. Such techniques are used to stimulate acupuncture points in cases in which the action of moxibustion is traditionally indicated or in which warming the point seems to be the most appropriate response. Older texts described the use of direct moxibustion on Leg Three Li and other acupuncture points as a method of health maintenance and prevention.

Indirect moxibustion involves the insertion of a mediating substance between the moxa fluff and the patient's skin. This gives the practitioner greater control over the amount of heat applied to the patient's body and offers the patient increased protection from burning, which allows for the treatment of delicate areas such as the face and back. Popular substances include ginger slices, garlic slices, and salt. The mediating substance is often chosen on the basis of its own medicinal properties and the way these combine with the properties of moxa. Ginger might be selected in patients with vacuity cold, whereas garlic is considered useful for treating hot and toxic conditions. Figure 28-4 shows a patient being treated for facial paralysis with indirect moxibustion using ginger slices.

During *pole moxibustion* a cigar-shaped roll of moxa wrapped in paper is used to warm the acupuncture points gently without touching the skin. This is a safe method

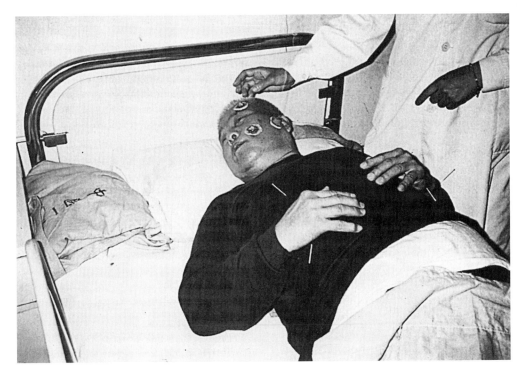

Figure 28-4 Patient receiving indirect moxa. (Courtesy Wind Horse, Marnae Ergil.)

of moxibustion that can be taught to patients for self-application.

The *warm needle method* is accomplished by first inserting an acupuncture needle into the point and then placing moxa fluff on its handle. After the moxa is ignited, it burns gradually, imparting a sensation of gentle warmth to the acupuncture point and channel. This method is especially useful for patients with arthritic joint pain.

Combined Therapy with Acupuncture

Together, moxibustion and acupuncture are used to treat, or at least ameliorate, a wide range of conditions and symptoms. On the basis of the simple premise that all disease involves the disruption of the flow of qi and that acupuncture and moxibustion regulate the movement of qi, all disease theoretically can benefit from these methods. A brief review of acupuncture texts provides ample evidence of the range of conditions for which acupuncture is considered appropriate. Over the years, efforts have been made outside of China to parse the range of conditions treatable by acupuncture, including that by a World Health Organization (WHO) interregional seminar in the late 1970s (Bannerman, 1979). More recently, the WHO established selection criteria for evaluating reports of controlled clinical trials of acupuncture as a basis for reporting on the use of acupuncture in the treatment of various diseases and disorders; Boxes 28-6 and 28-7 list partial results (World Health Organization, 2002). Although these lists

are comparatively short compared with the disorders enumerated in a clinical manual or acupuncture textbook, they are informative in terms of the routine application of acupuncture in China and elsewhere. It is also instructive to compare these two lists with the report of the National

BOX 28-7 *Diseases and Disorders for Which Acupuncture Shows Therapeutic Effects*[a]

Abdominal pain (in acute gastroenteritis or due to gastrointestinal spasm)	Neurodermatitis
Acne vulgaris	Obesity
Alcohol dependence and detoxification	Opium, cocaine, and heroin dependence
Bell palsy	Osteoarthritis
Bronchial asthma	Pain due to endoscopic examination
Cancer pain	Pain in thromboangiitis obliterans
Cardiac neurosis	Polycystic ovary syndrome (Stein-Leventhal syndrome)
Cholecystitis, chronic, with acute exacerbation	Postextubation in children
Cholelithiasis	Postoperative convalescence
Competition stress syndrome	Premenstrual syndrome
Craniocerebral injury, closed	Prostatitis, chronic
Diabetes mellitus, noninsulin dependent	Pruritus
Ear ache	Radicular and pseudoradicular pain syndrome
Epidemic hemorrhagic fever	Raynaud syndrome, primary
Epistaxis, simple (without generalized or local disease)	Recurrent lower urinary tract infection
Eye pain due to subconjunctival injection	Reflex sympathetic dystrophy
Facial spasm	Retention of urine, traumatic
Female infertility	Schizophrenia
Female urethral syndrome	Sialism, drug induced
Fibromyalgia and fasciitis	Sjögren syndrome
Gastrokinetic disturbance	Sore throat (including tonsillitis)
Gouty arthritis	Spine pain, acute
Hepatitis B virus carrier status	Stiff neck
Herpes zoster (human [alpha] herpes virus 3)	Temporomandibular joint dysfunction
Hyperlipemia	Tietze syndrome
Hypo-ovarianism	Tobacco dependence
Insomnia	Tourette syndrome
Labor pain	Ulcerative colitis, chronic
Lactation deficiency	Urolithiasis
Male sexual dysfunction, nonorganic	Vascular dementia
Ménière disease	Whooping cough (pertussis)
Neuralgia, postherpetic	

[a]Diseases, symptoms, or conditions for which the therapeutic effect of acupuncture has been shown but for which further proof of its effect is needed.

BOX 28-6 *Diseases and Disorders Effectively Treated with Acupuncture*[a]

Adverse reactions to radiotherapy and/or chemotherapy	Induction of labor
Allergic rhinitis (including hay fever)	Knee pain
	Leukopenia
Biliary colic	Low back pain
Depression (including depressive neurosis and depression following stroke)	Malposition of fetus, correction of
	Morning sickness
	Nausea and vomiting
Dysentery, acute bacillary	Neck pain
Dysmenorrhea, primary	Pain in dentistry (including dental pain and temporomandibular dysfunction)
Epigastralgia, acute (in peptic ulcer, acute and chronic gastritis, and gastrospasm)	
	Periarthritis of shoulder
Facial pain (including craniomandibular disorders)	Postoperative pain
	Renal colic
	Rheumatoid arthritis
Headache	Sciatica
Hypertension, essential	Sprain
	Stroke
Hypotension, primary	Tennis elbow

[a]Diseases, symptoms, or conditions for which acupuncture has been proved—through controlled trials—to be an effective treatment.

Institutes of Health (1997) Consensus Conference discussed later.

For further discussion of acupuncture and the adjunctive use of moxibustion, see Chapter 29.

CUPPING AND BLEEDING

Two methods important to the practice of Chinese medicine are cupping and bleeding. These may be used separately or together and are often used with other methods, such as moxibustion and acupuncture. *Cupping* involves inducing a vacuum in a small glass or bamboo cup and promptly applying it to the skin surface. This therapy brings blood and lymph to the skin surface under the cup, which increases local circulation. Cupping is often used to drain or remove cold and damp evils from the body or to assist blood circulation. *Bleeding* is done to drain a channel or to remove heat from the body at a specific location. Unlike the bloodletting practiced by Western physicians throughout the nineteenth century, this method expresses comparatively small amounts of blood, from a drop to a few centiliters. Figure 28-5 shows a patient receiving cupping and bleeding at an acupuncture point on the urinary bladder channel associated with the lungs.

CHINESE MASSAGE (*TUI NA*)

Literally "pushing and pulling," *tui na* refers to a system of massage, manual acupuncture point stimulation, and manipulation that is vast enough to warrant its own chapter. These methods have been practiced at least as long as moxibustion, but the first modern massage training class was instituted in Shanghai in 1956 (Wang et al, 1990:16). At present, this field of study can serve as a minor component of a traditional medical education or an area of extensive clinical specialization (see Chapter 17).

A distinct aspect of tui na is the extensive training of the hands necessary for clinical practice. The practitioner's hands are trained to accomplish focused and forceful movements that can be applied to various areas of the body. Techniques such as pushing, rolling, kneading, rubbing, and grasping are practiced repetitively until they become second nature (Figure 28-6). Students practice on a small bag of rice until their hands develop the necessary strength and dexterity.

Tui na often is applied to limited areas of the body, and the techniques can be quite forceful and intense. Tui na is applied routinely for orthopedic and neurological

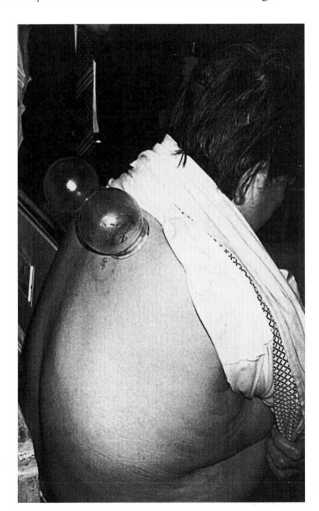

Figure 28-5 Cupping and bleeding. (Courtesy Wind Horse, Marnae Ergil.)

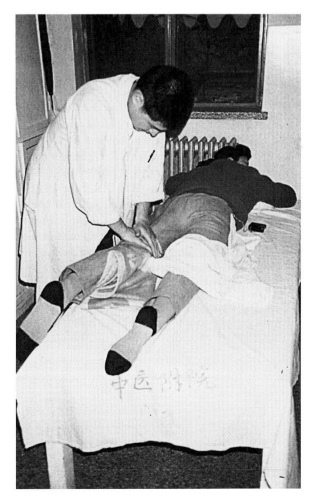

Figure 28-6 Tui na in clinical practice. (Courtesy Wind Horse, Marnae Ergil.)

conditions. It also is applied for conditions not usually viewed as susceptible to treatment through manipulation, such as asthma, dysmenorrhea, and chronic gastritis. Tui na is used as an adjunct to acupuncture to increase the range of motion of a joint or instead of acupuncture when needles are uncomfortable or inappropriate, such as in pediatric applications.

As with all aspects of Chinese medicine, regional styles and family lineages of massage practice abound. The formal tui na curriculum available in Chinese programs is extensive, but probably not a complete expression of the range of possibilities.

Qi Cultivation (Qigong)

Qigong is a term that literally embraces almost every aspect of the manipulation of qi by means of exercise, breathing, and the influence of the mind. Qigong includes practices ranging from the meditative systems of Daoist and Buddhist practitioners to the martial arts traditions of China. Qigong is relevant to medicine in three specific areas. First, it allows the practitioner to cultivate demeanor and stamina to perform the strenuous activities of tui na, to sustain the constant demands of clinical practice, and to quiet the mind to facilitate diagnostic perception. Second, qigong cultivates the practitioner's ability to transmit qi safely to the patient. Practitioners may direct qi to the patient either through the needles or directly through their hands. This activity may be the main focus of treatment or an adjunctive aspect, in which case the qi paradigm is expanded to include direct interaction between the patient's qi and the clinician's qi. Third, the patient may be taught to engage in specific qigong practices that are useful for the amelioration of the patient's illness.

Qi cultivation makes extensive use of the principles of traditional Chinese medicine, and its history is intertwined with that of famous physicians. The history of qi cultivation practices is considered to extend back into antiquity and to indicate the early recognition of the importance of exercise to the health of the body. In Lu's *Spring and Autumn Annals,* the following famous aphorism relates the importance of movement to the maintenance of health and function (Engelhardt 1989):

> Flowing water will never turn stale, the hinge of the door will never be eaten by worms. They never rest in their activity: that's why.

In this text, Lu described the role of dance and movement in correcting the movement of qi and yin within the body and benefiting the muscles (Zhang, 1990).

Descriptions of qi cultivation practices and exercises are attributed to the early Daoist masters. Zhuang Zi, writing in the fourth century BC, reveals the role of breathing and physical exercise in promoting longevity and describes a sage intent on extending his life (Despeux, 1989), as follows:

> To pant, to puff, to hail, to sip, to spit out the old breath and draw in the new, practicing bear hangings and bird-stretches, longevity his only concern. (Watson, 1968)

Among the texts recovered at Ma Huang Dui are a series of illustrated guides to the practice of conduction (*dao yin*) that provide guidance to the physical postures and therapeutic properties of this form of qi cultivation (Despeux, 1989:226).

The famous physician of second-century China, Hua Tuo, is credited with the creation of a series of exercises. These were based on the movements of the tiger, the deer, the bear, the monkey, and a bird and were to be practiced to ward off disease.

Zhang Zhong Jing, in his *Essential Prescription of the Golden Cabinet,* recommended the practices of dao yin or conduction and tui na or exhalation and inhalation to treat disease.

A wide variety of forms of qi cultivation were developed over the centuries, and many have achieved great popularity. Since the 1950s, qigong training programs have been implemented and sanatoria built, specializing in the therapeutic application of qigong to the treatment of disease.

Fundamental Concepts

Qi cultivation rests on several fundamental principles intended to support activity to enhance the movement of qi and to increase health. Most discussions of qi cultivation address the relaxation of the body, the regulation or control of breathing, and the calming of the mind. Qi cultivation generally is performed in a relaxed standing, sitting, or lying posture. Once the correct position is achieved, the practitioner begins to regulate breathing in concert with specific mental and physical exercises.

For example, one form of qigong involves the action of visualizing the internal and external pathways of the channels and imagining the movement of the qi along these channels in concert with the breath. As the practice develops, the practitioner begins to experience the sensation of qi traveling along the channel pathways. Traditionally, it is considered that the mind guides the qi to a specific area of the body and that the qi then guides the blood there as well, which improves circulation in the area. From this point of view, this particular exercise trains the qi and blood to move freely along the channel pathways, which leads to good health.

Another exercise involves the use of breath, visualization, and simple physical exercises to benefit the qi of the lungs. This therapeutic exercise is recommended for bronchitis, emphysema, and bronchial asthma. It is begun by assuming a relaxed posture, whether sitting, lying, or standing. The exercise is begun by breathing naturally and allowing the mind to become calm. The upper and lower teeth are then clicked together by closing the mouth gently 36 times. As saliva is produced, it is retained in the mouth, swirled with the tongue, and then swallowed in three parts while one imagines that it is flowing into the middle of the chest and then to an area about three finger-breadths below the navel (the *dan tian,* or cinnabar field). At this point, one imagines that one is sitting in front of a reservoir of white qi that enters the mouth on inhalation and is transmitted through the body as one exhales, first to the lungs, then to the dan tian, and finally out to the skin and body hair. This process of visualization is repeated 18 times.

This process makes use of the relationship between the mind and qi to strengthen the function of the lungs and to pattern regions of the body associated with the area where the qi governing the lungs and respiration is stored. This area is associated with the acupuncture point *dan zhong,* or chest center (Ren 17), which is located in the middle of the chest. Next, the qi is directed to the cinnabar field, which is associated with another location on the ren channel *qi hai,* or sea of qi (Ren 6), just below the umbilicus. This area is considered to be important to the production and storage of the body's qi and to the lungs on exhalation.

This exercise typifies the three aspects of a qigong exercise described previously: relaxation, mental tranquility, and breath control. It induces relaxation through mental concentration, because the exercise of focusing on breathing and the visualized process help remove distracting thoughts from the mind, and the patterning of the breath with visualization controls and regulates the breathing.

It should be stressed that although many forms of qigong exist, they share general principles of application and a relationship to Chinese medicine concepts.

CHINESE HERBAL MEDICINE (ZHONG YAO)

Since the legendary emperor Shen Nong tasted herbs and guided the Chinese people in herbal use, diet, and therapeutics, herbal medicine has been an integral part of Chinese culture and medical practice. The traditional Chinese materia medica includes much more than herbs; minerals and animal parts are listed as well. The number of substances currently identified is 5767, as recorded in the *Encyclopedia of Traditional Chinese Medicinal Substances (Zhong Yao Da Ci Dian)* published in 1977 by the Jiangsu College of New Medicine (Bensky & Gamble, 1986). This publication is the latest in a long line of definitive discussions of materia medica that have been produced in China over the millennia. The earliest known is the *Divine Husbandman's Classic of the Materia Medica,* reconstructed by Tao Hong Jing (AD 452-536). This text classified herbs into upper, middle, and lower grades and discussed the tastes, temperatures, toxicities, and medicinal properties of 364 substances.

Currently, substances are categorized systematically as expansions of the eight methods of therapy discussed earlier (Box 28-8). Subcategories exist within the basic categories into which substances are organized. Prescribing rules take into account the compatibilities and incompatibilities of substances, the traditional pairings of substances, and their combination for treatment of specific symptoms.

Both the Ma Wang Dui texts and the *Inner Classic* provide recommendations for the therapeutic combination of substances. Zhang Zhong Jing's work in systematizing herbal prescriptions as therapeutic approaches for specific diagnostic patterns based on yin and yang corre-

BOX 28-8 *Fundamental Categories of Chinese Materia Medica*

- Exterior resolving
- Heat clearing
- Ejection producing
- Precipitant
- Wind dispelling
- Water disinhibiting dampness percolating
- Interior warming
- Qi rectifying
- Food dispersing
- Worm expelling
- Blood rectifying
- Phlegm transforming, cough suppressing, panting-calming
- Spirit quieting
- Liver calming, wind extinguishing
- Orifice opening
- Supplementing
- Securing and astringing
- External use

BOX 28-9 *Fundamental Categories for Chinese Herbal Medicine*

- Exterior resolving
- Heat clearing
- Ejection producing
- Precipitant
- Harmonizing
- Dampness dispelling
- Interior warming
- Qi rectifying
- Dispersing
- Blood rectifying
- Phlegm transforming, cough suppressing, panting-calming
- Spirit quieting
- Tetany settling
- Orifice opening
- Supplementing
- Securing and astringing
- Oral formulas for sores
- External use

spondences was unusual for its time. It was not until physicians of the Sung dynasty became interested in relating herbal practice to a systematic theory and organizing diagnostics accordingly that interest was renewed in *On Cold Damage.* This book remains a significant resource for the current practitioner of Chinese herbal medicine. One of the most comprehensive English-language compilations of Chinese herbal prescriptions derives approximately 20% of its formulas from this source (Bensky & Barolet, 1990).

Not all herbal prescriptions or texts discussing application followed the lead of Zhang Zhong Jing. Many texts offered herbs or prescriptions for specific symptoms without reference to distinct theoretical structures or diagnostic principles. The general population probably applied herbs in exactly this manner. Even today, although the prescription of herbal formulas is primarily driven by traditional diagnostic theory and pattern diagnosis, extensive compilations of empirically derived herbal formulas with symptomatic indications are published.

Contemporary compilations of formulas follow an organization similar to that used for substances. The result is that both substances and formulas are organized in a manner that makes them accessible in terms of traditional theories (Box 28-9).

Let us examine the formula and its constituent substances that might be provided to our patient who has encountered a wind cold evil or who, in the pattern identification system described in *On Cold Damage,* would be said to have a "tai yang stage pattern." In either case, Ephedra Decoction *(ma huang tang)* would be an appropriate choice, particularly if the patient had a slight cough as well. The constituents and dosage of the formula are 9 g of ephedra *(ma huang),* 6 g of cinnamon twig *(gui zhi),* 9 g of apricot kernel *(xing ren),* and 3 g of licorice *(gan cao).* These ingredients are cooked together in water to make a slightly concentrated tea, which is drunk in successive doses. The tea is taken warm to induce sweating, a sign that the qi of the surface of the body that had been impeded by the cold evil is free to move and throw off the evil. The patient stops drinking the tea once sweat arrives.

A traditional system of organizing a formula is to identify ingredients as the ruler, minister, adjutant, and emissary. In this case the *ruler* of the formula is ephedra. The ruler sets the therapeutic direction of the formula. Acrid and warm, ephedra promotes sweating, dispels cold, and resolves the surface. (We examine ephedra again in the discussion of herbal research.) Cinnamon twig is the *minister,* working to assist the ruler in carrying out its objectives. As with ephedra, it too is said to warm the body. Apricot kernel is the *adjutant,* so it addresses the possible involvement of the lung and moderates the acrid flavor of the other two substances. Because the lung is the organ most immediately affected by wind cold or wind heat, the formula addresses the organ. Finally, licorice is the *emissary,* serving both to render the action of the other herbs harmonious and to distribute this action through the body.

The previous example is brief and simple but illustrates fundamental concepts. Chinese herbal therapeutics can be complex. Its practice is broad, and the range of conditions addressed is more extensive than with acupuncture. In terms of complexity and the diagnostic acumen required of the practitioner, it resembles the practice of internal medicine. Herbal therapy also encompasses the external applications of herbs and a variety of methods of preparation. Besides being prepared as the traditional water decoction, or tea, substances may be powdered or rendered into pills, pastes, or tinctures.

DIETETICS

Traditional dietetics encompasses the practice of herbal therapy but also addresses traditional Chinese foods in terms of the theoretical constructs of Chinese medicine. Five-phase theory has been applied to foods since the time of the *Inner Classic.* It is not unusual to see a classroom in a college of Chinese medicine equipped as a kitchen. In larger cities, special restaurants prepare meals with specific medicinal purposes. The practices of this field are deeply rooted in the cultural practices of China and cultural beliefs about diet. Many of the foods organized for use in therapy also are routinely prepared by families to promote health when the seasons change and when illness strikes, as well as to strengthen a woman after birth, to cause milk to fill the breasts of a new mother, or to nourish elderly persons in their declining years (see Chapter 26).

EAST ASIA: CHINESE MEDICINE "OVERSEAS"

China's traditional medicine is practiced in various forms all over the world. Sometimes its practice follows the contemporary patterns of *traditional Chinese medicine (zhong yi).* Sometimes its practice is deeply informed by local custom, preference, or regional elaborations.

CHINESE MEDICINE IN KOREA

A close relationship exists between China and Korea. Chinese medicine arrived in Korea during the Qin dynasty (221–207 BC). However, the textual basis of Korean medicine in the literary tradition of Chinese medicine seems to have been established during the Han and Tang dynasties (Hsu & Peacher, 1977), during a period of political domination by the Chinese. The closeness between China and Korea during the Kingdom of Silla (AD 400–700) facilitated this exchange of ideas. Formal medical instruction by government-appointed physicians began in AD 693. Texts such as the *Systematic Classic of Acupuncture (and Moxibustion)* were important to the development of the tradition. With the formation of the Liao dynasty (AD 907–1168), Korea established its independence from Chinese rule, but cultural and medical exchange continued. During the Li dynasty (1392–1910), many texts, including the *Illustrated Classic of Acupuncture Points as Found on the Bronze Model,* reached Korea (Chuang, 1982). Widely used techniques of acupuncture point selection based on five-phase theory have emerged from Korea, including those of the Buddhist priest Sa-am (1544–1610).

Korean Oriental Medicine (KOM) is the expression used to describe the South Korean approach to and adaptation of Chinese medicine. During the occupation of Korea by Japan (1910–1945), the Japanese government, following the Westernizing trends established during the Meiji Restoration, deprived KOM practitioners of practice rights and precipitated a decline in the tradition (Lee & Bae, 2008:18). The tradition revived in post-war Korea with KOM coming to be covered under the National Medical Insurance program in 1987 (Lee & Bae, 2008).

At least two comparatively recent innovations based on Chinese medicine have been developed in Korea and have become well known in other parts of the world. Korean *constitutional diagnosis* was developed initially by Jhema Lee (1836–1900) and based a system of herbal therapeutics on a system of diagnostic patterning that used the four divisions of yin and yang. In 1965, Dowon Kuan expanded the system to an eightfold classification and applied it to acupuncture (Hirsch, 1985). *Koryo sooji chim,* the system of Korean *hand and finger acupuncture,* was developed by Yoo Tae Woo and published in 1971. The system maps the channel pathways and acupuncture points of the entire body onto the hands, where they are stimulated using very short, fine needles and magnets. This system has gained a significant level of international exposure.

The continued development of KOM in South Korea has produced eleven KOM colleges variously offering masters or doctoral degrees, and a substantial expansion of research and publication on topics in KOM.

CHINESE MEDICINE IN JAPAN

The history of cultural exchange between China and Japan dates to at least AD 57. Kon Mu was the first physician to go to Japan and use Chinese methods; he was sent in AD 414 by the king of Silla, in southeast Korea, to treat the emperor Inkyo Tenno. This interaction continued; in 552, a Korean delegation brought a selection of Chinese medical texts to Japan (Bowers, 1970). In 562, Zhi Cong came from southern China with more than 100 books on the practice of Chinese medicine (Huard et al, 1968), including the *Systematic Classic of Acupuncture (and Moxibustion)* (Chuang, 1982). By the early eighth century, the influence of Chinese medicine was well established. With the adoption of the Taiho code in 702, provision was made for a ministry of health composed of specialists, physicians, students, and researchers (Lock, 1980). In 754, a Buddhist priest, Chien Chen, brought many medical texts from China to Japan. His influence was memorialized in a shrine in Nishinokyo (Chuang, 1982).

Chinese influences on Japanese medicine were derived primarily from the *Classic of Difficult Issues* and *Systematic Classic of Acupuncture (and Moxibustion)*. A revisionist movement in the late seventeenth century established *On Cold Damage (Shokanron)* as the core text of herbal medicine, or *kanpo* (Chinese method), in Japan (Lock, 1980).

Several factors have influenced the development of Chinese medicine in Japan, giving it a somewhat unique appearance. The scarcity of ingredients for the preparation of Chinese herbal formulas led to an emphasis on lower dosages in herbal prescriptions than are typical in China. An emphasis on palpatory diagnosis involving channel pathways and the abdomen also became well established. The use of finer-gauge needles and shallow insertion became typical of some styles of Japanese acupuncture.

In the mid-seventeenth century, Waichi Sugiyama, a blind man, began to train the blind in acupuncture using very fine needles and guide tubes. Because it had become customary in the earlier part of the Edo period for blind persons to do massage, both massage and acupuncture then became associated with blind practitioners (see Chapter 17). This association contributed to a lower social position for acupuncture practitioners and to specialization in medical practice. Kanpo physicians became primarily practitioners of herbal medicine (Lock, 1980).

This trend toward specialization has continued to the present, with the division of acupuncture, moxibustion, and massage into separately licensed practices (although many individuals hold all three licenses) and the actual practice of herbal medicine being retained in the hands of medical physicians. Interestingly, many Chinese herbal prescriptions are recognized as appropriate therapy for certain medical conditions according to regulations governing health care in Japan.

Japan has seen both focused specialization in and the innovative exploration and expansion of traditional acupuncture. The *Classic of Difficult Issues* often has been the focus for movements to revive the practices of traditional acupuncture. Its influence has contributed heavily to the comparatively recent development of groups of acupuncturists advocating *meridian therapy (keiraku chiryo)* based on the application of concepts in the *Classic of Difficult Issues* and their subsequent interpretation by later Chinese authors. A distinctive feature of meridian therapy is the application of five-phase theory to the transport points, a practice that has influenced the perception and adoption of five-phase theory by European practitioners (Kaptchuk, 1983).

The pioneering work of Yoshio Manaka (Manaka & Itaya, 1994) also has contributed dramatically to the practice of acupuncture. Manaka, a physician who experimented with acupuncture principles when medical supplies were lacking during World War II, became convinced of the efficacy and physiological relevance of traditional theories and continued to experiment and develop them throughout his life.

Japanese acupuncture practitioners have a broad range of practices and interests. Although some are particular partisans of specific schools of thought, including some based on contemporary Chinese medicine perspectives, many practitioners have adopted a comparatively eclectic approach.

CHINESE MEDICINE IN EUROPE

The history of Chinese medicine in Europe, particularly acupuncture, is both long-standing and broadly developed. The medical use of acupuncture in Europe dates from the middle of the sixteenth century (Peacher, 1975). The work of Willem Ten Rhyne (1647–1690) in this area culminated in the publication in 1683 of *Dissertatio de Arthritide: Mantissa Schematica: de Acupunctura: et Orationes Tres,* based on information gathered during his service in Japan as a physician for the Dutch East India Company. The German physician Kampfer, who also traveled with the Dutch East India Company and spent time in Japan, contributed his observations.

In France the Jesuit Du Halde published a text in 1735 that included a detailed discussion of Chinese medicine (Hsu, 1989). Soulié de Morant's publication of *L'Acupuncture Chinoise* was an extensive discussion of the practice of acupuncture based on direct translation, observation, and actual practice by the author. Published in 1939, the text was rooted in Soulié de Morant's exposure to the medicine of China in that country from 1901 to 1917.

England saw the publication of J.M. Churchill's *A Description of Surgical Operations Peculiar to Japanese and*

Chinese in 1825. Among early notable English acupuncturists were Drs. Felix Mann and Sidney Rose-Neil, both of whom began their explorations of acupuncture in the late 1950s and have influenced its development substantially in English-speaking countries. J.R. Worsley, a physical therapist, began his studies of acupuncture in 1962 and had a substantial impact on the perceptions of many English and U.S. practitioners. He visited Hong Kong and Taiwan for a brief period and then became a part of the study group established by Rose-Neil (Hsu & Peacher, 1977). Worsley went on to create the British College of Traditional Chinese Acupuncture and two U.S. schools.

CHINESE MEDICINE IN THE UNITED STATES

In 1826, Bache (Benjamin Franklin's great grandson) became one of the first American physicians to use acupuncture in his practice (Haller, 1973). Ten Rhyne's text was a part of Sir William Osler's library (Peacher, 1975), and in his *Principles and Practice of Medicine,* Osler prescribes acupuncture for lumbago (Osler, 1913).

Although only occasionally explored by the conventional U.S. medical community, the traditional medicine of China has been practiced in the United States since the middle of the nineteenth century. Herbal merchants, entrepreneurs, and physicians accompanied the Chinese who sold their labor in the United States. The practice of the China doctor of the town John Day, Oregon, named Doc Ing Hay, is one of the most famous (Barlow & Richardson, 1979). Ah Fong Chuck, who came to the United States in 1866, became the first licensed practitioner of traditional Chinese medicine in the United States in 1901, when he successfully won a medical license through legal action in Idaho (Muench, 1984). With the strengthening of medical practice acts throughout the United States, the interruption of the herb supply from China, and the advent of World War II, these practices disappeared or retreated into Chinatowns nationwide.

Substantial attention was focused on acupuncture, the traditional medicine of China, and its regional variants, as a result of James Reston's highly publicized appendectomy and postoperative care in 1971 and the subsequent opening of China by President Nixon. As a result, medical practices largely confined to Asia and the Chinatowns of America gained visibility throughout the United States. Increased visibility led to substantial public interest in acupuncture and gradually to licensure and the development of training programs in many states. Currently, 45 states (including the District of Columbia) license, certify, or register the practice of acupuncture and a range of other activities, including the practice of herbal medicine, by nonphysicians. More than 69 U.S. programs offer training in acupuncture and Oriental medicine.

Americans have a clear interest in the available range of expressions of Chinese medical tradition. In the United States, European interpretations of the application of five-phase theory, Korean constitutional acupuncture, traditional Chinese medicine (acupuncture, herbs, qigong, tui na), Japanese meridian therapy, and the approaches of special family lineages within the Chinese tradition all are taught and practiced. This willingness to accept and explore the traditional and contemporary interpretations of traditional Chinese medicine has led to the emergence of the concept of "Oriental medicine" as an umbrella term for the global domain of practice in this area.

The extent to which the practice of Chinese medicine has come to be viewed as an established therapeutic practice in the United States was recently illustrated by a regulatory action taken by the U.S. Food and Drug Administration (FDA). After a series of reports of adverse events surrounding the use of ephedra-containing supplements in support of weight loss regimens and athletic training, neither of which can be considered to constitute the practice of Chinese medicine, the FDA was compelled to act. In February 2004, the FDA issued a final rule prohibiting the sale of dietary supplements containing ephedrine alkaloids (ephedra), "because such supplements present an unreasonable risk of illness or injury" (U.S. Food and Drug Administration, 2004). Intriguingly, it was specifically stated that the "scope of the rule does not pertain to traditional Chinese herbal remedies." Although the logistics of honoring this exemption remain complicated, it is a definite acknowledgment of the professional practice of Chinese herbal medicine in the United States.

PRACTICE SETTINGS

In general, traditional Chinese medicine is practiced in a range of clinical settings. Large hospitals entirely devoted to its practice are common in China. In this setting, acupuncture, herbal medicine, and tui na are provided on both an inpatient and an outpatient basis. It is not unusual to see a large outpatient facility treating 20 patients simultaneously in the same space. Other settings include smaller practices and even roadside stands. Individual consultations and herbal formulations can be obtained from a Chinese herb store in most countries with a significant Chinese population. In Japan, small hospitals, large clinics, and private offices are typical settings.

In the United States and Europe, while private practice is the norm, hospital-based practice and innovative group treatment settings have emerged as well.

Wherever traditional Chinese medicine is practiced, the delivery settings are not significantly different from the environment in which biomedical services are provided, unless the practitioner wants to emphasize the distinctive character of the practice or the practice is marginalized through lack of regulation. In the United States, record-keeping processes, insurance billing, biomedical screening, and concerns about office hygiene often produce a setting that—except for such peculiarities as acupuncture needles, moxa fluff, and herbs—looks very much like a typical physician's office.

RESEARCH AND EVALUATION

Chinese medicine represents a large domain of clinical interventions including acupuncture, moxibustion, therapeutic massage, bone setting, herbal medicine, and qigong. While almost all aspects of Chinese medicine have been the subject of research studies, it is hard to find large-scale systematic research programs that seek to examine Chinese medical interventions in their own terms. Aspects of Chinese medicine have been the focus of concerted research efforts in China and Japan since the mid-twentieth century, or even earlier if one considers research into Chinese herbal medicine in Japan and China, which dates to the late nineteenth century.

Recently, substantial research initiatives in some areas of Chinese medicine have been undertaken in the United States, Europe, and Korea as well, developing rapidly in terms of quality and quantity in the last 20 years. However, both the actual and perceived quality of such research, in both the East and the West, can vary widely. As is the case with medical systems, research standards—and even the practice of scientific research—are subject to cultural influences. The randomized, placebo-controlled, and double-blind clinical trial is the definitive standard for an unambiguous biomedical recognition of pharmaceutical efficacy, and has come to be the standard for research that signals the efficacy of any clinical intervention. However, not all societies require or encourage their medical communities to establish knowledge in this manner. This is especially true when the therapies in question have been part of the cultural fabric of medical practice for millennia. In addition, the accessibility of research data is influenced by the language and location of its publication.

All of these issues can pose obstacles to the availability and use of research information. Therefore, research that is meaningful to members of a given scientific or clinical community in China, Japan, Korea, Europe, or the United States may vary in its relevance to and impact on other communities. Additionally, the motivations for undertaking research can vary as well. Is the purpose to validate a traditional system of knowledge or therapy? Is the goal drug discovery? Do the researchers wish to bring a product to market? Is the purpose to find the utility of an intervention independent of the way in which the medical system understands it?

The question of study design arises as well. Is our goal to examine a traditional therapy as an adjunct to conventional therapy or as an alternative? Do we wish to rule out the possibility that placebo effects and expectation contribute to the effectiveness of the intervention? Are we satisfied to know that the therapy works as well as or better than a conventional biomedical therapy? For some researchers in China, a study designed to demonstrate which acupuncture intervention is better may be important and meaningful. In the West an acupuncture study without a non-acupuncture control (and ideally a placebo control) would be meaningless.

BOX 28-10 *Examples of NIH-Funded Studies on Chinese Medicine*

Chinese Herbal Medicine

Alternative Medicine Approaches for Women with Temporomandibular Disorders

Consistency of Traditional Chinese Medicine Diagnoses and Herbal Prescriptions for Rheumatoid Arthritis

Herbal Treatment of Hepatitis C in Methadone Maintained Patients

T'ai Chi Ch'uan

Alternative Stress Management Approaches in HIV Disease

Complementary/Alternative Medicine for Abnormality in the Vestibular (Balance) System

Tai Chi Chih and Varicella Zoster Immunity

Qigong

Qigong Therapy for Heart Device Patients

Chinese Exercise Modalities in Parkinson's Disease

HIV, human immunodeficiency virus; NIH, National Institutes of Health.

In the United States the period from 1991 to 2010 was rich and diverse in terms of the volume of funded research on complementary therapies that involved aspects of Chinese medicine. Efforts by the Office of Alternative Medicine (OAM), created in 1991 under the National Institutes of Health (NIH), substantially contributed to this process (Box 28-10). The OAM hosted several conferences dealing with methodological considerations in the field of alternative medicine, and each event addressed aspects of traditional Chinese medicine. Other OAM-supported projects included funding of numerous small research grants, many in the area of Chinese or Oriental medicine. However, as the complexity of designing useful randomized controlled trials of acupuncture became apparent, the National Center for Complementary and Alternative Medicine (NCCAM) shifted its focus to imaging studies and research designed to understand acupuncture mechanisms. In a similar fashion, where there was once funding for studies of traditional Chinese herbal formulas, the focus has shifted to individual herbs and the actions of their constituents.

RESEARCH INTO SPECIFIC AREAS OF CHINESE MEDICINE

Research on fundamental concepts, or what might be called *fundamental theory*, includes the exploration of whether concepts such as qi, the channels, acupuncture points, the diagnostic aspects of the pulse, and aspects of pattern diagnosis actually can refer to reproducibly identifiable and quantifiable phenomena. All these areas have been or are being actively pursued in a number of countries. In some instances, this research resembles basic research in physiology and relies on the development of sophisticated models and the design of instrumentation to test these models.

Research questions derived from the search for the physiological basis of Chinese medical concepts have been pursued for some time in China. One such study investigated the nature of kidney yang and concluded that patients displaying a diagnostic pattern associated with kidney yang vacuity showed low levels of 17-hydroxy corticosteroids in their urine, which ultimately suggests a relationship between the concept of kidney yang and the adrenocortical system (Hao, 1983).

Research on the correlation between the force and waveforms of the radial artery and the diagnostic perceptions of clinicians and physical status of patients has long been pursued in China, the United States, Japan, and Korea (Broffman & McCulloch, 1986; Takashima, 1995; Zhu, 1991). Typically, this research depends on the use of pressure sensors that are pressed against the skin overlying the radial artery in a manner and location that replicates that of the finger position of the traditional clinician. Pulse patterns are recorded and correlated to observations made by the clinician in an effort to determine the physical features that must be present for a diagnostic perception (Guo et al, 2012, Wang & Cheng, 2005). Preliminary results are intriguing, but methodological questions concerning population size and standardization of measurement remain.

Other aspects of Chinese medicine diagnostics are the subject of inquiry as well. Pattern identification, discussed above, represents a historical effort to organize aspects of Chinese medicine diagnosis. Although there are tensions between advocates of "standardized" diagnosis and more flexible approaches, both camps agree that pattern identification is an important part of the diagnostic process. Some studies have attempted to investigate the prevalence of certain patterns in various clinical conditions (MacPherson et al, 2013). The relevance of patterns to increasing the efficacy or accuracy of treatment is also an area of exploration (Jiang et al, 2012; Borud et al, 2009). The consistency of the application of patterns and the criteria used by clinicians has been examined from the point of view of assessing inter-rater reliability. Based on a fairly limited number of studies, the relevance of patterns to planning distinctive interventions has been called into question; however, most of this work has been in the area of acupuncture.

MATERIA MEDICA AND TRADITIONAL PHARMACOLOGY

Investigations of materia medica and traditional pharmacology have been ongoing since the early part of the twentieth century, in both China and Japan. This area of research continues unabated in China, the Republic of China, Japan, and Korea, and to a lesser extent in the West. This research can be divided into two areas of examination: the pharmacological properties of traditional materia medica, particularly their constituents, and the clinical efficacy of traditional pharmacology. The first area does not differ from the typical concerns of pharmacological research. In vitro studies and exploration of traditional use can suggest the potential usefulness of certain substances. If one becomes aware of a substance that is alleged to have pharmacological properties, it is comparatively easy to conduct studies to assess the presence of these properties and to isolate apparently active compounds.

A famous case in point is the first herb listed in the Chinese materia medica: *herba ephedra,* known botanically as *Ephedra sinica* Stapf (ma huang). Herba ephedra is recorded in the *Divine Husbandman's Classic of Materia Medica.* Its chief active component, ephedrine, was isolated in 1887 in Japan but remained largely unexplored for 35 years, until C.F. Schmidt from the University of Pennsylvania and K.K. Chen began to explore its pharmacological effects at the Peking Union Medical College, where the department of pharmacology was beginning a systematic exploration of the Chinese materia medica (Chen, 1977).

These explorations revealed that ephedrine was a sympathomimetic with properties of epinephrine, causing an increase in blood pressure, vasoconstriction, and bronchodilation. Clinically, ephedrine had several distinct advantages over epinephrine; ephedrine could be used orally, had a long duration of action, and was less toxic. It also was found to be useful in the management of bronchial asthma and hay fever and to support the patient's vital signs during the administration of spinal anesthesia. *Ephedra sinica* Stapf contains several physiologically active sympathomimetic alkaloids. One of these, pseudoephedrine, a diastereomer of ephedrine, is now synthesized and found in a number of pharmaceuticals, including over-the-counter products such as Sudafed and Actifed.

Historically and clinically, herba ephedra has been applied in a similar fashion in Chinese medicine, except for spinal anesthesia. As mentioned earlier, it is a principal ingredient in the herbal formula Ephedra Decoction. This herb also figures prominently in formulas used to address presentations that relate to asthma and allergy. The study of herba ephedra represents an early and impressive example of pharmacological research in the Chinese materia medica. Other single herbs for which the traditional clinical applications are supported in recent clinical experimentation include *herba artemisiae (yin chen hao)* for hepatitis and *caulis mu tong (mu tong)* for urinary tract infections. Extensive compilations discussing identified active constituents, clinical studies, and toxicity of large numbers of substances have been prepared (Chang, 1986).

Explorations of traditional pharmacology are somewhat more complex, although they too are amenable to the methods of double-blinding and placebo control that are critical to recognition in the biomedical world. However, given the breadth of possible substances that may be applied clinically (more than 5000) and the number of possible permutations for their combination in formulas, the scope of the inquiry becomes quite large. In addition, there is the question of whether to include the traditional considerations that surround diagnosis and pattern identification in the process of prescription and selection of herbal formulas for investigation.

Some contemporary studies are designed to take this issue into account, with the traditional clinician being able to assign individuals to specific treatment groups on the basis of symptoms while still being blinded with regard to the actual constituents of the substances administered to the patients. An example of this approach can be seen in a randomized clinical trial of the use of Chinese herbal medicine for the treatment of irritable bowel syndrome conducted by Alan Bensoussan under the auspices of the Research Unit for Complementary Medicine at the University of Western Sydney. This study, in which patients were randomly assigned to one of three treatment groups—placebo, standard formula, and individualized formula—showed that Chinese herbal medicine provided significant reduction in the symptoms of irritable bowel syndrome (Bensoussan et al, 1998).

Because Chinese researchers and journals have engaged the indexing process, the availability of published studies on Chinese herbal medicine has increased over time. Many of the publications are in English. Additionally, the engagement of Chinese medicine researchers with the Cochrane process—carrying out systematic reviews and, where possible, meta-analyses—has facilitated assessment of the existing literature. While interesting, these reviews are often unsatisfying or inconclusive. This can be due the inclusion criteria used by the reviewers, the quality of the studies reviewed, the choice of controls, disparate outcome measures, and the fact that it can be hard to compare the diverse herbal interventions that are used to treat even one clinical condition in Chinese medicine. Thus, although it is easy enough to conceptualize a study of any given Chinese herbal medicine intervention for a given condition, the diversity of therapeutic interventions available in Chinese medicine can render the results inconclusive in the context of the systematic review.

For example, Gan et al (2010) conducted a review of traditional Chinese medicine herbs for stopping bleeding from hemorrhoids, examining the results of nine trials that included 1822 patients with bleeding hemorrhoids. The authors characterized the trials they reviewed as "generally not of high quality." They did find that the Chinese medicine herbs "showed a statistically significant difference for the improvement in the general curative effects or total grade of symptoms in six trials . . . of hematochezia in three trials . . . and of inflammation of perianal mucosa in one trial" (Gan et al, 2010) with no evidence of adverse effects. The adverse effects reported were not serious and were scarce. However, because of the heterogeneity and low quality of the studies, they concluded that there was not strong evidence for the use of Chinese herbal preparations in stopping bleeding from hemorrhoids.

The authors did, however, conclude that the inclusion of some specific herbs in the formulas *Radix Sanguisorbae, Radix Rehmanniae, Fructus Sophorae, Radix Angelicae Sinensis,*

and *Radix Scutellariae* might contribute to the observed therapeutic effects.

Because herbal formulas are complex interventions, and because even assessing the therapeutic effects of a single herb, let alone a collection of them, can be challenging, some systematic reviews bear little fruit.

A review that examined Tianma Gouteng Yin formula for treating primary hypertension (Zhang et al, 2012) found no studies that met their standard for inclusion in their review. The formula Tian Ma Gou Teng Yin (Gastrodia and Uncaria Drink) is well regarded in the practice of Chinese medicine for the treatment of hypertension. However, after reviewing 59 papers in Chinese or English, none of the studies were included for review because of an absence of a control, the use of a hypertensive as a control, the use of multiple arms, or problems in randomization. Although the lack of a control and improper randomization are good reasons to reject a study from a review, many Chinese medicine reviews will consider multi-armed studies and controls that consist of conventional therapy. In either case, this review illustrates the challenges of applying the method of systematic reviews to Chinese medicine.

In cases where a traditional Chinese medicine has been developed as a standardized prepared medicine and evaluated as a pharmaceutical, the outcomes of such reviews can be a bit different. The standardized product Xiong Shao Capsule contains two "blood quickening" herbs in concentrated form, being roughly equivalent to 30 g Chuanxiong and 15 g Chishao (Xu et al, 2001). This product has been assessed in four trials to determine whether it would be helpful in preventing restenosis after percutaneous cardiac intervention and stenting. Restenosis is a consequence of inflammation processes interacting with the vascular wall that can lead to complications after percutaneous cardiac intervention. Zheng et al (2013) evaluated the trials in question, which examined the use of Xiong Shao Capsule as an adjunct to conventional pharmacotherapy in preventing restenosis. The authors concluded there was a protective effect produced by the Xiong Shao Capsule. It should be noted that the use of a single standardized version of an herbal formula and its application, in the context of conventional care, to a carefully defined clinical problem led to somewhat more compelling results.

This brief survey provides a glimpse of the richness and complexity of research into Chinese pharmacotherapeutics, and shows why this domain should remain a fertile area of inquiry for years to come.

ACUPUNCTURE

Research into the theoretical basis, safety, and therapeutic effects of acupuncture is discussed in Chapter 29.

Acknowledgments

This presentation owes a heavy debt to the work of Paul Unschuld and Nigel Wiseman. The scholarship and enterprise of these two individuals is reflected in their work and the help that they have provided to students of Chinese medicine such as me. Marnae Ergil, my wife and colleague, contributed enormously by reviewing text, answering questions, and being willing to check technical points in Chinese-language materials at any hour of the day or night. This project would not have been possible without the institutional commitment to scholarship and the support provided by the Pacific College of Oriental Medicine, later by Touro College and by the Finger Lakes School of Acupuncture and Oriental Medicine of NYCC.

References

Auteroche B, Gervais G, Auteroche M, et al: *Acupuncture and moxibustion: a guide to clinical practice*, Edinburgh, 1992, Churchill Livingstone.

Bannerman RH: The World Health Organization viewpoint on acupuncture, *World Health* 24, 1979.

Barlow J, Richardson C: *China doctor of John Day*, Portland, Ore, 1979, Binford & Mort.

Bensky D, Barolet R: *Chinese herbal medicine: formulas and strategies*, Seattle, 1990, Eastland Press.

Bensky D, Gamble A: *Chinese herbal medicine: materia medica*, rev ed, Seattle, 1986, Eastland Press.

Bensoussan A, Talley NJ, Hing M, et al: Treatment of irritable bowel syndrome with Chinese herbal medicine: a randomized clinical trial, *JAMA* 280(18):1585, 1998.

Birch S: A historical study of radial pulse six position diagnosis: naming the unnameable, *J Acupunct Soc N Y* 1(3-4):19, 1994.

Borud EK, Alræk T, White A, Grimsgaard S: 2009 The acupuncture treatment for postmenopausal hot flushes (Acuflash) study: traditional Chinese medicine diagnoses and acupuncture points used, and their relation to the treatment response, *Acupunct Med* 27(3):101-108, 2009.

Bowers JZ: *Western medical pioneers in feudal Japan*, Baltimore, 1970, Johns Hopkins University Press.

Broffman M, McCulloch M: Instrument-assisted pulse evaluation in the acupuncture practice, *Am J Acupunct* 14(3):255, 1986.

Chang HM: *Pharmacology and applications of Chinese materia medica*, Singapore, 1986, World Scientific (translated by SC Yao, LL Wang, CS Yeung).

Chen KK: Half a century of ephedrine. In Kao FF, Kao JJ, editors: *Chinese medicine—new medicine*, New York, 1977, Neale Watson Academic, p 21.

Chuang Y: *The historical development of acupuncture*, Los Angeles, 1982, Oriental Healing Arts Institute.

Despeux C: Gymnastics: the ancient tradition. In Kohn L, editor: *Taoist meditation and longevity techniques*, Ann Arbor, Mich, 1989, University of Michigan, Center for Chinese Studies, p 225.

Engelhardt U: Qi for life: longevity in the tang. In Kohn L, editor: *Taoist meditation and longevity techniques*, Ann Arbor, Mich, 1989, University of Michigan, Center for Chinese Studies, p 263.

Ergil KV: Chinese specific condition review: urinary tract infections, *Protocol J Botan Med* 1(1):130, 1995a.

Ergil KV: Where tradition matters: identifying epistemological and terminological issues in research design. In *Proceedings of the Second Symposium of the Society for Acupuncture Research*, Boston, 1995b, Society for Acupuncture Research, p 59.

Ergil MC: Medical education in China, *CCAOM News* 1(1):3, 1994.

Farquhar J: Problems of knowledge in contemporary Chinese medical discourse, *Soc Sci Med* 24(12):1013, 1987.

Gan Tao, Liu Yue-dong, Wang Yiping, Yang Jinlin: Traditional Chinese Medicine herbs for stopping bleeding from haemorrhoids, *Cochrane Database Syst Rev* 2010.

Guo R, Wang Y, Yan J, Yan H: Recurrence quantification analysis on pulse morphological changes in patients with coronary heart disease, *J Tradit Chin Med* 32(4):571-577, 2012.

Haller JS: Acupuncture in nineteenth century western medicine, *N Y State J Med* 73(10):1213, 1973.

Hao LZ: An attempt to understand the substance of kidney and its disorders, *J Am Coll Tradit Chin Med* (3):82, 1983 (translated by CS Cheung).

Hirsch RC: Korean constitutional nutrition, *J Am Coll Tradit Chin Med* (1):24, 1985.

Hsu E: Outline of the history of acupuncture in Europe, *J Chin Med* 29(1):28, 1989.

Hsu H, Peacher W: *Chen's history of Chinese medical science*, Taipei, 1977, Modern Drug Publishers.

Huang B, Di F, Li X, et al: *Syndromes of traditional Chinese medicine*, Heilongjiang, China, 1993, Heilongjiang Education Press (translated by D Ma, W Guo'en, S Sun, et al).

Huard P, Wong M: *Chinese medicine*, New York, 1968, McGraw-Hill, World University Library.

Jiang M, Lu C, Zhang C, et al: Syndrome differentiation in modern research of traditional Chinese medicine, *J Ethnopharmacol* 140(3):634-642, 2012. [Epub 2012 Feb 1].

Kaptchuk TJ: *The web that has no weaver: understanding Chinese medicine*, New York, 1983, Congdon & Weed.

Kleinman A: *Social origins of distress and disease: depression, neurasthenia, and pain in modern China*, New Haven, Conn, 1986, Yale University Press.

Lee JK, Bae SKB: *Korean acupuncture*, Seoul, 2008, Ko Mun Sa.

Lin Y: Laotse, the book of Tao. In Lin Y, editor: *The wisdom of China and India*, New York, 1942, Modern Library, p 578.

Lock M: *East Asian medicine in urban Japan: comparative studies of health systems*, vol 4, Berkeley, Calif, 1980, University of California Press.

Maciocia G: *The foundations of Chinese medicine*, Edinburgh, 1989, Churchill Livingstone.

MacPherson H, Elliot B, Hopton A, et al: Acupuncture for Depression: Patterns of Diagnosis and Treatment within a Randomised Controlled Trial Evid Based Complement Alternat Med. 2013. [Published online 2013 June 27].

Manaka Y, Itaya K: Acupuncture as intervention in the biological information system, *J Acupunct Soc N Y* 1(3-4):19, 1994.

Muench C: One hundred years of medicine: the ah-fong physicians of Idaho. In Schwarz HG, editor: *Chinese medicine on the Golden Mountain: an interpretive guide*, Seattle, 1984, Washington Commission for the Humanities, p 51.

National Institutes of Health: Acupuncture, *NIH Consens Statement* 15(5):1, 1997.

Osler W: *The principles and practice of medicine*, New York, 1913, Appleton.

Peacher W: Adverse reactions, contraindications and complications of acupuncture and moxibustion, *Am J Chin Med* 3(1):35, 1975.

Qiu XI: *Chinese acupuncture and moxibustion*, New York, 1993, Churchill Livingstone.

Sivin N: Traditional medicine in contemporary China. In *Science, medicine and technology in East Asia*, vol 2, Ann Arbor, Mich, 1987, University of Michigan, Center for Chinese Studies.

Takashima M: Pulse research, personal communication, 1995.

Unschuld P: *Medicine in China: a history of ideas*, Berkeley, Calif, 1985, University of California Press.

U.S. Food and Drug Administration: FDA issues regulation prohibiting sale of dietary supplements containing ephedrine alkaloids and reiterates its advice that consumers stop using these products, *FDA News* 4, 2004.

Veith I, translator: *The Yellow Emperor's classic of internal medicine*, Berkeley, Calif, 1972, University of California Press.

Wang G, Fan Y, Guan Z: Chinese massage. In Zhang E, editor: *A practical English-Chinese library of traditional Chinese medicine*, Shanghai, 1990, College of Traditional Chinese Medicine, Publishing House of Shanghai.

Wang H, Cheng Y: 2005 A quantitative system for pulse diagnosis in Traditional Chinese Medicine, *Conf Proc IEEE Eng Med Biol Soc* 6:5676–5679, 2005.

Wang X: Research on the origin and development of Chinese acupuncture and moxibustion. In Xiangtong Z, editor: *Research on acupuncture, moxibustion and acupuncture anesthesia*, New York, 1986, Springer-Verlag, p 783.

Watson B: *The complete works of Chuang-tzu*, New York, 1968, Columbia University Press.

Wilhelm R: *The I Ching*, Princeton, NJ, 1967, Princeton University Press (translated by CF Baynes).

Wiseman N: *A list of Chinese formulas*, unpublished manuscript, Taiwan, 1993.

Wiseman N, Boss K: *Glossary of Chinese medical terms and acupuncture points*, Brookline, Mass, 1990, Paradigm.

Wiseman N, Ellis A, Zmiewski P, et al: *Fundamentals of Chinese medicine*, Brookline, Mass, 1985, Paradigm.

Wiseman N, Ellis A, Zmiewski P, et al: *Fundamentals of Chinese medicine*, Taipei, 1993, Southern Materials Center.

Wiseman N, Ellis A, Zmiewski P, et al: *Fundamentals of Chinese medicine*, rev ed, Brookline, Mass, 1995, Paradigm.

Wong CK, Wu TL: *History of Chinese medicine: being a chronicle of medical happenings in China from ancient times to the present period*, Taipei, 1985, Southern Materials Center.

World Health Organization: *Acupuncture: review and analysis of reports on controlled clinical trials*, Geneva, 2002, The Organization. Available at: http://www.who.int/medicines/library/trm/acupuncture/acupuncture_trials.doc.

Xu H, Shi DZ, Chen KJ: Effect of xiongshao capsule on vascular remodeling in porcine coronary balloon injury model, 2001.

Zhang E: Clinic of traditional Chinese medicine. I. In Zhang E, editor: *A practical English-Chinese library of traditional Chinese medicine*, Shanghai, 1990, College of Traditional Chinese Medicine, Publishing House of Shanghai.

Zhang HW, Tong J, Zhou G, et al: Tianma Gouteng Yin Formula for treating primary hypertension, *Cochrane Library* (6):2012.

Zheng GH, Liu JP, Chu JF, et al: Xiongshao for restenosis after percutaneous coronary intervention in patients with coronary heart disease, *Cochrane Library* 2013(5):2013.

Zhu B: *Pulse research in China*, personal communication, 1991.

Suggested Readings

Agren H: A new approach to Chinese traditional medicine, *Am J Chin Med* 3(3):207, 1975.

Aloysio DD, Penacchioni P: Morning sickness control in early pregnancy by Neiguan point acupressure, *Obstet Gynecol* 80(5):852, 1992.

Becker RO: *The body electric: electromagnetism and the foundation of life*, New York, 1985, Quill/William Morrow.

Berman BM, Singh BB, Lao L, et al: randomized trial of acupuncture as an adjunctive therapy in osteoarthritis of the knee, *Rheumatology (Oxford)* 38(4):346, 1999.

Birch S: A biophysical basis for acupuncture. In Birsh S, editor: *Proceedings of the Second Symposium of the Society for Acupuncture Research*, Boston, 1995, Society for Acupuncture Research, p 274.

Birch S, Hammerschlag R: *Acupuncture efficacy: a summary of controlled clinical trials*, Tarrytown, NY, 1996, National Academy of Acupuncture and Oriental Medicine.

Cherkin DC, Sherman KJ, Deyo RA, et al: A review of the evidence for the effectiveness, safety, and cost of acupuncture, massage therapy, and spinal manipulation for back pain, *Ann Intern Med* 138(11):898, 2003.

Christensen BV, Iuhl IU, Vilbe KH, et al: Acupuncture treatment of severe knee osteoarthritis, *Acta Anaesthesiol Scand* 36:519, 1992.

Coan R, Wong GT, Ku S-L, et al: The acupuncture treatment of low back pain: a randomized controlled study, *Am J Chin Med* 8(2):181, 1980.

Delis K, Morris M: Clinical trials in acupuncture. In Birch S, editor: *Proceedings of the First Symposium of the Society for Acupuncture Research*, Boston, 1993, Society for Acupuncture Research, p 68.

Dickens W, Lewith G: A single-blind, controlled and randomised clinical trial to evaluate the effect of acupuncture in the treatment of trapeziometacarpal osteoarthritis, *Complement Med Res* 3:5, 1989.

Dundee JW, Ghaly RG, Fitzpatrick KTJ, et al: Acupuncture prophylaxis of cancer chemotherapy induced sickness, *J R Soc Med* 82:268, 1989.

Ellis A, Wiseman N, Boss K: *Fundamentals of Chinese acupuncture*, Brookline, Mass, 1991, Paradigm.

Foreman J: What the research shows, *Boston Globe* 22/5(25):27, 1995.

Ghaly RG, Fitzpatrick KTJ, Dundee JW: *Anesthesia* 42:1108, 1987.

Hammerschlag R: Acupuncture: on what should its evidence be based?, *Altern Ther* 9(5):34, 2003.

Helms JM: Acupuncture for the management of primary dysmenorrhea, *Obstet Gynecol* 69(1):51, 1987.

Jobst K: A critical analysis of acupuncture in pulmonary disease: efficacy and safety of the acupuncture needle, *J Altern Complement Med* 1:57, 1995.

Junnila SYT: Acupuncture superior to piroxicam in the treatment of osteoarthritis, *Am J Acupunct* 10:341, 1982.

Kiresuk TJ, Culliton PD: *Overview of substance abuse acupuncture treatment research*, 1994, Workshop on Acupuncture.

Langevin HM, Churchill DL, Wu J, et al: Evidence of connective tissue involvement in acupuncture, *FASEB J* 16(8):872, 2002. Available at: http://www.fasebj.org/cgi/reprint/16/8/872.

Lao L, Bergman S, Hamilton GR, et al: Evaluation of acupuncture for pain control after oral surgery: a placebo-controlled trial, *Arch Otolaryngol Head Neck Surg* 125(5):567, 1999.

Lao L, Bergman S, Langenberg P, et al: Efficacy of Chinese acupuncture on postoperative oral surgery pain, *Oral Surg Oral Med Oral Pathol Oral Radiol Endod* 79:423, 1995.

Lee Hyun-Ji, Wang Jun, Hong Seung-Pyo: Alternative Modernity: The Revival of Korean Oriental Medicine in Modern South Korea Amercian Acupuncturist Winter, 2008.

Naeser MA, Michael PA, Stiassny-Eder D, et al: Real versus sham acupuncture in the treatment of paralysis in acute stroke patients: a CT scan lesion study, *J Neurol Rehabil* 6:163, 1992.

Oschman J: A biophysical basis for acupuncture. In Birch S, editor: *Proceedings of the First Symposium of the Society for Acupuncture Research*, Boston, 1993, Society for Acupuncture Research, p 141.

Patel M, Gutzwiller F, Paccand F, et al: A meta-analysis of acupuncture for chronic pain, *Int J Epidemiol* 18(4):900, 1989.

Payer L: *Medicine and culture: varieties of treatment in the United States, England, West Germany, and France*, New York, 1988, Henry Holt.

Pomeranz B: Scientific basis of acupuncture. In Stux G, editor: *The basics of acupuncture*, New York, 1988, Springer-Verlag, p 4.

Reichmanis M, Marino AA, Becker RO: Electrical correlates of acupuncture points, *Intern J Acupunct Electrother* 17:75, 1975.

Ryu H, Jun CD, Lee BS, et al: Effect of qigong training on proportions of T lymphocyte subsets in human peripheral blood, *Am J Chin Med* 23:27, 1995.

Sancier K: Medical applications of qigong, *Altern Ther Health Med* 2(1):40, 1996.

Seto A, Kusaka S, Nakazatio W, et al: Detection of extraordinary large bio-magnetic field strength from human hand, *Acupunct Electrother Res Int J* 17:75, 1992.

Shanghai College of Traditional Chinese Medicine: *Acupuncture: a comprehensive text*, Seattle, 1981, Eastland Press (translated by J O'Connor, D Bensky).

Tang KC: Qigong therapy—its effectiveness and regulation, *Am J Chin Med* 22:235, 1994.

ter Riet G, Kleijnen J, Knipschild P: Acupuncture and chronic pain: a criteria-based meta-analysis, *J Clin Epidemiol* 43:1191, 1990.

Thomas M, Eriksson SV, Lundeberg T: A comparative study of diazepam and acupuncture in patients with osteoarthritis pain: a placebo controlled study, *Am J Chin Med* 19: 95, 1991.

Vincent CA: A controlled trial of the treatment of migraine by acupuncture, *Clin J Pain* 5:305, 1989.

Vincent CA: Acupuncture as a treatment for chronic pain. In Lewith GT, Aldridge D, editors: *Clinical research methodology for complementary therapies*, London, 1993, Hodder & Stoughton, p 289.

Chronology of Chinese and East Asian Medicine

Dynasty	Time period	Medical literature and technology
Xia	2100–1600 BC	
Shang	1766–1121 BC	Magico-religious, shamans, oracle bones, ancestors
Zhou	1122–221 BC	Magico-religious, shamanism
Warring States	220–205 BC	*Kong Fu Zi* (Confucius)
Qin	221–206 BC	*Lao Zi* (Daoism); Great Wall of China
Han	206 BC–AD 220	Herbalism; *Shen nong*; *The Divine Husbandman's Classic of Materia Medica*; acupuncture and moxibustion; Qigong; compilation of *Yellow Emperor's Inner Classic*
Daoist Rebellion and Interregnum	AD 221–265	
Jin	AD 266–420	
Sui	581–618	
Tang (see also Han Dynasty)	618–907	*Classic of Spells*; *The Classic of Difficult Issues*
Sung	960–1279	Formal medical education, medical specialization
Yuan	1280–1367	Advances in acupuncture; herbalism; *Treatise on Cold Diseases*; "modern" Chinese medicine
Ming	1368–1644	Naturalistic theories; peak of acupuncture and moxibustion; *Discourse on Warm Epidemics*; *Great Compilations of Acupuncture and Moxibustion*
Qing (Manchu)	1644–1911	Decline in acupuncture
Republic of China	1912–1936	Emphasis on twentieth-century Western medicine
Manchukuo	1936–1945	Japanese influence
Civil War	1945–1949	Nationalist (*Chiang Kai Shek*) vs. Communist (*Mao Zedong*) China
People's Republic of China	1949–	Traditional Chinese medicine; *A Barefoot Doctor's Manual*
Republic of China (continued in Taiwan, formerly Formosa)	1949–	

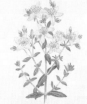

CLASSICAL ACUPUNCTURE

KEVIN V. ERGIL

MARNAE C. ERGIL

THE IDEA OF ACUPUNCTURE

Acupuncture, literally "sharp puncture," simultaneously invokes impressions of simplicity and complexity. A sharp object, a needle, is simple, whereas the body, its object, is complex. The surface of the body, when compared in area with the point of the needle, provides an almost limitless number of locations in which the needle might be inserted. The needle is "yang" in its sharp, metallic, focused, and intrusive form. The body is "yin," comparatively soft, organic, expansive, and complex.

Acupuncture, however, is not just about the yang and yin of a needle and a body, but rather the system of ideas, understood relationships, and practices that inform the clinician about where the needle, or needles, might be placed. How many, of what diameter and length, for how long, at what angle, with what movements, and with what intentions and intentionality? What other interventions might be applied to warm and/or stimulate the surface of the body? All these aspects, then, are part of acupuncture.

This chapter gives a detailed overview of acupuncture theory to provide the reader with a strong conceptual understanding of the fundamental ideas and practices from which acupuncture emerges. Particular attention is paid to the acupuncture channels and networks (meridians) themselves, the significance of which frequently goes unexplored even in many of the popular contemporary acupuncture texts. Models for acupuncture point selection and the use of associated techniques are discussed. The way in which these models inform the diverse traditions in acupuncture is explored, and, finally, acupuncture research and the relationship (or the lack of one) between this research and acupuncture theory are examined.

This chapter is designed to be read after finishing Chapter 28 on Traditional Medicine of China and East Asia. Many of the ideas developed in the following discussion rely on or refer to concepts already presented in that chapter. Although certain points are amplified here, the reader should be familiar with the basic concepts discussed in that chapter, such as historical developments in Chinese medicine, important text sources, the idea of yin and yang, the five phases, the six evils, the viscera and bowels, and disease causation.

The word *acupuncture* has attained a meaning in the West that allows the term to float free of its cultural and historical moorings, even in popular texts that purport to teach acupuncture, and appear as an independent modality that can be qualified in any number of ways removed from its obligatory context. The first decontextualizing movement is the separation of acupuncture from moxibustion. In both ancient and modern China, "acupuncture," in the sense that the term is used in the West, is actually known as *zhen jiu* (针灸), meaning "needle moxibustion." This expression recognizes that, although acupuncture needles and moxibustion fluff or floss are often used independently of each other, they are so closely associated in theoretical and therapeutic terms that they are inextricably linked. A similar construction is found in Japan, where the expression *shin kyu* (針灸) has the same meaning. In the West, although the use of moxibustion may occasionally be implicit in the use of the term *acupuncture*, it remains unstated, and so a critical component of the tradition vanishes from view. Thus, the practice of acupuncture in the West from the start is fundamentally diluted (see Chapter 3) by the frequent or routine absence of moxibustion.

"Acupuncture" then becomes qualified in a variety of ways that appear to add meaning to the term but often obscure as much as clarify. "Medical acupuncture," "Western acupuncture," "Chinese acupuncture," "Japanese acupuncture," "Korean acupuncture," "Vietnamese acupuncture," "new American acupuncture," "five-element acupuncture," "traditional Chinese medicine (TCM) acupuncture," "Taoist acupuncture," and "classical Chinese acupuncture" is a nonexhaustive list of some common types or styles of acupuncture represented in schools, workshops, publications, and scientific literature, and on the Internet.

Regardless of the way in which the term *acupuncture* is qualified, the basic framework for all practices described under these varying rubrics derives entirely and uniquely from acupuncture principles and concepts articulated in the great classics of Chinese medicine—the *Yellow Emperor's Inner Classic (Huang Di Nei Jing)* comprising the *Spiritual Axis (Ling Shu)* and *Simple Questions (Su Wen)*, ca. 200 to 100 BC; the *Classic of Difficult Issues (Nan Jing)*, ca. AD 200; and the *Systematic Classic of Acupuncture and Moxibustion (Zhen Jiu Jia Yi Jing)*, AD 282—and from later books based on these, such as the *Great Compendium of Acupuncture and Moxibustion (Zhen Jiu Da Cheng)*.

This chapter expands the exploration of acupuncture concepts begun in Chapter 28 to provide a detailed foundation of the core acupuncture concepts that form the basis for all contemporary acupuncture traditions or practice styles. Later in this chapter these various types or traditions of acupuncture are examined in greater detail. At this point, however, it is important to establish what might be termed the common conceptual sources of acupuncture (or acupuncture and moxibustion) theory and practice. These ideas, except for minor refinements, represent the core of acupuncture theory that was well established in China by the third century AD and have continued to provide the basis of theoretical elaboration and incremental development through to modern times. Although there are many innovative approaches to acupuncture therapeutics, all innovation and all traditions can be and ideally should be understood in reference to this conceptual core.

CORE ACUPUNCTURE THEORY AND PRACTICE

Core acupuncture theory is based on the principles of yin and yang; the five phases; the vital substances of the body (qi, blood, and fluids); the viscera and bowels, which act to produce, distribute, and store these vital substances; and the channels and networks that permit the flow and distribution of these substances throughout the body.

CHANNEL AND NETWORK THEORY

The channels and networks are the pathways that carry qi, blood, and body fluids throughout the body, including to the surface and to the internal organs. They are the paths of communication between all parts of the body. When qi and blood flow through the channels smoothly, the body is properly nourished and healthy. The organs, the skin and

body hair, the sinews and flesh, the bones, and all other tissues rely on the free flow of qi and blood through the channels. Ultimately, it is the channels and networks that create a unified body in which all parts are interacting and interdependent.

As we have seen in Chapter 28, the channels appear to have historical primacy over the points or holes through which the movement of qi and blood is manipulated by means of acupuncture and other techniques. Clear descriptions of acupuncture points appear well after the ancient methods of stimulating channels with heat or stones are described. Channels, then, are equivalent in importance to acupuncture points in acupuncture theory and are typically presented first in standard acupuncture texts. Although acupuncture points often seem to be the primary object of therapy (and can be the subject of intense care in the process of point location in which palpation, anatomical location, and measurement are used to establish a point for treatment), the channels are the basis for all relations among points and body regions.

Functions of the Channel and Network System

There are five major functions of the channel and network system: transporting, regulating, protective and diagnostic, therapeutic, and integrating (Table 29-1). These functions inform clinical practice. For example, when an evil invades the exterior of the body, it first enters the skin and body hair. If not expelled it may enter various levels of the channels or network vessels. Eventually it may even reach the internal organs. Understanding the path that an evil may take into the body helps the clinician to assess where the evil is and how best to treat it. Similarly, the channels can reflect the relative vacuity of the body's correct qi or the replete condition of an organ or body region due to illness. By observing changes to the channels and their nature and location, by palpating the channels, and by understanding channel relationships, the clinician can choose appropriate points to use to treat the condition.

Structure of the Channel and Network System

The pathways through which qi and blood flow are divided into two types: the channels and the networks. The channels are bilateral and symmetrical; they travel vertically through the body and are relatively deep within the body. The networks are branches of the channels. They connect interiorly–exteriorly related organs, and they connect channels. The networks are also bilateral, but they travel in all directions, and relative to the regular channels, they are more superficial.

The 12 Regular Channels

The 12 regular channels are the most well-known and frequently discussed channels. They contain the preponderance of acupuncture points that are located on channels, and each corresponds to one of the 12 organs of Chinese medicine. They are best known by their surface pathways.

Distribution and nomenclature: There are six yang and six yin channels, which are distributed bilaterally on the

TABLE 29-1 *Functions of the Channel System*

Function	Clinical relevance of channel system function
Transportation	The channel system encompasses all of the pathways for the circulation of qi and blood throughout the body, thus providing qi and blood to all of the organs and tissues for nourishment and moistening
Regulation	The channel system maintains the flow of qi and blood through the pathways, which then maintains the balance of yin and yang to regulate the functions of the organs
Protection and diagnosis	The channel system protects the body against the invasion of evils
	If evils invade or are internally generated, then the channel system reflects the signs and symptoms of the disease. This might include observable signs such as color change, rashes, and so forth; palpable signs such as changes in resistance, lumps, and so forth; or subjective changes such as pain, numbness, and so forth, along a pathway
Therapy	The signs and symptoms of disease are reflected in the channel (diagnosis), and then treatment is based on the selection of points along the channels that have a direct impact on the affected organ systems
Integration	The channel system connects the viscera and bowels with each other and with the limbs and body surface. It also connects the internal and external parts of the body, including the organs of the five senses, tissues, bone, sinew, muscle, and orifices

body. The yin channels run along the inner side of the limbs (three on the arms and three on the legs) and across the chest and abdomen. Each yin channel is associated with specific viscera. With the exception of the stomach channel, the yang channels run along the outer side of the limbs (three on the arms and three on the legs) and along the buttocks and back. Each yang channel is associated with a specific bowel.

Within the classification of yin and yang, the channels are further divided based on their relative location on the anterior, midline, or posterior aspect of the limb. The yin channels include the greater yin, located on the anterior, medial aspect of the limbs; the lesser yin, located on the posterior, medial aspect of the limbs; and the reverting yin, located on the midline of the medial aspect of the limbs. The yang channels include the yang brightness, located on the anterior lateral aspect of the limbs; the greater yang, located on the posterior lateral aspect of the limbs; and the lesser yang, located on the midline of the lateral aspect of the limbs.

The name of each of the channels is based on three features: (1) the distribution of the channel along either the upper limbs (the hand channels) or the lower limbs (the foot channels); (2) the yin-yang classification of the channel; and (3) the organ with which the channel is directly associated. Thus, the channel associated with the lung is referred to as the hand greater yin lung channel, because it runs from the interior of the abdomen out to the tip of the thumb, it runs along the anterior medial aspect of the arm, and it is directly associated with the lung.

The flow of qi in the 12 regular channels: In addition to being directly associated with one of the internal organs, each of the six yin channels is paired with its interiorly–exteriorly related yang channel. This pairing expresses an important physiological connection between the associated viscera and bowel and an anatomical relation between the channels. In addition, each hand channel is associated with a foot channel based on its yin-yang classification and location.

These two ways of pairing the channels are expressed in three circuits of the flow of qi through the 12 regular channels. The flow of qi in each circuit begins in a yin channel on the chest and passes to the interiorly–exteriorly related yang channel at the hand. It then ascends along the yang channel to the face, where it passes into the hand yang channel's paired foot yang channel. It then descends to the foot, where it passes to the interiorly–exteriorly related yin channel and ascends back to the chest to begin a new circuit. Thus, the qi passes from the chest to the hand to the face to the foot and back to the chest three times, traversing a complete circuit through the body and covering both the yin (anterior) and yang (posterior) aspects of the body before it completes its circuit of the 12 channels (Figure 29-1).

The directionality of qi flow is often exploited by means of specialized needling techniques. To drain qi and so to reduce activity in a channel, the direction of the flow is opposed. To strengthen or supplement the qi in a channel or organ, the needle can be oriented in the direction of flow (Table 29-2).

The three hand yang and three foot yang channels all meet in the head. The head is the most yang aspect of the body. Many of the diseases that manifest in the head, certain types of headache, acne, and so on, are caused by repletion of yang qi. Because yang is active and upbearing, the repletion will often rise via the yang channels to the head. Treatment entails down-bearing the yang qi and draining the repletion. Often points located on the ends of the hands and feet will be used to drain the repletion down and out of the head.

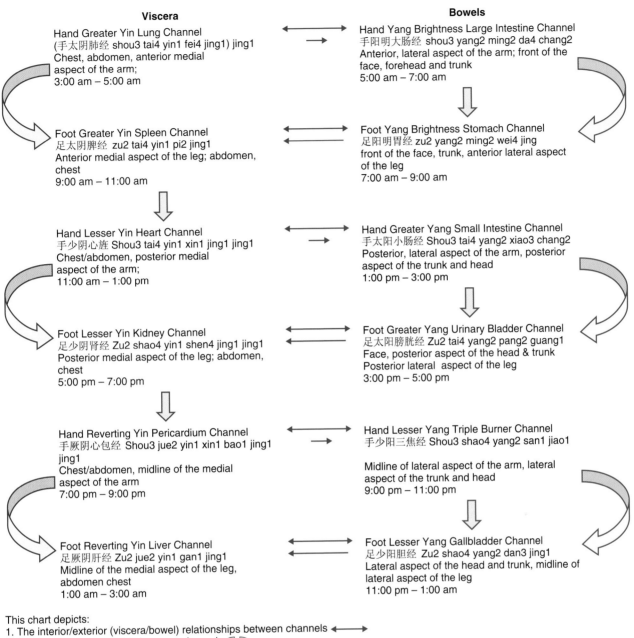

Viscera

Hand Greater Yin Lung Channel
(手太阴肺经 shou3 tai4 yin1 fei4 jing1) jing1
Chest, abdomen, anterior medial
aspect of the arm;
3:00 am – 5:00 am

Foot Greater Yin Spleen Channel
足太阴脾经 zu2 tai4 yin1 pi2 jing1
Anterior medial aspect of the leg; abdomen,
chest
9:00 am – 11:00 am

Hand Lesser Yin Heart Channel
手少阴心旌 Shou3 tai4 yin1 xin1 jing1 jing1
Chest/abdomen, posterior medial
aspect of the arm;
11:00 am – 1:00 pm

Foot Lesser Yin Kidney Channel
足少阴肾经 Zu2 shao4 yin1 shen4 jing1 jing1
Posterior medial aspect of the leg; abdomen,
chest
5:00 pm – 7:00 pm

Hand Reverting Yin Pericardium Channel
手厥阴心包经 Shou3 jue2 yin1 xin1 bao1 jing1
jing1
Chest/abdomen, midline of the medial
aspect of the arm
7:00 pm – 9:00 pm

Foot Reverting Yin Liver Channel
足厥阴肝经 Zu2 jue2 yin1 gan1 jing1
Midline of the medial aspect of the leg,
abdomen chest
1:00 am – 3:00 am

Bowels

Hand Yang Brightness Large Intestine Channel
手阳明大肠经 shou3 yang2 ming2 da4 chang2
Anterior, lateral aspect of the arm; front of the
face, forehead and trunk
5:00 am – 7:00 am

Foot Yang Brightness Stomach Channel
足阳明胃经 zu2 yang2 ming2 wei4 jing
front of the face, trunk, anterior lateral aspect
of the leg
7:00 am – 9:00 am

Hand Greater Yang Small Intestine Channel
手太阳小肠经 Shou3 tai4 yang2 xiao3 chang2
Posterior, lateral aspect of the arm, posterior
aspect of the trunk and head
1:00 pm – 3:00 pm

Foot Greater Yang Urinary Bladder Channel
足太阳膀胱经 Zu2 tai4 yang2 pang2 guang1
Face, posterior aspect of the head & trunk
Posterior lateral aspect of the leg
3:00 pm – 5:00 pm

Hand Lesser Yang Triple Burner Channel
手少阳三焦经 Shou3 shao4 yang2 san1 jiao1
Midline of lateral aspect of the arm, lateral
aspect of the trunk and head
9:00 pm – 11:00 pm

Foot Lesser Yang Gallbladder Channel
足少阳胆经 Zu2 shao4 yang2 dan3 jing1
Lateral aspect of the head and trunk, midline of
lateral aspect of the leg
11:00 pm – 1:00 am

This chart depicts:
1. The interior/exterior (viscera/bowel) relationships between channels ⟷
2. The hand/foot relationship between channels ↺↻
3. The flow of qi from one channel to the next ⟶
4. The 3 loops of the body (chest – hand – face – abdomen) that the qi completes in one day
5. The relative location of each channel on the limbs of the body
6. The time of day during which the qi is said to pass through each channel

Figure 29-1 Flow in channels and organs. (Courtesy Marnae Ergil.)

> The three hand yin and the three foot yin channels all meet in the chest and abdomen. The chest and abdomen are the place where all of the organs of the body reside.
> The yin and yang channels of the hand meet on the hands.
> The yin and yang channels of the feet meet on the feet. ∾

Qi and blood circulate through the body via the channels ceaselessly, from one channel to the next. Before returning to the beginning of the circuit, the qi and blood pass through the body in three loops. Over the course of one 24-hour period, the qi and blood in the channels pass through the entire body in the following sequence:

LU → LI → ST → SP → HT → SI → UB → KI → PC → SJ → GB → LR

where LU = lung; LI = large intestine; ST = stomach; SP = spleen; HT = heart; SI = small intestine; UB = urinary

TABLE 29-2 *Direction of Qi Flow in the Twelve Regular Channels*

Channels	Direction of qi flow
The three yin channels of the hand (LU, HT, PC)	Start in the chest and run along the medial aspect of the arms to the hands, where they meet and join their internally–externally paired yang channel. For example, the hand greater yin lung channel meets the hand yang brightness large intestine channel on the hand
The three yang channels of the hand (LI, SI, SJ)	Start on the hands and run along the lateral aspect of the arms to the head and face, where they meet their paired foot yang channel. For example, the hand yang brightness large intestine channel meets the foot yang brightness stomach channel on the face
The three yang channels of the feet (ST, BL, GB)	Start from the head and face and descend to the feet to meet their internally–externally paired yin channels. For example, the foot greater yang stomach channel meets the foot greater yin spleen channel on the foot.
The three yin channels of the feet (SP, KI, LR)	Start at the toes and ascend to the abdomen or chest to meet the three yin channels of the hands. For example, the foot greater yin spleen channel ascends to the abdomen, where it meets the hand lesser yin heart channel

Note: In each channel, the qi is said to flow in a particular direction.

BL, Bladder; GB, gallbladder; HT, heart; KI, kidney; LI, large intestine; LR, liver; LU, lung; PC, pericardium; SI, small intestine; SJ, triple burner (san jiao); SP, spleen; ST, stomach.

bladder; KI = kidney; PC = pericardium; SJ = triple burner (san jiao); GB = gallbladder; and LR = liver.

The flow of qi is cyclic. At any given time of day, as determined by ancient Chinese time-measuring methods of 2-hour increments, the flow of qi will be strongest in one specific organ. This idea can be used in both diagnosis and treatment. In the course of 1 day, the strength of qi will pass one time through each of the 12 channels. When the qi is passing through a given channel, the organ associated with that channel is considered to be at its strongest. The qi of the organ associated with the channel on the opposite side of the diurnal clock is considered to be at its weakest. Thus, from 3:00 AM to 5:00 AM, the qi of the lung is at its strongest and the qi of the urinary bladder is at its weakest.

Clinically, this information might be applied in several ways. For example, if an asthmatic patient consistently wakes between 3:00 and 5:00 in the morning with an asthmatic attack, one might think that the qi of the lung, which should be especially strong at this time, is instead exceptionally weak, which creates a circumstance in which the patient cannot breathe easily and other organs, the liver in particular, take advantage of this weakness and overwhelm the lung, causing an asthmatic attack. Or, if an elderly person wakes between 5:00 and 7:00 in the morning with an immediate need to move the bowels, one might suspect that the qi of the large intestine (5:00 to 7:00 AM) is weak and the qi of the kidney (5:00 to 7:00 PM), which is responsible for securing the loss of substances from the body, is also weak and unable to restrain the large intestine.

Pathology and treatment of the 12 regular channels Each of the channels has its own pathological symptoms and signs that guide the practitioner in determining a diagnosis and in choosing points for treatment. Pathology that is specific to the channel may present as pain, tension, rashes, and so on, that manifests along a specific channel pathway. For example, a patient who has shoulder and arm pain that covers the posterior portion of the shoulder, crosses over the scapula and trapezius muscle, and goes down the posterior aspect of the arm might be diagnosed with stagnation of qi and blood in the small intestine channel, which engenders pain.

Because the internal pathways of the channels connect directly to the associated organs, channel pathology may also be a reflection of organ pathology. For example, a patient who experiences constipation might also experience shoulder and neck pain along the pathway of the large intestine. Although the patient may not make the connection, through inquiry, a good diagnostician might learn that when the bowels move, the pain diminishes and both the pain and the constipation improve when there is less stress. Often, the patient will complain only of the shoulder pain and then be pleasantly surprised when both the shoulder pain and the constipation clear up. Thus, when discussing channel pathology, we refer not only to what is visible or what is manifesting along the exterior portion of the pathway, but also to the internal pathway and its organ connections (Table 29-3).

The internal branches of the channels also need to be considered when inquiring about symptomatology and when coming to a diagnostic conclusion. For example, an internal branch of the foot greater yin spleen channel travels to the underside of the tongue and spreads over the entire area. Thus, when the tongue is examined, if the bottom is especially pale, one might consider the possibility of blood vacuity as a result of dysfunction of the spleen in producing blood. An internal branch of the foot reverting yin liver channel travels up to the tissues surrounding the eyes and to the vertex of the head. Clinically, symptoms such as vertex headaches might be indicative of repletion of yang qi in the liver channel. All of the 12 regular channels

TABLE 29-3 *Signs of the External and Internal Pathways of the Channels*

Channel	External channel pathway signs	Internal channel pathway signs
Lung	Heat effusion and aversion to cold, nasal congestion, headache, pain along the channel pathway	Cough, panting, wheezing, rapid breathing, fullness in the chest, expectoration of phlegm, dry throat, change in urine color
Large intestine	Heat effusion, parched mouth, thirst, sore throat, nosebleed, toothache, swelling of the neck, pain along the channel pathway	Lower abdominal pain, wandering abdominal pain, rumbling intestines, sloppy stool, and excretion of thick, slimy yellow matter
Stomach	High fever, red face, sweating, delirium, manic agitation, pain in the eyes, dry nose, nosebleed, lip and mouth sores, deviated mouth, pain along the channel pathway	Abdominal distention and fullness, water swelling, vexation and discomfort while active or recumbent, mania and withdrawal, swift digestion and rapid hungering, yellow urine
Spleen	Heaviness in the head or body, weak limbs, motor impairment of the tongue, cold along the inside of the thigh and knee, swelling of the legs and feet	Pain in the stomach duct, sloppy diarrhea, stool containing untransformed food, rumbling intestines, nausea, reduced foot intake, jaundice
Heart	Headache, eye pain, pain in the chest and back muscles, dry throat, thirst with desire to drink, hot or painful palms, pain in the scapular region and/or the medial aspect of the forearm	Heart pain, fullness and pain in the chest, pain in the hypochondriac region, heat vexation, rapid breathing, discomfort in the lying posture, dizziness with fainting spells, mental diseases
Small intestine	Erosion of the glossal and oral mucosa, pain in the cheeks, tearing, pain along the channel pathway	Lower abdominal pain and distention with the pain stretching around to the lumbus or into the testicles, diarrhea, stomach pain with dry feces
Urinary bladder	Heat effusion and aversion to cold, headache, stiff neck, pain in the lumbar spine, eye pain and tearing, pain along the channel pathway	Lower abdominal pain and distention, inhibited urination, urinary block, enuresis, mental disorders, arched-back rigidity
Kidney	Lumbar pain, weak legs, dry mouth, pain along the channel pathway	Dizziness, facial swelling, blurred vision, gray facial complexion, shortness of breath, enduring diarrhea, sloppy stool, dry stool, impotence
Pericardium	Stiffness of the neck, spasm in the limbs, red complexion, pain in the eyes, pain along the channel pathway	Delirious speech, heat vexation, fullness and oppression in the chest and rib-side, heart palpitations, heart pain, constant laughing
Triple burner	Sore throat, pain in the cheeks, red painful eyes, deafness, pain behind the ears and along the channel pathway	Abdominal distention and fullness, hardness and fullness in the lower abdomen, urinary frequency, enuresis, edema
Gallbladder	Alternating heat effusion and aversion to cold, headache, malaria, eye pain, deafness, pain along the channel pathway	Rib-side pain, vomiting, bitter taste in the mouth, chest pain
Liver	Headache, dizziness, blurred vision, tinnitus, heat effusion	Fullness, distention, and pain in the ribs

have several of these internal pathways, along which there are no specific points that can be accessed but which must be considered in relation to diagnosis and treatment.

In addition to the 12 regular channel pathways, there are 4 additional types of channels that are directly associated with the 12 regular channels and similarly named. These are the 12 cutaneous regions, the 12 channel sinews, and the 12 channel divergences.

The 12 Cutaneous Regions

The 12 cutaneous regions are the most superficial of the channel pathways and divide the surface of the body into 12 segments. Their distribution follows the course of the regular channels; however, their pathway is distributed entirely over the body surface. They do not distribute interiorly, and they have no starting or terminating points and no directional flow. These are very broad pathways that cover a much larger area than any of the other channel pathways.

The cutaneous regions function to circulate defense qi and blood to the body surface, regulate the function of the skin and pores, and strengthen the body's resistance to disease and injury. All of these functions are related to the functions of the lung system. Thus, if the lung system is functioning well, then the cutaneous regions are well nourished, and there is sufficient defense qi on the surface of the body to keep the pores regulated and prevent the loss of qi through sweat or the invasion of an evil into the body.

Although specific descriptions of pathology of the 12 cutaneous regions do not exist, clinically skin disorders (rashes, discolorations, growths) may indicate a disorder of the related regular channel or organ. Channel obstruction manifesting as specific pain conditions can also show signs in the cutaneous regions. In addition, a patient who is susceptible to colds or who feels easily chilled on the exterior of the body might be showing signs of an insufficiency of defense qi circulating in the cutaneous regions.

The cutaneous regions also remind us that, although there is better or worse channel stimulation and more and less accurate point location, no place exists on the body at which a needle is not providing some degree of stimulation to associated organs or channels. Acupuncture points may be very specific in their locations, but the body as described by classical acupuncture theory is not a switchboard or a wiring diagram. Specificity in location of points is necessary when needling so as to obtain qi in the regular channel. But a stimulus can still be provided to the channel even when the site of stimulation is not exact. In fact, several techniques have been developed to treat the cutaneous channels and to stimulate broader areas. Some of these are gua sha, plum blossom or seven-star needling, moxibustion, cupping, shiatsu, and tui na.

The 12 Channel Sinews

The channel sinews are also relatively superficial channels, although somewhat deeper than the cutaneous regions. They follow approximately the same pathways as the regular channels with which they share their names; however, they do not travel internally at all. They are called "channel sinews" because they travel across the sinews, which include what we refer to as muscles, tendons, and ligaments. The channel sinews all branch off from the regular channels at the tips of the fingers or toes, then travel upward and inward across the body.

As surface channels, the channel sinews are said to contain only defense qi, and thus, like the cutaneous regions, they defend the body against the invasion of evils. If the defense qi in the channel sinews is overcome by the invasion of evil qi from the exterior, it may travel down the channel sinew to the tips of the fingers, where the channel sinews meet the regular channels, and from there enter the regular channels and travel internally.

For example, often when one is first catching a cold, one might experience pain, stiffness, or discomfort in the neck and shoulders. This muscular discomfort is indicative of the presence of a cold evil lodged in the channel sinews of the urinary bladder and small intestine channels. The presence of this evil may simply lead to a common cold. However, if the evil is able to invade into the urinary bladder or small intestine regular channel, and from there progress to the organ, then, in addition to the cold, the patient may develop signs such as scanty, dark urine and short or even painful urination: signs of a urinary tract infection. Thus, it is always best to treat signs of dysfunction in the channel sinews early, before the dysfunction progresses to more serious or complicated conditions.

In addition, the channel sinews supplement the regular channels by emphasizing the circulation of qi and blood to the muscles, tissues, joints, and body surface. They connect the muscles, tendons, and ligaments to the joints; link the structures of the body; and facilitate articulation and normal movement as well as protecting the bones.

The 12 channel sinews may reflect symptomatology of their associated organs, but in general, pathology in these channels will manifest as impediment patterns (associated with pain from obstruction of qi and blood and seen in conditions such as osteoarthritis), trauma, muscle strain due to overuse, or muscle tension and contraction, which may be caused by long-standing emotional or physical stressors. The primary symptom of all of these pathologies is pain. Whether the condition is replete or vacuous is determined by the presentation. Repletion conditions present with muscle spasms or contracture, edema, inflammation, and relatively sharp or severe pain, especially with light pressure. Vacuity conditions manifest with atony, dull pain or numbness that is often very deep and elicited with deep pressure, a lack of skin tone, poor motor control, and paleness or coldness of the skin.

Because the 12 channel sinews do not have their own points, it is necessary to use points on the associated regular channel or to think about other types of points. *Ah shi* ("That's it!") points are frequently needled to release the stagnation of qi and blood in the sinew channels. Ah shi points are essentially points that are tender and painful to the touch and are located by palpation. In addition to being clearly sensitive to the patient when palpated, these points are also identifiable to the practitioner by their distinct qualities (tension, stiffness, contraction) on palpation. Ah shi points may be located on or off the regular channels and are frequently found some distance from established acupuncture points. The concept of a "trigger point" used in the West since the 1960s has a great deal of similarity to the ah shi point, which formally emerged in Chinese medical thought around the seventh century AD. Cutaneous stimulation is also useful. The points located on the tips of the fingers and toes (the well points) as well as other points that are local, adjacent, and distal to the site of pain may be used. To effectively course a channel sinew, one might choose to use the first and last points on the associated regular channel pathways along with other points.

The 12 Channel Divergences

Channel divergence is a general term for 12 major branches of the 12 regular channels. These channels are distributed inside the body and have no points of their own. They are called "divergences" because they break off or diverge from the regular pathway and conduct qi and blood to different areas of the body. These channels make important internal linkages that may not be made by the primary channels and so serve to explain the actions and indications of many of the channel points.

TABLE 29-4 *Comparison of the Various Parts of the Channel System*

	12 Regular channels	12 Cutaneous regions	12 Channel sinews	12 Channel divergences
Pathways	Bilateral Internal and external pathways Have points to access qi	Bilateral Mostly superficial Divide the body into 12 broad regions	Bilateral Superficial, follow the regular channels but broader, cover muscle areas	Bilateral Travel from the limbs to the interior of the body and the head
Flow of qi	From chest to hand, hand to head, head to foot, foot to abdomen/chest	Nondirectional	From tips of fingers/toes inward along regular channel pathway	From elbows/knees, internally and then up to head
Functions	Transport Regulate Protect and aid diagnosis Treat Integrate	Circulate defense qi and blood to the body surface Regulate the function of the skin and pores Strengthen immunity	Defend the body against evils Supplement the regular channels' circulation of qi and blood to the muscles, tissues, joints, and body surface	Supply defense qi to the viscera and bowels Act as a secondary line of defense against the invasion of evil Strengthen the connection channels and organs Integrate areas of the body that are not covered by the main pathways
Pathology	Varied	Skin disorders (rashes, discolorations, growths)	Pain Symptoms reflecting symptomatology of associated organ	No clear description of pathology; symptoms are often intermittent or cyclic and one-sided
Treatment	Acupuncture points	Gua sha, plum blossom or seven-star needling, moxibustion, cupping, shiatsu, tui na	Ah shi ("That's It!") points Cutaneous stimulation First and last channel points	Regular channel points Diverging and merging points

The 12 channel divergences separate from the regular channel at a relatively superficial level of the body, usually at a spot near the elbow or knee joints. The yin and yang internally–externally related pair then merge together and enter the chest and abdomen to travel to the viscera and bowels. Together, they emerge from the body cavity at the neck or head, and finally merge with the regular yang channel of a yin-yang pair.

Like the channel sinews, the channel divergences run from the extremities to the trunk, face, and head, with the exception of the triple burner channel divergence, which runs from the vertex of the head down the body to the middle burner. Like the cutaneous regions and channel sinews, the 12 channel divergences contain only defense qi.

The channel divergences have three major functions: (1) they supply defense qi to the viscera and bowels and act as a secondary line of defense against the invasion of evil; (2) they strengthen the connection between organs and channels; and (3) they integrate areas of the body that are not covered by the main pathways.

Although the channel divergences are mentioned in the *Inner Classic*, there is no clear description of channel divergence pathology. Generally, the channel divergences are thought to share the same pathologies as the regular channels. However, when disease has entered the channel divergences, the symptoms produced are often intermittent or cyclic and one-sided. Divergent channel symptoms are produced by the pathogen's encounter with the defense qi, and thus as the defense qi waxes and wanes in flow, there will be an exacerbation or amelioration of symptoms. The point where the divergent channels separate from the regular channel and the point where they merge with the regular yang channel are the most important points for treatment of divergent channel pathology (Table 29-4).

The Eight Extraordinary Vessels

Although often discussed as an entirely different category of channels, the eight extraordinary vessels actually are a part of the general channel system. They are "extraordinary" because they do not fit the pattern of the other major channels. There are two primary differences between the eight extraordinary vessels and the 12 regular channels:

1. The eight extraordinary vessels do not have a continuous, interlinking pattern of circulation. In other words, although they have connections with each other and with the 12 major channels, they do not link one to the next as do the 12 regular channels.

2. The eight extraordinary vessels are not each associated with a specific organ system as are the 12 regular channels. Rather, the eight extraordinary vessels are associated with specific types of disorders based on their location and functions.

The eight extraordinary vessels function as reservoirs of qi and blood. They fill and empty in response to changing conditions and pathologies of the regular channels or of the organ systems, and they exert a regulating effect on the regular channels. All of the eight extraordinary vessels are considered to be very closely related to the functions of the liver and kidney systems and also to the functioning of the uterus and the brain (Table 29-5).

The basic functions of the eight extraordinary vessels are:

- To provide additional interconnections among the major channels and the organ systems and
- To regulate the flow of qi and blood in the regular channels. Surplus qi or blood from the regular channels may be stored in the eight extraordinary vessels and released when required.

Like the regular channels, each of the eight extraordinary vessels has its own distinct pathway. However, only two of the eight extraordinary vessels (the controlling vessel and the governing vessel) have acupuncture points. These two channels traverse the midline of the body, and the functions of their points are often associated with the functions of the organs lying in proximity to them.

Not only are specific points located on the controlling and governing vessels, but all of the eight extraordinary vessels are closely associated with a specific point on one of the 12 regular channels. This point, called a "confluent point," is used to access the qi and blood of the extraordinary vessel and make it available for use by the organ systems. Clinically, each of the eight extraordinary vessels is paired with another, which makes four couplets. Typically, when the confluent point on one channel is used, the confluent point of its paired channel is also used.

The Network Vessels

As discussed earlier, there are two types of major pathways in the body. All of the various types of channels have already been reviewed. The other major pathways are the network vessels. These are branches of the channels; however, they also have their own functions and pathologies. They connect interiorly-exteriorly related organs and they connect channels. Like the regular channels, the network vessels are bilateral, but they travel in all directions and are relatively superficial. As a general function, with the rest of the channel system, the network vessels form a network of pathways that integrate the entire body and distribute qi and blood, especially to the surface of the body.

There are two types of network vessels: (1) the network divergences; and (2) the superficial network vessels, also called the "grandchild network vessels" or the "blood network vessels." The network divergences can also be divided into two subcategories, the undefined or transverse network vessels, which connect an interiorly-exteriorly related channel pair, and the defined or longitudinal network vessels, which separate from the regular channels and have their own specific symptomatology.

Network divergences According to the *Inner Classic,* the undefined and the defined network vessels are one vessel with multiple pathways. However, their pathways are sufficiently distinct, and the functions and related symptomatologies different enough, that it is useful to separate them for discussion.

There are 12 undefined network vessels. These pathways are not definitively mapped, but they run from the network point on each channel to its interiorly-exteriorly related channel. Thus, the lung network vessel breaks off from the lung network point and travels to the large intestine channel, and the large intestine network vessel breaks off from the large intestine network point and travels to the lung channel. Clinically, through the use of these network vessels and the associated network and source points of the channels, the qi and blood in a channel can be balanced or harmonized. Essentially, these rather short pathways serve as a direct connection between the yin and yang channels of an internally-externally related pair. This direct connection through the network vessels strengthens the relationship between internally-externally related channels. Through a "source-network point" treatment, replete qi in one channel of a pair can be drained into the other, or a vacuity of qi in one channel of a pair can be supplemented through the use of the qi of its pair.

There are 16 defined network divergences, 1 for each of the 12 regular channels, 1 for the governing vessel, and 1 for the controlling vessel, as well as the great network of the spleen and the great network of the stomach. As with the undefined network vessels, these vessels break off from the network points of their named channels. Often, acupuncturists will forget about or be unaware of the pathways or symptomatology of the defined network divergences. However, awareness of these pathways and their associated symptoms can aid the acupuncturist in determining appropriate treatment. The defined network divergences are treated using the network point of the affected channel.

Grandchild network vessels The grandchild network vessels, also called the "superficial network vessels," are the small branches of the network divergences that appear on the surface of the skin. These are small veins and venules. Should these superficial network vessels change in color and become dark or stagnant, or should there be another need to treat them, a technique called "network vessel pricking" is used. In this method, a three-edged needle is used to prick the superficial network vessels and release blood.

Summing Up Channel Theory

If there is any single major misconception concerning acupuncture theory in the West, it is that acupuncture is

TABLE 29-5 *Eight Extraordinary Vessels*

Extraordinary vessel	Functions of the extraordinary vessel	Common clinical conditions indicating disharmony of the extraordinary vessel
Governing Vessel Confluent point: SI3 Paired vessel: yang springing	Sea of the yang channels Regulates all yang channels Sea of marrow Homes to the brain Reflects physiology and pathology of the brain and the spinal fluid	Pain and stiffness in the back, heavy-headedness, hemorrhoids, infertility, malaria, mental disorders Points along the channel influence areas and organs of the body located near the point
Controlling Vessel Confluent point: LU7 Paired vessel: yin springing	Sea of yin channels Regulates all yin channels Regulates menstruation and nurtures the fetus	Menstrual irregularities, menstrual block, miscarriage, infertility, enuresis, abdominal masses Points along the channel influence areas and organs of the body located near the point.
Penetrating Vessel Confluent point: SP4 Paired vessel: yin linking	Sea of the regular channels Regulates the 12 regular channels Sea of blood Regulates menstruation	Women: Uterine bleeding, miscarriage, menstrual block, menstrual irregularities, scant breast milk, lower abdominal pain, facial hair Men: Seminal emission, impotence, prostatitis, urethritis, orchitis
Girdling Vessel Confluent point: GB41 Paired vessel: yang linking	Binds all the channels running up and down the trunk Regulates the balance between upward and downward flow of qi Wraps around the body; the only channel to not travel vertically up and down the body	Vaginal discharge, prolapse of the uterus, abdominal distention and fullness, limpness, weakness or pain in the low back
Yang Springing Vessel Confluent point: UB62 Paired vessel: governing	Control opening and closing of the eyes Control the ascent of fluids and the descent of qi Balance the yin and yang qi of the body Balance gait and movement of the legs	Eye problems, insomnia, muscle spasms along the lateral aspect of the lower leg with flaccidity on the medial aspect
Yin Springing Vessel Confluent point: KI6 Paired channel: controlling	Control opening and closing of the eyes Control the ascent of fluids and the descent of qi Balance the yin and yang qi of the body Balance gait and movement of the legs	Eye problems, somnolence, lower abdominal or genital pain, muscle spasms along the medial aspect of the lower leg with flaccidity on the lateral aspect
Yang Linking Vessel Confluent point: SJ5 Paired channel: girdling	Unites all the major yang channels Compensates for superabundance or insufficiency in channel circulation Regulates yang channel activity Governs the exterior of the body	Exterior invasion, especially of heat
Yin Linking Vessel Confluent point: PC6 Paired channel: penetrating/chong	Unites all the major yin channels Regulates yin channel activity Governs the interior of the body Balances the emotions	Used for many different internal conditions

GB, Gallbladder; KI, kidney; LU, lung; PC, pericardium; SI, small intestine; SJ, triple burner (san jiao); SP, spleen; UB, urinary bladder.
Adapted from Ellis A, Wiseman N, Boss, K: *Fundamentals of Chinese acupuncture*, Brookline, Mass, 1991, Paradigm; Wiseman, 1998; Ni, 1996.

primarily about the points, the location where a needle or other therapeutic tool is applied. Perhaps because points are the locus of therapeutic action, they figure prominently in the mind of the Westerner encountering acupuncture. Channels and networks are, however, the complex substrate that organizes and provides meaning to acupuncture points. As we have seen, channel theory is rich and complex, although very often completely ignored when the West encounters acupuncture. It may be that the early translation of the terms *channels* and *networks* as "meridians" and *holes* as "points" provided the sense that both were imaginary constructs inscribed on the surface of the body and, as such, only vague and imaginary markings engraved on an anatomically established body. However, channels and holes are tangible entities and the objects of vivid experience as documented in the classical texts of acupuncture. Although there is no reason to privilege them as a form of distinct or alternate anatomy, it is unwise, if we wish to understand acupuncture as an object of clinical and scientific inquiry, to ignore them as merely abstractions.

The acupuncture point or hole is where the classics tell us we can touch and influence the qi, blood, and spirit of the patient. Why and where we would wish to do this is guided entirely by channel theory and the characteristics of the holes themselves.

ACUPUNCTURE POINT CATEGORIES, GROUPINGS, AND ASSOCIATIONS

Just as the specific pathway of each of the channels and networks discussed earlier is well beyond the scope of this chapter, so is an exhaustive discussion of individual acupuncture points. There are some 361 acupuncture points associated with the 12 regular channels and the governing and controlling vessels. In addition, there are numerous extra points, special reflex system points, and ah shi points. As we have discussed, an acupuncture point can best be considered as a hole where qi and blood can be manipulated in relation to a channel, organ, or body region. Historically the locations of acupuncture points have been described with varying degrees of precision and accuracy depending on the ease of fixing their locations by means of anatomical landmarks or measurement methods. Opinions about these have varied to some extent in the classics. Over the last half-century, efforts of the State Administration of TCM in China, the World Health Organization (WHO), and other bodies have been devoted to determining standard reference locations. However, the existence of standard locations should not negate the opinions of various traditions of practice or clinicians, because, in the end, the location of an acupuncture point is established by its ability to summon qi, to influence the body, and to cure illness. In some instances, precise location of acupuncture points in terms of anatomy and measurement is critical; in others, the dynamics of the response of the point to touch, the presence of qi, is the determining factor in establishing location.

Altogether, the points or holes on the 12 regular channels and on the governing and controlling vessels of the eight extraordinary vessels total 361.

12 Regular Channels (listed in order of the flow of qi)
   Lung channel: 11 points
   Large intestine channel: 20 points
   Stomach channel: 45 points
   Spleen channel: 21 points
   Heart channel: 9 points
   Small intestine channel: 19 points
   Urinary bladder channel: 67 points
   Kidney channel: 27 points
   Pericardium channel: 9 points
   Triple burner channel: 23 points
   Gallbladder channel: 44 points
   Liver channel: 14 points
Extraordinary Vessels:
   Governing vessel: 28 points
   Controlling vessel: 24 points

As we shall see later, many points belong to special point groupings that help to define their clinical efficacy. However, generalizations can also be made about points on specific channels or groups of channels. So, for example, points on the three hand yin channels all treat disorders of the chest, but on each individual channel the points treat signs and symptoms associated with the organ for which the channel is named (Table 29-6).

Special Point Categories and Groups

One of the most important parts of the acupuncture treatment planning process is to understand the clinical significance of special group points. Every individual point has specific functions and is able to help treat specific symptoms or conditions. Many points also belong to special groups. Membership in a special group helps to define the functions of a given point. A summary of the more commonly used special groups can be found in Table 29-7. Points that belong to special groups tend to be used more commonly than many other points. A good working knowledge of what these special groups are, what points belong in each group, and how that group affects a point's function is essential to designing clear, well-delineated point prescriptions. In the following sections a few of the special groups are described in detail to help the reader to understand their importance.

Five transport points (five-phase points) Perhaps the most powerful and certainly the most commonly used points on the body are the transport points. These points, located on the arms and legs below the elbow or knee, are associated with the five phases. Beginning at the tip of the finger or toe and moving up to the elbow or knee are five points on each channel that are associated with the five phases, for a total of 80 points. The five points are the jing-well, ying-spring, shu-stream, jing-river, and he-uniting (sea) points. The category name for each of these points is

TABLE 29-6 *Clinical Applications of Major Points on the Four Limbs*

Channel categorization	Channel/organ name	General clinical applications	Specific system clinical applications
Three hand yin channels	Lung	Chest disorders	Respiratory conditions, throat, nose, exterior patterns
	Pericardium		Mental-emotional conditions, heart conditions, stomach distress (nausea, vomiting)
	Heart		Mental-emotional conditions, heart conditions (angina, palpitations, etc.), eye conditions
Three hand yang channels	Large intestine	Face, head, sense organs, febrile diseases	Front of the face and head, including frontal headaches, nasal congestion, tooth pain, sores on the gums
	Small intestine		Occipital headaches, neck soreness, stiffness and pain, scapular pain
	Triple burner		Temporal headaches, earaches, ear congestion, pain, swelling or discomfort on the sides of the head or face, pain in the hypochondriac region
Three foot yin channels	Spleen	Urogenital, abdomen, and chest disorders	Digestive disorders such as nausea, poor appetite, loose stools
	Kidney		Urinary disorders such as incontinence, infertility conditions
	Liver		Liver and gallbladder conditions such as insomnia, anger, menstrual irregularities, genital sores or itching
Three foot yang channels	Stomach	Mental disorders, febrile diseases, eye problems	Pain on the frontal aspect of the face or head, acne, acid reflux, mania
	Urinary bladder Pain in the occipital area or nape, back, and lumbus; urinary problems such as incontinence, dysuria		
	Gallbladder		Temporal headaches, migraine headaches; pain or discomfort of the side of the head and face, hypochondriac region, or hip

Adapted from Ellis A, Wiseman N, Boss, K: *Fundamentals of Chinese acupuncture,* Brookline, Mass, 1991, Paradigm, p 57.

associated with the flow of water, which is used as a metaphor for the flow of qi through the body and for the depth of the qi at these points. The qi flows from the well points, on the tips of the fingers and toes (the tips of the mountains), where the qi is said to be "shallow and meek," to the next proximal point, the spring, where the qi has a "gushing quality." From the spring, the qi travels to the stream points, where the flow pours from shallow to deep. From the stream, flow continues to the river, where the force becomes more powerful and the qi is found at a deeper level. Finally, the qi reaches the uniting (sea) points at the knees and elbows. At the uniting points, the qi unites with its home organ, just as a river reaches its final destination, the sea. The names of the points describe the nature of the qi at each of the points. This description of the nature of the qi is not the same as the directional flow of qi through the channels.

There are two major ways in which these points are used clinically and which inform point selection.

In the *Classic of Difficult Issues,* the points that held membership in each of these point categories were identified as being especially effective in treating certain types of conditions (Table 29-8). Thus, the appropriate point on a given channel might be selected to treat the corresponding condition manifesting in a particular organ.

These points are also frequently selected according to their five-phase correspondences (see Table 29-8). Each of the transport points is related to a specific phase (as is the organ of the channel on which the points lie). These relationships are used in theory-based treatment models that, when taken to their fullest extreme, can become quite complex.

Using the five-phase organizational scheme, on a basic level vacuity conditions are treated by supplementing the

TABLE 29-7 *Point Categories*

Category	Description of point category
Source points	Called "source points" because these are points at which the source qi of the associated organ collects. There is one source point for each channel. The source qi is stored by the kidneys and spread throughout the body by the triple burner. Used to promote the flow of source qi and regulate the function of the internal organs. Often used in a treatment that entails the appropriate draining or supplementing of the source and the network point to treat simultaneously affected internally–externally related channels.
Network (luo) points	The site on a channel where the network vessel splits from the regular channel. There are 16 of these points: one for each regular channel, one on the controlling vessel, one on the governing vessel, and one each for the great luo of the spleen and the great luo of the stomach. Used to treat interiorly–exteriorly related organs and the specific symptomatology of the defined network vessel. Frequently, these points are combined with source points to treat internally–externally related channels.
Eight meeting (influential) points	Each of the eight points is associated with a specific substance or tissue. The substances with which the points are associated include qi, blood, viscera, bowels, sinews, marrow, bones, and vessels. These are very general points and can treat any aspect of disharmony in their related tissue or substance. They are generally combined with other points to increase their specificity.
Four command points	These points are especially effective in treating disorders located in a particular anatomical area of the body. Each point is associated with a specific area of the body. The areas covered are the abdomen, the back, the head and back of the neck, and the face and mouth. Whenever one of these areas is involved in a patient's complaint, it would be appropriate to use the command point for that area.
Eight confluent points	Each of the eight extraordinary channels has a single point on one of the 12 regular channels that is said to be confluent with the associated extraordinary channel and to open or access that channel (see discussion in "The Eight Extraordinary Vessels").
Cleft points	As qi and blood circulate through the channels, they accumulate in the cleft points. Palpation and observation of these points can indicate repletion or vacuity in the channel. Sharp or intense pain on pressure or redness and swelling indicates repletion, and dull or mild pain or a depression indicates vacuity. They are used for both stubborn and acute conditions. They are also thought to be good for the treatment of bleeding conditions associated with the organ.
Ma Dan Yang's 12 heavenly star points	These are 12 points that Song dynasty physician Ma Dan Yang considered to be extremely useful. The points were compiled into song form by his students to be passed down through the generations. The 12 points are not used together. Among the 12 points are many that that belong to other point categories and so are generally recognized as very useful.
Window of heaven points	A list of 10 points first mentioned in the *Inner Classic (Nei Jing)*. They were never well explicated, and all but two of the points are located on the neck. Analysis of the points and their actions indicates that they seem to be useful for treating conditions that manifest primarily in the head or the sense organs but are the result of a disharmony of the movement of qi between the head and the body.
Nine needles for returning yang	A set of nine points that, when needled together, are indicated for yang desertion manifesting as loss of consciousness, generalized cold, counterflow cold of the limbs, cyanosis, etc.
13 Ghost points	Thirteen points compiled by the seventh-century physician and ethicist Sun Si Miao for the treatment of mental conditions. The original names of the points all contained the character *gui* (鬼), which means ghost or demon.
Points of the four seas	The four seas, first described in the *Inner Classic,* are the sea of qi, the sea of blood, the sea of water and grain, and the sea of marrow. There are several points that are directly associated with one of the four seas and are thought to be especially useful for treatment of disorders of the particular sea.
Extra points	Extra points, also called "new" points, are points that have specific locations but are not a part of the channel and network system. This category of points continues to grow as more points are found with specific uses.
Crossing points or intersection points	These are points where two or three channels meet. Because channels meet here, these points have a strong therapeutic effect on any of the channels that cross. Use of these points can eliminate the need to use multiple points when more than one channel is affected.
Ah shi ("That's it!") points	These are nonspecific points on the body that are particularly sensitive to palpation. There is no defined location for these points, they are simply tender spots that are most often used to treat disorders in their immediate vicinity.

TABLE 29-8 *Nature and Location of the Transport Points and Their Classical Clinical Actions*

Point location	Point category	Phase relationship on a yin channel	Phase relationship on a yang channel	Representation of qi	Classical clinical actions
Near the end of finger or toe	Jing-well	Wood	Metal	Shallow and meek	Revive clouded spirit Clear heat
Second most distal point on the channel	Ying-spring	Fire	Water	Like a small spring with somewhat more force	Treat externally contracted heat conditions
Usually the third most distal point on the channel	Shu-stream	Earth	Wood	Pouring down from a shallow place to a deeper one	Treat pain in the joints
On the wrists or ankles	Jing-river	Metal	Fire	Free flowing like the water in a river	Treat cough and panting
At the elbow or knee	He-uniting (sea)	Water	Earth	Large and deep as it unites with the organ of the home channel	Correct bowel patterns

mother of the affected channel/organ, and repletion conditions are addressed by draining the child of the affected channel/organ. Thus, if there is a vacuity in the fire phase, then the mother point on the fire channel might be supplemented (the wood point on the heart channel). In addition, one can supplement the same-phase points on the mother channel (wood point on the liver channel).

Alternatively, if there is a repletion condition in the fire phase, then one could drain the child point on the fire channel (the earth point on the heart channel) or the same-phase point on the child channel (the earth point on the spleen channel).

Some classic point selection texts discuss variants of these techniques, originally suggested by the theoretical discussions in the *Classic of Difficult Issues*. These approaches became very popular in the 1930s and again in the 1950s when there was a revival of interest, especially in Japan, in the acupuncture theories of the *Classic of Difficult Issues*. Contemporary schools of clinical thought in Japan, such as *"meridian therapy,"* use transport points extensively based on a five-phase paradigm. This approach to acupuncture point selection is also practiced in Korea (notably in the Korean *four-point method*) and elaborated in China with the *six-point method*. Essentially, the theory is that if a particular phase is vacuous or replete, then the relationships of the engendering and restraining cycles can be used to supplement or drain the affected phase as needed.

For example, a patient comes for treatment with loose stools and nausea that are exacerbated by stress. One might diagnose this as spleen qi vacuity with the liver overacting on the spleen. First, one would focus on supplementing the spleen by supplementing the mother point on the affected channel, the spleen channel. The spleen is associated with earth, thus its mother would be fire. This means that the fire point (the ying-spring point) on the spleen channel would be supplemented. In addition, the fire point on the fire channel would be supplemented. This would be the ying-spring point on the heart channel. Taken further, one would drain the controlling phase on the affected channel, which in this case would be the wood point (the jing-well point) on the spleen channel and drain the wood point on the controlling channel or the jing-well point on the liver channel. (See Table 29-9 for a summary of the Korean four-point and Chinese six-point treatments.)

Five-phase approaches to treatment have had a substantial influence on some portions of the English and American acupuncture communities through the work of J.R. Worsley. Worsley's studies with exponents of meridian therapy led him to develop an approach to acupuncture diagnosis and treatment based almost exclusively on five-phase correspondences and the use of phase-associated transport points.

The use of the five-phase points in point selection entails a much more complex theoretical structure and understanding than is needed for use of most of the other point categories. The *Classic of Difficult Issues* discusses the alarm mu points and the back transport points together in the 67th difficult issue. Frequently the alarm mu and the back transport points will be used together in treatment or they will be used in alternate treatments.

Alarm mu points Alarm mu points are points on the chest and abdomen where qi collects. There is 1 alarm point associated with and named for each of the 12 organs. These points may be palpated for tenderness, lumps, gatherings, depressions, and so forth, and also used to treat their associated organs. If, for example, a patient were to have either diarrhea or constipation, the practitioner would be likely to palpate and probably use the alarm point of the large intestine, which is located on the stomach channel, just lateral to the umbilicus. All of the alarm points are located in close proximity to the organ with which they are associated, but generally not on the channel associated with that organ. In fact, many of the alarm points are located on the controlling vessel, because that channel crosses over the

TABLE 29-9 *Korean Four-Point and Chinese Six-Point Treatment Strategy*

Vacuity Conditions

Korean four point	Supplement the mother point on the channel of the affected organ
	Supplement the phase point on the mother channel
	Drain the controlling phase point (the grandmother point) on the affected organ's channel
	Drain the phase point on the controlling phase (the grandmother channel)
Chinese six point	Drain the phase controlled by the affected phase (the grandchild point) on the channel of the affected organ
	Drain the phase point on the channel controlled by the affected phase (the grandchild channel)

Repletion Conditions

Korean four point	Drain the child of the affected phase on the channel of the affected organ
	Drain the phase point on the child channel of the affected organ
	Supplement the phase point on the channel that controls the affected organ (the grandmother channel)
	Supplement the control point (the grandmother point) on the channel of the affected organ
Chinese six point	Supplement the phase controlled by the affected phase (the grandchild point) on the channel of the affected organ
	Supplement the phase point on the channel controlled by the affected phase (the grandchild channel)

entire abdomen and chest, passing through many of the organs.

Back transport points Back transport points are points that are all located on the urinary bladder channel, lateral to the spine. There is one back transport point for each organ, and the qi of that organ runs through the point. In addition, there are back transport points for the governing vessel, for the diaphragm, for the sea of qi, and for other concepts in Chinese medicine. These points are regulating points, so they can be used to treat vacuity or repletion in the associated organ. Back transport points are frequently combined with alarm mu points to treat diseases of the viscera and bowels.

As noted earlier, a good working knowledge of what the point categories are, what points belong in each category, and how that category influences a point's function is essential to designing clear, well-delineated point prescriptions. Without this knowledge it is difficult to design a point prescription that will effectively and efficiently treat the presenting condition. This underscores the importance of a thorough understanding of the channel and network

theory and of point theory for the practitioner. Without it, one begins to practice acupuncture as simply a technique that is not associated with a specific medical paradigm rather than as a part of a larger medical system that works best when used within its defined paradigm.

ACUPUNCTURE TREATMENT PLANNING

The classical Chinese therapeutic goal of acupuncture is to regulate qi and blood. Qi and blood flow through the body, its organs, and the channel pathways. When they flow freely, the body is healthy. When some cause, such as an evil, an emotion, trauma, and so on, disrupts the flow of qi or blood, illness or pain can result. Or, if the body does not have enough qi or blood, then symptoms such as fatigue, poor appetite, and so on, may appear. Acupuncture may be used to remove evils, to direct qi to where it is insufficient, to move obstructions and allow qi to flow, or to boost the functions of organs to produce more qi or blood.

Today, stimulation of acupuncture points is accomplished using a wide variety of tools and methods, but the most common is the filiform needle. The needle itself can vary significantly in structure, diameter, and length.

A typical acupuncture needle has a shaft that is 1 to 1.5 inches (25.4 to 38.1 mm) long and a handle of approximately 1 inch. The distinctive part of the needle is the tip, which is round and moderately sharp, much like the tip of a pine needle. The acupuncture needle is solid and gently tapered; it does not have the lumen or cutting edge of the hypodermic needle. The length of an acupuncture needle can vary from as little as 0.25 inch (6.4 mm) for very specialized applications to as much as 7 inches (17.8 cm). The shortest typical length is 0.5 inch (12.7 mm) for use in auricular acupuncture. Needles may be as long as 7 inches or more for transverse or very deep needle insertion. Typical long needles are about 5 inches (12.7 cm) for deep insertion at points in the gluteal region.

The diameter of the acupuncture needle can range from as little as 0.12 mm to as much as 0.46 mm. Typically needles used for medium (0.25 to 1 inch), deep, and very deep insertive techniques range from about 0.22 mm to 0.46 mm, whereas needles used for shallow and minimally insertive techniques (often seen in certain Japanese styles) are in the 0.12- to 0.20-mm range. The diameter most commonly used by American practitioners of medium and deep insertion is 0.25 mm (Figures 29-2 and 29-3).

From a classical and modern Chinese acupuncture point of view, the aim of the acupuncturist is to obtain qi at the site of insertion. The obtaining of qi may be seen or felt by the practitioner, the patient, or both parties. The practitioner seeks either an objective or subjective indication that the qi has arrived. The arrival of qi may be experienced by the practitioner as sensations felt by the hands as the needle is manipulated or through observation of color changes or of skin appearance at the site of insertion. The sensation of the arrival of qi often is felt by the practitioner as a gentle grasping of the needle at the site, as if one is fishing and one's line has suddenly been seized by the fish.

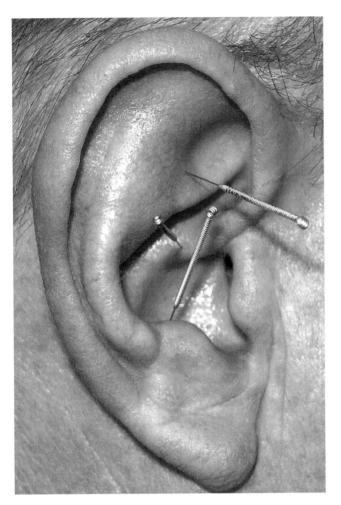

Figure 29-2 Example of ear acupuncture. (From Oleson T: *Auriculotherapy manual: Chinese and Western systems of ear acupuncture,* ed 3, Edinburgh, 2003, Churchill Livingstone.)

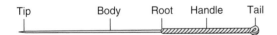

Figure 29-3 The structure of the filiform needle. (From Qiu ML: *Chinese acupuncture and moxibustion,* Edinburgh, 1993, Churchill Livingstone.)

The patient may feel the arrival of qi as a sensation of itching, numbness, soreness, or a swollen or distended feeling, or the patient might experience local temperature changes or an "electrical" sensation. Sometimes, the patient may not have any sensation, but the practitioner will be aware that qi has arrived, or the patient may be aware of the arrival of qi before the practitioner. Although the sensation or observation of the arrival of qi is not absolutely necessary for a successful treatment, it is considered to be one of the goals of traditional needling styles.

Perspectives on qi arrival, its signs and significance, and detection of qi by the practitioner, patient, or both can vary with the tradition of practice. In some styles of practice emerging out of the Japanese tradition, insertion of the

needle is very minimal (or nonexistent) and the arrival of qi is to be detected by the clinician and not experienced by the patient, at least not as a distinct local sensation.

For the purposes of this section, acupuncture techniques are presented from a primarily Chinese perspective. Although many of the concepts and practices described apply to other traditions, schools, or styles, there may be variations from what is presented here.

When a site for insertion has been determined, the needle is rapidly inserted and then adjusted to an appropriate depth. Many considerations will alter the angle and depth of insertion, methods of manipulation, and length of retention. A twelfth-century text, *Ode of the Subtleties of Flow,* states, "Insert the needle with noble speed then proceed (to the point) slowly, withdraw the needle with noble slowness as haste will cause injury" (Shanghai College of Traditional Chinese Medicine, 1981).

Once a point has been needled and qi obtained, the practitioner may manipulate the needle to achieve a specific therapeutic effect. Methods of manipulation range from simply inserting the needle and leaving it, to using techniques that involve slow or rapid insertion, to performing deeper or shallower insertions. Rotation of the needle will influence the therapeutic effect, as will other, more complex manipulations. The needle may be withdrawn immediately after qi arrives or may be retained for 20 to 30 minutes, or a very short, fine needle (known as an *intradermal*) may be retained for several days. In all cases, the goal of the clinician is to influence the flow or production of qi.

Practitioners use different methods to select acupuncture points for a particular patient or condition. Points may be chosen on the basis of the trajectory of the channel on which they lie, on the basis of membership in a particular traditional point category, or through an empirical understanding of what points work best for a given condition, based on the experience of generations of practitioners. Points may also be selected based on sensitivity to palpation or changes in texture that are perceived by the practitioner. Each of these methods gives the practitioner information about a particular point and should be considered when creating a treatment plan (Box 29-1).

To correctly determine the appropriate points to be used in treatment, a correct Chinese medicine diagnosis must be reached, using the methods discussed in Chapter 28. Some practitioners will choose points to treat the presenting symptoms of a specific biomedical condition. Although these points may give some symptomatic relief of the condition, they generally will not treat the root cause of the symptoms, and thus the condition will not be resolved. For example, if a patient comes for treatment of chronic low back pain, there are many points that might be chosen to treat the pain. However, there are several different possible Chinese medicine diagnoses for low back pain. If the practitioner does not concern himself or herself with the diagnosis, the techniques employed and even some of the points used to "treat" the low back pain at best

BOX 29-1 *Acupuncture Treatment Planning in Chinese Medicine*

A. Point matching: determining a large set of potentially appropriate points
   1. Diagnosis
   2. Treatment principle and method
   3. Matching of points to fulfill the treatment principle based on:
      a. Channel theory and channel pathways
      b. Areas of effect
      c. Special group points
      d. Pathology-condition points
B. Point selection: creating specific treatment plans
   1. Address tip and root
   2. Ensure balance
      a. Yin and yang channels
      b. Front and back of the body
      c. Top and bottom of the body
      d. Left and right sides of the body
   3. Include local, adjacent, and distal points
   4. Determine the overall purpose of each point prescription
   5. Determine the appropriate size of a point prescription
   6. Choose appropriate adjunctive techniques
      a. Moxibustion
      b. Cupping
      c. Bleeding
      d. Plum blossom (seven-star) needling
      e. Gua sha
      f. Electroacupuncture
      g. Laser
      h. Magnets
      i. Bodywork/tui na
      j. Microsystems

might be inappropriate and at worst might worsen the condition.

Once a Chinese medicine diagnosis has been determined, the practitioner begins the process of choosing a set of points to treat the condition. The process begins with *point matching*. Point matching entails creating a large set of points (usually 20 to 40 points) that might possibly be appropriate for the given diagnosis. These points should address both the root cause of the condition and the presenting symptoms. This large set of points is chosen based on an understanding of channel theory and knowledge of the areas that different channels affect, on a clear knowledge of point categories and how points in specific categories affect areas of the body or substances in the body, on knowledge of specific channel points and how they differ, and on knowledge about empirical points that might be appropriate for a given diagnosis or condition.

Point Selection

Once the large set of points has been created, from this set two to five smaller acupuncture prescriptions are developed. This is a process called *point selection*. When creating

the smaller prescriptions, the practitioner must be mindful of additional considerations.

First, a point prescription must address both the tip and the root of the problem. For example, if a patient arrives with a chief complaint of loose stools, the practitioner must develop a point prescription that will treat the root cause of the loose stools, which might be spleen qi vacuity, kidney yang vacuity, damp heat, and so forth. The prescription should also address the presenting symptom of the loose stools. If the focus is entirely on the root, it may be that for several weeks there will be no improvement in the stools. But if the focus is entirely on the tip, the loose stools, then although there may be temporary improvement, the condition will not be fully resolved.

Second, a point prescription must be balanced. Achieving balance includes balancing points between the upper and lower portions of the body, balancing points between the left and right sides of the body, balancing points between the front and the back of the body, and balancing points between yin and yang channels. Frequently students of acupuncture will, for example, create a point prescription that consists of only yin channel points or only points on the legs with no arm points, and so on. This type of treatment may leave the patient feeling unbalanced or as if the treatment was incomplete.

Third, point selection is based on choice of local, adjacent, and distal points. For low back pain, one might choose several local points on the lower back. In addition, one would choose points near the site of the pain (e.g., in the hip, the sacrum). Finally, one would choose appropriate distal points on the four limbs. For loose stools, one might choose several local points directly over the large intestine on the abdomen, adjacent points on the upper abdomen associated with the spleen and stomach, and, again, distal points on the leg to address the root of the loose stools. This process gives a balance to the prescription and allows the qi to move or be acted upon so that it will address both the clinical problem or symptom (the tip) and its cause (the root).

Finally, the elements of function and size of the treatment must be considered. Each individual point chosen has its own functions and indications; however, the overall point prescription should also have a general function or purpose. If the cause of the low back pain is qi and blood stagnation due to trauma, then the points chosen should act together to move the qi and blood to reduce the pain and improve healing. If the cause is a kidney vacuity, then the points chosen should still move the qi, albeit more gently; however, points should also be chosen to boost the kidneys, and adjunctive techniques such as moxibustion might be appropriate. Essentially, the function of the point prescription should match the treatment principle that is determined by the diagnosis.

The number of needles being inserted is an important consideration. Some practitioners say that no more than eight needles should be inserted. Others say that about eight bilateral points (16 needles) should be used. There is no absolute rule about the number of needles used, but choosing points that might work on several aspects of treatment is often more effective than choosing points that act only on one symptom. The age, constitution, and gender of the patient should also be considered when determining the number of needles. Some treatments might require a higher number of needles, but if, for example, the patient is elderly or debilitated, use of a large number of needles could cause the patient to become extremely tired or uncomfortable. As few needles as possible should be used on children, and fewer needles are generally desirable on menstruating women.

The frequency of treatment, as well as the various techniques to be used, is also addressed when thinking about point selection. In China, a typical course of treatment is 10 treatments, which are usually given every day or every other day for 10 to 20 days, followed by a break for 10 days. Then, if necessary, treatment recommences. In the West, although 10 treatments may be considered an appropriate course of treatment, practitioners tend to treat once a week for 10 weeks. This method is probably not as effective for treating pain conditions as more frequent sessions would be. Techniques vary widely depending on the style in which the practitioner is trained, whether it be TCM, one of the many systems coming out of Japan or Korea, or one of the schools or styles developed outside of Asia.

Adjunctive Techniques

All of the techniques described in what follows are important elements of the training of an acupuncturist. Although they may or may not involve the insertion of a needle, they are all forms of stimulation that can be used over large areas of the body, over channel pathways, or over specific points to achieve a therapeutic effect. They might be used by themselves or in conjunction with acupuncture. In some traditions or schools, they have been very highly developed as specialized and independently utilized stimulation techniques, whereas in others they are used as adjunctive techniques to complement and support the acupuncture treatment. The discussion here is provided primarily from the point of view of the Chinese tradition and is necessarily very cursory.

Moxibustion Moxibustion refers to the burning of dried, powdered leaves of *Artemisia vulgaris* (*ai ye,* or mug-wort), either on or close to the skin, to affect the flow of qi in the channel. Artemisia is acrid and bitter, and it warms and enters the channels. References to warming techniques appear in very early materials, including the Ma Wang tomb texts (Unschuld, 1985). As mentioned at the beginning of this chapter, the term *zhen jiu* literally means "needle moxibustion," although in the West we typically use simply the term *acupuncture* when referring to these techniques.

Moxibustion can be applied to the body in many ways. *Direct moxibustion* involves burning a small amount of moxa (about the size of a small grain of rice) directly on the skin. The moxa can be allowed to burn down to the skin, causing a blister or scar, or it can be removed before it has burned down to the skin. This technique is used less frequently in the West than other techniques because of the scarring.

Indirect moxibustion involves putting a substance between the moxa and the patient's skin. This gives the practitioner greater control over the amount of heat and helps to protect the patient from burns. Some frequently used substances are ginger slices, garlic slices, and salt. The overall action of the technique changes slightly depending on the medium used. For example, moxa on salt is more astringent and is used to help stop diarrhea, whereas moxa on ginger is more warming.

Other techniques include pole moxa and warm needle moxa. In *pole moxa,* a cigar-shaped roll of moxa wrapped in paper is used to gently warm an area without touching the skin. This is a very safe method of moxibustion that can be taught to patients for self-application. The *warm needle method* is accomplished by inserting an acupuncture needle and then placing moxa on its handle. After the moxa is ignited, it burns slowly, giving a gentle sensation of warmth to the acupuncture point and to the channel.

Any of these techniques might be used to stimulate acupuncture points or areas of the body, especially when warming is appropriate. For example, if a patient is suffering from joint pain that worsens in cold, damp weather, applying moxa either directly or indirectly to the affected area will help to relieve the pain by warming the area and allowing the qi to flow more smoothly. In some places, most notably Japan, moxibustion techniques are highly developed, and specialized training is required to become a moxibustion practitioner (Figure 29-4).

Cupping In *cupping,* once known as "horning" because animal horns were traditionally employed, a flame is used to induce a vacuum in a small glass or bamboo cup, which is then applied to the skin. The subsequent suction on the skin helps to drain or remove cold and damp evils from the body or to assist blood circulation. For example, if a patient arrives with a common cold accompanied by cough and sore muscles on the upper back, cupping might be performed on the upper back to move the qi and dispel the evil. The cups may remain static on the area to which they

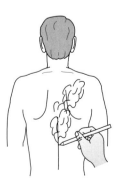

Figure 29-4 Moxibustion. (From Wang Y: *Microacupuncture in practice*, St. Louis, 2009, Churchill Livingstone.)

are applied or a medium may be applied to the body and the cups then drawn over the medium to cover a larger area. When the cups are removed, the patient is usually left with discoloration at the site of the vacuum. Today, some practitioners use small glass or plastic cups with a suction valve and then attach a hand-held vacuum to remove the air.

Gua sha Usually thought of as a folk technique, *gua sha,* literally "sand scraping," is used throughout Asia. It entails applying an oily medium to the skin and then using a spoon, a horn, or some other smooth utensil to scrape along the surface of the skin. Although the resulting marks on the skin look quite painful, patients describe the sensation as like having a very deep itch that they have been unable to scratch scratched. The release of the sha from the muscles releases evils from the muscle layer of the body, allows qi and blood to flow more freely, and often reduces muscular pain and stiffness. The technique is primarily used to release external evils or to relieve muscular pain, stiffness, and tension.

Bleeding *Bleeding* is done to drain a channel or to remove heat from the body. In this method small amounts of blood are expressed, from a drop to a few centiliters. It is commonly used on points that are located on the tips of the fingers or toes or over areas where there is a large vessel. On the tips of the fingers or toes, it is used to release acute heat that might be causing a sore throat or a severe headache. On the back of the knee, or in the crease of the elbow, it might be used to release heat that is causing a skin condition such as eczema or acne. Bleeding the tip of the ear can cause a rapid drop in blood pressure and is an emergency technique for preventing stroke. Bleeding may also be performed where there has been an injury and blood stasis has developed, causing chronic sharp pain.

Electroacupuncture A relatively modern acupuncture technique involves the application of a small electrical current to needles that have been inserted into the body. The intensity of the stimulus provided is determined by the patient and the patient's condition. The purpose of the technique is to apply continual stimulation to the needle throughout treatment. Electroacupuncture is particularly useful in the treatment of pain conditions and is frequently used for wind stroke. The electrical stimulus may be applied to regular body points as well as to auricular points, facial points, or the head. The technique is also frequently used in acupuncture anesthesia.

Plum blossom needling (seven-star needling) A plum blossom or seven-star needle was traditionally made by binding five or seven sewing needles to a bamboo stick. Today, five or seven very small needles are attached to a metal or plastic hammer. The hammer is used to lightly tap the skin. The technique may be used on a particular area of the body, on a specific point, or over the pathway of a channel. It is used to treat areas of numbness or paralysis, and even to treat balding. It is also used as a treatment for children or individuals who are hesitant about being needled.

Tui na Bodywork is an important part of many health care systems. The technique developed in China is called *tui na,* literally "pushing and pulling." In China, many practitioners specialize in tui na and become practitioners of tui na alone. The techniques are varied. They include rubbing pressing, pinching, pulling, rolling, and so on. Like the other techniques described here, tui na may be used over large areas of the body, over channel pathways, or simply at a specific point. In some cases, a patient may receive a full-body tui na treatment. Traditionally, the art of bone setting was also a part of the practice of a tui na practitioner. In fact, many of the tui na techniques bear a close resemblance to some of the techniques used today by osteopaths or chiropractors (see Chapters 18 and 19).

MICROSYSTEMS

All of the various microsystems that are used in the context of acupuncture treatment are comparatively modern developments. Almost all claim roots in classical Chinese acupuncture theory; however, in most cases there is little evidence of anything in the classics supporting the degree of elaboration seen in contemporary systems. Almost all of the microsystems can be considered as reflex zones, specific and bounded areas of the body that can be stimulated to influence all regions of the body itself. They are essentially maps of the body and its organ systems drawn on various specific areas of the body, which can then be used to treat the entire system.

The theoretical rationale for the reflex zones that comprise most microsystems is typically based on interpreted neurology or developmental biology, and thus they are usually connected with contemporary ideas about neurology, development, and anatomy. However, the idea that a bounded region of the body can relate directly to all body regions is seen in the diagnostic principles described in classical texts (particularly face and tongue diagnosis), and thus the principle of reflex zones is not without its classical antecedents.

The reflex zones are typically used in one of three ways: (1) Chinese medicine theory may be applied to the choice of points (i.e., for a diagnosis of kidney qi vacuity, the kidney points in a given system might be chosen); (2) biomedical concepts may be applied to choose the points (i.e., if there is a problem with the pancreas, then the pancreas region in a given system might be chosen); or (3) the points in the reflex zone might be used symptomatically (i.e., if there is pain in the back and knees, then the back and knee region in a given system might be chosen for stimulation).

A number of different microsystems have been developed. The ear and scalp microsystems are particularly biomedicalized, whereas hand, foot, nose, face, and abdomen systems are perhaps a little less so. Although some microsystems are relatively obscure and the province of specialists with expertise in their application, the use of others is comparatively common in clinical settings. Almost all require some degree of specialized training to use effectively. In general, the microsystems are used in conjunction with conventional acupuncture points, but some, such as the Korean hand acupuncture system, are intended to be used as independent acupuncture systems. Two common systems, auricular acupuncture and scalp acupuncture, are discussed here.

Auricular Acupuncture

Auricular or ear acupuncture is a widely used acupuncture microsystem. In 1951, Dr. Paul Nogier, a French physician, encountered patients who had been treated for sciatica by the application of cautery to specific areas of the ear as part of a folk tradition. These patients claimed reduction of their symptoms (Nogier, 1983a, 1983b). Nogier became interested and began a deep exploration of the therapeutic stimulation of the ear to treat medical conditions. He used a number of stimulus methods, including acupuncture, which was well known to French physicians. Nogier's work led him to describe a pattern of reflex areas that corresponded with an inverted homunculus mapped onto the human ear.

Subsequent to the initial publication of his ideas in 1957, his work was translated into Chinese and republished in 1958. Based on Nogier's publications and subsequent work in China, the academy of TCM in Beijing published its version of an auricular acupuncture chart in 1977, blending Nogier's model with Chinese additions. It is from this point that auricular therapy can be said to be an important aspect of Chinese acupuncture. It has become so integrated with Chinese acupuncture practice that both Chinese and Western practitioners are often surprised to learn of its European roots.

Ear acupuncture is used as an adjunct to group and behavioral therapies in supporting patients who are addressing substance abuse issues. Typically, in what is known as the National Acupuncture Detoxification Association (NADA) protocol, the *shen men*, liver, kidney, lung, and sympathetic ear points are needled bilaterally on a daily basis for several weeks. The NADA protocol is also used to address post-traumatic stress disorder.

Scalp Acupuncture

Standard acupuncture theory posits that all of the qi of the organs rises to the head via the various channel pathways; thus the flourishing of qi and blood is reflected in the head. In the 1950s and 1960s, based on knowledge gained from cerebral cortex mapping, a system of acupuncture was developed to treat central nervous system (CNS) conditions. Over the past 50+ years, other scalp systems have also been developed, but all are based on the areas of the brain associated with specific functions. Some use very carefully defined and measured lines as the locations for needle insertion, whereas others use more general zones to identify needling locations.

The earliest system identified lines on the scalp that corresponded with areas of the brain associated with motor skills and sensory perceptions. In addition, there are lines for tremors, for vertigo and hearing, for speech, for vision, and for balance, as well as several others. Based on the understanding of the crossing of the spinal nerves, contralateral needling is done for conditions affecting one limb. Bilateral needling is done for conditions affecting both limbs or for systemic conditions. Relatively thick (0.30 or 0.28 mm) needles are inserted horizontally into the scalp and then manipulated with strong continuous stimulation for 3 to 4 minutes. After manipulation, the needles are retained for several more minutes.

Scalp acupuncture appears to be quite useful for treatment of conditions such as poststroke paralysis, Parkinson disease, and other conditions related to balance and movement, and is frequently used when acupuncture is focused on rehabilitation.

TRADITIONS, SCHOOLS, STYLES, AND SYSTEMS

The idea that *acupuncture* is a term that floats freely and that may be distinguished by the addition of various qualifiers was introduced earlier. This section examines a range of approaches to acupuncture that are bound together through their common engagement with elements of the core traditions of Chinese medicine and are, at the same time, distinctive with regard to specific aspects of their approaches to therapy. Although it is tempting simply to refer to all of these approaches as particular "styles" of acupuncture, as does Ahn et al (2008), it may be helpful to draw a distinction of scale regarding what constitutes a tradition, a school, a style, and a system to clarify some of what is seen in the field of acupuncture.

When this scalar approach is used (see Chapter 5), an acupuncture *tradition* can be said to be organized so broadly that it has only a limited degree of central focus and may, in fact, contain diverse schools and systems within it. At the same time, any distinct elements of the tradition will still have characteristics in common. Very often traditions will have regional associations and characteristics (like regional styles of cooking within Chinese cuisine). From this point of view, what is termed "traditional Chinese medicine" or "Chinese medicine," as well as "Japanese acupuncture," can be said to be acupuncture traditions in their own right.

Acupuncture *schools* are approaches to practice that are organized around a central figure or organization. A school promulgates a distinctive doctrine that guides practice and insists on some degree of conformity to its methods, although it may exist within a larger tradition. Toyohari and keiraku chiryo within the Japanese tradition represent schools in that sense, as does five-element acupuncture.

A *style* involves the appropriation or rejection of the elements of a tradition or school and the assertion of a kind of distinctiveness, without the requirement for a great deal of clarity about the antecedents or basis for its assertions. "Western acupuncture," or "medical acupuncture," exemplifies an acupuncture style from this point of view.

TABLE 29-10 *Scalars in Acupuncture Practice*

Tradition	A regionally distinct approach or set of approaches that can be characterized by regional developments
School	Approach to practice organized around a central figure or organization (e.g., meridian therapy, toyohari, five-element acupuncture)
Style	Appropriation or rejection of a school or tradition, with the assertion of distinctiveness but with limited development of a distinctive theory of application (e.g., Western acupuncture, medical acupuncture, Japanese-style acupuncture)
System	Specific highly structured approaches to treatment not requiring adherence to a specific school or tradition and easily incorporated into different practice styles (e.g., five-step treatment protocol, auricular acupuncture, Korean hand acupuncture, abdominal needling)

Finally, *systems* involve specific and highly structured approaches to treatment that do not require a commitment to any specific school or tradition and can be easily incorporated into different styles of practice. Ryodaraku, Yoshio Manaka's five-step treatment protocol, auricular acupuncture, and Master Dong's points are examples of acupuncture systems (Table 29-10).

The ideas presented in the sections addressing channels, networks, and points represent the common core of the East Asian acupuncture traditions that have developed in China, Japan, Korea, and Vietnam, as well as most of those to be found in the West. This core pertains even to those systems that overtly eschew any engagement with core theory (such as Western acupuncture) and simply use acupuncture points removed from any traditional context, because the points themselves would not exist as objects of knowledge without the centuries of exploration contributed by the ancient Chinese. In this sense, then, there is no acupuncture tradition that is not, in essence, based on the originating contributions of the Chinese.

Even within China, however, and certainly in Japan, Korea, Vietnam, Europe, and the United States, there have been shifts of emphasis, theoretical elaborations, clinical developments, and refinements in technique that have produced approaches to acupuncture that seem so distinctive to their developers or their adherents that they have come to be identified as specific schools or systems of acupuncture. This is definitely the case with the wide range of practices that are subsumed under the general heading of "Japanese acupuncture," in which myriad distinctive schools of practice show both a strong relationship to the acupuncture traditions and texts of China, and regional innovation and development.

Intriguingly, many of these systems that have developed outside China and East Asia often seek to contrast their practice methodologies with what is seen as the dominant, even hegemonic, paradigm of TCM. In China, however, divergent or distinctive practice styles are always understood to be part of the greater "Chinese medicine" or "acupuncture and moxibustion" paradigms, even when they break truly new ground or diverge significantly from traditional approaches to practice. There are many possible reasons for this contrast in attitudes between those within China and those without. The two most apparent are the following: In some cases a degree of national pride suggests that it is important to demonstrate that the distinctive practice was developed outside of China, whereas exponents of the Chinese tradition may wish to point clearly to the Chinese origins of every acupuncture practice. In other instances, an attempt to brand acupuncture is occurring, and the acupuncture style in question may make an effort to distinguish itself from standard professional acupuncture by asserting engagement with more authentic practices, development of areas said to be neglected by TCM, or rejection of practices attributed to TCM.

This section proposes no evaluation of the merits of competing claims, nor will we pronounce on the validity of differing practice styles. The goal here is to provide the reader with some guidance to the significance of some of the common qualifiers applied to the term *acupuncture*. We make no claim to providing an exhaustive list of traditions, schools, systems, and styles of acupuncture practice, but rather offer a window into the diversity of approaches to clinical practice by presenting some of the commonly encountered models for delivering acupuncture therapy.

CHINESE ACUPUNCTURE STYLES AND SYSTEMS

Readers of Chapter 28 should recall that there is exceptional conceptual flexibility in theoretical approaches to Chinese medical practice. Even today in China, during one of the comparatively most standardized periods of acupuncture practice in Chinese history, the diversity of practice styles and schools as one departs from the standard curricula of academic institutions and enters private and institutional practice settings is immense. However, the persistence of the Chinese cultural tendency to integrate, incorporate, and retain tends to cause even proponents of the most radical departures from "standard" Chinese medicine to find that their distinctive school or system has been absorbed into the greater paradigm of the Chinese tradition.

For all intents and purposes, *Chinese acupuncture, traditional Chinese acupuncture,* and *TCM acupuncture* can be considered virtually synonymous terms that convey the acupuncture practiced in the dominant paradigm of modern China. "Classical Chinese acupuncture" is an expression that tries to assert a distinction between itself and the modern practice traditions of China, but that in actuality conveys nothing, because it refers to the same classical texts and traditions as the predominant paradigm.

"Daoist acupuncture" is an expression that has emerged over the years. What seems to be meant is a repertoire of acupuncture point selection strategies associated with Daoist physicians or traditions of Daoist ritual practice. There are also texts that assert a "Daoist" lineage for their acupuncture practices (Liu, 1999) and even training programs in the United States that claim a privileged connection between the traditions of Daoism and their instructional content. The problem is that a great number of physicians in China were, in fact, Daoists (and often Buddhists and Confucians as well), and so a great deal of "standard"—that is, classically derived and widely disseminated—acupuncture theory can be attributed to texts that are associated with Daoist traditions. Many of the most notable "Daoist" components are systems of acupuncture point selection based on the *I Ching (Yi Jing)* or on the stems and branches (traditional calendrics). However, all these methods are practiced in the context of standard acupuncture theory and so distinguish themselves mainly in the details.

JAPANESE ACUPUNCTURE SCHOOLS AND SYSTEMS

As discussed in Chapter 28, the recorded history of cultural exchange between China and Japan dates back to at least AD 57 (obviously there were important contacts in prehistory as well), and the exchange has been a long and productive one, especially in the field of medicine. Today, acupuncture in Japan encompasses a wide range of schools and systems. The typical Japanese acupuncturist draws from the many different schools and systems of practice in an eclectic fashion. Alternatively, some practitioners adhere closely to the tenets of a particular school. For this reason it is not entirely accurate to generalize about Japanese acupuncture except, perhaps, as a tradition of practice. Rather, it is more useful to speak of the schools and systems that have emerged from Japan. Japan has seen both focused specialization in, and the innovative exploration and expansion of, acupuncture practice.

Meridian Therapy

The *Classic of Difficult Issues* has historically been the focus for movements to revive the practices of "traditional" acupuncture in Japan. The text was an important influence in the development of meridian therapy (keiraku chiryo), a school of acupuncture developed in the 1930s based on the application of concepts in the *Classic of Difficult Issues* and their subsequent interpretation by later Chinese authors. A distinctive feature of meridian therapy is the application of five-phase theory to the transport points, a practice that has influenced the perception and adoption of five-phase theory by European practitioners (Kaptchuk, 1983).

Toyohari

Toyohari is a distinctive school of acupuncture practice that grew out of meridian therapy. Like meridian therapy, it is built on the foundations of the *Classic of Difficult Issues* and uses the approach of pulse and abdominal diagnoses to select acupuncture points based on five-phase concepts. It is distinguished by an exceptionally gentle needling technique that can range from minimally insertive to entirely noninsertive (the effectiveness of noninsertive acupuncture fundamentally calls into question the mechanisms of action that have been proposed by Western biomedicine, which essentially relate to the physiology of skin puncture). Many of Japan's toyohari practitioners are blind, which links them closely with the historical tradition of acupuncture as a field of practice for the blind, as with shiatsu (see Chapters 17 and 28). In the mid-seventeenth century, Waichi Sugiyama, a blind man, began to train the blind in acupuncture using very fine needles and guide tubes. Practitioners of toyohari cultivate special sensitivity to the sensations felt by the practitioner with the arrival of qi, which is summoned to the acupuncture points with little if any needle insertion.

Yoshio Manaka

An interesting system of acupuncture therapy is the pioneering work of Yoshio Manaka. Manaka, a physician who experimented with acupuncture principles during a period when medical supplies were unavailable during World War II, became convinced of the efficacy and physiological relevance of traditional theories and continued to experiment and develop them throughout his life. His work, specifically his five-step protocol and the use of ion pumping cords, has contributed dramatically to the practice of acupuncture.

The variety of systems emerging from Japan also include systems such as shoni shin (literally "pediatric needles"), akabane, and many others. Each of these systems is quite unique, and yet the term *Japanese acupuncture* has been used to cover all of them. This misnomer leads one to believe that a specific tradition developed in Japan, when in fact all of the systems emerging from Japan are grounded in the core texts of the Chinese tradition and the core acupuncture theory of China.

KOREAN SCHOOLS AND SYSTEMS

Widely used techniques of acupuncture point selection based on five-phase theory have emerged from Korea, including those of the Buddhist priest Sa-am (1544-1610). Although these are known as Korean four-point (eight-needle) techniques, the method has been established for so long that it has become integrated into many other acupuncture traditions and schools.

Two comparatively recent acupuncture systems developed in Korea have become relatively well known in other parts of the world. Korean constitutional diagnosis was developed initially by Jhema Lee (1836-1900). It based a system of herbal therapeutics on a set of diagnostic patterns using the four divisions of yin and yang. In 1965, Dowon Kuan expanded Jhema Lee's system to an eightfold classification and applied it to acupuncture (Hirsch, 1985). This system became known as *Korean constitutional acupuncture.*

Another influential contemporary system is *koryo sooji chim,* the system of Korean hand and finger acupuncture developed by Yoo Tae Woo and published in 1971. This system has gained a significant level of international exposure. Koryo sooji chim maps the channel pathways and acupuncture points of the entire body onto the hands, where they are stimulated using very short, fine needles and magnets. Specialized tools are required to insert the small needles into very specific areas on the hands and fingers.

WESTERN EUROPEAN TRADITIONS AND STYLES

"Medical acupuncture" is an expression with a wide and slightly contrasting range of uses. Its primary meaning is any form of acupuncture (tradition, school, style, or system) practiced by an individual who is a licensed physician.

The American Association of Medical Acupuncture (n.d.) defines medical acupuncture as "the clinical discipline of acupuncture as practiced by a physician who is also trained and licensed in Western biomedicine. Founded on medical texts of ancient China, the interpretation and application of acupuncture within the context of contemporary medicine is an extension of the physician's biomedical training. The medical acupuncture physician uniquely offers a comprehensive approach to healthcare, which combines classic and modern forms of acupuncture with conventional biomedicine."

In this context, the term *medical acupuncture* distinguishes only the professional status of the person performing the acupuncture, and this form of acupuncture relies substantially on a wide range of practice traditions and schools.

A somewhat less frequently encountered meaning of "medical acupuncture" is that of a system of acupuncture that typically (but not always) retains the acupuncture points derived from the Chinese tradition but seeks to describe a bioscience-based paradigm for their application (Filshie & White, 1998; Jin et al, 2006). In some cases, acupuncture points are renamed and reorganized to provide a less traditional, more "scientific" appearance (Ma et al, 2005).

Western acupuncture and *Western-style acupuncture* are terms that appears periodically in the literature, typically in descriptions of research in which the acupuncture to be provided is "Western," which seems to mean that it involves acupuncture stimulation of both standard acupuncture points and "trigger points" in the presence of a Western medical diagnosis but without, in some instances, any described process for determining the points selected for treatment.

Occasionally the term *dry needling* is used in association with the concept of Western acupuncture. Strictly speaking, dry needling is done with a hypodermic needle, not an acupuncture needle. The needle is different in that it has a lumen and a cutting edge. The technique emerged from Travell's approach to the treatment of myofascial trigger points (MTrPs) by injection (of lidocaine, saline, etc.), using a "wet needle" containing a substance to be injected. Some clinicians concluded that the use of a needle without injection of any substance was sufficient, hence "dry" needling. The term *dry needling* then implies (1) the use of a hypodermic needle inserted into (2) a trigger point. In the sense that a needle and a type of acupuncture point (the ah shi point) are involved, this could be said to be acupuncture, but the acupuncture paradigm is otherwise entirely absent from the method, and the use of the cutting needle creates different effects as well.

French Energetic Acupuncture

Several distinct influences shaped what might be termed a collection of acupuncture styles rooted in classical Chinese acupuncture theory and early twentieth-century Chinese acupuncture practice. The French diplomat George Soulié de Morant, who studied acupuncture in China from 1901 through 1917 and was recognized as a physician by the Chinese, produced several very influential texts in France during the 1930s and 1950s. His work substantially influenced the development of acupuncture in modern France and provided the basis for the engagement of French acupuncture with post–World War II Japanese and Vietnamese perspectives on acupuncture practice. The fact that Soulié de Morant chose to translate *qi* as energy and that his collaborator (and later nemesis) Niboyet chose to integrate acupuncture closely with homeopathy seems to have contributed substantially to the "energetic" orientation of this style.

Five-Element Acupuncture

J.R. Worsley, a physical therapist who began his studies of acupuncture in 1962, came to have a substantial impact on the perceptions of many practitioners in England and the United States. He visited Hong Kong and Taiwan for a brief period and then became a part of the study group established by Rose-Neil (Hsu & Peacher, 1977). Worsley went on to create the College of Traditional Chinese Acupuncture in the United Kingdom and two institutions in the United States. Worsley's five-element acupuncture constitutes a school of practice blending elements of Japanese acupuncture traditions, notably meridian therapy and akabane, with a very broadly developed interpretation of five-element theory based on ideas expressed in the *Yellow Emperor's Inner Classic.* Since the death of its founder and the appropriation of Worsley's five-element model of practice by others, there can also be said to be five-element styles.

Throughout Asia and Europe, a variety of schools, systems, and styles of acupuncture have developed. And yet, with few exceptions, all of them refer back to the classical texts that emerged out of the Han dynasty in China. The basic core acupuncture theory that we have discussed in this chapter continues to be the core of almost all of the traditions, schools, systems, and styles, for without that core theory, there is no structure for understanding the actions of individual points or for developing different methods of point selection.

ACUPUNCTURE RESEARCH

What we might term the "modern" history of acupuncture research in the West has a scope of just under 40 years (and perhaps 60 years in East Asia). That is not to say there are not earlier instances of research activities in both East Asia and the West. However, those early efforts were distinct, isolated, and comparatively limited and certainly not part of the system of internationalized research communication that constitutes what we term "modern."

Ongoing lines of scientific inquiry into acupuncture have focused primarily on three specific types of questions: (1) Are there physiological processes that can, at least partially, explain acupuncture effects such as pain control? (2) Is acupuncture safe? (3) Can acupuncture be shown to treat specific clinical conditions effectively?

The answer to questions 1 and 2 is yes, and the answer to question 3 is a qualified yes for many clinical conditions. This section reviews work done on each of these questions to give the reader an understanding of the complexity of the questions and the amount of research that has been done over the last 40+ years.

ANATOMY AND PHYSIOLOGY OF ACUPUNCTURE EFFECTS

One of the advantages of acupuncture, as its practitioners and advocates seek to increase its acceptance into mainstream health care, is that its primary therapeutic tools and methods are not abstract in any sense. The acupuncture needle is a tangible object that is introduced into or adjacent to tissue. That simple physicality has formed the basis for many intriguing ideas and investigations into the basic physiology of acupuncture. Kaptchuk (1983, 2002) states that acupuncture, in his opinion, is the "most credible" of complementary therapies in terms of acceptance by the medical community. He proposes that this greater acceptance may be the result of the existence of a substantial body of data showing that acupuncture in the laboratory has measurable and replicable physiological effects that can begin to offer plausible mechanisms for the presumed actions. This point is echoed by Filshie and White (1998) when they tell us, "Acupuncture owes much of its respectability to the discovery that it releases opiate peptides" (pp. 3–4). The fact that acupuncture can point to a body of basic research that provides a number of scientifically derived hypotheses for many of its clinically observed effects has been helpful in supporting its acceptance in a variety of medical settings.

TABLE 29-11 *Comparison of Biomechanistic Model and Acupuncture Model*

Reductionist science-based model	Acupuncture theory model
Events attributed to observed or hypothesized physiological processes	Events attributed to described system (based on observations of results of physiological processes)
Narrowly described	Broadly described
Incomplete	Comprehensive
Implicit reductionism	Implicit holism
Developing model	Static model

The contrast between ancient and traditional models of acupuncture and contemporary biomechanistic models is quite distinct. As we have seen, the classical constructs of acupuncture theory model a system that has been described through the observation of the body in health and disease and the body's response to stimulus. Although these models are explanatory, they were not developed in the context of the linearity and reductionism of the currently popular positivist, reductionist scientific enterprise. Instead they were developed on the basis of observation and an effort to describe observed relations systematically. They capture a diverse range of information in very broad and general terms (Table 29-11).

Contemporary biomechanistic models are constructed on the basis of currently established understandings of anatomy and physiology. The most prevalent models apply concepts derived from studying the neurophysiology of pain and accordingly seek to explain acupuncture in terms of what is already "known" about the body. Newer models have actually used traditional descriptions of physical responses to acupuncture stimulation to develop experiments that have led to new understandings of the way the body, particularly connective tissue, responds to acupuncture. From an acupuncturist's perspective, 30 years of basic science research into acupuncture using a biomechanistic model has furnished valid and valuable insight into many acupuncture phenomena, but cannot yet fully explain the range of observed acupuncture phenomena. There is, in fact, no reason that it should be expected to do so. Science consists of a rigorous process of investigation and explanation that relies on careful descriptions of observable processes. The methodology of science derives its power from the strict limitations placed on its methods. Scientific knowledge is continually developing, and so we should expect two things from proposed scientific models of acupuncture: (1) that they will be limited or incomplete because the current state of our knowledge about the body is incomplete, and (2) that they will continue to develop as our understanding develops.

Acupuncture theories, on the other hand, are based on observations of the results of processes that are then organized in very general terms and in terms that make sense of observable results, but not the underlying processes (see Table 29-11). It should not surprise us at all when acupuncture theories are not entirely captured by current scientific models or, to put it another way, when scientific models fail to capture all aspects of acupuncture theory.

What we can see when we investigate some of the basic science underlying our understanding of acupuncture is that acupuncture exploits a wide range of bodily responses to stimulation in a systematic fashion. No single physiological process fully explains all of acupuncture's effects, and at this time, acupuncture theory may offer a more coherent model for organizing and using (while not describing the causes of) acupuncture effects.

For instance, there are now two very suggestive theories concerning the significance of channels from a scientific point of view. One theory suggests that there is a detectable difference in the electrical impedance of channels compared with that of surrounding tissue. Another suggests that described channels may correspond to the distribution and spatial organization of fascia (connective tissue) and that the network formed by interstitial connective tissue throughout the body may form the basis of the communicating channels and networks described by acupuncture (Langevin & Yandow, 2002:263). Although both theories are highly suggestive, neither of these theories has been completely demonstrated to be correct, nor would they fully explain all of acupuncture's observed effects.

This situation should not surprise us. Acupuncturists have been thinking about acupuncture for over 2000 years, whereas scientists have been thinking about it for perhaps 100 years. This is not to say that all acupuncture theory is "true" in scientific terms, but that a rush to reduce its meaning to a few very basic physiological processes may ultimately limit our understanding of both acupuncture and physiology.

Are Channels and Points "Real"?

The contrast between scientific understanding and the traditional forms of knowledge associated with acupuncture becomes vividly clear when we contemplate the two most well-known acupuncture concepts: points and the external pathways of the regular channels. Depending on the approach guiding the research—and, perhaps, the disposition of the researcher or the interpreter of the data—it can be concluded that either there is no such thing as an acupuncture point or channel at all, or that channel theory represents a reasonably accurate description of a collection of interacting structures and processes.

From a reductionistic point of view, the impulse is to clearly establish an absolute physical structure that correlates precisely to all aspects of the acupuncture model. It was this impulse that led to the tragedy and travesty of the Korean researcher Bong Han, who became a virtual cultural hero in Korea during the 1960s because of his reported discovery of Bong Han corpuscles, distinct tissue

structures that were found only at acupuncture points and along channels. These were later shown to be artifacts of microscopic slide preparation, and Bong Han committed suicide. Of course, the entire modern practice of pathology, for example, is based on the systematic artifacts introduced when devitalized tissues removed from the living body are manipulated by chemical and mechanical processes and rendered in a two-dimensional plane of microscopic slide preparations.

Although there is research suggesting that the areas defined as acupuncture points and external channels may have features associated with them that are distinctive (and that distinguish them from other areas of the body's surface), there is nothing to suggest that there are any specific physical structures corresponding precisely to points and channels. Instead there is research indicating that: (1) the regions described by acupuncture points are particularly rich in nerve bundles and small blood vessels; (2) the tissues specified by channels and points may have different electrical characteristics than surrounding tissues; and (3) the organization of fascia shows distinctive characteristics underneath many acupuncture points and along channel pathways (Langevin et al, 2001a, 2002).

The idea that there are differentials in the electrical resistance of acupuncture points and channels is a comparatively old one, dating to research efforts as far back as 1950 (MacPherson et al, 2008). The work of Becker (1985) and Tiller (1997) has been very influential in suggesting that the activity of acupuncture channels and points may be closely related to their electrical properties. It is hypothesized by clinicians applying these ideas that variations in the electrical activity of acupuncture points and channels in disease states may aid in diagnosis of disease states, or that variations among acupuncture points, channels, and surrounding skin surface can be detected by measuring differences in electrical resistance. Although these concepts have given rise to the production, sale, and use of a vast array of electrodiagnostic devices and "point detectors," the present state of the science does not support their clinical use.

All of these devices work by measuring galvanic current, the standing current produced by the normal skin surface. The measurement of galvanic current is achieved with what is essentially an ohmmeter. The subject holds an electrode in one hand and a probe is applied to a desired area of the skin surface. Typically, direct current is supplied through the probe and measured by the meter. However, even slight variation in the pressure with which the probe is applied can cause significant fluctuations in current flow (resistance), which essentially causes a point to be detected wherever the probe is pressed firmly against the skin. For this reason, although the few well-designed studies of these phenomena are very suggestive, conclusive statements about the electrodermal properties of acupuncture channels and points remain elusive.

The idea that fascia might have a distinctive role in acupuncture phenomena has become very well established as a consequence of the work of Helene Langevin and her research team at the University of Vermont Medical School. Langevin began with a question concerning the physical basis of *de qi,* the sensation of the needle's being "grabbed" on insertion that is associated in many acupuncture traditions with the arrival of qi. She asked if there could be an actual anatomical event associated with the sensation reported by practitioners over centuries of acupuncture practice. Her initial hypotheses were that the "needle grasp," or the gripping associated with de qi phenomenon, was caused by the winding of connective tissue around the needle during rotation. And that the manipulation of the needle, now coupled with connective tissue, "transmits a mechanical signal to connective tissue cells via mechanotransduction" (Langevin et al, 2001a: 2275).

She was able to demonstrate that the increased pull-out force associated with rotated needles was 18% greater at acupuncture points than at control points (Langevin et al, 2001b). She simultaneously proposed a mechanism through which the physical stimulation of connective tissue at the needling site might produce a variety of "downstream" changes in interstitial connective tissue that might be implicated in acupuncture effects. A later paper demonstrated a close relation between channel pathways and connective tissue and between acupuncture points and areas where intermuscular and intramuscular connective tissue was particularly dense (Langevin & Yandow, 2002).

Her work demonstrates the potential existence of a nonneural signaling system, the course and structure of which parallels ancient observations concerning channels and networks. At present the data are only suggestive. Langevin's work substantially supports the ideas of other authors who have proposed that acupuncture effects not attributable to neural events may be related to connective tissue signaling systems (Oschman, 1993).

Intriguingly, the concept of MTrPs is often presented as a science-based and medically established version of the idea of acupuncture points. MTrPs have a long history of conceptual development based on the palpation of tender regions in the musculature of patients with pain. Travell and Simons (1983) substantially organized the concept and coined the term, which is applied to points that are located on palpation and are exquisitely tender on palpation (and are typically found in areas where the patient is experiencing pain). Unlike the locations of channel and extra points, which are substantially fixed, the described locations of MTrPs are areas where MTrPs may be found if they are present. The presence of an MTrP is evidenced by acute tenderness on palpation and, in the case of an active MTrP, by local pain as well.

As is the case with acupuncture points, there is no clear evidence of any distinctive anatomical features specific to MTrPs; however, because they are conceptualized within the biomedical model, and because there are bioscience-based hypotheses concerning their production and action, MTrPs are considered to be a scientifically developed idea. The publication in 1977 by Melzack (of the Melzack-Wall

gate theory of pain) of a paper claiming a 71% correlation between acupuncture points and these "trigger points" seemed to suggest that acupuncture points formed part of a well-described domain in the neurobiology of pain (Melzack et al, 1977). Since publication of this paper, MTrPs originally described in relation to the diagnosis and treatment of myofascial pain are frequently invoked to explain or dismiss effects or models described in traditional acupuncture theory (Baldrey, 1993, 1998; Bowsher, 1998).

Ironically, as Steve Birch has been careful to point out, some 6 years after the publication of Melzack's article, Travell and Simons's textbook on trigger points contained an analysis of the Melzack et al study. Their conclusion: "Acupuncture points and trigger points are derived from vastly different concepts. The fact that a number of pain points overlap does not change that basic difference. The two terms should not be used interchangeably" (Travell et al, 1983, cited in Birch 2008:343).

Although it is clear from our earlier discussion that a region that is tender on palpation, or an ah shi point, is an important category of point in acupuncture therapy, it is not so clear that many, or even a majority, of acupuncture points used in the treatment of pain are equivalent to trigger points. This issue has been well demonstrated. A careful analysis of Melzack's assertions (Birch, 2003; Birch & Felt, 1999) suggests that the actual correlation between trigger points and the acupuncture points examined by Melzack that are actually used for the treatment of pain is approximately 18%.

As suggested by Birch, however, the desire to establish that acupuncture points fall fully within the domain described by MTrPs seems to be deeply compelling to segments of the medical community. The unsuccessful attempt by Dorsher (2008) to rebut Birch's analysis of Melzack et al by insisting that the majority of acupuncture points are directly equivalent to trigger points is an example of this determination.

In the end it is important to remember that acupuncture points may be channel points, extra points, or ah shi points. It is clear that the ah shi point and the MTrP are almost exactly equivalent in concept. They both are present when they elicit pain on palpation and are not present when they do not. Channel points or extra points may be painful on palpation and may even act as ah shi points, but their clinical application is not limited to pain, nor are they present only when painful. From this point of view, acupuncture and trigger point therapy exploit similar physical observations with regard to exceptionally tender myofascial points. The close agreement of the trigger point theory and the theory of ah shi points suggests that an equivalent physiological phenomena has been independently observed by two very different traditions of clinical practice. However, the conceptualization of acupuncture points as purely MTrPs limits the complete understanding of acupuncture channels, channel points, and extra points.

BOX 29-2 *The "Splinter" Effect*

Splinter or needle pierces skin

Vasoconstriction commences to halt blood loss and prevent circulation of any microorganisms carried on the object (duration 20 minutes)

Slightly later vasodilation increases local circulation to allow white blood cells and other cells to enter the area to assist in infection control and tissue repair (duration 2 to 3 hours)

Vasomotion begins after 1 hour. This is the pumping of microscopic vessels to allow flushing away of damaged cells and blood (duration 1 hour)

Birch's splinter effect (Birch & Felt, 1999) describes a series of vascular changes that support defensive, tissue repair, and metabolic processes that are typical of the body's response to a wound and illustrate the immediate vascular changes associated with acupuncture

BOX 29-3 *Seven Local and Central Reactions to Needling an Acupuncture Point*

1. Skin and tissue reactions at needle site, including induction of "current of injury"
2. Interaction between needle shaft and connective tissue
3. Relaxation of contracted muscle, increased circulation to site
4. Nociception and motor neuronal activation, neuroendocrine activation via central nervous system, segmental, and nonsegmental pathways
5. Blood coagulation, lymphatic circulation
6. Local immune response
7. Tissue repair (DNA synthesis) at site of injury (needling)

Although it is very clear that acupuncture channels and points as traditionally described do not define new or distinct structures unknown to science, it is quite likely that they describe relations among existing tissue and processes that may cooperate and interact in ways that are not presently completely understood.

How Does Acupuncture Work?

Acupuncture, like any therapy, must interact with existing anatomy and physiology to produce its effects. There are a number of well-described and scientifically demonstrated models of the way in which acupuncture might achieve its effects. It is very clear that acupuncture effects are the consequence not of a single physiological process, but rather of a complex dynamic of local tissue, vascular, and CNS-mediated neuroendocrine events.

Birch's description of the "splinter effect" (Birch & Felt, 1999:163) illustrates the complex range of vascular events that occur when the body encounters a common injury. This model suggests that many of the physiological responses to acupuncture are quite common to the body's response to injury with any sharp object, hence the splinter effect. The splinter effect captures the potential complexity surrounding such an obviously "simple" event as insertion of an acupuncture needle. Birch presents his concept of the splinter effect to illustrate a range of local and regional vascular effects that can occur with acupuncture (Box 29-2). The splinter effect involves a series of vascular responses to acupuncture that are equivalent to the changes provoked by any tissue damage with a sharp object. Local vascular effects are only one set of the many changes provoked by acupuncture.

Based on his interpretation of the research data, Ma has created a useful description of seven specific events or "chain reactions" that acupuncture activates in both local tissue and the CNS (Ma et al, 2005:26). Although most of these are local, central responses are also described, because Ma correctly considers local and central responses to be

"physiologically inseparable" (Box 29-3). Ma's outline captures the elements of Birch's splinter effect and points out some additional interesting features of the physiological events provoked by acupuncture. His observations capture complex local effects such as "current of injury," which refers to the creation of a current flow produced by any lesion in tissue. In this case the acupuncture needle produces a very focused lesion with a small current (10 mA) that supports tissue growth and healing (Ma et al, 2005: 27).

Ma's inclusion of nociception and motorneuronal activation and neuroendocrine activation via CNS, segmental, and nonsegmental pathways captures the idea that acupuncture needling which provides a detectable level of stimulus (some styles do not), invokes a complex of neurophysiological responses that diminish pain. In particular, acupuncture is considered to invoke descending pain regulation by stimulating the production of the body's own chemical messengers for pain control.

The Nobel Prize–winning discovery in 1975 by Solomon Snyder and Candace Pert of opiate neuropeptides, which have come to be known as endorphins, shed a great deal of light on certain aspects of the process of pain control. This discovery occurred coincident with recently emergent medical interest in acupuncture and acupuncture effects in pain control. By 1977, published studies strongly suggested that acupuncture effects in pain control or acupuncture analgesia might be linked to the activity of endorphins (Mayer et al, 1977; Pomeranz & Chiu, 1976). These studies showed that the effects of acupuncture analgesia, induced both by manual stimulation of acupuncture needles and by electrical stimulation, could be blocked by the administration of the opiate antagonist naloxone. This finding suggested that acupuncture's ability to control pain relied, at least in part, on its ability to trigger the release of endogenous opiates. Responding later to criticism that the reversal of acupuncture analgesia by the administration of naloxone was insufficient to validate the hypothesis that acupuncture analgesia was produced by endorphins, Pomeranz (1988) provided a list of 17 distinct

BOX 29-4 *Examples of Experimental Evidence Supporting the Endorphin Hypothesis for Acupuncture Analgesia*

· Different opiate antagonists block acupuncture analgesia
· Rats with endorphin deficiency show poor acupuncture analgesia
· Mice with genetic deficiency in opiate receptors show poor acupuncture analgesia
· When endorphins are protected from enzymatic degradation, acupuncture analgesia is enhanced
· Transference or cross circulation of cerebral spinal fluid from an animal with induced acupuncture analgesia to a second animal will produce acupuncture analgesia, and this effect is blocked by naloxone
· Lesions of the periaqueductal gray, an important endorphin site, eliminates acupuncture analgesia

Adapted from Pomeranz B, Stux G: *Basics of acupuncture*, Springer-Verlag, 1998.

lines of experimental evidence that support the acupuncture analgesia–endorphin hypothesis. Six examples of these lines of experimentation are provided in Box 29-4.

Based on these data, it is conventionally accepted that many of acupuncture's perceived effects in the direct reduction of pain are likely mediated by the production of endogenous opiates. This conclusion may be overly general in light of the specific nature of the evidence that supports it; however, the assertion that endorphin secretion lies at the root of acupuncture effects is still a popular one.

Functional magnetic resonance imaging (fMRI) has been applied to the investigation of acupuncture since the late 1990s. Within the limitations of the technology, which includes limited access to the body and the need for the subject to remain immobile during data collection, fMRI studies of acupuncture have produced intriguing results. One of the key studies presented the dramatic conclusion that there might be a direct correlation between the stimulation of an acupuncture point and cortical activation (Cho et al, 2006). What appeared initially to be evidence of the specificity of the action of acupuncture points, as demonstrated by regional neural activation, was later seen to be a comparatively typical response to needling. Over the years, the preponderance of evidence has suggested that acupuncture effects revealed by fMRI need to be understood in terms of the role of the CNS in processing the signals produced by the acupuncture stimulus.

Other research has suggested that traditional Chinese needling techniques that elicit "de qi" can create neural deactivation of the limbic system in a way that can benefit patients with chronic pain (Hui et al, 2000, 2005).

This line of inquiry has produced research showing that patients with carpal tunnel syndrome respond to acupuncture very differently than do healthy subjects. Patients experiencing the pain of carpal tunnel syndrome have been shown to respond to acupuncture stimulation with neural deactivation of the limbic system, which can be hyperactivated in chronic pain conditions (Napadow et al, 2007). Concurrent activation of the lateral hypothalamic area, a region critical to the release of endogenous opiates (a pain control system) also occurs. This information has been interpreted to suggest that patients with pain respond differently to acupuncture than do healthy individuals.

TABLE 29-12 *Acupuncture Adverse Events*

Minor	Serious
Bleeding or bruising	Organ puncture (pneumothorax)
Pain	Infection (*Staphylococcus,* hepatitis B virus)
Transient nerve damage	Spinal lesions
Feelings of tiredness	Syncope

SAFETY OF ACUPUNCTURE

In a clinical setting, patient safety is of critical importance. Although substantial work remains to be done to demonstrate the efficacy of acupuncture treatment in all areas to the degree that it has been demonstrated in the treatment of postextraction dental pain or the nausea and vomiting associated with cancer chemotherapy, the data on the clinical safety of acupuncture are exceptionally strong. A recent analysis (Birch, 2004; Birch et al, 2004) of published reviews of acupuncture safety conducted between 1993 and 2003 indicates that acupuncture is a comparatively safe therapy. This is not to suggest that serious adverse events cannot occur with acupuncture, but these are quite rare. Pneumothorax, for example, was found to have occurred twice in the course of approximately one-quarter million treatments (Ernst & White, 2001).

Although a comprehensive review of findings in relation to acupuncture safety lies beyond the scope of this chapter, it is important to point out that emerging data continue to confirm the safety of clinical acupuncture. A recent study presented to the Society for Integrative Oncology at its 2006 Boston meetings demonstrated the safety of acupuncture in patient populations with exceptionally low platelet counts (well below $50\,\mu\text{Mol/mL}$), a population typically excluded from acupuncture based on surgical guidelines applied to acupuncture without clinical evidence (Taormina et al, 2006) (Table 29-12).

Considering the number of patients treated (estimated 9–12 million treatments per year [in the United States]) and the number of needles used per treatment (estimated average of 6–8), "there are . . . remarkably few serious complications" (American Medical Association Council on Scientific Affairs, 1982).

From Lytle (1993), cited in Birch et al (2004).

One of the advantages of acupuncture is that the incidence of adverse effects is substantially lower than that of many drugs or other accepted medical procedures used for the same conditions. As an example, musculoskeletal conditions, such as fibromyalgia, myofascial pain, and tennis elbow, or epicondylitis, are conditions for which acupuncture may be beneficial. These painful conditions are often treated with, among other approaches, anti-inflammatory medications (aspirin, ibuprofen, etc.) or with steroid injections. Both medical interventions have a potential for deleterious side effects but are still widely used and are considered acceptable treatments. The evidence supporting these therapies is no better than that for acupuncture.

From National Institutes of Health: Acupuncture, NIH Consensus Statement 15(5):9, 1997.

Clinical Efficacy of Acupuncture

The clinical application of acupuncture has been the object of concerted research efforts in China and Japan since the mid-twentieth century. More recently, substantial research initiatives in this area have been undertaken in the United States and Europe as well, and these have developed rapidly in terms of quality and quantity in the last 30 years, with a corresponding increase in the volume of publication on acupuncture research.

The actual and perceived quality of such research can vary widely. As is the case for medical systems, research standards—even for scientific research—are subject to cultural influences. Whereas the randomized, placebo-controlled, double-blind clinical trial is the definitive standard for an unambiguous biomedical recognition of pharmaceutical efficacy, not all societies require or encourage their medical communities to secure knowledge in this fashion. In addition, the simple matter of the accessibility of research data, and the more complex issue of the acceptability of such data, are both deeply influenced by the language and location of data publication. All of these factors can present challenges and obstacles to the effective design, availability, and use of research.

There is a history of productive acupuncture research in the United States dating from the early 1970s as the diplomatic and cultural exchange was restored with President Nixon's visit to China. Acupuncture piqued the imaginations of American physicians and researchers, especially in relation to pain control, and basic science research and small clinical studies were carried out. The establishment in the United States of the Office of Alternative Medicine (OAM) in 1991 under the National Institutes of Health (NIH) led to a distinct increase in the quality and scope of acupuncture research, particularly clinical research, in the United States and, to some extent, abroad.

The OAM hosted conferences dealt with methodological considerations in the field of alternative medicine, and

at each of these, acupuncture research occupied an important place. The Workshop on Acupuncture sponsored by the OAM in cooperation with the U.S. Food and Drug Administration (FDA) in 1994 was crucial to the continued development of acupuncture in the United States. The event was research based, and members of the acupuncture medical and scientific community gave presentations detailing the safety of acupuncture needles and the apparent clinical efficacy of acupuncture. These presentations formed the core of a petition that led, in March 1996, to the re-classification of acupuncture needles by the FDA from a class III or experimental device to a class II or medical device for use by qualified practitioners with special controls (sterility and single use). To aid in this effort, the editor of this textbook was asked by scientists at FDA to provide copies of computer discs with hundreds of references on acupuncture that had been compiled in connection with his early editorial work. The FDA scientists (including several Asian-Americans) had volunteered to work on their own time to move the re-classification forward. As such, they did not have access to government clerical assistance (a mixed blessing in any case) for re-entering the citations.

In November 1997 the NIH convened a Consensus Development Conference on Acupuncture that included 2 days of presentations of the evidence for the safety and efficacy of acupuncture for the treatment of specific conditions. This evidence was presented by experts in the field to a panel that reviewed reports of research on the use of acupuncture in the treatment of a wide variety of conditions. The panel reached the following formal conclusion:

> Acupuncture as a therapeutic intervention is widely practiced in the United States. Although there have been many studies of its potential usefulness, many of these studies provide equivocal results because of design, sample size, and other factors. The issue is further complicated by inherent difficulties in the use of appropriate controls, such as placebos and sham acupuncture groups. However, promising results have emerged, for example, showing efficacy of acupuncture in adult postoperative and chemotherapy nausea and vomiting and in postoperative dental pain. There are other situations such as addiction, stroke rehabilitation, headache, menstrual cramps, tennis elbow, fibromyalgia, myofascial pain, osteoarthritis, low back pain, carpal tunnel syndrome, and asthma, in which acupuncture may be useful as an adjunct treatment or an acceptable alternative or be included in a comprehensive management program. Further research is likely to uncover additional areas where acupuncture interventions will be useful. (National Institutes of Health, 1997)

Given that less than 2 years previously acupuncture needles had still been considered an experimental device in the eyes of the federal government, this marked a significant degree of progress for acupuncture in the West.

Many of the studies presented at the Workshop on Acupuncture sponsored by the OAM in 1994 were also presented at the consensus development workshop in 1997.

BOX 29-5 *Conditions for which Acupuncture Is Proven Effective*

1. Adult postoperative and chemotherapy-induced nausea and vomiting
2. Postoperative dental pain
3. Addiction
4. Stroke rehabilitation
5. Headache
6. Menstrual cramps
7. Tennis elbow
8. Fibromyalgia
9. Myofascial pain
10. Osteoarthritis
11. Low back pain
12. Carpal tunnel syndrome
13. Asthma

The consensus statement developed at the 1997 Consensus Development Conference on Acupuncture mentioned 13 clinical conditions for which acupuncture showed either efficacy or usefulness as an adjunctive or alternative treatment. Of these, only three—addiction, postoperative dental pain, and osteoarthritis—had been targets of National Institutes of Health–funded research. By 2007 an additional seven areas had been examined by NIH-funded studies: carpal tunnel syndrome, fibromyalgia, headache, low back pain, menstrual cramps, myofascial pain, and nausea and vomiting (MacPherson et al, 2008).

For the most part, the best clinical research could be clustered into five specific areas that seemed to represent the best and most positive research related to acupuncture. These areas were: (1) antiemesis treatment; (2) the management of acute and chronic pain; (3) substance abuse treatment; (4) the treatment of paralysis caused by stroke; and (5) the treatment of respiratory disease. In addition, there are areas such as female infertility, breech presentation, menopause, depression, and urinary dysfunction in which acupuncture was able to show good clinical results (Birch & Hammerschlag, 1996) (Box 29-5).

A review of the list of clinical conditions presented in the consensus statement reveals that all but four are pain conditions. Pain control is the one application of acupuncture that has been well accepted by the conventional medical community in Europe and the United States for many years. This area became very visible in the United States in the 1970s as a result of Chinese reports on acupuncture anesthesia (more correctly termed *acupuncture analgesia*) that were coincident with the restoration of diplomatic relations with China. The fact that the effects of acupuncture on pain appeared to be readily explainable in terms of familiar Western constructs already associated with the understanding of pain (e.g., gate-control theory, counterirritation, trigger points, and the actions of endorphins) provided an acceptable mechanism for acupuncture's effects on pain and further legitimized this area of exploration. As a result, this is one of the most widely researched applications of acupuncture. However, it has not been without problems.

Some of the problems that are typical of research on acupuncture treatments for pain, as well as acupuncture therapy in general, are exemplified by the results of two early meta-analyses of studies that examined the use of acupuncture in the management of chronic pain. The first was conducted by pooling data from 14 studies that carried out randomized controlled trials of acupuncture to treat chronic pain and that measured their outcomes in terms of the number of patients whose condition was improved (Patel et al, 1989). This meta-analysis reached a number of conclusions concerning the relationship of study design to research outcomes and concluded that acupuncture compared favorably with placebo and conventional treatment.

A second meta-analysis reviewed 51 studies and compared the quality of published controlled clinical trials in terms of research design and other specific factors, including randomization, single and double blinding, and numbers of subjects. This meta-analysis concluded that, of the studies reviewed, those with results favorable to acupuncture were more poorly designed than those that found negative results for acupuncture. The evidence suggested that the efficacy of acupuncture as a treatment for chronic pain is doubtful (ter Riet et al, 1990).

A careful review of the ter Reit et al meta-analysis by Delis and Morris (1993) suggested that its authors had "included studies which did not meet their criteria," such as a study that was not controlled and a study in which laser light was used instead of acupuncture needles. This finding prompted Delis and Morris to conduct their own analysis and to reanalyze the studies examined by ter Riet et al in relation to a number of factors, including investigator training and the appropriateness of treatment. Their meta-analysis showed a trend toward improvement in study design over time, which suggested that many poorly designed acupuncture studies might best be viewed as preliminary efforts by investigators who were insufficiently familiar with the modality to design effective studies.

All three of these meta-analyses pointed out significant issues in relation to acupuncture study design. Besides questions concerning randomization, blinding, placebo control, and sample size, a variety of questions emerged pertinent to the practice of acupuncture as a distinct modality. Is the investigator trained in acupuncture? Is the acupuncture treatment appropriate for the condition? Does the study allow for adjusting the treatment to the individual patient's needs according to traditional diagnostics? Are outcome measures clear? Is placebo or sham acupuncture used, and how is it administered?

Of all the debated areas in acupuncture research, the question of "sham" acupuncture for experimental control has received the most attention. The problem of how to provide a sham treatment in acupuncture is a vexing one. In drug or herbal studies, a capsule of inert material that appears similar to the capsule of the medication being investigated can be provided to the patient. Because the patient cannot tell the difference between the two capsules, he or she is effectively blinded to the use of a placebo. In acupuncture the problem becomes rather more complex. This is because the patient may be able to observe and feel all the sensations associated with either a true or a false treatment.

Proposed solutions vary from comparing real acupuncture with other modalities to carefully selecting a treatment with few effects (Vincent, 1993) or selecting acupuncture points that are entirely irrelevant (BRITS method) to the conditions being treated. In addition, methods of providing simulated acupuncture have been used successfully (Lao et al, 1999).

If a clinical trial compares acupuncture to an inactive treatment that does not involve the insertion of needles, the trial may be criticized because the act of simply inserting needles into a subject may have a greater placebo effect than other inactive interventions. Thus the study might not be able to determine whether the observed effects of acupuncture were greater than those of a placebo because the effects observed in the study might only be the result of acupuncture's being a better placebo. A second criticism leveled at failure to test acupuncture against a control that involves an insertive sham is that hypothesized effects such as diffuse noxious inhibitory control (an aspect of descending pain regulation systems) might be the actual cause of the observed effects rather than any specific acupuncture treatment.

The level of sophistication at which the problem of designing studies with appropriate inactive treatments, shams, or placebo acupuncture has been addressed has increased dramatically over the years. However, the essential characteristics of the problem remain. Some studies have produced results that show the selected form of "sham" acupuncture to have clinical effects that are essentially equivalent to those of "real" acupuncture, and these will be discussed later.

Understanding of the criteria for study design has improved substantially. The publication of Birch's paper presenting 64 critical points that must be assessed in the design or review of controlled trials of acupuncture, the routine application of standards such as the Jadad score to published studies in meta-analyses, and the improvement of the quality of meta-analyses (and the resultant improvement of study design) as a consequence of the work of the Cochrane Collaboration have all produced improvements in the quality of acupuncture research (Birch, 2004).

Acupuncture and Pain

The control of pain is considered to be a major area for the clinical application of acupuncture, and although some of the research in this area has been problematic, a number of studies strongly indicate the importance of acupuncture in pain management. As we have seen, one of the conclusions of the Consensus Development Conference on Acupunc-

ture was that acupuncture could be demonstrated to be efficacious for reduction of postoperative dental pain. One study showed that patients receiving acupuncture required less postoperative analgesia after oral surgery than a group receiving a sham acupuncture treatment (Lao et al, 1995).

Although patients frequently seek out acupuncture for low back pain and acupuncturists regard low back pain as an area in which they provide effective treatment, the research evidence produced over the years remains equivocal. A systematic review of randomized controlled trials determined that "acupuncture for acute back pain has not been well studied" and that the value of acupuncture in treating chronic back pain "remains in question" (Cherkin et al, 2003:905). Birch's review of reviews found that only two out of the seven reviews examined indicated that acupuncture had been shown to be effective for low back pain. The remaining reviews found promising or contradictory results (Birch et al, 2004).

A 2005 meta-analysis concluded that acupuncture provided short-term relief of chronic low back pain (Manheimer et al, 2005). In addition, it was concluded that true acupuncture worked better than sham acupuncture. The authors also stated that they could not reach a conclusion about the effectiveness of acupuncture compared with other active treatments.

It is against this background that published results of the findings of the German acupuncture trials are particularly striking (Haake et al, 2007). These trials were conducted from 2001 through 2005 and involved 340 outpatient practices. In all, 1162 patients were treated for low back pain and received ten 30-minute sessions of acupuncture each week. The study offered acupuncture delivered according to TCM principles (administered by physicians trained in acupuncture) and two control treatments. One of the control treatments was sham acupuncture, which was provided by needling areas that were identified as "nonacupuncture points" (Molsberger et al, 2006), and the other was conventional therapy consisting of drugs, physical therapy, or exercise.

At the end of the study when patients were assessed 6 months after concluding treatment, the response rate for acupuncture was 48%, whereas the response rate for conventional therapy was 27%. These statistically significant results demonstrated unequivocally that acupuncture could be more effective than conventional therapy in the treatment of low back pain. The greatest surprise lay in the patient response to sham acupuncture, which was 44%, almost as high as the response to true acupuncture treatment. These results, while substantiating acupuncture's claim to therapeutic effectiveness, have raised significant questions about the importance of specific point location in effective acupuncture treatment.

Because the points chosen for sham acupuncture were typically 5 cm away from any described acupuncture points and were needled shallowly (only 3 mm), the results of this study strongly suggest that there may be little importance to needling at traditionally described needling sites or that, at least, the degree of specificity implied by traditional locations is not relevant to this acupuncture effect. These findings are provocative.

Over the years, a number of studies have suggested that the joint pain of osteoarthritis seems to respond well to acupuncture (Dickens & Lewith, 1989; Junnila, 1982; Thomas et al, 1991), and one study suggested a significant cost benefit when the use of acupuncture removed the need for surgical intervention (Christensen et al, 1992). The implications of these studies have led to the increased commitment of resources to the investigation of the potential role of acupuncture in the management of osteoarthritis and the production of promising clinical data (Berman et al, 1999). This work culminated in 2004 with publication of the results of a large-scale trial of acupuncture involving 570 subjects who received acupuncture, sham acupuncture, or patient education. The study's authors concluded that acupuncture provided improvement in function and pain relief when used as an adjunctive therapy for osteoarthritis (Berman et al, 2004).

Headache pain is often treated with acupuncture. In 1989 a controlled trial of the use of acupuncture in the management of migraines was conducted that enrolled 30 patients who had chronic migraine headaches. Acupuncture was significantly effective in controlling the pain of migraine headaches (Vincent, 1989). A more recent pragmatic trial of acupuncture for chronic headache and migraine demonstrated clinical benefits for patients and low costs (Vickers et al, 2004).

Other Clinical Applications

The 1997 Consensus Development Conference concluded that acupuncture has been demonstrated to be efficacious for the treatment of adult postoperative and chemotherapy-related nausea and vomiting. Research in the area of anti-emesis revolves around the use of the acupuncture point "inner gate" (neiguan, P6) to control nausea and vomiting. The use of this point in acupressure to control nausea and vomiting is well known. Its use to control the nausea of pregnancy with pressure bands has been determined to be effective as well (Aloysio & Penacchioni, 1992).

Consumer products are even available that exploit this effect by applying light pressure to the acupuncture point in question, although their clinical usefulness remains in question. The inner gate point also has been investigated in relation to its use to control perioperative emesis resulting from premedication and anesthetic agents (Ghaly et al, 1987) and nausea and vomiting induced by cancer chemotherapy (Dundee et al, 1989; Ezzo et al, 2006). Today, the inner gate point forms the basis of many clinical acupuncture interventions to provide relief to patients receiving chemotherapy in hospital-based oncology services. The application of acupuncture in this context is so routine that in at least one metropolitan area biomedical clinicians refer to P6 as "the Sloane point," using the name of a hospital with a pioneering application of acupuncture in its oncology service.

On the basis of clinical experiences in China, acupuncture is used extensively in the United States for the management of symptoms associated with withdrawal from a variety of substances, including alcohol and cocaine. The summary conclusion reached by presenters at the 1994 OAM Workshop on Acupuncture panel on substance abuse was that early trials and empirical findings suggested positive treatment effects (Kiresuk & Culliton, 1994). Although acupuncture continues to be widely used in this area, the research evidence remains equivocal.

Asthma continues to be a complex area in which to assess acupuncture's effectiveness. An early extensive review of acupuncture in the treatment of pulmonary disease led its author to conclude that acupuncture produced favorable effects in the management of patients with bronchial asthma, chronic bronchitis, and chronic disabling breathlessness (Jobst, 1995). Since 1996, only 12 randomized controlled trials examining acupuncture in the treatment of asthma have been conducted. Although earlier trials focused on lung function as a primary outcome measure, more recent randomized controlled trials have also evaluated acupuncture's effects on the patient's quality of life and inflammatory response.

These randomized controlled trials have demonstrated significant reduction in irritability and anxiety (Mehl-Madrona et al, 2007), which may trigger asthma; reduction in days of "acute febrile disease" (Stockert et al, 2007); and reduced medication use (e.g., Mehl-Madrona et al, 2007). The use of acupuncture for asthma management still fares somewhat poorly in systematic reviews (McCarney et al, 2007; Passalacqua et al, 2005). McCarney et al declared that "more pilot data" should be acquired before investigators proceed to any large-scale randomized trials in this clinical area and spoke to the difficulty of developing "objective comparisons between different acupuncture types" on the basis of existing data.

A study conducted at a private fertility center in Denmark examined the timing of acupuncture treatment in *in vitro* fertilization to maximize the likelihood of pregnancy. The study showed that pregnancy rates were significantly higher when acupuncture was received on the day of embryo transfer. Although the control group had an ongoing pregnancy rate of 22%, the acupuncture group had a rate of 36% (Westergaard et al, 2006). Acupuncture also has shown promise in reducing the pain associated with *in vitro* fertilization (Sator-Katzenschlager et al, 2006) and improving its clinical outcomes.

What Acupuncture Can Treat

Although the preceding discussion reviews recent developments in clinical research into acupuncture, it may be helpful to explore the question of what conditions acupuncture can treat. The answer to this question may be very broad or a very narrow depending on who provides the response. From the perspective of the acupuncturist, there are very few clinical conditions that acupuncture cannot at least palliate or make more tolerable for the patient. Based on the strictest standard of clinical efficacy, perhaps only conditions such as postextraction dental pain or chemotherapy-associated nausea and vomiting can be said, unequivocally, to be extremely well treated by acupuncture.

The middle ground can be captured based on an examination of two wide-ranging systematic reviews. One was completed by the WHO (2002) and included Chinese-language sources, and the other was completed by Birch (Birch, 2004; Birch et al, 2004). Neither of these can be considered complete. The WHO document is a systematic review of controlled clinical trials for which results were published through early 1999. The Birch et al reviews are essentially reviews of reviews, and thus consolidate the data from several very rigorous reviews of acupuncture trials from the English-language literature.

Both reviews assessed the research in similar ways and described acupuncture as either "effective" or "promising" in treating a given condition. Table 29-13 summarizes the findings of the two reviews. The WHO reviewers evaluated 30 of 46 specific conditions examined as ones in which acupuncture had a proven or demonstrated therapeutic effect. Birch et al's stringent assessment of the evidence gleaned by other reviewers entirely omits Chinese-language publications and is purely a review of systematic reviews of randomized controlled trials. Their more stringent criteria rated acupuncture as "effective" for 4 of the 46 conditions and as "promising" for 8.

This analysis is limited, and it could appropriately be criticized on the basis of either what it has included or what it has failed to include. There are numerous promising studies, some of which have been examined here, that would support arguments for a broader and more inclusive list. The clinical experience of many acupuncturists would also support broadening this list. On the other hand, it is likely that rigorously constructed meta-analyses could fail to find compelling evidence for the usefulness of acupuncture in the management of many of these conditions. On this basis, then, the list in Table 29-13 provides a roster of the clinical domains for which comparatively robust clinical research data exist to support the use of acupuncture.

LOOKING FORWARD

The way forward in acupuncture research includes an emergent effort to examine acupuncture in pragmatic terms. Many clinical trials of acupuncture, in order to isolate its effects, reduce variables, and control for placebo effects, apply a clinical research model—the randomized controlled trial—that is designed to establish the "efficacy" of a pharmaceutical agent, not a "hands-on" therapy where both patient and practitioner are unavoidably aware of an ongoing therapeutic process. Although such trials can help us learn more about what aspects or components of acupuncture treatment do or do not have specific effects, they do not offer much guidance to the clinician or the patient, because the acupuncture treatments they examine are

TABLE 29-13 *What Acupuncture Treats*

	WHO[a]	Birch[b]
Acute and Chronic Pain		
Abdominal pain	2	
Acute postoperative dental pain	1	1
Back pain (chronic low back pain)	1	1
Biliary colic	1	
Bursitis, tendonitis	1	
Cancer pain	2	
Carpal tunnel syndrome		2
Facial pain	1	
Fibromyalgia	2	2
Joint pain related to bursitis, tendonitis, or arthritis	1, 2	2
Neck pain	1	
Neuralgias (trigeminal, herpes zoster, postherpetic)	1, 2	
Pain associated with sprains, contusions, fractures	1	
Post-traumatic or postoperative pain	1	
Sciatica	1	
Tennis elbow	1	2
Other Conditions		
Allergic rhinitis	1	
Asthma	2	2
Bell palsy	2	
Dysmenorrhea	1	2
Functional gastrointestinal disorders	1, 2	
Headache	1	1
Hypertension	1	
Insomnia	2	
Mild depression	1	
Muscle spasms, tremors, tics, and contractures	2	
Nausea and/or vomiting	1	
Premenstrual syndrome	1	
Sequelae of cerebrovascular accidents (aphasia, hemiplegia)		2
Substance abuse	2	2
Temporomandibular joint dysfunction, bruxism	2	1
Overweight	2	

Acupuncture is considered to be effective in treating or ameliorating those conditions marked 1 and to show promise of clinical effectiveness in treating those marked 2.
[a]Data summarized from World Health Organization: Acupuncture: review and analysis of reports on controlled clinical trials, Geneva, 2002, The Organization. Available at http://www.who.int/medicines/library/trm/acupuncture/acupuncture_trials.doc.
[b]Data summarized from Birch S, Keppel Hesselink J, Jonkman F, et al: Clinical research on acupuncture. Part 1. What have reviews of the efficacy and safety of acupuncture told us so far? *J Altern Complement Med* 10(3):468–480, 2004; and Birch S: Clinical research on acupuncture. Part 2. Controlled clinical trials, an overview of their methods, *J Altern Complement Med* 10:481–498, 2004.

often different from the acupuncture therapy that occurs in normal practice.

Hammerschlag (2003) speaks to the heart of this matter when he asserts the need to reassess the importance of a central tenet of evidence based medicine: that acupuncture should outperform placebo and suggests that it is time to think about research that considers whole systems of care rather than isolated modalities.

Many researchers see pragmatic trials as a potential solution that addresses this issue. These trials examine interventions that are very close to normal treatment approaches and typically involve comparisons with conventional therapy. This type of trial provides information that is valuable to patients and clinicians. The findings of German acupuncture trials, which compared acupuncture with conventional care, resulted in acupuncture's becoming a covered/reimbursed therapy for chronic low back pain in Germany, based on the clear demonstration of acupuncture's superiority to conventional care. This result occurred even though the trials problematized the question of the specific location of acupuncture points, which suggests that shallow needling might be as effective as deeper needling, and failed to control for nonspecific effects.

During the past few decades of acupuncture research, deeper insights have been afforded by technological advances demonstrating greater knowledge of human anatomy and physiology. These advances also broaden our appreciation of the complex models advanced by acupuncture theory. It remains too early to determine whether all propositions of the systems described in the first section of this chapter are based on "real" anatomical or physiological processes. Recent discoveries emerging from research into the properties of fascial tissue and into neural activation based on MRI suggest the existence of complex and interacting systems that may ultimately validate many of the insights provided by acupuncture theory.

The challenge we confront is simultaneously pursuing scientific inquiry while maintaining comprehensive engagement with traditions of acupuncture theory and practice.

References

Ahn AC, Colbert AP, Anderson BJ, et al: Electrical properties of acupuncture points and meridians: a systematic review, *Bioelectromagnetics* 29(4):245, 2008.

Aloysio DD, Penacchioni P: Morning sickness control in early pregnancy by Neiguan point acupressure, *Obstet Gynecol* 80(5): 852, 1992.

American Association of Medical Acupuncture: AAMA position paper, n.d., available at http://www.medicalacupuncture.org/aama_marf/position.html.

American Medical Association Council on Scientific Affairs: *Reports of the Council on Scientific Affairs of the American Medical Association, 1981*, Chicago, 1982, The Association.

Baldrey PE: *Acupuncture, trigger points and musculo-skeletal pain*, London, 1993, Churchill Livingstone.

Baldrey PE: Trigger point acupuncture. In *Filshie and White's Medical Acupuncture*, London, 1998, Churchill Livingstone.

Becker RO: *The body electric: electromagnetism and the foundation of life*, New York, 1985, Quill/William Morrow.

Berman BM, Lao L, Langenberg P, et al: Effectiveness of acupuncture as adjunctive therapy in osteoarthritis of the knee, *Ann Intern Med* 141(12):901–910, 2004.

Berman BM, Singh BB, Lao L, et al: Randomized trial of acupuncture as an adjunctive therapy in osteoarthritis of the knee, *Rheumatology (Oxford)* 38(4):346, 1999.

Birch S: Trigger point-acupuncture point correlations revisited, *J Altern Complement Med* 9(1):91–103, 2003.

Birch S, Keppel Hesselink J, Jonkman F, et al: Clinical research on acupuncture. Part 1. What have reviews of the efficacy and safety of acupuncture told us so far? *J Altern Complement Med* 10(3):468–480, 2004.

Birch S: Clinical research on acupuncture. Part 2. Controlled clinical trials, an overview of their methods, *J Altern Complement Med* 10:481–498, 2004.

Birch S: Trigger points should not be confused with acupoints, *J Altern Complement Med* 14:1184–1185, 2008.

Birch S, Felt R: *Understanding acupuncture*, London, 1999, Churchill Livingstone.

Birch S, Hammerschlag R: *Acupuncture efficacy: a summary of controlled clinical trials*, Tarrytown, NY, 1996, National Academy of Acupuncture and Oriental Medicine.

Bowsher D: Mechanisms of acupuncture. In *Filshie & White's medical acupuncture*, London, 1998, Churchill Livingstone.

Cherkin DC, Sherman KJ, Deyo RA, et al: A review of the evidence for the effectiveness, safety, and cost of acupuncture, massage therapy, and spinal manipulation for back pain, *Ann Intern Med* 138(11):898, 2003.

Cho ZH, Hwang SC, Wong EK, et al: Neural substrates, experimental evidences and functional hypothesis of acupuncture mechanisms, *Acta Neurol Scand* 113(6):370, 2006.

Christensen BV, Iuhl IU, Vilbe KH, et al: Acupuncture treatment of severe knee osteoarthritis, *Acta Anaesthesiol Scand* 36:519, 1992.

Delis K, Morris M: Clinical trials in acupuncture. In Birch S, editor: *Proceedings of the First Symposium of the Society of Acupuncture Research*, Boston, 1993, Society for Acupuncture Research, p 68.

Dickens W, Lewith G: A single-blind, controlled and randomised clinical trial to evaluate the effect of acupuncture in the treatment of trapeziometacarpal osteoarthritis, *Complement Med Res* 3:5, 1989.

Dorsher PT: Can Classical acupuncture points and trigger points be compared in the treatment of pain disorders? Birch's analysis revisited, *J Altern Complement Med* 14(4):353–359, 2008.

Dundee JW, Ghaly RG, Fitzpatrick KTJ, et al: Acupuncture prophylaxis of cancer chemotherapy induced sickness, *J R Soc Med* 82:268, 1989.

Ernst E, White A: *Acupuncture: a scientific appraisal*, St Louis, 2001, Elsevier reprint.

Ezzo JM, Richardson MA, Vickers A, et al: Acupuncture-point stimulation for chemotherapy-induced nausea or vomiting, *Cochrane Database Syst Rev* (2):CD002285, 2006.

Filshie J, White A: *Medical acupuncture: a Western scientific approach*, London, 1998, Churchill Livingstone.

Ghaly RG, Fitzpatrick KTJ, Dundee JW: Antiemetic studies with traditional Chinese acupuncture: a comparison of manual needling with electrical stimulation and commonly used anti-emetics, *Anaesthesia* 42:1108, 1987.

Hammerschlag R: Acupuncture: on what should its evidence be based? *Altern Ther Health Med* 9:5, 2003.

Haake M, Muller H, Schade-Brittinger C, et al: German Acupuncture Trials (GERAC) for chronic low back pain: randomized, multicenter, blinded, parallel-group trial with 3 groups, *Arch Intern Med* 167:1892–1898, 2007.

Hirsch RC: Korean constitutional nutrition, *J Am Coll Tradit Chin Med* (1):24, 1985.

Hui KK, Liu J, Makris N, et al: Acupuncture modulates the limbic system and subcortical gray structures of the human brain: evidence from fMRI studies in normal subjects, *Hum Brain Mapp* 9(1):13, 2000.

Hui KK, Liu J, Marina O, et al: The integrated response of the human cerebro-cerebellar and limbic systems to acupuncture stimulation at ST 36 as evidenced by fMRI, *Neuroimage* 27(3):479, 2005.

Hsu H, Peacher W: *Chen's history of Chinese medical science*, Taipei, 1977, Modern Drug Publishers.

Jin GY, Xiang JJ, Jin L: *Contemporary medical acupuncture: a systems approach*, 2006, Springer-Verlag.

Jobst K: A critical analysis of acupuncture in pulmonary disease: efficacy and safety of the acupuncture needle, *J Altern Complement Med* 1(1):57, 1995.

Junnila SYT: Acupuncture superior to piroxicam in the treatment of osteoarthritis, *Am J Acupunct* 10:341, 1982.

Kiresuk TJ, Culliton PD 1994. *Overview of substance abuse acupuncture treatment research*. Workshop on Acupuncture. pp 1-17, 21/4.

Kaptchuk TJ: *The web that has no weaver: understanding Chinese medicine*, New York, 1983, Congdon & Weed.

Kaptchuk TJ: Acupuncture: theory, efficacy, and practice, *Ann Intern Med* 136(5):374–383, 2002.

Langevin HM, Churchill DL, Cipolla MJ: Mechanical signaling through connective tissue: a mechanism for the therapeutic effect of acupuncture, *FASEB J* 15(12):2275, 2001a.

Langevin HM, Churchill DL, Fox JR, et al: Biomechanical response to acupuncture needling in humans, *J Appl Physiol* 91:2471, 2001b.

Langevin HM, Churchill DL, Wu J, et al: Evidence of connective tissue involvement in acupuncture, *FASEB J* 16(8):872, 2002. Available at: http://www.fasebj.org/cgi/reprint/16/8/872. [Epub April 10, 2002].

Langevin HM, Yandow JA: Relationship of acupuncture points and meridians to connective tissue planes, *Anat Rec* 269(6):257, 2002.

Lao L, Bergman S, Hamilton GR, et al: Evaluation of acupuncture for pain control after oral surgery: a placebo-controlled trial, *Arch Otolaryngol Head Neck Surg* 125(5):567, 1999.

Lao L, Bergman S, Langenberg P, et al: Efficacy of Chinese acupuncture on postoperative oral surgery pain, *Oral Surg Oral Med Oral Pathol Oral Radiol Endod* 79:423, 1995.

Liu C: *Study of Daoist acupuncture and moxibustion*, Boulder, CO, 1999, Blue Poppy Press.

Ma Y, Ma M, Cho Z: *Biomedical acupuncture for pain management: an integrative approach*, London, 2005, Churchill Livingstone.

MacPherson H, Thomas K, Armstrong B, et al: Developing research strategies in complementary and alternative medicine, *Comp Ther Med* 16:359–362, 2008.

Manheimer E, White A, Berman B, et al: Meta-analysis: acupuncture for low back pain, *Ann Intern Med* 142:651–663, 2005.

Mayer DJ, Price DD, Rafii A: Antagonism of acupuncture analgesia in man by the narcotic antagonist naloxone, *Brain Res* 121(2):368, 1977.

McCarney RW, Lasserson TJ, Linde K, et al: Acupuncture for chronic asthma, *Cochrane Database Syst Rev* 2007.

Mehl-Madrona L, Kligler B, Silverman S, et al: The impact of acupuncture and craniosacral therapy interventions on clinical outcomes in adults with asthma, *Explore* 3(1):28, 2007.

Melzack R, Stillwell DM, Fox EJ: Trigger points and acupuncture points for pain: correlations and implications, *Pain* 3:3, 1977.

Molsberger AF, Boewing G, Diener HC, et al: Designing an acupuncture study: the nationwide, randomized, controlled, German acupuncture trials on migraine and tension-type headache, *J Altern Complement Med* 12:237–245, 2006.

Napadow V, Kettner N, Liu J, et al: Hypothalamus and amygdala response to acupuncture stimuli in carpal tunnel syndrome, *Pain* 130(3):254, 2007. [Epub January 19, 2007].

National Institutes of Health: Acupuncture, *NIH Consens Statement* 15(5):1, 1997.

Nogier P: Face to face with auriculotherapy, *Acupunct Electrother Res* 8:99–100, 1983a.

Nogier P: *From auriculotherapy to auriculomedicine*, 1983b, Maionneuve.

Oschman J: A biophysical basis for acupuncture. In Birch S, editor: *Proceedings of the First Symposium of the Society for Acupuncture Research*, Boston, 1993, Society for Acupuncture Research, p 141.

Passalacqua GB, Bousquet P, Carlsen K, et al: ARIA update: I— Systematic review of complementary and alternative medicine for rhinitis and asthma, *J Clin Immunol* 117(5):1054, 2005.

Patel M, Gutzwiller F, Paccand F, et al: A meta-analysis of acupuncture for chronic pain, *Int J Epidemiol* 18(4):900, 1989.

Pomeranz B: Scientific basis of acupuncture. In Stux G, editor: *The basics of acupuncture*, New York, 1988, Springer-Verlag, p 4.

Pomeranz B, Stux G: *Basics of acupuncture*, 1998, Springer-Verlag.

Pomeranz B, Chiu D: Naloxone blockade of acupuncture analgesia: endorphin implicated, *Life Sci* 19:1757–1762, 1976.

Sator-Katzenschlager SM, Wölfler MM, Kozek-Langenecker SA, et al: Auricular electro-acupuncture as an additional perioperative analgesic method during oocyte aspiration in IVF treatment, *Hum Reprod* 21(8):2114, 2006. Epub May 5, 2006.

Shanghai College of Traditional Chinese Medicine: *Acupuncture: a comprehensive text*, Seattle, 1981, Eastland Press. (translated by J O'Connor, D Bensky).

Stockert K, Schneider B, Porenta G, et al: Laser acupuncture and probiotics in school age children with asthma: a randomized, placebo-controlled pilot study of therapy guided by principles of traditional Chinese medicine, *Pediatric Allergy Immunology* 17:160–166, 2007.

Taormina K, Rooney D, Ladas EJ, et al: Abstract #62: *A retrospective review investigating the feasibility of acupuncture as a supportive care agent in a pediatric oncology service*, Society for Integrative Oncology Meeting, Boston 2006.

ter Riet G, Kleijnen J, Knipschild P: Acupuncture and chronic pain: a criteria-based meta-analysis, *J Clin Epidemiol* 43:1191, 1990.

Thomas M, Eriksson SV, Lundeberg T: A comparative study of diazepam and acupuncture in patients with osteoarthritis pain: a placebo controlled study, *Am J Chin Med* 19:95, 1991.

Tiller WA: *Science and human transformation: subtle energies, intentionality and consciousness*, Walnut Creek, Calif, 1997, Pavior.

Travell JG, Simons DG: *Myofascial pain and dysfunction: trigger point manual*, Media, Pa, 1983, Williams & Wilkins.

Unschuld P: *Medicine in China: a history of ideas*, Berkeley, 1985, University of California Press.

Vickers A, Rees R, Zollman K, et al: Acupuncture for chronic headache in primary care: large, pragmatic, randomized trial, *BMJ* 328:744, 2004.

Vincent CA: A controlled trial of the treatment of migraine by acupuncture, *Clin J Pain* 5:305, 1989.

Vincent CA: Acupuncture as a treatment for chronic pain. In Lewith GT, Aldridge D, editors: *Clinical research methodology for complementary therapies*, London, 1993, Hodder & Stoughton, p 289.

Westergaard LG, Mao Q, Krogslund M, et al: Acupuncture on the day of embryo transfer significantly improves the reproductive outcome in infertile women: a prospective, randomized trial, *Fertil Steril* 85(5):1341, 2006.

World Health Organization: *Acupuncture: review and analysis of reports on controlled clinical trials*, Geneva, 2002, The Organization. Available at: http://www.who.int/medicines/library/trm/acupuncture/acupuncture_trials.doc.

Suggested Readings

Agren H: A new approach to Chinese traditional medicine, *Am J Chin Med* 3(3):207, 1975.

Bensoussan A, Talley NJ, Hing M, et al: Treatment of irritable bowel syndrome with Chinese herbal medicine: a randomized clinical trial, *JAMA* 280(18):1585, 1998.

Birch S: A historical study of radial pulse six position diagnosis: naming the unnameable, *J Acupunct Soc N Y* 1(3–4):19, 1994.

Coan R, Wong GT, Ku S-L, et al: The acupuncture treatment of low back pain: a randomized controlled study, *Am J Chin Med* 8(2):181, 1980.

Ellis A, Wiseman N, Boss K: *Fundamentals of Chinese acupuncture*, Brookline, Mass, 1991, Paradigm.

Hao LZ: An attempt to understand the substance of kidney and its disorders, *J Am Coll Tradit Chin Med* (3):82, 1983 (translated by CS Cheung).

Helms JM: Acupuncture for the management of primary dysmenorrhea, *Obstet Gynecol* 69(1):51, 1987.

Huang B, Di F, Li X, et al: Syndromes of traditional Chinese medicine. In Huang B, editor: *Thousand Formulas and Thousand Herbs of Traditional Chinese Medicine*, Heilongjiang, China, 1993, Heilongjiang Education Press.

Jobst K, Kim A: *J Altern Complement Med* 2(1):179, 1996.

MacPherson H, Hammerschlag R, Lewith G, et al: *Acupuncture research strategies for building evidence bases*, London, 2007, Churchill Livingstone.

Manaka Y, Itaya K: Acupuncture as intervention in the biological information system, *J Acupunct Soc N Y* 1(3–4):19, 1994.

Naeser MA, Michael PA, Stiassny-Eder D, et al: Real versus sham acupuncture in the treatment of paralysis in acute stroke patients: a CT scan lesion study, *J Neurol Rehabil* 6(4):163–174, 1992.

Reichmanis M, Marino AA, Becker RO: Electrical correlates of acupuncture points, *IEEE Trans Biome Eng* 22(6):533, 1975.

Ryu H, Jun CD, Lee BS, et al: Effect of qigong training on proportions of T lymphocyte subsets in human peripheral blood, *Am J Chin Med* 23:27, 1995.

Sancier K: Medical applications of qigong alternative therapies, *Altern Ther Health Med* 2(1):40, 1996.

Wang X: Research on the origin and development of Chinese acupuncture and moxibustion. In Xiangtong Z, editor: *Research on acupuncture, moxibustion and acupuncture anesthesia*, New York, 1986, Springer-Verlag, p 783.

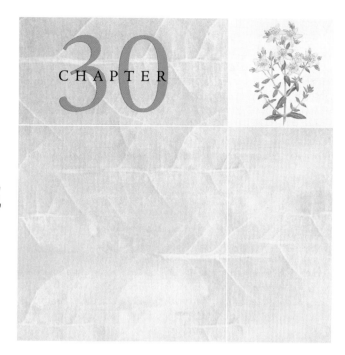

CHAPTER 30

TIBETAN MEDICINE

KEVIN V. ERGIL

Practitioners of the Tibetan system of medicine, the *science of healing* (*gso.ba.rig.pa*), can trace a lineage of practice and precept back through the centuries. As with many aspects of Tibetan cultural practices, the Tibetan medical system manifests the thoughtful mixture of aspects of Indic traditions and those of other cultures with indigenous practices. Tibetan medicine is deeply rooted in the worldview of Buddhism and is organized primarily around concepts of the body, which it shares with Ayurveda, India's *science of life* (see Chapter 31).

Tibetan medicine is a rich and literate tradition (since the eighth century AD), with diverse practice lineages, specialized knowledge, and regional variation. Tibetan medicine manifests a remarkable syncretism and adaptability, and its spiritual history, with its links to the origins of Buddhism, reminds its practitioners of the fundamental meaning of the practice of medicine: *compassion.*

From a historical perspective, the circumstances that shaped Tibetan medicine are to a great extent a circum-

stance of geopolitical factors. Geographically, the region known as Tibet lies to the south of what became known as the "Silk Road." By the second century BC, this route allowed materials of value to be traded along its length. Precious medicinals, such as rhubarb, found their way west to Greece and Rome. This trading route, which provided markets for silk, spice, medicines, produce, gold, and gemstones, also furnished a conduit for the exchange of knowledge and ideas between East and West.

The understanding within Tibetan medicine concerning the origins of medical knowledge in general and of the knowledge contained within the Four Tantras in particular is intriguing. It is an understanding that simultaneously asserts the primacy of Buddhist medical knowledge and implicitly asserts that all healing traditions share the ultimate goal of providing compassionate care to suffering beings.

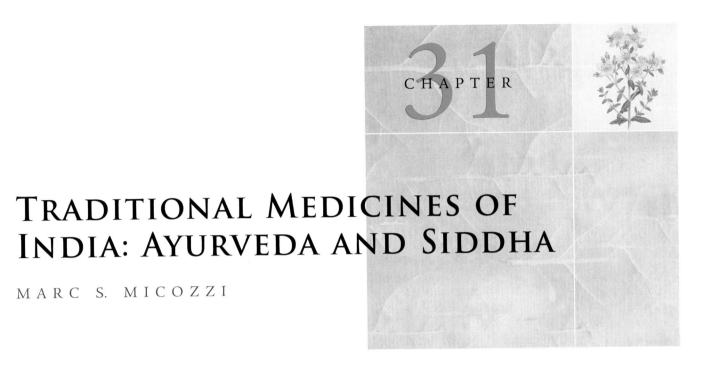

TRADITIONAL MEDICINES OF INDIA: AYURVEDA AND SIDDHA

M A R C   S.   M I C O Z Z I

Three traditional medicinal systems predominate in modern India: Ayurveda, Siddha, and Unani. Ayurveda is found mostly in northern India and in Kerala in the south. Siddha medicine is found mostly in Tamil Nadu and in parts of Kerala. Unani is found throughout India and Pakistan, mainly in the urban areas, and actually derives from Greco-Arabic medicine, rather than Indian sources (see Chapter 32).

This chapter describes Ayurveda, and other, related traditional systems, Siddha medicine, yoga (see Chapter 21), and the contemporary development of Maharishi Ayurveda in India and the West. Yoga is a meditative and devotional practice that originated in India. It is not part of Ayurveda and is discussed in a separate chapter because its focus in the West is primarily through its physical aspects as expressed in *Hatha* Yoga, for example (see Chapter 21).

Traditional medicine, in addition to being a highly developed and complex form of "ethnomedicine," remains in living use as an available form of primary health care in India; it is also becoming more available in the West as a "complementary/alternative" medical system that is sometimes accessed in the practice of "integrative medicine."

THE SCIENCE OF LIFE

Ayurveda is, literally, the science of life, or longevity. As with any popular development, aspects of this Indian medical system and its cures have sometimes been appropriated by individuals (such as popular "gurus" in the west) not wholly familiar with the basic assumptions of Ayurveda as a science of longevity. However, scholars have undertaken serious study of this ancient healing tradition. The fundamental principles and practices of traditional Ayurveda may be understood from their work on the

classical Sanskrit sources and from accounts from traditional Indian practitioners.

FOUR PHASES

On the basis of available literary sources, the history of Indian medicine occurred in four main phases (Zysk, 1991, 1993). The first, or Vedic, phase dates from about 1200 to 800 BC. Information about medicine during this period is obtained from numerous curative incantations and references to healing that are found in the *Atharvaveda* and the *Rigveda,* two religious scriptures that reveal a "magico-religious" approach to healing (Zysk, 1993). The second, or classical, phase is marked by the advent of the first Sanskrit medical treatises, the *Caraka Samhita* (Sharma, 1981–1994) and *Sushruta Samhita* (Bhishagratna, 1983), which probably dates from a few centuries before to several centuries after the start of the common era. This period includes all medical treatises dating from before the Muslim invasions of India at the beginning of the eleventh century. These works tend to follow the earlier classical compilations closely, and provide the basis of traditional Ayurveda. The third, or syncretic, phase is marked by clear influences from Unani, Siddha, and other nonclassical medical systems in India. Bhavamishra's sixteenth-century *Bhavaprakasha* is one text that reveals the results of these influences, such as diagnosis by examination of pulse or urine (Upadhyay, 1986). This phase extends from the time of the Muslim incursions to the present era.

The fourth phase is phrased as "New Age Ayurveda," wherein the classical paradigm is being adapted to the world of modern science and technology, including quantum physics, mind–body science, and advanced biomedical science. This recent manifestation of Ayurveda is

TABLE 31-1 *Medical Traditions of South Asia and the Middle East*

Phase	Dates	Sources	Modalities
I. Vedic	1200–800 BC	*Atharvaveda, Rigveda*	Magico-religious
II. Classic	700 BC–AD 400	Sanskrit texts: *Caraka, Sushruta, Samhita*	Herbal medicines
III. Syncretic	1000–1980	Muslim influences, Unani, Siddha, *Bhavaprakasha*	Pulse, urine diagnosis
IV. New Age	1980–2010	Maharishi Ayurveda	Quantum physics

most visible in the Western world, although there are indications that it is filtering back to India in its worldwide reach. These four phases of Indian medical history provide a simple chronological grid for understanding the development of this ancient system of medicine (Table 31-1). A more comprehensive chronology of historical developments relating to traditional Indian medicines in the region of Middle Asia is given in the Chronology of Indian Medicines table.

From its beginnings during the Vedic era, Indian medicine always has adhered closely to the principle of a fundamental connection between the microcosm and macrocosm as in Western traditions until the modern era (Chapter 1). Human beings are minute representations of the universe, and contain within them everything that makes up the surrounding world. Comprehending the world is crucial to comprehending the human, and, conversely, understanding the human is necessary to understanding the world.

THE FIVE ELEMENTS

According to Ayurveda, the cosmos consists of five basic elements: earth, air, fire, water, and space. Certain forces cause these elements to interact, giving rise to all that exists. In human beings these five elements occur and combine as the three *doshas,* forces that, along with the seven *dhatus* (tissues) and three *malas* (waste products), make up the human body.

THE THREE *DOSHAS*

When in equilibrium, the three *doshas* maintain health, but when an imbalance occurs among them, they defile the normal functioning of the body, leading to the manifestation of disease. An imbalance indicates an increase or decrease in one, two, or all three of the *doshas*. The three *doshas* are *Vata, Pitta,* and *Kapha* (Svoboda, 1984) (Table 31-2).

Vata or *Vayu,* meaning "wind," is composed of the elements air and space. It is the principle of kinetic energy and is responsible for all bodily movement and nervous functions. It is located below the navel, in the bladder, large intestines, nervous system, pelvic region, thighs, bone marrow, and legs; its principal seat is the colon. When disrupted, its primary manifestations are gas and muscular or nervous energy, leading to pain.

Pitta, or bile, is made up of the elements fire and water. It governs enzymes and hormones, and is responsible for

digestion, pigmentation, body temperature, hunger, thirst, sight, courage, and mental activity. It is located between the navel and the chest, in the stomach, small intestines, liver, spleen, skin, and blood; its principal seat is the stomach. When disrupted, its primary manifestations are acid and bile, leading to inflammation.

Kapha, meaning "phlegm," is made up of the elements of earth and water. It connotes the principle of cohesion and stability. It regulates *Vata* and *Pitta* and is responsible for keeping the body lubricated, and maintaining its solid nature, tissues, sexual power, and strength. It also controls patience. Its normal locations are the upper part of the body, the thorax, head, neck, upper portion of the stomach, pleural cavity, fat tissues, and areas between joints; its principal seat is the lungs. When it is disrupted, its primary manifestations are liquid and mucus, leading to swelling, with or without discharge.

The attributes of each *dosha* help determine an individual's basic bodily and mental makeup and to isolate which *dosha* is responsible for a disease. *Vata* is dry, cold, light, irregular, mobile, rough, and abundant. Dryness occurs when *Vata* is disturbed, and is a side effect of motion. Too much dryness produces irregularity in the body and mind. *Pitta* is hot, light, intense, fluid, liquid, putrid, pungent, and sour. Heat appears when *Pitta* is disturbed, and produces irritability in the body and mind. *Kapha* is heavy, unctuous, cold, stable, dense, soft, and smooth. Heaviness occurs when *Kapha* is disturbed, and produces slowness in body and mind.

THE SEVEN DHATUS

The seven *dhatus,* or tissues, are responsible for sustaining the body. Each dhatu is responsible for the one that comes next in the following order, according to Zysk (1993).

1. *Rasa,* meaning sap or juice, includes the tissue fluids, bile, lymph, and plasma, and functions as nourishment. It comes from digested food.
2. Blood includes the red blood cells and functions to invigorate the body.
3. Flesh includes muscle tissue and functions as stabilization.
4. Fat includes adipose tissue and functions as lubrication.
5. Bone includes bone and cartilage and functions as support.

TABLE 31-2 *The Three Doshas: Vata, Pitta, Kapha*

Dosha	Effect of balanced *dosha*	Effect of imbalanced *dosha*	Factors aggravating
Vata	Exhilaration Clear and alert mind Perfect functioning of bowels and urinary tract Proper formation of all bodily tissues Sound sleep Excellent vitality and immunity	Rough skin Weight loss Anxiety, worry Restlessness Constipation Decreased strength **Arthritis** **Hypertension** Rheumatic disorder Cardiac arrhythmia Insomnia **Irritable bowel syndrome**	Excessive exercise Wakefulness Falling, bone fractures Tuberculosis Suppression of natural urges Cold Fear or grief Agitation or anger Fasting Pungent, astringent, or bitter foods In USA: Late autumn and winter In India: Summer and rainy season
Pitta	Lustrous complexion Contentment Perfect digestion Softness of body Perfectly balanced heat and thirst mechanisms Balanced intellect	Yellowish complexion Excessive body heat Insufficient sleep Weak digestion Inflammation Inflammatory bowel diseases Skin diseases Heartburn **Peptic ulcer** Anger	Anger Strong sunshine Burning sensations Fasting Sesame products, linseed Yogurt Wine, vinegar Pungent, sour, or salty foods In USA: Summer and early autumn In India: Rainy season and autumn
Kapha	Strength Normal joints Stability of mind Dignity Affectionate, forgiving nature Strong and properly proportioned body Courage Vitality	Pale complexion Coldness Laziness, dullness Excessive sleep Sinusitis Respiratory diseases, **asthma** Excessive weight gain Loose joints Depression	Sleeping during daytime Heavy food Sweet, sour, or salty foods Milk products Sugar In USA: Spring In India: Late winter and spring

6. Marrow includes red and yellow bone marrow and functions as filling for the bones.
7. *Shukra* includes male and female sexual fluids and functions in reproduction and immunity.

THE THREE MALAS

The *malas* are the waste products of digestion. Ayurveda delineates three principal malas: urine, feces, and sweat. A fourth category of other waste products includes fatty excretions from the skin and intestines, cebum (ear wax), mucus of the nose, saliva, tears, hair, and nails. According to Ayurveda, an individual should evacuate the bowels once a day and eliminate urine six times a day.

The Importance of Digestion

Ayurveda considers digestion to be the most important function that takes place in the human body. It provides all that is required to sustain the organism and is the principal cause for all maladies from which an individual suffers. The process of digestion and assimilation of nutrients is discussed under the topics of the Agnis (enzymes), Ama (improperly digested food and drink), and the Srotas (channels of circulation).

THE THREE AGNIS

The Agnis, or enzymes, assist in the digestion and assimilation of food and are divided into three types according to Zysk (1993):

1. *Jatharagni* is active in the mouth, stomach, and gastrointestinal tract and helps break down food. The waste product of feces results from this activity.
2. *Bhutagnis* are five enzymes located in the liver. They adapt the broken down food into a homologous chyle in accordance with the five elements, and assist the chyle to assimilate with the corresponding elements in the body. The homologous chyle circulates in the blood channels as rasa, nourishing the body and supplying the seven dhatus.
3. *Dhatvagnis* are seven enzymes that synthesize the seven dhatus from the assimilated chyle homologized with the five elements. The remaining waste products result from this activity.

AMA

Ama is the chief cause of disease and is formed when there is a decrease in enzyme activity. A product of improperly digested food and drink, it takes the form of a liquid sludge that travels through the same channels as the chyle. Because of its density, however, it lodges in different parts of the body, blocking the channels. It often mixes with the *doshas* that circulate through the same pathways, and it gravitates to a weak or stressed organ or to a site of a disease manifestation. Because all diseases invariably come from ama, the word *Amaya,* meaning "coming from Ama," is a synonym for disease. Internal diseases begin with ama, and external diseases produce ama. In general, ama can be detected by a coating on the tongue; turbid urine with foul odor; and feces that is passed with undigested food, an offensive odor, and abundant gas. The principal course of treatment in Ayurveda involves the elimination of ama and the restoration of the balance of the *doshas.*

THE THIRTEEN KINDS OF SROTAS

The Srotas are the vessels or channels of the body through which all substances circulate. They are either large, such as the large and small intestines, uterus, arteries, and veins, or small, such as the capillaries. A healthy body has open and free-flowing channels. Blockage of the channels, usually by ama, results in disease (Zysk, 1993).

1. Pranavahasrotas convey vitality and vital breath (*prana*), and originate in the heart and alimentary tract.
2. Udakavahasrotas convey water and fluids, and originate in the palate and pancreas.
3. Annavahasrotas convey food from the outside, and originate in the stomach.
4. Rasavahasrotas convey chyle, lymph, and plasma, and originate in the heart and in the 10 vessels connected with the heart. Ama primarily accumulates within them.
5. Raktavahasrotas convey red blood cells, and originate in the liver and spleen.
6. Mamsavahasrotas convey ingredients for muscle tissue, and originate in the tendons, ligaments, and skin.
7. Medovahasrotas convey ingredients for fat tissue, and originate in the kidneys and fat tissues of the abdomen.
8. Asthavahasrotas convey ingredients for bone tissue, and originate in hip bone.
9. Majjavahasrotas convey ingredients for marrow, and originate in the bones and joints.
10. Shukravahasrotas convey ingredients for the male and female reproductive tissues, and originate in the testicles and ovaries.
11. Mutravahasrotas convey urine, and originate in the kidney and bladder.
12. Purishavahasrotas convey feces, and originate in the colon and rectum.
13. Svedavahasrotas convey sweat, and originate in the fat tissues and hair follicles.

CONSTITUTIONAL TYPES

This broad outline presents the Ayurvedic view that the human body's anatomical parts are composed of the five basic elements, which have undergone a process of metabolism and assimilation in the body. Human beings differ in their normal bodily constitution (*prakriti*), which is determined at the moment of conception, and remains so until death. The four factors that influence constitutional type include the father, the mother (particularly her food intake), the womb, and the season of the year. A large imbalance of the *doshas* in the mother will affect the growth of the embryo and fetus, and a moderate excess of one or two of the *doshas* will affect the constitution of the child.

PRAKRITI

There are seven normal body constitutions (*prakriti*) based on the three *doshas: Vata, Pitta, Kapha, Vata-Pitta, Pitta-Kapha, Vata-Kapha,* and *sama.* The latter is triple balanced, which is best but extremely rare. Most people are a combination of *doshas,* in which one *dosha* predominates. The classic characteristics of *doshas* are outlined in Box 31-1 and Table 31-3. In general, *Vata*-type people tend to be anxious and fearful, exhibit light and "airy" characteristics, and are prone to *Vata*-diseases. *Pitta*-type people are aggressive and impatient, exhibit fiery and hot-headed characteristics, and are prone to *Pitta*-diseases. *Kapha*-type people are stable and entrenched; exhibit heavy, wet, and earthy characteristics; and are prone to *Kapha*-diseases (Svoboda, 1984).

These are the principal factors that help the Ayurvedic physician determine the correct course of treatment to be administered to a patient for a particular ailment.

TABLE 31-3 *Times of Day, Seasons, and Life Cycle Classified According to the Doshas*

Kapha time	Approximately 6 AM (sunrise) to 10 AM, and 6 PM to 10 PM
Kapha season	In USA, Spring; In India, Late winter and spring
Kapha period in life cycle	Childhood
Pitta time	Approximately 10 AM to 2 PM, and 10 PM to 2 AM
Pitta season	In USA, Summer and early autumn; In India, Rainy season and autumn
Pitta period in life cycle	Adulthood
Vata time	Approximately 2 AM to 6 AM (sunrise), and 2 PM to 6 PM
Vata season	In USA, Late autumn and winter; In India, Summer and Rainy season
Vata period in life cycle	Old age

BOX 31-1 *Classic Characteristics of Vata, Pitta, and Kapha*

Vata (ectomorphic constitution)

· Light, thin build
· Performs activity quickly
· Tendency to dry skin
· Aversion to cold weather
· Irregular hunger and digestion
· Quick to grasp new information, also quick to forget
· Tendency toward worry
· Tendency toward constipation
· Tendency toward light and interrupted sleep

Pitta (mesomorphic constitution)

· Moderate build
· Performs activity with medium speed
· Aversion to hot weather
· Sharp hunger and digestion
· Medium time to grasp new information
· Medium memory
· Tendency toward irritability and temper
· Enterprising and sharp in character
· Prefers cold foods and drinks
· Cannot skip meals
· Good speakers
· Tendency toward reddish complexion and hair, moles, and freckles

Kapha (endomorphic constitution)

· Solid, heavier build
· Greater strength and endurance
· Slow, methodical in activity
· Oily, smooth skin
· Tranquil, steady personality
· Slow to grasp new information, slow to forget
· Slow to become excited or irritated
· Sleep is heavy and for long periods
· Hair is plentiful, tends to be dark color
· Slow digestion, mild hunger

MENTAL STATES

In addition to physical constitution, Ayurveda understands that an individual is influenced by three mental states, based on the three qualities (*gunas*) of balance (*sattva*), energy (*rajas*), and inertia (*tamas*). In the state of balance the mind is in equilibrium and can discriminate correctly. In the state of energy the mind is excessively active, causing weakness in discrimination. In the state of inertia the mind is excessively inactive, also creating weak discrimination.

Ayurveda always has recognized that the body and the mind interact to create a healthy, normal (*prakriti*), or unhealthy, abnormal (*vikriti*) condition. A good Ayurvedic physician will determine both the mental and physical condition of the patient before proceeding with any form of diagnosis and treatment.

THE NAMING OF DISEASE

Aspects of the Ayurvedic understanding of disease have been mentioned above. These understandings provide a basis for the Ayurvedic classification of disease, the naming of disease, and the manifestations of disease (Dash, 1980; Dash & Kashyap, 1980).

Ayurveda identifies three broad categories of disease, on the basis of causative factors (Zysk, 1993):

1. *Adhyatmika* diseases originate within the body, and may be subdivided into hereditary diseases, congenital diseases, and diseases caused by one or a combination of the *doshas*.
2. *Adhibhautika* diseases originate outside the body, and include injuries from accidents or mishaps, and, in the terminology of the modern era, from germs, viruses, and bacteria.
3. *Adhidaivika* diseases originate from supernatural sources, including diseases that are otherwise inexplicable, such as maladies stemming from providential causes, planetary influences, curses, and seasonal changes.

A six-step process determines the manner by which a *dosha* becomes aggravated and moves through the different channels to produce disease. An accumulation of a *dosha* leads to its aggravation, which causes it to spread through the channels until it lodges in a particular organ of the body, bringing about a manifestation of disease. Once a general form of the disease appears, it progressively divides into specific varieties. As in systems of medicine worldwide, many patients consult an Ayurvedic physician only after the disease appears.

Ayurveda delineates seven basic varieties of disease on the basis of the *doshas*: diseases involving a single *dosha*, diseases involving two *doshas*, and diseases involving all three *doshas* together.

In Ayurveda, diseases receive their names in one of six ways. A disease is named for the condition it produces (fever, or *Jvara*), its chief symptom (diarrhea, or *Atisara*), its chief physical sign (jaundice, or *Pandu*), its principal nature (piles, or *Arshas*), the chief *dosha(s)* involved (wind-disease, or *Vata-roga*), or the chief organ involved (disease of the duodenum, or *Grahani*). Regardless of its given name, most diseases are understood to involve one or more of the *doshas*.

During the course of a disease, an Ayurvedic physician seeks to identify its site of origin, its path of transportation, and its site of manifestation. The site of manifestation of a disease usually differs from its site of origin. Recognizing this distinction enables the physician to determine the correct course of treatment.

Ayurveda describes the manifestation of all diseases in the same fundamental way. Causative factors (e.g., food, drink, regimen, season, mental state) suppress digestive (enzyme) activity in the body, leading to the formation of ama. The circulating ama blocks the channels. The site of the disease's origin is where the blockage occurs. The circulating ama, often combining with one or more of the *doshas,* then takes a divergent course, referred to as the *path of transportation.* Finally, the *dosha(s)* and ama mixture comes to rest in and afflicts a certain body part, which is known as the *site of disease manifestation.* Treatment entails correction of all the steps in the process resulting in disease manifestation, thus restoring the entire person to his or her particular balanced state (Zysk, 1993).

DIAGNOSIS AND TREATMENT

In Ayurveda, restoring a person to health is not viewed simply as the eradication of disease. It entails a complete process of diagnosis and therapeutics that takes into account both mental and physical components integrated with the social and physical worlds in which the patient lives. It begins with Ayurvedic diagnosis, examination of the disease, and types of therapeutics (Jolly, 1977; Lad, 1990; Sen Gupta, 1984).

Ayurveda uses a detailed system of diagnosis, involving examination of pulse, urine, and physical features.

After a preliminary examination by means of visual observation, touch, and interrogation, the Ayurvedic physician undertakes an eightfold method of detailed examination to determine the patient's type of physical constitution and mental status and to get an indication of any abnormality.

FEELING THE PULSE: SNAKE, FROG, AND BIRD

The first mention of pulse examination is in a medical treatise from the late thirteenth to early fourteenth century of the common era. It is a highly specialized art and all Ayurvedic physicians do not use pulse examination. The diagnostic process involves evenly placing the index, middle, and ring fingers of the right hand on the radial artery of the right hand of men and the left hand of women, just at the base of the thumb. A pulse resembling the movement of a snake at the index finger indicates a predominance of *Vata;* a pulse resembling the movement of a frog at the middle finger indicates a predominance of *Pitta;* a pulse resembling the movement of a swan or peacock at the ring finger indicates a predominance of *Kapha;* and a pulse resembling the pecking of a woodpecker in all three fingers indicates a predominance of all three *doshas.* To get an accurate reading, the physician must keep in mind the times when each of the *doshas* are normally excited, and should take the pulse at least three times, making sure to wash his or her hands after each reading. Optimum timing for the reading is early in the morning when the stomach is empty, or 3 hours after eating in the afternoon (Upadhyay, 1986).

URINE EXAMINATION: THE SHAPES OF DROPS

Like pulse examination, urine examination probably was formalized in the syncretic phase (see Table 31-1). After collecting a midstream urine evacuation in a clear glass container, after sunrise, the physician submits the urine to two kinds of examination. First, the physician studies it in the container to determine its color and degree of transparency. Pale-yellow and oily urine indicates *Vata;* intense yellow, reddish, or blue urine indicates *Pitta;* white, foamy, and muddy urine indicates *Kapha;* urine with a blackish tinge indicates a combination of *doshas;* and urine resembling lime juice or vinegar indicates ama. The physician also puts a few drops of sesame oil in the urine and examines it in sunlight. The shape, movement, and diffusion of the oil in the urine indicate the prognosis of the disease. The shape of the drops also reveals which *dosha(s)* is/are involved. A snakelike shape indicates *Vata;* umbrella shape, *Pitta;* and pearl shape, *Kapha.*

EXAMINING THE BODY

The physician concludes his diagnostic examination with careful scrutiny of the tongue, skin, nails, and physical features to determine which *dosha(s)* is/are affected. Using the basic characteristics of each of the *doshas,* the physician will examine the different parts of the body. Coldness, dryness, roughness, and cracking indicate *Vata;* hotness and redness indicate *Pitta;* and wetness, whiteness, and coldness indicate *Kapha.*

Having completed this phase of the diagnosis, the Ayurvedic physician proceeds to examine any malady present.

FIVE STEPS

A detailed examination of the disease involves a *five-step process,* leading to a complete understanding of the abnormality (Zysk, 1993).

1. *Finding the cause.* A disease is *caused* by one or several of the following factors: mental imbalances resulting from the effects of past actions (*karma*); unbalanced contact between the senses and the objects of the senses affecting the body and the mind; effects of the seasons on the mental and doshic balance; the immediate causes of diet, regimen, and microorganisms; *doshas* and ama; and the interaction of individual components such as *doshas* and tissues or *doshas* and microorganisms.

2. *Early signs and symptoms* appear before the onset of disease and provide clues to the diagnosis. Proper diet and administration of medicine can avert disease if it is recognized early enough.

3. *Manifest signs and symptoms.* The most crucial step in the diagnostic process involves determining the site of origin, site of disease manifestation, and the path of transportation of the ama and *dosha(s).* Most signs and symptoms are associated with the site of manifestation, from which the physician must work his or her way back to the site of origin to effect a complete cure. Although symptomatic treatment was largely absent in traditional Ayurveda, modern medicine in India has introduced Ayurvedic physicians to techniques of symptomatic treatment in cases of acute disease.

4. *Exploratory therapy.* This step involves 18 different experiments that use herbs, diet, and regimens to determine the precise nature of the malady and suitable therapy by allopathic and homeopathic means.
5. *Prognosis.* Because Ayurvedic physicians traditionally did not treat persons with incurable diseases, it was important for the physician to know precisely the patient's chances of recovery. Therefore, a disease is classified as one of three types. It is (1) easily curable, (2) palliative, or (3) incurable or difficult to cure.

The three categories of prognosis are similar to those described in ancient Egyptian medicine as laid out in the Edwin Smith papyrus, for diseases of the head and neck, as "diseases I will treat," implying the expectation of cure, "diseases with which I will contend," implying the expectation to alleviate suffering, and "diseases I will not treat," implying the incurable (van Houten & Micozzi, 1981).

In general, if the disease type (*Vata, Pitta, Kapha*) is different from the person's normal physical constitution, the disease is easy to cure. If the disease and constitution are the same, the disease is difficult to cure. If the disease, constitution, and season correspond to doshic type, the disease is nearly impossible to cure (Singhal, 1972-1993).

Having determined the patient's normal constitution, diagnosed his or her illness, and established a prognosis for recovery, the Ayurvedic physician can begin a proper course of treatment.

CONTINUOUS HEALING

Ayurveda recognizes two courses of treatment on the basis of the condition of the patient. The first is prevention, for the healthy person who wants to maintain a normal condition based on his or her physical constitution and to prevent disease. The second is therapy, for an ill person who requires health to be restored. Once healthy, Ayurveda recommends continuous prophylaxis based on diet, regimen, medicines, and regular therapeutic purification procedures.

When a person is diagnosed with a doshic imbalance, either purification therapy, alleviation therapy, or a combination of these is prescribed.

PURIFICATION: THE FIVE ACTIONS

Purification therapy involves the fundamental Five Actions, or *Pañchakarma,* treatment. This fivefold process varies slightly in different traditions and regions of India, but a standard regimen generally is followed. All five procedures can be performed, or a selection of procedures can be chosen on the basis of different factors such as the physical constitution of the patient, his or her condition, the season, and the nature of the disease.

- Before any action is taken, the patient is given oil internally and externally (with massage) and is sweated to loosen and soften the *dosha(s)* and ama.
- An appropriate diet of food and drink is prescribed.

After this two-part preparatory treatment, called *Purvakarma,* the five therapies are administered in sequence over the period of about a week.

The patient is advised to set aside time for treatment in light of the profound effects on the mind and body. First, the patient might be given an emetic to induce vomiting until bilious matter is produced, thus removing *Kapha.* Second, a purgative is given until mucous material appears, thus removing *Pitta.* Third, an enema, either of oil or decocted medicines, is administered, flushing the bowels, to remove excess *Vata.* Fourth, head purgation is given in the form of smoke inhalation or nasal drops to eradicate the *dosha(s)* that have accumulated in the head and sinuses. Fifth, leeches may be applied and bloodletting performed to purify the blood. Some physicians do not consider bloodletting in the five therapies of *Pañchakarma,* instead counting oily and dry (decocted medicine) enemas as two separate forms (Singh, 1992).

Alleviation therapy uses the basic condiments honey, butter or ghee, and sesame oil or castor oil to eliminate *Kapha, Pitta,* and *Vata,* respectively. This therapy and *Pañchakarma* are often employed in conjunction with one another. It is becoming increasing difficult to find ghee (or clarified butter).

HERBAL REMEDIES

Ayurveda prescribes a rich store of natural medicines that have been collected, tested, and recorded in medical treatises from ancient times. The tradition of collecting and preserving information about medicines in recipe books, called *Nighantus,* continued to the twentieth century (Nadkarni, 1908). The most traditional source of Ayurvedic medicine is the kitchen garden. From an early stage of development, Indian medical and culinary traditions worked hand in hand with each other.

In light of the close association between food and medicine, Ayurveda classifies foods and drugs (usually vegetal) by the taste on the tongue, potency, and taste after digestion (Tables 31-4 and 31-5).

Rasa, taste by the tongue, is categorized into six separate tastes, with their individual elemental composition and energetic effects on the three *doshas* (Zysk, 1993):
1. Sweet, composed of earth and water, increases *Kapha* and decreases *Pitta* and *Vata.*
2. Sour, composed of earth and fire, increases *Kapha* and *Pitta* and decreases *Vata.*
3. Saline, composed of water and fire, increases *Kapha* and *Pitta* and decreases *Vata.*
4. Pungent, composed of wind and fire, increases *Pitta* and *Vata* and decreases *Kapha.*
5. Bitter, composed of wind and space, increases *Vata* and decreases *Pitta* and *Kapha.*
6. Astringent, composed of wind and earth, increases *Vata* and decreases *Pitta* and *Kapha.*

Virya, potency, comprises eight types that are divided into four pairs: hot-cold, unctuous-dry, heavy-light, and dull-sharp.

TABLE 31-4 *Tastes and Food Qualities: Effects on the Doshas*

Tastes	
Decrease *Vata*	Increase *Vata*
Sweet	Pungent
Sour	Bitter
Salty	Astringent
Decrease *Pitta*	Increase *Pitta*
Sweet	Pungent
Bitter	Sour
Astringent	Salty
Decrease *Kapha*	Increase *Kapha*
Pungent	Sweet
Bitter	Sour
Astringent	Salty
Major food qualities	
Decrease *Vata*	Increase *Vata*
Heavy	Light
Oily	Dry
Hot	Cold
Decrease *Pitta*	Increase *Pitta*
Cold	Hot
Heavy	Light
Oily	Dry
Decrease *Kapha*	Increase *Kapha*
Light	Heavy
Dry	Oily
Hot	Cold

TABLE 31-5 *Common Examples of the Six Tastes and Major Food Qualities*

Six tastes	Common examples
Sweet	Sugar, milk, butter, rice, breads
Sour	Yogurt, lemon, cheese
Salty	Salt
Pungent	Spicy foods, peppers, ginger, cumin
Bitter	Spinach, other green leafy vegetables
Astringent	Beans, pomegranate
Six major food qualities	Common examples
Heavy	Cheese, yogurt, wheat products
Light	Barley, corn, spinach, apples
Oily	Dairy products, fatty foods, oils
Dry	Barley, corn, potato, beans
Hot	Hot (temperature) foods and drinks
Cold	Cold foods and drinks

Vipaka, postdigestive taste, identifies three kinds of aftertaste: sweet, sour, and pungent.

Contrary foods and drugs are always to be avoided. For instance, clarified butter and honey should not be taken in equal quantities, alkalis and salt must not be taken for a long period, milk and fish should not be consumed together, and honey should not be put in hot drinks.

Compounding

Four important criteria are considered when compounding plant substances and other ingredients into medical recipes. The substances that make up the recipe should have many attributes that enable it to cure several diseases; they should be usable in many pharmaceutical preparations, they should be suitable for the recipe and not cause unwanted side effects, and they should be culturally appropriate to the patients and their customs. Every medicine should be able to treat the disease's site of origin, site of manifestation, and its spread simultaneously.

A brief survey of the different kinds of medical preparations indicates the depth and content of Ayurvedic pharmaceuticals. The botanically based medicines derive largely from the Ayurvedic medical tradition, whereas the mineral and inorganic-based drugs derive from the Indian alchemical traditions, called *Rasashastra* (Zysk, 1993).

- Juices are cold-presses and extractions made from plants.
- Powders are prepared from parts of plants that have been dried in the shade and other dried ingredients.
- Infusions are parts of plants and herbs that have been steeped in water and strained. Cold infusions are parts of plants and herbs that were soaked in water overnight and filtered the next morning. Decoctions are vegetal products boiled in a quantity of water proportionate to the hardness of the plant part and then reduced by a fourth. It is then filtered and often used with butter, honey, or oils.
- Medicated pastes and oils. Often the plant and herbal extracts are combined with other ingredients and formed into pastes, plasters, and oils. Used externally, pastes and plasters are applied for joint, muscular, and skin conditions, and oil is used for hair and head problems. Medicated oils also are used for massages and enemas.
- Large and small pills and suppositories. Plant and herbal extracts are also formed into pills and suppositories to be used internally.
- Alcoholic preparations are made by fermentation or distillation. Two preparations are delineated: one requires the drug to be boiled before it is fermented or distilled, and in the other the drug is simply added to the preparation. Fifteen percent is the maximum allowable amount of alcohol content in a drug.

Several Ayurvedic medicines are prepared from minerals and metals ultimately derived from ancient traditions (Zysk, 1993). Sublimates are prepared by an elaborate method leading to the sublimation of sulfur in a glass container. They are found in recipes (*Rasayanas*) used in rejuvenation therapies.

- *Bhasmas* are ash residues produced from the calcination of metals, gems, plants, and animal products. Most are metals and minerals that are first detoxified and then purified. An important bhasma is prepared from mercury, which undergoes an 18-stage detoxification and purification process. Ayurveda maintains that bhasmas are quickly absorbed in the blood and increase the red blood cells.
- *Pishtis* are fine powders made by trituration of gems with juices and extracts.
- Collyrium is made from antimony powder, lead oxide, or the soot from lamps burned with castor oil. Collyrium is used especially to improve vision.

Of the hundreds of plants, minerals, and metals mentioned in various Ayurvedic treatises, only a small selection are commonly used by the typical Ayurvedic physicians today. Similar emphasis and some shared traditions are illustrated in the practices of Siddha medicine in Southern India, the subject of the next section of this chapter.

SIDDHA MEDICINE OF SOUTH INDIA

Unlike Ayurveda, which has a long and detailed textual tradition in Sanskrit dating from thousands of years ago, Siddha medicine's textual history, in the Tamil language of South India, remains vague and uncertain until about the thirteenth century of the common era, when there begins evidence of medical treatises. Most of our knowledge about Siddha medicine comes from modern-day practitioners, who often maintain an unverified history of the development of their own tradition, and who, in light of the modern upsurge of Tamil pride, make fantastic claims about the age and importance of Siddha medicine *vis-à-vis* its closest rival in India, Ayurveda.

Based on the evidence of written secondary sources and the reports of fieldworkers in Siddha medicine, Siddha and Ayurveda share a common theoretic foundation, but differ in their respective forms of therapy. This disparity suggests an original form of Siddha medicine may have consisted primarily of a series of treatments for specific ailments. These individual therapeutic prescriptions were then later overlaid with a theoretical component from Ayurveda. In addition, diagnosis by pulse and urine, based on Ayurveda, and perhaps also Unani (see Chapter 32), could well have been the source, in turn, for the same means of pulse and urine diagnosis.

The same pattern of medical development, which involves empirical practice first, followed by theory, may also apply to other forms of Indian medicine, beginning with Ayurveda itself, and including the more recent Visha Vaidya tradition of Kerala.

Siddha medicine is also distinctive in its use of *alchemy*, with fundamental principles that conform to the alchemical traditions of ancient Greece and China, and of Arabic alchemy, as reflected, for example, in Unani medicine. Siddha alchemy might well have been derived from one or a combination of these older traditions.

Just as Ayurveda eventually left India and found fertile ground in the West (Chapter 7), and where alternative and complementary forms of healing have become popular in recent decades, there are signs on the horizon that Siddha medicine may follow the same course. Indian systems of medicine must undergo changes and adaptations to be accommodated in a foreign environment, as in the case of Maharishi Ayurveda in the West (see Chapters 3, 7). Some of these modifications find their way back to India, where they become integrated into the indigenous systems. Such has been the pattern of traditional medicine in most parts of the world, so that the final chapter on the history of a particular medical system can never be written. In fact, an understanding of Siddha's medical history can only be revealed in light of change and adaptation over time.

SOUTHERN SOURCES

Looking into Siddha medicine in Tamil Nadu, Southern India, presents challenges to understanding this medical system and its history. A central problem lies with the limited availability of primary sources (akin to the "Classics" of traditional Ayurvedic or Chinese medicine) and the reliability of secondary sources prepared primarily by modern Tamil Siddha doctors. Little research on the subject has been carried out by Western students and scholars of India and Indian medicine. Even in the twenty-first century much of this mysterious medical tradition remains to be discovered.

Along with increased awareness of the Tamil language's Dravidian roots, in the second half of the twentieth century, a strong nationalist movement has grown up in Tamil Nadu. Tamils consider their cultural and linguistic heritage to be older and more important than that of the Indo-Aryans of northern India; some even claim their ancestors comprised the first civilization on the planet. This controversy has recently been kindled by a debate centering on the still-to-be-deciphered script of the so-called Indus Valley Civilization. This ancient urban culture, which predated the Hindu civilization of the Ganges River Valley, extended along the Indus River and its tributaries in what is now Pakistan. It resembled the great civilizations of ancient Egypt and Mesopotamia in size, development, and age. One side of the debate maintains that the script represents a language probably of Dravidian origin, whereas the other side claims that it does not represent a language at all. Tamils, whose language is Dravidian, are anxiously following the debate, for if the former side prevails, it would confirm their antiquity on the Indian subcontinent. The lens through which Tamils look at their own history influences the image in favor of Tamil superiority and antiquity.

References to Ayurveda occur early in Tamil literature. Already in the mid-fifth century text *Cilappatikara*, there is reference to Ayurveda (Tamil: *āyulvetar*). Mention of the three humors (Tamil: *tiritocam*; Sanskrit: *tridosha*) occurs in the *Tirukural*, a collection of poems that dates from around 450–550.

MIDDLE EAST CONNECTIONS

The first Tamil Siddha text is the *Tirumandiram*, written by Tirumular and dated probably to around the sixth or seventh century. There is mention of alchemy used to transform iron into gold, but no specific references to Tamil medicinal doctrines. The major sources of Siddha medicine belong to religious groups called Kayasiddhas. They seek the "perfection of the body" by means of yoga, alchemy, medicine, and certain types of Tantric religious rituals. Their works date from about the thirteenth to the fourteenth century, and are attributed to numerous authors, including Akattiyar (Sanskrit: *Agastya*), the traditional founder of Siddha medicine and Teraiyar (ca. late seventeenth century), who is said to have written 12 works on medicine. His famous disciple, Iramatevar, travelled to Mecca in the late seventeenth or early eighteenth century, where he studied, converted to Islam, and took on the name Yakkopu (i.e., Jacob). The numerous texts on Siddha medicine that present it as a system of healing are probably not older than the sixteenth century. Therefore, Tamil Siddha medicine, as it is now exists in both theory and practice, began in Tamil Nadu around the sixteenth century, but elements of healing practices that became part of Siddha medicine, including those they hold in common with Ayurveda, came from an earlier period.

BUDDHIST CONNECTIONS

Tamil folklore surrounding healing shares a common origin with Buddhism from northern India. Legend holds that Akattiyar performed a trephination on a sage in order to remove a toad (*terai*) from inside his skull. Akattiyar's disciple made the toad jump into a bowl of water. Because of his skill in removing the toad, Akattiyar gave the disciple the name Teraiyar, who is, however, a different person from the late seventeenth century medical author of the same name.

This legend is interesting because there is a similar account in Buddhist literature, and the legend of the toad and the cranium is a popular motif of Buddhist art and sculpture. In its earliest version found in the Pali texts of the Buddhist Canon, a skilled physician opened the cranium of a merchant from Rajagriha and removed two centipedes by touching them with a hot poker. The merchant made a full recovery. Versions of this folk story also occur in the Sanskrit literature of later Mahayana Buddhism and were translated into Tibetan and Chinese. The uniqueness of the story and its spread throughout Buddhist Asia demonstrates the influence of Buddhism in the dissemination of medical knowledge in pre-modern India.

DIVINE SOURCES

Like all systems of Hindu knowledge, Siddha medicine attributes its origin to a divine source; hence its knowledge is sacred and eternal, passed down to humans for the benefit of all humanity. According to Hindu tradition, the god Shiva transmitted the knowledge of medicine to his wife, Parvati, who in turn passed it on to Nandi, from whom it was given to the first practitioners of Siddha medicine. Tradition lists a total number of 18 Siddhar practitioners, beginning with Nandi and the legendary Agattiyar through to the final Siddhar, Kudhambai.

They are the acknowledged semi-mythical transmitters of Siddha medical doctrines and practices. By attributing a divine or extra-human origin to its medicine, the Tamil Siddhars have assured Siddha medicine a legitimate place in the corpus of Hindu knowledge. Although the transmission begins with Nandi, who in the form of a bull is Shiva's mode of transportation, tradition attributes the origin of medicine as well as of the Tamil language to Agattiyar.

SHIVA AND SHAKTI

According to Siddha cosmology, all matter is composed of two primal forces: matter (*shiva*) and energy (*shakti*). These two principles of existence operate in humans as well as nature, and connect the microcosm with the macrocosm. This connection is expressed by the association between the human body and the signs of the zodiac in Indian astrology, or *jyotish*. The formulation of the sequence of body parts is interesting because it follows a Babylonian and Greco-Roman system of head-to-toe correspondence (see also Unani medicine, Chapter 32) rather than an Indian one, which begins at the toes moves upwards. This formulation is illustrated in the following list, using Latin-based zodiac names, according to Zysk (2000):

♈ Áries (0°) = the neck
♉ Taurus (30°) = the shoulders
♊ Gémini (60°) = the arms and hands
♋ Cancer (90°) = the chest
♌ Leo (120°) = the heart and the stomach
♍ Virgo (150°) = the intestines
♎ Libra (180°) = the kidneys
♏ Scórpio (210°) = the genitals
♐ Sagittárius (240°) = the hips
♑ Capricornus (270°) = the knees
♒ Aquárius (300°) = the legs
♓ Pisces (330°) = the feet.

In addition to this cosmic connection, which occurs in all traditions of Indian astrology (or *jyotish*), Siddha medicine relied on Ayurveda for the medical doctrines that bridge the natural world and the human body. In modern-day Siddha practice, evidence of that genealogy is not always acknowledged.

There are five elements (*pañcamahabhutam*), which make up the entire natural world: solid/earth, fluid/water, radiance/fire, gas/wind, and ether/space. These elements combine in specific ways to grant the three bodily humors, called *muppini* in modern Tamil. They are said to be in the proportion of 1 part wind to $\frac{1}{2}$ part bile to $\frac{1}{4}$ part phlegm, according to Zysk (2000):

1. *Wind* (Tamil: *vatham*; Sanskrit: *Vata*) is a combination of space and wind, and is responsible for nervous actions, movement, activity, sensations, etc. It is found in the form of the five bodily winds.
2. *Bile* (Tamil: *pittam*; Sanskrit: *pitta*) is made up of fire alone and governs metabolism, digestion, assimilation, warmth, etc. Its principal seat is in the alimentary canal, from the cardiac region to small intestines. Some Ayurvedic formulations state that bile is a combination of the elements fire and water.
3. *Phlegm* (Tamil: *siletuman*; Sanskrit: *shleshman, Kapha*) is a combination of earth and water and is responsible for stability in the body. Its principal seats are in the chest, throat, head, and joints.

Next, there is the shared doctrine of the seven tissues (Tamil: *dhatu*) of the body: lymph/chyle, blood, muscle, fat, bone, marrow, and sperm and ovum. Finally, there are the five winds (Tamil: *vatham*; Sanskrit: *prana*) that circulate in the body and initiate and carry out bodily functions: *pranam* is the inhaled breath and brings about swallowing; *apanam* is the exhaled breath and is responsible for expulsion, ejection, and excretion; *samanam* helps digestion; *vyanam* aids circulation of blood and nutrients; and *udanam* functions in the upper respiratory passages. There are also five secondary winds: *nagam*, the air of higher intellectual functions; *kurmam*, the air of yawning; *kirukaram*, the air of salivation; *devadhattham*, the air of laziness; and *dhananjayam*, the air that acts on death.

Like Ayurveda, Siddha medicine maintains that the three humors predominate in humans in accordance with their nature and stage of life, and that they vary with the seasons. Every individual is born with a unique configuration of the three humors, which is called the individual's basic nature (Sanskrit: *prakriti*). It is fixed at birth and forms the basis of his or her normal, healthy state. However, during the three different stages of life and during the different seasons, one humor usually predominates. This pattern is normal, but domination by a humor must be understood in relation to the person's fundamental nature in order to maintain the balance that is the individual's basic natural state. The classification of the humors according to stages of life and seasons in Siddha differs from that found in Ayurveda. In the case of the seasons, the variation is attributed simply to the different climatic conditions that occur in the different parts of the year in the northern inland areas and the southern, Tamil coastal and inland environments.

According to Siddha, wind predominates in the first third of life, bile in the second third, and phlegm in the last third of life, while in Ayurveda phlegm dominates the first third and wind the last third of life. In terms of climate in the Indian subcontinent, the north is colder in the winter (December and January) than is the south, and the west coast has rain in June and July (with prevailing westerly winds in the northern hemisphere), when the east coast is extremely hot. A dry, cold climate is rare in the south, but it is precisely that climate that increases wind. Bile and phlegm, on the other hand, are increased when it is hot and wet.

DIAGNOSIS: THE EIGHT FEATURES

The diagnosis of disease in Siddha medicine relies on the examination of eight anatomical features (*envagi thaervu*), which are evaluated in terms of the three humors, according to Zysk (2000):
1. *Tongue:* black indicates wind, yellow or red bile, and white phlegm; an ulcerated tongue points to anemia.
2. *Complexion:* dark indicates wind, yellow or red bile, and pale phlegm.
3. *Voice*: normal indicates wind, high-pitched bile, and low-pitched phlegm.
4. *Eyes:* muddy colored indicates wind, yellowish or red bile, and pale phlegm.
5. *Touch*: dryness indicates wind, warm bile, and cold, clammy phlegm.
6. *Stool:* black indicates wind, yellow bile, and pale phlegm.
7. *Pulse:* a complex system described below.
8. *Urine:* also described in detail below.

Pulse examination is the most emphasized diagnostic approach for modern Siddha doctors. Both diagnosis and prognosis can be obtained through this one process. These methods of diagnosis also occur in Ayurveda, but only after the fourteenth century, perhaps influenced by the introduction of Unani medicine (see Chapter 32) with the arrival of the Mogul (Persians converted to Islam) in northern India. Prior to this time, and in the Ayurvedic classical literature, diagnosis of disease was determined by vitiation of one or more of the humors based on observation, touch, and interrogation.

Siddha pulse diagnosis (Tamil: *natiparitchai*; Sanskrit: *nadipariksha*), like that found in Ayurveda, probably owes it origins to Unani medicine. It requires a highly developed sense of touch and refined subjective awareness. According to Siddha, the following conditions must not be present in the patient when doing a reading of the pulse: emotional distress, exhaustion, full stomach or hunger, or oily hands.

If readings cannot be taken on the hand, other arterial points may be used, such as the ankle, neck, or ear lobes. It is also advised to read the pulse at different times of the day and during different seasons of the year, since the body and mind change during the course of the day and climatic conditions affect the person's psychological and physiological states.

The pulse is felt on the female's left and male's right hand by the doctor's opposite hand, a few centimeters below the wrist joint, using the index, middle, and ring fingers. Pressure should be applied by one finger after the other beginning with the index finger. Each finger detects a particular humor, which in normal conditions has a movement representative of certain animals. The index finger feels the windy humor, which should have the movement of a swan, a cock, or a peacock; the middle finger feels the bilious humor, which should have the movement of a tortoise or a leech; and ring finger feels the phlegmatic humor, which should have the movement of a frog or a snake. Any deviation from these normal movements indicates which humor or humors are disturbed. If all humors are affected, the pulse is usually rapid with a good deal more volume than normal. After long periods of practice under the guidance of a skilled teacher, a student can begin to detect subtle differences in the flow, volume, and speed of the pulse at the point of each of the three fingers. These changes correspond to abnormalities in particular parts of the body, which the skilled Siddha doctor can pin-point, and for which the appropriate cure can be prescribed (Zysk, 2000).

Urine examination (*muthira paritchai*) is another form of diagnosis in Siddha medicine. Not an original part of Ayurveda, urine examination probably derived from Unani medicine, where this form of diagnosis is described in early Arabic and Persian medical literature; it is also important in Tibetan medicine. Siddha practice examines the urine for its color, smell, and texture, and further uses a technique for determining the vitiated humor by reading the distribution of a drop of gingili (sesame) oil added to the urine. The meaning of the drop's configuration is as follows: longitudinal dispersal indicates windy humor; dispersal in a ring, bilious humor; and lack of dispersal points to phlegmatic humor. A combination of two types of dispersal means that two humors are involved. Prognosis is determined by such reading as well: A slow dispersal of a drop in a circular form, or a drop that forms the shape of an umbrella, a wheel, or a jasmine or lotus blossom indicates positive prognosis. A drop that sinks, spreads rapidly with froth, splits into smaller drops and spreads rapidly, mixes with the urine, or spreads so that its pattern is that of an arrow, a sword, a spear, a pestle, a bull, or an elephant indicates a poor prognosis.

Finally, as in Ayurveda and Unani, the *conditions of the eyes* show which of the humors is vitiated, as well as the patient's mental and emotional state: shifty, dry eyes point to wind; yellow eyes with photophobia indicate bile; watery, oily eyes devoid of brightness reveal that phlegm is affected; and red, inflamed eyes show that all three humors are vitiated.

TREATMENT

According to traditional Siddha, a physician must be knowledgeable in alchemy, astrology, and philosophy. He must be able to apply intuition and imagination. He must not seek fame or fortune from healing. He must not treat a patient before a proper diagnosis has been reached. And he must use only medicines that *he has prepared himself.*

Treatment and pharmaceutics are two areas where Siddha differs considerably from Ayurveda. As in yoga (described in Chapter 21), the principal aim of Siddha medicine is to make the body perfect, not vulnerable to decay, so that the maximum term of life can be achieved. Like Ayurveda, Siddha places emphasis on positive health, so that the object of the medicine is disease prevention and health promotion.

While traditional Ayurveda lists the following eight branches of medicine: general medicine, pediatrics, surgery, treatment of ailments above the neck, toxicology, treatment of mental disorders due to seizure by evil spirits, rejuvenation therapy, and potency therapy, Siddha medicine developed expertise in five particular branches of medicine: general medicine, pediatrics, toxicology, ophthalmology, and rejuvenation. Further, Ayurveda prescribes a therapeutic regimen involving the *Pañchakarma*, purification, or "five purifying actions" (including emetics, nasal therapies, purgatives, enemas, and bloodletting [these same approaches were also independently employed in the practice of "regular medicine" in the West up to the twentieth century—see Chapters 1 and 2]). Siddha employs only purgation for purification purposes.

General Medicine

In Ayurveda, surgical practice forms a separate school of medicine but surgery *per se* is not a significant part of Siddha medicine. Medicated oils and pastes are applied to treat wounds and ulcers, but the use of a knife is rarely encountered at all.

Closely connected with the tradition of the martial arts in South India, there developed a type of acupressure treatment based on the vital points in the human body, known as *varmam* (Sanskrit: *marman*). There are 108 points mentioned in the Ayurvedic classics, which identify them and explain that if they are injured, death can ensue. In Siddha medicine, the number of important *varmam* points is also 108 (some say 107) out of a total of 400. Siddha doctors developed techniques of applying pressure to special points, called *Varmakkalai*, to remove certain ailments and of massaging the points to cure diseases. They also specialized in bone-setting and often practiced an Indian form of the martial arts, called *cilampam* or *silambattam*, which involved a kind of dueling with staffs.

According to the French Institute in Pondicherry, India, the art of *varmam* is particularly widespread among the hereditary Siddha practitioners belonging to the Natar caste in the district of Kanyakumari in Tamil Nadu. The development of this special form of healing appears to have evolved naturally from the fact that the men of this caste, while carrying out their task of climbing coconut and *borassus* trees to collect the fruits and sap for toddy, occasionally fell from great heights. In order to repair the injury or save the life of a fall victim, skills of bone-setting and reviving an unconscious patient by massage developed among certain families within the caste, who have passed down their secret art from generation to generation by word of mouth. In the past, rulers employed members of this caste to cure injuries incurred in battle and to overpower their enemies by their knowledge of the Indian martial arts.

Toxicology

Toxicology as part of Siddha medicine seems to be closely linked to indigenous systems of treating snake bites and other forms of poisoning. It may have some affinity to the

Visha Vaidya (poison-doctor) tradition practiced by certain Nambudiri Brahmins of Kerala. Similar to this Keralan toxicological tradition, Siddha has adopted the Ayurvedic system of the three humors in order to explain the different effects of poisons; but it remains fundamentally an indigenous and local toxicological tradition. It classifies the severity and cure by means of the number of teeth or fang marks left in the victim. Four, the most severe, is incurable; it implies two complete bites. One fang mark, the least severe, is cured by cold water baths and fomentation on the site of the bite. Even the bite of a venomous snake may not carry venom; the more fang marks the greater likelihood that venom was injected.

Ophthalmology

Siddha medicine excels in ophthalmology. It has two separate treatises devoted to the treatment of 96 different eye diseases. This focus may be related to the strength of Arabic optics from the Unani tradition that was evidently introduced.

Rejuvenation Therapy

Closely connected with Siddha Yoga, the Siddha system of rejuvenation therapy, known as *Kayakalpa* (from Sanskrit, meaning "making the body competent for long life"), marks a distinctive feature of Siddha medicine. It involves a five-step process for rejuvenating the body and prolonging life, according to Zysk (2000):

1. Preservation of vital energy via breath control (Tamil: *vasiyogam*; Sanskrit: *pranayama*) and yoga.
2. Conservation of male semen and female sexual secretions.
3. Use of *muppu,* or rare earth salts.
4. Use of calcinated powders (Tamil: *chunnam*; Sanskrit: *bhasma*) prepared from metals and minerals.
5. Use of drugs prepared from plants special to each Siddha doctor.

The esoteric substance called *muppu* is particular to Siddha medicine. It may be considered Siddha's equivalent of the "philosopher's stone." Its preparation is hidden in secrecy, known only by the guru, and taught only when the student is deemed qualified to accept it. It is generally thought to consist of three salts (*mu-uppu*), called *puniru, kallupu,* and *vediyuppu,* which correspond respectively to the sun, moon, and fire. *Puniru* is said to be a certain kind of limestone composed of globules that are found underneath a type of clay called Fuller's Earth, which contains heavy metals. In early Europe, Fuller's Earth was used by *fullers,* or those who prepared and preserved wool to weave into cloth. It is collected only on the full-moon night in April, when it is said to bubble out from the limestone. It is then purified with the use of a special herb. *Kallupu* is hard salt or stone salt (i.e., rock salt) that is dug up from mines under the earth, obtained from saline deposits under the sea, or gathered from the froth of sea water that carries the undersea salt. Kallupu is considered to be useful in the consolidation of mercury and other metals. Finally, *vediyuppu* is potassium nitrate, which is cleaned seven times and purified with alum.

This magical-religious form of therapy is a common component of Siddha alchemical practice and provides a basis for the rich assortment of alchemical preparations comprising the pharmacopoeia of Siddha medicine.

PHARMACOPOEIA

The precise origin of the system of Siddha pharmacology is not known, but it seems to have been closely linked to the Tantric religious movement, which can be traced back to the sixth century of the common era in North India, and influenced both Buddhism and Hinduism. It was strongly anti-Brahminical, and stressed ascetic practices and religious rituals that involved "forbidden" foods and sexual practices, and often included the use of alchemical preparations.

The alchemical part of Siddha is present from at least the time of Tirumular's *Tirumandiram* (sixth or seventh century AD). Alchemy is also found in Sanskrit texts from North India, but only from about the sixth or seventh century. It later became an integral part of Ayurvedic medicine, called *Rasashastra,* "traditional knowledge about mercury." In the classical treatises of Ayurveda, however, mention of alchemy is absent, and only certain metals and minerals are mentioned in late classical texts from the seventh century. Since alchemy reached a far greater level of development in Siddha medicine than in Ayurveda, it is believed that medical alchemy may well have begun in South India among the Siddha yogins and ascetics, and was later assimilated into Ayurveda.

There are three groups of drugs in Siddha medicine: (1) inorganic substances (*thatuvargam*); (2) plant products (*mulavargam*); and (3) animal products (*jivavargam*). These drugs are all characterized by means of taste (*rasa*), quality (*guna*), potency (*virya*), postdigestive taste (*vipaka*), and specific action (*prabhava*).

Siddha has further classified the inorganic substances into six types, according to Zysk (2000):

1. *Uppu*: 25 or 31 varieties of salts and alkalis, which are water soluble and give out vapor when heated;
2. *Pashanam*: 64 varieties (32 natural, 32 artificial) of non-water-soluble substances that emit vapor when heated;
3. *Uparasam*: seven types of non-water-soluble substances that emit vapor when heated, including mica, magnetic iron, antimony, zinc sulfate, iron pyrites, ferrous sulfate, and asafoetida (*hingu*);
4. *Loham*: six varieties of metals and metallic alloys that are insoluble, but melt when heated and solidify when cooled, including gold, silver, copper, iron, tin, and lead;
5. *Rasam*: drugs that are soft and sublime when heated, transforming into small crystals or amorphous powders such as mercury, amalgams and compounds of mercury, and arsenic;

6. *Gandhakam*: sulfur that is insoluble in water and burns off when heated.

Rasam and *gandhakam* combine to make *kattu*, which is a "bound" substance, i.e., a substance whose ingredients are united by a process of heating.

In addition, there are 13 varieties of gems and minerals, 16 varieties of mud and siliceous earth, 35 varieties of animals, and 24 varieties of rocks. This variety resembles in some respects the remedies of homeopathic medicine as developed in Europe during the eighteenth century.

The cornerstones of Siddha pharmacology are mercury and sulfur, which are equated to the deity Shiva and his consort Parvati, and are combined to make mercuric sulfide. Mercury, or quicksilver, is the crucial ingredient in almost every Siddha alchemical preparation. It is used in five forms (*panchasthuta*): pure mercury (*rasa*), red sulfide of mercury (*lingam*), mercuric perchloride (*viram*), mercurous chloride (*puram*), and red oxide of mercury (*rasacheduram*). Although mercury plays a key role in both the Siddha and Ayurvedic forms of medical alchemy, mercury in its pure form is not found in India and, therefore, must have become available through trade with the Roman and Byzantine empires and, subsequently, the Italian city-states of the Middle Ages. As an aside, mercury was a popular remedy in Europe until the middle of the nineteenth century, where its German name "quacksalber" gave origin to the term "quack," for those who practiced dangerous and ineffective medicine.

Siddha pharmacology combines substances that from a natural affinity to each other—such as borax and ammonia sulfate—to create a compound greater than the sum of the individual parts. This combination is called *nadabindu*, where *nada* is acidic and *bindu* is alkaline, or, in the Siddha cosmology, the female Shakti mated with the male Shiva. The most important mixture of this kind is alkaline mercury and acidic sulfur. Similarly, Siddha medicine has devised a classification of drugs as friends and foes. The former increase the curative effect, whereas the latter reduce it.

Six pharmaceutical preparations are common to both Siddha and Ayurveda. They can be administered internally or on the skin. They include: calcinated metals and minerals (*chunnam*), powders (*churanam*), decoctions (*kudinir*), pastes (*karkam*), medicated clarified butter (*nei*), and medicated oils (*ennai*). Particular to Siddha medicine, however, are three special formulations: *chunnam*, metallic preparations that become alkaline, yielding calcium hydroxide, which must always be taken with another more palatable substance (*anupana*, "after drink"); *mezhugu*, waxy preparations that combine both metals and minerals; and *kattu*, inextricably bound preparations, which are impervious to water and flame. Sulfur and mercury or mercuric salts are combined to make them resistant to heat. While on the fire, certain juices are added by drops to empower the substance. The drug can be kept for long periods and given in small doses once a day. It should not, however, be completely turned into a powder, but should be rubbed on a sandal stone so as to yield only a few grains of the powerful substance (Zysk, 2000).

Both Ayurveda's Rasashastra, or traditional knowledge of mercury, and Siddha's alchemy have devised different methods for purifying or detoxifying metals and minerals, called *shodhana* in Sanskrit, and *suddhi murai* in Tamil, before they are reduced to ash (Sanskrit: *bhasman*; Tamil: *chunnam*). Purification is accomplished by one of two methods. One involves repeatedly heating sheets of metal and plunging them into various vegetable juices and decoctions. The other method, called "killing" (*marana*), entails destroying the metal or mineral by the use of powerful herbs, so that is loses its identity and becomes converted into fine powders with the natures of oxides or sulfides, which can be processed by the intestinal juices. After this purification procedure, the metal or mineral is combined with its appropriate acid or alkaline, and is prepared for its final transformation into an ash, or *bhasman*, by incineration in special furnaces made of cow-dung cakes (replaced by electric ovens in modern establishments!).

According to Zysk (2000), there are nine principles that must be followed in the calcination of metals and minerals:

1. There is no alchemical process without mercury.
2. There is no fixation without alkali.
3. There is no coloring without sulfur.
4. There is no quintessence without copper sulfate.
5. There is no animation without conflagration.
6. There is no calcination without corrosive lime.
7. There is no compound without correct blowing.
8. There is no fusion without suitable flux.
9. There is no strong fluid without salammoniac.

The traditional incineration process may vary slightly among different Siddha doctors, but all procedures require repeated heating in a fire fuelled by dung patties. The number of burnings can reach one hundred for certain preparations. In traditional Ayurveda, the duration and intensity of the heat is regulated by the size of the pile of dung, called a *puta* in Sanskrit. Siddha medicine devised a method with a special substance made of inorganic salts, in Tamil called *jayani*, which reduces the number of burnings to only three or four. In order to increase the potency of the ash (*chunnam*), Siddha practitioners add the esoteric substance *muppu*, which seems to vary in individual composition from one Siddha doctor to another. Other ingredients added to increase a *chunnam*'s potency are healthy human urine (*amuri*), or urine salts (*amuriuppu*) obtained from the evaporation of large quantities of urine. Neither of these additives is found in Ayurveda's Rasashastra.

According to Zysk (2000), in modern Siddha medicine, different metals have different healing effects:

- *Mercury* is antibacterial and antisyphilitic (and was used for this purpose in the West until the early twentieth century).
- *Sulfur* is used against scabies and skin diseases, rheumatoid arthritis, spasmodic asthma, jaundice, blood poisoning, and internally as a stool softener.

- *Gold* is effective against rheumatoid arthritis, and as a nervine tonic, an antidote, and a sexual stimulant.
- *Arsenic* cures all fevers, asthma, and anemia.
- *Copper* is used to treat leprosy, skin diseases, and to improve the blood.
- *Iron* is effective against anemia, jaundice, and as a general tonic for toning the body.

This kind of knowledge about the healing properties of various minerals was ultimately carried into the use of mineral baths, spas, and water therapies in the West.

Despite the scientific evidence that shows many of these inorganic substances—minerals and metals—to be toxic to the human body, both Siddha and Ayurvedic practitioners continue to use them in their everyday treatment of patients. They claim that their respective traditions have provided special techniques to detoxify the metals and minerals and to render them safe and extremely potent. Again, as in the practice of homeopathy, certain biologically active substances that are toxic in one form or dose may be prepared so that its beneficial effects predominate.

Plant Products

In terms of herbal drugs, Siddha practitioners draw upon a materia medica of over 100 plants and plant products, some of which are imported from as far away as the Himalaya (see Chapter 30). These herbal remedies are used for three purposes in Siddha medicine. First, as mentioned earlier, certain drugs purify the minerals and metals before they are transformed into ash. Second, many plants and plant substances are used to eliminate waste products from the body through a process of body purification involving purgation of the nose and throat, enemas and laxatives, and the removal of toxins from the skin by the application of medicated pastes. This procedure resembles the process of the five methods of purification (Sanskrit: *pañcakarman*) in Ayurveda. Third, plants are used to treat specific ailments, and for the general toning or tonification of the body.

Animal Products

Siddha doctors also used animal products, such as human and canine skulls and bones, in the preparation of a special "ash" or *chunnam* (Tamil: *peranda chunnam*), which is said to be effective against mental disorders. The preparation of bone ash would serve to alkalinize (make basic vs. acidic) any mixtures and unbind various active principles that might otherwise not be metabolically available. A clear example from American Indian ethnomedicine is the use of ash, or mineral lime from seashells, to alkalinize (make basic vs. acidic) maize, allowing the B vitamins such as niacin to become unbound and available for metabolism when ingested.

Ayurvedic pharmaceutical manufacturers in India have begun to adopt the Western system of "good manufacturing procedures," and to resort to Ayurveda's rich pharmacopoeia of plant-based medicines, in order to make their products more accessible to a Western clientele. Such is not the case with Siddha medicine, which has yet to experience the financial rewards that come from serving Western markets.

Both Siddha and Ayurveda are sophisticated systems of medicine, practiced in India for more than 2500 years. Traditional medicine in India focuses on the whole organism and its relation to the external world to re-establish and maintain the harmonious balance that exists within the body and between the body and its environment. Few reliable sources for traditional Ayurveda have been available in English. Most of the accurate works are by and for specialists, and are virtually inaccessible to the reader without knowledge of Sanskrit (e.g., Meulenbeld, 1974; Srikanta Murthy, 1984). This circumstance suggests that many of the mysteries of Ayurvedic and Siddha healing are yet to be uncovered, and may hold yet greater promise than has yet been realized.

HERBS COMMONLY USED IN SOUTH AND SOUTHEAST ASIA

The use of many versatile herbs included in Ayurvedic and Siddha traditions spread throughout the ancient historical region of Further India (see Chapter 35). The "Spice Islands" of Southeast Asia are within the realm of Further India and were also a valuable source of many medicinal plants that were used as and considered spices in indigenous as well as European food preparation (and preservation). Their medicinal properties are commonly available today in the West.

The plant chemicals present in herbs and spices are able to protect the plant from the oxidizing effects of the sun, from microbes, and from insect and animal predators, as well as allowing them to compete with other plants for soil, water, and nutrients. The biologically active plant chemicals in turn have properties as anti-oxidants, antibiotics, and other medicinal activities (see also Chapter 27). These properties made spices invaluable in being able to preserve meats and foods, making them precious to Europeans in the era before refrigeration or canning of foods. They offer many of the same properties that make them safe and effective herbal remedies today. See Table 31-6 for a summary of herbal remedies.

Allium sativum **(Garlic)** Garlic has long been used as a medicinal food. In modern herbal medicine, it was initially used as an *anti-infective* agent and subsequently became popular for its antihypertensive and *lipid-lowering* effects. In the United States, the sales of garlic products have soared in recent years, generating over $60 million in the year 2000 alone. Garlic has lipid-lowering, antithrombotic, antihypertensive, antioxidant, and immune-modulatory properties.

Several trials have shown the effectiveness of garlic in reducing total and low-density lipoprotein (LDL) cholesterol. Garlic's reported antiplatelet, fibrinolytic, and anti-atherosclerotic effects in some studies need to be better defined and understood in terms of their benefits in various

TABLE 31-6 *Summary of Herbal Remedies*

Genus, species (common English name)	Conditions and results
Allium sativum (garlic)	Hyperlipidemia: results in improved levels of lipids. (lipid lowering, antithrombotic, antihypertensive, immunomodulatory)
Boswellia serrata (frankincense)	Arthritis: solid reports of beneficial effects. (anti-inflammatory)
Capsicum annuum (chili pepper, paprika)	Cluster headaches, neuropathy, and arthritis: improvement reported in several studies. External: rubifacient, blocks pain neurotransmitter substance P, depletes substance P, desensitizes the sensory neurons. Internal: reduces platelet aggregation and triglycerides, and improves blood flow
Curcuma longa (turmeric)	Functional gallbladder problems (increase in secretin and bicarbonate output), hyperlipidemia: studies report improvement in cholesterol levels (fatty acid metabolism alteration and decrease in serum lipid peroxide levels). Osteoarthritis: studies report positive results. (anti-inflammatory)
Commiphora guggulu (guggul lipid)	Hyperlipidemia: improved lipid levels noted (antagonist of farnesoid X receptors)
Withania somnifera (winter cherry)	Arthritis: studies report improvement. (anti-inflammatory)
Zingeber officinale (ginger)	Antiemetic (carminative, local effect on stomach): reduces nausea Osteoarthritis: studies report benefit (anti-inflammatory, inhibits cyclo-oxygenase pathways, prostaglandin E2 [PGE2] and leukotriene [LTB4] synthesis)

neurological and cerebrovascular conditions. In a recent analysis performed by the Agency for Healthcare Research and Quality (AHRQ), it was concluded that garlic may have short-term, positive lipid-lowering and encouraging antithrombotic effects. All these effects can be expected to *reduce the risk of cardiovascular diseases and heart attack and stroke* (see also Chapter 24).

***Bosweillia serrata* (Frankincense)** *Bosweillia* is a commonly used ingredient in herbal preparations. It comes from a gum tree that grows in South and Middle Asia. In Christian belief it was one of the traditional gifts brought from the East by the Three Magi at Epiphany. During the Crusades it was brought back to Europe, including by the famous Germanic (Frankish) crusader Frederick Barbarossa (or "Red Beard"), thus acquiring the common name "frank incense," or frankincense. Its immune effects are similar to those of corticosteroid anti-inflammatory drugs, but without the side effects. Boswellic acids are reported to have significant analgesic, anti-inflammatory and complement-inhibitory properties. In one study involving 30 patients with *osteoarthritis* of the knee, those who received *Boswellia* tree extract reported a significant improvement in their knee pain, range of motion, and walking distance. In another study of *rheumatoid arthritis* patients, a special gum extract of *Bosweillia serrata* resulted in a significant improvement of symptoms of pain and swelling. These results are promising.

***Capsicum annuum* (Chili Pepper)** Common names of this plant/herb include cayenne pepper, paprika, red pepper, bird pepper, and Peruvian pepper. The preparations of this plant are used in topical creams and ointments. It is commonly used for pain related to *herpes zoster* and *diabetic neuropathy*. Many use it for *osteoarthritis* pain. Some basic science studies have shown that it reduces *pain* by depleting substance P, a chemical pain transmitter. There are also reports of the herb desensitizing neurons.

***Curcuma longa* (Tumeric)** The active ingredient, *curcumin*, of this commonly used spice in South and Southeast Asian curry dishes has *anti-inflammatory* and *lipid-lowering* effects. It is one of the three components of traditional curry spices, together with *coriander* and *cumin*, and sometimes *chili pepper* (see above). Curcumin's lipid-lowering effects observed in animal experiments are attributed to changes in fatty acid metabolism and facilitating the conversion of cholesterol to bile acids. There are also reports of its benefit in patients with *osteoarthritis*. The benefits of tumeric are not conclusively proven, but its use as a spice in an overall healthy diet is prudent.

***Withania somnifera* (Winter Cherry)** Basic science studies suggest that this herb may have anti-inflammatory, antioxidant, immune-modulatory, and hematopoietic as well as *anti-aging* properties. It may also have a positive influence on the endocrine and central nervous systems. The mechanisms of these proposed actions require additional clarification. Several observational and randomized studies have reported its usefulness in the treatment of *arthritic* conditions.

***Zingiber officinale* (Ginger)** Ginger is widely used throughout Asia and the Middle East, most commonly for control of *nausea* and *osteoarthritis* pain. Several studies have shown its benefit in controlling nausea associated with pregnancy, motion sickness, and anesthesia, and some studies have demonstrated its usefulness in the treatment of osteoarthritis.

Memory, Cognitive Improvement, and "Anti-Aging" Effects

Many of these plants and their products, as well as berberine (from the barberry bush), have been reported to have "anti-aging" effects. Examples of these effects include improvements in memory and cognition. Based on the available scientific information, these herbs or their extracts are promising and additional studies are in progress to validate their reported benefits.

CLINICAL TREATMENTS

There are clinical protocols available from traditional Indian medicines that are useful for many of today's common medical problems. Approaches derived directly from the ancient Sanskrit texts of Ayurveda are provided here for allergies and asthma, arthritis, cancer, fever, headache, high blood pressure, and peptic ulcer that can help prevent the development of these disorders and provide relief for those already suffering from these medical conditions.

Furthermore, they offer help without the risks of side effects and complications that are unfortunately common with high-powered drugs, surgery, and medical procedures of mainstream treatments. And beyond, these remedies also offer natural enhancements that help improve quality of life, longevity, and probably relationships with your fellow human beings.

As we said at the beginning of this book, because such approaches treat the causes and not just the symptoms of diseases, they are effective at preventing as well as treating these problems (see Chapter 2). In addition to what is offered here, ancient Sanskrit remedies are available for many other medical problems, such as diabetes mellitus and viral hepatitis, but require treatment with complex herbal preparations (available today from trusted sources) that are beyond the scope of this book.

ALLERGIES AND ASTHMA

Astyma is the Sanskrit term for allergies, from which the English word *asthma* is derived. Ayurveda views allergies as altered reactivity caused by weakened metabolism in one or more of the seven tissues of the body. They are categorized according to the three constitutional types: *Vata, Pitta,* and *Kapha.*

Immediate allergic reactions (*anaphylactic* reactions, from the Greek *ana-*, meaning not or without, *phylaxis,* meaning defense or protection) are seen as related to *Pitta. Intermittent* allergies (pets, foods) are *Vata-Pitta* or *Vata-Kapha* types, and delayed allergies (seasonal) are *Kapha.*

Vata allergic symptoms include aches and pains, coughing, gas, sneezing, and sensitivity to dirt, dust, and pollens. Symptoms may also include heart palpitations, muscle allergies, and wheezing (a symptom associated with the constriction of the airways found in asthma). People having these *Vata*-type allergies may find they are sensitive to plants from the Solanaceae family, for example, eggplant, potato, tomato, and deadly nightshade (the source of the drug atropine, or *bella donna,* from the Italian, meaning "beautiful woman," because women during the 1700s, a time when Italy was a "fashion capital" of Europe, placed atropine in their eyes to cause dilation of the pupils, producing that "doe-eyed" look, due to the toxic effects on the autonomic nervous system affecting the ciliary muscles of the eyes). Other *Vata*-type food sensitivities may include black beans, chick peas (garbanzo beans, for making *houmus*), and other beans. These allergies can often be managed with a *Vata*-pacifying diet and *Vata*-reducing herbs.

Pitta-type allergic symptoms include acne, contact dermatitis, eczema, and sensitivity to heat and light, insect bites, foam (as in pillows and mattresses), formaldehyde, and preservatives. Food sensitivities include bananas, eggs, carrots, grapefruit, garlic, pork, onions, and certain cheeses and spicy foods.

A *Pitta*-pacifying diet and herbs are recommended.

Kapha-type allergies include asthma, allergic rhinitis, hay fever and pollen sensitivities, and latent spring fever, causing symptoms of colds, runny nose and teary eyes, as well as laryngeal edema (swelling of the throat), and possibly generalized edema. Food sensitivities may include avocado, bananas, beef, dairy, cucumbers, lemons, lamb, pork, peanuts, and watermelon. A *Kapha*-reducing diet with hot, green teas (with methyl xanthenes such as caffeine and theophylline, which are natural treatments for decongestion and expansion of airways) and herbal teas are recommended.

The thymus gland and spleen are seen in Ayurveda as important to the immune system. In fact, the thymus gland, which is active in childhood and shrinks at adulthood, is important in development of the "T-cell" lymphocytes, or white blood cells, as part of the immune system. The spleen has an important role in filtering the blood and houses large numbers of white blood cells, as well as a reserve of red blood cells. The *heating* factor of the thymus helps to maintain immunity in proper balance, and weakness may be a cause of *Kapha*-type allergy. The spleen is understood as the *root* of the blood-forming system of the body and as a reservoir for blood (indeed it has this role during fetal development and early childhood, and acts as a reserve for blood cells during adulthood). The spleen also is said to contain components that destroy foreign particles and microbes, which is indeed an important function of the spleen as part of the immune system.

Weakness in the spleen is detectable in the pulse and likely to be present in individuals prone to allergies.

ARTHRITIS

Arthritis is known as *amavata* in Sanskrit, which implies the involvement of *ama* in the digestion and the *Vata dosha* (wind). No distinction is made between rheumatoid arthritis (rheumatism) and osteodegenerative arthritis. The cause is seen as all factors leading to poor digestion, with formation of ama: poor digestive function, excessive intake of fatty foods and meats, insufficient exercise, and generally unhealthy foods and habits. In arthritis, ama is said to build up and leave the digestive tract, spilling over and accumulating in the joints and the heart (which are indeed involved in acute rheumatic fever). As implied by the name, *Vata* is the principal *dosha* affected, aggravation of which causes indigestion, joint pain, and rough skin. If *Pitta* is also involved, a burning sensation may spread throughout the body, especially in the joints (like some of the complaints in the mysterious modern syndromes of chronic fatigue and fibromyalgia, thought to be a rheumatoid illness). If *Kapha* is further involved, the victim gradually becomes crippled. Less pain is experienced in the morning because at that time, ama is just beginning to move.

Treatments involve using diet, herbal remedies, and physical modalities and procedures to reduce ama and alleviate *Vata*. The first line of treatment is

- Mild fasting
- Herbs with bitter taste, hot potency, and pungent, post-digestive aftertaste for stimulation of the digestion (bitter-tasting herbs stimulate release of bile from the gallbladder into the intestines—a powerful digestant)
- Sweating.

The second line then proceeds to the formal purification therapy of *Pañchakarma*:

- Preparation with oleation (oil treatments) and sweating
- Comprehensive, five-part, classic purification therapy protocol over five days, including enema, herbal decoctions, and oil.

Third, the patient should then adopt a healthy regimen:

- Avoid sleep during the day and after meals (to help stimulate digestion)
- Avoid heavy foods
- Regular massage.

Modern medical research has also shown the importance of meditation and yoga at increasing movement and reducing symptoms in arthritis. These steps are also generally helpful at preventing the development of arthritis. Effective ongoing treatments of arthritis, including childhood arthritic conditions (juvenile arthritis), involve wet massages in conjunction with enemas for digestion and detoxification. Affected joints can be given *tapotement* (massage term for light tapping or patting) with a cloth bag filled with rice cooked with milk and herbs—delivering heat and physical therapy to the joints. Simple massage with oils is also helpful.

There is no denying the benefits of these approaches for arthritis. One of the reasons that Western biomedicine is so often ineffective at treating arthritis may be related to missing the insight into the digestive system, and missing the connection to diet and digestion (or the rheumatologist sending the patient to the gastroenterologist—and never "putting it together"). The importance of exercise and physical activity may or may not be addressed, and ignoring the importance of sleep patterns can generally be assumed, in Western medicine.

CANCER

There is no Sanskrit equivalent for the word cancer in classic Ayurveda. This omission may be consistent with findings from paleopathology that demonstrate the exceeding rarity, in prehistoric and ancient times, of most of today's common cancers (Micozzi, 1991, 2007). If cancer did not exist to any appreciable extent in ancient Sanskrit civilization, the opportunities to describe it in cultural terms would not present themselves. Nonetheless, as fundamental metabolic disruption is evident in cancer (*cachexia*), there are Ayurvedic approaches to restoring metabolic balance in cancer patients, cancer survivors, and those at high risk of developing cancer due to family history or genetics. Ayurveda also recognizes the importance of the immune system here, which is seen as critical in modern cancer studies of the "immune surveillance" theory of cancer.

Under the influence of cancer, the three *doshas* function to destroy, rather than to preserve and nourish, the body. *Vata* causes normal cells to proliferate and become cancerous; *Pitta* steals nutrients away from other tissues to feed cancer cells; and *Kapha* allows these cancer cells to continue multiplying unchecked. Although it affects all three, it usually begins by dominating one of the *doshas*. This imbalance, together with accumulation of ama toxins and inadequate digestive function or *fire*, sets the stage for cancer to appear.

Further, as a mind–body medicine, Ayurveda recognizes the intimate connection between suppressed emotion and suppressed immunity—another contributor to development and spread of cancer. Other factors recognized by Ayurveda include devitalized foods, chemical, and radiation exposure long term (which, of course, is itself the typical "*treatment*" of cancer in Western biomedicine), sedentary lifestyle, and even a lack of spiritual purpose in life.

Because ama toxins are seen as the primary problem in cancer, of course, the classic detoxification therapy of *Pañchakarma* is applied as the primary treatment. Patients are also given potent blood-cleansing herbs, immune-strengthening herbs, circulatory stimulants, and special *dosha*-dispelling herbs according to the types of cancer. These Ayurvedic remedies have been subjected to testing in the laboratory, which demonstrates effects at immune stimulation and re-differentiation of cancer cells literally back to normal cells (in distinction to Western chemotherapy, which is entirely based on "cytotoxicity" or killing cancer cells, which harm all normal cells as well). These therapies are monitored clinically according to the patient's skin tone and color (not the grey of chemotherapy patients), and general demeanor among the other diagnostic procedures available in Ayurveda. In addition, remedies are given by *dosha* type, together with the anticancer herbs:

- *Vata*: fresh ginger
- *Pitta*: aloe gel
- *Kapha*: honey and black pepper.

HEADACHE

The common complaint of headache (or head pain; Sanskrit, *Shira Shula*), according to Ayurveda, has many different causes, including cold and flu, indigestion, lack of sleep, muscle tension, overwork, and stress. Migraine headache specifically is thought to relate to inborn constitutional factors and are most commonly caused by *Vata* and/or *Pitta* imbalances.

Diagnosis is based upon presence of symptoms associated with each of the three *doshas*.

- *Vata*: extreme pain, constipation, dry skin, and depression and anxiety:
  - worsens with excessive activity, irregular lifestyle, stress and worry.
- *Pitta*: anger, burning sensation, irritability, light sensitivity, redness of eyes and face, nosebleeds:
  - may be accompanied by liver problems or blood toxicity.
- *Kapha*: dull ache, heaviness, fatigue:
  - may be accompanied by excess phlegm and salivation, nausea and vomiting, or lung problems; accumulation of *Kapha* in the head.

Treatments for both general headache and migraine are similar.

- Sinus and congestive headaches (*Vata* and *Kapha* types) are usually associated with allergies, common colds and coughs due to colds. They are given decongestant and expectorant herbs:
  - angelica, bayberry, calamus, ginger, and wild ginger.
- Effective soothing volatile oils are provided by:
  - camphor, holy basil (also as tea), eucalyptus, tulsi, wintergreen.
- In addition, therapies are added depending upon the *dosha* type:
  - *Vata*: purgation, herbal sedatives for restorative sleep
  - *Pitta*: liver cleansing with aloe powder or rhubarb root, cooling the head with sandalwood oil and avoiding heat and sun, internal gotu kola, inhalation of aromatic oils of rose or lotus.
- Application of medicated oils to the head and in the nose are recommended for all forms of headache, including migraine.

Meditation and yoga are also helpful for tension headaches and migraine. In addition, Ayurvedic *Marma* therapy provides 107 points on the body that are sensitive to touch and may be stimulated to restore balance among the *doshas*. These points are accessed on the skin and specifically associated with enhancing immunity, raising serotonin levels, and increasing secretion of hormones associated with the pineal gland (the vestigial "third eye," sometimes associated with the *chakra* in the head). Five sets of points are specifically used in the treatment of headache:

- Base of eyes (above the tear ducts, at the medial epicanthal folds)
- Either side of the nose (one-third of the way down from bridge to nostrils)
- Above the upper lip (mid-way between the margin of the upper lip and the base of the septum)
- Top of the head (crown)
- At the pineal gland (third eye).

HIGH BLOOD PRESSURE (HYPERTENSION)

Ayurveda understands that both high venous blood pressure and arterial blood pressure (the latter typically measured as the "normal" 120/80 in Western medicine) relate directly to the functioning of the heart and circulatory system. While high venous blood pressure (or congestion of the veins) is associated with heart failure (the typical congestive heart failure effectively treated with the herbally derived drug digitalis), this section addresses the arterial blood pressure elevation that is common and commonly known as hypertension in Western biomedicine.

Ayurveda considers it to be caused by imbalances in any of the three *doshas*:

- *Vata*: accumulation of toxins in digestive tract, absorbed into the blood, causing constriction of blood vessels:
  - rapid rise and fall in blood pressure ("labile hypertension"), accordingly, irregular heart rate and erratic pulse (as the heart responds to changes in BP), dry tongue, insomnia, puffiness ("bags") under the eyes, constipation
  - primary treatments of colonic cleansing, medicated enemas
  - secondary *Vata*-balancing diet of fish, fat-soluble vitamins A, D, E, garlic taken with milk.
- *Pitta*: toxins from poor digestion cause increased blood viscosity, redness of eyes, flushing of face, nosebleed, violent headache; anger, irritability, or burning sensation; sensitivity to light:
  - both systolic (first reading) and diastolic (second reading) pressures increased
  - treatment with bitter herbs, including aloe vera gel, bayberry, *Katuka*; and purgation
  - calming the mind with gotu kola; and other herbs to pacify *Pitta*.
- *Kapha*: thought to originate in stomach, mucosal secretions produce elevated triglycerides and cholesterol, eventually contributing to atherosclerosis of the arteries:
  - associated with edema, fatigue and hypothyroidism, obesity
  - both systolic and diastolic pressures elevated, but diastolic may not rise as much as in *Pitta*
  - treated by elimination of dairy and fatty foods, and administration of herbs: cayenne (red) pepper, garlic, hawthorn berries, motherwort, myrrh.
  - use of diuretics recommended only in *Kapha*-type hypertension.

All three forms of high blood pressure are benefitted by:

- Reduction of caffeine, salt, sugar, and fatty and fried foods

- Deep breathing exercises (the first step toward meditation)
- Meditation and yoga daily (proven by modern research as effective and cost effective without side effects, but many side benefits)
- Moderate physical activity daily, for example, walking three miles.

FEVER

Ayurveda sees fever (*Jvara Roga*) as both a disease and a symptom. We read in Chapter 2 that fever is simply a physiologic response by the body to arrest the multiplication of infectious disease-causing microbes, until the immune system can naturally overcome the infection (see Figure 2-3). Accordingly, fever is viewed as a positive sign in AV because it is said to loosen and release ama, the cause of illness. It is often, therefore, allowed to run its course, letting the fever "break," unless one or more of the following danger signs are present:

- Both high and prolonged elevation in body temperature
- History of prior seizure due to fever in a child
- Rapid "depletion" of patient.

In addition to infection, causes are seen to be wrong combinations of food, for example, mixing hot with cold (fruit with starch, bananas with milk—a typical Western breakfast), excessive emotion such as anger or fear, stress from overwork. Fever is classified according to the three *doshas*:

- *Vata*: during *Vata* time of day (dawn or dusk), or season (fall), begins in colon, pushes digestive fire into channels for transporting lymph, chyle and plasma, and heating the blood:
  - primary: body ache, headache, shivering, tremors
  - secondary: backache, constipation, fatigue, insomnia
- *Pitta*: mid-day and midnight, and during summer, onset like *Vata* fever:
  - primary: diarrhea, nausea and vomiting, rash, red eyes, perspiration, sensitivity to light
  - secondary: severe dehydration and reduction in blood pressure (fever with severe dehydration is typical of cholera, for example, which has been a historic problem in India and persists to this day in areas like Calcutta)
  - it may also be caused by alcohol abuse or very sour foods, or fermented beverages. Aspirin is not given because it may damage the stomach, which is already involved in this condition
- *Kapha*: morning and evening, and late winter and spring, production of excessive secretions, which dampen digestive fires and cause undigested food to accumulate, increasing ama and forcing it out into the body:
  - primary (prodromal): cold, congestion, runny nose
  - low grade fever, chest pain, cough, shortness of breath
  - laryngitis, sinusitis, sinus congestion, and sinus headache

- loss of appetite, cold and clammy skin, heavy and dull feeling
- causes may be overexposure to cold, improper combinations of foods, especially involving milk.

Ayurveda is able to make further distinctions among fevers caused by intestinal parasites, and continuous vs. fluctuating, or remittent, fevers (such as malaria, another historic problem in India).

PEPTIC ULCER (STOMACH AND DUODENUM)

Peptic ulcers (*Parinama Shula* in Ayurveda) are often associated with excess stomach acid and have been linked to the presence of specific bacteria in the stomach. Ulcers also appear in patients who have suffered shock, severe burns, and head injuries. The following prodromal symptoms are addressed in Ayurvedic texts:

- Belching of sour taste
- Heartburn
- May be accompanied by nausea and vomiting.

Symptoms are brought on by overeating, alcohol, or greasy, sour or spicy foods. Hyperacidity may be accompanied by migraine headache.

Vomiting may alleviate symptoms. With a gastric ulcer, there is more pain between meals, which is alleviated by eating and neutralizing excess acid. A duodenal ulcer is painful after eating as acidic stomach contents are emptied into the intestines.

Each of the three *doshas* are associated with stomach ulcers:

- *Vata*: excessive mental activity and nervousness lead to stress and overwork, causing ulcer; more gas in the stomach with radiating pain outward.
- *Pitta*: aggression, frustration, and anger cause high acid secretion in stomach and lead to ulcers; localized, sharp, penetrating pain can cause waking in the middle of the night; more likely to lead to perforated ulcer.
- *Kapha*: deficiency of protective mucus secretions of stomach permit stomach acids to burn through the lining of the stomach, even in the presence of normal or low stomach acidity; deep, dull, but bearable pain.

For all types of ulcers, a *Pitta*-pacifying diet is given, excluding citrus, sour and spicy foods, and including ghee (clarified butter), milk, and whole grains, such as basmati rice. Alcohol and smoking is avoided.

Specific herbal compounds are recommended before (*Avipattikara*) and after (*Jatamamsi, Kamadudha, Shatavari*) meals. For a bleeding ulcer, the remedy *Sat Isabgol* is taken with milk before sleep. If blood is seen passing into the stool (duodenal ulcer), other specific herbal remedies may be applied.

INDIVIDUALIZED MEDICAL PROFILE ACCORDING TO AYUVEDA

In Chapter 10 we described the use of psychometric profiling to match personality types to susceptibility to diseases and to treatments. Ayurveda uses constitutional types to match personalities, propensities, susceptibilities, and treatment as well. The information in this section on medical conditions can be used with the charts below. Ayurvedic therapies are designed to rebalance and reintegrate the individual based upon constitutional type and the type of the disorder from which patients suffer or are at risk. Every remedy is seen as either *tonifying* (or nourishing) a deficiency or a weakness in the organ(s) involved, and/or to *detoxify* (or reduce) aggravation of the *doshas*. *Reducing* the specific problem usually comes first, followed by *rejuvenation* to generally rebuild strength.

Reduction of the condition usually consists of *palliation*, followed by *purification*.

Palliation involves strengthening the digestive fires, reducing ama, and calming excess *dosha*. Purification involves the five-step classic therapy of *Pañchakarma*.

All these approaches emphasize the natural, self-healing abilities of the patient while providing individually tailored treatments for the person and the disorder.

Acknowledgments

Acknowledgment is given for the contributions in prior editions of Kenneth Zysk, PhD, and Georgia Tetlow, MD.

References

Bhishagratna KK (trans): *An English Translation of the Sushruta Samhita Based on Original Sanskrit Text*, 3 Vols. 1907-16, Reprint. Varanasi, India, 1983, The Chowkhamba Sanskrit Series Office.

Dash B, Kashyap L: *Basic Principles of Ayurveda Based on Ayurveda Saukhyam of Todarananda*, New Delhi, India, 1980, Concept Publishing Company.

Dash B: *Fundamentals of Ayurvedic Medicine*, Delhi, India, 1980, Bansal & Co.

Jolly J: *Indian Medicine*, Kashikar GC (trans), New Delhi, 1977, Munshiram Manoharlal.

Lad V: *Ayurveda. The Science of Self-Healing*, Wilmot, Wisconsin, 1990, Lotus Press.

Micozzi MS: Disease in antiquity: The case of cancer, *Arch Pathol Lab Med* 115:838-844, 1991.

Micozzi M: *Complementary & Integrative Medicine in Cancer Care and Prevention*, New York, 2007, Springer.

Meulenbeld GJ: *The Madhavanidana and Its Chief Commentary*, Leiden, Germany, 1974, EJ Brill.

Nadkarni AK: *Dr. K. M. Nadkarni's Indian Materia Medica*, 3rd ed, Bombay(Mumbai), India, 1908, Popular Prakashan. Reprint.

Sen Gupta KN: *The Ayurvedic System of Medicine*, New Delhi, India, 1984, Logos Press. 1906, Reprint.

Sharma PV (trans): *Caraka-Samhita. Agnivesha's Treatise Refined and Annotated by Caraka and Redacted by Dridhabala*, 4 Vols. Varanasi, India, 1981-1994, Chaukhamba Orientalia.

Singh RH: *Pañchakarma Therapy*, Varanasi, India, 1992, Chowkhamba Sanskrit Series Office.

Singhal GD, et al (trans): *Ancient Indian Surgery. [Sushruta Samhita]*, 10 Vols, Varanasi, India, 1972-1993, Singhal Publications.

Srikanta Murthy KR (trans): *Sharngadharasamhita of Shrangadhara*, Chaukhamba Orientalia, 1984, Varanasi, India.

Svoboda RE: *Prakruti. Your Ayurvedic Constitution*, Albuquerque, New Mexico, 1984, Geocom.

Upadhyay SD: *Nadivijana (Ancient Pulse Science)*, Delhi, India, 1986, Chaukhamba Sanskrit Pratisthan.

van Houten T, Micozzi MS: *The Edwin Smith Papyrus, Museum Applied Science Center for Art and Archaeology*, Philadelphia, 1981, University of Pennsylvania.

Zysk KG: *Asceticism and Healing in Ancient India. Medicine in the Buddhist Monastery*, New York, 1991, Oxford University Press.

Zysk KG: *Religious Medicine. The History and Evolution of Indian Medicine*, New Brunswick, New Jersey, 1993, Transaction Publishers.

Zysk KG: *Asceticism and healing in ancient India*, Delhi, 2000, Motilal Banarsidass. 1991; rpt.

Suggested Readings

Hausman GJ: *Siddhars Alchemy and the Abyss of Tradition: 'Traditional' Tamil Medical Knowledge in 'Modern' Practice*, Ann Arbor, 1996, University of Michigan.

Narayanaswami V: *Introduction to the Siddha system of medicine*, Madras, 1975, Pandit S.S., Anandam Research Institute of Siddha Medicine.

Natarajan K: 'Divine Semen' and the Alchemical Conversion of Iramatevar, *J Mediev Hist* 7(2):255-278, 2004.

Niranjana D: *Medicine in South India*, Chennai, 2006, Eswar Press.

Scharfe H: The doctrine of the three humours in traditional Indian medicine and the alleged antiquity of Tamil Siddha medicine, *J Am Orient Soc* 119(4):609-636, 1999.

Shanmugavelan A, Sundararajan A, editors: *Siddhar's Source of Longevity and Kalpa Medicine in India*, Madras, 1992, Directorate of Indian Medicine and Homoeopathy.

Subramania SV, Madhavan VR: *Heritage of the Tamils. Siddha Medicine*, Madras, 1984, International Institute of Tamil Studies.

Uthamaroyan CS, Anandan AR, editors: *A compendium of Siddha medicine*, Chennai, 2005, Department of Indian Medicine & Homoeopathy, Government of Tamilnadu.

Venkatraman R: *A history of the Tamil Siddha Cult*, Mandurai, 1990, N.S. Ennes Publications.

Zvelebil KV: *The Siddha quest for immortality*, Oxford, 2003, Mandrake of Oxford.

Chronological Phases of Indian and Middle Asian Medicine, with Sanskrit, Vedic, Buddhist, Muslim, Unani, British Colonial, Nationalist, and New Age Influences

Indus River Valley Civilization		2500 BC	Developed public health and medical practices; exchanged with Mesopotamia
Vedic Period		1500–1100 BC	Vedic texts; first medical classics
		1100–700 BC	Brahmana and Upanishads
Buddha		560–480 BC	Jivaka, founder of Indian surgery
Nanda Dynasty		350–320 BC	
Alexander the Great		327–325 BC	Development of Ayurvedic medicine
Maurya Dynasty		320–185 BC	Greek observations and documentation of human and veterinary medicine in India
Sunga Dynasty		185–75 BC	
Kusana Dynasty		AD 1–300	Samhitas of Caraka and Sushruta[a] in use
Gupta Dynasty		AD 320–500	Peak of Ayurvedic medicine
Reign of Harsha		AD 606–647	Vagbhata's Astangdahrdayasamhita
Muslim Conquest of Sind		AD 712	
Local Princely States		AD 800–1200	Madhava's *Treatise on Etiology* Vranda's & Vanagsena's therapeutics
Muslim Conquest of India		1200–1300	Introduction of Unani (Greco-Arabic) medicine
Sultanate of Delhi		1300–1500	
	Khalji Dynasty	1290–1320	Sarangadhara's *A Treatise on Medicine* Ayurvedic concept of circulation
	Tughluq Dynasty	1320–1413	Diya Mohammed's *Majmu'e Diya'e* Madanapala's *Materia Medica of Ayurveda*
	Sayyid and Lodi Dynasties	1414–1526	
Mogul Dynasty		1500–1700	Golden Age of Unani medicine Bhava Mishra's *Treatise on Ayurveda*
British Empire		1700–1947	Introduction of Western medicine Recovery of traditional medicines
Indian Republic		1947	Research on traditional medicine; clinical and pharmacological studies
Maharishi Ayurveda		1967	Rejuvenation of traditional Ayurveda Introduction of twentieth-century physics and "consciousness model" of Ayurveda

---

[a]Sushruta is considered the founder of anatomy. Jivaka came later, during the time of Buddha. Sushruta's dates are controversial but said to be 1000 BC or earlier, according to Hessler's Latin edition of Sushruta Samhita.

CHAPTER 32

UNANI MEDICINE

HAKIMA AMRI
MONES S. ABU-ASAB

Looking back we may say that Islamic medicine and science reflected the light of the Hellenic sun, when its day had fled, and that they shone like a moon, illuminating the darkest night of the European Middle Ages; that some bright stars lent their own light, and that moon and stars alike faded at the dawn of a new day—the Renaissance. Since they had their share in the direction and introduction of that great movement, it may reasonably be claimed that they are with us yet.
—ARNOLD AND GUILLAUME (1931)

The Eastern Mediterranean region, known as the Levant, was the site of several milestones in the history of humanity. It is where early crops and animals were first domesticated, alphabetical letters were invented and used, and many sciences and religions were developed and studied. It is likewise the home of an ancient system of Greco-Arabic medicine known worldwide today as Unani medicine. This medical system may be seen at once as a bridge between East and West and between ancient and modern. The word *Unani* is an Arabic adjective that means "Greek," referring mainly to the medical works of Hippocrates and Galen, which Arab and Muslim scholars translated from the Greek. However, as documented, the roots of the practice go back to Egypt and Mesopotamia (Nunn, 2002).

In the West, modern writers have always thought of Greece as part of European civilization and not as an integral part of North African, Middle Eastern, and Arabic regions—the Levant. Perhaps the European Renaissance was instigated by ancient Greek knowledge with no realization of its contemporary connections to the rest of the Levant. However, culturally, ethnically, and historically, Greece is part of the Eastern Mediterranean continuum (Bernal, 1987). When one studies Unani medical traditions, one can trace the continuity of medical knowledge

from ancient Egypt to Greece and Turkey, to Syria and Iraq, and back to Egypt. This comprehensive traditional medical system that developed over thousands of years is now known by the name Unani medicine, or by its Arabic common name, *Tibb*. It is practiced in several parts of the world, with a continued strong presence in India and Pakistan.

Unani medicine is recognized by the World Health Organization as one of the alternative systems of medicines (Bannerman et al, 1983; World Health Organization, 2002). As a medical system, Unani practices can be traced back a few thousand years to their roots in Egypt and Mesopotamia, where the great Greek physician Hippocrates (ca. 460–370 BC) probably traveled at a young age and where Galen (ca. AD 129–199) studied and practiced medicine (King, 2001). Aside from some fragmented records from the walls of the Egyptian temples and burial sites and Egyptian papyri (such as the Edwin Smith papyrus), as well as some Sumerian clay tablets, the works of Hippocrates and Galen remain the most extensive ancient medical writings that have survived, mainly through the translations of Arab and Muslim scholars during the Middle Ages.

Their works were further expanded by Arab and Muslim physicians such as Rhazes* and Avicenna,[†] who contributed from their own experience and pertinent observation.

---

*Abū Bakr Muhammad ibn Zakariyā Rāzī was a chemist, physician, philosopher, and scholar. Razi was born in Rayy, Iran, in the year AD 865 (251 AH) and died there in AD 925 (313 AH).
[†]Abū 'Alī al-Husayn ibn 'Abd Allah ibn Sīnā was born ca. AD 980 near Bukhara, Khorasan, and died in 1037 in Hamedan. He is also known as Ibn Seena.

They corrected misconceptions and recorded their own discoveries, such as (1) the alcohol extraction of medicinal plants and distillation of rose oil, described for the first time in the greatest detail; (2) the distinctions between diseases such as smallpox and measles; and (3) explanations for the first time of meningitis and pleurisy. Rhazes focused on infectious diseases, whereas Avicenna identified over 750 drugs and emphasized preventive medicine, exercise, diet, and mental health. Rhazes and Avicenna authored *Al-Hawi* (Razi, 1955) and *Al-Qanoon* (Avicenna, 1993), respectively. The former is considered the largest medical encyclopedia to date, and the latter became the standard medical textbook for hundreds of years throughout most of the Old World, until the development of chemistry and the rise of modern medicine. Unani medicine can be considered the catalyst for the revival, modernization, and systematization of ancient Egypto-Greco-Roman medicine that laid the foundation for modern medicine (Porter, 1999).

Unani medicine has profoundly influenced medicine in the West. The allopathic Western medical system in Europe evolved from the Unani tradition, and during the eighteenth and nineteenth centuries, Unani medicine provided a source for other natural, holistic, and alternative practices such as homeopathy, naturopathy, and chiropractic in Europe and the United States.

The Unani medical system is also distinguished by including mental evaluation in patient examination (an early approach to mind–body medicine). In addition to physical signs, Unani physicians use both mental and emotional characteristics to determine the temperament of the patient. They also attribute certain symptoms to mental causes and treat them as such.

The technically rudimentary methods of diagnosis of traditional medical systems do not imply that their medical knowledge and practice are primitive and unsophisticated. To the contrary, they represent an excellent understanding of biological systems and states of health and disease. These traditional systems, with their simple methods of patient examination, offer the most cost-effective real-time evaluation of patient status of any known method, one in which the caregiver does not have to rely on calibrated machines and delayed test results to treat an illness.

THEORETICAL BASIS OF UNANI MEDICINE

All traditional medical systems seek to harmonize the health of the individual with the universal elements of nature and the cosmos; they all aim for a balance between opposite, but complementary, elements of the human system. Similar to other traditional medical systems such as Chinese medicine and Ayurveda, Unani adheres to a holistic and balanced approach to health maintenance, diagnosis of illness, and restoration of health. As a holistic medical system, it aims to assist the natural recuperative power of the body; it recognizes all factors that contribute

to human health status; and it avoids harming sound parts of the body when pursuing treatment options for a disease (Osborn, 2008).

Unani's theoretical basis encompasses the theory of naturals (*tabie'iat*), which is a unifying explanation of humans and nature. It explains the shared natural building elements of the universe and humans and classifies normal constituents and functions of a healthy individual. Unani practice is based on the theory of causes (*mousabibat*), which identifies the elements underlying illness, and the theory of signs (*'alamat*), which identifies diagnostic symptoms (Chishti, 1991; Abu-Asab, Amri, & Micozzi, 2013).

THE NATURALS OF UNANI (*TABIE'IAT*)

Avicenna defined Unani medicine as a branch of knowledge that is based on physical laws—the naturals—and not on dogma or superstition (Abu-Asab, Amri, & Micozzi, 2013). There are seven main sets of naturals that form the essential constituents and the working principles of the body: the elements or phases (*arkan*), temperaments (*mizaj*), humors (*akhlat*), organs (*a'dha*), spirits (*arwah*), faculties (*quwa*), and functions (*af'al*).

The Elements or Phases (*Arkan*)

The elements are also known in Arabic as the basics, or origins (*ousoul*). The four elements are earth, water, air, and fire. A fifth energetic element, the ether, is considered the source of the other four but is not used in Unani medicine (Figure 32-1). The ancient philosophers of the Levant

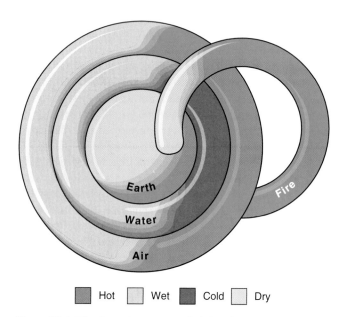

Hot ■ Wet □ Cold ■ Dry □

Figure 32-1 The four elements and their relation to each other as described by Avicenna and illustrated by the authors. The earth element is surrounded by water, which is enveloped by air, whereas fire connects all of them. The shades are indicative of the two natures (temperaments) characterizing each element: earth is dry and cold, water is cold and wet-moist, air is wet-moist and hot, and fire is hot and dry. (Copyright © Hakima Amri and Abu-Asab Mones.)

attempted to formulate a unifying theory that explains all natural phenomena; however, because in their time they lacked the tools for molecular and atomic investigations, they used symbolism to hypothesize, predict, and substitute for the unknown, and referred to things by their characteristics rather than their constitutions. For example, the elements also represent all physical phases of matter: solid, liquid, gas, and energy. These physical phases were considered to be the elements that form the ingredients of everything in the universe, including humans; their usage in medicine means that they confer their characteristics to the body, its organs, and its energies.

Avicenna described the earth element as "a simple motionless heavy object that occupies the center in a group of elements. It helps life forms attain cohesiveness, shape, and stability" (anticipating the Newtonian concept of gravity). He also described the physical relationships among the elements: "the water element engulfs the earth, and the two are surrounded by air." He placed the fire element as the connector between the other three elements (see Figure 32-1) and attributed to it the ability to bring earth and water from their elemental states into compounds by reducing their inertia. His characterization of the fire element is similar to a modern description of free energy. Furthermore, he pointed out that air and fire are constituents of the life energies or spirits (see section on the spirits later).

Each element is associated with fixed qualitative characteristics (nature or temperament) called the "elemental powers": these are hot, cold, wet or moist, and dry. Each element possesses two natures; earth is cold and dry, water is cold and wet–moist, air is hot and wet–moist, and fire is hot and dry (Bakar, 1990). In addition, earth and water are associated with heaviness, and fire and air with lightness. Heavy elements are thought of as strong, negative, passive, and female, whereas light elements are thought of as weak, positive, active, heavenly, and male.

The four elements are dynamic, interacting and resulting in a continuous change within the human body. This change is either cyclical or directional. The food and water cycles are examples of cyclical change, whereas abnormal growth of a tumor represents a directional change. Because the elements must exist in equilibrium to maintain health, any change in the elements is monitored to assess the health status of each part of the body. This requirement for assessment necessitated the development of a monitoring classification called the "*temperaments*" (*mizaj*).

The Temperaments (*Mizaj*)

The literal meaning of *mizaj* is the quality or qualities of a mixture; its classic use means that it is a product of the opposite physical qualities of the four elements (hot, cold, wet, and dry). Temperament, as it is usually called in the literature, is the sum quality of the body or any of its organs, resulting from the actions and reactions of the elements. Its definition can encompass the metabolic, behavioral, and mental profile of the individual; it can also be thought of as a physical state or phenotype. In modern interpretation, we have established that the individual acquires a temperamental phenotype during his or her life based on genotype, environmental effects, and lifestyle choices. The individual's genetic predisposition plays a role in the type of temperamental phenotype acquired. As explained in the section on Unani diagnosis (see below), it is important to understand the theory of the temperaments because certain conditions are associated with one particular temperament, signs that are normal for one temperament are abnormal for others, and the temperamental phenotype determines the suitability of a treatment and dosage of medication.

There are four basic temperaments: hot, cold, wet, and dry. Because these four can also occur in combination, however, the total number of temperaments is nine, although other sources like Al-Antaki* mention 17 (Antaki, 1982). These are classified into eight imbalanced and one balanced temperament. The eight imbalanced temperaments result from the unequal presence of opposing qualities. These include four single temperaments—hot, cold, wet, and dry—and four composite temperaments—hot and dry, hot and wet, cold and dry, and cold and wet. Because the elements are constantly interacting, the normal balanced state has a range and is not a strict point. Humans have a body temperament range that differs from that of animals; age groups and geographically based populations have their own ranges; and healthy ranges are different from ranges during illness. In addition, each organ has its own temperament, with ranges of heat and cold, as well as wetness and dryness. For example, the hottest are breath, blood, liver, flesh, and muscles; the coldest are phlegm humor, hair, bones, cartilage, and ligaments; the wettest are phlegm humor, blood, oil, fat, and brain; and the driest are hair, bone, cartilage, ligaments, and tendons.

The Humors (*Akhlat*)

The term *humor* is derived from the Greek *chymos* (χυμός; juice or sap); however, the humoral theory is ancient and cannot be attributed to a single person. Most of the humoral descriptions reference Hippocrates, whose writing on the subject has survived to this day. The four humors are present in the bloodstream in different quantities and are considered the essential components of the body that occupy the vascular system. Later, Avicenna concurred with Hippocrates and added the tissue fluids (intercellular and intracellular) as the secondary humors.

Balanced humors are considered the source of health, and restoring the humoral balance is the *modus operandi* of Unani treatment to restore the health of sick individuals. Unani adheres to the humoral theory with four humors in the body: blood (*dam*), phlegm (*balgham*), yellow bile (*safra'*), and black bile (*sauda*). Ancient Greek medicine used only three humors—blood, phlegm, and bile—until Thales of Miletus (ca. 640-546 BC), who had been educated in ancient

---

*Antākī, Dā'ūdibn'Umar, died in Mecca in AD 1599 (1008 AH).

Egypt, suggested bringing Greek traditions in line with Egyptian medical concepts by adding the fourth humor, black bile (Osborn, 2008). Like the elements, each humor has two natures: blood is hot and humid, phlegm is cold and humid, yellow bile is hot and dry, and black bile is cold and dry. Thus, there is a parallelism between the natures of the human body and the natures of objects in the physical world.

The temperament of the individual is the net result of the proportions of the four humors. There are four types of temperaments that are named after the predominant humor: sanguine (blood humor predominates; *damawi*), phlegmatic (phlegm humor predominates; *balghami*), bilious or choleric (yellow bile humor predominates; *safrawi*), and melancholic (black bile humor predominates; *saudawi*).

In the healthy state, each individual has a unique equilibrium of the humors that is maintained by the vital forces or powers, called *quwa*, which may be considered the metabolic strength and functions of organs (see section on the faculties, below). Although strong emphasis is placed on diet and digestion for the restoration of humoral balance and health, the restorative power of quwa is considered very important, and quwa is usually fortified by the prescribed medications.

The Organs (*A'dha*)

Based on structure, organs are classified into two types: simple and compound. The simple organs are homogeneous in structure, such as bones, nerves, tendons, veins, and arteries; the compound ones are heterogeneous and are composed of several other organs, such as the head. Unani medicine assigns four organs primary importance; these are the heart, brain, liver, and gonads. The heart is the essential distributor of the two vital energies (*pneuma* and *ignis*; see next section). The brain controls the mental faculties, senses, and movement. The liver carries out the nutritive and cleansing processes. The gonads give the masculine and feminine characteristics and temperaments and form the reproductive elements.

The Spirits: Life Energies (*Arwah*)

The spirits here differ from the theological and mystical ones; they are purely physical and refer to the "energies of life." The term is used in Unani medicine to signify the driving forces or energies that help the faculties carry out their functions and also connect between them (see next paragraph). Arab-Muslim and Greek physicians divided spirits into two types: (1) *pneuma* (breath; *nafas*), which is homologous to the oxygen needed for cellular aerobic respiration; and (2) *ignis* (fire; *hararah*), the thermal energy produced by physiological respiration needed for digestion and metabolism. Pneuma was described as "pure, warm, light, and mobile air," whereas ignis was described as being responsible for providing the heat or energy needed to carry out metabolic processes.

Lungs take out pneuma from the air, mix it with blood, and send it to the heart, from which it is distributed throughout the body organs and facilitates various functions by these organs. Unani physicians attributed various physiological functions to pneuma, not different organs, and divided pneuma into three forms in the human body on the basis of source and function: the vital, the psychic, and the natural. The vital or animalistic spirit (Greek, *pneuma zoticon*; Arabic, *hayawaniyyah*) stems from the heart and functions to preserve life by preparing suitable conditions for the other two spirits. The psychic spirit (*pneuma psychicon*; *nafsaniyyah*) originates in the brain, stimulating sensation and perception through the cognitive faculty and triggering movement through the motivation faculty. The natural spirit (*pneuma physicon*; *tab'iyyah*) derives from the liver and is associated with the nutritional and reproductive processes that are performed by the natural faculties.

Ignis is the fire or energy produced in the presence of air; therefore, it does not exist without pneuma. It is the energy that drives all metabolic processes within the body and is also responsible for the body's innate heat emanated during these metabolic processes. Ignis occurs within the same major organs as pneuma and assumes similar names.

There is a striking similarity between this ancient explanation of the body's energies and our current knowledge of respiration physiology. In a modern scientific interpretation, the pneuma and ignis are equivalent to oxygen intake and the important functional role of oxygen as the electron acceptor in the mitochondria, without which respiration-generated free heat and chemical energy in the form of adenosine triphosphate, the cell's energy currency, will not occur.

The Faculties (*Quwa*): Psychophysical Drives

A faculty is an ability or a potentiality. The faculties constitute the biological systems of organs and their physiological processes. There are three major faculties: the vital or animalistic (*hayawaniyyah*), the psychic (*nafsaniyyah*), and the natural or physical (*tab'iyyah*) (Figure 32-2). Each of these faculties carries out its functions under its corresponding spirit (see previous section), and the locations of the faculties are also identical with those of their spirits.

Vital faculties are the source of the motive energy (the life force that is referred to as *thymos* by classical Greeks). They are either the active type that is involuntary, such as heartbeat, or are acted upon (voluntary), such as the emotions of anger, happiness, and contempt.

Psychic faculties represent the conscious and unconscious mind. The psychic faculties perform three functions: they underlie behavior, they stimulate voluntary movement, and they generate sensation.

The natural faculties have a hierarchical relationship because they fall into those that serve other faculties and those that are served by others. For example, as the chart of faculties shows (see Figure 32-2), the nutritive faculty is served by four others: the attractive, the retentive, the digestive, and the expulsive. These four serving faculties

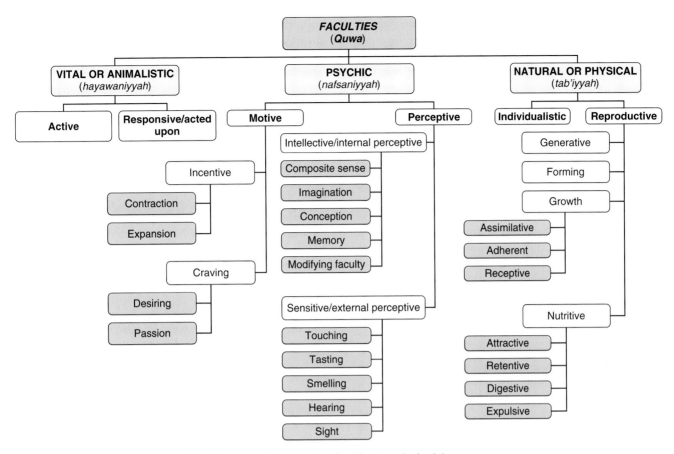

Figure 32-2 The three faculties and their characteristics as described by Unani physicians.

serve the nutritive faculty by attracting, retaining, digesting, and expelling. The nutritive faculty serves the growth faculty, which in turn, with the forming faculty, serves the generative faculty.

The Functions (*Af'al*)

The functions complement the faculties, and each faculty has its specific functions based on its specific organ. Avicenna classifies functions into single (such as digestion) and compound (such as eating, which requires the desire for food, taste, and swallowing).

UNANI VIEW OF DISEASE

Causes (Mousabibat/Alasbab)

For humans to maintain good health, six essential factors have to be present: (1) fresh clean air, (2) food and drink, (3) movement and rest, (4) sleep and wakefulness, (5) eating and excreting, and (6) healthy mental state. A long-term disruption of these essential factors results in illness. Illness is a state that affects the functions of the vital, psychic, or natural faculties because of an imbalance or obstruction of a temperament (dystemperament) or a combination of functions and temperaments. Unani physicians state that the body has three health conditions: (1) healthy (i.e., disease-free), (2) ill or diseased, and (3) a continuum between the two—situations in which the disease is still in its asymptomatic phase (which may manifest as a

functional complaint or disorder before the detection of pathology) or the body is recuperating from a disease. The third state may manifest in three forms: (1) disease affects only one organ but the rest of the body is healthy; (2) the healthy state is not optimal, as in aging individuals; and (3) health and illness alternate in a temporal fashion, as in individuals with a hot temperament who are ill in the summer but well during the winter, or vice versa.

Dystemperament is either local or systemic and involves one or more of the four basic qualities of hot, cold, wet, and dry. The effect is usually caused by an outside and often unexpected source. On the other hand, humoral illness involves metabolic disorder, which results in imbalances in or corruptions of (or both) one or more of the four humors. The disorder is either quantitative (excess or deficiency), qualitative, or both simultaneously. Most humoral disorders originate internally due to metabolic errors that result in either excess (anabolism), such as high levels of triglycerides, or wasting (catabolism), such as degenerative diseases.

According to Al-Antaki, there are four states in which the disease condition is not the result of an imbalance or a dystemperament (Antaki, 1982). Such diseases are of the following types: (1) congenital malformations and defects; (2) accidents (internal: poisoning; external: burn, fracture, wounds, etc.); (3) quantitative abnormality, organ enlargement or atrophy; and (4) dislocation, displaced organs.

Unani medicine (like Ayurveda) considers the origin of most illnesses to be the corruption of the *pepsis*: the digestive and metabolic processes (generation and distribution of the humors). Arab-Muslim medical literature is full of famous quotations that emphasize this point. According to Alkindi,* "the stomach is the house of all illness," and he also advised not to eat when angry and not to bathe on a full stomach. The conditions under which digestion occurs are as important as the diets that are consumed.

On a daily basis, the individual encounters potentially pathogenic stresses; however, most of these fail to cause illness. They succeed only when the individual's resistance and adaptive responses have been weakened or compromised and the virulence of the pathogen overwhelms the host's defenses, or the pathogen is able to establish itself through a weakness in the host systems.

Signs of Imbalance ('*Alamat*)

Evaluation of an individual's health should take into consideration some innate traits (*lawazem*) such as age, gender, race, skin complexion, and geographic adaptations. Traits attributable to the long-term multigenerational adaptation to living in a particular geographic area should not be confused with signs of temperamental imbalance. For example, people from the warm equatorial parts of the world have hot temperaments as well as dark complexions, eyes, and hair, whereas those from temperate zones have cold temperaments as well as light skin, eyes, and hair. Thus the cold temperament of the northerners is not an indication of a phlegmatic state.

Age also dictates different assessments, depending on its phase. Four phases of life are recognized: youth (from birth to 28 years of age), adulthood (ends at 40), maturity (ends at 60), and elderliness (ends at death). Because bodily functions vary in their efficiency during each phase, each is also associated with its own innate temperament: youth is hot and wet; adulthood is hot and dry; maturity is cold and dry; and elderliness is cold and—strangely—wet. Therefore, *age temperament* should be considered before an *organ's temperament,* and prescribed diet and herbal treatments should be suitable for the age group. There are also some traits that develop in association with age progression that should not be confused with symptoms of illness. For example, hair thinning and a desire for naps are associated with the phases of maturity and elderliness and are not indicative of an imbalance. These are life changes that should be accepted as normal with aging, rather than considered to require medical intervention.

Avicenna described a set of traits to be examined by the *hakim,* or Unani physician, to determine the temperamental status (Avicenna, 1993). These included the quality of skin texture and complexion (should be slightly moist, warm, smooth, elastic, and between white and red), the balance of muscle and fat, hair characteristics (should be full, thick, between straight and curly, with balanced growth in location and length), organ configuration, reaction time of the faculties, dreams, and the balance of sleep and waking. Also, the hakim looks for signs of humoral excesses in which all the humors are overabundant or one is in excess at the expense of another humor. Other focuses of observation are characteristics of stool and urine, stomach growling, mouth odor, shape of the nails, cheek color, involuntary movements (e.g., cough, spasm, shivering), congestion and blockage, gas formation and blockage, and tumors. Special attention is given to fevers, tongue color and texture, pain, pulse, and the eyes.

Imbalance of temperaments (dystemperament). The first diagnostic feature a hakim looks for is a dystemperament of the ailing organ or system. There are four main dystemperaments: hot (hotter than usual, but not moister or drier); cold (colder than usual, but not moister or drier); dry (drier than usual, but not hotter or colder); and moist (moister than usual, but not hotter or colder). These are dynamic, never static, dystemperaments that are constantly changing and interacting. In addition, there are four possible compound dystemperaments that develop when a simple dystemperament persists long enough to affect a second one. For example, a hot dystemperament expels moisture, which leads to a dry dystemperament; this produces a compound dystemperament. The four possible compound dystemperaments are hotter and moister, hotter and drier, colder and moister, and colder and drier.

Dystemperament can affect an organ, tissue, or system and may include any of the humors or a combination of them. A dystemperament of a humor differs from a humoral disorder because the humoral essence is not affected in this case and the humor or humors remain balanced. On the other hand, a humoral disorder progresses, ripens, and reveals itself after a period of time.

Dystemperaments are determined by the signs of the body or an organ. They are either qualitative (indicative of a disease) or material–spatial (indicative of the location). A dystemperament is qualitative if it is not located within an organ directly (as with a fever) and material if it is within an organ and causing changes there (e.g., a cold liver will produce pale urine and light-colored stool).

It is only after gathering as much information as possible about the patient that the hakim tries to identify the form of humoral imbalance.

Imbalance of humors. Humoral disorders result from the corruption of the pepsis processes (digestion and metabolism within the body), which fall under the natural faculty. It is also important to add that, nowadays, industrial chemical pollutants can cause humoral disorders if they enter and persist in the body. When the metabolic process is weak, the humors are undersupplied and underperforming, which leads to problems in the functions of the systems and organs. Underperforming humors tend to generate more phlegm and less blood. On the other hand, an overactive metabolic process corrupts the humors with an unbalanced oversupply of metabolites, which is toxic to

---

*Abū Yusūf Ya'qūb ibn Ishāq al-Kindī, ca. AD 801–873, known in the West as Alkindus.

BOX 32-1 *Signs of Humoral Imbalance*

Blood humor

Angina, bleeding disorders, canker sores, constant erection and spasm of penis, coughing, cracked nails, delirium, diphtheria, enlarged tongue, excessive menstrual flow, gout, headache, heart disease, hemorrhoids, high blood pressure, lethargy, loose teeth, migraine, nosebleed, nose itching, pleurisy, poor vision, slackness of uvula, swelling of liver, swollen palate, swollen testicles, tooth spaces, trembling lips, uremia, weak limbs

Phlegm humor

Acne, arthritis, atonic dyspepsia, asthma, backache, bad breath, bad taste in mouth, baldness, boils, canker sores, chronic bronchitis, colic, conjunctivitis, constipation, constriction of throat, continuous trembling, convulsion of stomach, convulsions, corrupt appetite, cough, dandruff, dandruff of eyelids, deficient appetite, dilation of pupils, diphtheria, dull feeling in teeth, enlarged tongue, erectile dysfunction, forgetfulness, foul odor from nose, grippe, headache, heart feels as if being pulled downward, insomnia, itching of anus, joint ache, lethargy, madness, melancholy, muscular tension, obstruction of liver, paralysis, pimples, pleurisy, respiratory allergies, retention of urine, ringing in ears, scabs, sebaceous cysts, severe perspiration, severe thirst, shedding eyelashes, sour mother's milk, styes, swelling of bladder, swelling of lips, swelling of liver, swelling of lymph nodes, swelling of spleen, swelling of testicles, swelling of uvula, swelling of womb, swollen eyelids, swollen palate, trembling limbs, ulcers of gums, ulcers of kidneys, upset stomach, vomiting, weak limbs, weak nail growth, whiteness of lips

Yellow bile humor

Anal ulcer, biliousness and biliary congestion, boils on eyelid, burning urination, canker sores, cough, delirium, discolored teeth, dull teeth, excessive appetite, excessive menstrual flow, feeling of "smoke" in chest, gallstones, gastric and duodenal ulcers, gastritis, grippe, hard eyelids, headache, heart attack, hemorrhoids, hyperacidity and acid reflux, insomnia, jaundice, migraine, nose itching, photophobia, pleurisy, rheumatoid arthritis, swelling of liver, swelling of testicles, tendonitis, vomiting, yellowed nails

Black bile humor

Abnormal growths and hard tumors, arthritis, cancer, canker sores, clots and embolisms, colic, constipation, delirium, diphtheria, excessive appetite, excessive libido, flatulence, grippe, hallucinations, headache, heartburn, insomnia, insufficient mother's milk, intestinal obstruction, irritable bowel, neuralgia, seizures and convulsions, skin cancer, stiffness, swelling of bladder, swelling of liver, swelling of spleen, swelling of stomach, swelling of womb, thickened nails, varicose veins, vomiting

---

the system. This toxic accumulation loads the body with black and yellow biles.

Although humoral disorders are metabolic in nature, the humors may be affected by dystemperament like any other part or organ of the body. Coldness, dryness, and wetness slow them down, whereas heat puts them into overdrive.

The symptoms and diseases that are usually associated with each of the humors are summarized in Box 32-1 (Chishti, 1991; Osborn, 2008).

PRACTICAL BASIS OF UNANI MEDICINE

UNANI DIAGNOSIS (*TASHKHEES*)

Accurate diagnosis is the path to a successful treatment. The hakim relies on his or her senses, knowledge, reasoning, and experience to gather all signs of imbalance and reach a diagnosis. In addition to taking the medical history of the patient, the hakim, through observation and physical examination, gathers the physical and mental signs of imbalance. The examination encompasses the tongue, nails, pulse, urine, and feces, and it notes the presence of pain and fever.

Determination of the Patient's Temperament

As mentioned earlier, there are four types of temperaments in humans. The hakim determines the patient's temperament from three sets of characteristics: (1) appearance (complexion, build, touch, and hair), (2) physiological features (movement, diet preferences, seasonal preferences, sleep, and pulse), and (3) emotions (calm, angry, nervous, etc.).

The patient's humoral imbalance manifests itself in the patient's mental status, behavior, and mannerisms. Characteristics related to these aspects can be attributed to one of the four humors. A sanguine personality is usually balanced, stylish, refined, passionate, positive, genial, inquisitive, playful, sensual, and indulgent. A phlegmatic personality is calm, good-natured, trusting, sluggish, inactive, sentimental, sensitive, loving, subjective, self-absorbed, and steady. A choleric personality is forceful, energetic, flamboyant, expressive, dramatic, bold, fidgety, short-tempered, angry, and argumentative. A melancholic personality is quiet, cool, aloof, detached, objective, withdrawn, cautious, prudent, frugal, stoic, stiff, inflexible, lonely, unhappy, thoughtful, and grumpy. A patient showing signs of mental fatigue or compulsiveness should be considered for examination. The hakim is usually on the lookout for behavioral signs that may provide a clue to the patient's illness.

Examination of Bodily Functions

Major traditional medical systems of the Old World use the same techniques to detect the signs of deviation from the normal range in order to determine the malfunctioning organ(s). Examinations of the pulse, tongue, urine, and feces are employed as diagnostic tools. Their usage is described briefly in the following sections.

Pulse (*nabd*). The heart is the distributor of pneuma to the rest of the body and directly determines the vitality of the system (the production of free energy and chemical energy); therefore, its health is of prime importance in Unani medicine. The current system of pulse diagnosis used in Unani medicine was developed by Avicenna. He studied all the available pulse information of his time and then integrated it all in his synthesis. Galen and Avicenna understood the challenging nature of pulse diagnosis, as is evident in their writings. Practicing hakims admit that it is the hardest part of Tibb to master.

A pulse is composed of two movements (systole and diastole), and two rests following each of the movements (Box 32-2). The pulse is felt at the radial artery near the wrist, where it is closer to the skin surface and easily accessible. To examine the pulse, the hakim places the middle finger on the radial artery, directly between the carpus and the prominence of the radius, with the two adjoining fingers next to it in their natural positions and the index finger proximal to the heart. It is recommended that the pulse be examined on the right hand for a female and on the left hand for a male, with the individual's palm turned upward for both.

Avicenna's description of pulse variation is very detailed and comprehensive. For example, he explained the underlying reasons for the natural heterogeneity of the pulse; the variation between male and female pulses; and pulse characteristics related to age, temperaments, seasons, geographical adaptations, food, sleep, sports, bathing, pain, tumors, and female gender.

A hot temperament, in a state of health, is associated with "great pulse," the best type of pulse, whereas a cold temperament is associated with a weaker pulse. A wet temperament produces a wavy and wide pulse, and a dry one is associated with tightness and stiffness and produces a spasmodic and shaky pulse. Furthermore, a sanguine temperament (hot and moist) is characterized by a moderate to slightly rapid pulse that is moderately soft and relaxed; a phlegmatic temperament (cold and wet) is associated with a deep, slow, and soft pulse; a melancholic temperament (cold and dry) produces a slow to weak, tense or constricted, thin, and well-defined pulse; and a choleric temperament (hot and dry) is associated with a strong, rapid, and well-defined pulse.

Tongue (*lisan*). There are two areas of interest with regard to the tongue: the body and the coat. The tongue body reflects the temperament and blood supply in the body in general, whereas the tongue coat reveals the health of digestive and metabolic processes and humoral imbalances.

The tongue body texture is indicative of systemic or chronic conditions that are severe. The texture can be dry or rough, cracked, raw, rumpled, or wet and glossy. These characteristics may indicate lack of body moisture, nervousness, advanced sickness, inefficient digestion, and excess moisture, respectively.

The color, size, and texture of the tongue's coat are all taken into consideration in diagnosis. The coat reflects the health status of digestion, the digestive tract, and metabolism, and the surface location of the coat reflects the affected part of the system (e.g., pancreas, intestine, stomach, liver). An absent or thin coat denotes good digestive and metabolic health, whereas an increase in coat thickness reflects poor digestion, and the thickness is proportional to the accumulation of metabolic toxins in the body. Coat color indicates the nature of the buildup (e.g., phlegmatic, choleric), and its texture reflects moisture content.

Urine (*boul*). The urine provides a window on the metabolic status of the individual. Avicenna stated that the urine is indicative of the health of the liver, urinary tracts, and blood vessels. He stressed several specifics for urine collection to ensure accurate assessment. For example, the sample should be the first collection of the day before the individual eats any food, and the patient should have had no food the night before that may color the urine, should not have had intercourse, and should have been resting for a while before urination. Hakims assess the urine within

---

BOX 32-2 *Ten Characteristics of Pulse Evaluation*

Avicenna listed 10 characteristics of pulse evaluation. The first seven determine whether the pulse of an individual is regular. These are as follows:

The first seven

1. Dimensions of expansion (length, width, and depth)
2. Strength as a force felt against the finger (strong, moderate, weak)
3. Speed (fast, moderate, slow)
4. Compressibility (soft, hard, and in between)
5. Turgor: tension of the artery between pulses—fullness (full, empty, and in between)
6. Temperature of the pulse (hot, cold, and in between)
7. Duration of diastole (short, long, and in between)

The next three

8. Regularity (regular in all preceding characteristics) or irregular
9. Order and disorder in irregularity
10. Rhythm, specific to the individual and usually measured as the ratio between the two movements and the two rests

Avicenna further classified the irregular pulse into *seven compound pulse types:*
a. Gazelle
b. Wavy
c. Wormy/cordlike/twisting
d. Antlike
e. Sawlike
f. Mouse tail
g. Snake tongue, needlelike/flickering

the first hour of its collection by evaluating its quantity, color, foaminess, texture, clarity, and sediment. Avicenna eliminated touching and tasting the urine as part of the evaluation.

Urine may have one of several colors, depending on the individual's state of health, ingested food, water intake, and use of drugs. It can be yellow, red, green, black, or white. Shades of yellow, for example, may range from straw yellow to lemon yellow to blond yellow to orange yellow to fiery yellow (saturated yellow) to saffron yellow with a tinge of red. The first two indicate a normal heat temperament, whereas the rest indicate increased heat or may be generated by extreme exercise, pain, hunger, or thirst.

The thick part of the urine is present and floats on the surface, particles suspended in the liquid, or sediment at the bottom. Foamy floats in urine are attributed to moisture and gases, especially in individuals with gaseous bloating. Abundance, persistence, and large bubble size of floats indicate an increase in viscosity caused by bad humor and cold. Thick elements of the other two types are referred to as sediment. Normal sediment is white, uniform, cohesive, and smooth, and it readily precipitates. Suspended turbid sediment, however, denotes immature intermediates of metabolism.

It is axiomatic among hakims that the urine odor of an ill patient differs from that of healthy individuals. However, odorless urine signifies cold humor, immature digestion, acute sickness, and diminished metabolic vitality. A foul odor of the urine is caused mostly by infections and ulcers in the urinary tract. Acidic urine is produced by cold temperament that is affected by abnormal metabolism, but extreme acidity is a sign of death due to diminished innate heat. A sweet odor of the urine indicates the dominance of sanguine temperament, an extremely foul odor is produced by choleric temperament, and an acidic foul odor is caused by melancholic temperament.

Feces or Stool (bouraz). Feces, also called "alvine discharge," have characteristics that are indicative of the individual's pepsis and health. Normal feces are yellowish and cohesive with uniform softness, similar in consistency to unfiltered honey. They come out easily without burning sensation, air sounds, or foam. The quantity of feces is compared with the amount of food ingested. A reduced amount is thought to be due to retention in the intestinal tract, and an increase points to the presence of humors. Wet feces (as in diarrhea) indicate weak digestion, weak absorption, or blockage, whereas hard feces (as in dehydration) may point to excessive urination, ingestion of dry food, prolonged retention, or fiery heat within the system. The color of the feces specifies the affecting humor; for example, a dark or black color is a sign of maturation of a melancholic disease, but only if one can exclude excessive heat or consumption of colored foods or a drink that produces black bile.

Pain (waja'). Pain is an unnatural transitory condition for the human body. It is usually caused by a dystemperament or an injury—loss of continuity (Box 32-3). Pain weakens

---

BOX 32-3 *The Fifteen Types of Pains and Their Causes*

Avicenna listed 15 types of *pains* and their causes:
1. Itching (*hakak*), caused by a humor that is bitter or salty
2. Rough (*khashin*), caused by a rough humor
3. Stabbing (*nakhes*), caused by a humor that extends the muscle membrane and separates it
4. Flattening or extended (*moumaded*), caused by a humor or gas that pulls the nerve or muscle from two opposite ends
5. Pressing (*daghet*), caused by a substance that engulfs the organ and presses on it
6. Splitting (*moufasekh*), caused by a substance that seeps out of the muscle or its membrane and separates the two
7. Breaking (*moukaser*), caused by a substance, gas, or coldness in between the bone and its membrane
8. Softening (*rakhou*), caused by extension of only the muscle without the tendon
9. Boring (*thaqeb*), caused by the trapping of gas or a substance between the tissues of a hard organ such as the colon
10. Piercing (*masalee*), caused by the boring of a hard organ by a gas or substance
11. Dull (*khader*), caused by a cold temperament or obstruction of blood supply
12. Throbbing (*dharabani*), caused by hot inflammation next to an organ
13. Heavy (*thaqeel*), a sense of heaviness in an insensitive organ such as the lung, kidney, or spleen caused by inflammation or tumor, or by the tumor's disabling of the pain sensation, such as in cancer in the mouth or the stomach
14. Tiring (*a `ya `i*), could be caused by fatigue or by an extending humor, gas, or ulcerative humor
15. Biting or incisive (*lathe'*), caused by a sour humor

---

the organ and halts its function. It warms the organ initially but later cools it down and saps its energy. Removal of the cause will halt the pain and is the preferred method of treatment (e.g., by applying a poultice of linseed [*Linum usitatissimum*] or dill [*Anethum graveolens*], or by applying wet sedatives [alcohols] or cold anesthetics [all narcotics]).

Fever (homa [sing.], homiat [pl.]). In the fourth volume of his *Al-Qanoon*, Avicenna wrote a detailed study of fever types, symptoms, causes, and treatments. Fever is an unnatural heat "centered within the heart and spirits" (i.e., involving pneuma and ignis energies) and carried throughout the body by blood and the vascular system; it is a disquieting sign of corruption and imbalance that requires attention. On the basis of origin, there are two main classes of fevers: (1) fevers associated with infections (*waba'yah*), and (2) transient fevers associated with warming effects, foul humor, hyperplasia, and blockage. Based on their causes and locations, the second class has three subtypes of fevers: (1) ephemeral fevers (*homa youm*), (2) humoral fevers/putrefactive fevers (*homa khalt/'of ounah*), and (3) organ fevers/hectic fevers (*homa daq*).

Avicenna attributed infection and its associated fever to the contamination of air and water with "malevolent soil objects" that are taken into the body. These "objects" corrupt the body's "spirit" and produce unnatural heat that spreads throughout the body. However, he ascribed the infection's success to the presence of corrupt humors that permits the infection to take place.

All of the *ephemeral fevers* are caused by external warming effects: the sun's heat, exhaustion, hot food and medications, sports, and emotional tension. These fevers usually last one day (hence the name *youm,* which means "a day" in Arabic) and, rarely, up to three days. The persistence of a fever beyond three days, however, signifies that it has spread to an organ or a humor and could turn into a putrefactive or hectic type.

Putrefactive fevers are caused by corruption of the humors. They arise in the body due to the ingestion of contaminated food and the effects of its by-products, consumption of high-moisture fruits, incomplete digestion, and lack of oxygen and proper breathing. Putrefaction may affect the whole body, an organ, or a humor. Because putrefactive fevers are associated with humors, they are classified according to the affected humor: (1) *alghibb* fever is alternating fever, day on/day off, caused by the putrefaction of yellow bile humor; (2) *mutbiqah* fever is consistent and caused by the putrefaction of blood humor; (3) *na'bbah* fever is caused by the putrefaction of phlegm humor; (4) *alroub'* fever recurs in cycles of one day on and two days off and is caused by the putrefaction of black bile humor.

Organ fever (or *hectic fever*) may follow after the other fever types mentioned previously. It is considered difficult to diagnose but easy to treat at its incipience, easy to diagnose but difficult to treat at its end, and untreatable if the patient withers. Organ fever affects the moisture at three stages: at the first stage it reduces moisture in the vessels; at the second stage it reduces moisture between the tissues and produces wilting (*thoubool*); and at the third stage it is decomposing (*moufatit*) and reduces moisture within the tissues.

HEALTH MAINTENANCE, PREVENTION, AND TREATMENT OF DISEASE

Unani medicine emphasizes healthy practices of exercise and diet for health maintenance and prevention of sickness. Avicenna divided medicine into theoretical and practical and further subdivided the practical into two sections: (1) management of healthy bodies, which he also called the "science of health preservation"; and (2) management of sick bodies (Figure 32-3).

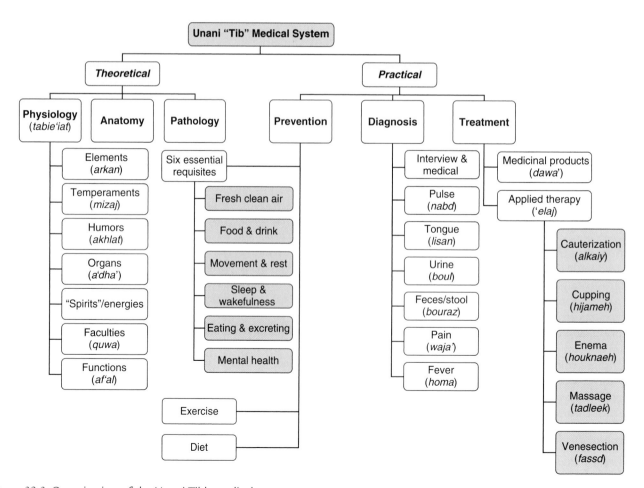

Figure 32-3 Organization of the Unani Tibb medical system.

Health is maintained by the proper internal balance of heat and moisture that allows the innate heat to be generated and participate in the proper functioning of the body. The body uses food to generate its needed energy and to provide building blocks to maintain structural integrity of the body.

Exercise (*Riyadhah*)

Avicenna placed exercise at the forefront as the most effective means for health maintenance. He claimed that regular exercise prevents dregs from accumulating in the body. In addition, exercise increases the innate heat, lightens the body, and strengthens muscles and tendons. It also prepares the organs to take in nutrients, reduces their stiffness, and prevents their weakness.

The *Al-Qanoon* section on exercise is extensive and lists a large number of general physical exercises such as running, archery, speed walking, jumping, horseback riding, wrestling, and rowing, as well as specific organ exercises such as exercises for the eye and ear. It also instructs on the time of exercise and on preparation for it, and goes on to describe the types of fatigue and other conditions that result from exercise and the methods to treat them. This section also encompasses the use of massage and steam baths.

Diet for Health and Healing (*Alghitha'*)

Health is also maintained by food that is balanced in quality and quantity. However, excretion does not get rid of all unutilized food material; there are residues that remain in the body that keep accumulating over time. These dregs have bad effects on the body: their by-products will harm the body, their accumulation in larger quantity leads to dystemperament, and their overload will produce the diseases of excesses. Accumulation of dregs in an organ produces tissue enlargement, and their spread throughout the tissues corrupts the ignis. Expulsion of dregs is accomplished with poisonous drugs most of the time or by detoxification. When humoral imbalance is addressed, a ripening of the humoral substances is performed first, usually with laxatives, followed by purging.

The process of detoxification is carried out to rid the body of the accumulated dregs (toxins, superfluous matter). Over a period of a few days, the individual deviates from the regular daily diet and takes in food and drink that will induce detoxification. The process culminates in a "healing crisis" or catharsis of elimination in which the elimination may occur as diarrhea, nosebleed, perspiration, urination, or vomiting. There are many recipes for detoxification by food ingestion or administration of enemas; however, detoxification should not be carried out more than once a year.

Recognizing that humans have different needs at their various life stages, Avicenna described the types of diets that should be followed for infants, pregnant and breastfeeding women, adults, and elderly individuals. He also described and treated the various conditions that may arise from the diet because of excesses or imbalances for each age group.

The therapeutic diet of Unani medicine is used to restore balance by providing the proper food that suits the individual's temperament and that of his or her digestive system. Such a diet entails the elimination of unsuitable food, low-quality or contaminated food, excesses of one type of food and unhealthful mixtures; reduction in the number of meals; and the introduction of foods stimulating digestion, breathing, circulation, and innate heat such as spices, vegetables, and oils.

Medicinal products (*Dawa'*)

Treating with medications (botanical, zoological, and metallic substances) is the second choice for treatment after diet. Unani use of herbs is extensive and is well documented in many old texts that are still in current use (Antaki, 1982; Avicenna, 1993; Levey et al, 1967). These treatments cover almost all known diseases. Unani hakims use single and compound formulas as well as internal and external applications.

There are three rules to treating with medications: the first is to know the temperament of the medication (hot, cold, moist, dry); the second, to determine the quantity to be given to the patient and its effect (warming or cooling, drying or wetting); and the third, to determine the most effective time of its administration. Selection of the medication follows the diagnosis of illness, and as a rule, the medication is opposite in its temperament to that of the disease. The characteristics of the diseased organ, however, determine the quantity of the medication. These include its temperament, architecture, position, and strength. For example, the quantity of the medication should correspond to the amount of deviation from the normal temperament. Additional factors are also considered in calculating the quantity, such as the patient's strength, gender, and age, as well as time of the year (season), and geographic location.

Food and medications are ranked according to their power to affect the human body, into eight classes: four degrees for hot food and medications and four degrees for cold ones. Unani formularies always give the power degree; for example, a medication may be followed by "hot in the second degree" or "cold in the third degree." Table 32-1 summarizes the various degrees of action.

Use of aromatic oil and alcohol extracts is featured prominently in Unani treatments. Avicenna invented steam distillation of rose oil; alcohol extraction and preservation of active ingredients of botanicals had been discovered earlier by Arab chemists and put to use by hakims. Herbal treatments can be delivered in a number of ways, including capsules, conserve, decoction, essence, fomentation, infusion, ointment, oxymel, plaster, poultice, salve, suppository, syrup, and tincture (Avicenna, 1993; Chishti, 1991).

Applied and Manual Therapy (*'elaj*)

Cupping (*hijameh*) is the external application of vacuum suction to the skin to draw humors to the surface, away

TABLE 32-1 *Summary of the Degrees of Action of Food and Drugs on the Metabolism*

Hot food and medications (increase metabolism)	Cold food and medications (decrease metabolism)
First Degree Mostly neutral in its effect, but has a light stimulative action on the body if applied in large amount or repeated, e.g., hot water, chamomile (*Anthemis nobilis*).	*First Degree* Mostly neutral in its effect, but has a light suppressive action on the body if applied in large amount or repeated, e.g., cold water, cistus (*Cistus landaniferus*).
Second Degree Stimulates metabolism without adverse effects, e.g., ginger.	*Second Degree* Suppresses metabolism without adverse effects, e.g., Syrian rhubarb (*Rheum ribes*).
Third Degree Overwhelming in its action and effects but does not cause death except in overdose or repeated use. Most medications fall within this category, e.g., senna.	*Third Degree* Downregulates metabolism in a substantial manner but does not cause death except in overdose or repeated use, e.g., resin of cypress (*Cupressus sempervirens*).
Fourth Degree Hot poisons. Corrupt the metabolic process and bring death, e.g., hemlock and belladonna. Used only in small amounts by a hakim.	*Fourth Degree* Cold poisons. Bring metabolism to a halt and cause death, e.g., narcotics such as opium or heavy metals like arsenic. Administered by a hakim only in measured quantity.

from an organ or an area of the body. It is used for treatment of an inflammation and for detoxification. The type of disease determines the location of cupping; for example, cupping on the heels is beneficial for amenorrhea, varicose veins, and gout, whereas cupping on the sides of the neck affects the organs of the head. Cupping is not advised for people over 60 years of age.

Enema (*houknaeh*) is an effective method for emptying the intestines (especially after vomiting), reducing kidney and bladder pain and enlargement and detoxifying the upper organs. A harsh enema, however, may weaken the liver and produce fever.

Massage (*tadleek*) and bathing (*istihmam*) are ancient traditions in the Old World that can be considered one integral activity. It takes place in a warm bathhouse, the *hammam,* which is usually built on a freshwater source, and starts with a vigorous cleansing rub with a soapy loofa (*leefeh*), usually from a dried fruit of the *Luffa* plant, or a linen mitt. After a good rinse, an oil massage is performed

with the fingers and palm, using various pressures, depending on the treatment goals.

Blood humor is purged through bloodletting from a vein, a procedure called *venesection* (*fassd*). There are two main conditions that require venesection: (1) excess of blood, and (2) low quality of blood. However, venesection also should be carried out at the early signs of some diseases such as varicose vein, gout, joint pain, high blood pressure, epilepsy, and melancholy. Use of leeches (*al'alaq*) is another method of bloodletting. Leeches are placed on the skin of the patient. They attach to the skin by their oral suckers, remain there until they are full, and then fall off to digest the blood. This method is still in use today in both Eastern and Western countries (Munshi et al, 2008).

Cauterization (*alkaiy*) is the application of heated metal or a corrosive directly to the skin surface. It is considered a treatment of last resort because of its harsh effects. One of the main purposes of its use is to prevent disease from spreading to healthy parts of the body. However, it is also applied to infected areas and unhealthy flesh and is used to strengthen weak parts.

UNANI VIEW ON TUMORS (*AWRAM*) AND CANCER (*SARATAN*)

Avicenna placed tumors, both benign and malignant, into the category of the compound diseases that are multicausal, and he emphasized that they are rarely homogenous. He declared that, developmentally, tumors recapitulate all known disease types: dystemperament due to corrupting substance, disfigurement of histology and shape, and discontinuity. He also stated that there is no clear cause of cancer, but he speculated that it may be caused by a harmful humor that is usually kept in check by good humors and then carries out its harmful action when humors become imbalanced, or it may be caused by the movement of a substance from one organ to another.

There are six types of tumors, based on origin: tumors originating from the four humors as well as aqueous (*ma'yeh*) tumors and gaseous (*reehia*) tumors. Hot tumors originate from a sanguine or choleric humor and are named after their humors. The purely sanguine tumors are called *phalghamonia*, the purely choleric tumors, *jamra,* and the combination of the two, *kharaj.* The last type, if it occurs in soft tissues such as under the axilla or behind the ears, is termed *ta'oon.*

There are four origins for cold tumors: melancholic, phlegmatic, aqueous, and gaseous. Avicenna attributed cold melancholic tumor formation to a corrupt black bile that originated from yellow bile, or a substance containing yellow bile, and its fast growth to the abundance of nutrients. There are three types of melancholic tumors: solid, cancerous, and glandular. The latter are tumors that have glandular secretory contents at their inception, such as those of the neck lymph nodes, termed *khanazeer,* and cutaneous glands, termed *sal'.* Solid tumors begin as localized, painless, and slowly developing solid growths, whereas cancers are mobile, fast growing, and begin within the organs, thus destroying sensation and eventually the organ itself. Phlegmatic tumors are of two types: soft tumors (*rakhu*) that are mixed and indistinct and soft, encapsulated, glandular tumors (*sal' layen*).

Cancerous tumors separate from the organ and develop their own vascular supply. Avicenna concurred with Hippocrates that it is best not to disturb an internal tumor because it may lead eventually to death, and he suggested that a cold and moist diet of barley water, ground fish, and hard-boiled egg yolk may prolong the life of the patient. For a tumor that is accompanied by fever, however, he advised the intake of filtered cow's buttermilk, legumes, and a type of gourd called cucurbits. Small tumors can be cut out; however, the best treatment for them is an aggressive surgery. Surgery was developed and practiced by several hakims for virtually all parts of the body, including the brain and nerves (Rahimi et al, 2007).

Aqueous tumors develop due to the accumulation of liquids in cysts or within the tissues. Gaseous tumors result from the accumulation of gas in the organ's cavity or within the organ's tissue.

Unani Medicine, CAM and Contemporary Biomedical Science

It is important to note that several of the concepts emphasized in Unani medicine still hold ground today in the modern world and are compatible with our scientific knowledge. The millennium-old Unani medicine reported the following:

- Malevolent bodies present in the soil cause infection (i.e., germs)
- Energy is generated by breathing light bodies in the air (i.e., oxygen) and by ingesting food (i.e., chemical or metabolic energy) (Amri & Abu-Asab, 2011)
- Disease is the corruption of the energy of the body, and each organ has its own level of energy (i.e., most diseases today are attributed to dysfunctional mitochondria, and organs have variable numbers of mitochondria) (Bereiter-Hahn, 2013; Davila & Zamorano, 2013)
- Diseases are the dystemperaments of the humors and temperaments (i.e., homeostasis and allostasis)

In addition, the approach to healing and treating disease resonates so profoundly with today's slogans of personalized and preventive medicine. Biomedicine realized a few years ago that males and females develop different sets of symptoms and recently started a dialogue about population genetics. The Unani medical system has been offering personalized treatment plans based on gender, age, geographical location, season, state of health, and stage of disease for hundreds of years.

Furthermore, this ancient medical system emphasizes six essential requirements for health (as explained above), and these are as follows: (1) fresh clean air, (2) food and drink, (3) movement and rest, (4) sleep and wakefulness, (5) eating and exercising, and (6) healthy mental states. These factors are the pillars of today's programs for healthy living and preventing disease—something that modern integrative physicians are trying to implement. The wisdom and knowledge of this medical system had not been fully articulated and expressed, in terms of accurate and precise translation of both the Arabic language and technical content, until a new modern translation of Ibn Sina's *The Canon of Medicine* became available recently. His numerous insights will benefit our health care and should be seriously considered by the medical community.

SUMMARY AND CONCLUSION

It is important to recognize that the contributions of Arab and Muslim scholars to modern medicine originally involved translation of the Greco-Roman medical texts but evolved to encompass development of independent methodical approaches to the following:

- Disease etiology, prognosis, and diagnosis
- Systematization of medical practice
- Construction of organized hospitals and clinics
- Expansion of the repertoires of drugs and catalogues of surgical instruments
- Establishment of a professional ethical code

Unani medicine thus represents a vital link, fertile ground, and a prerequisite to the modern medicine that developed later in the West during the decline of the Arab-Muslim era.

Despite the comprehensive compendia and encyclopedic books transcribed by Unani Tibb physicians and the widespread practice and teaching of Unani medicine in the West as well as other parts of the world for centuries, the Unani medical system today is restricted to South Asia, Nepal, and West China, where it survives alongside Ayurveda, Siddha, and Chinese medicine. The recognition of Unani Tibb as a traditional medical system by the West today was lagging, probably because of the lack of scholarly endeavors and inadequacy of translations, as well as the interests of South Asian countries in developing and exporting Ayurveda.

Unani and Ayurveda, like all systems of natural medicine, have similarities, but they also have fundamental differences. The two systems share some similarities on the practical side, but the theoretical as well as some philosophical aspects of Unani medicine are different from those of Ayurveda. A synthesis of the relevant chapters in this book will help delineate the commonalities and differences of the two systems.

The reader's view should also be informed by the general perception that Unani is not just a Greco-*Muslim*, or even a Greco-*Arabic* medical system. Unani physicians and scientists were not all Arabs, and not all Muslims, but also included Jews (Rabbi Moses ben Maimon, 1134–1204, known as **Maimonides**), Christians (Hunayn Ibn Ishaq, 808–873, known as **Johannitus**), and Persians who wrote and practiced in Arabic, such as Ibn Sina or **Avicenna** (see above). Arabic was the language of the political elite and of the sciences in the golden age of the Arab-Muslim civilization that extended from Spain, through North Africa, to Central and Southeast Asia for over 700 years. Arabic was also the language of the Muslim religion, which highly praised knowledge and tolerance at the time. Among traditional medical systems, Unani represents a complete system of practice with a highly developed system of physical diagnosis. It is time, and there is now an opportunity, to embrace it again and benefit from its valuable body of knowledge.

References

Abu-Asab M, Amri H, Micozzi MS: *Avicenna's Medicine: A New Translation of the 11th-Century Canon with Practical Applications for Integrative Medicine*, Rochester VT, 2013, Healing Arts Press/Inner Tradtions.

Amri H, Abu-Asab M: Physiology of Qi. In Mayor DF, Micozzi MS, editors: *Energy Medicine East and West: A Natural History of Qi*, London, 2011, Churchill Livingstone Elsevier.

Antaki DiU: *Tadhkirat 'uli al-albab wa-al-jami' lilajab al-'ujab*, ed Last Edition, Cairo, 1982, Sharikat Maktabah wa-Matbaah Mustafa al-Babi al-Halabi.

Arnold T, Guillaume A: *The Legacy of Islam*, Oxford, UK, 1931, Oxford University Press.

Avicenna: *al-Qanoon fi tibb*, New Delhi, 1993, Dept. of Islamic Studies, Jamia Hamdard.

Bakar O: The philosophy of Islamic medicine and its relevance to the modern world, *MAAS J Islam Sci* 6(1):39–58, 1990.

Bannerman RHO, Ch'en W-C, Burton J: *World Health Organization. Traditional medicine and health care coverage: a reader for health administrators and practitioners*, Geneva, 1983, World Health Organization; [Albany, N.Y.: WHO Publications Centre USA, distributor].

Bereiter-Hahn J: Do we age because we have mitochondria? *Protoplasma* 251(1):3–23, 2013. doi: 10.1007/s00709-013-0515-x. 2014 Jan.

Bernal M: *Black Athena: The Afroasiatic roots of classical civilization*, New Brunswick, N.J., 1987, Rutgers University Press.

Chishti GM: *The traditional healer's handbook: a classic guide to the medicine of Avicenna*, Rochester, Vt., 1991, Healing Arts Press; Distributed to the book trade in the U.S. by American International Distribution Corp.

Davila AF, Zamorano P: Mitochondria and the eveolutionary roots of cancer, *Phys Biol* 10:2013. doi: 10.1088/1478-3975/10/2/026008.

King H: *Greek and Roman Medicine*, London, 2001, Duckworth Publishers.

Levey M, Khaledy N: *The medical formulary of al-Samarqandi and the relation of early Arabic simples to those found in the indigenous medicine of the Near East and India*, Philadelphia, 1967, University of Pennsylvania Press.

Munshi Y, Ara I, Rafique H, Ahmad Z: Leeching in the history—a review, *Pak J Biol Sci* 11(13):1650–1653, 2008.

Nunn J: *Ancient Egyptian Medicine*, London, 2002, University of Oklahoma Press ed: British Museum Press.

Osborn DK: Greek Medicine, 2008. Available from: www.greekmedicine.com. Accessed September 2008.

Porter R: *The Greatest Benefit to Mankind: A Medical History of Humanity*, New York, 1999, W. W. Norton & Company.

Rahimi SY, McDonnell DE, Ahmadian A, Vender JR: Medieval neurosurgery: contributions from the Middle East, Spain, and Persia, *Neurosurg Focus* 23(1):E14, 2007.

Razi A: *Kitab al-hawi fi al-tibb*, Haydarabad al-Dakkan, 1955, Matbat Majlis Dairat al-Ma'arif al-Uthmaniyah.

World Health Organization: *WHO traditional medicine strategy, 2002–2005*, Geneva, 2002, World Health Organization.

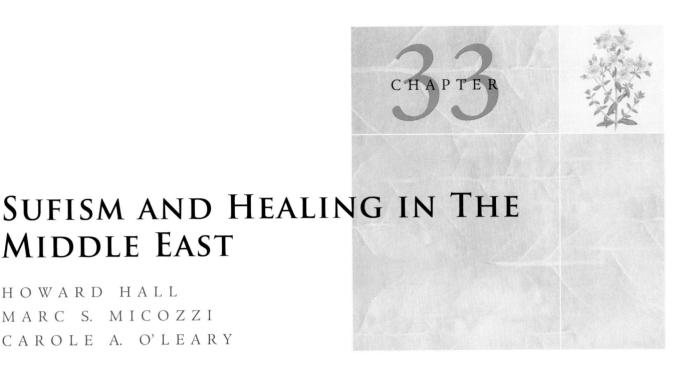

CHAPTER 33

SUFISM AND HEALING IN THE MIDDLE EAST

HOWARD HALL

MARC S. MICOZZI

CAROLE A. O'LEARY

Sufism is a devotional branch of Islam, with various orders that date back to the Middle Ages or earlier (some say even pre-Islamic) and has many followers today throughout the Middle East, in the West, and globally. These orders are perhaps best known to Western observers, for example, for the "Whirling Dervishes" derived from the old Persian word *darwish*, for a supplicant—"one who goes door-to-door"—now referring to a Sufi aspirant. The term is also used for a mystical "holy man" (a term not used in orthodox Islam) by which each order is led. Members of this particular "Dervish" order, the *Naqshbandi*, are geographically found from North Africa, the Arabian Peninsula, Turkey, Afghanistan, and into Southeast Asia.

Sufism also crosses ethnic lines among Muslims from North African Berbers, to Arabs, Turks, and Persians. One origin of the word *Sufi* means "thread," like a mystical woolen thread or pathway leading to the divine, but as an internal search for the divine. It may also have connections with the Greek word for wisdom, *sophia*. There are some similarities to the traditional, devotional forms of yoga in India (see Chapter 21), which of course predate Islam.

The orthodox practices of Islam at various times in history were not accepted as outward practice by various Sufi orders. Some Sufi orders are also notable for their practice of deliberately caused bodily damage (DCBD) as a devotional practice. Under such circumstances, remarkable healing has been observed. Sufism has at times been criticized by orthodox Islam for using such metaphors as being "drunk on divine love," or referring to sexual intercourse to describe a sublime, transcendent love of the divine. (Here one may discern a pattern connected to *Tantra* yoga.) Such states of consciousness may be colloquially described as "feeling no pain," for reasons that will become apparent in the next section of this chapter.

SUFISM AND RAPID HEALING

The Sufi Islamic school of mysticism in Baghdad, Iraq, is one of the largest Sufi schools in the Middle East (Hussein et al, 1994a, 1994b, 1994c, 1997). Followers (dervishes) of this Sufi school have demonstrated instantaneous healing of DCBD. For example, dervishes have inserted a variety of sharp instruments (e.g., spikes, skewers) into the body, hammered daggers into the skull bone and clavicle, and chewed and swallowed glass and sharp razor blades without harm to the body and with complete control over pain, bleeding, and infection, as well as rapid wound healing within 4 to 10 seconds (Figure 33-1).

The Tariqa Kasnazaniyah School of Sufism has described extraordinary phenomena of instantaneous healing of wounds from DCBD. This Sufi school's name, Tariqa Kasnazaniyah, can be attributed to three of its senior scholars, i.e., Imam Ali bin Abi Talib; Shaikh Abd al-Quadir al-Gaylani; and Shaikh Abd al-Karim al-Kasnazan.

Linguistically and historically, *Al-Kasnazan* is a Kurdish (Eastern Turkey and Syria, and Northern Iraq and Iran) word that means "no one knows" (similar to a meaning taken for Zen). It was first associated with Shaikh Abd al Karim, as a title when he spent four years in seclusion, meditating and worshiping Allah (God) in the Qara Dagh (Black Mountains in Kurdistan, Iraq).

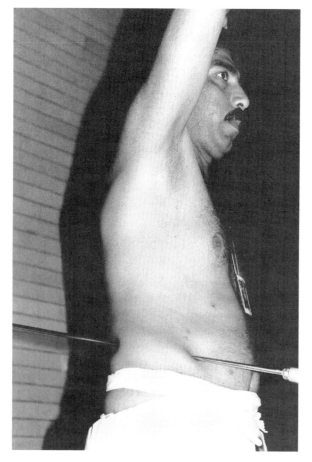

Figure 33-1   A dervish at the major Sufi school in Baghdad demonstrating Sufi wound healing.

NO ONE KNOWS

During that period of isolation, Shaikh Abd al Karim experienced the sublime joy and love of drawing nearer to Allah. Following his period of isolation, dedication, and worshiping Allah, Allah's messenger, the Prophet Muhammad, gave him a blessing of a great secret. This revelation was the extraordinary ability to tolerate without harm strong electrical shocks, immunity against snake and scorpions, rapid healing from being stabbed or shot, protection against being burned, as well as healing of clinical conditions such as cancers, heart disease, infertility, depression, and psychosis.

During his absence, when anyone would ask about the shaikh, the answer was "Kasnazan," meaning that no one knew where he was. With the passage of time, this word turned into a title for that revered shaikh and his path. Thus, the expression "Al-Tariqa" has the added meaning of the way of the secret that no one knows of the glorious Quran, the course of the Prophet, and his pious companions. Also, *Al-Kasnazania* became a family title associated with his descendants as well as a name of Tariqa. After reviewing early and updated research, this chapter introduces new clinical applications of Tariqa Kasnazaniyah Sufi spiritual healing without DCBD.

EARLY RESEARCH

Researchers reported that such extraordinary abilities are accessible to anyone and are not restricted to only a few talented individuals who have spent years in special training. These unusual healing phenomena have also been reproduced under controlled laboratory conditions, and are not similar to hypnosis (Hall et al, 2001).

Similar DCBD phenomena have been observed in various parts of the world in a variety of religious and nonreligious contexts (Don et al, 2000; Hussein et al, 1997). For example, trance surgeons in Brazil have employed sharp instruments to cut, pierce, or inject substances into a patient's body for therapeutic purposes. Laboratory electroencephalographic (EEG) investigation of trance surgeons has shown that this "state of spirit possession" of the healers was associated with a hyperaroused brain state (waves in the 30- to 50-Hz band) (Don et al, 2000). In the United States, little scientific attention has been given to the investigation of these claims of rapid healing. In fact, claims of extraordinary healing abilities have been met with scorn and have been challenged by so-called skeptic groups such as the Committee for the Scientific Investigation of Claims of the Paranormal. These groups offer monetary incentives to discredit such claims in unscientific and dangerous settings (Mulacz, 1998; Posner, 1998; see Dossey, 1999, and Fatoohi, 1999a,b, for a response), sometimes employing the services of career magicians who make their living as illusionists, not scientists.

"OTHERS HEALING" PHENOMENON

Followers of the Tariqa Kasnazaniyah School of Sufism describe the ability to accomplish DCBD healing as an "others-healing phenomenon" within the context of healing energies (Hussein et al, 1994a, 1994b, 1994c). This "higher energy" is alleged to be instantly transferable, mediated through a spiritual link from the current shaikh of the Sufi school and through the chain of masters to Muhammad (P) and ultimately to Allah (Hussein et al, 1997). As noted in the Quran, "The Prophet is closer to the Believers than their own selves" (33:6). In Chapter 15, this Sufi "higher energy" might be characterized as a "biophysical" phenomenon.

When we became aware of DCBD phenomena, the first question that naturally arose was: How might Western scientists empirically investigate such unusual claims of healing? From a scientific perspective, this process would demand a series of systematic observations of the Sufi rapid wound healing phenomenon in both field and laboratory settings. Of course, the first question that needed to be addressed was whether this phenomenon was real. This would require a field trip to directly observe, video record, and possibly even experience DCBD healing. If these initial observations showed the phenomenon to be genuine, then the question would become, Can the phenomenon be explained by traditional paradigms, such as hypnosis or the placebo effect?

SUGGESTIBILITY

Because one of us (Hall) had conducted research in hypnosis and psychoneuroimmunology (Hall, Minnes, Tosi, et al, 1992; Hall, Mumma, Longo, et al, 1992; Hall, 1982, 1989; Hall, Minnes, & Olness, 1993; Hall, Papas, Tosi, et al, 1996) as well as clinical work in hypnosis for over 25 years, it was of interest to compare this rapid healing with hypnotic phenomena during a visit to Iraq for field observations and direct experience of DCBD healing. It was an impression following that visit that what had been seen and experienced represented a phenomenon that went beyond classical Newtonian mechanics and argued for explanations for DCBD healing involving psychological factors that influence healing, such as the placebo effect, hypnosis, or altered states of consciousness (Hall, 2000).

The next question in systematic observation was, Can this unusual healing phenomenon be exported to the United States and observed within a traditional medical setting? If the phenomenon could be brought to the United States, what measures should be employed to help us understand underlying processes of DCBD healing, particularly if it represented a new paradigm as defined by Thomas Kuhn (1970), for example, in describing the structure of scientific revolutions? After we found that DCBD healing could be transported to the United States, we then undertook a series of structured observations of the phenomenon to explore possible underlying mechanisms, using both traditional and novel instruments and measures.

LABORATORY STUDIES

These systematic observations laid the foundation for more traditional follow-up laboratory studies that can be conducted with randomized control groups (or what Kuhn [1970] might refer to as the puzzle-solving process of "normal science." Kuhn does caution, however, that anomalous observations that do not fit within existing paradigms can result in a crisis and lead to the revolutionary process of a paradigm shift.) The ultimate interest may lie in the more important area of the translational application of this research to the healing of clinical conditions. Normal science in general has been criticized for its typical lack of interest in translating basic science into practical applications (Shapley & Roy, 1985). Translating anomalous findings into practical use is an exciting venture and opportunity to expand our views of health and healing.

FIELD INVESTIGATIONS

In 1998, with an invitation from the shaikh of the Tariqa Kasnazaniyah School of Sufism in Baghdad and support from the Kairos Foundation in Illinois, one of us (Hall) traveled alone to Baghdad to meet with the spiritual leader of this group, Shaikh Muhammad Al-Kasnazani, and witnessed a group demonstration of DCBD healing at their major school (Hall, 2000). At this meeting, which was professionally videotaped, there was an opportunity to examine firsthand the objects that were employed during the DCBD demonstrations, such as knives, razor blades, and glass, and observe them being inserted into various parts of the body. What was witnessed and recorded is consistent with the extraordinary claims made by this group about rapid wound healing and lack of apparent pain.

Although there was no evidence of a ruse, some skeptics might question whether the observer had somehow been deluded, even with video footage. Thus, one of us (Hall) had requested permission, while at this demonstration, to experience DCBD healing by having my cheek pierced (Hall, 2000). After witnessing several demonstrations of DCBD healing, an assistant asked me to face the shaikh to ask permission to allow the healing energy for rapid wound healing. The shaikh nodded, indicating that I had his permission. What was most striking was that I did not feel any different or in an altered state, and my cheek was not numb. The assistant then inserted a metal ice pick through the inside of my left cheek to the outside. It felt like a poke, but with no pain (Figure 33-2). I walked around the group circle with the ice pick in my cheek, introspecting on how it was not hurting, bleeding, or numb. I could feel the weight of the object and notice the metal taste in my mouth, but I felt no discomfort. Again, consistent with the reports, my cheek healed rapidly in minutes with only a couple of drops of blood. This personal experience was compelling to me, despite my considerable doubt and my dislike of pain. Nonetheless, I still imagined that skeptics would question whether such practices could be demonstrated outside this religious context and exported to the West.

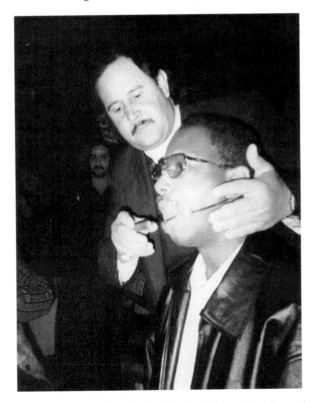

Figure 33-2 The author having his cheek pierced at the major Sufi school in Baghdad.

BIOMEDICAL PERSPECTIVES

A demonstration of such rapid wound healing was clearly needed within a Western medical setting, given the scientific implications of such healing. If such spiritually based healing approaches are genuine, they hold much promise for addressing some of today's most serious medical issues.

The investigation of such unusual healing phenomena in the West raises many questions. What should be measured within a scientific context? Would standard measures of brain and immune activity be associated with changes in rapid wound healing, or should standard measures, such as EEG activity, be used in less standard ways? Would high-frequency EEG activity need to be examined for hyperaroused brain states? Would new approaches be needed to detect "fields of consciousness," such as the examination of changes in the output of a random event generator (REG)?

Case Study

With the support of the Kairos Foundation of Wilmette, Illinois, a Sufi practitioner (J.H.) was invited from the Middle East to a local radiology facility in Cleveland, Ohio, on July 1, 1999. He had permission from the shaikh of the Kasnazaniyah Sufi School to perform a demonstration of rapid wound healing after insertion of an unsterilized metal skewer, 0.38 cm ($\frac{5}{32}$ inch) thick and approximately 13 cm (5$\frac{1}{6}$ inch) long, while being videotaped by a film crew in the presence of scientists and health care professionals (Hall et al, 2001). This was apparently the first demonstration by a practitioner from this Sufi school in the United States. The practitioner consented to sign a release of liability for the medical facility and personnel against claims from possible injuries. Emergency medical technicians were present. The major goal of this demonstration was to observe the authenticity of rapid wound healing following a deliberately caused injury within a medical setting.

The demonstration was also conducted with radiological, immunological, and EEG evaluations, as well as a Zener noise diode random event generator (REG), similar to equipment employed at Princeton University by Dr. Robert Jahn and colleagues. Based on previous studies in Brazil with healer–mediums engaged in quasi-surgical practices, it was hypothesized that DCBD healing would be accompanied by alterations in brain waves and effects on REGs. The alterations in brain waves found in the Brazilian healer–mediums showed statistically significant enhancement of broadband 40-Hz brain rhythms (Don & Moura, 2000). A statistically significant deviation from random behavior in REGs was found in a test run covertly, while the Brazilian healer–mediums were in a trance. This methodology was developed by Robert Jahn and associates at the Princeton Engineering Anomalies Research (PEAR) Laboratory (Nelson et al, 1996, 1998). Such energy fields have been considered to be theoretically associated with rapid wound healing (Don & Moura, 2000).

Nineteen-channel EEGs were recorded during baseline resting conditions, while the dervish inserted the skewer through his cheek and immediately after removal of the instrument.

An REG, plugged into the serial port of a computer, was run in the background without informing the dervish. The distribution of binary digits was tested for possible significant deviations from random behavior. Data were acquired before and after the self-insertion, as well as during the self-insertion. Before insertion of the skewer and about one hour after the piercing, blood was collected from the practitioner and from three volunteers (used as control subjects) for an immunological analysis of the percent change in white blood cell CD4, CD8, and total T-cell counts.

Results

Radiological images were made while the skewer was inserted. Computed axial tomographic images through the lower mandibular region showed artifact from dental metal. In addition, a horizontally oriented metallic bar elevated the left lateral soft tissues just anterior to the muscles of mastication. There was no associated underlying mass. A single frontal fluoroscopic image showed the presence of EEG leads over the maxilla and mandibular regions. A transverse piece of metal was superimposed, extending from the soft tissues on the right through to the left without interval break.

Because of movement and scalp muscle artifacts throughout the experimental self-insertion condition, it was impossible to assess the EEG for the hypothesized 40-Hz brain rhythms. The frequency spectrum of scalp muscle discharge overlaps the 40-Hz EEG frequency band of interest.

The REG output during baseline periods did not differ significantly from random behavior. However, during the self-insertion condition, there was a trend toward significant nonrandomness. The chi-square test result was 3.052, $df = 1$, and P was approximately .07.

Field of Consciousness

The behavior of the REG was in the predicted direction of nonrandomness. This finding has been interpreted by our laboratory and the PEAR laboratory as being associated with states of heightened attention and emotion. Further, the PEAR group has proposed that a "field of consciousness" is associated with such nonrandomness. Unfortunately, the 40-Hz brain wave hypothesis was not testable because of the excessive amount of scalp artifact and thus awaits further exploration. The presence of increased theta rhythms after the insertion condition (and a slight decrease in average alpha power) suggests a mild hypoaroused altered state of consciousness. The Sufi practitioner performing this feat was doing so for the first time. With further practice or with testing of more experienced subjects, it may be feasible to obtain EEG data without large amounts of scalp artifact. Because the subject reported no perceived pain during the self-insertion, preliminary relaxation exercises might eliminate all or most of the artifact. This circumstance would enable us to test the 40-Hz hypothesis definitively. Clearly, further work is indicated.

The immunologic analysis did not reveal any major difference between the Sufi practitioner and the control subjects. These data suggest that the variation found in the practitioner was not different from that of normal controls.

The radiological film documented that the skewer had actually penetrated both cheeks, which addresses the arguments of skeptic groups that such practices are the result of "fakery." After the removal of the skewer, there was a slight trickle of blood, which stopped with application of pressure to the cheek, using clean gauze. The physicians and scientists present documented that the wound healed rapidly within a few moments. The practitioner also reported that there was no pain associated with the insertion or removal of the metal skewer. This demonstration was conducted outside the traditional religious context, where chanting, drumming, and head movements (which would compromise some scientific measurements) are generally part of the ceremony when it is done in the Middle East. Thus, our case study argues against the view that a religious context, with its accompanying state of consciousness, is important to the successful outcome of such a demonstration. This case study also demonstrated that DCBD healing could be done when a large distance separated the dervish from the master (from Baghdad to Cleveland). This condition would suggest a robust phenomenon independent of the distance separating the source and the scene where the DCBD phenomenon occurs.

It should also be noted that the skewer stayed in the dervish's cheeks for more than 35 minutes, longer than the few minutes I had observed during my field observations at the major school of Tariqa Kasnazaniyah. Thus, this case study argues against the necessity of a brief piercing for a successful outcome of rapid healing following DCBD. Further, the dervish in this demonstration reported that there was no pain associated with the piercing, minimal bleeding, and no postprocedural infection. Finally, about a half-hour after the completion of the demonstration, the dervish, along with seven other people who had witnessed the DCBD event, had dinner together.

EXPERIENCE OF RAPID WOUND HEALING

After witnessing rapid wound healing in the Middle East and experiencing it there myself, I was initiated into the Sufi order with the ritualistic handshake, which took about two to three minutes. After a subsequent visit with the shaikh in the United Kingdom in June 2000, I was given a license to perform DCBD rapid healing.

I first requested permission from the shaikh in Baghdad to perform a cheek piercing on myself in May at the 2001 World Congress on Complementary Therapies in Medicine in Washington, DC, chaired by the editor of this textbook. After lecturing on DCBD rapid healing, I informed

the audience that I needed to take an earlier flight home because of a family medical emergency in Cleveland. Skipping a break, I went right into the cheek piercing for the first time on my own. My mind was on the family medical crisis back home, but I was instructed to focus on connecting with the shaikh, asking mentally for spiritual energy for rapid wound healing before the piercing. This process took about a minute. One physician in the audience was particularly skeptical, so I invited him to stand next to me when I did the piercing. Please note that this was about four months before September 11, 2001, so I had been able to bring a meat skewer from my kitchen drawer (to be used for the demonstration) in my carry-on luggage.

After the one-minute mental connection with the energy from the shaikh, and with much nervousness, I pushed a very dull skewer through my left cheek. Yes, I was quite worried about the medical situation at home. The most difficult aspect of this experience was getting this dull object through my cheek. Eventually it went through with no pain. My skeptical medical colleague was very quiet after that. I pulled it out and there were a couple of drops of blood, which I blotted with a tissue until the bleeding stopped. From there, I had a friend take me directly to the airport.

The second time I demonstrated DCBD healing on myself (making this my third experience with DCBD healing including Baghdad) was at the Fifth World Congress on Qigong in November 2002. Because this was after September 11, 2001, I had to shop locally at my destination for a better piercing instrument. This demonstration was preceded by a video interview by some of the leading scientists in the field of energy healing attending the conference. The video camera was then set on a stand by my left cheek. I again focused on connecting with the energy of the shaikh for rapid wound healing. I did not feel different, but I had faith that the connection was there, despite the distance in space. Again, I found that pushing the metal pick through my cheek was very difficult. After some effort (*jihad*), both physical and mental, it went through. I also spoke on camera about how I was feeling, with the object through my cheek. After the interview, I pulled the pick out and padded a tissue against my cheek to absorb the few drops of blood. The wound closing was also documented on film for the first time. I had cut myself shaving early in the morning of the previous day, before flying to the conference. Immediately after the demonstration, the shaving cut was more noticeable than the piercing. I was able to enjoy a late dinner after this demonstration.

BIOPHYSICAL PERSPECTIVES

The next day after the demonstration, I had the opportunity to meet and be evaluated by Dr. Konstantin Korotkov, professor of physics at St. Petersburg State Technical University in Russia, using his gas discharge visualization (GDV) technique, which measures human energy fields as did the earlier Kirlian photography (Korotkov, 2002, 2004;

Korotkov et al, 2005) (see Chapter 15). Dr. Korotkov first took a baseline measure of my energy field from my fingers and displayed the results on a screen to the audience. He then asked me to invoke the Sufi energy. I again took about a minute and requested energy from the shaikh for this demonstration. It should be noted that I had not planned this energy reading nor had I obtained prior permission from the shaikh for this energy demonstration. After about one minute, I said I was ready for the second (after-energy) measure. Dr. Korotkov outwardly expressed surprise at how quickly I had invoked energy. This time when he took the energy reading from my hand, the computer malfunctioned, and another one had to be brought in. After the new computer was in place, the GDV reading revealed a major increase in my energy field after the one-minute energy invocation.

My fourth experience with DCBD healing occurred in response to a request by National Geographic Television and Film (Washington, DC) to participate in a program to be aired for the cable network series *Is It Real?*, titled "Superhuman Powers," in 2005. This demonstration was performed in collaboration with Gary Schwartz, PhD, at his Human Energy Systems Laboratory, Center for Frontier Medicine in Biofield Science, at the University of Arizona in Tucson (Hall & Schwartz, 2004). Again I obtained permission from the shaikh to conduct another DCBD demonstration, and we also explored whether there were any changes in brain activity associated with this process or any changes in my energy field or aura as indicated by the GDV measures. A 19-channel EEG, along with GDV recordings, were taken before and after I pierced my left cheek with a 5-inch ice pick and while being filmed by National Geographic. This demonstration took about 90 minutes to complete as I connected with the current shaikh and other masters who are part of this Sufi school's chain of shaikhs (i.e., silsila).

During the demonstration, my mind did reach a more relaxed state as measured by EEG recordings. There was, however, no anomalous neurological activity, such as seizure, sleep, or hyperaroused brain patterns. Pre- versus post-piercing changes on GDV measures did show, for the first time ever, a selective decrease in the energy field where the cheek was pierced, revealing a gaping hole in my "aura" in that area. As with my prior experiences with DCBD healing, there were a few drops of blood after the ice pick was removed, but the wound healed very quickly and was not noticeable after a few minutes. Again, even with these additional scientific measures, traditional paradigms offered little insight to account for the rapid wound healing phenomenon.

Such an observation was consistent with the results of the demonstration involving the Sufi practitioner from the Middle East, described earlier in the case report, in which we also failed to find any correlations between DCBD healing and any of the blood tests or imaging studies. The only hints of associations were the GDV energy measures and the trend of the REG output, which also suggested some change in the energy field. Work in this area might take us beyond Newton's classical mechanics to quantum mechanics and quantum physics to account for possible subtle energy constructs. Our colleague Eric Leskowitz (2005) proposes a multidimensional model of wound healing, incorporating energy concepts to help shift our current paradigm of wound healing beyond the physical and psychological dimensions or, as he describes it, from biology to spirit as well as to biophysical aspects of healing (see Chapter 15).

CURRENT RESEARCH

The most recent research on Sufi rapid wound healing was done in collaboration with Jay Gunkelman, Erik Peper, Tom Collura, and a Sufi living in Europe. For this project, we measured the impact of Sufi rapid healing from a skewer going from inside the bottom of the mouth to the outside of the throat, with EEG analysis. The most interesting finding that will be outlined in a separate report is that the Sufi demonstrated an extreme state of relaxation despite having a skewer through his throat, and he was able to selectively disengage a broad-based brain network that may be related to attention.

Tariqa Kasnazaniyah Spiritual Healing (Clinical Applications of Sufi Rapid Healing without DCBD)

Al-Shaikh Muhammad Al-Kasnazani has granted spiritual healing for a variety of medical conditions. To receive this spiritual healing, the person is invited to become spiritually connected to the shaikh by taking *bay'a*, a brief ceremony that pledges allegiance to Allah, the Prophet Muhammad, and the chain of shaikhs down to the present master. The other major part of bay'a is also having one repent for one's shortcomings. Although bay'a may appear to be very simple, it entails many spiritual secrets. A male who wants to take bay'a puts his dominant hand in the right hand of the master or one of his caliphs or deputies. A female would hold the caliph's beads instead of his hand.

Bay'a is not restricted to men but is open to women and adolescents, as well as individuals from other religious paths. Regarding spiritual healing, some describe bay'a as being a spiritual touch from the disciple's soul connecting to that of the master, who is connected to the chain of masters who preceded the current master, leading to the Prophet Muhammad, and ultimately to Allah. Bay'a existed during the time of the prophet of Islam, and after his departure, Iman Ali inherited the spiritual touch as well as the succession of caliphs, down to the present master. Thus, this unbroken chain of spiritual healing remains intact today as it existed at the time of the prophet.

Once bay'a is taken, the new Sufi is instructed in frequent meditation, or "remembrance," as it is known in Sufism. Much healing can result from such remembrances and sometimes the shaikh will prescribe a specific Quran remembrance for a particular number of reputation for a particular person.

MEDITATION

> When you neglect your meditation, you contract with pain. This is God's way of telling you that your inner pain can become visible. Don't ignore it.
>
> —RUMI (1991)

Meditation is one of the most important Sufi tools for drawing nearer to Allah, by "remembering" God and thus treating one's inner heart that has become distant, diseased, and hardened. Worshipful meditation is an integral part of Sufism and is also known as "Divine Remembrance," *Dhikr*, or *Zekr* (Chishti, 1991). As noted in the Quran, "Then do ye remember Me, I will remember you" (2:152). The place of worship or the *takiya* is also known as the "house of remembrance." These Sufi meditation practices are above and beyond the traditional prayers.

Such meditation practices involve a prescribed number of recitations of verses from the Quran using prayer beads (i.e., a rosary to keep count), such as "la illaha illa Allah," or "there is no god but Allah (the God)" (Ansha, 1991), or other remembrances, such as "the beautiful names" of Allah. For some *tariqas* (school or order, e.g., Tariqa Kasnazaniyah), this recitation is done aloud with accompanying head movements symbolizing a hammer slamming a heart that has become "hardened like a stone." The remoteness from Allah causes this hardness, and the remembrance is the remedy. As noted in the Quran (2:74), "Thenceforth were your hearts hardened: they became like a rock and even worse in hardness." Other tariqas use silent remembrances or employ different movements altogether.

Meditation has been suggested to help treat diseases. To do so, it has been recommended that the number of recitations end with a zero (e.g., 100, 300) (Chishti, 1991). Again, from the Sufi perspective, worshipful meditation is a means of drawing near to Allah, and with that connection may come transcendent healing outcomes.

Research has documented the many health and physiological benefits of meditation, including decrease in blood pressure, rate of breathing, heart rate, and oxygen consumption (see Chapter 10). The positive effects of meditation are associated with the production of a physiological "relaxation response" that is opposite to the "fight-or-flight response" (Benson, 1975). Thus, Sufi remembrances may play an important role in contributions to increased health.

WATER AND HEALING

Water has been employed as a medium for the biophysical properties of Tariqa Kasnazaniyah spiritual healing. For example, the shaikh has given individuals a small stone that has been blessed, to be dropped in a large container of water for a few minutes. After removing the stone, the person is asked to drink a cup of that water several times a day for several weeks. In other instances, instead of using a stone, Kasnazaniyah remembrances are taped to a bottle of water, with instructions to drink several times a day. It should be noted that the shaikh discourages drinking very cold water because that can have a nullifying effect on the meditation practices. It might be speculated that water may respond to our thoughts, as Masaru Emoto (2001) has suggested in his book, *The Hidden Messages in Water*.

Not only has water been employed in Tariqa Kasnazaniyah Spiritual Healing, but also the eating of blessed dates as a treatment of infertility in women and men, where both partners are treated. There is a reference in the Quran 19:21-26, where the Virgin Mary, mother of Jesus, was suffering from the anguish of childbirth. When she cried out to Allah for help, God commanded her to eat a date.

In 2013, the shaikh gave permission for a Sufi dervish to travel to India to heal people, as needed, following the shaikh's spiritual/intuitive guidance. I met with him in Amman, Jordan, to hear his report of this journey. For example, dozens of individuals with dengue fever were reported to be cured by drinking water from a large tub of blessed water. He also discussed how he treated individuals with various cancers after they took bay'a, did remembrances, and drank blessed water.

HOW DOES SUFISM EXPLAIN HOW SPIRITUAL HEALING CAN OCCUR?

Sufism can form a unified theory for mechanistic, mind-body, and spiritual healing. Traditional Islamic theology recognizes that Allah (God) created a world that can apparently operate under mechanistic and Newtonian principles. As noted in the Quran (6:95-99), Allah created order in this world, causing seeds to sprout, the sun to rise and set, and the rain to fall. "Such is the judgment and ordering of (Him) the exalted in Power, the Omniscient" (6:96).

This view is consistent with the mechanistic Newtonian view of the world and humans. Thus, there is no rejection of mechanistic views in traditional Islamic philosophy. Sufi philosophy goes further, noting that mechanistic views can also be explained within a vitalistic perspective. From this point of view, Sufism can predict the biophysical aspects of Sufi healing phenomena in ways that Newtonian models cannot.

Sufi Shaikh Gaylani explains it as follows:

> The belief of the followers of the Book and the Sunna of the Messenger of Allah (Salla Allah ta'ala 'alayhi wa sallam) is that the sword does not cut because of its nature, but it is rather Allah ('Azza wa Jall) who cuts with it, that the fire does not burn because of its nature, but it is rather Allah ('Azza wa Jall) who burns with it, that food does not satisfy hunger because of its nature, but it is rather Allah ('Azza wa Jall) who satisfies hunger with it and that water does not quench thirst because of its nature, but it is rather Allah ('Azza wa Jall) who quenches thirst with it. The same applies to things of all kinds; it is Allah ('Azza wa Jall) who uses them to produce their effects and they are only instruments in His hand with which He does whatever He wills. (Al-Kasnazani al-Husseini, 1999, p. 42)

Thus, most of the time, the world operates by mechanistic laws allowed by Allah, but mediation by a Sufi shaikh, based on the shaikh's nearness to Allah and through Allah, would allow for fire not to burn or a knife not to cut, so that mechanistic laws are suspended. The Quran is clear in several verses that so-called natural laws can be suspended by Allah. For example, 2:117 says, "when He (Allah) decreeth a matter, he saith to it: 'Be,' and it is."

The goal of the Sufi and all spiritual paths is nearness to God. In Sufism, this goal is pursued by following the Sufi path, practicing remembrances, and engaging in jihad or struggling against the lower self or *nafs* (see Chapter 32). It is the lower self that keeps humans distant from God. Islam and Sufism are about surrendering to the will of God by following this path. Once this nearness to God has been achieved, alterations of mechanistic laws may occur. This nearness to Allah is the explanation for "miracles" performed within religious contexts in ancient times and today.

Rapid wound healing is a very impressive phenomenon to observe and experience, but Islam and Sufism teach that one's heart is the center of one's being, and it becomes diseased (5:52) and hardened (6:43) from wrong acts (sins). Sufism, however, offers healing for the heart, as noted in the Quran: "O mankind! There hath come to you a direction from your Lord and a healing for the (diseases) in your hearts—and for those who believe a guidance and a Mercy" (10:57). Thus, when the heart has been purified through remembrances, and jihad, the nearness and true healing will occur.

SUFISM AND COMPLEMENTARY AND ALTERNATIVE MEDICINE

Sufism is a mystical tradition and devotional practice within Islam, based on drawing nearer to Allah through the spirituality of Muhammad. Masters of present-day Sufi schools trace their origins back to Muhammad through a chain of masters. Sufism can be described as a path or way of attaining nearness to Allah with its possible paranormal powers, knowledge, and healing. The psychology of Sufism is geared toward this attainment. The Sufi way involves following orthodox Islamic practices such as daily prayer, fasting, and some dietary prohibitions, as well as frequent worshipful meditation (i.e., remembrances). These practices may have not only spiritual purposes, but also many positive health implications.

Although Sufism generally is focused on spiritual development, some Sufi schools have focused on healing. This healing is a blend of Sufi philosophy and other Islamic healing traditions. Paranormal Sufi healing abilities have been observed and explained on the basis of a spiritual link mediated by the Sufi master back to the Prophet and Allah. Such phenomena from the Sufi way do not appear to result from meditative or altered states of consciousness but may be caused by a higher consciousness.

The implications of Sufism for integrative health is that Western high-tech medicine can be helpful for medical and surgical emergencies but may not be as helpful for chronic non–life-threatening conditions. What is needed today is a blending of "high tech" with "high touch." Sufism is one of the least-studied approaches that offer an integration of earlier eras of medicine.

The Sufi way is a universal path for spiritual traditions, including prayer, fasting, and meditation; avoidance of intoxicants, pork, and sex outside marriage; engagement in *jihad* (or battle against the lower self); and ultimate attainment of nearness to God (Allah) through remembrances.

Acknowledgments

We would like to acknowledge Carole O'Leary, Ph.D., for her help on researching the historical and cultural background of Sufism in the Middle East.

References

Al-Kasnazani al-Husseini M: *Jila'al-khatir: purification of the mind*, Philadelphia, 1999, Alminar Books.

Ansha N: *Principles of Sufism*, Fremont, Calif, 1991, Asian Humanities Press.

Benson H: *The relaxation response*, New York, 1975, Avon.

Chishti HM: *The book of Sufi healing*, Rochester, NY, 1991, Inner Traditions International.

Don NS, Moura G: Trance surgery in Brazil, *Altern Ther Health Med* 6(4):39, 2000.

Dossey L: Response to Peter Mulacz, *J Soc Psychical Res* 63(856):246, 1999 (letter to the editor).

Emoto M: *The Hidden Messages in Water*, New York, 2001, Atria Books.

Fatoohi L: Response to Peter Mulacz, *J Soc Psychical Res* 63(855):179, 1999 (letter to the editor).

Hall H: Deliberately caused bodily damage: metahypnotic phenomena? *J Soc Psychical Res* 64(861):211, 2000.

Hall H, Don NS, Hussein JN, et al: The scientific study of unusual rapid wound healing: a case report, *Adv Mind Body Med* 17:203, 2001.

Hall H, Minnes L, Olness K: The psychophysiology of voluntary immunomodulation, *Int J Neurosci* 69(1–4):221, 1993.

Hall H, Papas A, Tosi M, et al: Directional changes in neutrophil adherence following passive resting versus active imagery, *Int J Neurosci* 85(3–4):185, 1996.

Hall H, Schwartz G: Rapid wound healing: a Sufi perspective, *Semin Integr Med* 2(3):116, 2004.

Hall HR: Hypnosis and the immune system: a review with implications for cancer and the psychology of healing, *Am J Clin Hypn* 25(2–3):92, 1982.

Hall HR: Research in the area of voluntary immunomodulation: complexities, consistencies and future research considerations, *Int J Neurosci* 47(1–2):81, 1989.

Hall HR, Minnes L, Tosi M, et al: Voluntary modulation of neutrophil adhesiveness using a cyberphysiologic strategy, *Int J Neurosci* 63(3–4):287, 1992.

Hall HR, Mumma GH, Longo S, et al: Voluntary immunomodulation: a preliminary study, *Int J Neurosci* 63(3–4):275, 1992.

Hussein JN, Fatoohi LJ, Al-Dargazelli SS, et al: Deliberately caused bodily damage phenomena: mind, body, energy or what? *Int J Altern Complement Med* 12(9 Pt 1):9, 1994a.

Hussein JN, Fatoohi LJ, Al-Dargazelli SS, et al: Deliberately caused bodily damage phenomena: mind, body, energy or what? *Int J Altern Complement Med* 12(10 Pt 2):21, 1994b.

Hussein JN, Fatoohi LJ, Al-Dargazelli SS, et al: Deliberately caused bodily damage phenomena: mind, body, energy or what? *Int J Altern Complement Med* 12(11 Pt 3):25, 1994c.

Hussein JN, Fatoohi LJ, Hall H, et al: Deliberately caused bodily damage phenomena, *J Soc Psychical Res* 62:97, 1997.

Korotkov K: *Human energy field: study with GDV bioelectrography*, Fair Lawn, NJ, 2002, Backbone Publishing.

Korotkov K: *Measuring energy fields: state-of-the-science*, Fair Lawn, NJ, 2004, Backbone Publishing.

Korotkov KB, Bundzen PV, Bronnikov VM, Lognikova LU: Bio-electrographic correlates of the direct vision phenomenon, *J Altern Complement Med* 11(5):885, 2005.

Kuhn TS: *The structure of scientific revolutions*, ed 2, Chicago, 1970, University of Chicago Press.

Leskowitz E: From biology to spirit: The multidimensional model of wound healing, *Semin Integr Med* 3(1):21, 2005.

Mulacz WP: Deliberately caused bodily damage (DCBD) phenomena: a different perspective, *J Soc Psychical Res* 62:434, 1998.

Nelson RD, Bradish GJ, Dobyns YH, et al: Field REG anomalies in group situations, *J Sci Explor* 10(1):111, 1996.

Nelson RD, Bradish GJ, Dobyns YH, et al: Field REG II: consciousness field effects—replications and explorations, *J Sci Explor* 12(3):425, 1998.

Posner G: Taking a stab at a paranormal claim, 1995, available at http://www.csicop.org/sb/show/taking_a_stab_at_a_paranormal_claim. Accessed July 9, 2014.

Rumi J: *Feeling the shoulder of the lion*, Putney, Vt, 1991, Threshold Books.

Shapley D, Roy R: *Lost at the frontier: U.S. science and technology policy adrift*, Philadelphia, 1985, ISI Press.

Suggested Readings

Abdalati H: *Islam in focus*, Plainfield, Ind, 1996, American Trust Publications.

Alexander FM: *Man's supreme inheritance: conscious guidance and control in relation to human evolution in civilization*, London, 1910, Chatterson.

Armstrong K: *Muhammad: a biography of the prophet*, San Francisco, 1993, HarperCollins.

Benor D: *Spiritual healing: scientific validation of a healing revolution*, Southfield, Mich, 2001, Vision Publications.

Clarke PB, editor: *The world's religions: understanding the living faiths*, Pleasantville, NY, 1993, Reader's Digest Books.

Dewey J: *Human nature and conduct*, New York, 1922, Henry Holt.

Dossey L: *Healing words*, New York, 1993, HarperSanFrancisco.

Dossey L: *Prayer is good medicine*, New York, 1996, Harper SanFrancisco.

Dossey L: *Healing beyond the body: medicine and the infinite reach of the mind*, Boston, 2001, Shambhala.

Eisenberg D, Davis RB, Ettner SL, et al: Trends in alternative medicine use in the United States, 1990-1997, *JAMA* 280(18):1569, 1998.

Eisenberg D, Kessler R, Foster C, et al: Unconventional medicine in the United States: prevalence, costs, and patterns of use, *N Engl J Med* 328(4):246, 1993.

Ergil KV: Chinese medicine. In Micozzi M, editor: *Fundamentals of complementary and alternative medicine*, ed 2, New York, 1996, Churchill Livingstone, p 303.

Farez S, Morley RS: Potential animal health hazards of pork and pork products, *Rev Sci Tech* 16(1):65, 1997.

Fatoohi L, Al-Dargazelli S: *History testifies to the infallibility of the Qur'an*, Kuala Lumpur, Malaysia, 1999, AS Noordem.

Fatoohi L: *Jihad in the Qur'an*, Kuala Lumpur, Malaysia, 2002, AS Noordem.

Friend MB: Group hypnotherapy treatment. Hospital treatment of alcoholism: a comparative, experimental study, *Menninger Clin Monogr Ser* 11:77, 1957.

Gessner BD, Beller M: Protective effect of conventional cooking versus use of microwave ovens in an outbreak of salmonellosis, *Am J Epidemiol* 139(9):903, 1994.

Hall H: Handwashing in medicine: infrequent use of an ancient practice, *Int J Psychosom* 42(1–4):44, 1995.

Khan HI: *The music of life*, New Lebanon, NY, 1983, Omega Publications.

Lang J: *Even angels ask: a journey to Islam in America*, Beltsville, Md, 2000, Amana Publications.

Lings M: *What is Sufism?* Berkeley, 1977, University of California Press.

McGee CT, Sancier K, Chow EPY: Qigong in traditional Chinese medicine. In Micozzi M, editor: *Fundamentals of complementary and alternative medicine*, New York, 1996, Churchill Livingstone, p 225.

McKercher PD, Hess WR, Hamdy F: Residual viruses in pork products, *Appl Environ Microbiol* 16(1):65, 1978.

Muhaiyaddeen MRB: *Questions of life, answers of wisdom by the contemporary Sufi M.R. Bawa Muhaiyaddeen*, vol 1, Philadelphia, 1991, Fellowship Press.

Murray M, Pizzorno J: *Encyclopedia of natural medicine*, Rocklin, Calif, 1991, Prima Publishing.

Oschman J: *Energy medicine: the scientific basis*, Philadelphia, 2000, Elsevier.

Starfield B: Is US health really the best in the world? *JAMA* 284(4):483, 2000.

Tauxe RV: Emerging foodborne diseases: an evolving public health challenge, *Emerg Infect Dis* 3(4):425, 1997.

Walford RL: *Maximum life span*, New York, 1983, Avon.

Woodward MR: Healing and morality: a Javanese example, *Soc Sci Med* 21:1007, 1985.

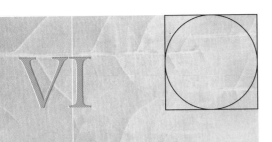

VI

GLOBAL ETHNOMEDICAL SYSTEMS: AFRICA, THE AMERICAS, AND THE PACIFIC

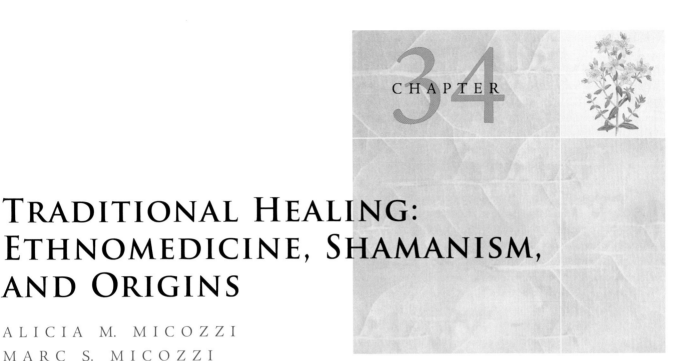

CHAPTER 34

TRADITIONAL HEALING: ETHNOMEDICINE, SHAMANISM, AND ORIGINS

ALICIA M. MICOZZI

MARC S. MICOZZI

SCIENTIFIC STUDY OF ETHNOMEDICINE AND SHAMANISM

Ethnomedicine and shamanism are scientifically studied by anthropologists, or ethnologists, and more recently by the subdiscipline of medical anthropology. Medical anthropology is both a scientific, academic discipline and an applied professional field of practice. First, as an academic discipline, medical anthropology is a subject that draws upon the theory, methodology, principles, and practices of its parent discipline, anthropology. Anthropology is in turn a relatively recent discipline. Taking the perspective of George Stocking, an anthropologist and historian, we can see how anthropology evolved relatively recently in the academic arena to study peoples, times, and places that had not already been "claimed" by other established academic disciplines by the early twentieth century. From a contemporary standpoint, most scholars that we think of as "historians" consider themselves *social historians*, while they think of anthropologists as *cultural historians*. More specifically, among historians, there is the field of *documentary history* based upon written documents that recorded and preserved information and knowledge that could be passed down to future generations. Regarding medical traditions, the great "classics" of Indian, Chinese, Unani, and Islamic medicine, discussed in preceding Section V, provide this kind of "historical" or classical background to the theory and practice of these medical systems.

The idea of *culture* arose on a different basis from social or documentary history and was introduced from the work of anthropologists as a new discipline in the late nine-teenth century. The whole concept of culture itself can be seen as a uniquely American contribution to the field of anthropology and, more broadly, the social sciences (see below). This feature (culture) also distinguished American anthropology from British-European social anthropology during the early twentieth century (until British anthropologist Anthony Radcliffe-Brown came to teach at the University of Chicago and began building a bridge between the two during the 1930s).

STUDY OF "PRE-HISTORIC" PRACTICES

With the appearance of *anthropology* on the scene as an academic discipline, it emerged in the world of learning long after *historians* had begun studying the past through their analysis of documentary records and "classics" from different ancient civilizations (documentary history) and where early *archaeologists* were unearthing cultural materials from the past (before "culture" became the underlying theory of archaeology itself in the 1960s and 1970s).

Thus, one domain of early anthropology became the study of "pre-historic," i.e., before *history*, "man." That is, the study of the biology and, where possible, culture of humans who existed before written languages—technically, "prehistory," or at the dawn of history. Human societies that predated written languages or records became a domain of study for anthropology. For these, there are no documents for documentary historians to study, and the past must be understood through material records. Recovery of early fossils of hominid human ancestors provided a basis to study biology, and archaeology's ability to recover artifacts, such as stone tools, etc., became a basis for the study of prehistoric technology and culture.

During the twentieth century, anthropology found its niche among the prior academic disciplines of history, Oriental studies, classics, and other pillars of academia. Since anthropology was able to study human biology and culture from "prehistoric" humans, a logical extension was to "preliterate" or "primitive" peoples in the contemporary world of the late nineteenth century, where there were likewise no documents or written records available. Therefore, the spoken language (versus written records) became another route to understanding through the development of anthropological *linguistics*. The colonial experiences of Great Britain, France, Germany, and other European nations during this era provided ample opportunity for European anthropologists to study "primitive" peoples where there were no written records. Thus the work of Bronislaw Malinowski in the Trobriand Islands of the **South Pacific**, for example, anticipated the appearance of the "pop" American anthropologist Margaret Mead in Samoa.

At the end of the nineteenth century, the United States presented a different picture from that of Europe and its colonies in **Africa** and **Asia**. In the United States, **Native Americans** were a fast-disappearing people who also did not have written records, thus lending themselves to study by the new field of anthropology.

CAPTURING CULTURAL TRADITIONS

Franz Boas was an immigrant to the United States from Europe and became known as the "founder" of American anthropology. He studied both **biology** and **culture** and made no distinction between the two in what he studied (a useful alliance for medical anthropology). In contrast to European social anthropology, which sought *generalizable rules* for the **structure** and **function** of human societies (which also theoretically conferred the ability to understand and *control* them), Boas and American anthropologists encountered peoples and societies that were fast disappearing from the earth and became interested in capturing and documenting the *unique features* of each group or tribe—thus the concept of **culture** and of *ethnography,* **the study of cultures**.

The early methods of American anthropology relied on the *"informant interview,"* reflected as early as the publications of the Bureau of American Ethnology in the 1880s. In describing interviews with the **Lakota Sioux** (see Chapter 37), for example, there is a repeating footnote: "But *Two Crows* denied this," in distinction to what other members of his tribe generally answered to questions regarding their customs. While building a consensual view of what constituted culture as *shared, learned knowledge and behavior*, there was room even at the dawn of ethnography for this kind of variation *within* the culture.

Not all differences in beliefs and behaviors can be explained by culture. This insight opened the door to the eventual anthropological study of personality within culture, famously by Ruth Benedict during World War II, a student of Alfred Kroeber at University of California,

Berkeley, who in turn had been a student of Boas. Her classic studies of Japanese culture and personality, including *The Chrysanthemum and the Sword*, were very important to American military and diplomatic personnel during World War II and the subsequent U.S. military governance of Japan under General Douglas MacArthur.

The centrality of the **informant interview** methodology was illustrated by Boas himself at the turn of the twentieth century. He was studying the **Native Americans** of the northwest coast of North America, who are unique in representing a culture that practiced *sedentism*, that is, living in permanent shelters, and not nomadic encampments, but without practicing agriculture. Usually sedentism and agriculture, instead of hunting-gathering, go together. His field notes have an entry to the effect that: Today was wasted . . . could not talk to anyone because they all went to a *potlatch*. In the later development of the methodology of **participant observation,** watching the potlatch itself would become central in understanding the culture and social functioning of these peoples in addition to simply asking them about their beliefs and behaviors (see also Chapter 2).

THEORY AND METHODOLOGY

Through the evolution of anthropological study it came to have these attributes:

- Theory: humans have biology and culture (and both have been and are evolving)
- Methodology: informant interview, participant observation
- Principles: through biology and culture, humans interact with and adapt to their environments
- Practices: understanding human biology and culture, and their interplay, in ways that enhance human success at sustenance, subsistence, reproduction, and health (and the counterargument that some human behavior is not adaptive for the species—but in fact may be protective for other species on earth—is addressed in the *Gaia Hypothesis*) (see Chapter 27)

These academic approaches can be applied specifically to the study of health and disease. Taking the approach of physical anthropology to human biology and evolutionary biology, biological attributes can be seen as adaptations to the environment in what is now called *health ecology*. Academic critics, who typically do not understand biology, decry such an approach as *"environmental determinism."*

A particular emphasis on human biology—understanding biological evolution—is known as *evolutionary biology* or *Darwinian biology*. These academic orientations add to our understanding of human health, complementing the essentially typological approach of modern, reductionist biomedical science (see Chapters 1, 2). (In fact, the study of human variation is a major field within human biology.)

Because humans have both *biology* and *culture,* a complete practice of medical anthropology would take both into account. Given the way that the academic field of anthropology is currently taught and practiced, however, departments, professors, and students tend to overspecialize in one or the other (analogous to some of the problems of modern biomedicine). The old "four fields" approach (physical anthropology/human biology, cultural anthropology/ethnography, archaeology, and linguistics) is out of favor at all but a few university programs (e.g., University of Pennsylvania, University of Arizona). From what can be observed today, younger anthropology faculty are generally incapable of teaching (well) outside the narrow confines of their own subspeciality. This same kind of problem (overspecialization) is also one of the major factors, though not the only one, contributing to the frequently problematic care that is now provided by Western biomedicine (see Chapter 3).

Therefore, medical anthropology ranges from an academic subdiscipline of either physical anthropology or cultural anthropology or both. At a meeting of the American Anthropological Association in Denver in 1986, the distinguished ethnographer George Foster stated, *"Medical anthropologists contribute most to anthropological theory and method when they write good, detailed ethnographies."* (Foster wrote the seminal ethnography *The Image of Limited Good* in 1965 to explain beliefs about health and wellness, and "good fortune," in agrarian, peasant societies.) At this end of the spectrum, medical anthropology is simply seen as just another domain for the extension of "ivory tower" academic anthropology into human health and medical practices, to test theories and methods important to the field of anthropology itself. At the other end of the spectrum is the *application* of medical anthropology to help improve the health of the world's peoples, including now dealing with some of the problems of the contemporary Western health care system.

APPLYING MEDICAL ANTHROPOLOGY

Medical anthropology as *applied anthropology* involves those with the academic training in anthropological theory, methods, and principles (1) studying the health of specific populations, (2) using those studies to improve access to health care, and (3) improving the health and nutritional status of human populations. Medical anthropologists can also work as part of health care teams in *clinical anthropology* to help deliver care with *cultural competence* to those from cultural traditions outside contemporary North America and Europe. In a general sense, through their studies of population health, medical anthropologists can help formulate national health policies and bilateral and multilateral international health assistance programs. There is also the influence from human biology on growth and development—standards and guidelines vary by ethnicity, gender, body size, and climate.

Health care dominates over 18% of our economy. It is seen as a social institution and as an instrument of social policy. Health care is a creation of the application of medical sciences. The gaps between our medical science and our health care largely lie in social, cultural, and economic issues. Many health issues may be said to be behavioral.

The influence of behaviors (e.g., smoking, physical activity, overeating and undereating) on health and disease can explain much about risk of disease and quality of life.

ALTERNATIVE MEDICINE AS ETHNOMEDICINE

The development of ethnoscience and ethnomedicine in the 1960s provided a basis for seeing indigenous health traditions as part of cultural and empirical systems of knowledge that are rational and adaptive to the local environment. Thus, early Western perceptions moved away from ethnomedicine as "superstition, myth and magic" in, for example, Sir James Frazer's *The Golden Bough*, in the late nineteenth century. W. H. R. Rivers, the British anthropologist and physician (a common combination at that time), established as early as the 1920s that what we call ethnomedicine today represents an internally ordered, rational system of beliefs about health and disease. This system is generally adaptive to a given environment and provides a society with tools to cope with illness and disease as part of its culture.

These tools almost always include the use of materia medica, primarily plants, from the local environment that are biologically active and have medicinal properties. It is a premise of *ethnobotany* that, just as it is adaptive for peoples to learn to harvest or grow plants for foods, they learn as part of culture to harvest or grow plants for medicines. Ethnomedicine includes the capability both to *diagnose* and to *treat* illnesses. Ethnomedical theories of disease and illness include the development of classification typologies based on the causation of diseases. In the mind–body continuum of ethnomedicine, disease causation systems may be based upon *naturalistic* causes (as we would find analogies in Western biomedicine) or *personalistic* (or *supernatural*) causes (or both).

Ideas about disease originating from curses, voodoo deaths (which have actually been documented in Western medicine [Jawer and Micozzi, 2009]), and envy as a source of illness, are *personalistic* causes. George Foster's *Image of Limited Good* (1965) describes how curses arise from envy; the admiring eye is the "Evil Eye," so that "good" must be either hidden or shared. A heavy emphasis on the ethos of sharing in a culture may underlie a deep-seated image of limited good. Disorders in the division of good(s) lead to illness; a disorder in the community, or the **cosmos**, leads to a disorder in the human body.

There are also diseases that literally, or figuratively, "blow into" the body, such as *hangin, or* "wind sickness" of Southeast Asia, and *susto*, or "startle response" (Chapters 6, 35, 40). These causations may straddle the *personalistic* and the *natural* origins of disease causation. A paper by Charles O. Frake from his work in the 1950s, "Classification of Skin Diseases Among the Subanum," illustrates several features (Chapter 40). Although the Subanum, a traditional tribe living in the Southern Philippines, generally agreed amongst themselves as to the categories of skin diseases, there was frequently disagreement as to how to categorize a specific example of skin diseases. Therefore, knowledge of the categories was part of the culture—learned behavior that is passed down and shared, but the ability to apply the knowledge varied based upon the abilities and experiences of individual members of the cultural group.

The **"natural" healers** are those gifted with the ability to use this cultural knowledge to diagnose and treat.

Having a disease classification system based upon causation of disease—either *natural* or *supernatural* (*personalistic*) causes—does not make a health care system by itself. The "diagnostic" system of disease classification may confer a benefit to a culture in understanding, in its own terms, disease as a result of disorder within the **cosmos** or within the **community.** As shared knowledge, passed down, disease classification forms part of culture. The development of a health care system (see below) is based upon **cultural** ideas about health and healing but also represents part of the larger **social** structure (Table 34-1).

MIND–BODY SINGULARITY VERSUS DUALISM

In ethnomedical systems, there is no distinction between the mind and the body (a division dating back in Western philosophy to the "Cartesian" duality, splitting the study of mind from the study of the body). Therefore, for example, what we call a psychological problem may literally be manifested as a somatic pain felt in the body itself, or "*somatization,*" in indigenous societies. The mind–body unity of ethnomedicine sometimes contributes to its perception by Western biomedicine as being overtly "spiritual" or even "magico-religious" (as initially labeled by Frazer in the late nineteenth century). While the practice of Western biomedicine has divided both diagnoses and treatments of mental versus physical diseases into the professional practices of psychology and psychiatry versus internal medicine, respectively, ethnomedicine engenders healing both for mental disorders through physical interventions and for physical disorders through "spiritual" interventions. It is now being recognized in Western science that the mind and the body are connected through neurological, endocrinological, and immunological pathways, documented by science (so-called, psychoneuroimmunology, or PNI; see Chapter 8).

HEALTH CARE AS A SOCIAL–CULTURAL SYSTEM

In addition to shared knowledge or beliefs about health and medicine (which exist at two levels: the *common knowledge,* or **"folk medicine,"** and the professional knowledge of healers and doctors), the society as a whole maintains mechanisms, structures, and technologies for the practice of medicine and the delivery of health care. The components of a health care system may be described as follows:

1. A developed theory of the body-person, known as the *explanatory model.* This theory includes the causes of

TABLE 34-1 *Ethnomedical Classification of Illness and Health Care Systems*

Social type	Subsistence	Illness causation	Healers
Nomadic	Hunter–gatherer, foraging	Self, ancestors, deity, "outsiders"	Shamans, diviners
Village	Simple horticulture	Community members, simple ethnopathology	Shamans, magico-religious healers, spiritual mediums, herbalists
Nomadic Pastoralists	Herding, animal domestication	Imbalances in hot and cold	Healers, spiritual mediums, exorcists
Chiefdoms	Sedentary agriculture	Imbalances in "humors"	Healers, spiritual mediums, herbalists, shamans
Early states	Complex agriculture	Imbalances	Same as above, plus priests
Civilizations	Irrigation agriculture	Individual behavior, moral failings, imbalances, elaborate ethnopathology	Priests, physicians, folk and religious healers
Modern, Industrial	Mechanized	Germs, genes, lifestyles, elaborate pathologies	Physicians, folk healers, alternative practitioners
Postmodern	Information	Mind–body, imbalances, "humors"	"Integration"

Adapted from Fabrega H Jr: *Evolution of healing and sickness,* Berkeley, 1997, University of California Press.

malfunctions as well as appropriate ways to address them

2. Plans to educate and train new practitioners through apprenticeship, schooling, or both. Or in the case of many indigenous societies, healers are selected through a process of divination to determine who has the attributes to become a healer (Fabrega, 1977)

3. A health care subsystem that delivers care to the needy

4. Associated means of producing substances or technologies necessary to delivery systems and educational subsystems

5. Professional organizations of practitioners who monitor each other's practices and promote the system to potential users

6. Legal mandate that provides for the official recognition of practitioners and maintains standards of quality based upon intellectual and moral authority, knowledge and ethical codes

7. Social mandate that informally reveals levels of social acceptance, for example, by frequency of use, willingness to pay, and stereotypes about practitioners (see Chapter 5)

HIERARCHY OF RESORT

In the contemporary world of global medicine, many people in cosmopolitan societies have access to more than one type of health care. These alternatives range, through scales of complexity (see Chapter 5), from an entire system of health care and medical practice (such as traditional Chinese medicine [TCM]) to a particular therapy or technique (such as bee venom therapy or the style of inserting acupuncture needles in TCM). Anthropologists have described a *hierarchy of resort* (e.g., Young's *Medical Choice in a Mexican Village*), whereby individuals and members of distinct social/cultural groups make decisions about where to get their care for what types of medical problems.

Sometimes decisions are based on *economic access*—ability to pay for the care or ability to get to the sources of care. At other times and in other circumstances, decisions are based on *cultural access*—that is, what does a given person believe will be the best or appropriate treatment, or source of care, for a given illness or problem. In modern Western society, the old consensual belief in **natural (cosmos)** and **supernatural (deity)** causes and cures has been largely supplanted by a *faith in technology*. The modern Western "magico-religious" belief is that new technologies will solve all problems of nature and human nature. Thus the "white coat," "black bag," "prescription pad," and, more recently, "biotech" have become the modern talismans of healing in Western biomedicine. The existence and ability to access different therapies and practices (such as complementary and alternative medicine [CAM] and "integrative" medicine in the modern West) and practitioners from among different healing traditions (as

enumerated above), and the coexistence of these different traditions side by side in a given society, is one definition of *medical pluralism*.

MEDICAL PLURALISM

The United States, Canada, Europe, Australia, and New Zealand, as well as large segments of the societies in India, Japan, South Africa, and parts of South America, for example, today provide rich examples of medical pluralism, where different medical traditions exist together, side by side. This phenomenon has also been labeled alternative, complementary, and integrative medicine.

The introduction of ethnomedical practices and therapies into the United States, for example, has long been part of health care for disadvantaged **immigrant** populations, who often use them because mainstream medicine is unaffordable, incomprehensible, or otherwise inaccessible.

At the other end of the spectrum, alternative therapies have been offered as part of **"elite"** medicine (patients pay out of pocket), partly because it is exotic but mostly because it works. The criteria for selection of practitioners may differ extremely between "immigrant" medicine and "elite" medicine. For example, in Chinatown, immigrants will not visit an acupuncturist unless he or she is a sixth-generation acupuncturist, whereas in modern suburbia, a licensed medical physician can become a licensed acupuncturist in most states by taking a six-week course—a difference of *six generations* versus *six weeks*. However, the medical doctor has the ability to provide acupuncture in a white coat and in a sterile environment. Any medicine works best when it meets cultural expectations.

In the middle ground, there is now widespread acceptance and availability of "CAM" among consumers and increasing practice of "integrative medicine" among physicians, nurses, and other health care practitioners in the United States *Alternative* implies an exclusivity of choosing one system or another, whereas *complementary* describes more accurately the situation in the West where patients pick and choose among a variety of therapies and practitioners. The term *integrative medicine* implies an active effort to sort through the evidence regarding CAM therapies to make them available as part of the continuum of care, together with regular or mainstream medicine, as appropriate, to individual patients for their conditions. However, like most medical practice, integrative medicine remains driven by finances and fashion, while education, research, and practice in integrative medicine remain too often painfully disconnected from each other.

Thus, the CAM movement has been a consumer-driven phenomenon based upon the desire and need for people to take a more "holistic" approach to their chronic health problems, combining mind and body, as is typically true of the ethnomedical traditions from which much of the common CAM modalities are drawn. This pathway has led to the *informal* incorporation of traditional ethnomedicine into some of Western medical practice (often in the form of holistic medicine, natural medicine, or wellness, or even reflected in consumer-based models, such as women's health).

Today, the beneficiaries of CAM in the United States are those who are described by the following:

- Have a desire for affiliation and therefore want a relational style of health care
- Want to alleviate symptoms gently and safely, with few side effects
- Will not take "hopeless" or "incurable" for an answer with serious diseases
- Want to prevent disease and enhance wellness
- Interpret the body-person as having more than a physical aspect and address the energetic, psychosocial, and spiritual bodies when receiving or delivering health care
- Are concerned with the end-state focus and invasiveness of typical biomedical care (see Chapter 5).

The *formal* introduction of ethnomedical therapies into Western medicine is being led by self-selected, and often isolated, health care practitioners who are doing research, developing treatment protocols, and creating facilities and practice for the delivery of CAM. Biomedical science requires "controlled clinical trials" to test the evidence for effectiveness of alternative therapies from ethnomedical traditions, although the trial methodology is designed for testing drugs and not for testing ethnomedical healing. Thus, *medical pluralism* in the United States is ultimately restrained by the medical paradigm (as well as the generally cited issues of safety and dosing, regulations, etc.).

Conversely, there have also been many attempts to introduce Western biomedicine to the rest of the world. The initial assumption was that high-tech Western medicine was the "best" medicine. This attitude conveniently benefits the purveyors of Western drugs and technology, while it has become understood in the international health community that health care on a global basis does best and is more affordable when it recognizes and utilizes traditional ethnomedical resources and practitioners (such as traditional birth attendants-midwives, herbalists, shamans). This indigenous care is not only more affordable, it is culturally more accessible. In the international development arena it has become known as *appropriate technology*. Enlightened "technology transfer" includes consideration of the indigenous culture and ethnomedical resources.

With the long stalemate in the "war on cancer," the re-emergence of infectious diseases that are resistant to antibiotics ("magic bullets" have become "friendly fire"), the inability of Western medicine to deal effectively with disorders of the mind–body, and the costs of biomedicine, there is now a more sober assessment of the ultimate benefits of Western biomedicine. We are now witnessing a "reverse technology transfer," in which the knowledge and wisdom of ethnomedical traditions are being incorporated

into Western health care as effective, affordable, "whole" health care, labeled as *CAM*.

GOVERNMENT-INDUSTRIALIZED MEDICINE AS AN ECONOMIC SYSTEM

There has been a tremendous social investment in biomedical research and technology in the West. Much of the basic research for the pharmaceutical industry has been undertaken by the U.S. National Institutes of Health (NIH) and other federally supported research. The ambitious doubling of the NIH budget over 10 years at the turn of the twenty-first century coincided with the pharmaceutical industry spending more "research and development" funds, not just on basic laboratory and clinical science, but on "market research" and direct-to-consumer marketing, turning patients themselves into drug detail men and women, in addition to hiring former cheerleaders as drug salespeople to help get the attention of physician prescribers.

This approach had led to a generation of "blockbuster" drugs to treat "risk factors," such as elevated cholesterol; questionable or quasimedical problems, such as "restless legs," male impotence, and "low-T" or low testosterone (in post–reproductive-age men); and questionable drug treatments (such as Prozac) for arguably "spiritual" problems such as depression. A popular book, blithely entitled *Listening to Prozac*, seems to encourage us to pay more attention to this chemical drug rather than to the underlying reasons why people are depressed. Perhaps the state of health care today is a good reason to be depressed. The leadership of the pharmaceutical industry (and in fact, of federal health agencies and the health care industry as a whole) has now passed from physicians, nurses, scientists, and pharmacists, to businesspeople, opportunists, career bureaucrats, and politicians. This development increasingly leaves public health largely out of the equation of Western biomedicine, and we have lost a generation of true therapeutic breakthroughs that would have allowed our potent medical sciences to result in better, safer medical treatments for more people. Instead, a 2013 study from Harvard University found that 90% of new drugs approved by the FDA during the prior 30 years are not more effective than prior drugs and that 50% are less safe (see Chapter 1).

Arguably, because of the economic interests of Western biomedical pharma and medical technology to seek the universal application of drugs to all problems and life events, there has been a "*medicalization*" of prevention, wellness, birth, life, and death. For every person who actually has a disease, there are many who as yet have only risk factors for the disease—the market to treat *risk factors* is much larger than the market to treat actual disease. The pharmaceutical companies have discovered this arithmetic and often appear more interested in selling drugs to the multitudes who are not sick, but only *at risk*, versus providing therapeutic advancements to the smaller numbers of those who are actually sick.

This *medicalized* model of disease prevention, by taking a pill, leaves out the more holistic aspects of the mind–body, spiritual health, and wellness (and alignment with the *cosmos*) offered by ethnomedical approaches. Likewise, for a person to be depressed or anxious in the modern world may be a sign to do something proactive and progressive in a more traditional behaviorist model of psychology, rather than being tranquilized by an antidepressant pill. Perhaps as a society, indeed, instead of "listening to Prozac," we would be well served to "*listen to depression*" and what it is telling us about the frequent disharmony of life in the modern world with nature and human nature.

There is widespread recognition that the drug-therapy model is limited, although presenting potentially unlimited opportunity for financial gain (which has also upended other segments of our economy and society). Now, Western, "magico-religious" faith in technology beckons to "biotech" as the next generation of biomedical cures. The promise of biotech over the past three decades has been a chimera. With its emphasis on materialistic, reductionist approaches to therapy, it compounds the error of drug therapy by eliminating the holistic, humanistic, energetic, mind–body dimensions recognized by ethnomedicine at the other end of the (human) scale. The economic and ethical problems have yet to be resolved. And, after three decades, there are no real biotech "cures" in terms of replacing "defective" genes. Modern molecular medicine is, however, demonstrating how vitamins and minerals (well beyond their putative roles as "antioxidants") have such profound effects in the body by regulating gene expression. Herbert Benson and colleagues have even shown that mind–body therapies, such as relaxation therapy, also influence gene expression, having profound effects on human physiology (see Chapters 9, 10).

There are no cures for the human condition, no matter how much human life is medicalized. The problem lies in the philosophy (or *paradigm*) of Western medicine. We now have modern, cutting-edge medical technologies guided by nineteenth-century Western philosophies of health and healing and uninformed by the traditional wisdom of ethnomedicine, which was conveniently discarded in the twentieth century only to see its resurgence in the twenty-first.

Medical anthropology provides a disciplined approach (literally, as an academic discipline and as a field of practice) to understanding human biology and culture and human nature in the context of nature, which provide a window to *understanding the original, traditional approaches to healing, in harmony with the cosmos, as practiced by shamans and other indigenous healers*. These approaches have tremendous value in understanding those aspects of medical practice and health care that are compelled, or chosen, and those that represent true alternatives on a global basis. While biomedical science and clinical trials may not hold all the answers to human medicine, ethnomedicine provides another resource whereby other kinds of knowledge about

health and medicine may be brought to bear, in a modern world clamoring for true *health care reform,* instead of the contemporary political pablum that institutionalizes and government-mandates, in the twenty-first century, everything that went wrong with twentieth-century medicine. Traditional healing in Asia, Africa, the Americas, and the Pacific (discussed in Sections V and VI) is closer to the source and may still help offer useful insights and solutions.

ORIGINS OF SHAMANISM: CENTRAL ASIA AND ANCIENT CHINA

The previous section of this book (Section V) presented the background, practice, and science of classical Chinese medicine and its pervasive influence in Asia and throughout the world. However, in prehistoric times, Chinese medicine had not yet become concerned with channeling revealed knowledge from semimythical emperors for health and healing. Rather, it was concerned with battling demonic forces that caused illness and disease. This primordial battle against disease-causing demons was not yet informed by the later developments in Chinese medical theory that seek balance and harmony.

In this regard, prehistoric Chinese medicine was essentially shamanism—the kind of traditional healing that the later, organized, systematic, celestial healing of Chinese medicine (derived from the three semimythical divine emperors) would later encounter in Southeast Asia during its own expansion (see Chapter 35).

In fact, the concept and the very term *shamanism* originated with reference to traditional spirit healers, or medicine men, of North Central Asia—what is today Siberia, in Russia, and Manchuria, in China, and the northern Korean Peninsula. Perhaps holdovers from the very type of prehistoric Chinese "medicine men" that held sway before the advent of more modern, naturalistic concepts of health and healing.

Thus, Chinese medicine itself started as "shamanic healing," with oracle bones and demon-exorcising *Wu,* or *shamans.* Later, it had become a more organized and theoretically sophisticated and systematic form of medicine, when it again encountered shamanic healing traditions in the jungles of Southeast Asia and grafted its more organized views on the claimed celestial origins of medical knowledge and practice onto the more individuated "primitive" practices of demon-haunted Southeast Asia.

Shamanism has now taken on a wider meaning, among scholars as well as in popular culture. It provides recognition that indigenous societies have "spiritual" practitioners outside the confines of recognized, organized "religions." Although its origin has a specific definition relating to societies in Central Asia, such as **Siberia and Manchuria**, the general usage of the term fulfills the need to describe a widespread cultural phenomenon among indigenous peoples in traditional societies worldwide beyond the confines of Siberia, Manchuria, or ancient China.

Taking the Word Shaman *Out of Cold Storage*

Shaman is a word that comes from the *Tungas* language of Central **Siberia**. The term incorporates men and women as religious leaders who serve their community by use of drums to call spirit allies. It is a priestly calling and cannot typically be "learned," as most shamans are born into such a life. It is important to note this definition as a basic point because the term has drawn many different false definitions and people have misused the word (see also Chapter 42).

There is evidence in ancient China reflecting concern with human illness and disease dating back to 1500 BC. The first thousand years of evidence, prior to the origination or compilation of classic Chinese medical texts, reflects concerns with oracular therapy, demonic medicine, and religious healing. Eventually, with the development of Chinese medicine proper, these "demons" would be exorcised and banished to the far reaches of the Malaysian Peninsula, Indonesian Archipelago, and Philippine Islands, where they would flourish through their later encounter with the official medicines of Greater China, as well as further India during different eras and Islam (Chapter 35).

In prehistoric China, the causation of illness and disease was seen to be by supernatural phenomena more than by natural causes. These causes were ancestors, spirits and demons, gods, and transcendental law. These associations reflect general observations about disease and medicine as related to the stage of evolution of a human society (Table 34-1).

The civilization of the Shang Chinese arose along the midcourse of the Yellow River in modern Hunan province in the period from 1800 to 1600 BC. Information about this period draws largely from archaeology, although there was a written language that used some of the Chinese pictographs that are still in use today.

A great number of inscribed bones and tortoise shells—"oracle bones"—have been recovered over the past century from this era. Although the great mass of people still lived with Stone Age technology, metallurgy was advanced into the Bronze and Iron Ages. The origin and purpose of a number of large bronze pots has remained a mystery to experts on ancient Chinese civilization, but the editor of this book has proposed that these pots were used for boiling animal remains to derive oracle bones, and represents the best method to do so. Initially the bones of cattle, then of tortoises, were used to communicate with the ancestors. Heating the bones caused cracks to appear, and the patterns of these cracks could then be interpreted as signaling the answers and intentions of these ancestors.

When it came to illness and disease, pathophysiologic phenomena were observed and systematically labeled as "blow of a demon" (heart attack), or the more versatile "curse of an ancestor," which covered toothache, headache, abdominal distention, or leg pains. The ultimate balance to be achieved for the avoidance of illness and disease was harmony between the living and the dead ancestors. The notion of balance within the individual or between the individual and nature was to come later.

However, the Shang also believed in other causes for illness, which the ancestors nonetheless understood, such as "malignant wind" from wind spirits. According to bone inscriptions, the *Wu* (ancient Chinese shaman) could control the forces of the wind. Evil wind may have acted in its own right or been used a tool by evil ancestors. The theme of wind sickness from ancient China is widespread throughout modern Southeast Asia. Among Chinese communities in Hong Kong and Taiwan, for example, the desire to this day to have their ancestors' bones passed by good "wind and water" (modern *feng-shui*) is an echo of these ancient winds of the Shang.

Finally, Shang oracle bones sometimes showed a pictographic character (subsequently used since the Han period) as a representation for "black magic," that is, deliberate illness-causing intentions of one person against another.

The interventions of the Wu with the ancestors did not directly involve any real contact with the "patient." Healers who actually dealt with the physical aspects of the individual with the illness had not yet appeared in favor of the purely "social therapy" conducted by the Wu. This social therapy has strong parallels in the communal healing rituals found throughout Southeast Asia to this day.

The Shang Dynasty gave way to the Zhou, a seminomadic group from the northwest, who settled down to develop communally managed irrigation agriculture, granting an advantage. The Zhou Dynasty manifests certain political parallels to the era of feudalism in Europe. There was a long period of blood strife, giving way to what is known as the "*Warring States*" period throughout much of China. Ultimately, the Qi Dynasty was able to subdue all rivals in the third century BC but effectively rejected what might be called the code of "chivalry" in favor of "total war." Finally. these excesses led to eradication of the Qin by 200 BC in favor of the Han Dynasty, whose fourth emperor, Emperor Wu, brought to China a period of peace and stability and a social-political system that was to be characteristic of the next two thousand years.

Thus, it is not surprising that during the Zhou period, the "demons were loosed" and were seen to be responsible for everyday misfortunes, including illness and diminishing the role of the ancestors. The Wu of the Shang period were adopted as leaders who were believed to possess magical powers. The pictograph for Wu shows a dancer at its core. With the temporary breakdown of the old system of the earth and the ancestors, rifts opened between the realms of the living and the dead, creating myths about the role of demons in exerting influences over the living. Exorcism became the chief responsibility of the Wu. The ancestors had lost control over the living descendants, whose fates were cast into the hands of demons, who could freely roam from one person to another. In contrast to both the prior ancestor medicine, and the Confucian system about to come, the cause of disease during the Warring States period may best be described as "all against all." Typical demonic illnesses were labeled as follows:

- "Assaulted by demons"
- "Possessed by the hostile (influences of demonic guests)"
- "Struck by evil"

The efforts of the Wu were directed to expelling demons, often by thrusting spears into the air, or more dramatically, into unfortunate political prisoners. The Chinese pictographic character used for "*healing*" and "*healer*" shows the character for Wu in the lower half, with a quiver with an arrow, and a lance or spear, in the upper half. Breath magic, including blowing, spitting, and shouting, was believed to be like blowing out the stream of fire to the spiritual world. Likewise, burning of talismans transferred the written word to a spiritual destination.

The entire population also wore talismans, of wood, jade, or gold, depending upon the means of the wearer. Wu exorcists prepared talismans in the form of official state documents that would "command" demons to leave. These may have been the first prescriptions. Incantations had the same purpose. Of interest is the manipulation of what is believed to have been acupuncture points—at this time labeled "demon camp," "demon heart," "demon path," "demon bed," and "demon hall." The needles used to penetrate "demon heart" were analogous to the spears used by exorcists. Although there is no written reference to therapeutic acupuncture needling prior to the first century BC under the Han, the possibility that acupuncture originally had a purely "demonic medicine" function cannot be ruled out. The long persistence of many of these practices may ultimately be better explained by their resonance with social and political developments in ancient China than by their consistency with later Buddhist and Daoist philosophies.

Ultimately as time went by, spiritual powers began to be seen as emanating from celestial sources (characteristic of later Chinese civilization) and the *Chu*, priests or supplicants, supplanted the Wu, supernatural demon practitioners. The Chu no longer held the power like the Wu had, but simply tried to access the divine sources of power, which ultimately were associated with the semimythical emperors and their brethren. As for the demons, they apparently sought the warmer climes of Southeast Asia, where a shamanic system of traditional healing persisted long after the development of Chinese medicine proper.

These traditional healing systems, and their centuries-long interplay with Chinese Medicine and other Asian medical traditions, as well as shamanism, are discussed in the next chapters on Southeast Asia: Vietnam, Indo-China, Malaysia, Indonesia (Chapter 35) and Burma, Thailand, and Nepal (Chapter 36). This same geopolitical–cultural sphere has also been referred to as "Greater China" as well as "Further India," reflecting these influences that extend to health and medical practices.

References

Fabrega H Jr: Evolution of healing and sickness. In Landy David H, editor: *Medical Anthropology*, Berkeley, 1977, University of California Press.

Foster G: *Image of Limited Good*, Berkeley, 1965, University of California Press.

Frake Charles O: Classification of Skin Diseases Among the Subanum. In Landy David H, editor: *Medical Anthropology*, Berkeley, 1977, University of California Press.

Jawer M, Micozzi MS: *The Spiritual Anatomy of Emotion*, Rochester, 2009, Park Street Press.

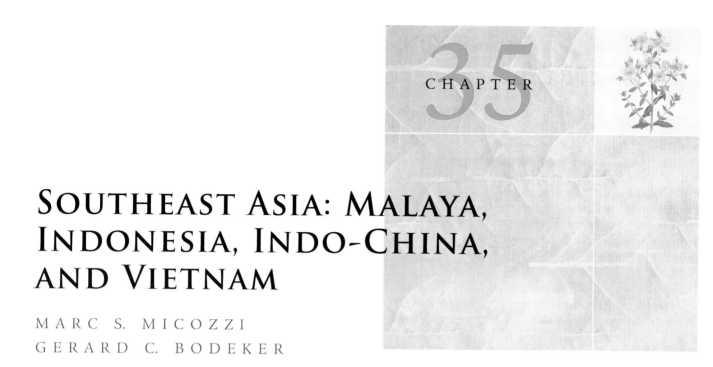

CHAPTER 35

Southeast Asia: Malaya, Indonesia, Indo-China, and Vietnam

MARC S. MICOZZI

GERARD C. BODEKER

INTRODUCTION

Concepts of energy, mind, and spirit that appear common among traditional medicines are evident with the spread of Indian and Chinese influences, and their encounter with indigenous healing, throughout Southeast Asia. When considering the medical traditions of Southeast Asia, it is useful to recognize that almost all these territories came under the influence of two of the earliest civilizations at the dawn of history. The cultural diffusion of first what have been called **"Further India,"** and then **"Greater China,"** represented succeeding waves of influence emanating from the great river valleys of the Indus and the Yellow River, respectively, carrying along common discoveries and understandings of the nature of human life and health.

Scholars of prehistoric humans locate the original center of Indian or Hindu culture and Sanskrit language texts in the Indus River Valley (modern-day Pakistan) in the second millennium BC. These Indo-European (or Aryan) peoples were once considered to have originated in the Caucasus Mountains of Central Asia (thus, the popular term "Caucasian"), based upon earlier typological approaches to population studies, which have since been supplanted by modern genetic studies (see below). This population group expanded east and south into the Indian subcontinent, establishing a new center in the Ganges River Valley, at the foot of the Himalaya Mountains, during the first millennium BC, carrying the Sanskrit texts and knowledge with them.

This Vedic civilization (which we associate with Ayurvedic medicine and the related but separate practice of yoga) encountered the Dravidian peoples, whom we associ-

ate with Siddha medicine, now prevalent on the southeastern tip of India and on the island of Ceylon, or Sri Lanka. Most Indian groups descend from a mixture of two genetically divergent populations: Ancestral North Indians (ANI), related to Central Asians, Middle Easterners, Caucasians, and Europeans; and Ancestral South Indians (ASI), not closely related to groups outside the subcontinent. The date of mixture is unknown, but results of genetic studies show that India experienced a demographic transformation several thousand years ago, from a region in which major population mixture was common to one in which mixture even between closely related groups became rare because of a shift to endogamy, which has in turn been related to the beginning of the *caste system*.

One may see the subsequent outgrowth of **Buddhism** from the Hindu Prince Siddhartha Gautama (the Buddha) as a manifestation of another wave of influence from "Further India" giving birth to the new wave in **Greater China, East Asia,** and **Southeast Asia,** including **Indo-China** (today's **Vietnam, Laos,** and **Cambodia**). The very name **Indo-China** implies this *intersection* of **India** and **China.**

Ultimately a third wave, **Islam,** spread during the 700 years from AD 750 to 1450, all the way to the western border of North Africa and east through India, the **Malay** region, and the southern **Philippines,** and throughout Indonesia. **Islam** also carried along Greek-Roman (*Unani,* Arabic for "Greek") concepts of health and healing, which it had incorporated and preserved following the ancient Classical Era in the West, and to which it added many important insights and practices (see Chapter 32). Islam also helped carry Ayurveda to Southeast Asia, as the first Muslims going to the region were Indian converts who had been traveling there as Hindus and Buddhists for centuries before the advent of Islam.

Bali, in the center of **Indonesia**, is a place that remained substantially uninfluenced by Islam. The Balinese fended off Islamization from Java and offered a home to large numbers of Javanese who fled forced Islamization during the fourteenth and fifteenth centuries, when Java came under Islamic influence from the Batam Regency near Singapore, on the Malay Peninsula. Thus Bali retained its Indian Vedic roots, with a substantial Buddhist influence merged in, as well. Sri Lanka, off the far southeast coast of India, and **Timor,** at the far eastern edge of **Indonesia**, represent socio-cultural "fault lines" that have had serious repercussions on traditional medicine, as well as geopolitical consequences in the twentieth century.

All three of these great successive traditions of Hindu-Buddhist, Chinese, and Islamic-Unani influences placed emphasis on the concept of **vital energy, mind, and spirit** as central to health and healing.

In India, in the geographic center of the southern half of Asia, there were centuries of foreign rule, beginning in the fifteenth century, when invaders from Persia (modern-day Iran) occupied neighboring parts of India, carrying the banner of Islam. They established the Mogul Empire, which was dominant especially in Northern India until the period of European colonization in Asia (See Chronological Phases of Indian and Middle Asian Medicine table after ch 31).

(HEMI) SPHERES OF INFLUENCE

Initially, in the sixteenth century, the **Portuguese** established missions in south, **southeast,** and **east Asia** under the dominions established by the Roman Catholic Pope Alexander VI by the Treaty of Tordesillas in 1494. This decree divided the globe into two hemispheres, along a line of longitude through the Atlantic Ocean (and in 1529 around the other side of the globe through the Pacific) between the "eastern" half, under **Portuguese** influence, and the "western" half, under **Spanish** influence, for purposes of trade and evangelization.

The borders of these *hemi-spheres of influence* extended longitudinally around and over the globe such that the **Portuguese** had an outpost in Brazil in the New World at the western end of its eastern half of the world, while the **Spanish** developed a foothold in the **Philippines** in Asia at the far western end of its western half of the world. India, **Malaya,** and **Indonesia** (the "Spice Islands," of interest to the mercantile trade of that time) were firmly in the **Portuguese** half, as evidenced by the development of settlements from **Goa** at the western end, **Malacca** in the middle on the Malay Peninsula, to **Timor** at the eastern end of Indonesia, of this vast sweep across Asia. All became active Portuguese Roman Catholic settlements. Malacca doesn't remain so—there is a small population of Portuguese-Malay residents remaining—but Islam is firmly established as the dominant tradition, followed by Chinese Buddhists.

The longtime influence of the Spanish in **the Philippines** led to the development of a syncretic brand of faith healing, intermingling Asian concepts of **vital energy** with Roman Catholic **charismatic** religious and **spiritual** practices. After the Spanish–American War of 1898, and the 25-year effort to "pacify" the southern, Islamic, half of the Philippine Islands by the United States, there also remained many pockets of traditional Islamic and ethnomedical practices well into the second half of the twentieth century (studied by the authors), while the vast majority of the national population were practicing Roman Catholics (with ethnomedical traditions as discussed in Chapter 40).

GOING DUTCH (AND OTHER EUROPEANS)

During the seventeenth century, the dominance of Portugal and Spain in global trade and colonization slowly gave way to **Dutch** rule in **Malaya** and **Indonesia**. The Dutch continued to focus their interests in the ancient territories of so-called Further India in the Indonesian archipelago, where **Bali** still stands as a remnant of ancient Hindu and Buddhist civilization, among a sea of subsequent influences from Islam.

Then, during the eighteenth century, influence passed to the **French** in parts of India (Pondicherry) and Indo-China (**Vietnam, Laos,** and **Cambodia**), and to the **British** in India, Burma, and **Malaya,** with European footholds in **Chinese** treaty ports, such as **Hong Kong (Great Britain), Macao (Portugal),** and **Port Arthur (Germany)**. Ultimately, European influence parcelled itself out by the nineteenth century, such that India, Burma, and **Malaya** were in the sphere of **Great Britain**; Indo-China (**Cambodia, Laos,** and **Vietnam**) was in the sphere of **France**; **Indonesia** remained with the **Dutch**; and the **Philippines** remained with **Spain** (with occasional forays by the British). The **Portuguese** became relegated to their few remaining footholds in Goa, Macao, Malacca, and Timor (at the eastern edge of Indonesia). The ancient **Buddhist** kingdom of Siam (**Thailand**) always remained independent as a *de facto* buffer zone between Britain and France, its influence extending to the Lao people of northwest Indo-China (**Laos**).

The long-independent **Thailand** was a political state with a divine, **celestial** ruler (as in ancient China), and strong **Buddhist** influences derived from **Ashokan India** via **Burma** in the second century BC. These influences fostered a distinctive medical practice (see Chapter 36). The remnants of Indian influence are not forgotten, as depicted in the representations and reenactments of the Ramayana epic, for example. The **celestial** rulers of **Thailand** remain in place to this day, while the "Last Emperor" of **China** survived only the first decade of the twentieth century (except for the brief period of rule in *Manchukuo*, the Japanese puppet state in Northern China, or **Manchuria**, before and during World War II).

PERSISTENT INFLUENCES OF CHINA

The role of energy, mind, and spirit are central in all these medical traditions, which also share the view that healing ultimately emanates from celestial or divine spiritual sources as articulated in the development of Chinese medicine. As we introduced earlier in the book, Chinese medicine has its influence in Southeast Asia through both (1) dissemination and diffusion of the concepts and theories of Chinese medicine, during historic periods, into the indigenous medical traditions, and (2) the presence of millions of "overseas Chinese," who came as immigrants during the eighteenth- to the nineteenth-century era of European colonialism in Southeast Asia and acted as emissaries, bringing Chinese medicine proper with them. In addition, as we have seen, Chinese immigrants to new lands brought back new materia medica for incorporation back into Chinese medicine itself (see Chapter 24). More than anything, it is this exchange that characterizes the concept of "Greater China" with respect to medicine and other key aspects of society.

As outlined above, these Chinese influences came to Southeast Asia on top of already established Indian traditions. They never replaced these traditions but fused with them in a secondary position in Malaysia and Indonesia, Thailand, Burma, Laos and Cambodia, and in primary position in Vietnam. The Chinese were trading with the Malay world—including the Indonesian Archipelago—from the second century AD. They settled in permanent trading communities beginning in the twelfth century AD. So these influences far predate the later nineteenth century and British colonial use of Chinese workers.

THE MALAY PENINSULA

A clear case in both points is that of **Malaysia** (Malaya prior to independence from Britain in 1962). In addition to indigenous **Malay** practices, there were early Indian and **Chinese** influences, followed by **Islamic** conversion, and then successive waves of Europeans: Portuguese, Dutch, and British. Further, under British control, **Malaya** again saw the immigration of more **Chinese** people, primarily to engage in local commerce and work in the rich tin mines, and **Indians**, to work on the agricultural plantations of palm oil, rubber (once it arrived from the Amazon Basin), and coconut. This migration of the nineteenth century witnessed the re-introduction of **Indian** and **Chinese** influences in a contemporary context. Today, Malaysia is approximately 50% Malay, 35% Chinese, and 10% Indian, with 5% of others. This rich mix shows the practice of many different medical traditions side by side (medical pluralism).

Throughout the Malay Peninsula and islands of **Southeast Asia**, there are also the **"Orang Asli,"** or "original men" in *Bahasa Malay*, which represent the indigenous peoples (probably related to the **Aborigines** of **Australia**). When the **proto-Malay** subsequently arrived in ancient times throughout the region, they pushed these original inhabitants to where, today, they can be found in the deep interior, high in the mountain regions (such as the **Semang,** or *"Negritos,"* in the center of Malaysia). The proto-Malay were then supplanted by the **Malay** of today, in turn pushing them into the hinterlands where they are found today, for example, as the *Manobo, Tiboli,* and *Subanum* of the southern Philippines (see Chapter 40), the *"Montagnards"* of Indo-China, the interior tribes of Formosa (Taiwan, Nationalist China, or ROC), and the "outer" islands of Japan, such as Okinawa in the south, and Hokkaido in the north.

Each tribe has its own ethnomedical traditions, typically drawing from the concepts common to medical traditions in Greater China and India and from local traditions. The antecedents in this great ancient population migration were not Chinese but native peoples such as the Ainu (now in the northern Japanese island of Hokkaido).

Early Ethnographic Connections

> Early East Asians include Buryats in Siberia and Mongolia, Han Chinese, Man Chinese, Korean Chinese, South Koreans, and Taiwanese indigenous populations, as well as regional populations in Japan, including Hondo, groups in the Ryukyu Islands, and Ainu (northern Honshu and Hokkaido). These populations, once classified typologically as "Mongoloid," are highly diversified, and several clusters, such as Northeast Asians, Southeast Asians, Oceanians, and Native Americans are observed genetically. Interestingly, an indigenous population in North Japan—Ainu—is placed relatively close to Native Americans in genetic correspondence analysis.
>
> Genes shared by Ainu and Native Americans are also commonly observed in Taiwanese indigenous populations, Maori in New Zealand, Orochon in Northeast China, Inuit, and Tlingit. These findings further support the genetic link between East Asians and Native Americans. Various ancestral populations in East Asia migrated and dispersed through multiple routes. Relatively small genetic distances between Ainu and Native Americans suggest that these populations are descendants of the same Upper Paleolithic (Stone Age) populations of East Asia.

In addition to these heritages, local practices are also influenced by utilizing local indigenous materia medica. While there are cultural boundaries among healing traditions, there is also commonality among them. Beyond cultural boundaries, natural boundaries also have influence over ethnomedical traditions in light of the varieties of plant life and materia medica.

NATURAL BOUNDARIES: THE WALLACE LINE

Throughout the last section of this book, we have illustrated that medical practices are guided by the concepts of **vital energy** and **celestial** revelation throughout **Greater**

China but are also influenced by the local **materia medica** as part of the ecology indigenous to each region. In addition to the historic political demarcation between Portugal and Spain that ran between the Pacific Ocean and Southeast Asia beginning in the sixteenth century, there is also another important line of demarcation relating to the native *flora* and *fauna* (the basis of materia medica). The **"Wallace Line"** runs generally north and south through the middle of the Southeast Asian Archipelago. Discovered by the nineteenth-century British natural scientist Alfred Russel Wallace, this line traces the divide between the region where the plants and animals are part of the Asian ecology versus the transition to a primarily Australian and Pacific type of distribution. Between these two ecological zones lies the richest and most exotic assortment of plants and animals (above water) anywhere on earth, including the legendary *Komodo dragon* and the *bird of paradise* (the bird itself; not the flower named after it), as well as unusual, highly nutritious fruits that cannot grow anywhere else on the planet (*durian, mangosteen, rambutan*). By studying this rich diversity, Wallace actually came to understand the principles of natural selection and evolution long before Charles Darwin was able to formulate his theory from his own observations on the Galapagos Islands during the much earlier voyage of the *HMS Beagle*. It was Wallace who finally convinced Darwin to come forward with the theory of evolution, decades later.

Wallace also had the opportunity to observe and document many ethnomedical practices as well as medicinal herbs and foods throughout the *Malay Archipelago*, reported in his famous book of the same name and dedicated to Charles Darwin.

Some of the "discoveries" he documented and recorded are shown in Table 31-6, as a practical guide to the reader.

MALAY PENINSULA AND INDONESIAN ARCHIPELAGO

The most recent form of social organization in the Malay Peninsula, prior to unification under the British Empire and then as an independent nation in 1962, were **Islamic Sultanates.** These endure to the present, where each of nine states has its own sultan, and each sultan rotates through the Kingship of Malaysia for a period of five years. These sultanates equate approximately with the provinces or states of modern-day Malaysia. In addition to the Malaysian Peninsula, the former sultanates of Sabah and Sarawak, on the northwestern coast of the large island of Borneo to the east, also form part of Malaysia. Borneo also contains the independent nation of Brunei and the large Kalimantan province of Indonesia.

Influences from Further India, Greater China, and Islam have mixed with the ethnomedical practices of the indigenous Malay people, which include a four-element theory identical to that of Ayurveda (minus the space element) and also identical to the four-element theory of Islamic medicine. The sultanates of Kelantan and Terengganu on the eastern coast of Malaysia are considered among those representing traditional Malay culture, as are Perak and Kedah, as well as Johor, to some extent, which is the heir to the Malacca Sultanate. Here, it is generally acknowledged that Western health care can do little for diseases of the *spirit* and that Western psychotherapy has little place. And illnesses involving the spirit are a major category of disease. Care of the spirit is the province of Imams, and less publicly of shamans, called **bomoh,** or faith healers.

In the traditional healing of Southeast Asia, the concept of the celestial origins of the knowledge of healing is evident, as in ancient China and India, and spiritual aspects of healing predominate. Like the ancient, prehistoric, or more "primitive" aspects of Chinese medicine (from even before the advent of acupuncture, tui na, and qigong) for the manipulation of vital energy, or Shintoism in Japan, traditional healing remains close to nature (Chapter 2). However, for example, Malay massage or *urut*, with its long strokes and use of oil, is much more akin to Ayurvedic abhyanga than to Chinese tui na, with its pressure points and hard short movements.

Naturalistic causes for illness and paths to healing are ascribed to observable natural phenomena like the wind, literally (versus the more symbolic representation of wind in five-elements Chinese medicine, for example). In fact, the idea that illness is carried "on the wind" has been likened by some Western observers to the idea of disease-causing germs or microbes (which only came to currency in Western thinking in the late nineteenth century) that may also be airborne.

The traditional healer channels energies from celestial sources for both diagnostic and therapeutic purposes. Thus, diagnoses and prescriptions in traditional medicine in the Malay world are *written on the wind*, and the process of healing has been likened to *taming the wind of desire*.

WRITTEN ON THE WIND

Three general types of illness are perceived in traditional Malayan ethnomedicine. *Sakit biyasa* is ordinary sickness, whereas *sakit hangin* is literally sickness (*sakit*) from the wind or moving air (*hangin*). The third variety of illness is intermediate between these two, also assigning spirit as a large component of illness. Beyond just "catching a cold" in a draft (as part of Western folklore; see Chapter 5), for example, the wind imagery has a literal meaning in the belief that air rushing into the body results in disease.

For example, in Malaysia and the Philippines (Chapter 40), the most widely used method of birth control was *coitus interruptus*, despite the popular understanding that it is detrimental to health. It is believed that in the process of intercourse, the woman's lower body becomes overheated so that, when the penis is abruptly withdrawn, air rushes into the womb, inflicting internal disturbances.

Aside from sexual desires, the wind imagery for sickness is also symbolic of a "*wind of desire*" in the heart, whereby continual denial of emotion leads to illness. The Malay attitude of "it is nothing only" (*walay lang*) to emotionally charged events, or the striving to "save face" in public, produces a denial of feelings that may eventually take its toll, potentially leading to either *sakit hangin*, internalizing the injury, or literally running *amok* (from the Malay word itself) and externalizing the injuries by inflicting them on other parties.

HEALERS AND HEALING RITUALS

Traditional Malay medicine is practiced by an estimated 2000 full-time and 20,000 part-time bomoh healers. Although bomohs share a number of characteristic skills, there is no single path for the training of these folk healers. Some have studied a few existing texts (mostly in Bahasa Malay of Javanese origin), but most learn from a special teacher, usually their father, or gain special knowledge by revelation through dreams, waking encounters, or inheriting a familiar, or helping spirit, such as a *hantu raya*.

Bomohs may be approximately categorized as spiritualists, herbalists, or traditional bonesetters, but there are no rigid specializations. Most bomohs use supernatural, or Islamic, incantations but also know a great deal about herbal remedies in treating a patient. Some also perform massages and special cleansing baths and place "charms" on their patients. The bomoh's *hantu raya*, in addition to helping heal, may also act as a threat against returning to bad habits that cause bad health.

For a healing ritual, a **bomoh** involves the entire community. A *konduri*, or ritual communal meal, is offered to the performers of the healing. The communal nature of this meal is exemplified by its conduct for courtships, contracts, or even car accidents, today, in addition to healing. Symbolic foods such as *betel* nuts and fish curry are prepared, and young coconuts are scored with spices and tobacco placed inside. The use of various indigenous materia medica draws on both the pharmacologic properties of the constituents, such as betel nut, curry (coriander, turmeric), tobacco (nicotine), as well as the symbolic significance of the ritual plants (equivalent to a "placebo effect") (Micozzi, 1983).

HEALING SOUNDS IN THE RAINFOREST

The bomoh goes into a trance in the company of a **mindok** partner who does not, however, go into trance. Instrumental groups are always present, often using the trancelike music of the *gamelan*. Emphasis is placed upon the ability of sounds, arranged in specific patterns, to heal—whether in the repeated *mantras* of meditation and yoga, or arranged in the repetitive music of the gamelan orchestra—especially in Ayurvedic healing traditions of **Further India**. Here, by noting the instruments of later Islamic origin, combined with the music and sounds of ancient India, we can observe these layers of influences as transposed into the indigenous healing practices of Southeast Asia.

The gamelan orchestra generally consists of the following **four** instruments: *ketak, kenong, kempul,* and *gong,*

arranged in a semicircle on the ground. The gong is used as a drum, striking it with the palm of the hand. These are essentially **Islamic** instruments, the knobbed gong of Malaysia and Indonesia being distinct from the flat gong of **China**. The music is played in *kulingtang* rhythmic mode rather than a musical note mode. There are no scores and no conductors (like a modern jazz jam session), just a sense of circular, perpetual motion to carry the players along. The scale is *anhemitonic* (five tones without half-steps) and the polyphonic stratification is typical of rice agriculture-based cultures. This music facilitates the trancelike state.

While in the trance, the bomoh manifests a marked resting tremor and may assume the spirits of the *Black Jin* (who represents the areas below the earth), the *Yellow Jin* (representing the mountains), and/or *Hanuman* (the white monkey of the *Ramayana*; *Presbytis entellus*, a monkey of Southern Asia, having bristly white hairs on the crown and the face; from the Sanskrit *hanumat*, "having jaws," from *hanu*, "jaw"). The manifestation of these spirits themselves draws from the **Sanskrit** roots of Further India, as well as the representations of the **Buddha's** healing realms of the mountains and under the earth, with the final gloss of taking the shapes of the *Jins* from **Islam.** Thus, in the *actual practice of the healing trance, in real time, we can observe the successive influences of Further India, Greater China, and later Islam* on the images of health and healing, as if converging on an ancient archetype.

These *spirits* speak, sing, and dance through the trance state with culturally significant gestures similar to those observed in the Malay opera and *Wayang Kulit* puppet theatre. The diagnosis is made by *divination*, which then may or may not lead to exorcism. However, it is stressed that the ill individual is not possessed by a spirit but simply made sick by one. The spiritual ritual is to "weld the patient back together" after the illness has caused him or her to come apart.

Attempts are made today to draw these rituals into the currently predominant Islamic religion. *Fatima*, the daughter of *Mohammed* the Prophet, is said to have conducted the first spirit ritual therapy. The four companions of Mohammed played the four instruments. When they finished, they threw the instruments into the sea from whence the Hebrews obtained them, going on to become the great healers of the ancient Islamic world.

The heritage of Adam and Eve, the original peoples of "the book," according to Islam, is also worked into the practice. In the Bible, the task of assigning names to the objects of nature is given to Adam and Eve, thereby allowing them to take part in this process of "creation." In the traditional formulation of disease causation, Satan gave birth only to the names of *Hontu* (superheated air) demons, which take on existence in the mind and go on to cause psychosomatic illness—the *spirit* component of disease. Also present is the Greco-Roman, Aristotelian concept of the four humors and the hot and cold qualities, ultimately incorporated into Arabic Unani medicine.

Despite these attempts to legitimize ethnomedical practices congruent with Islam, Muslim officials do not recognize these healing rituals as part of health care. The situation is complicated by government ministries, where some support the practice, others tolerate it, and still others oppose it. The attitude to traditional ethnomedical healing is very different in the country of Vietnam, for example, as we shall see in this chapter.

INDONESIA

The Indonesian Archipelago consists of tens of thousands of islands, ranging from the semicontinents of Java, Borneo (Kalimantan), and Sumatra, to "islands" within the islands, such as the Vedic Indian enclave of Bali. The indigenous populations and languages are similar to those of Malaya. Indonesia has the largest population of any Islamic country, numbering over 200 million, including the addition of millions of overseas Chinese and Indians, primarily in the urban areas.

Aside from prehistoric archaeological evidence of early humans (fossil "Java man"), relatively little is known of Indonesia before two thousand years ago, when it appears immigrants from Southeast Asia brought the technology of bronze metallurgy, irrigation agriculture, and animal domestication, together with the cult of animism.

Chinese merchants and mariners visited the islands in search of precious gems. In the first century AD, the Han Chinese emperor dispatched a delegation to Sumatra to obtain exotic zoological specimens, as recorded in Chinese texts. Written history in Indonesia (Figure 35-1) itself began only in the fifth century, with the early sequence of Hindu, Buddhist, and Islamic kingdoms, followed by the Portuguese, Spanish, and finally, Dutch. A representation of written medical knowledge is provided by books assembled from Lontaar leaves.

The Persistent Influences of Ayurveda and Islam

Islamic (including Sufi) philosophy plays a major role in influencing traditional medical practices in the Indonesian islands, of which the center of culture is Java. Indonesia was swept by the further reach of Islam in the fifteenth century, extending eastward to the island of Timor and northeast to the southern Philippines. The earlier Vedic influences of Further India were swept back to the island of Bali, where they can be observed today.

The Javanese medical system draws on a wide variety of symbols, roles, and interactional patterns which, as in the Malay communal healing rituals, are not strictly medical. Concepts of personal identity, cosmology, power, and knowledge are blended into a body of closely related theories explaining the origins of disease and motivating highly diverse treatment strategies. Medical pluralism is an inherent feature of Javanese traditional medicine. There are two primary modes of medical practice. One, practiced by holy men (Sufi *wali*), is based on Islamic mystical concepts of miracles and gnosis, clearly grafting the currently predominant Islamic religion onto healing practice. The other, practiced by *dukun* (curers), involves the use of sometimes morally suspect (by Islamic authorities) forms of magical power that has its own origins from celestial sources.

These two modes of medical practice can be seen to reflect a cosmological divide between light and dark, or in the predominant religion's terms, between animism and Islam.

VIETNAM

Vietnam is representative of the former French **Indo-China** (formerly Cambodia, Laos, and North and South Vietnam). For one thousand years, until AD 939, Vietnam was politically part of the Chinese Empire from the Han to the Sung Dynasties. Except for language, Vietnam adopted virtually all of China's culture, including Confucianism, which had come to light during this era. There continued a long period of mutual influence and respect with China because Vietnam did indeed have Chinese culture and had been part of the "Middle Kingdom." When Vietnam was invaded by the Mongols of Kublai Khan in 1288, then ruling China under the Yuan Dynasty, and again in 1427, under the succeeding Ming Dynasty, Vietnam fought them back but was careful to maintain political and cultural ties with China.

At the same time, Vietnam looked beyond China to the north, and expanded to the south, encountering the Khmer Civilization (in what became Cambodia). Throughout history, Vietnam remained largely an agrarian society, organized in villages where the communal good and the ethos of sharing were critical to maintaining health, as in Malaysia.

Despite the strong presence of Chinese medicine, the Vietnamese believe that being ill still means that one has offended a spirit. A spiritual healer prescribes medicine and conducts ritual healing. The Vietnamese also believe in the law of *karma*, where Buddhist teachings are invariably intermixed with those of Confucius. Good and evil influences can be projected and also can come home to roost, in terms of both illness and healing. "Projected vilification" is used to save face—for example, a woman scolding a dog in a village intends that her words are meant for another woman next door, inappropriately scolding and slapping her children. The only ones who did not know what was really happening were the naughty children and the poor dog.

In the nineteenth century, the French introduced Roman Catholicism and Western medicine.

Turning Back to Find a Way Forward

Developments in medicine were thence dominated by periods of armed conflict with Japan, ending in 1945, with France, ending at Dien Bien Phu in 1954, and with the United States, ending in 1975, after which North and South Vietnam became united. During these extended

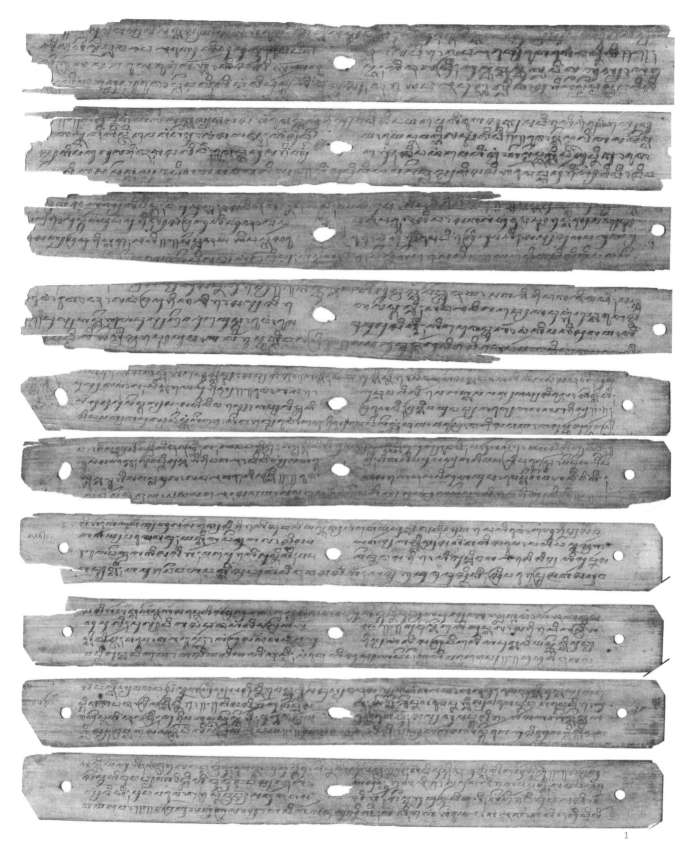

Figure 35-1 Lontaar book, leaf. (Courtesy Dr. Wine Langeraar, 2013.)

1

periods of conflict, Vietnam was unable to obtain Western medicines. Following Vietnam's war of independence from France, an official policy was first articulated by President Ho Chi Minh in 1954, asserting the importance of preserving and developing traditional medicine as a basic component of health care throughout the country because a significant proportion of the population could not afford or obtain modern medicine.

A national heritage program in traditional medicine was established to ensure that the medical knowledge of experienced practitioners was gathered, recorded, and passed on to future generations through formal training programs. Simultaneously, a policy was developed to promote the modernization of traditional medicine and to incorporate it into health service provision integrated with modern medicine. This policy was expanded and strengthened during the 1960s and 1970s, during the war between the North and the South. Emergency medical strategies were generated, including the development of a traditional medical program for the treatment of burns.

After several decades of pharmacognostic and toxicological research, the National Institute of Materia Medica in Hanoi developed a list of 1863 plants of known safety and efficacy in the treatment of common medical conditions. Traditional medicine now accounts for one third of all medical treatments provided (National Institute of Materia Medica, Hanoi, 1990).

Thus, during the U.S.–Vietnam War, for a full decade from 1965 to 1975, North Vietnam actively redeveloped traditional ethnomedical resources to substitute for the Western medicines it could not obtain. After the unification of Vietnam under a communist government and an extended period of political isolation from the West, the government continued to foster the use of traditional ethnomedicine. In light of the rich flora of Indo-China, many medicinal plants provide effective and cost-effective remedies. In addition to the understanding that herbal remedies can be useful for the management of chronic medical conditions, as now accepted in the West, circumstances in Vietnam demonstrated the effectiveness of "alternative" remedies in emergency care, urgent care, and acute care situations In many ways, the intentional and necessary *turning backward* of Vietnam toward ancient medical knowledge and recourses may actually represent *a way forward* for developing countries and for Western, industrialized countries as well.

APPROPRIATE MEDICAL TECHNOLOGY

In Vietnamese peasant communities, there is a common saying that traditional medicine costs one chicken, modern medicine costs one cow, and modern hospital treatment costs the whole herd. Rural people may have to travel for a day or more to reach a modern medical clinic or pharmacy. This requirement results in lost wages, compounded by the cost of transport and the relatively high cost of medicines themselves.

At the basis of global concern about the ever-increasing cost of health care lies the issue of sustainability. Unlike Vietnam, many developing countries are mired in health care systems based on expensive, imported medicines and technologies, and continued reliance on these systems results in health care costs consuming national finances and stifling national economic growth.

Also, industrialized countries are struggling with decisions over who pays for health care—state, employer, the public—and how the escalating costs of high-technology medicine can be controlled.

In the developing world, basic questions are now being asked about priorities in health expenditures and national economic development: How can countries address the health needs of their people without continuing to rely on expensive, imported pharmaceuticals? How can local, existing systems of health care be utilized to provide basic health services to rural and poor communities?

Increased attention is being paid to the potential of *locally available medicinal plants* and *inexpensive herbal medicines,* the keys to diverse and distinct medical practices in providing effective primary health care. This consideration has in turn raised concerns about the sustainable use of wild sources of medicinal plants, the conservation of biodiversity, appropriate forms of local cultivation and production, the safety and effectiveness of natural medicines, and the regulatory environment that should accompany the incorporation of traditional systems of health into national health care.

References

Micozzi M: Traditional Ethnomedicines: Four Levels of Effect, *Hum Organ* 42:351, 1983.

National Institute of Materia Medica, Hanoi, 1990.

Wallace AR: *The Malay Archipelago,* 1869 first published by MacMillan & Co., UK; 1983 unabridged reprint of the last revised edition published by Graham Brash (Pte) Ltd., Singapore.

Suggested Readings

Claver A: *Dutch Commerce and Chinese Merchants in Java: Colonial Relationships in Trade and Finance, 1800–1942,* Leiden, Netherlands, 2014, Brill.

Eiseman FB Jr: *Bali: Sekala & Niskala: Essays on Religion, Ritual, and Art,* North Clarendon, VT, 1990, Tuttle.

Hall KR: *A history of early Southeast Asia: Maritime trade and social development, 100–1500,* Plymouth, UK, 2011, Rowman & Littlefield.

Hanna WA: *Bali chronicles: A lively account of the island's history from early times to the 1970s,* Singapore, 2004, Periplus.

Harthawan ID: *Uang kepeng Cina dalam ritual masyarakat Bali,* Bali, 2013, Pustaka Larasan.

Heng D: *Sino-Malay trade and diplomacy from the Tenth through the Fourteenth Century,* Athens, OH, 2009, Ohio University Press.

Johnson CY: Genetic study finds caste system in ancient India began about 2,000 years ago, 2013, Boston Globe. Available at: http://www.boston.com/news/science/blogs/science-in-mind/2013/08/09/genetic-study-finds-caste-system-ancient-india

-began-about-years-ago/hu52rKxbmjJn3XUMNHS2LK/blog.html. Accessed July 9, 2014.

Johnson CY: Genetic study finds caste system in ancient India began about 2,000 years ago, 2013, Boston Globe. Available at:: http://www.boston.com/news/science/blogs/science-in-mind/2013/08/09/genetic-study-finds-caste-system-ancient-india-began-about-years-ago/hu52rKxbmjJn3XUMNHS2LK/blog.html. Accessed July 9, 2014.

Liu Y: *The Dutch East India Company's Tea Trade with China, 1757–1781*, Leiden, Netherlands, 2006, Brill.

Millburn W: *Oriental Commerce* (vol 2), London, 1813, Black, Parry & Co., pp 527–542.

Milner A: *The Malays*, Oxford, UK, 2011, Wiley-Blackwell.

Moorjani P, Thangaraj K, Patterson N, et al: Genetic Evidence for Recent Population Mixture in India, *Am J Hum Genet* 93(3):422–438, 2013. doi: 10.1016/j.ajhg.2013.07.006.

Munoz PM: *Early kingdoms of the Indonesian Archipelago and the Malay Peninsula*, Singapore, 2006, EDM.

Pringle R: *Understanding Islam in Indonesia: Politics and Diversity*, Singapore, 2010, EDM.

Pringle R: *Bali: Indonesia's Hindu realm*, Singapore, 2011, Talisman.

Ricklefs MC: *A history of modern Indonesia since c. 1200*, ed 3, Hampshire, UK, 2001, Palgrave.

Roger T: The domestic architecture of South Bali, *Bijdragen tot de Taal-, Land- en Volkenkunde Deel* 123:442–475, 1967. 4de Afl.

Rose S: *For all the tea in China*, London, UK, 2009, Arrow Books.

Short T: *A dissertation on the properties and nature of tea*, London, 1930, W. Bowyer, p 11.

Team Penulis Buku: *Mengenal Lebih Dekat, Tempat Ibadat Tri Dharma*, Singaraja, Bali, 2013, Ling Gwan Kiong dan Seng Hong Bio.

Tokunaga K, Ohashi J, Bannai M, Juji T: Genetic link between Asians and Native Americans: evidence from HLA genes and haplotypes, *Hum Immunol* 62(9):1001–1008, 2001.

Vickers A: *Bali: A paradise created*, Hong Kong, 2012, Tuttle.

Zheng Y: *China on the Sea: How the Maritime World Shaped Modern China*, Leiden, Netherlands, 2012, Brill.

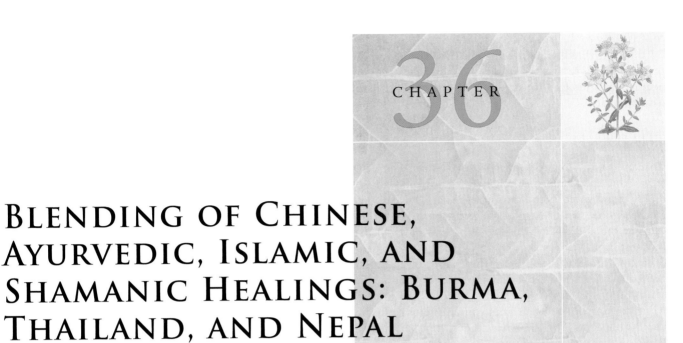

Blending of Chinese, Ayurvedic, Islamic, and Shamanic Healings: Burma, Thailand, and Nepal

LAUREL S. GABLER

MARC S. MICOZZI

Although, historically, China did not ultimately incorporate Burma, Cambodia, Laos, and Thailand into its Empire, as it had Vietnam, the influences of the Middle Kingdom were strong in practical matters such as weights and measures, kite flying, and medicine. Literature and art show the influences of Further India and the teachings of the Buddha, equally claimed by China and East Asia as well. For example, the traditional national Burmese dress, the *longyi*, consists of a wraparound skirt from India and a short formal jacket with three pockets and cloth buttons from China.

BURMA

The Burmese paid tribute to the Emperor of China through most of history. Adjacent to India, Burma became dominated by Britain during the nineteenth and first half of the twentieth centuries. But the Burmese were fiercely resentful of European colonization and became willing to change sides to the Japanese during World War II to drive out the British. They quickly regretted the move when they discovered the Japanese to be far worse than the British as rulers. Traditional medicine is very strong in Burma to this day and has its roots in Ayurveda (see Chapter 31).

ON THE BURMESE–THAI BORDER

In contrast to Thailand (see below), little is known today about the contemporary state of traditional medical practices in Burma, in light of the isolationist and repressive regime in power there since 1962 (what some have called a

"*Ne Win*" situation), aside from anthropological ethnographies from the 1930s and 1950s, by Edmund Leach and others. A recent example among Burmese refugees on the Thai border (which includes the River Kwai, made famous by David Lean's film about the World War II bridge built there by British prisoners of war) illustrates two principles that have been presented throughout this book: the importance of the local materia medica and the ability to adapt and incorporate new resources into medical practice.

Forced migration due to war or persecution of political dissidents can remove people from mainstream medical care and force increased reliance on medical practices from their own cultural traditions, even in the face of unfamiliar local materia medica. In one study of Burmese refugees at the Thai–Burma border, a high degree of traditional medicine use was found despite official views that there was little or no traditional medicine use among these displaced groups (Bodeker et al, 2005).

Surveys of outpatients at a refugee-run clinic at the Thai–Burma border revealed that 59 refugee respondents listed 271 traditional remedies used for common health conditions. Research on psychosocial health found that separation from ancestral spiritual practices and shrines in the home country may exacerbate and even prolong mental health conditions.

Bureaucratic Western refugee aid agencies set the global agenda for refugees and ultimately determine the fate of refugees' health and well-being. By not looking at traditional systems of health care, these agencies are also overlooking a valuable sustainable resource as well as contributing to the loss of important cultural knowledge. By contrast, through harnessing this knowledge and its practices, refugee health agencies could help facilitate new global strategies for coping and new prospects for development.

THAILAND

Thailand's past remains somewhat mysterious. There is a legend that the Thai people originally came from China to escape from Kublai Khan during the Yuan Dynasty. The Khmer civilization of Angkor Wat was overtaken by the Thai in the 1430s, and the Lao Kingdom by the Thai, Burmese, and Vietnamese. The original capital of Siam (Thailand) arose on the waters of the Chao Phraya River. In 1636, a Dutch trader described it as one of the largest cities south of China, "frequented by all Nations, and impregnable," but, after nearly half a millennium, it was sacked by the Burmese in 1767. The new center of Thai culture, Bangkok, was not founded until 1782.

Although Thailand (Siam) remained independent of Greater China, as well as subsequent British and French colonialism, massive immigration from China over the centuries has profoundly influenced Thai practices. The kings of Thailand's present dynasty have Chinese ancestry. Although a relatively recent dynasty in terms of Asian history, the Thai kings have combined the ancient Chinese traits of being considered divine, as well as compiling their histories retrospectively to cast great antiquity upon them. These attributes lend a celestial and spiritual aspect to cultural traditions such as the practice of Thai medicine. In addition, the immigration of millions of Chinese people have brought the systematic forms of Chinese medicine to widespread currency.

The spiritual and the practical exist side by side. A medical officer was practicing on the Gulf of Siam but saw his work endangered by communist insurgents in the late 1960s. He appealed to King Bhumibol at the royal palace and spoke of roads, crops, psychology, the importance of the community, and spirits. The king gave the doctor funds but also commanded him, "I forbid you to become discouraged," in the best tradition of the ancient Chinese emperors.

Spirits are seen to inhabit everything in Thailand. In Bangkok, where a six-lane thoroughfare intersects with an eight-lane highway, stands a shrine to the Hindu deity Brahma, creator of the world, on the site of Erawan Hotel, named for the three-headed elephant ridden by another deity. There had been problems with construction of the new hotel, and Brahma is the patron of builders, since after all, he built the world. The Thai are in awe of spirits—spirits of places and things, living beings, from animals to the semi-divine (such as the king), and spirits of the dead and ancestors, mixing with Chinese as well as Hindu ideas.

In medicine, the spiritual often overcomes the material. Village parents say they don't like to give medicines to their children that might offend them because it was better not

to hurt their feelings. Instead, babies only two weeks old are gently guided by their mothers to put their tiny palms together and raise them to the forehead in the traditional gesture of supplication. As the children grow older, they are taught elevation of the pressed palms to the different degrees: forehead for the Buddha and monks, the nose for superiors, and the chest for subordinates. Many ill children are treated by being taken to the Lord Abbott at the local wat, or Buddhist monastery. A fever is treated by the monk winding a thread around the child. Today, these Buddhist practices are as well established in Thailand as anywhere in the world.

Together with the spiritual emphasis, materia medica also has an important place in medical practice. A prized medicinal substance comes from birds' nests, the soup of which, in the Chinese pharmacopeia, is said to lower blood pressure. Considerable organization and effort is required to harvest them from the vast limestone caverns that tunnel the Thai panhandle and islands, housing hordes of swifts, which secrete a glue-like substance in their mouths to mold delicate nests, sticking them fast to the most remote heights. Collectors harvest the first two nests of the birds, leaving the third for raising their young.

THAI MEDICAL CONCEPTS

Traditional Thai medicine (TTM), as it is practiced today, lies at the intersection of many disparate medical traditions from Indian Ayurvedic and yogic traditions to traditional Chinese medical influences. It draws on each for inspiration, in the process carving out its own unique niche in the medical world. Some observers have tried to distinguish the tradition into formal "medical" and informal "folk healing" practices or tried to unify all of the distinct beliefs under a single theoretical umbrella. However, in actuality, Thai medicine is an amalgam of both formal practices, documented in writing and given credence by the royal court and the Thai government, as well as informal "folk" practices handed down orally and practiced outside of the government sphere. Its diversity and knowledge cannot be easily pigeonholed or grouped within Ayurvedic medicine or TCM.

The Thai notion is that of holistic being and the idea that human life is composed of three essences—body, **mind**/heart (*citta*), and **energy**—which constantly flow into each other and create the "Circle of Life." The body refers to the physical self, the *citta* encompasses the complete inner self—thoughts, emotions, and the spirit—and the energy is the glue that binds the two selves, somewhat analogous to the Chinese notion of *qi*. This energy is an intangible force that flows throughout the body along 72,000 different channels (*sen*) (Salguero, 2003). According to TTM, disease arises from an imbalance in these three interconnected essences. In this way, disease is not merely a physical phenomenon but also an emotional, psychological, and spiritual event. All diseases affect all three essences, and thus all TTM treatment must address all three in order to maintain a proper balance (Salguero, 2006). These three

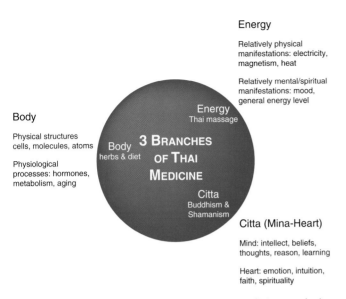

Figure 36-1 The three branches of Thai medicine and the "Circle of Life."

TABLE 36-1 *The Four Body Elements, Their Qualities, and the Organs They Affect*

Element	Quality	Organs
Earth	Solid	Skins, muscles, tendons, bones, viscera, fat, other solid organs
Water	Liquid	Blood, eyes, phlegm, saliva
Air	Movement	Respiration, digestion, excretion, motion of limbs and joints, sexuality, aging
Fire	Heat	Body temperature, circulatory system, metabolism

essences give rise to the three branches of Thai medicine, the goal of which is maintaining a physical, emotional, spiritual, and mental equilibrium (Figure 36-1).

Traditional Thai medicine resembles other Asian traditional medical practices with their holistic views of health and their focus on the relationships among the physical, spiritual, and emotional selves. It parallels Chinese medicine, where energy balance is accomplished through qigong, tai chi, or acupuncture, while *citta* balance is maintained through Mahayana Buddhist and Taoist practices. It also resembles Indian Ayurvedic medicine, where energy balance is maintained through yoga, while *citta* balance is maintained through Hindu practices. In TTM, body balance is maintained through herbal remedies and a proper diet, *citta* balance is maintained through the practice of Buddhism and Thai animism, while energy balance is maintained through Thai massage.

The exact ways in which each of these essences interacts and affects well-being is of little consequence to the TTM practitioner. He does not search for a scientific way of substantiating his beliefs, or seek to understand the rationale behind the various therapies, but takes them as a given. He instead works to help patients maintain existing balance or restore balance when it is disrupted, by prescribing herbal remedies, administering herbal ointments, offering manipulative massage therapies, or reciting various chants or incantations. Balance can be upset by a variety of different factors ranging from environmental or climate factors to dietary factors, from emotional factors to interpersonal relationship factors, from genetic factors to other physical factors. Different TTM practitioners, both formal and informal, are trained to address different aspects of the imbalance using different therapies to do so.

To become a full-fledged TTM doctor, as recognized by the Royal Court and the government, requires three years of official training in herbalism and traditional diagnostics. Massage therapy can be taken during a fourth optional year. In 2005 there were over 37,000 formally recognized TTM practitioners in Thailand, and over 80% of hospitals incorporated some form of TTM into their practice (Chokevivat, 2005a,b). In addition to formal TTM practitioners, there are also a host of different "folk" healers who operate outside of the formal realm to treat both natural and supernatural causes of disease using various ceremonies, charms, amulets, tattoos, and holy incantations (Brun, 2003; Chuakul, 1997). Both these formal and informal practitioners make up the pluralistic medical landscape of Thailand, allowing patients choices from among allopathic, traditional, or folk healers who best suit their spiritual, psychological, and physical needs.

THAI HERBALISM: TREATING THE BODY

The principal goal of Thai medicine is balancing, not only amongst the different essences, but also amongst the different elements that compose the physical body. According to Thai medicine, the physical body is composed of the same four elements that make up the universe—earth, fire, water, and air. The goal of herbalism is to ensure that each of these elements is kept in proper proportion to each other—that they are balanced. This concept is similar to the Ayurvedic notions of cosmology and the body constitutions. Each of the organs of the body can be broken down into various elemental categories based on their qualities and properties (Table 36-1).

Disease develops when any of these elements is in excess, depleted, or completely absent (Table 36-2).

These different elements provide the essential link between patient symptoms and herbal treatments. A patient's symptoms correspond to an excess or depletion of any of these elements, so once the element(s) involved is (or are) identified, the body systems involved can be identified and herbal remedies can be prescribed accordingly. In TTM practice, analogous to some Ayurvedic and Siddha practices in India as well as Chinese food and flavor guidelines, pharmacological substances are classified based on their flavors or tastes—astringent (*fat*), oily (*man*), salty (*khem*), sweet (*wan*), bitter (*khom*), toxic (*mao-buea*), sour

TABLE 36-2 *The Elements of the Body and an Example of What Occurs When They Are in Excess, Depleted, or Completely Absent*

Element (sample organ)	Excess	Depletion	Absence
Earth (Muscle)	Cramps, stress	Weakness, convulsions, poor elasticity in muscles	Inflammation, pain, bruising, spasms, fatigue, muscular atrophy, paralysis
Water (Saliva)	Excess saliva in mouth	Thick saliva, difficulty chewing and swallowing	Dry, painful, bloody mouth; bad breath; dry throat; extreme thirst
Wind (Circulation)	High blood pressure, headache	Low blood pressure, fatigue, faintness	Circulatory failure, unconsciousness, paralysis
Fire (Metabolism)	Fast deterioration of cells and organs	Thick skin and tongue	Bleeding and circulatory problems; blood vessel constriction; brain atrophy; heart failure; death

(*priao*), hot (*phet*), aromatic (*hom yen*), and bland. Each taste has a different effect (either increasing or decreasing) on each of the elements and hence a different effect on body functioning. Because herbs each have a distinctive taste associated with them, different herbal remedies can be used to treat different elemental imbalances (Table 36-3).

Symptoms often simultaneously manifest as both an excess **and** depletion of different elements that need to be teased apart in order for the proper treatments to be administered (Table 36-4). As a result, this process of elemental diagnosis is more of an art than a science, one reason why to be a certified TTM practitioner requires several years of training.

As in China, Thai herbalism practice rarely uses single herbs as a treatment. Rather, they are prescribed as compounds consisting of multiple different ingredients, classified as the main ingredients; *auxiliary* herbs, which support the action of the main ingredients; *controlling* herbs, which are used to reduce the toxicity of and control the compound and coloring; and *flavoring* herbs, which are used to make the concoction more palatable. Herbs can be made into fluid extracts, infusions, alcoholic macerates, pills, or tablets or delivered through an herbal sauna bath, each herb having a different ideal preparation.

Although there are a handful of different herbs unique to Thailand and the practice of TTM, the vast majority of herbs found in TTM texts are also found in the classic Ayurvedic pharmacopoeia. In fact, almost 80% of the herbs found in TTM texts are also found in Ayurvedic texts, while most of the remaining 20% come from popular Chinese remedies. In this way, Thai herbalism draws on multiple external influences, combining them in a multitude of different recipes, which make them uniquely Thai. Thai herbalism builds on existing Asian medical traditions but adds to them and the ways in which they can be used to diagnose and treat the physical body. The vast majority of Thai herbal recipes have been transmitted orally from one generation to the next. As in China and Vietnam, the government of Thailand has launched a massive effort to recover this evanescent Thai knowledge and record it before it is lost forever.

THAI MASSAGE: TREATING THE ENERGY

As Thai herbalism provides a way of balancing the elements of the physical body, Thai massage provides a way to maintain the flow of vital energy throughout that body and to ensure the continual connection between the physical and spiritual selves. Thai massage (*nuat boran*) is a unique blend of both Indian tantric yoga and Chinese acupressure and involves the therapist both manipulating the patient's body into various yogic positions and stimulating specific pressure points along the bodies "sen" or vessels. Although Thai herbalism practice has been standardized across the country, Thai massage differs drastically from one region to the next and from one school to the next. Each school teaches different "sen" lines and different massage techniques. Moreover, Thai massage is often practiced by informally trained healers who have learned the art orally without the theory behind it.

Thai massage can be used both as a preventative measure, to strengthen patients' immunity, increase circulation and lymphatic functioning, and ensure adequate energy flow, and as a form of treatment, by stimulating and relaxing a patient's mind and body to promote the natural healing process and free up trapped energy that may be preventing proper bodily functioning. It can also be used as an *adjunct* therapy to promote healing alongside herbal remedies or other allopathic treatments. Because massage is an art of working with energy, rather than with the body *per se*, traditional massage practitioners are not guided by anatomical structures but instead follow patients' energy meridians, guided by intangible forces.

Thai massage is governed by a Buddhist code of ethics that all practitioners must follow, both inside and outside of their practice. One of the most important aspects of the healing process is the compassionate *intent* of the healer, who must have a deep awareness of himself and his client in order to adequately perform the practice. This compassionate state of mind is referred to as *metta*, which translates directly into "loving kindness." This notion of *metta*, in conjunction with proper techniques, guides the healer in his massage performance. In order to conjure up this *metta*,

TABLE 36-3 *The Ten Tastes and Their Therapeutic Uses*

Taste	Action	For treatment of...	Contraindications
Astringent	Hemostatic, topical astringent, topical antiseptic, diuretic, hepatic, digestive, stomachic, antirheumatic	Internal bleeding wounds, dysentery and other diarrhea, pus, discharge, water retention, liver and stomach disease, sluggish digestion, arthritis	Constipation
Oily	Nutritive tonic	Impaired strength, energy, vitality, chronically low body temperature, stiff and sore joints, muscles and tendons, skin disease, itching	Obesity
Salty	Laxative, antiseptic	Constipation, flatulence, sluggish digestion, excessive mucus in digestive tract, mouth sores	Chronic thirst, dehydration
Sweet	Nutritive tonic, demulcent	Impaired strength, energy and vitality; chronic disease; low immunity; chronic fatigue and exhaustion; convalescence from disease or injury; asthma; sore throat; cough	Diabetes, hypoglycemia, gum disease, tooth decay
Bitter	Bitter tonic, tonic for blood and bile, antipyretic, alternative, cholagogue, heptic, lymphatic	Disease of blood and bile, parasites and infection in blood, fever, dengue, malaria, low immune system functioning	Chronic fatigue
Toxic	Detoxifier, anthelmintic, vermifuge, purgative, analgesic, antiseptic	Systemic infections, tetanus, venereal diseases, cholera, dysentery, diarrhea, gastrointestinal parasites, infections, festering wounds	These herbs have a nauseating taste and smell and should be used only with caution
Sour	Expectorant, pectoral, refrigerant, nervine, diuretic	Congested mucus, respiratory infections, asthma, bronchitis, cough, fever, infection of blood, lymph, sluggish circulation, clarity of mind and senses	
Hot	General stimulant, digestive, carminative, cardiac, expectorant, aphrodisiac, anti-inflammatory, antispasmodic, diaphoretic	Low immunity, chronic fatigue, sluggish digestion, indigestion, flatulence, constipation, sinusitis, common cold, nasal congestion, sore or cramping muscles	Fever, hypertension, cardiac disease
Aromatic	Cardiac tonic, hepatic, pectoral, nervine, sedative, calmative, stimulant, female tonic, detoxifier, diuretic	Heart disease, circulatory problems, disease of liver and lungs, chronic anxiety, tension or stress, hypertension, psychological and emotional imbalances, chronic fatigue, exhaustion, depression, mental clarity and well-being, post-partum depression	Aromatics are typically administered through sauna or steam, which should be avoided by those suffering from fever, heart disease, or high blood pressure
Bland		Food or chemical poisoning, chronic thirst	

TABLE 36-4 *Tastes and Their Effects on the Elements*

Taste	Increases	Decreases
Astringent	Air	Earth, water, fire
Oily (Nutty)	Earth, water, fire	Air
Salty	Earth, water, fire	Air
Sweet	Earth, water	Air, fire
Bitter	Air	Earth, water, fire

every practitioner begins his session with a prayer to Shivago Komarpaj, who was Buddha's doctor and is said to be the founder of TTM.

Whereas herbalism treats the patient's **body** and helps to restore physical balance, and Buddhist prayer treats the patient's **mind** and helps to restore **spiritual** and emotional balance, Thai massage deals with the patient's **energy** and helps to promote its flow throughout the body and mind.

COMBINING FORMAL AND FOLK PRACTICES

Thai herbalism and Thai massage only scratch the surface of the formal practice of TTM, which is documented in books and on stone tablets such as those found at Wat Pho in Bangkok. These formalized practices and the theories behind them draw heavily on influences from India, China, and other surrounding nations. In fact, in many respects these theories and traditions evolved in the way they did—to resemble Ayurvedic, yogic and Chinese practices—because of pressure by the Thai government to standardize them and legitimize them in the way these other medical practices have now been legitimized. By being grounded in theory and documented in books, TTM gained a credence it had once lacked and thus became a formal healing art. However, in the process of standardizing and formalizing TTM, a lot of important traditional "folk" practices were left out of the literature and out of the training. These "folk" practices have both shaped TTM and given it a unique flair, and set Thai medicine apart from Chinese medicine and Ayurveda.

On the one hand, formal TTM emphasizes the internal world and the internal balance amongst the different essences and amongst the different elements that comprise the physical body. In this way, disease is seen as an internal imbalance. On the other hand, TTM also deals, in a less formal sense, with the external world and the external spiritual forces that can cause disease or malady. This aspect of Thai medicine, dealing with the cosmos, like the ancient Shamanic traditions, is not the purview of formally trained TTM doctors but rather the realm of "folk" healers who use magical powers or spiritual allies to treat or protect patients. Together, these two brands of Thai medicine can address both the internal and external, and the supernatural and natural causes of disease. According to Thai beliefs, it is even possible for these external forces to upset internal balance, so it is important to understand not only the formal practices of Thai herbalism and Thai massage but also the informal practices of the *mo tjalo* (folk practitioners), *mo du* (fortune tellers), *mo song* (diviners), *mo phi* (spirit mediums), and *mo wicha* (controllers of magical powers).

While folk healing traditions are not based on learned ideas or coherent theories, beliefs about the supernatural realm are deeply entrenched in the fabric of Thai culture and thus play an important part in Thai medicine. Spirit mediums can be used to maintain harmony between the human and spirit worlds to ensure that the needs of spirits are met so they do not harm human beings. Other spirit mediums are said to have the ability to pacify ghosts or demons using consecrated water and holy chants to drive them from the bodies of possessed individuals. Still other folk healers are said to be able to call back a soul that has been dislodged or lost, and in doing so, restore health to that individual. *Tham khwan,* or calling of the soul, usually involves offerings, chanting, and the binding of the patient's right wrist with **consecrated thread** to metaphorically tie the soul to the body once it has returned.

It is not just folk healers, however, who use incantations or call on spirits to affect health. Even traditionally trained Thai herbalists recite sacred chants over their medicinal concoctions to give them additional spiritual potency, and Thai massage therapists call on the spirits of past teachers to guide them in their treatment work. Thai medicine is an amalgam of both formal practices, which require formal training and follow requisite courses, and informal, folk practices, which are practiced by village "folk" healers and transmitted orally. In making decisions about treatment options, a patient rarely sees the therapeutic options

available as mutually exclusive. It is often the case that people seek a multitude of different allopathic, folk, and formal TTM treatments in addressing their maladies—further blurring the lines that separate one practice from the next. So rather than lumping all TTM practices under a single unified theory, it helps to understand under what circumstances each practice is most suitable because, more often than not, dealing with ailments requires treatment of both the supernatural and natural causes of illness by restoring balance amongst all three essences and elements, using herbs, acupressure, chants, and allopathic medicines in succession.

In this way, Thai medicine embodies the merger of medical concepts and practices from Greater China with Further India, as well as relying upon local resources.

NEPAL

Cycling back to the Himalayas, northwest of Burma, brings one to **Nepal**, which is located between China and India. Nepal has endeavored to preserve a unique identity from that of its strong neighboring cultures. Although Nepal is not considered a part of Southeast Asia, Nepali traditional medicine has been influenced as much by Chinese medicine and Ayurvedic traditions as has TTM. It is one of the poorest countries in the world, but is also one of the most culturally diverse, with over a dozen distinct ethnic groups, each with its own traditions and languages. Traditional medicine is strongly influenced by surrounding Tibeto-Siberian and Indo-Shamanic traditions (Casper, 1979), as well as Tibetan (Chapter 30), Ayurvedic (Chapter 31), and Unani (Chapter 32) medical systems. The shamanic folk medical tradition illustrates both medical pluralism and a defined hierarchy of resort (Chapter 34). Nepal is as diverse in its practice and philosophy as the country itself.

This intersection of these traditions is apparent in the formal, scholarly system of traditional medicine in the country. First, there is a strong Ayurvedic presence, which manifests itself in the two central-level Ayurvedic hospitals, the fourteen zonal *Ayurvedalayas*, the 55 district Ayurvedic health centers, the 216 Ayurvedic health dispensaries, and the over 391 Ayurvedic physicians registered with the government (Dixit, 2005). The government runs an Ayurvedic production unit that manufactures over one hundred different Ayurvedic *churna* (powders), *vati/gutika* (pills and tablets), *avaleha* (semisolid concoctions), *asava/arishta* (fermented preparations), *bhasma/pisti* (ash and fine powders), and *taila/ghrita/malham* (medicated oils and ghee ointments) (Gewali, 2008).

As in India, the Nepali government has also recognized the formalization of homeopathic treatment through the creation of a six-bed homeopathic hospital, which treats 250 patients daily, and through the establishment of a homeopathy medical college, which graduates ten students per year (Gewali, 2008). The country recognizes and supports the large presence of Tibetan *Amchis*, which are financed through the *Himalayan Amchi Association* and trained through the *Lo Kunphen* school in far western Nepal. Finally, the country accepts Unani medicine through a government-sponsored Unani dispensary, staffed by *hakims* (Unani doctors trained in India) (Gewali, 2008).

While the formal traditional systems of medicine demonstrate the strong influence of India, Tibet, and Europe, in the realms of folk medicine and informal shamanic healing practices, Nepal differentiates itself. There is a multi-tiered public health infrastructure that extends into the rural communities and provides a host of free services to the population, including formalized, government-supported Ayurvedic, homeopathic, Amchi, and Unani programs. Nonetheless, a sizable number of rural Nepalese still seek care outside the governmental sector, either from unofficial faith healers or through self-treatment using herbs culled from their surroundings. In fact, there are more traditional healers (THs) in Nepal than there are certified health personnel. It has been estimated that there are between 400,000 and 800,000 people who render faith healing in the country, and they are found in almost every ward of every village in rural Nepal (Dixit, 2005; Neupane & Khanal, 2010).

More than just outnumbering medical professionals, THs are more physically accessible, as well as more culturally acceptable, to the vast majority of patients (Poudyal et al, 2003). At one point, the government started several training programs for THs in an attempt to extend the populace's embrace of these healers to increase the use of government health services (Oswald, 1983). Part of the reason for their acceptability is that they are aligned with many patients' belief systems and allow patients to address the spiritual, not just the physical, causes of ill health and to address what are perceived to be the deeper sources of illness (Dixit, 2005). The quotes in Table 36-5 illustrate the diversity of different etiology beliefs that Nepalese people hold.

In a pluralistic cultural setting like that in rural Nepal, multiple illness etiology beliefs abound, not only from one household to the next, but also within households or even within individuals. These beliefs range drastically from those in which personal responsibility is important, to those that relinquish all responsibility and focus solely on external factors or the foul play of others as the cause of illness. Certain diseases seem to lend themselves to particular belief systems dictated by the larger community in which an individual is embedded, but there remains diversity of opinions for specific illnesses as well. Some illnesses, like pneumonia, seem to engender greater consensus on their causes—cold weather or unsanitary environmental conditions—whereas other illnesses draw on a wide range of beliefs. The diversity of beliefs is associated naturally with a diversity of providers.

There is a host of different healers, each serving different purposes, each consulted for different illnesses by different ethnic groups. *Jhankris* and *dhamis* are spirit mediums who can put themselves or patients into trances by chanting and beating drums or use animal sacrifices and spells to break curses. *Ojha* are healers who can receive referrals only from other healers when those healers have failed to treat an illness. *Lamas, pundits, pujaris,* and *gubhajus* are all priestly healers who are said to diagnose and cure illnesses through Buddhist tantric prayers and rituals. *Jyotishis* are astrologers who use numerology and horoscopes to discern the effects of various *graha* (planets) on health and well-being. On the other hand, *Jadi* and *Buti Walas* are considered medical providers and use herbal elixirs and preparations for treatment of ailments (Dixit, 2005; Gewali, 2008; Gartoulla, 2008).

TABLE 36-5 *Etiology Beliefs Held by Nepalese People*

Etiology belief	Quote(s)
Evil Spirits	***Regarding a Sudden Loss of Consciousness:*** *Apparently an ox had died last year by falling off the same cliff. I lived because God held out his arms to catch me . . . There was probably an evil spirit roaming around there. There are evil spirits in that place. They say such things happen from time to time even now . . . It is said that there is something that makes people feel intoxicated, unconscious and causes them to fall. They say you don't realize you are falling. A villager around there told me this . . . What happens in places where evil spirits seize you and intoxicate you is that there is a "Hyo" [a kind of evil spirit]. That is what intoxicates you and makes you fall. If you fall, you have to kill or chase away the "Hyo" of the place where you fell. You have to kill it at either sunrise or sunset. (61, M)*
Curse/Evil Intentions of Others	***Regarding Pneumonia:*** *I asked what happened and he [TH] said it was due to "chuachut." He said that a woman had come to my house and she looked at him with evil intentions. I don't know if that is true or not. I don't know who came. (27, F)*
Eating/Food Habits	***Regarding Typhoid:*** *Food is the factor that causes typhoid. Apparently, it occurs if you drink alcohol and eat meat. I am also someone who drinks alcohol and eats meat. We never know when we have fever and as we continue to eat such things, we suffer from typhoid. (50, M)* ***Regarding Pneumonia:*** *It starts with cough and cold. Then the mother eats everything including the sour kind of food and that affects the baby . . . The mother eats carelessly . . . Whatever the mother eats goes into her milk, which the baby feeds on. (17, F)*

Continued

TABLE 36-5 *Etiology Beliefs Held by Nepalese People—cont'd*

Etiology belief	Quote(s)
Inadequate Diet/ Dirty Food	**Regarding Typhoid:** *It is "khaibigar." Once you have "khaibigar" you become weak. You can't digest anything you eat and you suffer from high fever . . . "Khaibigar" means there is something wrong with what you eat. One's strength wasn't adequate, blood circulation couldn't occur and the fever won over one's body . . . If dirt gets into the food, then people certainly fall ill. (54, F)*
Alcohol	**Regarding Tonsillitis:** *Well, the reason could be that we eat a lot of spicy food and drink alcohol. When there are festivals, we invite people, we get invited as friends, we celebrate together and when we celebrate we have to drink. That is probably why it's seen commonly. (38, F)*
"From Within"/ Eating Habits	**Regarding Abdominal Pain/Gastritis:** *Some people believe that witches or spirits cause illness, but I don't think such things happen. People have illnesses in their own bodies. So, why would one blame another for their illness? They should seek treatment instead . . . I should eat on time. Apparently, gastritis occurs if you don't eat regularly and on time, and it can be cured if you eat on time. (35, F)*
Changing Seasons	**Regarding Diarrhea:** *I think it happens mostly when the winter season ends and summer starts . . . We have to be careful during the months of Falgun, Chaitra, Baisakh, and Jestha [February to July]. (50, M)*
Cold Weather	**Regarding Migraines:** *I feel it might be because my head was hit by wind during the postnatal period . . . Cold wind. We have to walk around even during the period right after childbirth. In the village, we aren't allowed to rest inside our houses. We have to walk around like we would at any other time. Sometimes I think that is the reason. (41, F)*
	Regarding an upper respiratory tract infection (URTI): *He became ill because of the weather. You can't really control a child's behaviour. Even if you make him wear warm clothes and a hat, he removes them instantly. He doesn't know what's good for him and what's not. So I think he is suffering from this illness because of the cold weather. I haven't thought about any other reasons. (24, M)*
Hygiene/Unhygienic Environment	**Regarding Undiagnosed Uterine Problems:** *I think it might be because in the village we have to clean the cattle's dung and work in an unhygienic environment during our postnatal periods. (28, F)*
	Regarding Pneumonia: *Cleanliness could be a factor. The mother needs to take care of her child's cleanliness and hygiene no matter how busy she is . . . I thought I was careful about this. (27, F)*
External Environmental Factors: Smoke	**Regarding TB:** *I don't drink alcohol or smoke cigarettes. Perhaps because I make alcohol I am exposed to the smoke that is formed from the fire used while making alcohol. I feel that is the reason . . . I have TB because it developed in my own body. (42, F)*
External Factor/ Community Belief	**Regarding an Ear Infection:** *The elders used to say that when a mother feeds a baby her milk, the milk goes into the baby's ears and they get infected. I knew that but I don't know if milk has entered into my ears. (42, M)*
Physical Factor/ Heavy Work	**Regarding TB:** *I am thinking there is something wrong in my lungs . . . I also did work that involved lifting heavy loads (i.e., stones, wood) for around two months. I also feel that this might be the reason. (36, M)*
Bad Luck	**Regarding a Fall Injury from Top of Bus:** *It was bad luck. His daughter was also asking him to come inside, but he didn't . . . If he had listened to his daughter and sat inside . . . When one has evil luck, one can't really do much. (Respondent 1, 44, F)*
	Even if I had not fallen from the bus, I definitely would have been injured some other way. (46, M)
"From Within"	**Regarding Lower Abdominal Pain:** *I feel it develops from deep inside . . . I think it has developed from inside my body. I don't think it is due to external factors such as the cold weather and wind. (22, F)*
Emotional Problems/Stress/ Worry	**Regarding Schizophrenia:** *I think he's suffering from this illness because he lost a lot of money . . . He used to be very stressed about money. Someone else took his land so he has developed mental illness. He keeps thinking about the same thing over and over again. (18, M)*
	Regarding Anxiety: *Other than that, I was suffering from gastritis from before this illness started. It had been a month since I started taking medicines; I was worried about that too. Sometimes I wonder if that worry caused this illness. (18, M)*
Germs	**Regarding a URTI:** *There are germs in the surrounding air we don't know about that can cause sickness. (24, M)*
Other Natural Factors	**Regarding Eye Injury:** *My sisters say that because I did not go to the astrologer and consult with him when this house was built, such things are happening to me. I had actually gone to the astrologer and put the date this house was built on as Jestha 1. Yet my friends and sisters say that I didn't follow the proper procedure. Also, my buffalo died nine days ago. (33, F)*
Multiple Beliefs: Cleanliness, Weather, Transmission from Others	**Regarding Mumps:** *Perhaps it is due to lack of cleanliness; farmers are unable to look after their children very well . . . The weather is also probably a factor. If not, the illness should be occurring all the time . . . Perhaps because it is a communicable disease. When one child in the school gets it, all the others seem to get this illness . . . They say it transmits if you share food. They [son and daughter] eat from the same plate, being from the same household. (40, F)*

Traditional healing and allopathic medicine, however, are not mutually exclusive healing systems. Often people will consult THs to address the spiritual aspects and then consult allopathic care providers to address the physical aspects of their illness (Jimba et al, 2003). Despite their prominent role in the informal health care infrastructure of rural Nepal, and despite attempts to use them to facilitate referrals to allopathic providers, THs have yet to be fully incorporated into government health policies and are often neglected by the government as part of people's health-seeking pathways.

TRADITIONAL HEALING VERSUS ALLOPATHIC MEDICINE IN RURAL NEPAL[1]

But how do individuals living in such a complex, pluralistic medical environment make determinations about which providers to consult? As research in Makwanpur District has shown, there seems to be a set of rules to which most households subscribe—not so much to determine whether to use a TH or allopathic provider (referred to as "HP" or health post), but to help them determine the order in which to use them (hierarchy of resort; see Chapter 34).

Most of the decisions about whether or not to use TH or allopathic care first have to do with the nature of the disease. For many households, certain illnesses are the purview of the TH and others are the purview of allopathic medicine. Depending on which category an illness falls into, a specific provider is to be utilized first. Some of this decision process had to do with the specific symptoms an individual is experiencing. For example, illnesses that involve vomiting, dizziness, and sudden pain are for THs first, whereas headaches, coughs, and difficulty breathing are for allopathic providers.

> THs can only treat illnesses that are caused due to ghosts or spirits and for pain that occurs suddenly . . . When you feel your blood pressure is high and when you are vomiting, they can heal you. The THs are also important and so are doctors. When it is hurting somewhere, when one has a headache, a cough or difficulty breathing, one should go to a doctor. If one feels dizzy, one should go to a TH, and if that doesn't help, then go to a hospital. (46, M)

These rules are not just about specific categories of symptoms but also about the evolution of the symptoms. For example, if pain is localized, it is an illness for allopathic professionals, but if it radiates, THs should be consulted first.

> If pain starts suddenly in a certain part of the body and moves to other parts of the body gradually, then we consult the TH. If the pain doesn't move to parts of the body other than the initial part, then we go to the hospital. (24, M)

The decision is not solely restricted to the types of symptoms experienced, or to their progression, but also to the timing of their onset. Sudden illnesses are for THs first, whereas more gradual ones are for allopathic medicine.

> For sudden illness, it [TH] works quite well, but for other illnesses, not so much . . . I think one should go to the hospital. If someone has a sudden illness or vomits without any reason they should consult the TH. However, if the illness continues one to two days after consulting the TH, then they should either go to the hospital or the health post. (35, F)

> When someone suddenly faints and no one knows what caused it, then we seek a TH, suspecting the influence of spirits. If someone becomes sick gradually, then they go to the health post. But, if the illness comes suddenly with vomiting, then we suspect that spirits caused it. (25, F)

Still, the decision rules are not pertinent to symptoms alone, but also to etiology beliefs (which may manifest themselves in certain categories of symptoms). Illnesses thought to be brought about by external factors are for THs first; illnesses that arise from within are for allopathic medicine first.

> If a disease is generated inside your own body, then medicines from the HP will work, but sometimes evil spirits pass through the human body, which leads to heart pain and vomiting. So, to cure that, a TH is called . . . Both the services of the TH and the health post are equal, I guess. (43, F)

> I trust doctors more because they are able to cure inner diseases, but the TH is only able to cure diseases outside the body. I think, though, that the people who rely **only** on the TH, die. (33, F)

For some households, it is about the distinction between illnesses of the body—physical concerns (for allopathic care) and illnesses of the soul—emotional concerns (for TH care).

> If the body has already physically suffered, then THs cannot do anything. But, if you live with worries, then the doctors can't do anything. I think they are equal. (21, M)

For other households, it is about the illness severity. More severe illnesses also require the TH in addition to the hospital.

> If the illness is very serious, there is need of traditional healing, and we seek it. Otherwise, we just go to the hospital. (30, F)

For illnesses of children, these same decision rules hold up. For illnesses with an unknown cause—manifested as shock or continuous crying—people consult the TH first. For diseases or illnesses with a known origin or cause, people consult allopathic professionals.

> In the village we believe in both kinds of healing—traditional healing and healing using modern medicines. When it is the case of spirits, the TH can heal it, but in the case of a cough, the TH cannot . . . For example, if a child gets shock or frightened, experiences pain and cries

[1]The quotes and information from this section come from a qualitative study of health-seeking behaviors carried out in three villages in Makwanpur District in 2011 by a researcher at Oxford University.

continuously, we call a TH. However, when the child gets cold and cough or fractures its limbs, then we take the child to the hospital. (24, M)

So, too, are certain categories of symptoms in children also considered to be the domain of traditional healing, while others are the domain of allopathic medicine.

There are some cases in children that need TH's consultations, while other that need medicines. If they are vomiting, then they should be taken to the TH, and if they have a fever, cough etc., they should be given medicines. (29, F)

Together, THs and allopathic providers and services can cover the entire spectrum of symptoms, illness etiologies, and illness courses. As a result, most households felt that it was bad to use only one of them, and that both had to be trusted and used in combination.

I believe in both doctors and THs. As the TH has been able to cure my illness slightly, I believe in him too. The doctors are very important and THs are important in some ways. But the THs aren't as important as the doctors. (18, F).
He [TH] comes and examines the pulse, but I didn't depend on the TH only. The fever got aggravated and after that, no matter how much medicine I gave her, it didn't work. So, after that, I sought care from the TH and it worked. I think both treatments [TH and HP] help. It is not good to believe in only one type of treatment. (25, F)
I went to the TH after the health post. You can't completely have faith in the health post—I feel like you should also use the TH. (30, F)
The tradition passed from several generations of collecting herbs in the jungle to consulting THs to finally getting examined by doctors. I feel that doing both at the same time will cure me. (77, M)

Many households simply feel for whatever reasons that they cannot rely solely on one provider in isolation.

Sometimes it is possible [to be influenced by evil spirits], you know. But we cannot totally rely on the TH. It is okay to follow him once or twice with all those burning of incense and throwing of rice grains, but we have to visit the medical of the health post later. I feel that only relying on the health post, hospital or TH is also not enough. (44, F)

Taking people to multiple providers is thought to expedite the recovery process.

The patients here are usually taken to the TH first and then to the health post. I will take him [son] there [TH] and on my way back to the health post. I think it will help him recover quicker. (20, F)

In part, though, the reason for consulting with multiple providers may also be predicated on something more practical—not wanting to offend any individual provider.

We should see and consult here and there. We have to see and consult both ways [traditional and allopathic]. We should be cautious where we go because it might cause

heartache in one of the providers if we go to one and do not show the illness to the other. (28, F)

Or these consulting patterns may have something to do with the fact that the methods employed by both providers are distinct. THs simply do things doctors cannot, and doctors do things THs cannot—they complement one another.

There are certain traditional healers that until they put a spell on the people suffering from heartache, they don't get cured at all. For these types of cases only, they can do it. Those types of THs I believe in, but I also believe in doctors. (77, M)

Or the consultation process may be motivated by completely impractical reasons—a willingness to try anything and everything that could potentially help with the recovery.

If the treatment could heal you, then you have to understand it is a good influence. We have also gone there [to TH] because we like the treatment. But we did not only rely on the TH; that's why we also went for treatment [at pharmacy]. We took advice both from the TH and the medical. (28, F)

In many cases, though, when someone in a family is healed after having sought care from multiple providers, both are attributed with the recovery process.

The TH also helped her [daughter] get better. As did the medical. We need TH and we need medicals. Everything has to work out. (35, M)

So, while it helps to look at each provider in turn and determine the specific reasons why each household may have selected a specific provider, this approach creates a false dichotomy between traditional care and allopathic care that really does not exist in the majority of health decision-making within the Nepalese context (although this might be changing somewhat). Health decisions are usually not a zero sum equation, so even if a household opts for an allopathic provider, it does not mean that they do not believe in THs or that they will not use them later in their health pathways. These decision rules, however, which have been culturally and socially shaped and defined, make it easier for households to decide when to seek certain providers first. When dealing with THs versus allopathic medicine, this decision is usually predicated on the nature of the illness more than anything else.

Preserving Thai Medicine

With deforestation threatening to destroy important plant life, and with the ever-increasing emphasis placed on allopathic approaches to health, it is becoming more important than ever to preserve traditional medical practices lest they vanish. It is important not only to keep traditions intact, but also to continue to adapt

Preserving Thai Medicine—cont'd

them to the ever-changing societies and environments in which they will inevitably exist.

The Chaophya Abhaibhubejhr Hospital in Prachin-buri, Thailand (Figure 36-2), provides an ideal model for how to keep traditional medicine alive both as a distinct discipline and practice and as an integrated part of an increasingly Western medical establishment. Established in 1941, the 505-bed hospital is the pride and joy of Eastern Thailand. Not only does the hospital boast modern medical facilities and equipment, and over 600 technical staff, but it also offers a wide array of TTM treatment services ranging from Thai massage to integrated stroke rehabilitation services, all of which utilize herbal products produced on the hospital premises. One of the major focuses of the hospital over the past 22 years has been to encourage and revitalize the use of Thai herbal medicines in everyday practice. More than just accepting the efficacy of these herbs as they have been passed down from generation to generation, the hospital has devoted its efforts to scientific research to prove their efficacy and to enable them stand alongside modern pharmaceuticals. The hospital generates over $250,000 per month through the sales of its herbal medicines and cosmetics. In conjunction with local farmers, who provide and harvest all the raw herbal materials, the hospital produces more than 18 herbal medicines, 7 dietary supplements, 35 toiletries and cosmetics, and 7 health beverages, all of which are tested, packaged, and sold on the premises (Figure 36-3).

In addition to the TTM and allopathic services offered, the hospital also contributes both formally and informally to shaping the next generation of TTM practitioners through its Thai Traditional Medical College, outreach and education programs, hospital tour programs, and the Abhaibhubejhr Thai Traditional Medicine Museum, which presents its over 500 visitors per month with an overview of the history and philosophy of TTM.

Ban Dong Bang Village Herbal Farming Group

What started over 50 years ago as a failing rice farm today is home to one of the most successful, fully organic herb farms in all of Thailand. Spanning over 40 acres of land, the Ban Dong Bang Village farm is cooperatively run by 11 families. The farm grows over 40 different types of organic herbs, several of which are unique to Thailand. All of the herbs are harvested in accordance with the World Health Organization guidelines for Good Agricultural Practice (WHO, 2003) (Figure 36-4). Once they are cleaned and dried, the herbs are then sold to the hospital for the production of its medicines and products.

In an area where rice farming is not sufficient to keep local farms afloat, the hospital has single-handedly contributed to the economic stability of Prachinburi and its local farmers by partnering with them in the maintenance and modernization of TTM.

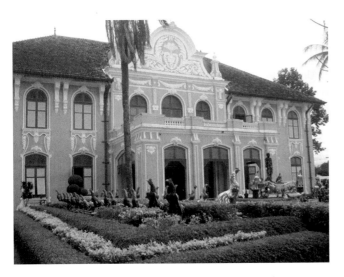

Figure 36-2 The Chaophya Abhaibhubejhr Hospital.

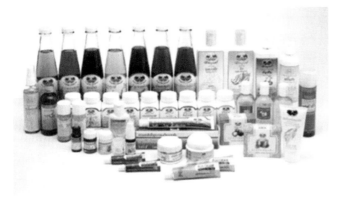

Figure 36-3 Products produced at the Chaophya Abhaibhube-jhr Hospital.

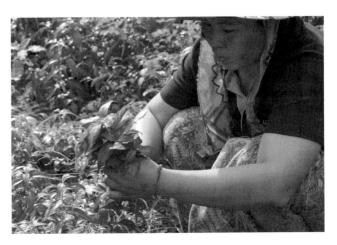

Figure 36-4 Herb harvesting.

References

Bodeker G, Neumann C, Lall P, Oo ZM: Traditional medicine use and healthworker training in a refugee setting at the Thai-Burma border, *J Refug Stud* 18(1):76–99, 2005.

Brun V: Tradtional Thai Medicine. In Selin H, Shapiro H, editors: *Medicine Across Cultures: History and Practice of Medicine in Non-Western Cultures*, Boston and London, 2003, Kluwer Academic Publishers.

Casper MJ: *Faith-healers in the Himalayas: an investigation of traditional healers and their festivals in Dolakha District of Nepal*, Kathmandu, 1979, Centre for Nepal and Asian Studies, Tribhuvan University.

Chokevivat V, Chuthaputti A: *The Role of Thai Traditional Medicine in Health Promotion*, Thailand, 2005a, Department for the Development of Thai Traditional and Alternative Medicine, Ministry of Public Health, 6GCHP Bangkok, pp 7–11.

Chokevivat V, Chuthaputti, A, Khumtrakul P: *The Use of Traditional Medicine in the Thai Health Care System*, Pyongyang, DPR Korea, 2005b, World Health Organization Regional Office for South East Asia: Regional Consultation on Development of Traditional Medicine in the South East Asia Region, pp 22–24. Document no. 9.

Chuakul W: *Medicinal Plants in Thailand* (vol 2), Bangkok, 1997, Department of Pharmaceutical Botany, Mahidol University.

Dixit H: *Nepal's Quest for Health*, Kathmandu, 2005, Educational Publishing House.

Gartoulla RP: *Textbook of Medical Sociology and Medical Anthropology*, Kathmandu, 2008, Research Centre for Integrated Development.

Gewali MB: *Aspects of Traditional Medicine in Nepal*, Toyama, 2008, Institute of Natural Medicine, University of Toyama.

Jimba M, Poudyal AK, Wakai S: The need for linking healthcare-seeking behaviors and health policy in rural Nepal, *Southeast Asian J Trop Med Public Health* 34(2):462–463, 2003.

Neupane D, Khanal V: *A Textbook of Health Service Management in Nepal*, Kathmandu, 2010, Vidyarthi Pustak Bhandar.

Oswald IH: Are traditional healers the solution to the failures of primary health care in rural Nepal? *Soc Sci Med* 17(5):255–257, 1983.

Poudyal AK, Jimba M, Murakami I, et al: A traditional healers' training model in rural Nepal: strengthening their roles in community health, *Trop Med Int Health* 8(10):956–960, 2003.

Salguero PC: *A Thai Herbal: Traditional Recipes for Health and Harmony*, Chiang Mai, 2003, Silkworm Books.

Salguero PC: *The Spiritual Healings of Traditional Thailand*, Scotland, 2006, Findhorn Press.

World Health Organization: *WHO Guidelines on Good Agricultural and Collection Practices (GACP) for Medicinal Plants*, Switzerland, 2003, World Health Organization. Available at: http://apps.who.int/medicinedocs/en/d/Js4928e/. Accessed July 14, 2014.

Suggested Readings

Chomchalow N, Bansiddhi J, MacBaine C: *Amazing Thai Medicinal Plants*, Bangkok, 2003, Horticultural Research Institute Department of Agriculture.

Micozzi MS: *Vital Healing: Energy Mind & Spirit in Traditional Medicine of India and Middle Asia*, London, 2011, Singing Dragon Press.

Mullholland J: Thai Traditional medicine: ancient thought and practice in a Thai context, *J Siam Soc* 67(2):80–115, 1979a.

Mullholland J: Traditional Thai medicine in Thailand, *Hemisphere* 23(4):224–229, 1979b.

Mullholland J: *Herbal Medicine in Paediatrics: Translation of a Thai Book of Genesis*, Canberra, 1989, Australian National University.

Salguero PC: *Encyclopedia of Thai Massage: A Complete Guide to Traditional Thai Massage Therapy and Acupressure*, Scotland, 2004, Findhorn Press.

Salguero PC: *Traditional Thai Medicine: Buddhism, Animism, Ayurveda*, Prescott, 2007, Hohm Press.

Saralamp P: *Medicinal Plants in Thailand* (vol 1), Bangkok, 1996, Department of Pharmaceutical Botany, Mahidol University.

Subcharoen S: *Thai Traditional Medicine: System and Practice*, 1989, Faculty of Graduate Studies, Mahidol University.

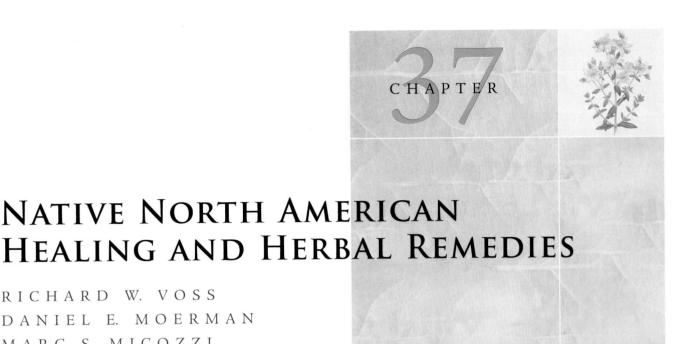

NATIVE NORTH AMERICAN HEALING AND HERBAL REMEDIES

RICHARD W. VOSS

DANIEL E. MOERMAN

MARC S. MICOZZI

Long before Columbus landed in what he thought was Hindustan (India) in 1492, the indigenous peoples of the Americas practiced a highly advanced medicine that was effective in combating diseases then common in the Americas. These medicine ways emphasized the "right order of things" in the **cosmos** and the **community** and viewed humans not as some higher intellectual being above lower animals, plants, and the earth, but as a kindred partner in the cosmos, relying on the other beings in creation for life itself.

The worldview of the new European visitors to the Americas prompted misunderstandings and exploitation of the peoples they called *Indios,* a corruption of the Spanish, derived from Columbus's perception of the people he encountered in the New World. He described them as *"una gente en Dios,"* which literally means "a people in with God."

Tragically, this early perception of the natural peacefulness, harmony, and ease of temperament of these "Indians" prompted Columbus to comment that "they would make excellent slaves," perhaps helping to set the stage for eventual degradation of the indigenous, or natural, peoples and cultures of the Americas. The "natural" style of these people was to be perceived as *"brutish"* and *"savage";* their attentiveness to primal experience would be perceived as *"primitive";* their understanding of the cosmos (all of creation) as infused with life and spirit would be seen as *"animistic."* In all these assessments, what was "Indian" was evaluated as inferior to the European cultural standards, including advanced technology and "higher" (theistic) religion(s).

That the single name *Indian* was imposed on the indigenous peoples of the Americas was erroneous because they were not a homogeneous group but rather distinct *"nations"* or "peoples" with different languages, beliefs, customs, social and political structures, and historical rivalries. The term *American Indian* is used today to talk about common values and a certain shared identity among many Native American people, and it is also used as the legal title of federally recognized tribes holding jurisdiction on reservation lands in the United States.

The indigenous people of Canada and the Six Nations' People (*Iroquois*) preferred the term *Natives,* which is the official term used by the Canadian government to identify indigenous people. The terms *American Indian, Native American,* and *Indian People* are used interchangeably throughout this chapter, with awareness of the complexity associated with these terms.

ANCIENT LIFEWAYS AND MEDICINE IN THE AMERICAS

For Indian people, *all* aspects of life were intimately connected to good health and well-being. The interconnections among family, tribe, or clan; moral, political, and ceremonial life all contributed to a sense of *harmony* and *balance* that was called *wicozani* (good total health) by the **Lakota** Sioux and *hozhon* (harmony, beauty, happiness, and health) by the **Navajo.**

Traditional Navajo healing practices revolve around the notion of *hozho,* a term that embodies the concepts of balance, harmony, and *spirituality.* When people achieve a life of *hozho,* they walk the "beauty way," and their lives are filled with peace, contentment, and positive health—physically, mentally, emotionally, and spiritually. Positive interconnections among family, clan, tribe, nature, all living things, and ceremonial life all contribute to a sense of harmony and balance, which is the achievement of *hozho*. When a Navajo medicine man performs a healing ceremony, a circle of healing is formed by the interconnection among the sick person, family, relatives, the spirits, and singers who help with ceremonial songs. For traditional Navajo, the world is a *dangerous place* requiring due caution and respect; there is an emphasis on preventing harm from occurring through ceremonies (*hozonji*) to better meet this dangerous world. Navajo healers (*Hatalie*) use sand paintings to cure the sick person (Figure 37-1). A

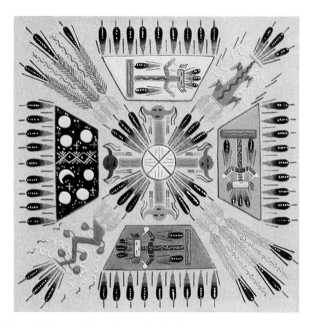

Figure 37-1 Traditional sand painting (Artist: Frank Martin). (Courtesy Penfield Gallery of Indian Arts, Albuquerque, NM, http://www.penfieldgallery.com.)

very stylized sand painting is drawn using various colors of sand; on its completion, the patient is instructed to sit on the painting while the healing ceremony is performed. Healing takes place as the sick person absorbs the power or spirits that exist in the sand painting.

EARLY DESCRIPTIONS OF NATIVE AMERICAN HEALING

As with all the societies described in this book, written records of medical practices were not kept or did not survive. Therefore, details about these practices are often provided by the accounts of early European explorers and settlers. One of the earliest accounts of a European observing an American Indian healing ceremony is in *William Penn's Own Account of the Lenni Lenape or Delaware Indians* in 1683 (Figure 37-2). William Penn was given the land grant for what became the Commonwealth of Pennsylvania (literally, "Penn's woods"). Penn was surveying his lands when he came across a *Lenape* man named Tenoughan involved in a healing sweat bath:

> I called upon an Indian of Note, whose Name was Tenoughan, the Captain General of the Clan of Indians of those Parts. I found him ill of a Fever, his Head and Limbs much affected with Pain, and at the same time his Wife preparing a *Bagnio* for him: The Bagnio resembled a large Oven, into which he crept, by a Door on the one side, while she put several red hot Stones in a small Door on the other side thereof, and fastened the Doors as closely from the Air as she could. Now while he was Sweating in this Bagnio, his Wife (for they disdain no Service) was, with an Ax, cutting her Husband a passage into the River, (being the Winter of 1683 the great Frost, and the Ice very thick) in order to the Immersing himself, after he should come out of his Bath.

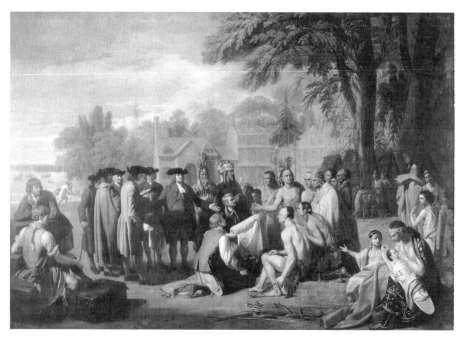

Figure 37-2 Benjamin West's painting of William Penn's treaty with the Indians. (Courtesy Pennsylvania Academy of the Fine Arts, Philadelphia, gift of Mrs. Joseph Harrison, Jr.)

In less than half an Hour, he was in so great a Sweat, that when he came out he was as wet, as if he had come out of a River, and the Reak or Steam of his Body so thick, that it was hard to discern any bodies Face that stood near him. In this condition, stark naked (his Breech-Clout only excepted) he ran into the River, which was about twenty Paces, and duck'd himself twice or thrice therein, and so return'd (passing only through his Bagnio to mitigate the immediate stroak of the Cold) to his own House, perhaps 20 Paces further, and wrapping himself in his woolen Mantle, lay down as his length near a long (but gentle) Fire in the midst of his Wigwam, or House, turning himself several times, till he was dry, and then he rose, and fell to getting us Dinner, seeming to be as easie, and well in Health, as at any other time. (Surveyor General Thomas Holme's letter, dated 5th Month [May] 7, 1688, concerning the running of a survey line)

Penn made this observation when he was on a surveying expedition of the "farthest northern region of his Provence," which was actually near Monocacy, Berks County, Pennsylvania, today about a 45-minute drive from Philadelphia (not in rush hour). The river would be the Schuylkill River, now polluted by a century of industrial contaminants and washoff from coal mines and agriculture farther inland to the north and west. Penn was not embarking to make observations of ethnomedical practices in 1683 but was intent on buying land from the Lenape people, when he stumbled on a healing bath taken by Tenoughan, a Lenape leader of some stature.

Penn was struck by the exotic and the unusual nature of the event he witnessed, as well as the apparent efficacy of the sweat bath on Tenoughan, but the observation lacks any real personal encounter between Penn and Tenoughan, although we read that *Tenoughan* served dinner for his guests after the sweat bath. As old and as minimally detailed as this account is, it illustrates a number of important insights into American Indian medicine.

First, the sweat bath was located near Tenoughan's home. It was familiar, literally in his backyard. Second, the practice included the assistance by a family member, Tenoughan's wife, who actually prepared the sweat bath for him, carried the red hot stones into the Bagnio, and assisted in closing the door securely.

"Powwow" Medicine: Pennsylvania Dutch Folk Healing

William Penn made a number of visits to Germany recruiting German farmers to his new experimental colony in America. These Germans became known as the Pennsylvania Dutch, or in their native dialect *die Pennsylvaanisch Deitsche*. Although today, many consider this use of "Dutch" to be a misnomer, it is derived from the 17th and 18th century English usage, which at one time applied to all culturally Germanic people, including the immigrants from Germany, Switzerland, parts of present-day France (Alsace), and other German-speaking regions. The immigrants were composed of two groups which persist in the present day: the "sectarians," who live in religious communities distinct from society at large, and worship in meetinghouses, and the "church people," who are comprised of members of Lutheran and Reformed congregational communities that were more worldly in their customs. Although members of this former group, such as the Old Order Amish and Mennonites, attract a certain level of attention from the American public because of their distinct culture, the sectarians are in fact a minority within the Pennsylvania Dutch community, while the majority is nearly indistinguishable from the rest of American culture today.

A number of years ago one of the contributors of this text box convened an informal inter-faith discussion with the help of a Mennonite friend who hosted a meeting at his home in rural Lancaster County, Pennsylvania, between a traditional Sicangu-Lakota medicine man and a group of about 8 community leaders from the Old Order Amish, Mennonite, and Church of the Brethern communities. The meeting began with a discussion with the elders followed by a dinner with the elders and their spouses. The children watched curiously from behind the stairway door. The purpose for convening such a meeting was to explore common elements of help and healing between these seemingly disparate traditions of the Lakota and the Pennsylvania Dutch particularly about what was understood as "Pow-wow" medicine, otherwise known as *Braucherei* (Donmoyer, 2012) a term from the dialect of the Pennsylvania Dutch.

While very different these traditions reflected interesting parallel elements, each a distinctive type of traditional medicine. Interest in exploring the traditions of the Pennsylvania Dutch was re-ignited recently upon the publication of an English edition of *Der Freund in der Noth* or *The Friend in Need, An Annotated Translation of an Early Pennsylvania Folk-Healing Manual*, by Johann Georg Hohman (Donmoyer, 2012) and subsequent discussions about Pennsylvania Dutch Folk Medicine. This section presents a brief look at the roots of Germanic folk medicine and current help and healing (folk) practices among the Pennsylvania Dutch today, and their implications for contemporary American community workers and healthcare professionals.

The word "Powwow" was a label given to Germanic folk medicine by the English speaking population of Pennsylvania, who likened the folk practices of the Pennsylvania Dutch to the traditions the Native Americans, although it is uncertain to what degree *Braucherei* was influenced by indigenous medicine. Despite this uncertainty, it is well known that the Pennsylvania Dutch, like every other early immigrant culture, adapted to their new surroundings with the assistance of their indigenous neighbors (see Chapter 1 and 34). To this day, some Amish contacts have noted that they know where the Lenape communities once were, and in fact, one said many generations ago his family knew about a Lenape band living on a section of their farm, leaving them undisturbed. The connections between these early

Continued

*"Powwow" Medicine: Pennsylvania Dutch Folk
Healing—cont'd*

German settlers and the Lenape were probably closer than we realize, providing many opportunities for continued research.

Although most health care professionals today are probably unaware of its presence in Pennsylvania, the Pennsylvania Dutch population has a well-developed tradition of folk medicine that was brought to the new world through the Germanic diaspora, and has persisted into the present day. This diverse tradition can inform health care professionals about cultural attitudes towards the nature of wellness and illness, the perceived sources of illness, and the non-conventional components of the healing experience. The climate in Pennsylvania for folk medicine is characterized by a spectrum of involvement. While many Pennsylvanians are distinctly self-aware about this tradition, many others are not particularly conscious of it, and while the latter may be very familiar with techniques and practices, for some there may be no single agreed-upon way of describing or communicating about the traditional practices for those who are not used to talking it. This spectrum demonstrates both a decline and a revival of the folk medicinal system simultaneously—evidence of a living tradition that continues to grow and change.

Braucherei in the Pennsylvania Dutch dialect, is a term that is absent from the modern Standard German language, meaning "traditions, customs, ceremonies, rituals, practices," also related to the verb *brauche*, "to need, to use, to employ." Some have used the transliterated phrase "The Necessary Tradition" to supply a meaningful English explanation. The bulk of these practices are prayerful and ritual in nature, and have been classified as a magico-religious tradition, combining verbal and gestural components, as well as the use of physical agents and herbs. These practices were imported from Europe, and were derived from formerly sanctioned Roman Catholic practices that were blended with ancient European medicine. While the tradition can be found in many European sources, the tradition has not survived intact as it has in rural Pennsylvania.

The term *Powwow* is the most popular word for the tradition today, and is an Algonquian loan-word derived from *Powan* meaning "he dreams"—a central component in the medicine of the Delaware Tribes, implying the role of a practitioner or medicine man. How this term came to be mixed with the Germanic folk medicine in Pennsylvania is the subject of debate. The Delaware population was strong in the formative years of Pennsylvania Dutch settlement in the 18th century, primarily through the Lenape who lived alongside many settlements such as Oley, in Berks County. There is little primary source information to determine exactly what portions of Pennsylvania Dutch medicine were influenced by their indigenous neighbors. However many of the very basic foundations of the medicinal practices are quite similar, such as the use of ritual, prayer, herbal components, as well as the implied use of visionary or ecstatic states used by the practitioner as a source of information and power. What is known about the term *Powwow* is that it was incorporated into English usage in the 17th century in New England, and it was later used as a derogatory slur to compare the ritual practices of the Germanic and Native practitioners. The term *Powwow* continues to be the most common word used today among English speaking populations.

In the Pennsylvania Dutch dialect, a folk practitioner is referred to as a *Braucher* if he is male, and a *Braucherin* if she is female. In English, the term "Pow-wow Doctor," "Pow-wower," and occasionally "Pow-wow" are used to describe male and female practitioners. In some areas, "Hex Doctor" is used, blending German and English words, due to the belief that a practitioner's role includes the removal of illness due to the presence of a curse or *hex*. The opposite of a healer in this cultural world-view is the *Hex*—literally meaning "witch or sorcerer," a mercenary practitioner of sinister craft who harms others for pay or amusement.

A person learns the tradition only from a member of the opposite sex, and usually from an older generation, although this protocol can occasionally vary. This form of transmission encourages cooperation and gender equality in the practice. These practices are ethically restricted (as in the Hippocratic tradition) to only those who wish to use them for the benefit of others—other reasons for learning are strongly discouraged.

The concept of a "practitioner" is not always clear-cut in Pennsylvania Dutch culture. A person may engage in ritualized behaviors and customs and not see themself as a practitioner at all, but merely acting according to cultural norms. This constitutes the most basic level of engagement with the folk practices. Secondly, non-professional practitioners often exists within families, usually a respected person of an older generation who may employ their healing methods within a circle of family or friends. A professional practitioner, however, is someone whose vocation is healing, and is often consulted by a variety of clients, ranging from family to complete strangers. These three roles are often blended, and also help to define what some ethnographers have called a "hierarchy of resort" (see Chapter 34) that characterizes the ways that traditional medicine was applied.

Within this cultural frame work, basic observations can be made about how medicine is applied. If a person perceives that they are ill, often a series of courses of action will be taken, that naturally vary according to severity of the illness, as well as from person to person. This "hierarchy of resort" characterizes how conventional and folk medicine are blended in application and practice. Normally, the first step is that an illness is allowed to incubate to see if it will go away on its own, followed often by the use of a home remedy. This can be of a ritual nature or through using herbal or physical compounds. At this stage, if the illness does not resolve, the next course of action varies according to history: If this occurred during a time when a conventional doctor

"Powwow" Medicine: Pennsylvania Dutch Folk Healing—cont'd

was available, often a visitation is made for treatment. If no doctor is available, or the conventional methods are not satisfying to the patient, a visit to a folk practitioner is made for a ritual cure.

Beginning in the late 19th century, when conventional doctors became more readily available, conventional and folk medicine were often blended, in cases where patients would visit both types of practitioners, and occasionally, where a conventional doctor also practiced folk medicine. In the 20th century, with the widespread establishment of medical societies and the standardization of medical education, folk practitioners were often consulted if conventional medicine proved ineffective or unsatisfying to patients.

In the 20th Century, many folk practitioners found themselves in the cross-fire between medical societies, conventional doctors, civic organizations, and educational institutions which aimed to eliminate folk medicine. Several early 20th-century confrontations between the justice system and folk practitioners were publicized by mainstream media through newspapers and radio, such as the famous trials of Dr. Hageman in Reading, and the infamous murder trial of John Blymire in York. These trials served to intimidate folk practitioners, and force large portions of the practice to become secretive, protected, and underground. As a result, the oral tradition is guarded from the public, and taboos about exposing the tradition or publishing it have become much more strict. At the same time, people who relied upon folk medicine often feared public criticism or were made to feel ashamed of their traditions.

In the present 21st century, the practice is experiencing somewhat of a revival. Many practitioners operate without fear of punishment from judicial, medical, or religious institutions, however the tendency towards secrecy or extreme humbleness is still very much alive. Practitioners exist in many positions and stations in life and are not restricted to the rural population, but are found in both urban and rural communities, among the rich and poor, as well as the educated and uneducated. Because practitioners are often difficult to find the practice has certainly diminished in widespread use, however many practitioners still continue to operate in the present day.

Despite apparent trends towards decline, Pennsylvania, while having more medical schools per capita than any other state, is still the home of thousands of people who use and apply folk medicine. This practice has historically been blended by patients who also receive treatment from conventional medicine. There is a tremendous opportunity for healthcare professionals to connect with their patients by forming a better understanding of local and regional cultural traditions relating to health and healing. The result of this dialogue is that professionals have the opportunity to 1) establish trust and rapport with patients through better understanding, 2) provide more comprehensive counseling for patients whose beliefs include folk medicine, 3) to explore folk methodology that may increase the efficacy of conventional medicine (a controversial idea, to be sure), and 4) establish stronger connections with the broader community.
—Patrick Donmoyer, Pennsylvania German Cultural Heritage Center, Kutztown University, Kutztown PA

Much of Indian medicine is *family* oriented; it is not something that is done by strangers. Medicine is a family matter; family is intimately involved and plays a significant role in the healing process. Later, Tenoughan's wife assisted in the arduous task of cutting a path through the ice for the "patient" to plunge into the river. Indian medicine often brings the patient into close interaction with the *natural world* and the elements. After the sweat bath, Tenoughan rests by the fire in his wigwam, and he then serves dinner to his guests. For many Indian people, stone, fire, air, water, food, spirits, and social and familial relationships are seen as part of the cosmic circle of medicine.

HEALERS AND NATURE

First, the concept of "professional healer" is foreign to traditional Indian peoples and has no precedent. The idea of "paid professionals" conflicts with the tradition that "helping other people" is a social responsibility for everyone, not just for a few. Today, professional, paid health care practitioners are often viewed with suspicion by some traditionalists. An Indian view of health care starts with the awareness of the power of the institutionalized systems to influence and assert social control, which, although aimed at "improved health care" or social well-being, may also reflect and enact the larger, more pervasive policies for exerting control over the individual. Government-sponsored or mandated health care carries this risk for all peoples.

Although no permanent or paid professional "health care providers" were traditionally among Indian bands or tribes, various individuals, groups, and societies provided health care functions to the people. In effect, every tribal member was expected to follow the "natural law of creation," or the *Wo'ope* for the **Lakota Sioux**, the unwritten natural law that guides life, which emphasizes unselfishness and generosity. The *Wo'ope* embodies the philosophy of *mitakuye oyas'in*, which, according to Lakota teacher White Hat, "is what keeps us together." It is the knowledge "that we come from one source, and we are all related." However, to make this work, "we must identify the good and evil in us, and practice what is good" (White Hat Sr., 1997).

Lakota philosophy does not separate good and evil, sickness and health, or right and wrong as distinct realities. They coexist in each person, in every creation; even in the most sacred thing there is good and evil (like the Chinese concept of the *yin* and *yang* in medicine). There is negative and the positive within everyone and everything, and to be responsible in one's life is to live in a good, moral, healthy way, in balance with all creation.

The **natural law** is the way nature acts. Understanding Lakota philosophy begins with understanding the natural law or the seven laws of the Creator. The "natural law," or the *Wo'ope*, required each person to exercise shared values, which, if acted on in one's life, gave the person, as well as the extended family (*tios'paye*) and the tribe (*wicozani*), what was understood as total or perfect health, balance and harmony, good social health, and well-being, which implies physical and spiritual health.

Another orienting value of healers among the Lakota is *nagi'ksapa*, or self-wisdom, the awareness of your aura or spirit. White Hat, Sr., translates and explains the *nagi'ksapa* as "one's spirit, the wise spirit in a person." He notes that "The Lakota are very much aware of the spirit within [us]—we talk to our spirit—we ask our spirit to be strong and to help us in our decisions" and life (1997). *Iha'kicikta* is the ability to look out for one another. If you move camp, you should be concerned that everyone is going to move together. You want to make sure there is enough water and food for everyone. *Wo'onsila* is the ability to have pity on each other. Albert White Hat, Sr., explains the word as "recognizing a specific need of someone or something, and you address that (specific) need." According to White Hat, Lakota philosophy does not encourage people to "stay stuck" or dependent. *Iyus'kiniya* is the ability to go do things with a happy attitude *Wi'ikt ceya* is the measure of wealth by how little one needs; it is the capacity to give to others; it is one's capacity for self-sacrifice. *Teki'ci'hilapi* is the ability to cherish, esteem, and treasure each other. Practicing these social values ensured good social functioning.

The primary orientation of traditional Indian medicine was *universalistic*. Health resources were made available to everyone through their family and community. Lakota society emphasized tribalism over individualism, social harmony over self-interest, and a commitment or loyalty to the people or the larger extended family relations over individual success. Health care functions were accomplished by one's extended family (*tios'paye*); it was the extended family that provided for the social support and material assistance of all its members. Wealth was distributed through the practice of the giveaway ceremony (*wopila*), which is still practiced by traditional Lakotas. This practice ensured that no one person's or one family's wealth or resources dominated.

Mental and physical health are viewed as inseparable from *spiritual and moral* health. The good balance of one's life in harmony with the *Wo'ope,* or natural law of creation, brings about *wicozani,* or good health, which was both individual and communal. Rather than viewing the individual as a mind–body split, which has influenced much of Western psychiatric thinking, traditional Lakota philosophy viewed the individual person as an unexplainable creation with four constituent dimensions of self. The *nagi* is one's individual soul, spirit; the shadow of anything, as of a man

(*wica nagi*) or of a house (*tinagi*). The *nagi la* is the divine spirit immanent in each human being. The *niya*, or *"the vital breath,"* gives life to the body and is responsible for the circulation of the blood and the breathing process. The fourth element of the person is the *sicun,* or "intellect." Albert White Hat, Sr., describes the *sicun* as "your (spirit's) presence [that] is felt on something or somebody." It is that in a man or thing which is spirit or spirit-like and guards him from birth against 'evil spirits.'" Often a person appeals to his *nagi la* for assistance. This is a power within each person that can help him or her overcome obstacles. When one goes on the *hanbleceya*, or *pipe fast*, one leaves the physical world as a *nagi.*

According to Gene Thin Elk, "We are not humans on a soul journey. We are nagi, "souls" who are making a journey through the material world (1995)." The *nagi la* has been described as the "little spirit," which is the "divine spirit immanent in each being." Existence in the material world is tenuous for the newborn, according to Lakota philosophy: Ms. Edna Little Elk commented, "The most important things for infants and little children are to eat good, sleep good and play good," and by doing so, the *nagi* of the child is persuaded to become more and more attached to its own body. Traditional Lakota philosophy sees abuse, rejection, or neglect affecting the child's *nagi*, where it may detach from the child's body and not come back. In this case, ceremonies are conducted by a medicine man to find the child's *nagi* and bring it back. Such a condition has been called *soul loss.* Thus, good mental or emotional health is intimately related to good spiritual, moral, and physical health; they cannot be separated.

HEALING PRACTICES

Although the sweat lodge, Sundance, and vision quest are all used by Lakotas, for example, for health and healing, not all were always conducted by "medicine women" or "medicine men." There was not exclusivity of these ceremonies, and in fact, there was considerable variation and scope for these practices, most of which were *family* oriented (Douville, 1997).

The sweat lodge (Figure 37-3) or "purification ceremony," for example, is very common and may be conducted by anyone who has "been on the hill" or completed the *hanbleceya*, often called the "vision quest." Although the English name emphasizes the physiological reaction of the "sweat," this ceremony of the common man (Lakota: *ikce wicasa*), it is really an encounter with one's spiritual self and one's spirit relatives. This is a purification that "gives life" (*inipi'kogapi*, "that which gives life") to the participants and represents a form of rebirth. This is a family-oriented ceremony and is an integral part of all other Lakota ceremonies. Participants enter a small lodge made of willow saplings (for support) and covered with heavy, dark canvas. Between 7 and 16 or more red-hot stones are brought into this little lodge, which can be 10 to 15 feet in diameter. The stones represent the "first creation" and have deep spiritual

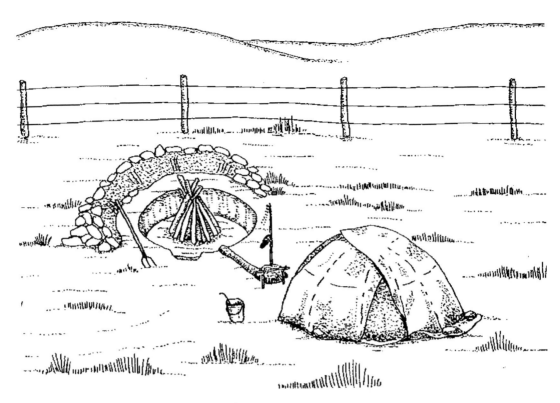

Figure 37-3 Sweat lodge. (Courtesy Sinte Gleska University.)

meaning in this ceremony. Water is poured over the stones by someone who is permitted to conduct this ceremony, and the steam from this generates intense heat. There is deep spiritual significance to this practice.

Usually, family members participate in this ceremony on a regular basis. Often, sweat lodges are located behind one's home. There is a prohibition that excludes menstruating women from ceremonies out of respect for the ceremony the woman's body is undergoing (i.e., menstruation, which is seen by Lakota people as a purification with its own proper spiritual power). This is often viewed by White culture as "discriminatory," but the tradition is not intended to be discriminatory. It is an affirmation of the natural feminine power, which White culture tends to minimize, often viewing menstruation as a handicap or a problem (e.g., premenstrual syndrome).

There are also different types of "medicine" people among the Lakota. It is difficult to generalize about the diverse functions using the English terms "medicine man" or "medicine woman." The Lakota practiced common medicines that included *herbal* remedies known to families whose primary medical care was prevention and geared to building up the immune system. The various common medicines included *teas*, *ointments*, and *smudging* (smoke from burning certain herbs, e.g., prairie sage or "flat cedar").

The first line of medical care was provided by knowledgeable family members or friends. When required, more spiritual consultations were sought from a *shaman* medicine man or an interpreter for the *Wakan Tanka* (the great mystery in all creation), which represents sacred medicine.

A "ceremony" may be requested by the patient and is usually held at night, with family members, close friends, and singers (see Figure 37-5). Usually, the patient presents a *sacred pipe* to the medicine man, who will smoke it if he accepts the request. The ceremony (which usually describes a *Lowanpi*, or spirit ceremony) takes place in a darkened room in the home. All furnishings are removed, and openings are covered. Certain ceremonial objects are used (e.g., various-colored flags, *tobacco* offerings, earth). During the ceremony, the spirits instruct the medicine man or interpreter on what remedies would be provided by *Unci Maka* ("Grandmother Earth") to heal the patient. This process is done with the support of the *tios'paye,* or the extended family, for the *wicozani* (good health) of the patient.

Along with these practices, family members actively participated in a ceremonial life, which revolved around the *Wo'ope,* or "natural law of creation," which included the behaviors and attitudes for right living. The *Wo'ope* is embodied in the philosophy of *mitakuye oyas'in,* which recognizes that all things, persons, and creations (both animate and inanimate, seen and unseen) are related (White Hat Sr., 1997). These laws are not written down; they are learned through observing the creation. These behaviors for "right living" were reinforced by the ceremonial life of the extended family system, or *tios'paye.*

Health care was primarily an extended family matter. Medical care was common and free to everyone who needed it because the herbs or materials for ceremonies used natural elements that could be harvested from nature's bounty. Although medical care was "free," it was not provided without cost because in Lakota philosophy, when someone gives you something, you are expected to return it fourfold in value. When treated by healers, the people who received help gave something back. The concept of receiving "something for nothing" is not part of Indian philosophy (White Hat Sr., 1997). The Lakota philosophy encourages self-reliance *and* mutual relations. Things changed when White man's medicine became institutionalized in the United States, emphasizing intervention over prevention, the individual over the tribe or extended family, materialism over spirituality, and the physical body over the spirit-body.

THE CIRCLE IS BROKEN

For Indian people, life is like a circle—continuous, harmonious, and cyclical—with no distinctions. Medicine was a coming together of all the elements in this circular pattern of life. The circle of healing was formed by the interconnections among the sick person, his or her extended family or relatives, the spirits, the singers who helped with the ceremonial songs, and the medicine practitioner (Figures 37-4 and 37-5).

After contact with European settlers, ceremonial practices were suppressed and the cultural fabric of Indian peoples was torn. Later, official U.S. government assimilation policies forced many traditional Indian medicine prac-

titioners "underground" for risk of being accused of "devil worship" and held up to public ridicule. Between 1890 and 1940, the Sundance, as well as all other native ceremonies, were forbidden under the *Indian Offenses Act. Fire Lame Deer* recalled:

> One could be jailed for just having an *inipi* (a sweatlodge ceremony) or praying in the *Lakota* way, as the government and the missionaries tried to stamp out our old beliefs in order to make us into slightly darker, "civilized" Christians. Many historians believe that during those fifty years no Sundances were performed, but they are wrong. The Sundance was held every year . . . but it had to be done in secret, in lonely places where no White man could spy on us. (1992, p. 230)

Luther Standing Bear reflected on the profound shift that was occurring as he recalled his experience traveling to the Carlisle Indian School as a boy:

> It was only about three years after the Custer battle, and the general opinion was that the Plains people merely infested the earth as nuisances, and our being there simply evidenced misjudgment on the part of *Wakan Tanka*. Whenever our train stopped at the railway stations, it was met by great numbers of White people who came to gaze upon the little Indian "savages." The shy little ones sat quietly at the car windows looking at the people who swarmed on the platform. Some of the children wrapped

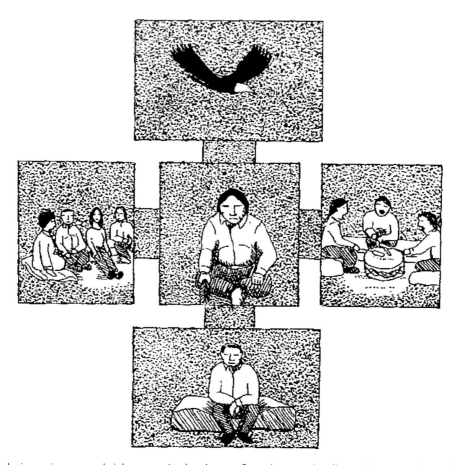

Figure 37-4 Spirits, relatives, singers, and sick person in the shape of two intersecting lines. (Courtesy Sinte Gleska University.)

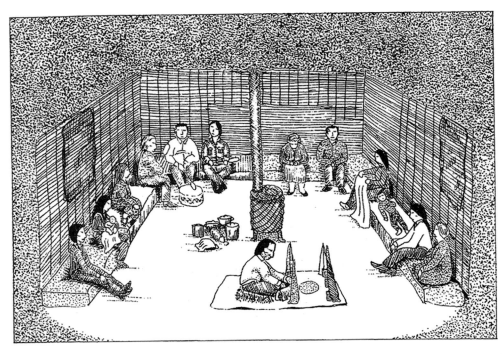

Figure 37-5 All of the elements from Figure 37-4 are depicted in this ceremony of the extended family in the healing process. The drawing shows a quiet gathering of people in a darkened room. (Courtesy Sinte Gleska University.)

themselves in their blankets, covering all but their eyes. At one place we were taken off the train and marched a distance down the street to a restaurant. We walked down the street between two rows of uniformed men whom we called soldiers, though I suppose they were policemen. This must have been done to protect us, for it was surely known that we boys and girls could do no harm. Back of the rows of uniformed men stood the white people craning their necks, talking, laughing, and making a great noise. They yelled and tried to mimic us by giving what they thought were war-whoops. We did not like this.

Often, students from Western tribes were sent east to the Carlisle Indian School at Carlisle, Pennsylvania, and students from eastern tribes were sent west. For example, the *Nanticokes* of Delaware were sent to the Haskell Indian School in Kansas. Other Indians whose behavior seemed odd or troublesome were sent to the infamous Hiawatha Insane Asylum for Indians, also known as the *Canton Insane Asylum*, which was the only segregated asylum built exclusively for American Indians in the United States, located in Canton, South Dakota. This institution was opened in 1902 as the second federal institution for the insane (predated by St. Elizabeth's Hospital in Washington, DC) to provide psychiatric care exclusively to Indian people by an act of Congress, despite opposition from the Department of the Interior and the superintendent of St. Elizabeth's Hospital when the bill was first passed by Congress in 1898. In December 1933, after further study, the Hiawatha Asylum for Indians was closed, its remaining 71 Indian patients transferred to St. Elizabeth's Hospital.

A Northern Hero of the US Civil War on Native Americans

Tosawi, chief of the Comanches, brought in the first band of Comanches to surrender to the U.S. army commander, Philip Sheridan, who had ravaged the Shenandoah Valley of Virginia as one of the closing acts of total war against the South during the American Civil War of 1861–1865. Addressing Sheridan, Tosawi spoke his own name and two words in English: "Tosawi, good Indian." Sheridan responded with the now-infamous words: "The only good Indians I ever saw were dead," which was shortened to the infamous aphorism, "The only good Indian is a dead Indian."

PLAGUES AND EPIDEMICS

In addition to the assault on Indian culture and spirituality, infectious diseases introduced by European settlers severely impacted their physical health. The massive and sudden losses of life during epidemics further contributed to breakdown of communities and lifeways, and it is important to keep in mind the devastation caused by exposure to Old World diseases (see also Chapter 40). Henry Dobyns (1983) estimated that Native people faced serious contagious diseases that caused significant mortality every four to five years, from 1520 to 1900. The pandemics affecting Indian people are often treated by White historians and others as types of "natural disasters" that were never intended to occur. However, in certain instances, "germ warfare" was conducted by military operations against them. One example often cited was the distribution of smallpox-infected blankets by the U.S. Army to *Mandan* (Indians) at Fort Clark on June 19, 1837, thought to be the source of the smallpox pandemic of 1837–1840.

After European contact, medical treatment and health care for American Indians was historically grossly inadequate and often seen as antagonistic with traditional Indian medicine ways. There was no supervision of agency doctors, and not until 1891 were physicians placed in a classified service and required to pass examinations in addition to having a medical degree. Charles Alexander Eastman, a Lakota Sioux Indian who served as an agency physician at Pine Ridge from 1890 to 1892, observed the practice of government-sponsored medical care. He wrote:

> The doctors who were in the service in those days had an easy time of it. They scarcely ever went outside of the agency enclosure, and issued their pills and compounds after the most casual inquiry. As late as 1890, when the Government sent me out as a physician to ten thousand Ogallalla Sioux and Northern Cheyennes at Pine Ridge Agency, I found my predecessor still practicing his profession through a small hole in the wall between his office and the general assembly room of the Indians. One of the first things I did was to close that hole; and I allowed no man to diagnose his own trouble or choose his own pills.

Physicians in the Indian Service had to use their own funds and gifts of money from friends to buy medicines and supplies. Drugs supplied to the Indians were "often obsolete in kind, and either stale or of the poorest quality" (DeMallie & Jahner, 1991). In 1893, Dr. Z.T. Daniel recommended that the procedures for Indian Service doctors be reappraised, modernized, and compiled in serviceable form. He also recommended that an agency physician be sent annually as a representative of the American Medical Association, and he urged that Indian Service doctors be supplied with medical textbooks and medical journals.

NATIVE AMERICAN MEDICINE IN THE "NEW AGE"

Shamanic traditions and healing practices are very active among traditional American Indians today and seem to be gaining ground after generations of official and unofficial prohibitions and sanctions (see Chapter 42 on neoshamanism). There is diversity among traditional Indian tribal practices. The Lakotas have been open and receptive to sharing knowledge and technology with other nations. Lakota medicine people rely on their spirit helpers to "give them permission" to treat people and conduct ceremonies. This permission is very specific; for example, a medicine man may be instructed to use certain herbal medicines for men only, women only, or people in general. The spirits work through the healer. The medicine man is only

as effective as the spirits "working through him." He is responsible and accountable to the spirits for everything (Figure 37-6).

Today, many of the old Indian healing traditions are experiencing a renaissance and are being viewed with a renewed sense of respect and credibility as an alternative to more invasive or secular Western medical models of treatment. For example, on the **Cheyenne** River Indian Reservation at Eagle Butte, the tribal council approved alcohol treatment programs and delinquency prevention programs based on traditional methods and approaches to helping people with alcoholism, which is viewed as a problem with social, emotional, physical, and spiritual dimensions (Red Dog, 1997). These traditional methods include the *inipi*, or purification ceremony (popularly called the sweat lodge); the *hanbleceya*, or pipe fast (often called the vision quest); and the *wiwang wacipi*, or the gazing-at-the-sun dance. The infusion of these ceremonies within the treatment process, collectively, has been called the *Red Road Approach* (Thin Elk, 1995).

However, within historical context, one can better perceive the basis for many Indian peoples' objections to the growing "popularity" of their traditional spirituality and healing practices among non-Indians—by the *wasicun*. This *Lakota* word describes the early White hunter's propensity to take the fatty, choice portion of the buffalo and leave the rest to rot. A wasicun is "one who takes things." This term is used today to express the perception of the narrow, materialistic, and destructive worldview of mainstream White culture. Interest among Whites in seeking out "Indian medicine men and *shamans*," and the resultant exploitation of Indian ceremonies (e.g., buying Indian spirituality in weekend or half-day workshops or seminars; paying fees for sweat lodge ceremonies), have prompted some Lakota leaders to issue a "declaration of war" against such exploitation. There are strong feelings about the contemporary curiosity of Whites about Indian medicine ways.

NATIVE AMERICAN MEDICINAL PLANTS

Native American peoples developed a sophisticated plant-based medical system in the millennia before the arrival of Europeans. There were also some non-plant substances that were used medicinally; *castoreum* from beaver was used for various conditions, and some minerals and clays were used as well. However, the preponderance of medicinal substances came from plants.

Many of the plants that these people used are familiar medicinal species and have taken a role in contemporary medicine. For example, echinacea is well known in Europe and increasingly well known in North America as a treatment for colds and particularly as an "immune system stimulant." The coneflowers, Native American species, were used in more than 100 ways by a dozen midwestern tribes (e.g., **Blackfoot, Cheyenne, Dakota, Omaha, Pawnee, Paiute**) to treat a variety of diseases and

WHAT IS A MEDICINE MAN?

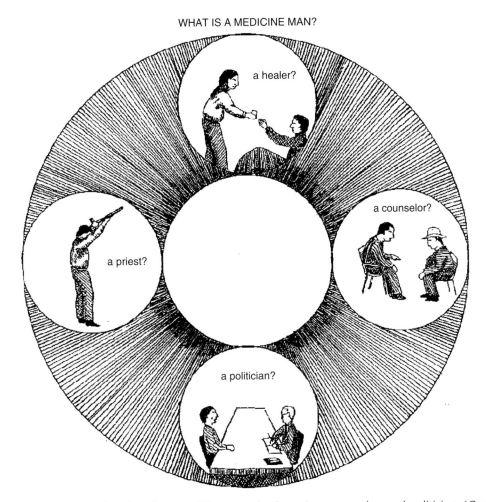

a healer?

a priest?

a counselor?

a politician?

Figure 37-6 Illustration of the multiple roles of the medicine man: healer, priest, counselor, and politician. (Courtesy Sinte Gleska University.)

conditions, including headaches, burns, and toothaches. The **Winnebago** used echinacea in an interesting way: fire handlers used the plant to make themselves insensitive to hot coals that they put in their mouths.

Another very interesting plant—*Podophyllum peltatum,* or mayapple—is less well known to the public but is probably more important medically than echinacea. Native Americans used the plant in many ways, but the most common use was as a laxative or purgative, which was a common use of the plant in early American medicine as well. For many years, podophyllum resin has been a standard treatment for venereal warts. Also, etoposide (VePesid), a semisynthetic derivative of podophyllotoxin, another mayapple constituent, is an effective treatment for refractory testicular tumors and for small cell lung cancer.

Plants used by Native Americans as medicinal species can also be dangerous. This danger is apparent with toxic species such as *Datura meteloides* (jimsonweed) and *Heracleum maximum* (cow parsnip), though others are less obviously dangerous. A classic case is ephedrine, derived from several species of the genus *Ephedra,* notably *E. sinica.* The American species, *E. viridis,* contains less ephedrine than

the Asian species. It was used by many Native American groups for the treatment of internal illnesses. It has a long use in the American Southwest as a stimulating drink known as "*teamster's tea*" or "*Mormon tea,*" and the drug and various synthetic variations (particularly pseudoephedrine) is a useful decongestant. In the recent past, herbal drug companies made capsules containing from 7 to more than 40 mg of ephedrine, along with other *Ephedra* alkaloids, and sold them under such names as "Herbal Ecstasy," "Ultimate Xphoria," and "Cloud 9." These drugs presumably mimic the action of the street drugs MDMA or STP —illegal in the United States—which produces euphoria; the street name of the drug is "ecstasy."

There are many such anecdotal stories about Native American medicinal plants and their modern uses, and these accounts are readily found. However, there are other, more systematic approaches to the medicinal plants of native North America. Although significant differences existed between the systems developed by the many native groups, there were also many broad similarities, providing a "pan-Indian" perspective. There are approximately 21,000 species of plants in North America. Native Americans used more than 2800 of them medicinally. Over the past 25 years, one of us (Moerman) has built a database with nearly 45,000 entries that lists the uses of plants by Native Americans as drugs, foods, dyes, fibers, etc. The database contains over 25,000 entries on uses of drugs, representing a total of nearly 3000 different species of plants. This figure rivals the ancient Chinese Pharmacopeia of medicinal plants.

Over 11,000 entries describe the uses of nearly 4000 species that were used as food. The database was constructed by gathering together several hundred published works on the ethnobotany of Native American people and coding all the information in a systematic way. Because many of these publications were originally obscure and often difficult to find, this database facilitates making such global statements about Native American plant use.

The used portion of the flora (the "medicinal flora") is a distinctly nonrandom assortment of available plants. The richest sources of medicines are the sunflower family (Asteraceae), the rose family (Rosaceae), and the mint family (Lamiaceae). By contrast, the grass family (Poaceae) and the rush family (Juncaceae) produce practically no medicinal species. This remarkable volume and extraordinary selectivity demonstrate the falseness of demeaning claims that suggest that Native American medicines were chosen at random, that they seemingly just used everything and stumbled on something useful (like echinacea or podophyllum) once in a while.

TREATING DISEASE, ILLNESS AND INJURY

To understand the character and effectiveness of a medical system, one must understand the health status of the people who use it. Native Americans were typically very healthy. They generally did not have the degenerative diseases of the heart and circulatory systems so common today; their diets were rich in fiber and carbohydrates and low in fats. They lived vigorous lives that provided hearty exercise on a daily basis. They experienced little cancer. Cancer is largely a modern disease of civilization; although the situation is complex, an apparently necessary condition for cancer is carcinogens, which are largely products manufactured by industrial societies (e.g., organic chemicals and dyes, nuclear radiation). Even current evidence indicates that the traditional **Navajo** still have lower rates of cancer than surrounding people.

In addition, Indian people had fewer classic infectious diseases, which had ravaged European society over the past two millennia. In large part, many such diseases (e.g., plague, typhoid, smallpox, cholera) are zoonoses, diseases of animals that, under conditions of domestication, underwent evolutionary change and subsequently affected the human keepers of these animals. Native Americans never domesticated animals to any significant degree. (The **guinea pig** and **llama** of Peru were apparently coming under domestication only in the few hundred years before European contact.) Confused Europeans during the seventeenth century, simultaneously exposed to new species

from Africa and the Americas, incorrectly identified the guinea pig as originating in West African Guinea (rather than America), just as the English thought the turkey came from Turkey and the French thought it from India (*oiseau d'Inde*, "bird of India," or simply *dinde*) instead of America.

Once infectious diseases were introduced into North America, they devastated native populations, which had no natural immunity to them (Dobyns, 1983). Until the sixteenth century, when Europeans underwent successive epidemics that regularly killed a quarter or half of the population, Native Americans were spared this devastation.

What medical problems did Native Americans face? In the Southeast and Southwest, evidence suggests a decline in health status after the switch to agriculture and sedentism (settling in one place), as the diet became simpler (less varied), which typically led to some deficiency diseases, and the crowded conditions of settlements, which facilitates transmission of infections.

Hunting and gathering people avoided that problem, but they, like Europeans, may have experienced some zoonotic infections, particularly from beavers and some trichinosis from bears. However, these infections would have been "direct" zoonoses that individuals contracted directly from the infected animal, not "remote" zoonoses, which, once passed to one human, were subsequently passed from person to person. As with rabies, a terrible disease for the individual who contracts it, these direct zoonoses are not serious threats to a whole society because they are not "contagious" in the ordinary sense of the term—from human to human.

Native Americans paid a price for the vigorous life they led—accidents, sprains, broken bones, cuts, lacerations, and other trauma were common. There was a range of arthritic conditions, with some probably the result of injury and some similar to rheumatoid arthritis. Ample evidence indicates that native peoples engaged in warfare, which would have been a source of serious medical problems. There was a range of occasional problems associated with menstruation, pregnancy, childbirth, and lactation that required attention. Living in smoky houses, it is not surprising that they had a wide range of treatments for irritated eyes and skin; they also treated colds, headaches, cold sores, and bruises, the normal insults of daily life.

To address this range of problems, Native Americans inevitably resorted to medicines based on various plants. Although a good deal of research has been done on this ethnobotany, much is difficult to find and use. Most of the research has been done on a "tribe-by-tribe" basis. This situation means that if you are interested in what plants the **Iroquois** used for medicines and how they used them, for example, you should look in James Herrick's doctoral dissertation, *Iroquois Medical Botany* (Herrick, 1977). However, if you are interested in how different cultural groups used the same plant, it is a much more challenging proposition. Moerman's database, described earlier, makes this work much more practical.

BOTANICAL PHARMACOPEIA

Every Native American group for which we have any information had a botanical pharmacopeia. Although some were quite small (the **Inuit** of the Arctic had few plant resources on which to rely, living in a subarctic region with limited plant life), most were quite elaborate, with hundreds of plant drugs used for a broad range of conditions.

Native American healers, or medicine men, even into the early twentieth century, regularly knew the identity of 200 or 300 medicinal plants, which they could readily distinguish from the 3000 to 5000 species that grow in any particular area. Among sophisticated and well-educated modern Americans or Europeans, few can identify 200 species of plants of any kind unless they are professional botanists. How did non-literate people, without reference to botanical keys or floras compiled by professionals, maintain this extraordinary amount of knowledge?

If a Native American person discovered, by whatever means, an effective medicinal plant that cured a child of a terrible rash, and if the plant was very rare and unusual, for example, an annual plant of uncertain origin, she might be hard pressed to find it a second time, and harder pressed yet to teach her daughter, or niece or neighbor, where to find it. Such a plant would be unlikely to become part of the common knowledge of the community. If the situation were compounded by the fact that the plant was drab, with no particularly visible flowers or leaves—an undistinguished, rare, annual forb, for example—it is even less likely that it would become part of common knowledge. Given such considerations, medicinal plants tend to have the following botanical characteristics:
- Abundant
- Perennial
- Large (e.g., trees rather than forbs)
- Widespread
- Distinctive—showy and visible

These criteria do not mean that a tiny, drab, undistinguished, rare annual occurring in one forest in Tennessee could not be part of the Native American medicinal flora. It means it is less likely to be used medicinally than a large, common, perennial tree found in 20 states.

ABUNDANCE

Incredibly, there is no available listing of the relative abundance of North American plants. One might question what the U.S. Department of the Interior and Department of Agriculture (USDA) have been doing all these years. However, medicinal plants do tend not to be rare and endangered species. This finding, in turn, has promising implications for the availability of medicinal plants as sources of effective medicines today.

The United States *Endangered Species Act* seeks to protect endangered and threatened species of plants and animals. To administer the act, the USDA maintains a list of such species (many of which are actually varieties or subspecies).

Currently, there are nearly 400 species (or subspecies or varieties) on the list, in four categories: (1) proposed threatened, (2) threatened, (3) proposed endangered, and (4) endangered. These species are all by definition found in limited areas, which are infrequent in their ranges. Two of 2572 medicinal species (about one-tenth of 1%) are on the list, whereas 387 of the remaining 28,543 species, subspecies, and varieties in North America (1.3%) are on the list. This difference is highly significant. By this admitted observation, medicinal plants tend not to be rare and unusual. If it were possible to measure directly the abundance of a good sample of American species, a much better test of this proposition could be performed.

DISTRIBUTION

In addition, evidence accumulated by the USDA is available for the distribution of **North American** plant species. There is information on the presence or absence of species in 60 states and territories and 10 **Canadian** provinces and 3 territories. Species used as drugs are found in an average of 16 states or provinces, whereas species not used as drugs are found in an average of only 5 states. Drug plants are much more widespread than are nondrug plants.

GROWTH HABITS AND FORMS

Evidence indicates, first, that among Native North Americans, a disproportionate share of medicinal plants have a perennial rather than annual growth habit. There are many more perennials (12,284) than annuals (3060); 16% of the perennials are used medicinally, whereas only 8.7% of the annuals are used medicinally.

The most commonly used growth form for medicinal plants is trees and shrubs, followed by forbs, vines, and grasses. Although these differences may not seem large, they are, again, highly statistically significant; a given tree or shrub is 30% more likely to be used as a medicine than is a given forb.

Flavor

Circumstantial evidence from a number of cases indicates that medicinal plants often have a distinctive and, in particular, bitter taste. This cannot be easily tested because no evidence is available on the flavors of plants *not* used as medicines (because botanists do not consider a plant's flavor to be an important characteristic).

Showiness

Finally, there is evidence that plants used for medicine by Native Americans are more showy or visible than other plants. This test is indirect. Most common garden plants **are** also medicinal plants. Why do we put one plant in a flower garden and not another one? In general, it is because the garden species has beautiful or unusual or colorful flowers, leaves, scent or growth habits, or a similar distinction; garden plants are typically recognizable and distinctive. Many "garden varieties" are much different from their wild ancestors, but the hybridizers rarely began with nothing. Native American medicinal plants are more likely to show up in gardens than would plants not used medicinally.

Ortho's Complete Guide to Successful Gardening has a 122-page encyclopedic chart of plants of value in a garden, alphabetically arranged from abelia to zoysia (Ferguson, 1983). Plant genera in the gardening book also appear in a standard list of the flora of North America (Kartesz, 1994). There are 3138 genera in this list, of which 852 appear as medicinal plants. In addition, there are 423 genera of plants listed in the garden book that appear on the Kartesz checklist (a few items in the book were not in the checklist because they do not appear outside of gardens). If all were distributed randomly, and if medicinal plants were not favored for use in the garden, we would predict that 115 of the garden plants would have appeared on the list of 852 medicinal species. However, there are actually almost twice that many, 213, again a highly significant difference. Medicinal plants tend to be visible, recognizable, and showy, helping traditional healers to find and identify them.

The medicinal knowledge of the native North American people is extraordinary. Just how this knowledge was developed remains a mystery. Native American peoples are thought to have come from Asia, and the flora of Asia is similar to that of North America in many ways. It is likely that the first migrants to the New World brought detailed knowledge of medical botany, much of which was applicable to this new flora. A detailed comparison of the ethnobotany of North America and China awaits scholarly attention. A preliminary account by James Duke (in Duke and Ayensu, 1985) is provocative.

Today, there is no significant, known, medicinal, indigenous American plant species that was not also actually used traditionally as medicine by one or another Native American group. An interesting example involves research on taxol, a substance of great potential medical value found in the common yew, *Taxus brevifolia*, and the Canadian yew, *Taxus canadensis*. Taxol has shown substantial effect in the treatment of tumors in several forms of cancer, particularly ovarian cancer, a highly refractory form. Native Americans did not use yew to treat cancer, since cancer was probably very rare (see previous discussion), but they did use it for a variety of other conditions, including skin problems, wounds, rheumatism, and colds.

In general, if one is interested in finding potentially useful botanical chemicals from the North American flora, it would be wise to focus first on that portion of the flora used by Native Americans. Their experience and knowledge still guides efforts to enhance human health.

COMMON NATIVE AMERICAN MEDICINAL PLANTS

Daucus carota (Queen Anne's Lace)

The wild European carrot, or Queen Anne's Lace, is a common medicine for Native Americans. Native Americans came to use a number of introduced species; other common European plants that became widely used are mullein (*Verbascum thapsus*), curly dock (*Rumex crispus*), catnip (*Nepeta cataria*), and the common tansy (*Tanacetum vulgare*). The Delaware and Mohegan used wild carrot to treat diabetes; the Iroquois used it as a diuretic; and the Cherokee used an infusion of the plant as a wash for swellings.

Echinacea angustifolia (Coneflower)

Echinacea, the coneflowers, represent 26 distinctly different use categories, such as "analgesic," "anti-rheumatic," and "cold remedy." There are 18 different tribes represented and 93 combinations of tribe and use (e.g., "Pawnee analgesic," "Crow cold remedy"). Nine different tribes are reported to have used echinacea as an analgesic. Some tribes used it several different ways: The Winnebago used it in a wash for pain from burns and also put it in a smoke treatment for headaches. The Ponca used it the same two ways.

Geranium maculatum (Wild Geranium)

Eight species of wild geraniums were used medicinally by Native American people (note that these are not the same as the common ornamental plants often called geraniums, which are actually members of the genus *Pelargonium*). The most widely used is *Geranium maculatum,* the wild cranesbill. This plant produces a long, pointed seed that has a series of small but distinct hooks on the end, which probably serve to catch the seeds in the fur of passing animals to aid in their dispersal. However, these hooks also provided the Iroquois with a rationale for using a poultice of the roots of this plant on chancre sores; the hooklike and ensnaring qualities of the plant (implied by its hooked seeds) are precisely what to use on a loose, running, everted sore. The plant is therefore a symbolically meaningful medicine for the Iroquois. The roots also contain substantial quantities of tannin, which would probably be an effective treatment for sores. Medicines typically have this double quality of symbolic *meaning* and *active chemistry* in all medical systems (Micozzi, 1983).

Serenoa repens (Saw Palmetto)

Long used by Native Americans for stomach ache, dysentery, sexual dysfunction, and other conditions, saw palmetto was prescribed by nineteenth- and early-twentieth-century Western physicians for prostate conditions, earning it the nickname "old man's friend." More recently, it was studied for use in improving sperm production, breast size, and sexual vigor. Today it is most popular for treating noncancerous enlargement of the prostate, known as benign prostatic hyperplasia.

Serenoa repens and *Sabal serrulata* are both used; the common name is *sabal*. The berries of this small palm tree are picked ripe and dried.

The most active components of saw palmetto are thought to be the sterols (including beta-sitosterol, campesterol, and stigmasterol), which are used in the synthesis of steroid hormones. The mechanism of action is thought to be the sterols' ability to decrease prostatic nuclear androgen (a steroid that controls masculine physical characteristics, such as hair growth) and estrogen receptors (which moderate female hormones).

Numerous recent investigations have studied the effects of saw palmetto on benign prostate enlargement. The *Journal of the American Medical Association* recently reported on a review of 18 randomized, placebo-controlled studies that involved nearly 3000 men. The researchers concluded that saw palmetto extract improved the comfort and volume of urination to a degree similar to the pharmaceutical finasteride, which is commonly prescribed for enlarged prostate, without the side effects (such as impotence) that can accompany the drug. A six-month study comparing saw palmetto to finasteride demonstrated similar results: participants taking saw palmetto experienced the same significant improvements in prostate symptoms, quality of life, and urinary flow as the group using finasteride, without the drug's side effects. In another study, pharmaceuticals proved more effective than saw palmetto.

The German Commission E approved saw palmetto for urination problems associated with benign prostate enlargement. The recommended dosage is 160 mg twice a day of an extract standardized to include 85% to 95% sterols and fatty acids. There are minimal, if any, side effects; occasionally users report mild gastrointestinal upset. Because saw palmetto can affect hormone levels, it may interfere with birth control medications and hormone replacement therapy (HRT).

Toxicodendron radicans (Poison Ivy)

Poison ivy is a common North American plant that causes serious, itchy rashes on many people. Children are taught "leaflets three; let it be." The toxic chemical urushiol is found throughout the plant: in the soft woody stem, the leaves, and the berries. It is particularly dangerous when burned with dead leaves in the fall; contact with the smoke can also cause serious allergic reactions. Several other members of this genus have similarly noxious properties, including *T. diversilobum* (Pacific poison oak), *T. pubescens* (Atlantic poison oak), and *T. vernix* (poison sumac).

It may be somewhat surprising, therefore, to discover that Native American people found this genus to be useful as a medicine. There are 57 listings of *Toxicodendron* as medicine. Although some of these listings indicate simply that the people recognized the plant as being poisonous, others found medicinal uses for the plants. The Yuki of California, for example, used Pacific poison oak to treat warts, whereas the Cherokee used a decoction of the bark of Atlantic poison oak as an emetic. The Kiowa Apache rubbed poison ivy leaves over boils or other skin eruptions, and the Houma of Louisiana took a decoction of the leaves as a tonic and "rejuvenator." In homeopathic preparations, *Toxicodendron* is a leading remedy for several common symptoms.

NOTE ON FURTHER READING

Many works on the medical systems of particular groups are available, although they are sometimes difficult to find. One is by James Herrick on the Iroquois (1977). For an overview of the range of forms of treatment and understanding of illness, see Vogel's classic work, *American Indian Medicine* (1970). The most comprehensive available listing of Native American medicinal plants is *Moerman's Medicinal Plants of Native America* (Moerman, 1986). For a more recent and much larger database, see Moerman's *Native American Ethnobotany* (1997). For a fascinating and controversial review of the impact of European diseases on Native Americans, see Calvin Martin's *Keepers of the Game* (Martin, 1978). The classic work on the zoonotic origins of modern diseases is R. N. Fiennes's *Zoonoses and the Origins and Ecology of Human Disease* (1978). A definitive treatment of non-Western botanical knowledge is provided in Brent Berlin's *Ethnobiological Classification* (1992); the best modern treatment of the problems of the origins of knowledge about food and drug plants is Timothy Johns's *With Bitter Herbs They Shall Eat It* (Johns, 1990); see also the USDA National Plants Database for further information. See **References** and **Suggested Readings** for full bibliographic details.

References

Berlin B: *Ethnobiological classification: principles of categorization of plants and animals in traditional societies*, Princeton, NJ, 1992, Princeton University Press.

DeMallie R, Jahner EA, editors: *Lakota Belief and Ritual*, Lincoln NE, 1991, University of Nebraska Press.

Dobyns HF: *Their Numbers Become Thinned*, Knoxville, 1983, University of Tennessee Press.

Donmoyer P: *Der Freund in der Roth Or: The Friend in Need. An Annotated Translation of an Early Pennsylvania Folk-Healing Manual by Johann Georg Hohman*, Morgantown, PA, 2012, Masthof Press.

Douville V: *Rosebud Sioux Tribe, Sinte Gleska University, Personal Communication*, Mission, SD, June 12, 1997.

Duke JA, Ayensu ES: *Medicinal plants of China*, Algonac, Mich, 1985, Reference Publications.

Ferguson B: *Ortho's complete guide to successful gardening*, The Woodlands, 1983, Ortho Press.

Fiennes RN: *Zoonoses and the origins and ecology of human diseases*, New York, 1978, Academic Press.

Herrick JW: *Iroquois Medical Botany*, Albany, 1977, State University of New York. PhD Thesis.

Johns T: *With bitter herbs they shall eat it: chemical ecology and the origins of human diet and medicine*, Tucson, 1990, University of Arizona Press.

Kartesz J: *Synonymized checklist of the flora of North America*, Portland, Ore, 1994, Timber Press.

Lame Deer FA, Erdoes R: *Gift of Power; the Life and Teachings of a Lakota Medicine Man*, Santa Fe NM, 1992, Bear & Co.

Martin C: *Keepers of the game: Indian-animal relationships and the fur trade*, Berkeley, 1978, University of California Press.

Micozzi MS: Traditional folk medicine and ethnopharmacology, *Hum Organ* 42(2):351–353, 1983.

Moerman DE: *Moerman's Medicinal Plants of Native America*, Ann Arbor, 1986, University of Michigan Museum of Anthropology Technical Reports No. 19.

Moerman DE: *Native American ethnobotany*, Portland, Ore, 1997, Timber Press.

Red Dog, Member of Cheyenne River Sioux Tribal Council, Eagle Butte, SD.

Thin Elk G: *The Red Road Approach*, Minneapolis, 1995, Little Turtle Press.

USDA (United States Department of Agriculture) USDA National Plants Database, Natural Resources Conservation Service, Retrieved from: http://plants.usda.gov. Accessed 7/14/2014.

Vogel VJ: *American Indian medicine*, Norman, 1970, University of Oklahoma Press.

White Hat Sr. A: *Reading and Writing the Lakota Language*, Salt Lake City, 1997, University of Utah Press.

Suggested Readings

Brower LP, Nelson CJ, Seiber JN, et al: Exaptation as an alternative to coevolution in the cardenolide-based chemical defense of monarch butterflies (*Danaus plexippus* L.) against avian predators. In Spencer KC, editor: *Chemical mediation of coevolution*, San Diego, 1988, Academic Press, pp 447–476.

Moerman DE: The medicinal flora of native North America: an analysis, *J Ethnopharmacol* 31:1–42, 1991.

Wrangham RW, Goodall J: Chimpanzee use of medicinal leaves. In Heltne PG, Marquardt L, editors: *Understanding chimpanzees*, Chicago, 1987, University of Chicago Press.

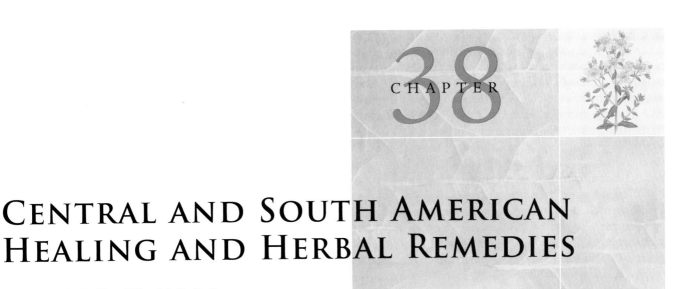

CHAPTER 38

CENTRAL AND SOUTH AMERICAN HEALING AND HERBAL REMEDIES

RICHARD W. VOSS

MARC S. MICOZZI

Traditional medicine in Mexico, Central America, and South America shows features in common with shamanic healing of Native North Americans and the importance of the use of medicinal plants in healing.

In addition, due to the effects of Spanish influence throughout the region for the past half-millennium, there are many examples of syncretic healing traditions that draw together indigenous practices with Roman Catholic spiritual ideas, as in the next chapter on Latin American *curanderismo*, and in Chapter 40 on the Philippine Islands.

Although we have emphasized that the indigenous peoples of the Americas are composed of many different tribes, bands, and nations, one practice that comes close to representing a *"pan-Indian"* healing practice is the *peyote* ritual, or religion deriving from ancient *Aztec* practices in Mexico and Central America.

PEYOTE

The term *Peyote religion* describes a wide range of spiritual practices, primarily from tribes of the American Southwest and Mexico, that have expanded into a kind of *pan-Indian* movement under the auspices of the Native American Church (NAC). Peyote religion is formally recognized, as the NAC incorporates the ritual use of peyote—the small, spineless peyote cactus *Lophophora williamsii*—into its spiritual and healing ceremonies. The peyote ceremony is led by a recognized practitioner, referred to as a *roadman*, who is sponsored by an individual or *family* requesting a ceremony, usually for some specific need or healing or to recognize some event, such as a birthday or an important life transition.

Derived from the Aztec word *péyotl*, the Peyote Way religions have expanded their spheres of influence from an area around the Rio Grande Valley, along the current U.S.-Mexico border, to indigenous groups throughout Central America and North America.

The ritual use of peyote has roots in antiquity. A ritually prepared peyote cactus was discovered at an archeological site that spans the U.S.-Mexico border dated to 5700 years ago. Other archeological evidence—paintings and ritual paraphernalia—indicates that the indigenous people of that region have been using both peyote and psychoactive *mescal* beans ritually for over 10,500 years.

The Peyote Way is a complex bio-psycho-social-spiritual phenomenon that encompasses much more than the pharmacology of the plant. The contemporary peyote practice found in North America and by *Mestizo* peoples in Mexico differs significantly from the older rites that continue to be practiced by the *Huichol*, the *Cora*, and the *Tarahumara* in Mexico. The forbears of the modern NAC were the **Lipan Apache**, who brought the practice from the Mexican side of the Rio Grande to their **Mescalero Apache** relatives around 1870. From the Mescalero it spread to the **Comanche** and **Kiowa** in Oklahoma and Texas. It then quickly spread to most of the Eastern Tribes that had been forcibly relocated to the Oklahoma Territory. To a considerable extent, the tribes in Oklahoma represented **Cherokee**, **Cree**, **Seminoles**, and other Southeastern U.S. tribes that had been forcibly relocated during the *Trail of Tears* marches under President Andrew Jackson in the 1830s. The quick spread from the Mescalero to most of the Oklahoma Tribes after the 1870s has been attributed to the loss of traditional religions, due to oppression and dislocations of the U.S. policy.

The psychedelic properties of peyote are just a part of the whole spiritual package; not to say that peyote does not facilitate visions, but rather that this is only one influence in a total religious setting. It is important to note that describing peyote as a *"psychedelic,"* while technically accurate, is fraught with problems, particularly when the Peyote religion is studied outside its indigenous context. Here, one needs to differentiate the ritual use of peyote by indigenous practitioners, called *roadmen*, and NAC, from its use or abuse by curiosity-seekers and experimenters who are simply seeking a "high" devoid of a ceremonial and cultural context. Peyote has been described as both a psychedelic as well as an *entheogen*. An entheogen is a chemical or botanical substance that produces the experience of God within an individual and has been argued to be an essential part of the study of religious experience. Elsewhere, an entheogen has been defined as a psychoactive sacramental plant or chemical substance taken to occasion primary religious experience (Anderson, 1996). Within such an understanding, the complementary use of peyote ceremony within the context of mental health treatment has been viewed as a form of cultural psychiatry. Other entheogens include *psilocybin* mushrooms and DMT-containing *ayahuasca* (see following section, below), which have also been used continuously for centuries by indigenous people of the Americas.

Mental health practitioners from across disciplines may view Peyote religion and the NAC with some degree of suspicion, if not downright skepticism. Mack (1986) discussed the medical dangers of peyote intoxication in the peer-reviewed *North Carolina Journal of Medicine*. Mack refers to the users of peyote as "the more primitive natives of our hemisphere" (p. 138), and gives repeated attention to details of nausea, vomiting, and bodily reactions that occur at doses (which he failed to mention) 150 to 400 times higher than the ceremonial amount reported nearly a century prior (Anderson, 1996).

Psychiatric researchers Blum, Futterman, and Pascarosa (1977) looked at the mildly psychedelic effects of the peyote, coupled with NAC ritual and exposure to positive images projected by the skillful use of folklore by the roadman. They found that these components facilitated an effective, therapeutic *catharsis*. Albaugh and Anderson (1974) hypothesized that the effects of peyote created a peak psychedelic experience that were similar to those found when using LSD as an adjunct to psychotherapy with alcoholics. In their study of a group of lifelong drug- and alcohol-abstaining **Navajo**, Halpern, Sherwood, et al (2005) found no evidence of psychological or cognitive deficits associated with regularly using peyote in a religious setting.

The placement of peyote, LSD, and other psychedelics on the U.S. Drug Enforcement Administration (DEA) Schedule 1 classification of drugs has eliminated public funding of psychedelic research and limited scientific inquiry on the effects. The current bio-medical opinion on efficacy of entheogens is inconclusive; yet there is limited evidence, and further study is warranted. Wright has suggested that the behavioral sciences should once again become open to the incorporation of mind-expanding substances in the psychiatric or psychotherapeutic treatment milieu. As science takes a more positive look at the effects of traditional healing practices and brain chemistry, new pathways for treatment and renewed discussions about traditional indigenous healing methods may be opened up for study.

AYAHUASCA OF THE RAIN FOREST

After falling out of favor in the United States (as described in Chapter 7), psychedelics made their way back into consciousness (or a version thereof) in the twenty-first century, with some researchers even asking, "Can psychedelics have a role in psychiatry?" (Sessa, 2005). On the legal front, the Supreme Court ruled in favor of the defendant, regarding freedom of religion, in the case of the *Alberto R. Gonzales, Attorney General, et al., v. O Centro Espirita Beneficente Uniao do Vegetal, et al*. The defendant was a New Mexico religious group affiliated with a **Brazilian** church by the same name, a syncretic religion, blending elements of Christianity and African religions with indigenous **Amazonian** shamanistic practices.

Many religious groups use *ayahuasca,* a psychedelic plant with origins in indigenous **South American shamanism**. The active ingredient in ayahuasca (sometimes called *Yagé*) is *N,N*-dimethyltryptamine (DMT), a potent, short-acting hallucinogenic agent also thought to be released during *near-death* experiences (Strassman, 2001). In the context of the religious healing ceremony, ayahuasca is more properly called an entheogen, a psychoactive sacramental plant or chemical substance taken to occasion primary religious experience (Council on Spiritual Practice, 2006).

Indigenous people in **South America** have used ayahuasca for centuries, and the ritual has become common among the *mestizo* populations in urban areas of the Amazon, particularly as a curing ritual for drug addiction (Dobkin de Rios, 1970). Like peyote in the United States, ayahuasca use amongst the indigenous people of the Amazon is a form of cultural "psychiatry." While entheogens are regularly being "discovered" by academic and popular presses, their use for spiritual and healing purposes, especially by indigenous people, has continued unabated. One mixed lineage Spanish and mestizo Indian *ayahuascera* in **Peru** has claimed a spiritual lineage extending 17,000 years.

During modern ceremonies there is a tendency of many of the Euro-Americans present to "do their own thing," whereas the Hispanic and indigenous people present tend to comply with the ritual instructions. Most notable is the recommendations regarding dietary restrictions, to abstain from foods high in salt or fat and eat only steamed vegetables and steamed fish. The shamans note that many physical problems could be solved by adopting these dietary recommendations on a permanent basis.

HEALING INTERACTIONS

The interactions between the healer and the participant are vital and important, and contextual meaning is lost when cultural and linguistic barriers are encountered. With ceremonial words, music, and phrases, **ayahuasca shamans** manipulate participants' consciousness (Dobkin de Rios & Katz, 1975). However, as with the peyote ceremony, the effects of ayahuasca in the context of the ritual environment produce a heightened sense of empathy.

An account of the ayahuasca is given by one witness:
A poignant example came the morning after a ritual. I had accompanied a friend who is in need of a healing, and since this was a serious healing of a physical problem (a tumor), the shaman took special note of the case. During his after-ceremony doctoring session, since I had accompanied the patient, I was asked to assist in the preparations. Since I understood very little Spanish, the interpreter joined us. As the shaman and I worked together for a while, the sense of being empathically connected heightened and at one point, I felt sufficiently connected that when the translator ran into words she did not know, I found myself able to tell her the meaning. Which echoed an experience we had had in the ceremony the night before. This experience came at the end of the ceremony and people were asked to share their experience with each other and with the shaman. Many shared experiences of psychedelic ecstasy, or deep soul-searching journeys; in my case it was a sense of super empathic connection, not so much with the group, but through the shaman and to the collective indigenous experience. To honor that experience I expressed my gratitude to the shaman in my best attempts, but in the Lakota (Sioux) language, not the local language. The translator was baffled, but I understood her to tell him that I was speaking in some indigenous language; his response was that he understood what I had said and proceeded to tell her what I had said and then gave the response he wanted for me.
—Robert Prue, MSW, PhD, assistant professor, University of Missouri, Kansas City; enrolled member, Rosebud Sioux Tribe

BRAIN, BIOLOGY, AND CHEMISTRY

A recent brain imaging study suggests ayahuasca interacts with neural systems central to interoception and emotional processing and point to a modulatory role of serotonergic neurotransmission in these processes (Riba et al, 2006, p. 93). Other types of psychedelics cause elevated blood levels of oxytocin and vasopressin (Jerome & Baggott, 2003), which have been linked to inhibited development of tolerance to opiates. Tolerance to drugs is a necessary part of drug addiction. Oxytocin also has social and emotional dynamics, being involved in pregnancy, labor, and breastfeeding, among other functions. Neurobiology research has highlighted the importance of this chemistry to the dynamics of falling in love and to commitment-making behaviors in primates, particularly playing a role in fostering monogamy. Social interactions are also known to produce increased levels of oxytocin. In a study of stress adaptation in humans, social interactions alone provided

better relief from stress than did the administration of oxytocin alone; however, the combination of the two provided the highest relief in that study group (Heinrichs, Baumgartner, Kirschbaum, & Ehlert, 2003). The administration of an oxytocin-producing substance during a culturally meaningful and often highly intimate social setting is but one element of the set and setting necessary to produce meaningful spiritual changes during entheogenic rituals.

The aim of this chapter is not to suggest that we adopt entheogens to assist in medical treatments or to ignore drug laws. We do well to remember Timothy Leary and Richard Alpert (who suffered a debilitating stroke and is now known as Ram Dass; see Chapter 7). Abuse problems with these types of substances tend to arise after entheogens have "passed from ceremonial to purely hedonic or recreational use" (Masters & Houston, 1966). The use of some types of entheogens is integral to some indigenous spiritual and healing practices. Indigenous healing systems have mechanisms by which one can stand to the status of shaman or facilitator of a healing ritual, a step that few, if any, Western practitioners observe or have risen to.

TALE OF THE SHAMAN'S APPRENTICE

Take the example of a shaman's apprentice, who assisted at two of the ayahuasca ceremonies attended by a witness and facilitated a third, solo:

Following my second meeting with her, I asked if she would be returning the following year, and her reply was "maybe?" She explained that the last ordeal she had to endure to become an independent ayahuasca practitioner was to live among the indigenous people in the rain forest for six months, under the tutelage of their shaman. She further indicated that if she had not properly learned the religion at the end of that six months she would not be allowed to leave, so closely did the indigenous people of the Amazon want to maintain their control of their intellectual property.

The issues of remedies from the rainforests, indigenous knowledge about remedies and healing, and protecting that knowledge and rainforests themselves are addressed in Chapters 34 and 43.

References

Albaugh BJ, Anderson PO: Peyote in the treatment of alcoholism among American Indians, *Am J Psychiatry* 131(11):1247–1250, 1974.

Anderson EF: *Peyote: the divine cactus*, Tucson, 1996, University of Arizona Press.

Blum K, Futterman SL, et al: Peyote, a potential ethnopharmacologic agent for alcoholism and other drug dependencies: Possible biochemical rationale, *Clin Toxicol* 11(4):459–472, 1977.

Council on Spiritual Practice, 2006. Available at: http://csp.org/.

Dobkin de Rios M: A Note on the Use of Ayahuasca among Urban Mestizo Populations in the Peruvian Amazon, *Am Anthropol* 72(6):1419–1422, 1970.

Dobkin de Rios M, Katz F: Some relationships between music and hallucinogenic ritual: The "jungle gym" in consciousness, *Ethos* 3(1):64–76, 1975.

Halpern JH, Sherwood AR, et al: Psychological and cognitive effects of long-term peyote use among Native Americans, *Biol Psychiatry* 58(8):624–631, 2005.

Heinrichs M, Baumgartner T, Kirschbaum C, Ehlert U: Social support and oxytocin interact to suppress cortisol and subjective responses to psychosocial stress, *Biol Psychiatry* 54:1389–1398, 2003.

Jerome L, Baggott M: *MAPS' MDMA investigator's Brochure Update #1: A review of research in humans and non-human animals*, 2003. from: www.maps.org. Retrieved 27 February 2006. 2006.

Mack RB: Marching to a different cactus: Peyote (mescaline) intoxication, *N C Med J* 47(3):137–138, 1986.

Masters REL, Houston J: *The varieties of psychedelic experience*, ed 1, New York, 1966, Holt.

Riba J, Romero S, Grasa E, et al: Increased frontal and paralimbic activation following ayahuasca, the pan-Amazonian inebriant, *Psychopharmacology (Berl)* 186(1):93–98, 2006.

Sessa B: Can psychedelics have a role in psychiatry once again?, *Br J Psychiatry* 186:457–458, 2005.

Strassman R: *DMT: the spirit molecule: a doctor's revolutionary research into the biology of near-death and mystical experiences*, Rochester, Vt., 2001, Park Street Press.

Suggested Readings

Bruhn JG, De Smet PAGM, et al: Mescaline use for 5700 years, *Lancet* 359(9320):1866, 2002.

Calabrese JD: Spiritual healing and human development in the Native American Church: Toward a cultural psychiatry of peyote, *Psychoanal Rev* 84(2):237–255, 1997.

Grof S: Spirituality, addiction, and Western science, *ReVision* 10(2):5–18, 1987.

Halpern JH: Research at Harvard Medical School, *Newsletter of the Multidisciplinary Association for Psychedelic Studies* 11(2):2, 2001.

Hwu H-G, Chen C-H: Association of 5HT2A receptor gene polymorphism and alcohol abuse with behavior problems, *Am J Med Genet* 96(6):797–800, 2000.

Marazziti D: The Neurobiology of Love, *Curr Psychiatry Rev* 1(3):331–335, 2005.

Mauro T: Religious liberty gets boost in hallucinogenic-tea case, *First Amendment Legal Center Bulletin*, 2005. Retrieved from: http://www.firstamendmentcenter.org/news.aspx?id=16524.

McKenna DJ: Clinical investigations of the therapeutic potential of ayahuasca: rationale and regulatory challenges, *Pharmacol Ther* 102:111–129, 2004.

Moir JJC: Shamanism, Traditional Medicine and Drug Dependency in the Peruvian Upper Amazon: A study of addiction therapy and rehabilitation at TAKIWASI centre Retrieved 3/02/02. 1998.

National Association of Social Workers: *Code of ethics (as revised)*, Washington, DC, 1999.

Roberts TJ, Hruby PJ: Toward an Entheogen Research Agenda, *J Humanist Psychol* 42(1):2002.

Sarnyai Z, Kovacs GL: Role of oxytocin in the neuroadaptation to drugs of abuse, *Psychoneuroendocrinology* 19(1):85–117, 1994.

Schaefer SB, Furst PT: *People of the peyote: Huichol Indian history, religion & survival*, Albuquerque, 1996, University of New Mexico Press.

Sherwood JN, Stolaroff MJ, et al: The psychedelic experience: A new concept in psychotherapy, *J Neuropsychiatr* 4(2):96–103, 1962.

Steinberg MK, Hobbs JJ, et al: *Dangerous harvest: drug plants and the transformation of indigenous landscapes*, New York, 2004, Oxford University Press.

Steinmetz, PB: *Pipe, Bible, and peyote among the Oglala Lakota: a study in religious identity*, Knoxville, 1990, University of Tennessee Press.

Tupper KW: Entheogens and existential intelligence: The use of plant teachers as cognitive tools, *Can J Educ* 27(4):499–516, 2002.

Weiskopf J, editor: *Yajé : el nuevo purgatorio*, ed 1, Bogotá, D.C., Colombia, 2002, Villegas Editores.

Wissler C: General discussion of shamanistic and dancing societies, *Anthropol Pap Am Mus Nat Hist* 11(12):853–876, 1916.

Young LJ, Wang Z, Insel TR: Neuroendocrine bases of monogamy, *Trends Neurosci* 21(2):71–75, 1998.

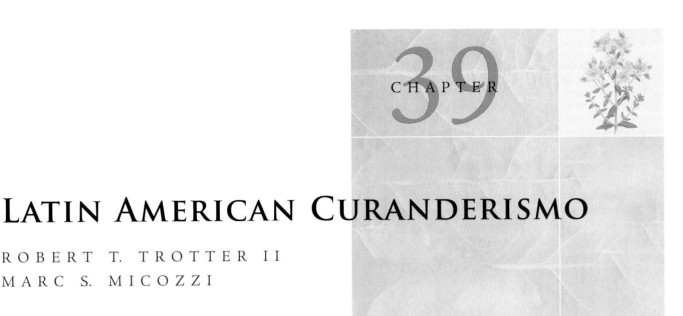

CHAPTER 39

LATIN AMERICAN CURANDERISMO

ROBERT T. TROTTER II

MARC S. MICOZZI

Curanderismo, from the Spanish verb *curar* (to heal), is a broad healing tradition found in in **Mexico** and **Mexican American** communities throughout the **United States**. It has many historical roots in common with traditional healing practices in **Puerto Rico** and **Cuba**, and in other Latin-American communities, as well as with traditional practices found throughout **Latin America**. At the same time, curanderismo has a history and a set of traditional medical practices that are unique to Mexican cultural history and to the Mexican American experience in the United States. It represents a blending (syncretism) of traditional indigenous practices of the **Aztec** civlization of ancient **Mexico** with **Spanish** influences from Medieval **Europe** and the Classical Period in Ancient **Greece-Rome**, as well as from modern biomedicine and even "complementary and alternative" medicine.

Curanderismo has *seven* cultural historical roots (Table 39-1). Its theoretical beliefs trace their origins partly to ancient **Greco-Roman** humoral medicine, also reflected in **Arabic** *Unani* medicine (Chapter 32), especially the emphasis on *balance* and the influence of *hot and cold* properties of food and medicines on the body. Many of the rituals in curanderismo date to healing practices that were contemporary to the beginning of the **Christian** tradition and even into earlier **Judaic** writings. Other healing practices derive from the European Middle Ages, including the use of traditional *medicinal plants* and *magical* healing practices in wide use at that time. The **Moorish** conquest of **Spain** is visible in the cultural expression of curanderismo (see Chapters 32 and 40). Some Mexican American concepts of folk illnesses originated in the **Near East** and then were transmitted throughout the Mediterranean, such as belief in *mal de ojo,* or the "evil eye" (the magical influence of

staring at someone). Homeopathic remedies for common health conditions such as earaches, constipation, anemia, cuts and bruises, and burns were later brought from **Germany** and **Europe** to the Americas to be passed down to the present time within curanderismo. There is also significant sharing of beliefs with **Aztec** and other **Native American** cultural traditions in Mexico (see Chapters 37 and 38). Some of the folk illnesses treated in pre-Columbian times, such as a fallen fontanelle (*caída de la mollera*) and perhaps the blockage of the intestines (*empacho*), are parts of this tradition. The pharmacopeia of the New World is also important in curanderismo (and added significantly to the plants available for treatment of diseases in Europe from the 1600s to the present). Some healers (*curanderos*) keep track of developments in parapsychology and **New Age** spirituality (see Chapter 42), as well as acupuncture and **Asian** healing traditions, and have incorporated these global perspectives into their own practices. Curanderismo is a deeply rooted traditional healing system that actively exists within the modern world. Western biomedical beliefs, treatments, and practices are very much a part of curanderismo and are supported by curanderos. On the border between the United States and Mexico, it is not unusual for healers to recommend the use of prescription medications (which can often be purchased in Mexico over the counter) for infections and other illnesses. These healers also use information obtained from television and other sources to provide the best advice on preventive efforts such as nutrition and exercise and on explanations for biomedical illnesses.

Individual healers vary greatly in their knowledge of the practices that stem from each of these seven historical sources. The overall system of curanderismo is complex

TABLE 39-1 *Seven Pillars of Curanderismo*

From Ancient Aztec	Folk illnesses, indigenous medicinal plants
From Spain:	
Ancient Greco-Roman	Balance of the four humors, hot and cold
Arabic (Moorish in Spain)	Malign magic, personalistic causes of illness
European Medieval	Herbal remedies, magical healing
From Europe and the United States:	
Germany	Homeopathy
United States	Prescription drugs available OTC
New Age	Spirituality, CAM, Asian medicine

and not only maintains its cultural link to the past but also evolves toward accommodation with the future (Table 39-1).

The earliest systematic research was done on curanderismo in the late 1950s, when modern biomedicine was either inaccessible or only recently available to significant segments of the Mexican American population. Since that time, modern medicine has become a more integrated part of the cultural system, although there are still many access barriers. These barriers to access are the same reason that the *holistic* health and *charismatic* healing movements are becoming increasingly popular. Although traditional healers in Mexican American communities now believe that modern medicine is as capable in certain types of healing, their experience shows that they can accomplish those same tasks better than modern medicine.

NATURAL AND SUPERNATURAL

Traditional Mexican American healers perceive health and illness to be related to a duality of "natural" and "supernatural" causes. This duality forms the theoretical base on which curanderismo is constructed. The *natural* source of illness is essentially seen as a biomedical construct that includes lay interpretations of some diseases inspired by Mexican culture; biomedical ideas such as the germ theory of disease, genetic disorders, psychological conditions, and dietary causes for medical conditions are accepted. These natural illnesses are treated with *herbal remedies*. Supernatural sources of illness are also recognized by this healing tradition. These illnesses are *not* considered amenable to treatment by the medical establishment. They can be repaired only by the supernatural manipulations of curanderos. The curanderos fault the scientific medical system for its failure to recognize the existence of *magic* or of supernatural causation. One curandero comments that as many as 10% of patients in mental institutions are really *embrujados* (hexed or bewitched), and because physicians

cannot recognize this condition, it goes untreated. This curandero is willing to test his theory scientifically in any way that the mental health professionals would be willing to set up as a research project. However, the mental health professionals are not willing to allow the tests to be conducted because of their negative attitudes toward curanderismo. In this case, it appears that curanderos have stronger belief and trust in *science*, even when directed at the *supernatural*, than do physicians and other health professionals.

Supernaturally induced illnesses are most often said to be initiated by either *espiritos malos* (evil spirits) or by *brujos* (individuals practicing malign magic; see also Chapter 42). These illnesses form a significant part of the curanderos' work; these healers explain that, theoretically, any particular illness experienced by a patient could be caused by either natural or supernatural processes. For example, they believe there is a natural form of diabetes and a form that is caused by a supernatural agent, such as a *brujo*. The same is true for alcoholism, cancer, and other diseases. Identifying the nature of the causal agent for a particular illness is a key problem for the curandero. Some identify more supernatural causes for illnesses, and others take a more biomedically balanced approach. In either case, there is much less separation of physical from social problems with curanderismo than with the medical care system. Curanderos routinely deal with problems of a social, psychological, and spiritual nature, as well as physical ailments. Many cases overlap into two or more categories. Bad luck in business is a common problem presented to curanderos. Other problems include marital disruptions, alcoholism or alcohol abuse, infidelity, supernatural manifestations, cancer, diabetes, and infertility. One healer distinguishes between the problems presented by women and men. The central focus of the problems brought by women is the husband; the husband drinks too much, does not work, does not give her money, or is seeing other women. Men bring problems of a more physical nature, such as stomach pain, headaches, weakness, and bladder dysfunction. Men also bring problems that deal directly with work; they need to find a job, cannot get along with people at work, or are having trouble setting up a business. The wife rarely is the focal point of their problems. The total list of problems presented to curanderos includes almost every situation that can be thought of as an uncomfortable human condition.

Curanderismo healers work by virtue of "a gift of healing" (*el don*) (Hudson, 1951; Madsen, 1965; Romano, 1965; Rubel, 1966, 1964, 1990). This inherent ability allows the healer to practice his or her work, especially in the supernatural arena. In the past this was believed to be a gift from God. However, a secular interpretation of the *don* is competing with the more traditional explanation. Many healers still refer to the *don* as a gift from God and support this premise with Biblical passages (Corinthians 12:7 and James 5:14), but other healers explain it as an inborn trait that is present in all humans, just like the ability to sing, run, or talk. Almost any person can do these things, but some do them better than others, and a few people can do them extremely well. Curanderos, according to this theory, are the individuals who are better at healing than the population as a whole. Healers refer to this concept as "developed abilities."

Another element common to Hispanic-based folk medicine is the *hot-cold* syndrome (Currier, 1966; Foster, 1953; Ingham, 1940), such as not eating citrus during menses, not ironing barefoot on a cement floor, or taking a cold shower after prolonged exposure to the sun. There is extensive knowledge and use of this system of classifying foods, treatments, and elements of illnesses to provide the basis for deciding which remedies apply to specific illnesses.

THREE LEVELS

The community-based practice of curanderismo has three primary areas of concentration, called *levels* (*niveles*) by the healers: the material level (*nivel material*), the spiritual level (*nivel espiritual*), and the mental level (*nivel mental*). More curanderos have the *don* for working at the material level, which is organized around the use of physical objects to heal or change the patient's environment. This theoretical area can be subdivided into physical and supernatural manipulations. Physical treatments are those that do not require supernatural intervention to ensure a successful outcome. *Parteras* (midwives), *hueseros* (bone setters), *yerberos* (herbalists), and *sobadores* (people who treat sprains and tense muscles) are healers who work on the *nivel material* and effect cures without any need for supernatural knowledge or practices. All the *remedios caseros* (home remedies) are part of this healing tradition.

The supernatural aspect of this level is involved in cures for common folk illnesses, such as *susto*, *empacho*, *caída de mollera*, *espanto*, and *mal de ojo*. These illnesses are unique to **Hispanic** cultural models of health and illness. This area of healing also includes the spells and incantations that are derived out of **medieval European** witchcraft (see Chapter 42) and earlier forms of magic, such as the *cabala*, that have been maintained as supernatural healing elements of curanderismo. Supernatural manipulations involve prayers and incantations in conjunction with such objects as candles, ribbons, water, fire, crucifixes, tree branches, herbs, oils, eggs, and live animals. These treatments use a combination of common objects and rituals to cure health problems.

The spiritual level (*nivel espiritual*) is parallel to the *channeling* found in **New Age** groups (neo-Shamanism) and in **shamanistic** healing rituals around the world (Macklin, 1967, 1974). Individuals enter a trancelike, *altered state of consciousness* and, according to the curanderos, make contact with the spirit world by one or all of the following means: opening their minds to spirit *voices*, sending their spirits out of the body to gain knowledge at a *distance*, and allowing spirits the use of the body to *communicate* with this world.

The mental level (*nivel mental*) is the least often encountered of the three levels. One healer described working with the mental level as the ability to transmit, channel, and focus mental vibrations (*vibraciones mentales*) in a way that would affect the patient's mental or physical condition directly. Both patients and healers are confident that the curanderos can effect a cure from a distance using this technique.

The three levels are discrete areas of knowledge and behavior, each necessitating the presence of a separate *gift for healing*. They involve different types of training and different methods of dealing with both the natural and the supernatural world. The *material* level involves the manipulations of traditional *magical* forces found in literature on Western witchcraft (in Chapter 42).

Spiritualism involves the manipulation of a complex spirit world that exists parallel to our own and the manipulation of *corrientes espirituales*, spiritual currents that can both heal and provide information or diagnosis from a distance. The mental level necessitates the control and use of the previously mentioned *vibraciones mentales*. Thus the levels are separate methods of diagnosing and treating human problems that are embedded in a single cultural tradition.

Common to the practices of all three levels is the use of **energy** to change the patient's health status. On the material level, this energy often is discussed in relation to the major ritual of that level, known as the *barrida* or *limpia* (a "sweeping" or "cleansing"). In this ritual a person is "swept" from head to foot with an object that is thought to either remove bad vibrations (*vibraciones malos*) or give positive energy (*vibraciones positives*) to the patient. The type of object used (e.g., egg, lemon, garlic, crucifix, broom) depends on the nature of the patient's problem and whether it is necessary to remove or to replace energy. On the spiritual level, the energy used for both diagnosis and healing is the previously mentioned *corrientes espirituales*. The mental level is almost totally oriented around generating and channeling *vibraciones mentales*.

The material level is the easiest of the three levels to describe; it is the most extensively practiced and the most widely reported. At this level the curandero manipulates physical objects and performs rituals (or *trabajas*, spells). The combination of objects and rituals is widely recognized by as having curative powers. Practitioners of the material level use common herbs, fruits, nuts, flowers, animals (chickens, doves), animal products (eggs), and spices. Religious symbols, such as the crucifix, pictures of saints, incense, candles, holy water, oils, and sweet fragrances, are widely used, as are secular items, such as cards, alum, and ribbons. The curandero allows the patients to rely extensively on their own resources by prescribing items that either are familiar or have strong cultural significance. Thus a significant characteristic of the objects used at the material level is that they are common items used for daily activities such as cooking and worship.

NATURAL ILLNESSES AND NATURAL CURES

Curanderos recognize that illnesses can be brought about by natural causes, such as dysfunction of the body, carelessness or the inability to perform proper self-care, and infection. Curanderos at the material level use medicinal herbs (*plantas medicinales*) to treat these natural ailments. Some traditional curanderos classify herbs as having the dichotomous properties considered essential for humoral medicine, based on a *hot-cold* classification system common throughout Latin America (Foster, 1953). They use these dual properties to prescribe an herb or combination of herbs, depending on the characteristics of the illness. If a person's illness is supposedly caused by excessive "heat," an herb with "cold" properties is given. Conversely, if a person's illness is believed to be caused by excessive "coldness and dryness," a combination of herbs having "hot and wet" properties is administered.

Other curanderos recognize herbs for their chemical properties, such as poisons (*yerba del coyote, Karwinskia humboldtuna* Roem. et Sch.), hallucinogens (*peyote, Lophaphora williamsii* Lem.), sedatives (*flor de tila, Talia mexicana* Schl.), stimulants (*yerba del trueno*), and purgatives (*cascara sagrada*). These individuals refer to the beneficial chemical properties of the herbs that allow them to treat natural illnesses.

Curanderos prescribe herbs most frequently as teas, baths, or poultices. *Borraja* (borage, *Borajo officialis* L.), for example, is taken to cut a fever; *flor de tila*, a mild sedative, is taken for insomnia; *yerba de la golondrina* (*Euphorbia prostrata* Ait.) is used as a douche for vaginal discharges; and *peilos de elote* are used for kidney problems. Herbal baths are usually prescribed to deal with skin diseases; *fresno* (ash tree, *Fraxinus* species) is used to treat scalp problems such as eczema, dandruff, and psoriasis; and *linaza* is prescribed for body sores. For specific sores such as boils, *malva* (probably a *Malvastrum*) leaves are boiled until soft and then applied to the sores as a poultice. Other herbs are used as decongestants. A handful of *oregano* (oregano, *Oregenum vulgare* L.) is placed in a humidifier to treat someone with a bad cold.

Some herbal lore is passed on as an **oral tradition**, and other information is available in **Spanish-language books** that are widely circulated among both curanderos and the public. These works describe and classify numerous herbs. Herbal remedies are so important to Mexican American folk medicine that often their use is confused with the art of curanderismo itself by the mass culture. Indeed, some curanderos, known as *yerberos* or *yerberas*, specialize in herbs, but their knowledge and skills go beyond the mere connection of one disease to one herbal formula. For curanderos to be genuine, even at the material level, an element of mysticism must be involved in their practice. Herbs are typically used for their spiritual or supernatural properties. Spiritual cleansings (*barridas*) often are given with *ruda* (*Ruta graveolens* L.), *romero* (rosemary, *Rosmarinus officinalis* L.), and *albacar* (sweet basil, *Ocimum basiticum* L.), among others. Herbs are used as amulets; *verbena* (verbena, *Verbena officinalis* L.), worn as an amulet, is used to help open a person's mind to learning and retaining knowledge.

Some curanderos have successful practices on the material level without resorting to the use of herbs. Some nonherbal treatments are described in the following section.

SUPERNATURAL ILLNESSES AND CEREMONIAL CURES

Supernatural illnesses, which occur when supernatural negative forces damage a person's health, can sometimes be confused with natural illnesses. One healer stated that these supernatural illnesses may manifest as ulcers, tuberculosis, rheumatism, or migraine headaches, but in reality, they are believed to be hexes that have been placed on the person by an enemy. Supernatural influences also disrupt a person's mental health and his or her living environment. Physicians cannot cure a supernatural illness. The curandero usually deals with social disruption, personality complexes, and sometimes, serious psychological disturbances.

Also, a number of illnesses are both supernaturally caused and of a supernatural nature but can be treated on the material level.

SWEEPING, "SMOKING," AND CONJURING

Curanderos use several types of rituals for supernatural cures. The *barrida* is one of the most common rituals. These cleansings are designed to remove negative forces while simultaneously giving the patient the spiritual strength necessary to enhance recovery. Patients are always "swept" from head to toe, with the curandero making sweeping or brushing motions with an egg, lemon, herb, or whatever object is deemed spiritually appropriate. Special emphasis is given to areas in pain. While sweeping the patient, the curandero recites specific prayers or invocations that appeal to God, saints, or other supernatural beings to restore health to the patient. The curandero may recite these prayers and invocations out loud or silently. Standard prayers include the Lord's Prayer, the Apostles' Creed, and *Las Doce Verdades del Mundo* (The Twelve Truths of the World). Many of the tools used in *barridas* are plants that are available in people's yards, while others can be purchased at local *yerberias* (*hierberias*) or *botanicas* (Figure 39-1).

The following description of a *barrida* illustrates how the material objects, the mystical power of these objects, the invocations, the curandero, and the patient come together to form a healing ritual designed for a specific patient and a specific illness:

In this case, five eggs, four lemons, some branches of *albacar* (sweet basil), and oil were used. To begin the healing process, the lemons and eggs were washed with alcohol and water to cleanse them spiritually. Before

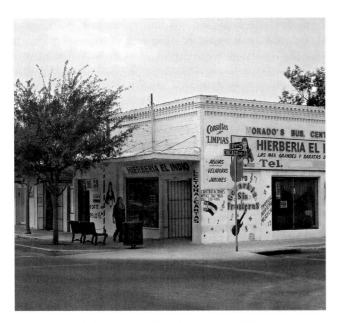

Figure 39-1 Hierberia (McAllen, Texas, June 2008).

beginning the ritual, the participants were instructed to take off their rings, watches, and other jewelry; high-frequency spiritual and mental vibrations can produce electrical discharges on the metal, which might disturb the healing process. The sweeping itself is done by interchanging an egg and a lemon successively. Sweeping with the egg is intended to transfer the problem from the patient to the egg by means of conjures (*conjuros*) and invocations (*rechasos*). The lemon is used to eliminate the *trabajo* (magical harm) that has been placed on the patient. The patient is swept once with *albacar* (sweet basil) that has been rinsed in *agua preparada* (prepared water). This sweeping purifies the patient, giving strength and comfort to his spiritual being. The ritual ends by making crosses with *aceite preparado* (specifically prepared oil) on the patient's principal joints, such as the neck, under the knees, and above the elbow. This oil serves to cut the negative currents and vibrations that surround the patient, which have been placed there by whoever is provoking the harm. The crosses protect against the continued effect of these negative vibrations. *Agua preparada* is then rubbed on the patient's forehead and occiput (*cerebro*) to tranquilize and to give mental strength. All the objects used in the *barrida* are then burned to destroy the negative influences or harm transferred from the patient.

Another common ritual is called a *sahumerio,* or "incensing." The *sahumerio* is a purification rite used primarily for treating businesses, households, farms, and other places of work or habitation. This ritual is performed by treating hot coals with an appropriate incense. The curandero may prepare his or her own incense or may prescribe some commercially prepared incense, such as *el sahumerio maravilloso* (miraculous incense). A pan with the smoking incense is carried throughout the building, making sure that all corners, closets, and hidden spaces, such as under the beds,

are properly filled with smoke. While incensing, the healer or someone else recites an appropriate prayer. If the *sahumerio maravilloso* is used, the prayer is often one to Santa Marta, requesting that peace and harmony be restored to the household. After the *sahumerio,* the healer may sprinkle holy water on the floor of every room in the house and light a white candle that stays lit for seven days. The *sahumerio* is an example of the curandero treating the general social environment, seeking to *change the conditions* of the people who live or work there. Incensing of a house removes negative influences such as bad luck (*salaciones*), marital disruptions, illness, or disharmony. For business and farms, incensing helps ensure success and growth and protects against jealous competitors. These rituals are designed to affect everyone in the environment that has been treated.

Another type of ritual, called a *sortilegio* (conjure), uses material objects such as ribbons to tie up the negative influences that harm the curandero's patients. These negative influences are often personal shortcomings, such as excessive drinking, infidelity, rebellious children, unemployment, or any other problem believed to be imposed by antisocial magic (*un trabajo*). One *sortilegio* required four ribbons in red, green, white, and black, each approximately 1 yard in length. The color of each ribbon represents a type of magic, which the curanderos can activate to deal with specific problems. Red magic involves domination, green deals with healing (green is the color associated with medicine in ancient Greece-Rome, spiritual healing in Islam, and is reflected in Western academic symbolism, as well as *Latino* practices today), white with general positive forces, and black with negative or debilitating forces.

When working with a specific area of magic, a curandero uses material objects that are the appropriate color naturally or that have been made that color artificially. The color-based division of magic is also carried over into another type of ritual system used on the material level, *velacione,* or *burning candles* to produce supernatural results. The *velaciones* and the colored material objects used in the *sortilegios* tie into the energy theme that runs throughout curanderismo, because the **colors** and objects are believed to have specific **vibratory** power or **energy** that can affect the patient when activated by the incantations used in conjunction with the objects. For example, blue candles are burned for serenity or tranquility; red candles are burned for health, power, or domination; pink candles are burned for good will; green candles are burned to remove a harmful or negative influence; and purple candles are burned to repel and attack bad spirits (*espiritus obscuros*) or strong magic. Once the proper color of candle has been chosen to produce the proper mental atmosphere, the candles are arranged in the correct physical formation and activated by the *conjuros y rechasos*. If patients ask for protection, the candles might be burned in a triangle, which is considered the strongest formation, one whose influence cannot be broken easily. If they want to dominate someone—a spouse, a lover, or an adversary—the candles might be burned in circles. Other formations include crosses, rectangles, and squares, depending on the results desired.

Another relatively common use of candles is to diagnose problems by studying the flame or the ridges that appear in the melted wax. A patient may be swept with a candle while the healer recites an invocation asking the patient's spirit to allow its material being to be investigated for any physical or spiritual problems that may be affecting the person. This ritual can also be performed by burning objects used in a *barrida*. Lighting the candle or burning the object after the *barrida* helps the curandero reveal the cause and extent of the patient's problems. Similarly, if a petitioner asks for candling, the wax of the candles burned for the *velacione* may be examined for figures or other messages that point to the source of a patient's problems.

One of the organizing principles of the material level of curanderismo is *synchronicity* with Christianity in general and the **Catholic Church** in particular. Special invocations often are directed at saints or spirits to bring about desired results. For example, San Martin de Porres is asked to relieve poverty, San Martin Caballero to ensure success in business, San Judas Tadeo to help in impossible situations, and Santa Marta to bring harmony to a household. Ritual materials used by the Church, such as *water, incense, oils,* and *candles,* are extensively used by **folk healers**. The ways in which these religious objects are used, and the theories for their efficacy, closely mirror concepts found within the healing ministry of the **Church**, which are actually not incompatible with **European witchcraft** (see Chapter 42), from which **curanderismo** partly derives.

THE SPIRITUAL LEVEL (NIVEL ESPIRITUAL)

There are fewer curanderos who have the *don* for working on the spiritual level (*nivel espiritual*) of curanderismo than those who work on the material level. These practitioners also must go through a developmental period (*desarrollo*) that can be somewhat traumatic. Spiritual practices in communities revolve around a belief in spiritual beings who inhabit another plane of existence but who are interested in making contact with the physical world periodically. Healers become a direct link between this plane of existence and that other world. In some cases the curanderos claim to control these spirit beings, and in other cases they merely act as a channel through which messages pass. Some of these practices are carried out by individual healers, whereas other activities occur in conjunction with spiritual centers (*centros espiritistas*) that are staffed by trance mediums and other individuals with occult abilities. These centers often work through two prominent folk saints: El Niño Fidencio from northern Mexico and Don Pedrito Jaramillo from southern Texas (Macklin, 1974). This trend in visiting spiritualist centers appears to be relatively recent, also extensively seen in Brazil now, not having been reported during the 1950s and 1960s by those doing research on Mexican American folk medicine.

Since the 1960s, other spiritualist centers have developed in Latin America, for example, in **Brazil**, under the auspices of "John of God." Through what is known explicitly as **Spiritism**, John of God and his disciples clearly describe that they are channeling healing energy from a divine source. Adherents see this approach as more appropriate for mental health than Western biomedical forms of psychotherapy, and more broadly, there is a movement that sees Spiritism as a global panacea for the health care system.

The practice of spiritualism rests on "soul concept," a belief in the existence of spirit entities derived from once-living humans. The soul is thought to be the immortal component, the life and personality force of humans, an entity that continues to exist after physical death on a plane of reality separate from the physical world. This concept is important not only to curanderismo but also to the religions and mystical beliefs found in all Western-derived cultures.

The soul is alternatively described by curanderos as a *force field*, ectoplasm, concentrated vibrations, or group of electrical charges that exist separately from the physical body. It is thought to retain the personality, knowledge, and motivations of the individual even after the death of the body. Under proper conditions the soul is ascribed the ability to contact and affect persons living in the physical world. Although souls occasionally can be seen as ghosts or apparitions by ordinary humans, they exist more often in the spiritual realm previously mentioned. Some people view this realm as having various divisions that are associated with positive or negative connotations (e.g., heaven, limbo, purgatory, hell). Other people see the spiritual realm as parallel to the physical world. They state that the spiritual is a more pleasant plane on which to live, but few attempt any suicidal test of this belief. One healer commented that "spirits" (*espiritos*) and "souls" (*almas*) are the same thing. These spirits' activities closely parallel their former activities in this world. Because the personality, knowledge, and motivation of the spirits are much the same as they were for the living being, there are both good and evil spirits, spirits who heal and spirits who harm, and both wise and foolish spirits.

These spirits might communicate with or act on the physical plane. Some have left tasks undone in their physical lives that they want to complete; others want to help or cause harm; and many want to communicate messages to friends and relatives, telling them of their happiness or discontent with their new existence. Therefore, curanderos with the ability to work on the spiritual realm become the link between these two worlds. Some curanderos believe that there are multitudes of spirits who want to communicate with the physical world, and they tend to hover around those who have the *don* to become a medium, waiting for an opportunity to enter their bodies and possess them. This situation explains the cases of spirit possession among various cultures. Individuals who become possessed are people with a strong potential to be trance mediums who have not had the opportunity to learn how to control this condition.

The ability to become a medium is thought to be centered in the *cerebro,* that portion of the brain found at the posterior base of the skull (anatomically, the cerebellum, which controls coordination and spatial orientation). Those with the gift are said to have a more fully developed cerebro, whereas those without it are said to have a weak cerebro (*un cerebro débil*). This weakness has no relationship either to the intelligence or to the moral nature of the individual, only to his or her ability to communicate with the spiritual realm. Weak cerebros represent a danger for anyone who wants to become a medium. Only rare individuals demonstrate mediumistic potential spontaneously and can practice as mediums without further training. Therefore, curanderos often test their patients and friends for this gift of healing, and those with the gift are encouraged to develop their ability.

The development of this ability is called *desarrollo* and is a fairly lengthy process that might last from two months to more than six months initially, with periodic refresher encounters often available from the *maestro* (teacher). *Desarrollo* is a gradual process of increasing an apprentice's contact with the spirit world, giving the apprentice more and more experiences in controlled trances and possessions, as well as the knowledge necessary to develop and protect the apprentice as a spiritualist. The teacher also is responsible for giving the apprentice knowledge at a safe pace. The curandero does not always explain what each sensation means; each person, as he or she develops, becomes more sensitive to the environment. The apprentice must expect to encounter odd sensations, such as bright lights, noises, changes in pressure, and other sensations associated with developing powers. At the end of these *desarrollo* sessions, the conversation reverts to social chatting for some time before the apprentice leaves. This developmental process continues, with variations, until the apprentice is a fully developed medium.

Fully developed mediums control how, where, and when they work, and several options are available to them. Some mediums work alone and treat only family problems Others might use their abilities only for their own knowledge and gratification. Some mediums work in groups with other mediums or with other persons whom they believe have complementary spiritual or psychic powers. Some mediums work in elaborate spiritual centers (*centros espiritistas*) that are formal churches, often dedicated to a particular spirit (e.g., Fidencio, Francisco Rojas, Don Pedrito Jaramillo). The spiritual centers and the activities surrounding them take on the major aspects of a formalized religion.

Sometimes a trance session is open to more than one person at the same time. This group session can be carried out by a lone curandero but more often is found at spiritual centers. Once a temple has been established, it may house from 1 to 20 mediums. The more mediums, the better; otherwise, a medium may have to let his or her body be used by too many different spirits, exhausting him or her, and laying the medium open to supernatural harm.

Larger temples might have four or five *videntes* (clairvoyants), as well as the mediums, and might be putting several apprentices through *desarrollo* at the same time. Some temples are located in *Espinazo,* the home of El Niño Fidencio and a center of pilgrimage for mediums practicing in his name, and others are in urban centers such as Tampico and Mexico City. Large numbers of people make pilgrimages to these healing centers in Mexico to deal with health care problems that they have not resolved in the United States.

One healing center is called *Roca Blanca,* after the spirit that speaks most often in that place. The owner, Lupita, founded it about 30 years ago, after discovering her ability to cure. She was granted permission to practice by a spiritual association.

These spiritual centers vary according to their size, their owners, and the spirits associated with them, but there is considerable regularity in the services they perform. Sometimes mediums prescribe simple herbal remedies for physical problems. These ingredients are virtually identical to the ones presented in the previous section on the material level, although, occasionally, it is said that a spirit will recommend a new use for an herb. The mediums might suggest that the patient perform the already familiar rituals of curanderismo, such as the *barrida*. The spirits are thought to be able to influence people's lives directly, in addition to imparting knowledge about remedies. The curanderos state that spirits control spiritual currents (*corrientes espirituales*) and mental vibrations (*vibraciones mentales*); they can manipulate patients' health by directing positive or negative forces at them from the spiritual realm.

THE MENTAL LEVEL

The mental level has the fewest rituals and outward, complex behaviors associated with it. To date, it also has the fewest practitioners. All the cases follow a similar pattern. For example:

> After the curandero chatted with the patient and asked about the basic problem. He asked the patient to state her complete name (*el nombre completo*). The curandero wrote the name on a piece of paper. Sitting behind the desk he used for consultations, he leaned his arms on the desk, bent forward slightly, closed his eyes, and concentrated on the piece of paper. After a few minutes, he opened his eyes, told the patient more about her problem, and stated that it was being resolved.

> The curandero stated that he had learned to use his mind as a transmitter through *desarrollo*. He could channel, focus, and direct *vibraciones mentales* at the patient. These mental vibrations worked in two ways—one physical, one behavioral. If he was working with a physical illness, such as cancer, he channeled the vibrations to the afflicted area, which he already had pinpointed, and used the vibrations to retard the growth of damaged cells and accelerate the growth of normal cells. In a case of desired behavioral changes, he sent the vibrations into the person's mind and manipulated these vibrations in a way that modified the

person's behavior. The curandero gave an example of one such case in which a husband had begun drinking excessively, was seeing other women, was being a poor father to his children, and was in danger of losing his job. The curandero stated that he dominated the man's thought processes and shifted them so that the husband stopped drinking to excess and became a model husband and father.

There also are a number of *syncretic* beliefs drawn from other alternative healing traditions—such as **New Age** practices, the "psychic sciences," and **Asian** philosophy—that have been incorporated into this area of curanderismo. For example, some healers state that they are able to perceive "*auras*" around people and that they can use these auras to diagnose problems that patients are encountering. They conduct the diagnosis on the basis of the color or shape of the patient's aura. Some state that they learned these practices from other healers, whereas others indicate that they learned them from books on parapsychology.

The mental level is practiced most often by individual healers working with individual patients, rather than in groups. It appears to be a new addition to this healing system and does not have, as yet, a codified body of ritual associated with it.

The three levels of curanderismo unify the theories of disease and illness found in the Mexican American folk medical model. The system emphasizes a *holistic* approach to treatment and relies heavily on the intimate nature of the referral system and the extensive personal knowledge of the patient's social environment that is normally held by the curandero. Christian symbols and theology provide both tools (candles, incense, water) and practice models (rituals, prayers, animistic concepts) for the material and the spiritual levels, but not to a similar degree for the mental level. An *energy* concept is the central idea that integrates the three levels and forms a systematic interrelationship among them. This energy concept derives from belief in forces, vibration, and currents that center in the mind of those who have the gift for healing and who can transmit to cause healing from a distance, by affecting the patient's social, physical, spiritual, or psychological environment.

All three levels of healing are still evolving. The variations in the practices of curanderismo can be explained partly by differences in the curanderos' personality, differences in their treatment preferences or abilities, and differences in their emphasis on theoretical or experiential approaches.

WHERE HEALING HAPPENS

Curanderismo is a **community**-based healing system. It is complex and widespread. In the United States, for example, it may be practiced in any area where Mexican Americans know about it. Part of this healing tradition is the information that is spread throughout the Mexican American culture on home treatments for common physical ailments (colds, flu, arthritis, asthma, diabetes) and for common

spiritual or "folk illnesses" (*susto*, *mal de ojo*, and *empacho*), analogous to the biomedical information that is spread throughout all European cultures, including the Mexican American culture, where the **home** is the first line of defense for the diagnosis of illnesses that eventually might necessitate a physician or hospital. On the other hand, some aspects of curanderismo require the use of special locations, preparations, and tools. This is especially true of spiritual practices on the spiritual level and for the effective treatment of supernatural harm on the material level.

The first setting where this knowledge is used is at **home**. When people become ill, they use their existing cultural model of health and illness to come up with solutions. One type of solution is home diagnosis and home treatment. Therefore, both biomedical concepts and folk medical concepts are applied immediately, and home treatments are attempted. In the case of curanderismo, this often results in the use of home remedies (*remedios caseros*) that have been part of the culture for generations, especially herbal cures. When the diagnosis identifies a magical or supernaturally caused illness, the illness results in a home-based ritual. These interventions are done by mothers, grandmothers, cousins, friends, or knowledgeable acquaintances.

Illnesses that appear to be too serious to handle at home, both natural and supernatural, are taken to **professional healers** who have a locally widespread reputation for being able to treat both biomedical and traditional health care problems. Most of these healers work in a silent, but positive, partnership with physicians, although often the physicians are unaware of the link. The curanderos consistently refer patients to modern health care services when they see the efficacy of that approach to be equal to or greater than their own. At the same time, they note significant differences in the models of health and illness between their own practices and modern medicine, especially in the areas of supernatural illnesses, in addressing social (marital, business, interpersonal) problems and in dealing with psychological problems.

In these cases the treatments take place either in the patient's home or work environment or in **special workrooms** established by the curanderos as part of their practices. The cure might call for working **directly in the environment** that is affected. In other cases the venue of choice is the curandero's area because the cure depends on careful preparation and protection from outside influences. These work areas contain altars, medicinal plants, tools for supernatural rituals, and other items, and the atmosphere is considered most beneficial for the healing process, particularly in the case of supernatural problems and treatments.

HOME REMEDIES

Herbal and chemical treatments for both natural and supernatural illnesses are common in Mexican American communities. More than 800 *remedios caseros* have been identified on the U.S.-Mexican border alone (Trotter, 1981). Many of the remedies have been tested for biochemical and therapeutic activities (Etkin, 1986; Trotter, 1981, 1983; Trotter & Logan, 1986). Overall, the remedies are not only biochemically active; more than 90% have demonstrated therapeutic actions that matched the folk medical model for their uses. At the same time, only a small proportion of the herbs have been tested. This lack of information is being overcome by an ongoing project to study the efficacy of the complete range of herbal cures available in Mexican American communities (Graham, 1994), by use of combined ethnographic and biomedical methods (Browner et al, 1988; Croom, 1983; Ortiz de Montellano & Browner, 1985; Trotter, 1985).

The exception to the general rule of efficacy is the use of remedies for illnesses such as the common cold, where the remedies relieve symptoms but do not directly treat the illness. The actions of these remedies, some of which are described earlier, include diuretics, treatments for constipation, abortifacients, analgesics, sedatives, stimulants, cough suppressants, antibacterial agents, coagulants and anticoagulants, vitamin and mineral supplements, and plants with antiparasitic actions. Most have proved safe and effective when used in the manner described and recommended by the curanderos. This area and the therapeutic, culturally competent counseling practices of the healers are the most clearly acceptable and useful approaches for articulation with modern medicine.

FOUR COMMON FOLK ILLNESSES

Of all the complex areas of Mexican American traditional healing, the one that has received the most research attention has been the study of common folk illnesses that are experienced and treated in Mexican American communities. The most frequently reported are *susto*, an illness caused by a frightening event; *mal de ojo*, an illness that can be traced to the Near East that involves a magically powerful glance taking away some of the vital essence of a susceptible person; *empacho*, a blockage of the intestines caused by eating the wrong type of food at the wrong time or by being forced to eat unwanted food; and *caída de la mollera*, a condition of fallen fontanelle in infants.

These illnesses have been well documented (Rubel, 1964; Weller et al, 1993) both singly and in combination (Baer et al, 1989; Weller et al, 1993). *Susto* is linked directly to serious illness patterns in Latin American communities and acts as an indicator that biomedical personnel should investigate multiple conditions and problems among patients complaining of its symptoms. *Caída de la mollera*, on investigation, is a folk medicine label that corresponds to severe dehydration in infants caused by gastrointestinal problems. It is life threatening and, when identified by parents, is an indicator that the child should be brought in immediately for medical care. *Empacho* is a severe form of constipation treated with numerous remedies that cause diarrhea. Because it is thought to be a blockage of the intestines, the purgative effect of these remedies signals that treatment has been effective. *Mal de ojo* has not been associated with a specific biomedical condition; however, symptoms include irritability, lethargy, and crying, and a connection to mental health may be made by such observations.

Latin American folk medicine contains useful, insightful, and culturally competent healing strategies that work well in Hispanic communities. These treatments range from proven herbal cures to culturally meaningful ways of labeling illness systems.

In light of the sophisticated means for identifying and addressing essentially *spiritual* problems as well, curanderismo appears to routinely exceed the limited ability of Western psychiatry and psychology to deal with chronic mental health conditions as well as alcohol and drug abuse. The practices of curanderismo to draw together meaningful influences from seven different sources of worldwide healing traditions also demonstrates its ability to incorporate and *integrate* culturally meaningful approaches in an era when *integration* of "alternative" therapies is the current fashion in recognizing age-old healing traditions in the Western world.

References

Baer R, Garcia de Alba DJ, Cueto LM: Lead based remedies for *empacho*: patterns and consequences, *Soc Sci Med* 29:1373–1379, 1989.

Browner CH, Ortiz de Montellano BR, Rubel AJ, et al: A new methodology for ethnomedicine, *Curr Anthro* 29:681–701, 1988.

Croom E: Documenting and evaluating herbal remedies, *Econ Botany* 37:13–127, 1983.

Currier RL: The hot-cold syndrome and symbolic balance in Mexican and Spanish American folk medicine, *Ethnology* 4:251–263, 1966.

Etkin N: *Plants used in indigenous medicine: biocultural approaches*, New York, 1986, Redgrave.

Foster GM: Relationships between Spanish and Spanish-American folk medicine, *J Amer Folkore* 66:201–247, 1953.

Graham JS: Mexican American herbal remedies, *Herbalgram* 31:34–35, 1994.

Hudson WM: The healer of Los Olmos and other Mexican lore, *Texas Folklore Society* XXIV, 1951.

Ingham IM: On Mexican folk medicine, *Am Anthropol* 42:76–87, 1940.

Macklin J: *El Nino Fidencio: un studio del Curanderismo en Nuevo Leon*, Anuario Huminitas, Centros de Estudios Humanisticos, Universidad de Nuevo Leon, Mexico, 1967.

Macklin J: Belief, ritual and healing: New England spiritualism and Mexican American spiritism compared. In Zaretsky IT, Leone MP, editors: *Religious movements in contemporary America*, Princeton NJ, 1974, Princeton University Press.

Madsen C: A case study of change in Mexican folk medicine, *Mid Amer Res Inst* 25:93–134, 1965.

Ortiz de Montellano BR, Browner CH: Chemical basis for medicinal plant use in Oxaca, Mexico, *J Enthnopharmacol* 13:57–88, 1985.

Romano O: Charismatic medicine, folk healing and folk saint-hood, *Am Anthropol* 67:1151–1173, 1965.

Rubel AJ: The epidemiology of a folk illness: Susto in Hispanic America, *Ethnology* 3:268–283, 1964.

Rubel AJ: *Across the tracks; Mexican Americans in a Texas City*, Austin, 1966, University of Texas Press.

Rubel AJ: Ethnomedicine. In Johnson TM, Sargent CF, editors: *Medical anthropology: contemporary theory and methods*, New York, 1990, Praeger, pp 120–122.

Trotter RT: Folk remedies as indicators of common illnesses, *J Ethnopharmacol* 4:207–221, 1981.

Trotter RT: Community morbidity patterns and Mexican American folk illness, *Med Anthropol* 7:33–44, 1983.

Trotter RT: A survey of episodic lead poisoning from a folk remedy. In Micozzi MS, editor: *Health Care*, vol 44, 1985, Human Organization, pp 64–71.

Trotter RT, Logan M: Informant Consensus: a new approach for identifying potentially effective medicinal plants. In Etkin N, editor: *Plants used in indigenous medicine; biocultural approach*, New York, 1986, Redgrave.

Weller S, Pachter LM, Trotter RT, Baer RM: Empacho in four Latino groups; study of intra- and inter-cultural variation in beliefs, *Med Anthropol* 15:109–136, 1993.

Suggested Readings

Bard CL: Medicine and surgery among the first Californians, *Touring Topics*, Los Angeles, 1930, Automobile Club of Southern California.

Bourke IH: Popular medicine customs and superstitions of the Rio Grande, *J Am Folklore* 7:119–146, 1894.

Cartou LSM: *Healing herbs of the Upper Rio Grande*, Santa Fe, 1947, Laboratory of Anthropology.

Chavez LR: Doctors, curanderos and brujos: health care delivery and Mexican immigration in San Diego, *Med Anthropol Q* 15(2):31–36, 1984.

Creson DL, McKinley C, Evans R: Folk medicine in Mexican American subculture, *Dis Nerv Syst* 30:264–266, 1969.

Davis J: Witchcraft and superstitions of Torrance County, *NM Histor Rev* 54:53–58, 1979.

Dodson R: Folk curing among the Mexicans. In *Toll the bell easy*, Texas Folklore Society, 1932, Southern Methodist University Press, Nacogdoches, TX.

Fabrega H Jr: On the specificity of folk illness, *Southwest J Anthropol* 26:305–315, 1970.

Gillin J: Witch doctor? A hexing case of dermatitis, *Cutis* 19(1):103–105, 1977.

Gobeil O: El susto: a descriptive analysis, *Int J Soc Psychiatry* 19:38–43, 1973.

Gudeman S: Saints, symbols and ceremonies, *Am Ethnol* 3(4):709–730, 1976.

Hamburger S: Profile of Curanderos: a study of Mexican folk practitioners, *Int J Soc Psychiatry* 24:19–25, 1978.

Johnson CA: Nursing and Mexican-American folk medicine, *Nurs Forum* 4:100–112, 1964.

Karno M, Edgerton RB: Perception of mental illness in a Mexican-American community, *Arch Gen Psychiatry* 20:233–238, 1969.

Klein J: Susto: the anthropological study of diseases of adaptation, *Soc Sci Med* 12:23–28, 1978.

Kreisman JJ: Curandero's apprentice: a therapeutic integration of folk and medical healing, *Am J Psychol* 132:81–83, 1975.

Madsen N: Anxiety and witchcraft in Mexican-American acculturation, *Anthropol Q* 39:110–127, 1966.

Maduro R: Curanderismo and Latino views of disease and curing, *West J Med* 139:868–874, 1983.

Marcos LR, Alpert M: Strategies and risks in psychotherapy with bilingual patients, *Am J Psychiatry* 113(11):1275–1278, 1976.

Marin BV, Marin G, Padilla AM: Utilization of traditional and nontraditional sources of health care among Hispanics, *Hispanic J Behav Sci* 5(1):65–80, 1983.

Montiel M: The social science myth of the Mexican-American family, *El Grito* 3:111, 1970.

Morales A: Mental health and public health issues: the case of the Mexican Americans in Los Angeles, *El Grito* 3(2):111, 1970.

Moustafa A, Weiss G: *Health status and practices of Mexican-Americans*, Berkeley, 1968, University of California Graduate School of Business.

Padilla AM: *Latino mental health: bibliography and abstracts*, Washington, DC, 1973, US Government Printing Office.

Paredes A: *Folk medicine and the intercultural jest in Spanish-speaking people in the U.S*, Seattle, 1968, University of Washington Press, pp 104–119.

Pattison M: Faith healing: a study of personality and function, *J Nerv Ment Dis* 157:397–409, 1973.

Press I: The urban Curandero, *Am Anthropol* 73:741–756, 1971.

Press I: Urban folk medicine, *Am Anthropol* 78(1):71–84, 1978.

Romano O: Donship in a Mexican-American community in Texas, *Am Anthropol* 62:966–976, 1960.

Romano O: The anthropology and sociology of the Mexican-American history, *El Grito* 2, 1969.

Rubel AJ: Ethnomedicine. In Johnson TM, Sargent CF, editors: *Medical anthropology: contemporary theory and methods*, New York, 1990, Praeger, pp 120–122.

Ruiz P, Langrod J: Psychiatry and folk healing: a dichotomy? *Am J Psychiatry* 133:95–97, 1976.

Samora J: Conceptions of disease among Spanish Americans, *Am Cath Soc Rev* 22:314–323, 1961.

Sanchez A: *Cultural differences and medical care: the case of the Spanish-speaking people of the Southwest*, New York, 1954, Russell Sage Foundation.

Sanchez A: The defined and the definers: a mental health issue, *El Sol* 4:10–32, 1971.

Saunders L, Hewes GW: Folk medicine and medical practice, *J Med Educ* 28:43–46, 1953.

Smithers WD: *Nature's pharmacy and the Curanderos*, Alpine, Texas, 1961, Sul Ross State College Bulletin.

Snow LF: Folk medical beliefs and their implications for care of patients, *Ann Intern Med* 81:82–96, 1974.

Trotter RT II: Folk medicine in the Southwest: myths and medical facts, *Postgrad Med* 78(8):167–179, 1986.

Uzzell D: Susto Revisited: illness as a strategic role, *Am Ethnol* 1(2):369–378, 1974.

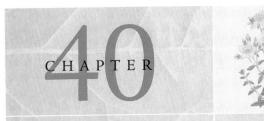

CHAPTER 40

HAWAII, SOUTH PACIFIC, AND PHILIPPINE ISLANDS; ALASKA AND PACIFIC NORTHWEST

MARC S. MICOZZI

ALICIA M. MICOZZI

Traditional healing practices and substances (materia medica) are prominent throughout Hawaii and the Pacific Islands, and in Alaska and the Pacific Northwest, including current and former foreign possessions, trusts, and territories of the United States, such as American Samoa and the Philippines, where health practitioners are likely to encounter them today.

HAWAII

There are many traditional medical experts in traditional Hawaiian culture (*kahuna lapa'au*). Like many traditional medical practices, they learned to approach cases differently based upon their prognosis (as in ancient Egyptian-Greco-Roman and Unani medicine, for example).

Practices among different healers are not identical, similar to the Subanun of Philippines (see also Chapters 34, 35). There are also different "specializations" among healers, one example of which is known as "internal medicine" (*kahuna lapa'au pa'ao'ao*).

There are also those healers who function as "revealers," who divine the causes of diseases (*kahuna kuni*). With this knowledge the revealer is often able to cure the disease as well. If the healer understands the disease but is uncertain about the prognosis, he may introduce other healers into the treatment of the patient. Other healers such as the kuni can be brought in to conduct divination by fire. There are then procedures for determining whether or not the patient could be successfully treated. If not, the healer drops the case, leaving the patient to other resources.

Part of the divination for some patients, includes identifying the patient's "guardian angels" or spirit guides or deities, including the shark, the serpent, the pig, the red fish, the owl, birds, and lizards.

Sometimes the cause of an illness can be attributed to the malevolent intentions of other person(s). If so, the healer may actually work to bring about the death of such person(s).

Through a system of trial and error, several specific disorders with appropriate treatments are developed. Some disorders with selected treatments are shown in Table 40-1.

There are other specific remedies for scrofula (TB of the neck), impetigo, boils, insanity, bone and skull fractures, deafness, swellings, and asthma. The number of different treatments that also have other uses in addition to asthma is notable.

The healer collects the appropriate herbal remedies. During the search the healer is not permitted to defecate or urinate (perhaps ensuring that the plant remedies will not be contaminated as well as having implications for the "purity" of the healing). In addition, he must not meet anyone on the way or be called after from behind (perhaps protecting the knowledge of the sources of remedies), and no bird may make a sound during the quest. Although these practices were looked upon with disdain by Christian missionaries, the rationale for their use in many cases is self-evident and they continued into modern times.

SAMOA

Samoa: Traditional use of *kava kava* (*Piper methysticum*)

TABLE 40-1 *Hawaiian Herbal Remedies*

Disorder	Treatment
Venomous bite	Papaya, Kowali[1] (*Ipomea dissecta*), internally
Headache	*Lomilomi* massage, water
Backache, fractures	Kowali[1] (*Ipomea dissecta*), topically
	Kukui (*Aleurites moluccana*)[2]
Skull fracture	Ilima (*Sida* sp.)
Cold, sore throat	*Lomilomi* massage, gargle with Uhaloa (*Waltheria americana*) root bark
Boils, ulcers	Ti (*Cordyline terminalis*) root
Asthma	Ti (*Cordyline terminalis*) inhalation
	Kukui (*Aleurites moluccana*)[2]
	Kalo[1] or taro (*Colocasia antiquorum*)
	Uhaloa (*Waltheria americana*)
Tuberculosis, involving organs of the neck (scrofula)	Clay, taro (*Colocasia antiquorum*), water
	Kukui (*Aleurites molucanna*)[2]
Lung congestion	Clay, foods, water
Hernia	Castor bean leaf (ricin)
Retained placenta	Hot stone (as in Malaya, Philippines, Indonesia)
Mental illness, debility, fatigue, insomnia	Awa/kava kava (*Piper methysticum*)[3]
	Kalo[1] (*Colocasia antiquorum*)

1. Kowali (*Ipomea dissecta*) and Kalo (*Colocasia antiquorum*) are also generally used as laxatives.
2. Kukui (*Aleuritis moluccana*) is used for stomach complaints; Kowali and Uhaloa (*Waltheria americana*) are used as "tonics" or adaptogens.
3. Awa, kava, or kava kava (**Piper methysticum**) (**Piper**: Latin for "pepper," **methysticum**: [Latinized] Greek for "intoxicating") is an ancient crop of the Western Pacific.

Located in the South Pacific, present-day Samoa includes American Samoa (Eastern Samoa, a trust territory of the United States) and Western Samoa (formerly German Samoa, ceded to New Zealand after World War I and granted independence in 1962).

In Samoa and other islands of the South Pacific, kava (also called kava kava) has a long history of use as a relaxing beverage consumed in rituals and ceremonies (McNally, 1998). Captain James Cook and his crew, arriving at the islands in 1768, were the first Westerners to sample the drink. In modern times, visiting dignitaries such as Pope John Paul II, Queen Elizabeth II, Lady Bird and Lyndon Johnson, and Bill and Hillary Clinton (Box 40-1) have drunk kava beverage as part of their welcome to the islands. In addition to its relaxing properties, kava was historically used for treating headaches, colds, rheumatism, and inflammation of the uterus, and as a sedative and an

BOX 40-1 *Kava Kava: Presidents and Politics*

Politicians and U.S. presidents from Lyndon Johnson to Bill Clinton have traveled to American Samoa (usually before elections) to partake in the ceremonial use of kava kava (also called *kava*). Kava is a psychoactive member of the pepper family. It has been used historically in Samoa and throughout the South Pacific Islands as a ceremonial and recreational tranquilizing beverage.

It is an approved medication in Germany under historical use (perhaps partially owing to the former political affiliation) for "states of nervous anxiety, tension, and agitation," in doses of 60 to 120 mg of kavalactones (compound in kava) for up to three months. Rather than implying any danger in continued use, the three-month limit is more likely a suggestion that one should explore other causes for the anxiety at that point, including those amenable to psychotherapy and stress-reduction techniques. A "scare" was created in Europe and the United States during the prior decade, when a few cases of liver toxicity were reported in association with the use of kava, which caused it to be pulled from the shelves for a time. However, careful analysis (Chapter 24) revealed that each case could be assigned to the concomitant use of hepatotoxic drugs or other conditions. (Meanwhile, for example, hundreds of deaths due to liver failure continue to occur in the United States annually over decades due to use of the over-the-counter medication acetaminophen.)

Kava is increasingly popular in the rest of world and the United States for short-term relief from anxiety and stress. It has been used successfully for stress and specific conditions such as fear of flying and performance anxiety. In one example, a 28-year-old Hollywood screenwriter reports that he took kava (2 x 60-mg caps) successfully to overcome presentation "nerves," with no impairment in his ability to concentrate and perform but without comment on the quality of the "product." The muscular relaxation effects also make kava useful for headaches, backaches, and tension-related pain.

Kava has also found use for women's health, regarding menopausal symptoms. A study of kava for menopausal symptoms in 40 women using doses of 30 to 60 mg per day for a minimum of 56 days found significant improvements in anxiety, hot flashes, sleep, and a sense of well-being, as well as in scores on the HAMA scale and Kupperman Index. In a follow-up study in 40 women (20 on placebo and 20 on 210 mg per day), similar effects were reported. In clinical practice it is highly effective for menopausal symptoms as well as for treating symptoms of premenstrual syndrome (see Chapter 24).

aphrodisiac. Kava has proven effective in counteracting anxiety, and is currently one of the most popular sleep aids in Europe. As of late 2014 Germany has removed restrictions on the use of kava that had been put into place due to specious claims of possible liver toxicity (Chapter 24).

Kava Kava (cont.)

- · Botanical name. *Piper methysticum* is its Latin name; common names are kava, kava kava, and awa.
- · How it works. Exactly how kava works is not fully understood. Some indicators suggest that the most active components are substances known as kavalactones, which may act primarily on receptors in the limbic system, deep in the brain.
- · Research. A German study published in 1999 demonstrated that kava's effects were equivalent to the antianxiety drugs oxazepam and bromazepam, with fewer side effects, no habit formation, and possible enhancement of vigilance and memory. A review of seven double-blind, placebo-controlled studies published in 2000 concluded that kava was effective in reducing anxiety as scored on the *Hamilton Anxiety Rating Scale*. Numerous research projects involving human subjects have demonstrated kava's effectiveness for insomnia and anxiety. One randomized, double-blind, placebo-controlled study demonstrated that after one week on kava, subjects had a significant reduction in anxiety as measured on the *Hamilton Anxiety Rating Scale*. Animal studies have demonstrated that, unlike standard antianxiety drugs, kava's effectiveness does not diminish with long-term use.
- · Uses. The German Commission E approved kava for treatment of nervous anxiety, stress, and anxiousness.
- · Dosage. The standard daily dosage is between 60 mg and 120 mg of kavalactones; kava should not be taken for more than three months without the advice of a physician.
- · Side effects. Kava rarely produces side effects. In a study involving 4049 patients, 1.5% experienced some gastrointestinal complaints or allergic skin reactions, which disappeared when kava was discontinued. Other research has indicated that prolonged, heavy use of kava may result in abnormal liver function, a yellow scaly rash, and an increase in cholesterol levels. It is possible for kava to impair motor reflexes and judgment, so tasks such as driving or operating heavy machinery should be avoided.
- · Interactions. Kava should not be taken with alcoholic beverages, barbiturates, benzodiazepines, or any other medications that depress the central nervous system, as kava may enhance the effects of these substances. The effectiveness of levodopa, a drug used in the treatment of Parkinson's disease, may be compromised when it is used in conjunction with kava.

THE PHILIPPINE ISLANDS

Chinese archaeological and historical records document extensive and ongoing contacts between the Philippine islands, largely through Chinese mariners and merchants. This contact increased after the Tang Dynasty (AD 618–906), when the overland Silk Road was impeded by incursions from the new Islamic wave emanating from Arabia (Chapter 35), and China increasingly relied on trade

overseas rather than overland. While trade expansion between Southeast Asia and China was due primarily to the spread of Chinese civilization for 1500 years, the arrival of Arab ships in China with goods from the Philippines began in AD 982.

Contacts with China were heavy during the Sung Dynasty (AD 960–1280) that followed. Contact also increased between the Philippines and Mainland Southeast Asia, still primarily through the intermediary of Chinese maritime trade. During the Ming Dynasty (1368–1644), contacts with the northern islands of the Philippines (e.g., Luzon) remained strong but the southern islands came directly under the influence of the expanding Islamic Empire from Indonesia (see Chapter 35). During the Late Ming and Qing Dynasties, trade contacts with China, and then the Americas, became dominated by the Spanish with their famous "Manila galleons." In 1898, following the Spanish-American War, the Philippines came under the temporary jurisdiction of the United States The plan for creating an independent nation was delayed by the Japanese Occupation during World War II, with independence finally coming after the war.

When the Spanish had first encountered the Malay peoples living in the Philippine Islands, they found a literate people who were versed in their own languages, with the ability to read and write. Their very first encounter with Ferdinand Magellan, a Portuguese mariner sailing for Spain, on his circumnavigation of the globe in 1521, was violent and ultimately fatal for Magellan at the hands of Chief Lapu-Lapu on the island of Cebu. Later, Spanish clerics such as Father Chirino would document the more peaceful, literary aspects of life in the Philippines. Nonetheless, not a single source of original Malay culture in the Philippines has remained. The materials used for writing on rice paper, banana leaves, coco palm, and bamboo were fragile and could not resist the constant humidity as well as periodic typhoons, frequent fires, and gnawing insects and rodents.

SPANISH AND ROMAN CATHOLIC SYNCRETISM

The Spanish clerics documented the practice of native healers they called *curanderos* (healers) and *herbolarios* (herbalists) but largely ignored the work of the mystic faith healers on the assumption that their *spiritual* work must somehow be associated with the devil (see Chapter 39). Therefore, the latter category of Philippine faith healing remained to be explored in the twentieth century, by which time the Filipinos themselves had melded traditional spiritual practices with the strong influence of the Roman Catholic Church brought by the Spanish in a kind of unique syncretic synthesis.

SPIRITUAL HEALING

The belief of the *Subanun*, an isolated tribe on the southernmost island of Mindanao, is fairly typical; illness was brought by *Pati-anak*, a demigod or devil that manifested as a beautiful child when held in the arms but assumed the form of a worm when let loose (see below, this paragraph; the form of demon *Ku* in Chinese medicine during the Zhou Dynasty) and to be avoided especially by pregnant women. The word *Pati-anak* is said to be derived from the Malay *pati*, meaning dead, and *anak*, child, although Blumentritt gives a Sanskrit origin to the word *pati*, again showing the ancient influence of Further India in this part of the world. The imagery of the worm may derive from the Chinese *Ku* from the Zhou Dynasty. The worm was thought to embody the demons that were considered the causes of illness.

Among those groups having more contact with outsiders over the course of history, this devil is called *Saitan*, *Sitan* (*Tagalogs*), or *Sidaan* (*Bisayas*), reflecting Islamic and Catholic influences for the name of the devil.

All these influences appear to converge around the legend of the demon *Kapre*, a cigar-smoking black giant (tobacco was introduced to the Philippines from the Americas by the Spanish in the 1500s). However, some folk healers are said to befriend the Kapre, which may actually bring good fortune. Although usually silent, they have been said to warn of impending typhoons. The Kapre is feared but has affinity with the "friendly" Arabian genie from Islamic folklore.

The Spanish, however, granted this demon its name, derived from the word *cafre*, referring to an infidel black African, or *kaffir*, from the Saracens, who occupied Spain from about AD 700 to 1480 (Moorish period). According to Jorge Luis Borges, the jinn (jinnee or genie, plural) was created by Allah by a black, smokeless fire, thousands of years before Adam. They may show themselves as clouds or vast pillars and can become visible in the shape of a man, jackal, wolf, lion, scorpion, or snake. Keeping with these ideas, the Kapre is dispelled by reciting the *Pater Noster* (Our Father), naming the three members of the Holy Family, or running their names together, such as *Susmariosep*, or even just *Mariosep* (Jesus, Mary, and Joseph).

Another demon is the *mutya*, identical with the Hindu word for gem or jewel. It may convey strength, invisibility, or fertility. Encounters with these demons may lead to *susto*, or the startle response, during which wind may enter the body, causing illness (Chapter 35).

SKIN DEEP

The Subanun were also the subject of a classic medical ethnography by Charles O. Frake, based on his field work conducted in the 1950s. Frake found that members of the Subanun all agreed on the types of skin diseases that exist (which can easily be seen on the surface of the body), but that individuals disagreed on the diagnosis of the specific type of skin disease present in a given patient. This finding is a key observation of ethnomedicine: *types of diseases that exist are generally known as part of the general knowledge of the culture, but the ability to correctly diagnose a specific disease in a given individual is highly dependent upon the skill of the individual who undertakes to treat the sick*—whether that skill is acquired by learning, apprenticeship, or divination. But there are healers in every society (see Chapter 34).

HEALING RITUALS

Healing rituals in the Philippines bear similarities to those described for Malaya (Chapter 35).

Here, a *Katalonan* invokes divine power of celestial origin before conducting a *magdiwang* for the sick. According to Pigafetta, more than one healer may participate. Offerings are shared in a communal meal, including pigs, chickens, fish, tortoise, oysters, rice, bananas, and aromatic spices. Often the most attractive girl is selected from among the participants to give a death blow to the sacrificial animal, perhaps like the Western myth of "beauty and the beast" and famously discussed in the pre-ethnomedical accounts of Sir James Frazer's *The Golden Bough* (Chapters 2, 34).

According to Fay-Cooper Cole, the healer enters a trancelike state and manifests resting tremors, as with the bomoh in Malaya (Chapter 35). Instead of a gong, the healer holds a plate by the fingertips of the left hand, striking it with a string of sea shells, making a bell-like sound.

Today many Filipino faith healers demonstrate syncretism with Roman Catholic religious concepts and figures (see Chapter 39).

HEALING HERBS

In the Philippines, there were also medicine men (*herbolarios*) skilled in the use of medicinal plants. In 1669, the Spanish Jesuit missionary Francisco Ignacio Alcina first documented this indigenous pharmacopeia, followed by the herbals of a Jesuit lay brother, Georg Joseph Camel, in 1704, and Jesuit Father Pablo Clain, in 1712. A series of works from 1751 to 1754 by Jesuit Father Juan Delgado addressed the botany of these medicinal plants. In 1768, the Dominicans added their contribution with an herbal by Fernando de Santa Maria, which was used as recently as 1923. The use of fly larvae (maggots) to treat infected wounds was among the effective knowledge of the herbolario that remained useful until this time.

The indigenous knowledge of the use of local herbs was considered appropriate and important by the Spanish, English (briefly), and later U.S. colonial rulers. The works of the Augustinian Father Ignacio de Mercado in 1879, Tissot's *Aviso al Pueblo* ("advice for the town," or essentially community public health, including the use of herbal medicines) in 1884, and Dr. Pardo de Tavera in 1892, were all published under Spanish royal patronage. With the arrival of the U.S. military in 1898, during and after the Spanish-American War, these works were translated into English by Captain Jerome Thomas, Assistant Surgeon General USA. Scientific studies on 17 selected medicinal plants were conducted by the first faculty of the University of the Philippines during the 1920s and 1930s. These remedies were found to be helpful for appendicitis, hydrophobia (former name for rabies), chronic ulcers, acute laryngitis, leprosy, and they even proved coconut and ylang-ylang oil effective as a hair tonic, the latter of which has not been lost on modern cosmetics manufacturers. A four-volume *Handbook on Philippine Medicinal Plants* is published by the University of the Philippines at Los Banos today.

ALASKA AND THE PACIFIC NORTHWEST

On the southeast coast of Alaska, as glaciers receded following the end of the "Little Ice Age" of the 1600s, new lands and passages were opened to the indigenous peoples of the northwest coast of North America. As indigenous peoples came into contact with new lands, they also came into increasing contact, and sometimes conflict, with European explorers seeking scientific knowledge and commercial exploitation. In the European perspective, the resources of nature were separate from the indigenous peoples who lived there. Eventually *preservation* of this rich *natural environment*; respect for traditional knowledge, such as ethnomedicine; as well as recognition of the *rights of indigenous peoples* would come to these lands. However, these two modern concepts are not always connected in terms of contemporary concerns about environmental preservation, biodiversity, and climate change, which affect the earth's lands and all its peoples.

THE LAND BRIDGE

It is thought that humans first came to North America from Asia approximately 50,000 years ago, across the land bridge of the Bering Strait, during the last major Ice Age, when sea levels were lower (see Chapters 35, 37). The northwest coast of North America provides a rare example in the history of human societies where many social groups became sedentary in the absence of agriculture. In the Old World, it was once thought that *sedentism* invariably accompanied *agriculture*, as human groups settled down in one place in order to engage in agricultural production as a means of subsistence. By contrast, the natural resources of the northwest coast of North America are so rich that human groups could settle there and enjoy high levels of subsistence from coastal resources *without* engaging in agriculture. During prehistory, the northwest coast of Europe had a very similar climate following the last great Ice Age 10,000 years ago, and it is even thought that these peoples may provide a model to explain human settlement patterns in Europe thousands of years ago. These indigenous peoples have been of great interest to anthropologists, including Franz Boas, often considered the founder of modern anthropology (see Chapter 34).

AT THE EDGE OF THE WORLD

During the age of European mercantile expansion, after expansion throughout Southeast Asia and the Pacific (see Chapter 35), North America became contested among the great European powers of Great Britain, France, Russia, and Spain. By the end of the eighteenth century, the northwest coast of North America remained an important area of interest. Animal furs were used and obtained there for clothing and for trade.

Alaska and the Pacific Northwest were simultaneously at the northern edge of New Spain and the eastern verge of the Russian Empire, which was also highly accessible to the naval powers of France and Great Britain, who struggled over the North American continent. During the 1750s, Great Britain and France had clashed in North America (today's Canada and USA) in what was known as the "French and Indian War" in North America and the "Seven Years' War" in Europe. The British expelled the French to holdings in Louisiana and parts of Canada, but the British victory was short lived. Within 20 years, their 13 American colonies were in open rebellion due to British taxes imposed to pay back that war's costs, and with trained militia, officers, and arms left from that earlier conflict. With the British expulsion from the new United States in 1781, the field for European exploration and exploitation in North America was becoming narrowed by the time of the expeditions of Captains Cook (1778) and Vancouver (1794) of England and La Pérouse of France (1786).

THE "LOST EXPEDITION"

The "Lost Expedition" of eighteenth-century French explorer La Pérouse documented scientific information about the natural features of these lands and their peoples, using the latest navigational equipment of *bousolle* (compass) and *astrolabe*, after which his two ships were named. After making their observations of North America, the expedition crossed the Pacific and was last heard from at Botany Bay (Australia).

After visiting North America, the expedition had crossed the Pacific Ocean. In Petropavlovsk, Siberia, La Pérouse entrusted a logbook and drawings to his Russian interpreter, Barthélemy de Lesseps, who carried them across Russia to King Louis XVI in Versailles by October 1788, on the eve of the French Revolution. (His journals were published for the first time by the French National Academy in 1798 [Bibliothèque Nationale, Paris, France].)

By this time, La Pérouse's two ships had mysteriously disappeared without a trace, one night in the South Pacific, in a cyclone off the island of Vanikoro in the Solomon Islands. (The wreckage was finally located there by the U.S. Navy after World War II.)

La Pérouse's final dispatch to reach France was written from Botany Bay (now Australia) in February 1788. Three years later the French National Assembly (under the revolutionary government) sponsored an expedition to search for La Pérouse's lost party and to publish his surviving journals, which had been sent by overland courier. The political situation complicated and delayed the process. Eventually, *A Voyage Around the World, Performed in the Years 1785, 1786, 1787 and 1788 by the Boussole (Compass) and the*

Astrolabe under the Command of JFG de la Pérouse was published in French in 1788 and translated into English in 1799.

The "Lost Expedition" of La Pérouse was later romanticized (and *Romanticized*) in mid–nineteenth-century France, in literature and art. It came to symbolize the "lost glory" of France, happening as it did at the time of the French Revolution and the end of the "Golden Age" of the French Bourbon Monarchy, and then followed by the failure of the First Empire under Napoleon I.

THE LOST "NOBLE SAVAGE"

The indigenous peoples of Alaska, and of all of North America, also came to be romanticized as the lost *"Noble savages"* (of Swiss-French, eighteenth-century Enlightenment social theorist Jean-Jacques Rousseau) as these populations died out, due to European contacts and succeeding waves of epidemic diseases:

- Smallpox: 1776, 1836, 1862
- Measles: 1800
- Typhoid: 1819, 1848, 1855

Two hundred years later, John Dunmore of New Zealand located the original journals of La Pérouse in a Parisian archive and prepared an updated translation. His contemporary translation updated the scientific data at the expense of ethnohistorical scholarship, thus replicating the "errors" (in retrospect) and perpetuating the misunderstandings of La Pérouse's ethnographic observations, thereby fossilizing the modern ethnography within an eighteenth-century perspective.

REVOLUTIONARY DEVELOPMENTS

Meanwhile, on the eastern coast of North America, the successful American Revolution (1776-1783) also introduced to the world the importance of the "rights of man," which soon provided a model for the French Revolution (1788-1793), and through the nineteenth and into the twentieth centuries, eventually increased global consciousness about the rights of indigenous peoples to their lands and cultures.

During the later nineteenth century, the Pacific Northwest region began to see a new concern for preservation of these lands and respect for indigenous peoples and their ethnomedical knowledge, especially about the land itself, including the local materia medica. The early American naturalist John Muir, with Samuel Hall Young, came to these lands in 1879 and 1880, interested in preserving the nature and "wilderness" areas without the imprint of people and promulgating a model of environmental preservation that was devoid of the indigenous peoples. One decade later, the English explorer Edward Glave came in 1890 and 1891 and was initially concerned about the indigenous peoples and preserving their knowledge. Eventually, Glave's work in Africa, probably influenced by his experiences in North America, helped bring about major reforms in the Belgian Congo and also helped raise the awareness of Europeans about the rights of indigenous peoples and respect for their ethnomedical knowledge.

The explorations and ethnographic observations of Edward Glave had an impact both contemporaneously in Africa, globally and contemporarily. Glave, described as "one of Stanley's Congo officers," also undertook explorations to the Congo before and after his visits to Alaska and Yukon, in an apparent attempt to establish for himself a life as an English Victorian "explorer." Under the offices of the Belgian *Association Internationale Africaine*, he arrived in the Congo in 1883 and again in 1889. Later, when he visited Alaska and Yukon as a putative "solitary explorer," he unconventionally used indigenous ***Tlingit*** names to identify landmarks, citing their crucial value both as directionals and as sources of (ethno) historical knowledge. When he then returned to Africa, he became concerned about corruption, slavery, and exploitation by King Leopold of Belgium, who was using the Congo as a private preserve for his personal wealth.

It remains a matter of debate whether Glave's initial appreciation of *Tlingit* customs and place-names in Alaska may have contributed to his subsequent passionate exposure of what are now called human rights abuses in what was then Belgian Congo. The situations in 1890s Alaska and in the Congo were comparable in some ways but not in others. Glave's influences can be seen in the twenty-first century in the human rights movement in Africa, colonial accountability by Belgium, and land claims in the indigenous *Tlingit* territories of Alaska and Yukon. In Glave's own era, eighteenth-century Enlightenment concepts of Nature and Culture had been exported from Europe through the expansion of the empire to places once considered to be at the edge of the globe, when "the sun never set on the British Empire," for example. The consequences of that Nature-Culture dualism continue to be felt in international debates about environmentalism, biodiversity, and global climate change as well.

The early ethnographic descriptions of La Pérouse and Glave have come down through academic and popular cultures. Glave's observations also crossed continents and still influence public discourse and policy. John Muir's observations of Nature in Alaska and elsewhere as ***separate from* humans** (and in fact his approach was deliberately ***to separate them***) also impact global environmental policy. However, often this separation results in the resources represented by Nature—"wilderness" and regions of great biological diversity—being seen as detached from the indigenous cultures that inhabit them (see Chapters 34, 43). This separation was inherent in the early approaches of European explorations of "the field" as a space of "scientific exploration" at the "edges of the world."

In central or southern Yukon, the face of the world was divided as if into the red summer world and the white winter world. The figures in the winter world are seen to be traveling in a boat. The theme of summer and winter worlds is reflected in several stories in their ethnomedical traditions.

European Expeditions to the Pacific

Capt. James Cook, England (1768-1771; 1776-1779)

Jean-Francois de La Pérouse, France (1786), "the lost expedition"

Capt. George Vancouver, England (1794)

Voyage of *The Beagle*, England (1838), with Charles Darwin, resulting in observations leading to theory of evolution

Commander John Wilkes, Exploring Expedition, United States (1838–40), resulting in founding museum collections for U.S. Smithsonian Institution

Erskine Scott Wood, England (1877)

John Muir, with Samuel Hall Young, United States (1879, 1880)

Edward Glave, England (1890, 1891)

Reference

McNally R, Cass H: Kava: *Nature's Answer to Stress, Anxiety, and Insomnia*, Roseville, 1998, Prima Lifestyles.

Suggested Reading

Pogue JF: *Rev. Moolelo of Ancient Hawaii* (trans. Charles Kenn), Honolulu, 1978, Topgallant Publishing.

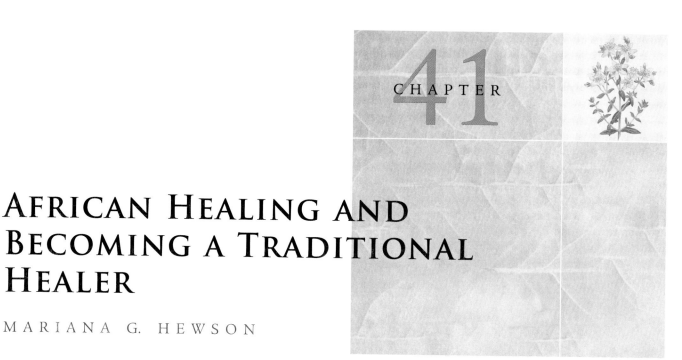

CHAPTER 41

AFRICAN HEALING AND BECOMING A TRADITIONAL HEALER

M A R I A N A   G.   H E W S O N

The vast African continent comprises a diverse array of healing traditions that well exemplify the ethnomedical concepts, as well as illustrate the process of becoming a traditional healer, in its purist form, persisting into the twentieth century.

Is traditional healing a profession? In the Western view, the medical profession consists of specialists who diagnose and prescribe in areas that draw on comprehensive knowledge and skills that transcend those available to nonspecialists. Education for the professions involves questions about legitimate knowledge, license to practice, arrangements for providing services, entry to education and training, the curriculum offered, standards of achievement, and assessment. Similarly, considerations of what constitutes a health care system are covered in Chapter 34. This chapter presents (1) the explanatory model of illness that underlies traditional healing in Africa, (2) the educational process of healers, (3) the professional accreditation of the practitioners, (4) the professional organization of practitioners who monitor and maintain standards of care, and (5) the social mandate through which the community influences the provision of care.

CONCEPTS OF HEALTH, ILLNESS, AND HEALING

Traditional healing in Africa existed long before the arrival of modern medicine, and it remains an intact system of caregiving among many African peoples. This system of healing is **shamanic** in nature. The term *shaman* refers to medicine men and women, and *shamanism* is a methodology (not a religion), originally used to describe the practices of healers in the regions of northern central Asia and

the North Pacific (see Chapter 40). Shamanism represents "the most widespread and ancient methodological system of healing known to humanity" (Harner, 1990, p. 40). This type of healing practice occurs all over the world, in areas as diverse as **Australia**, **New Zealand**, **North and South America**, Siberia, Central Asia, eastern and northern Europe, as well as **Africa**. This chapter refers specifically to healing practices found in African countries such as **Botswana**, **Lesotho**, **Swaziland**, **Mozambique**, **Zimbabwe**, and **South Africa**. In all these regions, the shaman is seen as "the great specialist of the human soul: he alone 'sees' it, for he knows its 'form' and its destiny" (Eliade, 1964, p. 8). Shamanic practitioners generally make use of "nonordinary reality" or controlled *entrancement* to access the information they seek on behalf of their patients, presumably from *cosmic* sources.

ORIGINS

Africa is also considered to be the cradle of humankind, but little has been written about its traditional healers. Traditional healers in Africa are not actually called "shamans," yet their practices are similar to those described by Eliade (1964) and Harner (1990). At present, their ancient practices coexist in a modern society that "officially" subscribes to and practices allopathic medicine. Despite regional differences throughout Africa, there appears to be a common system aimed at relieving illness and disease (feelings of being "out of sorts," or ill at ease, socially and spiritually).

In the African view, illness is thought to be caused by *Psycho-spiritual conflicts* or *disturbed social relationships* with persons living or dead. The accompanying disequilibrium is expressed as physical or mental problems (Frank, 1973).

Traditional healers believe that psycho-spiritual and social imbalances must be rectified before a patient can recover physically. Traditional healing thus focuses on psychological and *spiritual* suffering, as well as on physical suffering, and aims to correct the disequilibrium. Traditional healers view healing as the removal of impurities from the body or disequilibrium from the patient's mind, with the hope of reducing the anxieties it has produced. For example, a common concept of healing involves purification by draining the body of harmful substances, which results in wide use of *purgatives* and *emetics*. Healing also involves appeasing the patient's spirits (in particular the recently departed members of the family), who might be angry with the patient for some reason. Warding off bad spirits, such as the *tokoloshe* (a mischievous or evil spirit responsible for life's misadventures and accidents), curses from living people, or the ill will of angry ancestral spirits, constitutes a version of preventive medicine. Furthermore, in several southern African groups, such as the **Basotho of Lesotho**, the state of disequilibrium manifests in the form of being "hot" (not feverish) (Hewson & Hamlyn, 1985), and treating people who are "hot" involves cooling with appropriate agents such as ash, water plants, or aquatic animals. These views are quite distinct from modern allopathic medical concepts of disease as the malfunctioning of physiological systems.

TRADITIONAL HEALING PROCESSES

Traditional healers hold an esteemed and powerful position in society, especially in traditional African societies, and their role is a combination of physician, counselor, psychotherapist, and priest. Traditional healers prevent and treat illnesses mainly with **plant** and some **animal products** in combination with **divination**. There are two types of traditional healers: those who are mainly **herbalists** and those who use divination, or **diviners.** However, the distinction between the two is becoming increasingly blurred, and most traditional healers appear to practice both types of medicine. The majority of traditional healers are "called" to practice benevolently—their role is to serve their people. Sorcery (evil or malevolent actions for the purpose of harming others, e.g., for revenge) is practiced by some people in Africa and is considered further in Chapter 42 as a source of illness.

Traditional healers appear to work most successfully with illnesses that have a high psychological or emotional content related to envy, frustration, or guilt (Frank, 1973). In allopathic medicine, these might be called *psychosomatic illnesses.*

Currently, healers also appear to concentrate on illnesses for which allopathic medicine has little effective curative power, such as stroke, tuberculosis, cancer, and human immunodeficiency virus infection and acquired immunodeficiency syndrome (HIV/AIDS). Traditional healers claim to be effective in helping to treat pregnancy, malaise, arthritis, and social problems, especially those involving interpersonal disputes. The healers seem to be increasingly able to distinguish between those illnesses that need to be helped by Western medicine (e.g., broken bones, hernias) and those that respond to traditional healing methods. The claims to heal illnesses such as stroke, cancer, and HIV/AIDS appear to relate to the psychosocial and emotional components of the illness rather than the pathological or patho-physiological conditions. For example, traditional healers make no claims to be able to deal directly with bacterial or viral "impurities" but rather with the patient's ability to cope with and eliminate them as a host, similar to many alternative therapies. This view of healing suggests that if one takes care of the psychodynamics of illness, the body will heal, in contrast to the modern view that if one takes care of the body, the mind will heal itself.

As part of the *diagnostic* process, traditional healers "throw the bones." The "bones" consist of a set of 10 to 15 items, such as bones, shells, and various collectibles (e.g., dice, coins, bullets, domino pieces). These are usually thrown (like dice) in the belief that clues to the problem can be read in the configuration of the items when they come to rest. The bones are made up of an idiosyncratic collection of items that have *symbolic* meanings, depending on the context and meaning attributed by particular healers. Each item signifies an important aspect of a person's life (e.g., happiness, children, bad luck, ancestral spirits). The consistencies among these items are in the attributions for the items rather than in the items themselves. For example, a traditional healer from **Mozambique** had a red die signifying war (the country had experienced a civil war for many years), and a healer from **South Africa** had a bullet signifying death or misfortune (South Africa was, at that time, engulfed in violence).

Traditional healers use *drumming and dance* to augment the diagnostic and therapeutic processes. Drumming helps the healer enter nonordinary reality. Sustained dancing has the same effect. In nonordinary reality, healers use their dreams as manifestations of the higher wisdom of the spirits, especially their ancestors. The healers use their own spiritual powers, as well as those of the patient, to discern causes of the patient's spiritual, psychological, or social disequilibrium that cause physical ailments and bad luck. To encourage their own dreams, healers **wash with herbal** solutions, **drink herbal** potions, **smoke** a pipe, or use **snuff** (all of which appear to have psychotropic effects).

Healers prepare and prescribe therapeutic herbal remedies for their patients. A traditional healer must know the symptoms of a disorder and the conditions of the patient's life before prescribing a treatment. There is a lack of uniformity, however, about the prescribed remedies for particular illnesses. A medicine may be used for multiple problems. The actual prescription depends on the spiritual advice received by the healer through normal dreams and through the dreams of nonordinary reality or *entrancement.* Each prescription is driven by the particulars of the patient and the details of the situation in which the patient

TABLE 41-1 *Steps to Becoming a Professional in Traditional Healing and in Western Medicine*

Step	Traditional healing	Western medicine
Call to healing	Mysterious illness, significant dreams, interpreted and sanctioned by elders in community	Individual, personal "call" to become a clinician, family suggestion, augmented by academic counseling
Selection of trainees	Based on mysterious illness and recognizable evidence of healing capability and spiritual power	Based on standardized test scores, essay(s), and interviews with medical school personnel
Training	Rigorous, prolonged, relatively expensive; emphasis on subjective witness of healing powers by patients and/or trainers	Rigorous, prolonged, expensive; emphasis on objective measures of competence designed by professional boards
Accreditation	Approval by master healer, community members, and guidance from ancestral spirits	Approval on basis of national test scores in certifying/licensing examinations
Continuing education	Regular and frequent meetings and celebrations with other healers and regular ongoing communication with trainer	Regular and frequent conferences, with regulated continuing medical education accreditation
Professional relationships	Lifelong relationship with trainer and ongoing relationships with colleagues	Occasional mentors, ongoing relationships with professional colleagues, especially focused on research

became ill. The lack of a systematic, generalized approach to healing promotes *individuated* practices that often seem idiosyncratic to Westerners. This phenomenon is one of the reasons African traditional healing remains so mysterious to Western scientists.

Traditional healers seek causes for illness from a variety of areas. The common areas concern relationships with family, friends, and people at work. Healers are especially concerned about disturbed relationships involving jealousy, anger, loss, grief, and resentment. They seek to identify possible causes of illness from the following situations: someone wishes the patient ill; the patient wants something he or she does not or cannot have; the patient has known or unknown enemies; the patient experiences unrequited love or loss of a loved one; the patient has an unfaithful spouse or partner; the patient longs for progeny; and the patient's ancestors (the "recently departed") may be displeased with the patient for some reason, known or unknown. These motivations are reminiscent of the Image of Limited Good described by ethnographer George Foster for traditional societies. Good fortune must be hidden or shared to avoid envy. The "evil eye" that brings disease and misfortune is the admiring eye. Conversely, jealousy of the good fortune, or simply goods, of others is also a source of illness.

The healer inquires into every aspect of a patient's present and past activities, focusing on behaviors that would be most likely to provoke conflict with others in the community or even internal psychological conflict (e.g., in personal values). This is a process of divination commonly referred to as "seeing." A healer must "see" forward into the future as well as backward into the past. The process is similar to that used by shamans around the world (Harner, 1990). Although Africans make some use of **totemic animal spirits**, their emphasis is mainly focused on the

spiritual forces of recently departed family members. These ancestors are the source of key information and are powerful forces in the lives of their living family members.

If the *divination* process does not provide immediate answers, the process may take longer. In this situation the healer may say, "The bones are not talking today" and request subsequent visits. When healers cannot find an answer to the patient's problems, they will refer the patient to another traditional healer or to a Western physician. All healers are concerned with **truth and trust** in their relationship with a patient. If the healer discerns a lack of either, he or she will ask the patient to leave (Tables 41-1 and 41-2).

THE CALL TO BECOME A HEALER

Traditional healers are **"called" to become healers** and need to be validated by the group's elders, who check whether the call is real or not. First, the future healer experiences an unusual, mysterious *illness* that does not respond to usual herbal or allopathic treatment. Some examples include heart problems, lung problems, abdominal pain, swollen abdomen unrelated to pregnancy, amenorrhea, problems with feet, dizziness, headaches, mental problems (e.g., forgetfulness), pains throughout the body, and "fevers that are not real fevers" (which may relate to the cultural metaphor of being "hot"; see Hewson & Hamlyn, 1985).

The illness is often followed by *dreams* with significant, recognizable components. The future healer then asks his or her elders (e.g., parents, aunts, uncles, grandparents) about the dreams. If an elder recognizes the special components of the dream, the elder advises the future healer to consult a traditional healer. At the discretion of the traditional healer, the patient is then both treated and taken as an *apprentice* for several years.

TABLE 41-2 *Characteristics of the Practice of Traditional Healing and Western Medicine*

Step	Traditional healing	Western medicine
Concepts of curing the patient	Take care of the mind and the body will take care of itself	Take care of the body and the mind will take care of itself
Diagnosis	Use spiritual powers and psychological techniques involving nonordinary reality to "see" causes of spiritual, psychological, or social disequilibrium	Use technological and scientific tools to recognize directly or indirectly the pathology or pathophysiology. Use clinical reasoning and evidence-informed medicine
Prevention	Very important to ward off negative spirits and harmful circumstances	Increasing importance of preventive medicine
Treatment	Resolve disequilibrium and return person to harmonious state	Treat the biological causes of disease
Relationship to patient	Subjective, interpersonal involvement, counselor, confessor	Objective, scientific, rational, clinical relationship
Relationship to community and individual patients	Paternalistic relationship based on healers' spiritual and social status and reputation	Paternalistic relationship based on clinicians' accreditation level, social status, and reputation
Professional satisfaction and rewards for healing	Directly linked with patient satisfaction and monetary payment or in-kind gifts	Indirectly linked with patient satisfaction; salary negotiated with health care organization

To refuse this **calling by the ancestors** is to invite worse sickness, madness, and possible death. One healer recounted the story of a woman who had denied the call and had become "mad." A man in Cape Town, a renowned drunkard, believed he was being called to be a healer, but the elders of his family discouraged him from this idea, saying that his dreams and sickness were the consequence of alcohol. This story illustrates the importance of being able to distinguish by which *spirits* one is being called.

APPRENTICESHIP

After the call, becoming a healer then involves an **apprenticeship**, usually with a well-known master healer. If the master healer lives far away, the apprentices live in the master healer's compound (many small dwellings inhabited by extended family members) for the duration of the training. The art of the healer is thought to be transmitted through the *ancestral spirits* who speak to healers through *dreams*. Apprentices are encouraged to have dreams and to learn how to interpret them on behalf of their patients. Dreams can be induced by herbal potions, inhaled smoke, or snuff. As one traditional healer put it, "Through the dreams, your ancestors open your eyes to signs. I trust the dreams every time." Another said that anyone can learn about the practice of traditional healing, but "unless you have contact with the spirits through dreams, you cannot be a healer."

The master healer first demonstrates the use of herbs and animal parts and then teaches the apprentices how to administer them. Then, in a progressive weaning process, the master healer withdraws and expects the apprentices to perform independently. One healer described being taken into the bush by her teacher to find *muti* (medicinal

substances, such as herbs, roots, and barks, as well as animal parts, such as hooves, bones, and horns) that are used for healing. She had to rise at 4:30 AM "because the spirits only come early in the morning." She had to prepare herself to obtain the muti by bringing on the ancestral spirits. This she did by taking an herbal bath, drinking herbal concoctions, beating the drums, and dressing in a special outfit.

The training process is strenuous and challenges the mental and physical strength of the apprentices. One healer said, "I went to the bush for many days with my teacher to seek muti, with only *putu* (cornmeal porridge) and black tea. It was hard to live like that, but it is necessary for *nyangas* (healers) to suffer because this kind of work is *swarig*" (Afrikaans word for "heavy" or "burdensome"). Because this process is so exacting, not every apprentice completes the training. Confucius says, "from Great Suffering comes Great Enlightenment."

Apprentices help their master healers with patient consultations, seemingly acting as a team for the duration of the training program. Throughout training, apprentices are tested on their ability to find the location of objects, to identify and administer herbs, and to contact the ancestors through dreams to discern people's physical, psychological, or spiritual problems. Some of the objects to be found become part of the divining "bones," and others are used as medicines. The items that are needed are often given to the apprentice by patients, friends, or family members in recognition of the demonstrated healing skills and power of the apprentice. The master healer may also help the apprentices find things they need. For example, one healer described how, on occasion, the very item she had been instructed to find would be given to her by someone, apparently in a serendipitous manner (McCallum, 1992). Another described how she went to the beach with her teacher and collected the perfect shells for her set of bones. Other objects must be gleaned from the countryside, found in the bush, or purchased from stores that specialize in the healers' equipment and accoutrements.

The final test often involves finding a hidden object. For her final test, one healer had to find an unknown object that had been hidden somewhere in the vicinity of a village (McCallum, 1992). The final test also involves "finding" the animal(s) that will be slaughtered as part of the "graduation" ceremony, such as a chicken, goat, or cow. The apprentice first dreams about the animal(s) and notes the color and the type of spots or other distinguishing characteristics. This dream is viewed as a message from the ancestors, and it must be followed to the last detail. The procurement of these specific animals may involve gifting by the apprentice's family, friends, or satisfied patients. It is an additional social accreditation that represents faith and trust in the apprentice as a healer. The apprentice can also buy the animals from a market if none is given.

An apprentice "graduates" when the master healer is satisfied that he or she has passed all the tests (i.e., through dreams, the ancestral spirits have confirmed the apprentice's readiness) and the apprentice has paid the stipulated fees, including procuring the necessary animal(s) for slaughter. The master healer consults his or her own ancestral spirits concerning the sufficiency of each apprentice's knowledge and skills. When all the criteria have been satisfied, the master healer may give each apprentice a gift, such as a set of bones or a braided bracelet. Thus, both the teacher and the apprentice, and indirectly the community, assess the readiness for graduation. Patients also play a part in this judgment through their gifts.

More importantly, the ancestral spirits indicate, through dreams, when a trainee is ready. One healer explained that she knew that she was ready to graduate when she had a dream in which her ancestor (grandfather) "sent me to a *rondavel* (Afrikaans for 'small round dwelling') that had a half door made of glass. There was a man standing behind the door who asked, 'What do you want here? I don't know what you are doing here anymore.'" Then she heard the words coming from behind her, "Go and help people." At this point, she went through the final graduation ceremony, collected all her medicines and divining tools, and traveled back to her home, some 300 miles away.

Graduation often involves a final test of slaughtering an animal with the ceremonial spears. The apprentice drinks the animal's blood and selects various body parts, such as pieces of hoof or bone, to become part of his or her healer's tools (bones) or to be used as muti. For example, the skin of the slaughtered goat may be used as the mat for throwing bones, the animal's stomach may be used as a pouch for carrying other medicine, or a vertebra may become part of the divining tools. The rest of the animal is then consumed by the community to celebrate the occasion.

GATHERING TOGETHER

Traditional healers engage in meetings with other healers. One group described meetings that occurred on weekends, in which they would assemble, fully dressed in their ceremonial costumes (clothing, wigs, necklaces, anklets), to discuss healing matters, share their latest healing stories, and compare notes. The group may collectively criticize certain healers for dangerous or unwise practices. The regular meetings also include singing, dancing, drumming, drinking herbal potions, and engaging the ancestral spirits. These meetings are important social events in the lives of traditional healers.

The business of traditional healers includes their formal organization, their practice in the context of new diseases (e.g., HIV/AIDS), and their relationship with Western medicine. The World Health Organization has recognized traditional healers in **Mozambique** and elsewhere (see Chapter 43), and traditional healers are being increasingly recognized and incorporated into the general medical system.

Traditional healers typically maintain a lifelong relationship with their master healers, who serve as mentors. These relationships appear to be deep and profound. One healer from Maputo, in southern **Mozambique,** returned approximately once a year to visit her teacher in northern Mozambique. These visits were casual in nature, and the master healer might teach "depending on his mood. If he is not happy he doesn't teach anything!" This particular healer had trained five of her own apprentices, and she used the same methods as those used by her own teacher. She liked to teach, but reflected that to be a teacher, "You have to be happy all the time," which suggests that the essential relationship between teacher and learner involves enthusiasm and effort.

Mutual caring among healers becomes necessary under stressful or strained conditions, especially death. According to one healer, when a patient dies, the traditional healer becomes spiritually contaminated and loses his or her healing powers because the relationship with the patient has been broken, and the healer, of necessity, grieves. In this situation the healer removes his or her necklaces, ceremonial clothes, and artifacts and does not practice as a healer. This afflicted healer must be treated by another healer in a purification ceremony that restores the healing powers.

Being a traditional healer also carries dangers. One source of danger is that a healer may cure a patient of an intrusive spirit that has caused him or her to be sick, only to find that this spirit has entered the body of the healer. In such a case, the healer must be treated. *Professional jealousies* between healers concern access to patients as well as access to countryside *where they collect their herbs* for medicines. There are tacit agreements concerning the use of particular pieces of land by specific healers, but infringements are common. Healers thus may practice in a team context, which also provides them with a measure of protection in terms of the accuracy of their diagnoses and treatments. In addition, team practice helps protect a healer against the malevolent practices of other healers or sorcerers in this competitive field.

Community control is exerted through remuneration. Traditional healers are paid according to the type of service they provide. For straightforward dispensing of muti, patients pay over-the-counter fees for the medicines they receive. For diagnosis of physical, psychological, social, or spiritual problems, the patient must first open his or her pockets and pay a flat fee at the beginning of the process. This amount is prorated based on the approximate cost of one head of cattle and appears to be approximately one sixth of the total cost. When cured, the patient must pay an additional fee that appears to be independent of time spent or cost of medicines but is measured in proportion to the patient's satisfaction with the care, the cure, or both. Thus a moderately satisfied patient might provide a modest offering, such as food bought from a store (sugar, flour, or vegetables) or picked from a vegetable garden, whereas a highly satisfied patient might offer a live animal, such as a chicken or a goat. This offering would be ceremonially slaughtered at a later date. In urban areas, money is the usual mode of payment. The amount of money is often a loose translation of the worth of a cow, goat, sheep, chicken, or pumpkin.

For mentoring, an apprentice needs to pay a relatively large fee, equivalent to at least one head of cattle, and must also provide the animal(s) for the graduation ceremony. Apprentices are helped in paying the required fees by other people (patients, friends, family members), who pay or provide necessary items in proportion to their belief in the healing powers of the apprentice. This linking of the payment, patient satisfaction, and status provides a complex system of checks and balances in an otherwise unregulated system.

Healers refer to their own satisfaction in terms of "happiness." For example, one healer said that "to heal someone is to give life to that person," and when the person is healed, "both the traditional healer and the patient become happy." This happiness is manifest at a celebration in which the food offered is consumed in thanksgiving for the healing and for the continued goodwill of the spiritual beings whose power over the living is great.

THE ARCHETYPAL HEALER

Differences between traditional and allopathic professionalism are vast. Despite these differences, interesting phenomena characterize traditional healing and the professional training of the healers that are important to the fundamental, perhaps archetypal, contract between healer and patient.

SPIRITUAL CONTEXT

Spiritual powers are loosely defined within **African cosmology** as those spiritual powers that derive ultimately from God (within the African worldview) and that are present in decreasing amounts through the various levels of spirits of the *ancestors* (the forefathers) and the recently *departed family* members, living *people*, *animals*, *vegetation* (e.g., trees), and the *earth* itself (Mbiti, 1969).

Traditional healing relates to **spiritual powers** manifest through *an integrated conception of body and mind at all levels*. For example, in the call to be a healer, the person experiences a mysterious physical illness and has dreams that reveal a connection with ancestral spirits. In the mentoring process the apprentice learns both the physical skills of an *herbalist* and the *spiritual* skills of interpreting problems through dreams that involve the ancestral spirits. When traditional healers graduate, the tests involve knowledge and skills in both herbal medicine and spiritual healing.

The traditional system of healing is consistent with the **cosmology,** or worldview, of the peoples indigenous to this region. This worldview constitutes a paradigm that emphasizes some ways of thinking (e.g., **the body–mind connection**) and deemphasizes others (e.g., the objective, rational scientific approach). To be effective, traditional healing requires that patients who seek healing within this paradigm must subscribe to it. Thus, traditional healers are cautious in checking the adherence of patients to their traditional African way of thinking. In addition, there is the "dark side" to this practice: **malevolent sorcery**. For reasons similar to those that make benevolent traditional medicine effective, sorcery is powerful and greatly feared. Traditional healers need to discern the intentions of their patients, and they are alert to desires for "*dirty witch doctoring*." If a patient is thought to be untruthful or distrustful, the healer will send the patient away.

PSYCHOSOCIAL RELATIONS

Based on central premises concerning the connections between body and mind, and between the earthly and spiritual realms, traditional healing is a form of integrated psychosocial healing. The role of the healer is to "see" the cause of the problem that afflicts the patient, and this seeing includes spiritual dimensions. Healers pay close attention to the ways in which their patients describe their illnesses and to the contexts within which the illnesses occur. Healers concentrate on looking for signs that indicate the reasons for the disequilibrium that causes sickness. This holistic approach allows traditional healers to integrate body-mind phenomena and to provide healing, despite being extremely limited in terms of modern medical science.

In the training of traditional healers, patients have the opportunity to play a role in validating the apprentice through the voluntary gifts they make. To the extent that patients believe they are healed by a particular healer, they gift that healer. These gifts are often in the form of materials needed in the practice, for example, a special necklace or a medicine pouch. They may be worn to signify the healing power of the particular healer.

LIFELONG HEALING

Traditional healers in southern Africa appear to engage in lengthy apprenticeships with one master healer. Although the length of training may last from one to many years, the relationship with the master healer does not end at graduation. Instead, these relationships are treasured and maintained for life, which suggests that trainees benefit from the deeper, more sustained relationships, similar to those in traditional apprenticeships. The cross-fertilization of styles and standards of practice takes place at regular meetings of traditional healers. These gatherings can be seen as analogous to grand rounds and national and regional conferences.

The apprenticeships of traditional healers initially involve being shown how to do things (e.g., recognize herbs, interpret dreams) through role modeling and coaching. As the apprentice become more competent, the master healer allows the apprentice more independence and takes on a role more akin to that of an evaluator, in which the apprentice is tested for knowledge and skills and for evidence of the power of healing. At the same time the teacher personally rewards the apprentice with small, highly desired gifts that are needed as part of the prescribed collection of accoutrements (e.g., divining bones, various medications). In addition, the apprentice might wear some of the gifts from the master healer as a visible testament to the healer's skills.

This apprenticeship style of teaching is effective in developing professional competence. It makes use of several teaching approaches, such as role modeling (performing so that the learner can see what the teacher does) and coaching (helping the learner by providing assistance as well as feedback). The strategies also include experiential learning throughout the training process, such as collecting and preparing herbs and animals for medicines and helping with all patients seen by the master healer. The apprentices are expected to do much of the work around the master healer's practice. This includes helping the master healer to dress in ceremonial clothes, which often involve an elaborate ensemble of beads, skins, necklaces, anklets, and headdresses, as well as gathering and carrying the items needed for healing processes.

HARDSHIP AND HUMILITY

The training of traditional healers is strenuous because the practice of medicine is difficult. Healers are expected to lead a lifestyle characterized by a high level of personal and social responsibility, and their training is thus a test of physical and mental endurance. The requirement for this type of physical and mental testing is also present in the cultural initiation rites that take place at puberty for boys and girls in African cultures. Indeed, in **Xhosa**, the word for a healer-in-training is *mkweta,* the same word used for young boys and girls who undergo initiation.

In the practice of traditional medicine in Africa and the selection of traditional healers, there are substantial differences with Western medical practice and practitioners. Traditional healers lack the science and power of modern medicine; however, they are highly effective in a way that has stood the test of time for 20,000 to 30,000 years. As in modern medicine, the knowledge and skills of traditional healers are based on empirical experiences, and interesting similarities exist in the professional training of the practitioners. These similarities may influence perceptions of traditional healers and offer possibilities for a synergism between the two traditions, with potential mutual benefits for both types of healers, for the training of these healers, and ultimately for patients.

References

Eliade M: *Shamanism: archaic techniques of ecstasy,* Bollingen Series LXXVI, Princeton, NJ, 1964, Princeton University Press.
Frank JD: *Persuasion and healing: a comparative study of psychotherapy,* Baltimore, 1973, Johns Hopkins University Press, pp 46-77.
Harner M: *The way of the shaman,* San Francisco, 1990, Harper & Row.
Hewson MG, Hamlyn D: Cultural metaphors: some implications for science education, *Anthropol Educ Q* 16:31, 1985.
Mbiti JS: *African religions and philosophy,* ed 2, London, 1969, Heinemann Educational Books.
McCallum TG: *White woman witchdoctor: tales from the African life of Rae Graham,* as told by Rae Graham [to Taffy Gould McCallum], Miami, 1992, Fielden Books.

Suggested Readings

Hewson MG: Training in the traditional arts: some thoughts, *Med Encounter* 9(3):3, 1993.
Hewson MG: Traditional healers in southern Africa, *Ann Intern Med* 128:1029, 1998.

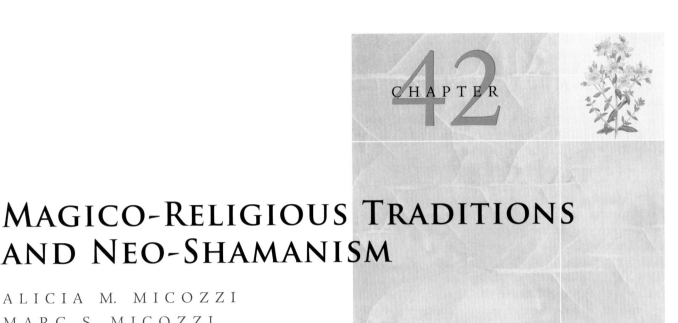

CHAPTER 42

MAGICO-RELIGIOUS TRADITIONS AND NEO-SHAMANISM

ALICIA M. MICOZZI
MARC S. MICOZZI

Throughout traditional societies worldwide, commonly observed folk beliefs make reference to malign magic, "evil eye," sorcery, and witchcraft as potential sources of disease, especially insofar as they reflect imbalances in the community and/or the cosmos. For example, in **West Africa** the practice of "witchcraft" (*djambe*) has been seen as a precarious **balance** between *leveling* and *accumulative* tendencies in a community. Balance is also a critical concept in understanding ethnomedicine as well as the place of humans in the **cosmos**. In addressing balance or imbalance, the benign "magic" of healers, and the malign magic of witches and sorcerers, may be seen as opposite sides of the same phenomenon.

There are tendencies for individuals in society to fly apart and for the society to fall apart, as each individual pursues his or her own interests (in **Africa**, as in Chinua Achebe's seminal novel, *Things Fall Apart*). There are also tendencies for societies to cohere insofar as the human nuclear family and extended family confer adaptive value to the society and have been generally seen as the basis for human social organization.

Addressing the balance between "leveling" and "accumulation" is appropriate as both of these tendencies are important in the development of complex human social organization and in the structure and function of those societies. This perspective is not just associated with modernity because these tendencies appear to have been a part of human experience from the earliest times when humans moved beyond being nomadic hunter-gatherers. The development of sedentism and agriculture appears to be strongly associated with the development of more complex, ranked, and stratified societies in which "accumulation" and "leveling" become major issues.

In agricultural societies, what appears at first to be a leveling phenomenon is actually another means of accumulation. For example, in a rural agricultural society where there may not be a banking system for accumulation of wealth, a farmer who has excess grain may hold a feast to distribute his surplus. Although this appears to represent leveling, the rich farmer is actually accumulating social obligations and social debt in place of the excess grain, which in any case is more than he can eat, and something that he cannot otherwise "bank."

Even in hunter-gatherer societies where there is an appearance of sharing, it may underlie a deep-seated fear of being envied or admired. Among the traditional hunter-gatherer !Kung Bushmen of the Kalahari Desert of **southern Africa**, a knife or metal object must either be jealously guarded or shared with the whole group. (In the context of witchcraft in a more complex society, such as *djambe* in **West Africa**, this admiration or envy is interpreted as a curse or the "evil eye.") For example, among the **Kalahari Bushmen** of **Botswana** and **South Africa**, a superior tool for hunting may be passed around, but only because the benefit or "wealth" represented by this item cannot practically be hidden away (or accumulated) under the circumstances of a hunter-gatherer society. Therefore, it is "shared."

THE AMBIGUITY OF DJAMBE

Concepts used in ethnography are sometimes imperfect analytical constructs that help to understand human belief and behavior. Witchcraft, similar to the terms *religion*, *totemism*, and *shamanism*, is one such imperfect concept. In describing *witchcraft* in **West Africa**, the term has a pejorative tenor and implies absolute opposition between good and evil where it does not exist.

Djambe is a force or being in a person's "belly" that incorporates good or evil intentions (in fact, good and evil don't adequately capture the complexity of human intention, where there is much gray). The conception of djambe is complex and ambiguous. Developed djambe can be used in constructive or destructive ways.

When Western anthropologists use the single term *djambe* to describe a complex set of social beliefs/behaviors relating to kinship, power, urban-rural, and socio-economic stratification, it almost necessarily results in ambiguous meanings. A positive, or constructive, aspect of djambe is that it represents a leveling force where there are other kinds of disparity, such as social, political, and economic inequality. It grants a kind of power to those who are otherwise powerless. Of course, that "leveling" is perceived as positive or constructive, and inequality as negative or destructive, may also be partially a bias in Western anthropology.

Social stratification (unleveling) may also serve some important purpose to the survival of the entire society. In a general sense, anthropological studies have also shown that the development of complex human societies and civilizations is invariably accompanied by ranked and stratified social organization, which is inherently not egalitarian. In fact, it can be argued that human social history has demonstrated that a purely egalitarian society has never existed naturally or, if developed, has never persisted. In the historical development of complex societies, there appears to be something fundamental about the ability of some people to accumulate that actually provides the engine for societies to progress.

Another of the forms of djambe is the ability to curse someone else through jealousy of the person's success. This form is interpreted as a negative, or destructive, form of djambe. However, this view actually presents a conundrum because leveling of inequality is seen as constructive, but cursing through envy, which is seen as destructive, is perhaps a means of accomplishing this leveling. Thus, the means of leveling inequality are seen as destructive, but the ends are seen as constructive—and in this case, the end does not justify the means in Western perspective. These issues are confounded by biases of the Western observer, and no such inconsistencies exist in the African view itself.

Finally, the powerful are said to use djambe against those who work for them and contribute to their success, turning them into "zombie" workers. So, there is also a balance in that djambe is accessible to the "bosses" and workers alike, in both creating inequality by "enslaving" workers, and by bringing about leveling between workers and bosses through the curse of envy. But in a different perspective, cursing those who are successful and wealthy may be in fact be destructive for the society, because these successful people are contributing to the economic advancement of the whole society in being able to provide employment to others. Perhaps the wealthy deserve their success and provide the means for moving the whole society into modernity—for better or worse.

The entire view that the successful turn their workers into "zombies" through djambe may be historically biased by the reluctance of indigenous people to work as organized labor on the plantations and refineries of European colonizers. In many parts of Africa, the British, for example (as they also did in Malaya), brought in laborers from their other colonies in India and China to provide labor for economic activities in the African colonies because the indigenous peoples could not be induced to do this work. One century later the peoples of China and India are seen as leading the entire world in terms of economic activity and economic growth, while Africa is still struggling with fundamental issues of economic, political, and social organization.

Human societies where everyone and everything is theoretically "leveled" on some "materialist basis," as in the former Soviet Union, Eastern Europe, Burma, and North Korea, have not proven to be very successful either in terms of material wealth or spiritual well-being of the society. Many contemporary academics who study human societies are generally biased by a view that a heretofore nonexistent, mythical, egalitarian society is somehow preferable to reality. This bias may cause these Western observers to place their own mystical or magical interpretations on phenomena for which there are more practical explanations. One example is interpreting the reluctance to work on European plantations in West Africa as some kind of political statement rather than simply not wanting to work hard under rigid conditions. It is always further assumed that European plantations were purely a systemized way of subjugating people without considering the economic reality of making land productive and feeding people in a society where males do not like to work. That circumstance is different from making the case that Europeans did not belong there in the first place.

BALANCE, POTENCY AND POWER

To consider the presence and potency of witchcraft as reflecting or resulting from inequality in the political body, it can be seen as imbalance in the physical body. Indeed, it may be "embodied" as a physical disorder—described as literally "being in the belly." The embodiment of a psychic disorder, or imbalance, in the physical body is known as "somatization," which has been a frequent observation in African societies.

Witchcraft can be used to confront political imbalance working traditionally through kinship. Kin represent the ally in village society. But *djambe* is described as the dark side of kinship in relation to political power. Because witchcraft is secret, occult, and hidden, it occupies a space in village life that is hidden from central authority and confers a kind of balance of power to the villagers.

The power elites become fearful of being "eaten" by villagers, not only through their political requests, but through witchcraft. (Use of the term "being eaten" in traditional societies can also mean consuming the spirit or soul of another, and has been connected and confounded with the practice of cannibalism.) Through witchcraft, villagers may still maintain local power against elites.

In the presence of inequality and imbalance, *djambe* may be seen as a leveling force restoring balance. However, there is also ambiguity or ambivalence because it also may represent a means of accumulation, creating imbalances and disparities in power or wealth (or both). Witchcraft is a double-edged sword because it grants power but also equates to danger. This view is common to most cultural perceptions of magic and witchcraft, like "playing with fire."

IMAGE OF LIMITED GOOD

A related concept is *limbo*, or jealousy, among the *Kako* (neighboring tribe in West Africa). Those who ascend socioeconomically must excuse themselves constantly to those who do not ascend (this is the same practice that has become *de rigeur* in the United States since 2008). This concern among traditional societies can be likened to the *Image of Limited Good* (George Foster, 1965), where the "evil eye" is the admiring eye.

Good fortune must be hidden (or shared) to avoid curse. For example, villagers may be reluctant to plant a cacao tree (potential source of cash crop) because they may not be alive to harvest it due to the malign effects of jealousy.

Witchcraft has also become associated with the accumulation of riches ("richcraft"?). Consumption and materialism are equated with modernity. While Western academics may view the "benefits" of mass consumption and materialism with irony, in West Africa they also tell jokes about accumulating goods. There is ambiguity in the appreciation of material goods but distrust of the source of material success ("the sorcery of success"). There is suspicion that the rich have used a new kind of witchcraft to force others to work for them (making them a kind of "zombie," and perhaps reflecting historical reluctance of the indigenous peoples to work for the plantations of German, British, and French colonizers).

MAGIC AND "ANTI-WITCHCRAFT"

In terms of modernity, the state political and judicial apparatus now takes an active "anti-witchcraft" stance (while former colonial administrators were reluctant to even take it seriously). The *nganga*, or traditional healers (perhaps reflecting the light side of magic), have been enlisted as expert witnesses against those accused of practicing magic, in the courts, and conduct active interventions in the communities. These traditional healers are highly adaptive, using the French term *"bricoleurs,"* which is translated as *inventors*, though it is more appropriately translated as *tinkerers* (Box 42-1).

The new witch trials in West Africa may be seen in relation to the European and American witch trials of the 1660s, when traditional societies confronted modernity,

BOX 42-1 *Translating Djambe*

Djambe requires at least two kinds of translation—cultural and linguistic—as well as transliteration. For example, some of the cultural concepts underlying *djambe* become translated into English terms that may be misleading, such as using magic to "consume" someone's parts. This interpretation is probably a mismatch in linguistic terms and by the fact that the modern English language does not have a lexicon for describing the vital energy, as opposed to physical anatomy, of the body. This problem may also be relevant in understanding somatization of psychic pain in African societies, for example, where a psychological pain is literally felt in the body because there are no indigenous African terms for psychiatric terminology.

and central authority developed increasing authority over village life (see "Sorcery and Witchcraft in the West," below). Historians relate social concepts of witchcraft to larger historical forces, while anthropologists focus on the particularistic aspects of the meaning and function of witchcraft in specific cultures and societies (which makes sense in terms of the analysis of George Stocking, for example, on the history of anthropology as an academic field of study; see Chapter 34).

The concept of *balance* remains important in terms of understanding the role of witchcraft in traditional societies. Mary Douglas's (1967) introduction to Evans-Pritchard's classic ethnography, *Witchcraft, Oracles and Magic Among the Azande*, reflects its importance in the study of African culture and culture and society in general. Witchcraft reflects both continuity and change in culture (an important issue in ethnographic studies, as articulated by Ward Goodenough [1963], in *Continuity and Change*, and other anthropologists).

RITUAL AND RELIGION

There are also issues of scale. For example, religious practice consists of many individual rituals but has a larger overall meaning. Also, for some, witchcraft is practiced as a religion in addition to having its separable rituals. In addition to ritual and religion, other terms have particular as well as general meanings. *Shamanism* describes a particular indigenous practice among traditional peoples of Siberia but is also used both by scholars and the general culture to embody groups of practices and practitioners that might formerly have been called "animistic," or said to be practicing "animism." These practices in turn were formerly termed "primitive" by Western observers (see Chapter 34).

The terms used are not just cultural constructs describing belief and behavior systems because they now appear to be attempts to describe a common human experiential phenomenon. What is called religious or spiritual experience appears now to involve an innate capacity of the human being and the human brain according to contemporary neuroscience research. Contemporary imaging studies have shown how meditative states, prayer, and religious practices (among Roman Catholic nuns and Buddhists, for example) create specific activity patterns in specific parts of the brain, using state-of-the-art neuroimaging techniques (see Chapter 10). Others have written about "the God gene," indicating that humans are "wired" for this kind of experience.

The authentic experience of spirituality is very powerful and can be transformative. These authentic experiences appear to occur among peoples at different times, among different societies, and within different cultures. Generally, the power of this authentic experience becomes channeled into some form of organized religion, relying upon ritual (and rote), as yet another means of exercising control by the powerful over the powerless. Thus, while anthropologists study religion and spirituality and the role of shamans, witchcraft, and magic, they are observing authentic spiritual experience only *after* it has been suborned and assimilated into the general power structure of that society.

Authentic religious experience is continuously being reborn as an innate human capacity. To this extent, the "new age" phenomenon is worthy of serious attention in our contemporary society, where it is not just a naked attempt to derive benefit from the spiritual needs and credulousness of certain people.

The ability to understand authentic religious experience at the point of origin and its "time of birth" is important—before it is seen as a threat and assimilated into general cultural forms that are acceptable to the power structure. Thus, rather than being spiritually liberating and enlightening, organized religion can ultimately become one more element used to control people in addition to the law and to economic needs.

SORCERY AND WITCHCRAFT IN THE WEST

While African witchcraft has ambiguous meanings in being able to either hurt or help the health of people or their communities, witchcraft came to have a pejorative meaning in the West. Witchcraft in the West is generally said to have grown out of pre-Christian pagan beliefs and popular common superstitions of the Middle Ages. Its beliefs included rituals, magic charms, love potions, demons, and spirits. Although witchcraft was illegal in the Middle Ages, the laws against it were not strictly enforced. Further, the village priests often tolerated some of the beliefs, or at least pretended to ignore them (see Chapter 39). To the ordinary villager who believed that spirits populated the world, the priests could often offer no better explanations of how the world worked. The priests were not the only people to whom the villagers turned in times of trouble.

They also looked to a so-called wise or cunning man or woman. This person, usually fairly old, was thought to have a special understanding of the way the world operated. Often, these elders had a knowledge of **medicinal herbs** gained from a lifetime of experience, or from local resources based upon **local folklore**. These "wise folk" were often called "good witches." However, if their relationships with their neighbors turned sour, "wise folk" might be accused of being "bad witches." In many cases, the person accused of witchcraft would be an elderly widow. Perhaps too weak to work, with no husband or family to support her, she would be the most defenseless person in the community and an easy target for attack.

In the fifteenth century, the Catholic Church, encouraged by the newly powerful political nation-states in Spain, France, and elsewhere, began an inquisition on "infidels" or nonbelievers in Christianity, such as the practice of Islam or Judaism and the practice of "witchcraft" in Europe. Witchcraft was declared a dangerous heresy and the people who practiced it were considered agents of the devil who wanted to destroy the church and work evil upon God's people. A witch was defined *by the church* as a person, usually a woman, who of her own free will rejected God and made a pact with the devil. When a number of witches met together to "worship the devil" and practice "diabolical magic," a witches' Sabbath took place. Stories about witches often became more sensational as they spread throughout the countryside.

Outrageous accusations were made; a person might be accused of flying on a broomstick. Some of the medicinal plants, containing potent ergot alkaloids, may have been rubbed on a broomstick, and "riding" on a broomstick (placed between the legs), could rapidly introduce these hallucinogens directly into the bloodstream through the vaginal mucosa, creating the sensation of "flying" (figuratively "getting high"). Sticking pins into dolls, or dancing with the devil in the woods at night, were other accusations. When the majority of people believed an accusation, the accused would be unable to convince a mob that the accusations were untrue.

Witchcraft was a crime punishable by execution, and normal rules of evidence and legal safeguards were regularly violated. Because it was done in God's name, torture was considered a proper tool to uncover witches. People accused of witchcraft were often considered guilty until they could prove their innocence, and many tests were devised to detect the guilty. In the water test, the accused would be thrown into a body of water. If the accused floated—as most did—it was taken as a sign of guilt and the person would be executed. If the person sank, he or she was considered innocent and hopefully rescued before the person drowned. Thumbscrews and boiling water were used to obtain confessions of guilt, and few people could withstand such torture. Many confessed to witchcraft in order to be executed quickly and put an end to the torture. These confessions became used, in turn, as proof of the existence of witchcraft. Convicted witches were often burned at the stake. In England, witches were usually hanged. In rare cases, the convicted might be spared death. Instead, a priest might perform a ceremony of exorcism to drive out the demon that was supposed to have taken over the witch's body.

"Witch hunting" signaled that the normal *balance* or harmony and cooperation of *community* life had broken down. No person was really safe from witch scares and witch hunts. Frequently, levelheaded people would let their emotions get the better of their common sense. Convictions would be obtained by weak and circumstantial evidence, and many well-meaning people were afraid to speak out and call attention to themselves in fear of being the next person accused of witchcraft. An enormous outburst of witch hunting broke out in Europe in the mid-1500s and lasted more than a century. Once started, it was virtually impossible to stop. Religious leaders were ready to attack witches because they were rivals for their own position as advisers in times of troubles. Political leaders were eager to use the law courts to prosecute witches and thus strengthen the power of the state.

In the American colonies, it is likely that traditional African beliefs and practices relating to such concepts as *djambe* and *lembo* were imported and gave substance to the perceived existence of witchcraft. This perceived African influence is illustrated in Arthur Miller's *The Crucible*, for example, in late seventeenth-century Salem, Massachusetts, where the African slave girl *Tituba* is the first to lead the adolescent girls into the woods to perform ritual dances in the nude. Rather than being punished, the young girls are induced to begin accusing old widows in the community of witchcraft, ultimately spreading the accusations to some of the community elders themselves. In the real history of the Salem witch trials, the local minister was eventually accused and escaped to Maine, where he was eventually found and hanged as a witch himself.

PERCEPTIONS OF SHAMANISM IN THE WEST

Observations of shamans is one of the major recurring topics in the study of religious and ethnomedical practices in tribal cultures. *Shamanism* is a term often associated with mere indigenous *mysticism*, with the concept being muddled and misused by academics who can be labeled as "armchair scholars" for their hands-off role in the study of shamanic practices. The widely held view of shamans as vestiges of a prehistoric religion that has never quite "developed" is a false generalization based on the poor accounts of academics who took little time (if any) to analyze a culture before making assumptions about it. This point is further supported by the analysis of certain societies that have been labeled "shamanic," but that, upon rudimentary inspection, are most definitely not akin to the tribes the term is meant to describe.

Cultural beliefs and practices can no longer be relegated to myth, superstition, and magic as presented 100 years ago by armchair Victorian scholars, as in Sir James Frazer's *The Golden Bough* (Chapter 34). As early as the 1920s, anthropologists began describing what we now call shamanic practices as logical constructs that make sense in terms of cultural cosmologies. By the 1960s, anthropologists were referring to and studying such practices as ethnomedicine, more specifically, in terms of shamanism. The origin of the term was in description of indigenous healers in Siberia and North Asia, and it came to be applied generally for the type of healing conducted in indigenous societies.

Aside from the misrepresentations visited upon them by Western culture, shamans are an integral part of northern Asian cultures, functioning as social leaders, religious vessels, voices of ancestors, medicinal healers, caregivers, and educational entertainers. They are not the metaphorical "wild men" praised by the new age movement, nor are they the dancing fools mocked by xenophobic academics and elites for hundreds of years. Their roles are important as functionaries that provide the societal backbone of each culture, with their practices imparting stories, social control, and a symbolic connection for all members of their tribe. Only by opening the perspective in which these men and women are viewed can Western anthropologists begin to understand the actual meaning of the term "shaman." This shift is necessary to facilitate the correct application of the word to the figures it actually represents without forming a biased opinion of the "other," due to a lack of knowledge of indigenous cultures.

Even before anthropological recognition of ethnoscience and ethnomedicine, Western scientists were studying comparative religions as an early aspect of psychology, for example, William James, *The Varieties of Religious Experience*. Nonetheless, as late as 1951, a book could appear with the title *Religion Among the Primitives* (Goode, 1951). Shamans, as in other traditional societies (see Fabrega, in David Landy, 1977), were selected through processes of divination because of their special abilities, which are being recognized by contemporary neuroscience on environmental sensitivity (see Jawer & Micozzi, 2009).

Because *shamanism* is used in the general sense described above, it can be misleading regarding the issue of gender. For example, women are now being shown biologically to be more "sensitive" or "empathic in some ways (see Jawer & Micozzi, 2009) and thus may have conferred upon them greater potential in this role. For example, in **Africa,** Hewson describes the role of the traditional "medicine man" as actually being more likely to be a woman in practice (see Chapter 41). It is more a Western view to confine the term *medicine man* to Native Americans (partially because of the problems of linguistic and cultural translation of *medicine*), and the general phenomenon is applicable to traditional societies across the globe. (see Chapter 1)

Academic disciplines have the goals of both (1) capturing and describing the individual, particular aspects of a culture (originally American cultural anthropology stemming from Boas and his students, Kroeber, Lowie, and others; and their students, such as Ruth Benedict) and (2) formulating general "laws" about the commonalities of human social organization (originally British-European social anthropology as brought to the University of Chicago by Alfred Radcliffe-Brown in the 1930s). Therefore, there should be no conflict in these approaches. In fact, understanding the scholarly history of cultural studies should be fundamental to formulating contemporary hypotheses that guide the design and conduct of new field studies.

THE MEANINGS OF SHAMANISM

Shamanism has taken on a meaning in the wider academic world as well as in the popular culture. It provides a recognition that indigenous societies have "spiritual" practitioners outside the confines of recognized, organized "religions." While its origin has a specific definition relating to societies in **Siberia**, the general usage of the term fulfills the need to have a descriptor for a widespread cultural phenomenon among indigenous peoples in traditional societies worldwide. It facilitates description about these practices and practitioners outside the confines of Siberian society.

Taking the Word Shaman Out of Cold Storage

> *Shaman* is a word that comes from the *Tungas* language of Central **Siberia**. The term incorporates men and women as religious leaders who serve their community by use of drums to call spirit allies. It is a priestly calling and cannot typically be "learned," as most shamans are born into such a life. It is important to note this definition as a base point for discussion because it has drawn many different false definitions, and people have misused the word.

"Neo-Shamanism"

Many today have made a living "selling shamanism," which is now put into the category of "New-Age spirituality." These purveyors come from all different areas of the world but have in common that they do *not* minister to their own communities but to strangers.

The phenomenon of neo-shamanism in the United States can be seen to have grown out of the more rational nature of mainstream contemporary Christianity. The three Abrahamic religions (Judaism, Christianity, and Islam) have all gone through cycles of rationalism and mysticism throughout their history. And, in fact, they coexist with charismatic Christianity, and fundamentalist Islam and Sufism (Chapter 33), in contemporary times.

As a religion becomes more rational or intellectual in its approach to justifying its beliefs and doctrines, at some point, practitioners begin to focus on received knowledge or wisdom rather than authentic religious experiences. Then, as people long to have a more emotional experience of spirituality, mystical or "charismatic" movements within the religion develop. However, a religion that becomes predominantly emotional may not appeal to some practitioners and leads unbelievers to comment on the lack of verification for the religion. Rational movements led by scholars writing academic treatises proving the religion's

veracity then develop. An example from Christianity would be the mysticism of women such as *Mechthild of Magdeburg*, *Julian of Norwich* and *Hildegard of Bingen* in the Middle Ages, followed by the rise of Scholasticism led by *Thomas Aquinas* in the later Middle Ages.

Contemporary mainstream Protestant and Catholic churches in the United States have been more rational and institutionalized for some time, which may be seen as ultimately contributing to the popularity of Pentecostal and other evangelical Protestant movements, both in the United States and in predominantly Roman Catholic areas of Latin America (e.g., *Iglesia ni Christo*). Likewise, *neo-shamanism*, focusing on a personal encounter with *friendly* (benign) spirits, attracts those disillusioned with mainstream religion and looking for spiritual experiences in nonordinary reality. However, the individualistic purposes of the shamanic journey for neo-shamanists distorts the role of shamans in traditional societies to one who communes with *dangerous* (malign) spirits on behalf of the whole clan, to bring healing, answers, and good fortune to everyone in the community.

New Agers have started teaching certain techniques, essentially reducing shamanic journeying to a basic technique that anyone can learn in a few hours, while sometimes even using recorded drum sounds. Is it right to homogenize practices forged in particular cultural histories and serve them up with a Western Romantic dressing? Is this teaching of shamanic technique exploitation of another culture's vast history, or is it just using the tools that have gotten shamans and their cultures through the centuries and that should in fact be passed on through different societies? And with that, how can we call something like the practices of shaman "new age" when they have been around for centuries? Is it new age, or "age old"?

Contemporary neuroscience is now discovering that *mystical experiences* and abilities are not so much supernatural but reflect *innate basic biological abilities* that relate to human physiology. The fact that traditional societies have found ways to recognize, honor, and utilize these abilities ends up being a subject for study among the "other" by Western social scientists as purely a cultural phenomenon rather than a human physiological characteristic. The traditional grounding of anthropology in both biology and culture should provide an advantage in understanding the full dimensions of these "shamanistic" phenomena, but anthropology, like all of academia, has become too overspecialized to be able to bring full studies to bear.

An element of cultural bias may also be seen in our manner of describing the shaman, including other societies, as "*primitive*." Cultural primitivism does more than exile non-Westerners from civilization. It seems that through the years, as Western society gets more technologically complex, we tend to view societies that are not participating in modernity as "baser" and "low technology societies." However, these societies are actually more appropriate technologically, and actually advanced, in that their technology is constructed from renewable, raw materials and relies to a greater extent on innate human capacities. Our society is unable to see shamans and their "primitive" societies as anything but the "others."

In the realm of medicine, it may well be that the ancient elders and shamans of "primitive" societies simply discovered old techniques of health and healing that may now be interpreted in light of new scientific discoveries regarding mind–body unity, bioenergy, and self-healing, and the relationships of our well-being to the social networks around us. How does Western medicine, so based on new technology, start to recognize these "others" as simply illustrating another way of living in the world?

References

Douglas M: Introduction. In *Witchcraft, Oracles and Magic Among the Azande*, New York, 1967, Oxford University Press.

Fabrega H Jr: Evolution of healing and sickness. In Landy DH, editor: *Culture, Disease, and Studies in Medical Anthropology*, Berkeley, 1977, University of California Press.

Foster G: Peasant Society and the Image of Limited Good, *Amer Anthropologist* 67(2):293–315, 1965.

Goode WJ: *Religion Among the Primitives*, Glencoe, IL, 1951, Free Press Publishers.

Goodenough WH: *Cooperation in Change*, New York, 1963, Russell Sage Foundation.

Jawer MA, Micozzi MS: *The Spiritual Anatomy of Emotion: How Feelings Link the Brain, the Body, and the Sixth Sense*, Rochester, 2009, Park Street Press.

Suggested Readings

Bonfanti L: *The Witchcraft Hysteria of 1692*, Burlington, 1977, Pride Publications.

Boyer P, Nissenbaum S: *Salem Possessed: The Social Origins of Witchcraft*, Oxford, 1976, Harvard University Press.

Brown DC: *A Guide to the Salem Witchcraft Hysteria of 1692*, Boston, 1984, David C. Brown.

Hansen C: *Witchcraft at Salem*, New York, 1985, George Braziller, Inc.

Micozzi MS: Implementation of health screening programs using ethnomedical resources, *Med Anthropol* 9(3):265–275, 1986.

Nevins WS: *Witchcraft in Salem Village in 1692*, New York, 1916, Salem Press Co.

Phillips JD: *Salem in the Seventeenth Century*, Boston, 1935, The Riverside Press.

Robinson EA: *The Devil Discovered, Salem Witchcraft 1692*, New York, 1991, Hippocrene Books.

Starkey ML: *The Devil in Massachusetts: A Modern Enquiry into the Salem Witch Trials*, New York, 1949, Alfred A. Knopf.

Upham CW: *Salem Witchcraft*, Boston, 1867, Wiggins and Lunt.

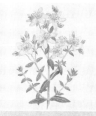

CHAPTER 43

MODERN ASIA, AFRICA, THE AMERICAS, AND THE PACIFIC

GERARD C. BODEKER

MARC S. MICOZZI

As we have seen, cultural factors play a significant role in the *continued reliance* on traditional medicine today. Often villagers seek symptomatic relief with modern medicine and turn to traditional medicine for treatment of what may be perceived as the "true cause of the condition" (Kleinman, 1980). The process by which villagers choose one type of care versus another is wonderfully described by Alan Young in his ethnography, *Medical Choice in a Mexican Village*. Traditional medical knowledge typically is coded into household cooking practices, home remedies, and health prevention and health maintenance beliefs and routines. The advice of family members or other significant members of a community has a strong influence on health behavior, including the type of treatment that is sought (Nichter, 1978).

THE AMERICAS

Decolonization and increased self-determination for indigenous groups has led some but not all countries to reevaluate and promote their traditional medical systems. At a 1993 **Pan-American Health Organization** conference on indigenous peoples and health, representatives from **South America** reported increasing activity and interest in traditional medicine in their countries (Zoll, 1993). Several Latin American countries have departments or divisions of traditional medicine within their health ministries. This meeting was followed by a gathering of traditional healers from both North and South America in Caracas, Venezuela, in September 1994, at the inception of the GIFTS of Health (Global Initiative for Traditional Systems of Health) program.

Mexico has undertaken an extensive program of revitalizing its indigenous medical traditions: over 1000 traditional medicines have been identified as a result of a program of ethnomedical and pharmacognostic research; training centers have been established by the government to pass traditional medical knowledge on to new generations of health care workers; and hospitals of traditional medicine have been established in a number of rural areas. The Constitution of Mexico was revised to include traditional medicine in the provision of national health care (Argueta, 1993). Nongovernmental organizations (NGOs) have played a strong role in revitalizing traditional health in Mexico, organizing national and international meetings on traditional approaches to health care. More than 50 different traditional medicine associations were represented at a 1992 meeting of the *Instituto Nacional Indigenista*. In the Amazon-Orinoco basin, the UN World Council of Indigenous Peoples has supported the functions of the *Organización Regional de Pueblos Indígenas del Amazonas* (ORPIA). ORPIA has representatives from eight tribes of the Upper Orinoco and Amazon basin. These groups are originally Neolithic (or "new stone age") tribes, without metallurgy, who are beginning to practice horticulture.

They have terrible problems with chloroquine-resistant malaria, which has reached the Amazon from its likely origin in Southeast Asia during the Vietnam War, where massive use of chloroquine against malaria led to the development of a resistant strain of this deadly parasite. But they cannot obtain costly Western drugs to treat this type of malaria from the cities in a timely fashion to reach the interior.

In addition to growing tobacco (which itself has medicinal properties as used traditionally in the Americas by indigenous peoples), they can grow *Artemisia* ("wormwood," as found in the West in vermouth, a traditional European medicinal for treating "worms," or internal

BOX 43-1 *Cinchona Bark in the Treatment of Malaria*

During Spanish explorations of the Amazon in the sixteenth century, missionaries came across an indigenous cure for so-called intermittent fevers, which we know today are caused by various strains of malaria. A crude extract of the bark of the cinchona tree was able to cure these fevers. Brought back to Europe, it proved a very popular remedy for malaria, which was still endemic throughout Southern Europe. Various genetic forms of hemoglobin and other red blood cell biochemicals (called *red cell polymorphisms*) evolved in Southern European populations as a protection against malaria. These genes provide protection against malaria when present in a single dose of the gene but cause disease when two doses of the gene are present in individuals (a minority) who carry the gene (such as thalassemia, from the Greek word for sea, *Thalassa*). Sickle cell anemia is an example of the same problem that afflicts Africans as a result of a similar adaptation to malaria.

This cinchona bark cure spread through Europe during the Age of Exploration and Colonization, initially known as *Spanish* bark or *Jesuit* bark, for those who brought it back to Europe. Eventually it found use as *quinine* throughout the British Royal Navy, which when mixed with gin and lime, provided a palatable protection against malaria, as well as scurvy (vitamin C from the lime to prevent deficiency), among the "limey" sailors of that day. A related compound, *quinidine*, is useful as a drug for the heart.

Although the tree was originally from the Amazon basin, by the twentieth century, commercial cultivation of cinchona for quinine against malaria was predominantly on British, Dutch, and French colonial plantations in tropical Southeast Asia, where this tree could grow. During World War II, the Japanese and Axis forces occupied these former European colonies (as well as two

of three European countries which had run these plantations).

By the time the United States entered World War II in late 1941, cinchona and quinine were unavailable to the Allied forces. The U.S. Army conducted a crash program to develop synthetic antimalarials to meet the need to protect 20 million Americans in uniform deployed around the world where malaria remained endemic, and they successfully developed a synthetic substitute. Subsequently, during the Korean War (1950-1953), it was noted that many American soldiers of Southern European and African descent had bad reactions to this synthetic substitute, for reasons having to do with the same red blood cell polymorphisms that normally protect against malaria. Eventually chloroquine was developed as an active drug against malaria. During the Vietnam War (1965-1975), the overuse of chloroquine in Southeast Asia led to the development of resistant strains of malaria against this drug, just as bacteria develop resistance from the overuse of antibiotics (turning these "*magic bullet*" drugs into "*friendly fire*," to use another concept borrowed from Vietnam). These resistant strains have now been introduced beyond Asia, into Africa and South America, as described in this chapter and book.

To come full circle, it has been noted that the *crude extract* of cinchona bark remained active against chloroquine-resistant malaria because the bark contains a synergistic *mixture* of active compounds against the parasite. This property of **synergy** among medicinal plants is a critical factor in the **potency of traditional remedies** for disease, compared to synthetic, single-ingredient chemical drugs, and represents a major advantage of medicines and foods in their **natural**, synergistic forms.

---

parasites) and aloe, which has been shown in West Africa to treat chloroquine-resistant malaria. Ironically, the crude extract of cinchona bark, which originally was found in the Upper Amazon basin and proved effective against malaria since the sixteenth century, is actually more difficult to cultivate (see Box 43-1).

Native North American communities have also been incorporating traditional forms of treatment into health programs for some years (see Chapter 37). In the United States, Indian Health Service (IHS) alcohol rehabilitation programs include traditional approaches to the treatment of alcoholism. An analysis of 190 IHS contract programs revealed that over 50% of these programs offered a **traditional sweat lodge** at their site or encouraged the use of sweat lodges (Hall, 1986). Treatment outcomes improved when a sweat lodge was available. Often these sweat lodges include the presence of **medicine men** or healers, and the presence of a traditional healer greatly improved the outcome when used in combination with the sweat lodge. In **northern Canada**, the **Inuit** Women's Association

developed a program to revitalize **traditional birth practices** (Flaherty, 1993) (Chapter 40). Women who were **midwives** in their own communities for many years were interviewed and recorded on videotape, and these tapes are being used to train young midwives in the use of traditional methods (see Micozzi, 1986).

NATIONAL CRISES

In addition to economic and cultural factors, **national crises** have spurred governments to evaluate their indigenous medical traditions as a means of providing affordable and available health care to their citizens. War and national epidemics are two common crises faced by these nations.

During the war in **Nicaragua**, there was an acute shortage of pharmaceutical supplies. In 1985, out of necessity, the country turned to its herbal traditions as a means of fulfilling the country's medical needs. A department was established within the health ministry to develop "popular and traditional medicine as a strategy in the search for a self-determined response to a difficult economic, military and political situation" (Castellon, 1992).

The department of traditional medicine initiated a program of ethnobotanical research in the midst of war. More than 20,000 people nationwide were interviewed regarding their use of traditional and popular remedies, the methods of preparing these remedies, and the sources of plant ingredients. Previously, nurses and health workers in rural areas frequently staffed outposts without medical supplies. They often were surrounded by medicinal herbs of which they knew nothing.

A national toxicology program was begun, based on the extensive survey. Over a period of six to seven years, pharmacognostic studies attempted to determine the chemistry and medicinal properties of commonly used plants. As a result of this effort, inexpensive medicines were produced locally and sustainably in rural areas to treat a wide range of conditions including respiratory ailments, skin problems, nervous disorders, diarrhea, and diabetes.

A historic example closer to home in the United States is provided during the Civil War (1861–1865), when the southern Confederate States of America could not obtain manufactured drugs from the North or from European countries due to the Northern Blockade. Confederate doctors turned to traditional folk remedies, and Native American medicinal plants, which were plentiful in the South and had been well documented in a series of popular *Herbals* written throughout the seventeenth, eighteenth, and early nineteenth centuries. These remedies can be found in the standard Confederate medical kits issued toward the end of the war.

AFRICA

In **Africa**, governments face huge drug bills for the growing AIDS crisis and are looking to their indigenous medical traditions and medicinal plants for inexpensive and effective methods of at least alleviating the suffering of AIDS victims. The health ministry of **Uganda** has been active in generating research into the role of traditional medical practitioners in treating people with AIDS. The Uganda AIDS Commission and the Joint Clinical Research Centre in Kampala have worked with traditional healer associations to evaluate several traditional treatments for opportunistic infections associated with HIV/AIDS. An official of the Uganda AIDS Commission commented on research findings, saying that traditional medicine is better suited to the treatment of some AIDS symptoms such as herpes, diarrhea, shingles, and weight loss (Kogozi, 1994).

As the AIDS crisis leads an increasing number of African countries to question their priorities in health expenditures, there is an emerging awareness that traditional health practitioners (THPs) can play an important role in delivering an AIDS prevention message. There is growing recognition that some THPs may be able to offer treatment for opportunistic infections. At the same time, there are concerns about unsafe practices and a growth in claims of traditional cures for AIDS. Partnerships between the modern and traditional health sectors (integration) are a cornerstone for building a comprehensive strategy to manage the AIDS crisis.

In **Uganda**, where there is only one doctor for every 20,000 people, there is one THP per 200 to 400 people (Green, 1994). In such settings, partnerships may be the only way that effective health care coverage can be achieved in managing the twin epidemics of AIDS and malaria. Clearly, such partnerships not only make good public health sense but, based on a growing body of pharmacological evidence, also may yield important preventative and treatment modalities.

AIDS

In light of the widespread availability of traditional health care services and the reliance of the population on these services, it is inevitable that people suffering from AIDS will turn to THPs for treatment. Collaborative AIDS programs have been established in many African countries, including **Malawi, Mozambique, Senegal, South Africa, Swaziland, Uganda, Zambia, and Zimbabwe**.

Information sharing and educational programs in **South Africa** have resulted in THPs providing correct HIV/AIDS advice as well as demonstrations of condom use. One such program trained 1510 THPs and it was calculated that during the first ten months, some 845,600 of their clients may have been reached with prevention messages about AIDS and sexually transmitted diseases (STDs). In similar programs in **Mozambique,** traditional healers learned that AIDS is transmitted by sexual contact, by blood, and by unsterile razor blades used in traditional practice. In a follow-up evaluation, over 80% of those trained reported that they had promoted condom use with at least their STD patients (Green, 1997).

One of the challenges in such workshop situations is to move beyond "training" to genuine information sharing. It has been noted that it is difficult to modify the manner in which health professionals teach about AIDS—a style that tends toward the didactic and use of scientific jargon. Removing communication barriers is a necessary first step in ensuring that training is an effective tool in mobilizing THPs as partners in AIDS control.

The **Ugandan** NGO, Traditional and Modern Health Practitioners Together Against AIDS (THETA), was established in 1992 to conduct research on potentially useful traditional medicines with HIV-related illness and to promote a mutually respectful collaboration between traditional and modern health workers in the fight against AIDS. THETA has conducted workshops to share knowledge on AIDS prevention and also treatment of opportunistic infections using local herbal remedies.

Traditional healers participating in clinical observational studies of their herbal medicines have subsequently sought training in prevention, education, and counseling issues as well as in basic clinical diagnostic skills. A 1998 UNAIDS-sponsored evaluation of THETA found that it had reached 125 THPs (44 women and 81 men) in five districts of Uganda. Fifty thousand people were found to have benefited from the improved services offered by THPs over a period of two years (Kabatesi, 1998).

MALARIA

The emergence of multidrug-resistant strains of malaria, which has accompanied each new class of antimalarial drugs, may be viewed as one of most significant threats to the health of people in tropical countries. Although there is widespread agreement that a fresh approach to the prevention and treatment of malaria is urgently needed, solutions have tended to focus on the development of new classes of drugs. More recently, there has been an emphasis on promoting combination therapy of existing drugs as a means of preventing resistance.

Historically, however, local communities in tropical regions have used local medicinal plants as a means of preventing and treating malaria (Kirby, 1997). It can be argued that these traditional medicines, based on the use of whole plants with multiple ingredients or of complex mixtures of plant materials, constitute combination therapies that may well combat the development of resistance to antimalarial therapy.

DRUG RESISTANCE, SYNERGISM, AND TRADITIONAL MEDICINES

Although combination therapy in malaria, cancer, and AIDS is based on the principle of synergistic action among multiple drugs, little significance has as yet being given to the obvious point that all of the major antimalarials have been derived from plants and that combinations existed in the traditional formulations before the process of extraction took place. For example, flavonoids in *Artemisia annua*, which are structurally unrelated to the antimalarial drug *artemisinin*, enhance the antimalarial activity of artemesinin (Phillipson et al, cited in Kirby, 1997).

Elsewhere, synergism has been observed between the alkaloids of the antimalarial plant *Ancistrocladus peltatum*. A total alkaloid extract of this plant had far greater antiparasitic activity than any of the six alkaloids isolated subsequently. In studies on antimalarial plants from **Madagascar**, the alkaloids bisbenzylisoquinoline, novel pavine, and benzyl tetrahydroisoquinolines all were found to potentiate the antiparasitic activity of chloroquine. Preparations of these plants are currently being tested as adjuvants to chloroquine therapy in Madagascar (Kirby, 1997). In Uganda, there are data from clinical case reports and a cohort study that a traditional Ugandan herbal remedy is effective against malaria (Bitawha et al, 1997; Willcox, 1999).

As they do with other conditions, people with malaria will often combine conventional drugs and traditional medicines, sometimes simultaneously or sequentially, as first- or second-line treatments (Agyepong et al, 1994; Bugmann, 2000; Gessler et al, 1995; Jayawardene, 1993; Lipowsky et al, 1992; McCombie, 1996; Pagnoni et al, 1997), with herbalists reporting their view that this combination gives an additional therapeutic effect (Rasoanaivo et al, 1994). Perceived efficacy is an important reason for people using traditional antimalarial medicines. Affordability is another. However, when patients themselves were asked why they choose traditional medicines over conventional drugs, a study in **Burkina Faso** (formerly Upper Volta) found that the cost of medicines accounted for only 50% of respondents' reasons. Lack of faith in doctors was the reason for the other 50% resorting to traditional medicine (Abyan & Osman, 1993). Elsewhere it has been reported that medical staff at Burkina Faso hospitals are less trusted as they are frequently young, do not speak the local languages, and are not courteous or welcoming to patients (Bugmann, 2000).

Several cohort studies have been conducted to evaluate the outcomes of traditional herbal treatments used by herbalists in managing malaria. A few of these studies have shown complete parasite clearance by day 7 (Mueller et al, 2000; Willcox, Bodeker, & Rasoanaivo, 2004), including one study that showed 100% parasite clearance in adults by a leaf extract of *Morinda lucida*. However, there was not full parasite clearance from infected children. Further preclinical and clinical studies on the antimalarial effects of plants have been reviewed in the book *Traditional Medicinal Plants and Malaria* (Willcox, Bodeker, & Rasoanaivo, 2004).

WORLD HEALTH ORGANIZATION

In response to rising demand for traditional medicines globally and the call from health ministries for formal regulation of this sector, the World Health Organization developed a Traditional Medicines Strategy (2002–2005), which focuses on four areas identified as requiring action if the potential of traditional medicine to play a role in public health is to be maximized. These areas are: policy; safety, efficacy, and quality; access; and rational use. Within these areas, WHO 2002–2005 identifies respective challenges for action.

National policy and regulation
- Lack of official recognition of traditional, complementary, and alternative medicine (TCAM) and TCAM providers
- Lack of regulatory and legal mechanisms
- TCAM not integrated into national health care systems
- Inequitable distribution of benefits in indigenous traditional medicine (TRM), knowledge, and products
- Inadequate allocation of resources for TCAM development and capacity building

Safety, efficacy, and quality
- Inadequate evidence base for TCAM therapies and products
- Lack of international and national standards for ensuring safety, efficacy, and quality control

- Lack of adequate regulation of herbal medicines
- Lack of registration of TCAM providers
- Inadequate support of research
- Lack of research methodology

Access

- Lack of data measuring access levels and affordability
- Lack of official recognition of role of TCAM providers
- Need to identify safe and effective practices
- Lack of cooperation between TCAM providers and allopathic practitioners
- Unsustainable use of medicinal plant resources

Rational use

- Lack of training for TCAM providers
- Lack of training for allopathic practitioners on TCAM
- Lack of communication between TCAM and allopathic practitioners and between allopathic practitioners and consumers
- Lack of information for the public on rational use of TCAM

The WHO Centre for Health Development has brought out the *World Health Organization Global Atlas of Traditional, Complementary and Alternative Medicine* to provide policymakers with a frame of reference on global utilization and policy trends and a set of country examples on policy development in this field (Bodeker et al, 2005b).

CONSERVING INTERNATIONAL BIODIVERSITY

Traditional health systems intersect with areas of the national economy other than health care—they interface with environmental concerns as well. Environmental factors such as land degradation through erosion or development have contributed to the loss of natural habitats. Loss of natural habitats can affect the availability of medicinal plants, and as a result, can affect local health standards. In countries where this loss has occurred, herb gatherers must walk increasingly longer distances to find herbs that previously grew nearby. This situation contributes to increasing the cost, availability, and sustainability of naturally occurring sources of medicines that traditionally provided basic health care to rural communities.

National economic development may be linked to the cultivation and use of traditional medicines. Wild harvesting of medicinal plants can provide an additional source of family income and also saves expenditure on other forms of medicine. However, overharvesting constitutes a serious threat to biodiversity. Overharvesting of medicinal plants occurs in China, where approximately 80% of the raw materials (animal and plant) for traditional medicines come from wild sources, raising the need for new policies to integrate health, environmental, and economic perspectives. Investments are needed to develop appropriate cultivation and harvesting strategies that will meet the demand for inexpensive and accessible medicines while ensuring the conservation of diverse biologic resources.

Most countries in Africa and the Americas lack the information and resources to apply the contemporary methods of studying the inventory of flora and fauna. It has not been possible to track resource depletion systematically in medicinal plants or in animal species that are used in traditional formulae. International collaboration in developing taxonomic capabilities of environmental and forestry departments is one means by which donor agencies can protect diverse medicinal plant species, thus influencing the long-term health of local populations in developing countries.

Although local health needs have constituted the primary beneficiary of the world's medicinal plant resources, there has been interest in traditional medicine from the international pharmaceutical industry, as well as from the natural product industry in Europe and America. Pharmaceutical industry interest has declined in the past decade as large pharmaceutical companies have shifted their interests to genetic and marine sources, due to challenges on intellectual property rights issues (Bodeker, 2007) and low yield of positive results from "culturally blind," high-throughput screenings programs.

The other source of interest in traditional medicine is the natural products industry in Europe and the United States. In Europe, where there is a large industry in phytomedicines, extracts of medicinal plants are sold in purified form to treat and prevent a wide variety of conditions.

These trends have led to a situation in which traditional medicine is viewed as a source for the production of other medicines, rather than in terms of its intrinsic value. These concerns have been expressed by the traditional medicine community. A prevailing view is that this trend does not contribute to the development of traditional medicine as a health care system for poor or rural communities, the main constituency of traditional medical care. Rather, the international drug development initiative is seen to take medicinal knowledge from these communities to serve the demand for new drugs in industrial countries. The drugs that are being developed are for the treatment of cancer and heart disease, which are the major killers in industrialized societies, rather than for the treatment of malaria and other endemic diseases that decimate the populations of the developing countries from which the knowledge derives.

There has been no attempt to date to develop a scientific understanding of the efficacy of medicinal plants in addressing the primary health care needs of the populations in the areas from which the plants derive. Some projects, however, have recognized this imbalance. The New York Botanical Garden's ethnobotany program in **Belize** (formerly British Honduras), for example, is addressing the situation through community-based projects to produce natural medicines for local consumption. In addition, this program is working to include knowledge of medicinal plants in school curricula as a means of conserving endangered traditional medical knowledge as well as to conserve medicinal plants and rainforest areas. The National Institutes of Health (NIH) is supporting research and policy evaluation on the role of traditional medicine in the provision of cost-effective primary health care in developing countries (National Center for Complementary and Alternative Medicine [NCCAM], www.nccam.nih.gov).

A broader economic perspective would recognize that the health status of developing countries is central to the economic health of those countries and thus to the world economy. Traditional medicine and medicinal plants play an important role in meeting the basic health needs of the majority of the world's population.

While the international community remains focused on preserving the great ecological regions of biodiversity, such as tropical rainforests in Africa and the Americas, it must be remembered that the indigenous peoples who have knowledge of their local medicinal plants are the true resource of knowledge for medicinal plants. As this author has often asked, based upon the old aphorism "If a tree falls in the forest, but nobody is there, does it make a sound," "If a medicinal plant grows in the forest, but nobody is there, does it make it make a cure?"

GLOBAL ETHNOMEDICINE IN THE TWENTY-FIRST CENTURY

Currently, there is wide variability in the consideration given by health planners to traditional health systems. In some countries, traditional medicine is incorporated routinely into health planning. However, this occurs in only a minority of cases, primarily in Asia. In most cases, the revival has come from NGOs. National and international funding is currently directed to the provision of Western-style health services in developing countries and indigenous communities. Research consistently links reductions in morbidity and mortality rates to economic conditions, educational levels—particularly to years of female education—and large-scale public health measures such as sanitation and water supply. While these factors—rather than the availability of Western medicines—have been found to lead to improved levels of health, health planners continue to operate under the view that Western medicine provides the primary means of improving health in these communities. This belief is not based on a scientific appraisal of the world's natural systems of health. Some traditional treatments are still more effective than modern treatments, as has been noted in this chapter.

While old and limited views of traditional systems of health continue to exist, there is an emerging intellectual and policy climate that is giving expression to a fresh perspective (Table 43-1). Whereas the old view favors the marginalization of traditional systems of health, the new view looks to them to provide complementary therapy, and in some cases, new solutions to major health crises. This new view is consonant with the ancient or traditional concepts of health and human potential that underlie many of the world's traditional systems of health.

TABLE 43-1 *Old Assumptions and New Perspectives on Complementary Medical Systems*

Old assumptions	New perspectives
"Primitive"	Holistic
Ineffective	Cost effective
Marginalized	Locally available
Extinct	Renewed
Should be regulated	Should be studied
Provides prospects for biomedicine	Valid in its own right
Active ingredient model	Synergistic activity

Finally, the global move toward a view of optimal health and well-being as the goal of health care has found expression through the wellness movement. According to the U.S. National Wellness Institute (NWI), wellness is "an active process through which people become aware of, and make choices towards, a more successful existence." NWI identifies six dimensions of wellness: social; occupational; spiritual; physical; emotional; and intellectual. Similarly, Lifestyles of Health and Sustainability (LOHAS) is a framework that focuses on "health and fitness, the environment, personal development, sustainable living, and social justice." Included is a strong nutritional emphasis and a focus on integrated health care and positive living. The size of this momentum is reflected in part by the growth of the global spa and "nature cure" industry into a $255 billion industry (see Chapters 2, 3).

From harnessing local forest herbs for everyday common ailments in rural parts of the developing world to the high use of standardized complementary medicines and licensed therapies in Europe and the United States, to the focus on wellness and healthy living through diet, natural products, and mind–body approaches to stress reduction, the CAM revolution appears to be maturing into an integrated and mainstream trend. Naturally, further clinical evidence is always desired and a global research endeavor is moving in this direction. The central shift has been that now consumers are active participants in management of their own health care. All health professionals do well to be aware of these trends in an effort to provide relevant, effective, affordable, and safe health care, and to develop successful practices, for all clients and consumers.

References

Abyan IM, Osman AA: Social and behavioural factors affecting malaria in Somalia. TDR/SER/PRS/11, Geneva, 1993, World Health Organization.

Agyepong IA, Manderson L: The diagnosis and management of fever at household level in the Greater Accra Region, Ghana, *Acta Trop* 58:317, 1994.

Argueta A: *Presentation to the World Bank Conference on Indigenous Knowledge and Sustainable Development*, Washington DC, 1993.

Bitawha N, Tumwesigye O, Kabariime P, et al: Herbal treatment of malaria—four case reports from the Rukararwe Partnership Workshop for Rural Development (Uganda), *Trop Doct* (Suppl 1):17, 1997.

Bodeker G: Intellectual property rights and traditional medical knowledge. In Bodeker G, Burford G, editors: *Public health and policy perspectives on traditional, complementary and alternative medicine*, London, 2007, Imperial College Press.

Bodeker G, Neumann C, Lall P, et al: Traditional medicine use and healthworker training in a refugee setting at the Thai-Burma border, *J Refugee Stud* 18(1):76–99, 2005a.

Bodeker G, Ong C-K, Grundy C, et al, editors: *WHO global atlas of traditional, complementary and alternative medicine*, Kobe, Japan, 2005b, World Health Organization, Centre for Health Development.

Bugmann N: *Le concept du paludisme, l'usage et l'efficacité in vivo de trois traitements traditionnels antipalustres dans la région de Dori, Burkina Faso, inaugural doctoral dissertation*, 2000, Faculty of Medicine, University of Basel.

Castellon U: *Report of the Fundación Centro Nacional de Medicina Popular Tradicional*, Nicaragua, 1992, Dr. Alejandro Dávila Bolaños.

Flaherty M: *Proceedings of the Conference on Indigenous Peoples and Health, Winnipeg, Canada, April 13–18, 1993*, Winnipeg, Saskatchewan, Canada, 1993, p 1.

Gessler MC, Msuya DE, Nkunya MH, Schar A, Heinrich M, Tanner M: Traditional healers in Tanzania: sociocultural profile and three short portraits, *J Ethnopharmacol* 48(3):145, 1995.

Green EC: *AIDS and STDs in Africa: bridging the gap between traditional healers and modern medicine*, Boulder, Colo, 1994, Westview Press (South African edition published by University of Natal Press, 1994).

Green EC: The participation of African traditional healers in AIDS/STD prevention programmes, *Trop Doct* 27(Suppl 1):56, 1997.

Hall RL: Alcohol treatment in American Indian communities: an indigenous treatment modality compared with traditional approaches, *Ann N Y Acad Sci* 472:168, 1986.

Jayawardene R: Illness perception: social cost and coping strategies of malaria cases, *Soc Sci Med* 37:1169, 1993.

Kabatesi D: Use of traditional treatments for AIDS-associated diseases in resource-constrained settings. In Robertson L, Bell K, Laypang L, et al, editors: *Health in the Commonwealth: challenges and solutions 1998/99*, London, 1998, Kensington Publications.

Kirby GC: Malaria and vector control, *Trop Doct* 27(Suppl 1):5, 1997.

Kleinman A: *Patients and healers in the context of cultures*, Berkeley, 1980, University of California Press.

Kogozi J: Herbalists open hospital, *The New Vision* (Kampala, Uganda) 14, 1994.

Lipowsky R, Kroeger A, Vazquez ML: Sociomedical aspects of malaria control in Colombia, *Soc Sci Med* 34:625, 1992.

McCombie SC: Treatment seeking for malaria: a review of recent research, *Soc Sci Med* 43:933, 1996.

Micozzi MS: Implementation of health screening programs using ethnomedical resources, *Med Anthropol* 9(3):265–275, 1986.

Mueller MS, Karhagomba IB, Hirt HM, Wemakor E. The potential of *Artemisia annua* L. as a locally produced remedy for malaria in the tropics: agricultural, chemical and clinical aspects, *J Ethnopharmacol* 73(3):487–493, 2000.

Nichter M: Patterns of curative resort and their significance for health planning in south Asia, *Med Anthropol* 2:29, 1978.

Pagnoni F, Convelbo N, Tiendrebeogo J, et al: A community-based programme to provide prompt and adequate treatment of presumptive malaria in children, *Trans R Soc Trop Med Hyg* 91:512, 1997.

Rasoanaivo P, Ratsimamanga-Urverg S, Milijaona R: In vitro and in vivo chloroquine-potentiating action of *Strychnos myrtoides* alkaloids against chloroquine-resistant strains of *Plasmodium* malaria, *Planta Med* 60:13, 1994.

Willcox M, Bodeker G, Rasoanaivo P, editors: *Traditional medicinal plants and malaria*, Boca Raton, Fla, 2004, CRC Press.

Willcox ML: A clinical trial of "AM," a Ugandan herbal remedy for malaria, *J Public Health Med* 21(3):318, 1999.

Zoll AC: Proceedings of the Conference on Indigenous Peoples and Health, Winnipeg, Canada, April 13–18, 1993.

Suggested Readings

Balick M: Conservation in today's world. In *Proceedings of WHO Symposium on the Utilization of Medicinal Plants, Philadelphia, April 19–21, 1993*, Philadelphia, 1995, University of Pennsylvania Press.

Bodeker G: Traditional health systems: valuing biodiversity for human health and well-being. In Posey D, editor: *Cultural and spiritual values in biodiversity*, Nairobi, Kenya, 2000, United Nations Environment Programme, p 261.

Bodeker G: Traditional medical knowledge, intellectual property rights and benefit sharing, *Cardozo J Int Comp Law* 11(2):785, 2003.

Bodeker G, Kronenberg F: A public health agenda for complementary, alternative and traditional (indigenous) medicine, *Am J Public Health* 92(10):1582, 2002.

Bodeker G, Kronenberg F, Burford G: Holistic, alternative and complementary medicine. In Heggenhougen K, Quah S, editors: *International encyclopedia of public health*, vol 3, San Diego, 2008, Academic Press, p 449.

Farnsworth N, Soejarto D: Potential consequences of plant extinction in the United States on the current and future availability of prescription drugs, *Econ Bot* 39:231, 1985.

Fellows LE: Pharmaceuticals from traditional medicine plants and others: future prospects. Paper presented at the New Drugs from Natural Sources Symposium, London, 1991, June 13-14.

Green EC, Zokwe B, Dupree JD: The experience of an AIDS prevention program focused on South African traditional healers, *Soc Sci Med* 40(4):503, 1995.

Honigsbaum M, Willcox ML: Cinchona. In Willcox M, Bodeker G, Rasoanaivo P, editors: *Traditional medicinal plants and malaria*, Boca Raton, Fla, 2004, CRC Press.

Institute of Burns: *Establishment of a new scientific center of Vietnam—the National Institute of Burns, named Le Huu Trac—that needs much support*, Hanoi, 1993, The Institute.

Institute of Materia Medica (Hanoi): *Medicinal plants in Viet Nam, WHO Regional Publications, Western Pacific Series No 3*, Manila, 1990, WHO Regional Office for the Western Pacific.

Kasilo OMJ, Soumbey-Alley E, Wambebe C: Regional overview: African region. In Bodeker G, Ong CK, Grundy C, Burford G, editors: *WHO global atlas of traditional, complementary and alternative medicine*, Kobe, Japan, 2005, World Health Organization, Centre for Health Development.

Koysooko R, Chuthaputti A. Promising practices in the use of medicinal plants in Thailand. Paper presented at the WHO Symposium on the Utilization of Medicinal Plants, Philadelphia, April 19–21, 1993.

Le Grand A, Wondergem P: *Herbal medicine and promotion*, Amsterdam, 1990, KIT Press Royal Tropical Institute.

Lei SH, Bodeker G: Changshan—ancient febrifuge and modern antimalarial: lessons for research from a forgotten tale. In Willcox M, Bodeker G, Rasoanaivo P, editors: *Traditional medicinal plants and malaria*, Boca Raton, Fla, 2004, CRC Press.

Micozzi MS: Implementation of health screening programs using ethnomedical resources, *Med Anthropol* 9(3):265–275, 1986.

Nations MK, de Souza MA: Umbanda healers as effective AIDS educators: case-control study in Brazilian urban slums (favelas), *Trop Doct* 27(Suppl 1):60, 1997.

Norbeck E, Lock M: *Health, illness and medical care in Japan*, Honolulu, 1987, University of Hawaii Press.

Patel V, Wang J, Shen RN, Sharma HM, Brahmi Z: Reduction of mouse Lewis lung carcinoma (LLC) by M-4 rasayana, *Nutr Res* 12:667, 1992.

Prasad KN, Edwards-Prasad J, Kentrotti S: Ayurvedic (Science of Life) herbal agents induced differentiation in murine neuroblastoma cells in culture, *Neuropharmacol* 31(6):599, 1992.

Reid W, Meyer CA, Gamez R, Sittenfeld A, editors: *Biodiversity prospecting*, Washington DC, 1993, World Resources Institute.

Sharma H: Effect of MAK (M4 & M5) on DMBA-induced mammary tumors, *Eur J Pharmacol* 183(2):193, 1990.

Sok CW: Country report. In *Proceedings of WHO Symposium on the Utilization of Medicinal Plants, Philadelphia, April 19–21, 1993*, Philadelphia, 1995, University of Pennsylvania Press.

Stepan J: Patterns of legislation concerning traditional medicine. In Bannerman R, editor: *Traditional medicine*, Geneva, 1983, World Health Organization.

World Bank: *World development report on health*, Washington DC, 1993, World Bank.

World Health Organization: *Traditional medicine*, Geneva, 1978, The Organization.

Wyler DJ: Bark, weeds and iron chelators—drugs for malaria, *N Engl J Med* 327(21):1519, 1992 (editorial).

Website

National Center for Complementary and Alternative Medicine: http://www.nccam.nih.gov.

Index

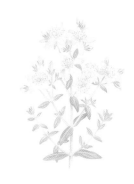

Page numbers followed by "f" indicate figures, "t" indicate tables, and "b" indicate boxes.